CHEMICAL DIAGNOSIS OF DISEASE

CHEMICAL DIAGNOSIS OF DISEASE

Edited by:

STANLEY S. BROWN

Head, Research and Development Subdivision and Deputy Head, Division of Clinical Chemistry, Medical Research Council Clinical Research Centre, Harrow, Middlesex HA1 3UJ, England

FREDERICK L. MITCHELL

Head, Division of Clinical Chemistry, Medical Research Council Clinical Research Centre, Harrow, Middlesex HA1 3UJ, England

and

DONALD S. YOUNG

Professor of Laboratory Medicine, Mayo Medical School and Head, Section of Clinical Chemistry, Mayo Clinic, Rochester, MN 55901, U.S.A.

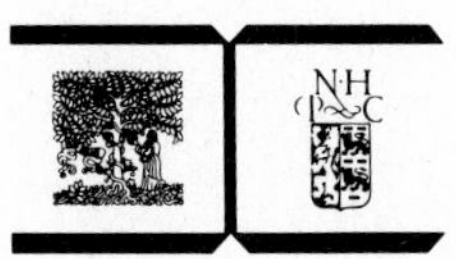

ELSEVIER/NORTH-HOLLAND BIOMEDICAL PRESS
AMSTERDAM · NEW YORK · OXFORD

ISBN 0-444-80089-1

1st edition 1979
2nd printing 1980

Published by:
Elsevier/North-Holland Biomedical Press
335 Jan van Galenstraat, P.O. Box 211
Amsterdam, The Netherlands

Sole distributors for the USA and Canada:
Elsevier North-Holland Inc.
52 Vanderbilt Avenue
New York, N.Y. 10017

Library of Congress Cataloging in Publication Data
Main entry under title:

Chemical diagnosis of disease.

Includes bibliographical references and index.
1. Chemistry, Clinical. 2. Diagnosis, Laboratory.
I. Brown, Stanley S. II. Mitchell, Frederick L.
III. Young, Donald S.
RB37.C458 616.07'56 79-9045
ISBN 0-444-80089-1

PRINTED IN THE NETHERLANDS

Preface

Some four years ago, the Editors canvassed opinion in several countries as to the need for an authoritative book on the interpretative aspects of clinical chemistry tests. It was felt that several detailed volumes on methodology were available, but similar depth of coverage of interpretation was incomplete or somewhat dated. All the individuals who were approached agreed on the value of an endeavour to gather together comprehensive surveys by authorities in all branches of the subject.

In seeking potential authors, we asked both physicians who were often faced with the problem of differential diagnosis of diseases and laboratory scientists who were commonly presented with isolated abnormal test values, to discuss the choice of tests and the interpretation of results from their different perspectives. Inevitably, this led to a certain measure of overlap, yet we felt that a dual approach was essential to provide adequate coverage of many different topics. We are grateful to the authors for minimizing duplication, but yet at the same time achieving thorough coverage of their own subjects. Strong efforts have been made not to overlook topics of actual or potential importance, but we would be grateful if readers could draw our attention to areas which they feel have been inadequately covered.

So far as possible, the material of each chapter has been organized in a uniformly systematic way, but the authors have been encouraged to adopt their own individual styles within this framework. Many of the chapters, and in some instances subsections of chapters, have been the subject of distinct monographs; and it has been essential to be highly selective. Undoubtedly on occasion the selection has been biased by the particular interests of the editors or the author concerned. However, a general attempt has been made to concentrate on the areas of major clinical importance; details of methodology have only been incorporated when they have an immediate bearing on the clinical interpretation of results. On matters over which there is still room for debate, authors have been aware in many instances of a need to cut corners by the use of dogmatic statements. This has been necessary to avoid a review format which attempts to mention all points of view and decide nothing.

Since the chapters have been written over a period during which moves towards the Système Internationale d'Unités have taken place, or are being considered in many countries, we have felt compelled to use both SI and traditional units throughout the book. An attempt has been made to implement many of the latest recommendations on nomenclature, and it is perhaps not surprising that problems have been encountered which may not have been appreciated by those making the recommendations.

In the past, it has sometimes been necessary to make clinical interpretations of results which were obtained by very dubious methodologies. Modern technology has rendered many of these interpretations obsolete and attention has been drawn to certain instances where the lack of specificity of an assay is likely to render the clinical interpretation of a result difficult or confusing.

It may be said by some that the title of the book should have incorporated the term "clinical chemistry", and indeed the book does concern a major aspect of this subject. Various definitions of clinical chemistry – or chemical pathology – have been proposed (IFCC Newsletters, Nos. 6–10, 1971–1974) which indicate three main divisions: analytical, fundamental research into the biochemistry of health and disease (in some countries termed clinical biochemistry), and the interpretation of results. It is this last – neglected – facet which is dealt with here. However, we hope that our readership will include both clinicians and laboratory scientists; the title of the book was chosen to emphasize that the interpretative role of clinical chemistry covers an area where clinicians and biochemists meet on common ground.

July 1979

Stanley S. Brown
Frederick L. Mitchell
Donald S. Young

List of affiliations

PAUL D. BERK, M.D., F.A.C.P.
Head, Division of Hematology, Department of Medicine, Mount Sinai School of Medicine, New York, NY 10029, U.S.A.

DOUGLAS A.K. BLACK, Kt., M.D., F.R.C.P.
Emeritus Professor of Medicine, University of Manchester and President, Royal College of Physicians of London, 11 St. Andrew's Place, Regent Park, London NW1 4LE, England

WILLIAM Z. BORER, M.S., M.D.
Clinical Chemistry Service, Clinical Pathology Department, National Institutes of Health, Bethesda, MD 20014, U.S.A.

STANLEY S. BROWN, Ph.D., F.R.I.C., M.R.C.Path.
Head, Research and Development Subdivision and Deputy Head, Division of Clinical Chemistry, M.R.C. Clinical Research Centre, Harrow, Middlesex HA1 3UJ, England

J. STEWART CAMERON, M.D., F.R.C.P.
Professor of Renal Medicine, Guy's Hospital Medical School, London Bridge, London SE1 9RT, England

ROBIN W. CARRELL, M.B., Ph.D., F.R.A.C.P., M.R.C.Path.
Professor of Clinical Biochemistry, Department of Pathology, Christchurch Hospital, Christchurch, New Zealand

ISRAEL CHANARIN, M.D., F.R.C.Path.
Head, Section of Haematology and Consultant Haematologist, M.R.C. Clinical Research Centre, Northwick Park Hospital, Harrow, Middlesex HA1 3UJ, England

KAY W. COLSTON, B.Sc., Ph.D.
Senior Research Officer, Endocrine Unit, Royal Postgraduate Medical School, Du Cane Road, London W12 0HS, England

JAMES B. ELDER, M.D., F.R.C.S.(Ed.), F.R.C.S.(Eng.)
Reader in Surgery, University of Manchester and Consultant Surgeon, The Royal Infirmary, Manchester M13 9WL, England

IMOGEN M.A. EVANS, M.D., Ph.D., F.R.C.P.(C.)
Honorary Consultant, Endocrine Unit, Royal Postgraduate Medical School, Du Cane Road, London W12 0HS, England

PROVASH C. GANGULI, M.B., F.R.C.P.
Senior Lecturer in Gastroenterology, University of Manchester and Consultant Physician, The Royal Infirmary, Manchester M13 9WL, England

PETER B. GREENBERG, M.D., Ph.D., F.R.A.C.P.
Physician, Royal Melbourne Hospital, Melbourne, Victoria, Australia

C. NICHOLAS HALES, M.A., M.D., Ph.D., M.R.C.Path, F.R.C.P.
Professor and Head of Department of Clinical Biochemistry, University of Cambridge, Addenbrooke's Hospital, Hills Road, Cambridge CB2 2QR, England

R. ANGUS HARKNESS, M.B., Ph.D., F.R.C.P.E., F.R.C.Path.
Deputy Head, Division of Perinatal Medicine, M.R.C. Clinical Research Centre and Honorary Consultant Chemical Pathologist, Northwick Park Hospital, Harrow, Middlesex HA1 3UJ, England

RAYMOND HOFFENBERG, M.D., Ph.D., F.R.C.P.
William Withering Professor of Medicine and Head of Department of Medicine, University of Birmingham, Birmingham B15 2TH, England

C. DEREK HOLDSWORTH, M.D., F.R.C.P.
Consultant Physician, Gastrointestinal Unit, Hallamshire Hospital, Sheffield S10 2JF, England

MOGENS HØRDER, Fr.Med.Sc., M.D.
Associate Professor in Clinical Chemistry at the University of Odense and Head, Department of Clinical Chemistry, Odense University Hospital, DK-5000 Odense, Denmark

VIVIAN H.T. JAMES, D.Sc., Ph.D., F.R.I.C., F.R.C.Path.
Professor of Chemical Pathology, Department of Chemical Pathology, St. Mary's Hospital Medical School, Paddington, London W2 1PG, England

E. ANTHONY JONES, M.D., M.R.C.P.
Head, Section of Diseases of the Liver, Digestive Diseases Branch, National Institute of Arthritis, Metabolism and Digestive Diseases, National Institutes of Health, Bethesda, MD 20205, U.S.A.

RICHARD G. LARKINS, M.D., Ph.D., F.R.A.C.P.
First Assistant, Department of Medicine, University of Melbourne, Repatriation General Hospital, Heidelberg, Victoria 3077, Australia

ALEXANDER A.H. LAWSON, M.D., F.R.C.P.E.
Consultant Physician, Milesmark Hospital, Dunfermline, and to the West Fife Group of Hospitals; Honorary Consultant Tutor, Department of Medicine, University of Edinburgh and Postgraduate Tutor for West Fife, Scotland

HERMANN LEHMANN, M.D., Sc.D., F.R.C.P., F.R.S., F.R.I.C., F.R.C.Path.
Emeritus Professor of Clinical Biochemistry, University of Cambridge, University Department of Biochemistry, Tennis Court Road, Cambridge CB2 1QW, England

BARRY LEWIS, M.D., Ph.D., F.R.C.P., M.R.C.Path.
Professor, Department of Chemical Pathology and Metabolic Disorders, St. Thomas' Hospital Medical School, London SE1 7EH, England

IAIN MacINTYRE, M.B., Ch.B., Ph.D., D.Sc., F.R.C.P., F.R.C.Path.
Professor of Endocrine Chemistry and Director, Endocrine Unit, Royal Postgraduate Medical School, Du Cane Road, London W12 0HS, England

ROBERT D.G. MILNER, M.A., M.D., Ph.D., F.R.C.P.
Professor and Head of Department of Paediatrics, University of Sheffield, Children's Hospital, Sheffield S10 2TH, England

FREDERICK L. MITCHELL, D.Sc., Ph.D., F.R.I.C., F.R.C.Path.
Head, Division of Clinical Chemistry, M.R.C. Clinical Research Centre, Harrow, Middlesex HA1 3UJ, England

HIPOLITO V. NIÑO, Ph.D.
Director of Research and Development, Diagnostics Operations, Beckman Instruments, Inc., Fullerton, CA 92634, U.S.A.

THEODORE PETERS, Jr., Ph.D.
Diplomate, American Board of Clinical Chemistry; Research Biochemist, The Mary Imogene Bassett Hospital, Cooperstown, NY 13326 and Adjunct Associate Professor of Biochemistry, College of Physicians and Surgeons, Columbia University, New York, NY, U.S.A.

D. NOEL RAINE, B.Sc., Ph.D., M.B., B.S., F.R.I.C., F.R.C.Path.
Consultant Chemical Pathologist and Head, Department of Clinical Chemistry, The Children's Hospital, Birmingham B16 8ET, England

COLIN R.J. RUTHVEN, Ph.D., M.Sc., F.R.I.C., C.Chem.
Top Grade Biochemist, Bernhard Baron Memorial Research Laboratories, Queen Charlotte's Maternity Hospital, London W6 0XG, England

MERTON SANDLER, M.D., F.R.C.P., F.R.C.Path.
Professor of Chemical Pathology, University of London, Institute of Obstetrics and Gynaecology, Queen Charlotte's Maternity Hospital, London W6 0XG, England

MORTON K. SCHWARTZ, Ph.D.
Vice President for Laboratory Affairs and Chairman, Department of Biochemistry, Memorial Sloan-Kettering Cancer Center, New York, NY 10021, U.S.A.

OLE SIGGAARD-ANDERSEN, M.D., Ph.D.
Professor of Clinical Chemistry, University of Copenhagen and Head, Department of Clinical Chemistry, Copenhagen County Hospital, Herlev, DK-2730 Herlev, Denmark

F. WILLIAM SUNDERMAN, Jr., M.D., F.A.C.P., F.C.A.P.
Professor and Chairman, Department of Laboratory Medicine, University of Connecticut School of Medicine, Farmington, CT 06032, U.S.A.

DONALD P. TSCHUDY, Ph.D.
Senior Investigator, Metabolism Branch, National Cancer Institute, National Institutes of Health, Bethesda, MD 20014, U.S.A.

RICHARD W.E. WATTS, M.D., D.Sc., Ph.D., F.R.C.P., F.R.I.C.
Head, Division of Inherited Metabolic Diseases, M.R.C. Clinical Research Centre and Honorary Consultant Physician, Northwick Park Hospital, Harrow, Middlesex HA1 3UJ, England

† J. HENRY WILKINSON, C.B.E., Ph.D., D.Sc., F.R.I.C., F.R.C.Path.
Professor of Chemical Pathology in the University of London at Charing Cross Hospital Medical School and Consultant Chemical Pathologist to Charing Cross Hospital, Department of Chemical Pathology, Charing Cross Hospital, Fulham Palace Road, London W6 8RF, England

† Died November 29th, 1977.

DONALD S. YOUNG, M.B., Ph.D.
Professor of Laboratory Medicine, Mayo Medical School and Head, Section of Clinical Chemistry, Mayo Clinic, Rochester, MN 55901, U.S.A.

Contents

CHAPTER 3: HYDROGEN IONS AND BLOOD GASES

CHAPTER 4: GLUCOSE METABOLISM

CHAPTER 5: LIPIDS

CHAPTER 6: PROTEINS

CHAPTER 7: ENZYMES

CHAPTER 8: CALCIUM AND MAGNESIUM

CHAPTER 9: RENAL FUNCTION

CHAPTER 21: PURINES AND NUCLEOTIDES
Richard W.E. Watts 1059

CHAPTER 22: VITAMINS
Hipolito V. Niño 1121

CHAPTER 23: TOXICOLOGY AND DRUG MONITORING
Stanley S. Brown and Alexander A.H. Lawson 1161

Chapter 1

Biological variability

Donald S. Young

Department of Laboratory Medicine, Mayo Clinic, Rochester, MN 55901, U.S.A.

CONTENTS

Chemical diagnosis of disease, edited by
S.S. Brown, F.L. Mitchell and D.S. Young

1.1. INTRODUCTION

Many factors, other than disease, cause alterations in the concentration of constituents in body fluids and must always be considered if correct interpretation of laboratory data is to be made. The factors may be grouped under several headings. Firstly, there are population factors that are characteristic of a specific group of which an individual is a member. These factors usually remain constant, although the extent of their influence may change with time. Other factors can be classified as long-term physiological influences, which include the ageing process, the geographical location and environment in which the individual normally resides, and his habitual diet. Short-term physiological influences such as the effect of recent food intake or smoking, the posture of the individual, or the time of day when the specimen was obtained, have an immediate effect on the composition of the blood before it is collected. The handling and processing of the specimen between collection and analysis may markedly influence its composition. The analytical methods used in the clinical laboratory, because of different degrees of accuracy, specificity and precision, may yield results that do not reflect the true composition of body fluids.

Disease, and its treatment, must be considered only as additional, although major, factors that may alter the composition of the body fluids. All test values are subject to non-disease influences, yet this has been recognized only recently, and many of the laboratory data that have been reported in past studies must be considered with suspicion unless supported by evidence of control of the physiological and analytical aspects of the work.

As with all biological systems, there is not necessarily a uniform response among individuals, so that while a response may be described as if it were typical of all individuals, several may respond in a different manner. Data are presented here typical of the majority response, but even then, particular experimental conditions may affect the response.

1.1.1. Composition of the body

The average water content of an adult is about 40 litres – 60% of the total body mass. In the obese individual, water comprises a lesser proportion of the body mass, and in lean individuals it is greater. In the newborn the contribution of water to the total body mass is much greater, but in the elderly adult both the absolute amount and the percentage of total water decrease below those of the younger adult. Of the total body water in the adult 70% is intracellular. It is this fraction that is most increased in the newborn. Approximately three-quarters of the extracellular water is extravascular, mainly interstitial, and the remainder is intravascular. The considerable differences in the composition of the major body fluids are summarized in Table 1.1.

The total body content of sodium is between 2.5 and 3.5 mol. Sodium exists in an exchangeable form, which is freely diffusible, and also, to a lesser extent, in a bound form in the skeleton, which is not exchangeable with the other elements in the extracellular compartment. Unlike the exchangeable sodium, the bound element is metabolically inactive. Total body sodium and chloride remain relatively constant in adult males but decline in women after age 60 years (Ellis et al., 1976). The total body content of potassium is between 3.0 and 4.0 mol, of which less than 0.1 mol is present intravascularly.

TABLE 1.1.

TYPICAL ELECTROLYTE COMPOSITION OF BODY FLUIDS (all values expressed in mmol/litre)

	Serum	Interstitial fluid	Intracellular fluid	Cerebrospinal fluid
Sodium	142	145	10	141
Potassium	4	4	150	3
Calcium	2.5	2.5	2	1
Magnesium	1	1	7.5	1
Chloride	101	114	10	122
Bicarbonate	27	31	10	24
Phosphate	2	2	90	1

About four-fifths of the potassium is present in muscle cells from which it is freely exchangeable. The total body potassium increases with an increase in body fat.

The body contains about 30 mol of calcium, almost all of which is incorporated into the skeleton, with only a small part in blood or other tissues. The absolute quantity of calcium may vary markedly between individuals. Thus the total body calcium may be as much as 40% less in women than men (Cohn et al., 1976a, b). The total body calcium, phosphorus and potassium decrease in both sexes with age. In women, the rate of loss of calcium from the body is approximately 0.4% per year until the menopause, at which time the rate of change increases to 1.1% annually. In men, there is little change until age 50 years but thereafter it decreases by 0.7% per year. The rates of loss of potassium and phosphorus are similar to that for calcium. The mechanisms for these changes are not established but may be related to modification of the effective use of food with age, or to decreased gonadal function, associated with reduced physical activity, which may affect both skeletal and muscular metabolism.

The composition of the lean body mass of individuals, i.e. the body mass less that due to fat, is quite constant from individual to individual. The lean body mass decreases with age to the extent of approximately 3 kg per decade in the mature adult, so that the elderly adult is shorter, with a reduced skeletal and muscular mass, than his younger counterpart (Forbes, 1976). The basal metabolic rate, oxygen consumption, and plasma and erythrocyte volumes are also decreased.

Approximately 16%, or 12 kg, of a healthy adult's mass is protein, of which one-third is collagen and metabolically inactive. At birth the protein constitutes less of the lean body mass than in the older child or adult. Most of the body protein is contained in skeletal muscle. This tissue is also the main store of carbohydrate in the form of glycogen. However, the total store of carbohydrate is generally only 0.5 kg, of which less than one-quarter is available for use as energy, i.e. less than one day's normal consumption (Passmore and Draper, 1970).

The quantity of body fat varies greatly from individual to individual. An average value of 14% of body weight has been obtained in young adult males and 26% in older men. In women, the values are approximately 10% higher in both age groups (Keys, 1955). The fat depots serve as the largest store of available energy in healthy adults.

1.1.2. The individual versus the population

The concept of biochemical individuality was first discussed extensively by Williams (1956). He attributed the differences in size of organs and composition of body fluids to genetic influences. However, the composition of fluids is also affected by an individual's life-style. Quite large differences in the concentration of constituents of blood and urine between different individuals can occur in the absence of disease. Thus comparison of the test values obtained from one individual may not be meaningful when assessed against values obtained from other people. Worse still, misinterpretations may arise.

Generally, the variation in the concentration of the constituents of serum or plasma is greater between individuals than within one person, even when measured over some time. This is illustrated in Table 1.2. It is apparent that even in a good laboratory, analytical variability may exceed physiological variability for several test constituents. Physiological variability, both within and between individuals, is quite small for most constituents except for glucose, cholesterol and several of the commonly measured enzyme activities. These constituents are among those most affected by the factors that are discussed later in this chapter.

As Williams (1967) has demonstrated, the variability of results for the same test constituent may be quite different in different individuals when measured over the same period of time. The point around which the data appear to vary is characteristic for each individual. Each individual has his own biological variability. Both set-point and variabil-

TABLE 1.2.

RELATIVE INFLUENCE OF ANALYTICAL, INTRAINDIVIDUAL AND INTERINDIVIDUAL FACTORS ON RESULTS OF SERUM TESTS EXPRESSED AS PERCENTAGE OF TOTAL VARIABILITY

The actual figures vary with the technique and instrument used. (Data reproduced, by permission, from Van Steirteghem, A.C., Robertson, E.A. and Young, D.S. (1978) Variance components of serum components in healthy individuals. Clinical Chemistry, 24, 212–222.)

Test	Analytical	Intraindividual	Interindividual
Albumin	20	16	64
Bilirubin	4	24	72
Calcium	47	15	38
Cholesterol	4	8	88
Creatinine	29	10	61
Sodium	88	12	0
Triglycerides	1	19	80
Urea	5	36	59
Uric Acid	11	19	71
Alanine Aminotransferase	10	12	79
Alkaline Phosphatase	3	5	92
Aspartate Aminotransferase	4	13	83
Creatine Kinase	3	57	39
Lactate Dehydrogenase	6	5	89

ity may be genetically determined. Even so, the set-point within one individual may not remain constant and may be influenced both by age and other physiological factors.

1.1.3. Reference values

Biological variability assumes clinical importance when laboratory tests are performed on a sick person. Test results are usually compared against what has been conventionally called a "normal range". In many institutions the origin of the range is obscure. In others, it has been derived from values obtained from the blood of laboratory personnel, medical students or nurses. The results are then used in their entirety, or after some statistical manipulation to remove outliers, to develop the "normal range". Yet this population differs in many respects from that which is typically the patient population in a hospital, or that which visits a physician or health screening clinic.

Dybkaer and Gräsbeck (1973), among others, have advanced the concept of reference values for correct interpretation of data. The reference values are obtained from a group matched in as many respects as possible to the individual on whom the data were obtained. This concept acknowledges that different physiological variables may have as much influence on laboratory data as genetic background. At present it is uncertain how many different factors should be considered in deriving a reference range and which of these are sufficiently important that they must always be considered. Many factors that affect laboratory data have been identified, but few appear to be so important that a physician would normally question a patient about them. In fact, considerable education of physicians is required to alert them to the influence of even some of the major factors.

1.1.4. Mathematically derived normal values

In general, it is impractical to obtain repeated laboratory data on a single individual under ideal conditions in order to develop his own reference values to be used for interpretation of his test values when he is ill. In the past, too few factors have been considered in the various studies of healthy populations to obtain enough data to produce adequate reference values.

Hoffman and Waid (1965) proposed the use of data obtained on a hospital population from which "normal" data could be extracted for use as a reference range by means of various statistical approaches. Many arguments have been produced against this. They include the biases introduced by different disease populations, the underlying reasons for performing the laboratory tests in the first instance and the frequency distribution of the test values, even in a healthy population. This approach has been commonly used to develop a reference range for complicated tests because of the expense involved in performing additional analyses. Yet it is particularly unwise to use such an approach when an expensive test is concerned because of the strong suspicion of abnormality that a physician would usually have before requesting such a test. The use of reference ranges developed mathematically from data from hospital patients has recently been thoroughly discussed by H.F. Martin et al. (1975).

1.2. GENETIC INFLUENCES

While it is widely believed that heredity has a major influence on the composition of body fluids, few studies have been undertaken to confirm this. It is always necessary to separate the influence of environment from that of heredity. Accordingly most studies have had to rely on differences between monozygotic and dizygotic twins. It has been shown, for example, that the enzymes involved in catecholamine metabolism show smaller differences in activities between monozygotic than dizygotic twins. This has been conclusively demonstrated for erythrocyte catechol-*O*-methyltransferase (EC 2.1.1.6), platelet monoamine oxidase (EC 1.4.3.4) and serum dopamine-β-hydroxylase (EC 1.14.17.1) (Weinshilboum et al., 1974). There is greater concordance between the plasma amino acids of monozygotic twins than between dizygotic twins (Scriver and Rosenberg, 1973).

The influence of heredity and environment may interact. Thus, while the difference between serum cholesterol concentrations in monozygotic twins is less than that between dizygotic twins when the pair live together, the difference between dizygotic twins is not significantly affected when they live apart. In contrast, the difference between monozygotic twins becomes significantly greater (Meyer, 1962). The concentrations of free cholesterol and of high- and low-density lipoproteins appear to be more affected by heredity than environment, yet the influence of environment is greater than heredity on the esterified cholesterol (Christian et al., 1976). The concentration of total cholesterol in plasma, and especially low-density lipoprotein cholesterol, is higher in individuals possessing the Lp(a) antigen than in other people, but the triglyceride concentration is less (Berg et al., 1976). Less variation of serum concentrations of total phospholipids, glyceride glycerol, and uric acid has been shown to occur in monozygotic twins than dizygotic twins (Jensen et al., 1965). This is also true for the fatty acid composition of plasma lipids and cholesterol esters (Kang et al., 1976). There is a signficant influence of heredity on the concentrations of plasma urea, urate and bilirubin, and there is also a significant effect on the plasma glucose concentration one hour after a glucose load (Havlik et al., 1977).

Obvious inherited influences on the composition of body fluids are apparent in certain situations of hypercholesterolaemia, hypophosphatasaemia, diabetes mellitus (Zonana and Rimoin, 1976), and in a family with a high serum concentration of zinc in the absence of a recognizable aetiological basis (J.C. Smith et al., 1976). Other trace elements may be affected in the same way. The existence of an atypical combination of biochemical findings in an inbred group is suggestive of a strong influence of heredity, although an important environmental influence cannot be excluded. The genetic influence probably predominates in the Masai tribe of East Africa who characteristically have low serum concentrations of cholesterol and β-lipoproteins despite a high dietary cholesterol intake (Biss et al., 1971). In these people the concentration of α_2-globulin is high, as is the concentration of immunoglobulin IgA. Further, the ratio of concentrations of phospholipid and bile acids to cholesterol in their bile is considerably higher than in other individuals.

Certain statistical correlations between blood groups and the concentrations of various compounds in serum have been demonstrated. Changes associated with blood group are relatively small, but include a higher concentration of uric acid in people of blood group

B and lower in group A. The concentration of α_1-antitrypsin is less in the plasma of men of group B than those of group O (Dawson et al., 1976). The intestinal component of alkaline phosphatase (EC 3.1.3.1) is rarely found in the serum of ABH non-secretors. Total alkaline phosphatase activity is higher in individuals with blood groups O or B than in group A. The activity of the enzyme in group AB individuals is intermediate between that of the other groups. Serum cholesterol concentration is generally slightly higher in men of blood group A than in those of other groups. The serum cholesterol ester concentration is greatest in group A individuals (Banerjee and Saha, 1969). Thus there appears to be an inverse relationship between the ABO-associated factors which affect serum cholesterol concentration and intestinal alkaline phosphatase activity.

1.3. LONG-TERM PHYSIOLOGICAL INFLUENCES

Under this heading are considered many of the in vivo factors that affect laboratory data. The differentiation between long-term and short-term physiological factors is somewhat arbitrary. The same factor, such as diet, may have both long- and short-term effects. The habitual diet is considered as a long-term effect whereas the influence of a single meal is considered as a short-term effect.

1.3.1. Ageing

Time not only alters the physical appearance of an individual but has a marked effect on the composition of his blood plasma. Shakespeare recognized seven ages of man but there are four critical periods as far as laboratory data are concerned. These are the newborn period with the immediate adaptation to extrauterine life, early childhood to puberty, puberty to the menopause in women and to middle age in men, and finally, old age. While puberty and the menopause may impose abrupt changes, there is generally a gradual change of test values within each of these four time periods for each individual. Hormonal influences more than chronological age affect test values, so that careful questioning is required to determine whether puberty or the menopause has actually occurred at the ages at which these events are likely to occur.

1.3.1.1. Newborn

Most physiological systems are involved in the infant's adjustment to extrauterine life. His ability to respond to a new independent existence is affected by his maturity at the time of birth. The amount of trauma at birth also has a major effect on the composition of his body fluids.

In the mature infant, much of the foetal haemoglobin (Haemoglobin F) has already been replaced by adult Haemoglobin A. At birth, the oxygen tension of the mature infant's umbilical vein may be as low as 20 mm Hg (2.7 kPa), but it is usually even less in the immature infant. Oxygen saturation of arterial blood is less in infants than in adults but the former are able to withstand a greater degree of unsaturation than would be tolerated by either older children or adults. In the first hour after birth the blood oxygen tension and saturation increase rapidly. While the pO_2 may still be as low as 60 mm Hg

(8.0 kPa) at this time, the oxygen saturation may be as high as 95%. Nevertheless it usually remains below the adult values for several weeks following birth (Oliver et al., 1961). Following a difficult birth, or if apnoea occurs following delivery, the blood pO_2 and degree of oxygen saturation may be much reduced below the normal values. Crying induces hyperventilation, and possibly respiratory alkalosis, which may create a false impression of a baby's blood gas status.

At birth, the mature infant has an adequate supply of erythrocytic carbonic anhydrase (EC 4.2.1.1) although the activity may only be one-third as much as in an adult. In a premature infant it may be only one-twentieth of the adult's concentration. Nevertheless, the pCO_2 and bicarbonate content of the infant's blood are only slightly lower than the values determined in a healthy adult. If the onset of respiration in a newborn is delayed there is a marked prompt rise of the blood pCO_2. The biochemical findings of the general stress response in adults (section 1.6.3.) are observed.

During life in utero, the blood pH of the foetus is higher than after birth. In a mature infant a metabolic acidosis, characterized by decreased pH, bicarbonate and buffer base, supervenes after birth although the acid–base state becomes similar to that of the adult within 24 hours (Pincus et al., 1956). In the premature infant the acidosis is more severe. Much of the acidosis is due to the accumulation and retention of organic anions, especially lactate. This is presumed to arise from imperfect metabolism of carbohydrate, but it may also arise from the mother during labour, and from anoxia in the infant. Even in the infant who is mature at birth, the blood lactate does not decrease to the adult concentration for about four days: in the premature infant it takes longer.

Within a few minutes of birth, fluid shifts out of the blood vessels into the extravascular tissues (Gairdner et al., 1958). With the exception of protein, the concentration of which is less, this fluid has a composition similar to that of plasma. This causes an increase in the plasma protein concentration, by as much as 20%, which is detectable within the first hour. This also causes an increase in the plasma osmotic pressure and stimulates the secretion of vasopressin. After this initial rise, the plasma protein concentration falls to a new level at 4 weeks, from which it gradually increases over the next 4 years. Fibrinogen and globulins decrease during the first month of extrauterine life. The decreased protein concentrations may be a manifestation of impaired ability of the liver to synthesize protein in the newborn period.

The concentrations of the immunoglobulins in an infant's blood at birth reflect the transfer of these from the maternal circulation. The changes that occur following birth result from the catabolism of these proteins, the de novo synthesis by the infant, and the different half-lives of the proteins. Premature infants usually have lower concentrations of antibodies and are less able to synthesize new antibodies than term infants. Yet at birth, the concentration of IgG is similar in the serum of infant and mother, but the infant's serum contains very little IgM and no detectable IgA. The concentration of IgG falls to its lowest level at age 3 to 6 months but reaches adult values between 1 and 4 years of age. The adult concentration of IgM is attained at about 6 months and that of IgA, after an initial rapid increase to 6 months, climbs more slowly to reach adult values during adolescence or later. IgD is not detectable in plasma of infants less than 6 months of age (Rowe et al., 1968).

In all infants, the concentration of bilirubin increases in the first few days of life to reach a peak in the term baby at the third to fifth day. In the premature infant, the concentration is usually higher and also peaks later. In newborn infants with reduced erythrocyte glutathione reductase (EC 1.6.4.2) activity, the plasma bilirubin curve is higher than in others (Lie-Injo et al., 1974). The serum iron concentration is considerably higher in the infant than the mother at birth but falls to the adult value in about 5 months. The serum transferrin concentration changes in an inverse manner.

The blood glucose concentration decreases from the adult value at birth to about 3.4 mmol/litre (60 mg/dl) in the first few days. The fall is usually greater in premature infants because of decreased hepatic glycogen reserves or inadequate gluconeogenesis. The adult concentration is regained by about 2 weeks after birth. At birth the concentration of all lipids is less than in the adult, but by 2 weeks all concentrations have increased substantially. The plasma cholesterol may be as much as 80% of the adult value within four days and constitutes a greater proportion of the total lipid than in the adult. The concentration tends to be higher in breast-fed than formula-fed infants because of the high cholesterol content of mother's milk (Friedman and Goldberg, 1975). The influence of a low cholesterol diet in infancy persists during childhood, with a lower serum cholesterol concentration being observed several years later (Hodgson et al., 1976).

In newborn infants the plasma concentration of vitamin E is low: in premature infants it is even less. The concentration of vitamin D is also low in premature infants because of a low concentration of binding protein. In term infants, the protein concentration of the binding protein is the same as in adults (Haddad and Walgate, 1976).

Although it is higher at birth than in the adult, the plasma sodium concentration decreases to that of the adult within 12 hours. In the premature infant the concentration is less than in the term baby, and hyponatraemia may persist for 2 weeks (Honour et al., 1977). After 36 hours the concentration rises in all mature infants to a value slightly higher than in the adult. The rise is probably associated with loss of water from the circulation to produce a relative haemoconcentration. In the newborn infant, renin activity is high and aldosterone secretion is low in spite of the hyponatraemia. The chloride concentration in the plasma of infants and adults is similar. The potassium concentration in cord blood plasma may be as much as 7 mmol/litre but it decreases rapidly after birth. The concentration is higher in the plasma of premature infants. In the foetus, the plasma potassium concentration is higher and falls steadily towards the end of pregnancy. The high potassium concentration at birth may be caused in part by the transient anoxia and acidosis that occurs with birth. The plasma phosphate is high at birth and increases further during the first few hours of life. This has been attributed to the utilization of glycogen and the release of bound phosphate. Later, the plasma calcium, which is also increased at birth, and phosphate decrease in parallel. The fall in calcium may be as much as 0.35 mmol/litre (0.7 mEq/litre) during the first day of life. The decrease may be related to a temporary dysfunction of the parathyroid glands or to the deposition of calcium phosphate in the bones. The change in composition of serum with respect to some of the commonly measured constituents, which occurs shortly after birth, is illustrated in Figure 1.1.

The serum activities of alkaline phosphatase, creatine kinase (EC 2.7.3.2), γ-glutamyltransferase (EC 2.3.2.2) and aspartate aminotransferase (EC 2.6.1.1) are high at birth, but that of alanine aminotransferase (EC 2.6.1.2) is low. At birth, the concentration of urea

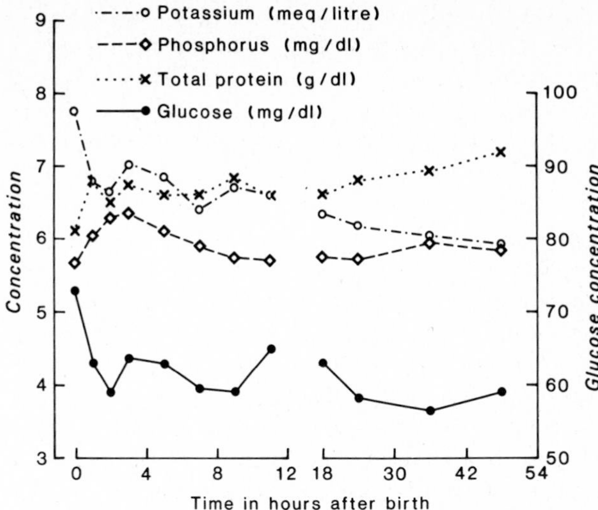

Figure 1.1. Change in composition of full-term infant's plasma during first 48 hours of life. SI Unit conversion for glucose, mg/dl × 0.056 = mmol/litre; for phosphate, mg/dl × 0.323 = mmol/litre. (Reproduced, by permission, from Acharya and Payne, 1965)

in cord blood is determined by the mother, but shortly afterwards the concentration of urea decreases in the newborn's blood as a result of the synthesis of protein. As tissue catabolism increases, the concentration of urea begins to rise. Although the plasma urate is high at birth its clearance is high in the first week of life so that the plasma urate concentration soon falls to a low value.

Shortly after birth the plasma aminoacid concentration falls. It is especially low in newborn infants. Plasma aminoacid concentration is low in infancy during the period of rapid growth. Aminoacid clearance is higher in infants than adults because of lower tubular reabsorption (Scriver and Rosenberg, 1973). In premature infants the aminoaciduria is generalized and urinary excretion may be as much as five times the adult excretion. In full-term babies the aminoaciduria is less pronounced but still much greater than in adults. The adult excretion pattern is normally achieved at 6 months. Taurine excretion is high during the first 7 days of extrauterine life. Iminoaciduria and glycinuria may persist for several months (Hill et al., 1976).

During the first week of extrauterine life, the newborn excretes large quantities of urinary oestrogens derived from the mother during pregnancy. At the same time the excretion of pregnanediol decreases so that the output is negligible by the seventh day. The plasma prolactin concentration increases within 30 minutes of birth, possibly in response to the secretion of thyrotrophin releasing hormone (Sack et al., 1976), but it then declines during the next week. The older infant, also when breast fed, excretes prolactin, probably ingested in mother's milk.

At birth the concentration of 17-oxosteroids is higher in the infant's plasma than in that of the mother: in premature infants it may be as much as ten times higher. During pregnancy the concentration of androgens in the mother's plasma is low but it rises in response to the stress of delivery. The higher concentration in infants may be due to direct placental transfer of the steroids or trophic hormones. However, the distribution of the androsterone and dehydroepiandrosterone fractions is quite different between mother and child, which implies that the infant's adrenals are actively functioning at birth. The mother's influence probably does produce some degree of hypocorticism in the infant which persists for several days after birth and is manifested by low concentrations of cortisol and other glucocorticoids in plasma. The hypocorticism is initially masked by the stress of labour and delivery which produces high concentrations of cortisol in both mother and infant. In infants delivered by Caesarean section, the plasma concentration of cortisol is much less than in infants delivered vaginally. The corticotrophin concentration is also less. The plasma corticotrophin is high two hours after birth but then falls to about one-third of this value at 24 hours (Cacciari et al., 1976). This probably occurs with the end of the stress induced by birth. During the neonatal period, the adrenals are reported to respond sluggishly to stimuli that normally provoke corticotrophin secretion. The plasma cortisol of the infant rises to the adult concentration about a week after birth. The plasma concentrations of growth hormone (somatotrophin), follicle stimulating hormone (FSH) and luteinizing hormone (LH) in the foetus are increased above the concentrations in adults during the last half of pregnancy (Fisher et al., 1973). The plasma growth hormone concentration remains markedly elevated in the neonate. Gastrin is actively secreted by the newborn infant and the plasma gastrin concentration is high, as is also the gastric acidity (von Berger et al., 1976).

At birth, the concentration of thyroxine in an infant's blood is only slightly less than in the mother, and is considerably greater than in the non-pregnant woman. Following birth, there is a prompt and dramatic secretion of thyroid-stimulating hormone (TSH, thyrotrophin) and the concentration of thyroxine in the infant's blood rises further. This physiological hyperthyroidism gradually declines over a year, at which time the adult concentration is reached. In the infants of a multiple birth, the plasma thyroxine concentration tends to be less than in a single baby. Free and total triiodothyronine (T_3) concentrations are low at birth but increase rapidly in response to TSH stimulation. The concentration of reverse T_3 may be increased by up to four times the adult concentration during the first month of life (Avruskin et al., 1976).

1.3.1.2. Childhood to puberty

As a child grows, the concentrations of almost all amino acids in the plasma decrease, but at puberty their concentrations increase to almost adult values. Urinary excretion increases in childhood until puberty. The alteration in aminoacid concentration is probably linked to skeletal muscle mass, as the changes are greater in boys than girls (Armstrong and Stave, 1973). Following the initial decrease in plasma protein concentration that occurs in the newborn period, the total protein concentration increases so that adult values are reached by age 10 years. The fractions generally increase in proportion to each other with the exception of γ-globulin, which appears to increase at the expense of α_2-globulin. Serum IgD concentration declines during adolescence from the high value of childhood. The changes in concentrations of other immunoglobulins with age are illustrated in Figure 1.2.

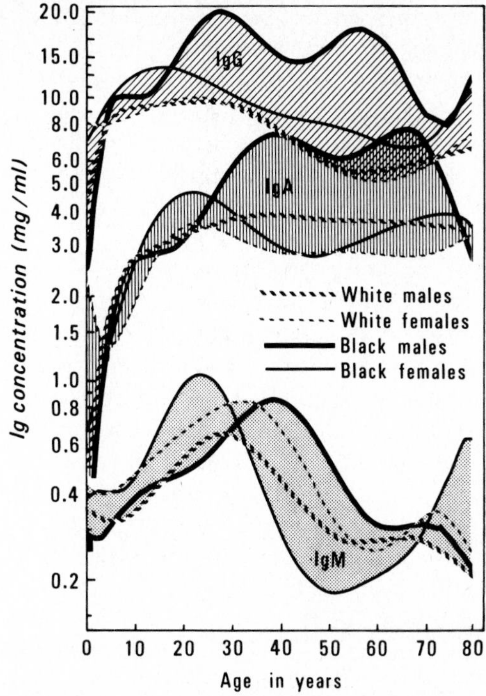

Figure 1.2. Differences in concentration of serum immunoglobulins with age, sex and race. (Reproduced, by permission, from Buckley and Dorsey, 1971)

Total body water, renal plasma flow, glomerular filtration rate and blood volume all increase relative to surface area with age until puberty (Krovetz, 1965). The serum creatinine concentration increases slowly from infancy to puberty, but is only slightly higher in males until puberty, at which time the sex difference becomes more marked. The serum concentration is closely correlated with body and muscle mass. Approximately 2% of body creatine – almost all of which is in skeletal muscle – is converted into creatinine each day (Cheek, 1968). The serum concentration of uric acid falls from its high value at birth to a nadir between ages 7 and 10 years, at which time it is lower in boys than girls. Thereafter, the concentration begins to rise rapidly in boys until age 16 years, at which time it becomes stable. Girls exhibit an increase also, but it is less pronounced. The increased serum concentration has been correlated with increased androgen secretion.

The activities in serum of several enzymes decrease during childhood. The rate of decrease is constant between ages 6 and 20 years for aspartate aminotransferase and is greater in girls than boys. The rate of decrease of lactate dehydrogenase activity is slight until puberty at which time it accelerates. During childhood, serum aldolase (EC 4.1.2.13) activity is only half of that at birth, but it still is greater than in the adult. The activity of creatine kinase and γ-glutamyltransferase falls rapidly during the first year, at the end of which values are similar to those in the adult. In contrast, serum activity of alanine aminotransferase increases in males from ages 6 to 50 years, although there is little change in females between ages 6 and 20 years. Serum 5′-nucleotidase (EC 3.1.3.5) activity is lowest around puberty (Goldberg, 1976).

Serum alkaline phosphatase activity is high in infancy and then decreases during childhood before increasing further to puberty. It peaks shortly afterwards at the time of maximum osteoblastic activity and bone growth. The correlation of alkaline phosphatase activity with changing sexual maturity is close, and activity decreases rapidly after puberty. The fall is more marked in girls whose growth ceases more rapidly. The serum phosphorus concentration decreases at the same time.

The plasma concentrations of urea, glucose, sodium, potassium, calcium and magnesium do not alter with age between 6 and 20 years. Between the ages of 2 and 6 years, the serum concentration of magnesium is low while that of calcium is high. The concentration of ionized calcium is highest between 6 and 16 years of age and shows a negative correlation with the serum parathyroid hormone concentration. The serum cholesterol concentration increases from birth, albeit slowly initially. The plasma folate concentration is higher in girls than boys. The concentration falls in both sexes with increasing maturity.

Prepubertal children secrete growth hormone during sleep only, whereas adolescents secrete it during periods of wakefulness also. Serum somatomedin activity rises steadily in children from one month of age until 15 years when adult values are reached (Pierson et al., 1976). The concentration of thyroxine in serum decreases to 6 years of age when adult values are reached. Serum triiodothyronine concentration is high in children (Westgren et al., 1976). The serum concentrations and urinary excretions, of FSH and LH increase during childhood until puberty. The adult concentration of FSH is reached at puberty. The concentration of LH in boys also reaches the adult values at this time, but in girls a further slight rise to the adult value occurs after puberty. The prepubertal oestradiol concentration is higher in girls than boys, but the oestrone concentrations are similar. With progression of puberty, oestrone and oestradiol concentrations rise in girls to a greater extent than in boys.

Peak values of pregnanetriol occur in both sexes between 16 and 20 years. Plasma testosterone concentration increases rapidly during puberty to reach adult values. The increase is less marked in girls than boys, the change in the former being due to increased adrenocortical activity. The growth spurt at puberty is not associated with increased secretion of growth hormone but with the increased secretion of androgens (Butenandt et al., 1976). An increased urinary excretion of 11-deoxy-17-oxosteroids occurs from 7 years of age and becomes more pronounced 2 to 3 years before clinical signs of puberty (Savage et al., 1975). The excretion is greater in boys than girls, indicative of a greater androgen secretion even before puberty. The rise continues beyond puberty until the adult concentration is reached. The excretion of 17-hydroxycorticosteroids and the α-ketolic metabolites of cortisol gradually rises with age and correlates with the individual's body mass. The α-ketolic metabolites of corticosterone are relatively high in infancy, but after 4 years their excretion correlates with body mass. The excretion of 17-oxosteroids and 17-hydroxycorticoids increases in both sexes until puberty but the excretion per gram of creatinine remains fairly constant throughout the growing years. The excretion in males increases steeply at this time while the increase in females is less marked. Adult values in males are not reached until after age 20 years. Peak values in women are reached between 16 and 20 years. Urinary total hydroxyproline excretion increases with age until puberty, then declines rapidly to the values observed in early childhood (Jones et al., 1964).

During childhood and adolescence there are gradual increases in the excretion of dihydrotestosterone, androstenedione, and dehydroepiandrosterone, all of which are precursors of oestrone in the adrenal. The plasma testosterone concentration increases rapidly during puberty to reach adult values (Reiter and Root, 1975). The plasma prolactin concentration falls to the adult value shortly after birth and is unaffected by growth and adolescence. In girls, the plasma prolactin and progesterone concentrations are unaffected by puberty until after the menarche (Lee et al., 1976). The excretion of catecholamines is low in infants but rises after 3 years. The excretion of homovanillic acid, vanillylmandelic acid and metanephrine is the same in children after puberty and adults.

1.3.1.3. Adult life

Between puberty and middle age, the changes in the plasma concentrations of most constituents are generally small. Indeed, reports are often conflicting about the direction and extent of the change. Serum total protein and albumin concentrations decrease slightly during this time. A slight decrease, or no change, has been reported for the serum calcium concentration in men; in women, there may be no change, or a slight decrease. The serum phosphorus decreases markedly after age 20 years in men and continues to fall at a lesser rate after this age. The phosphorus concentration decreases in women until just before the menopause, at which time it begins to rise. The change in serum phosphorus with the menopause may be related to reabsorption of bone. The serum alkaline phosphatase is less in adults than in children but during middle age there is little change in activity in either sex. After this time the activity rises in women so that in the elderly, alkaline phosphatase activity is higher in women than men. Serum magnesium concentration is unaffected by ageing.

Serum urea concentration increases in both sexes during middle age and uric acid increases in women, although there is little change in the concentration in men after puberty. Peak uric acid concentrations are usually reached in men in their third decade. Serum creatinine does not change with ageing in men, although it increases in women. The serum cholesterol concentration increases in both men and women with increasing age at a rate of approximately 0.05 mmol/litre (2 mg/dl) per year. The increase is greatest in the third decade in men, and the serum cholesterol concentration reaches a maximum between ages 50 and 60 years. There is actually little change in the absence of weight gain in men. In women, the serum cholesterol remains relatively constant until after the menopause. The serum triglyceride concentration increases with the rise in cholesterol. The serum bilirubin concentration increases after puberty but falls during the third decade to a new constant level. In both sexes the serum lactate dehydrogenase and aspartate aminotransferase activities are less than in adolescence. The alanine aminotransferase and creatine kinase activities fall with age in men. In women creatine kinase activity also tends to decrease. The concentration of glucose in plasma 1 hour after glucose administration rises about 0.45 mmol/litre (8 mg/dl) per decade. No differences in bromosulphthalein retention or galactose tolerance have been observed after age 20 years.

Pregnanediol and pregnanetriol excretion continue to increase in both men and women after puberty. Pregnanediol excretion peaks at about age 20 years in both sexes but falls thereafter. Pregnanetriol peaks a little earlier in women and the rate of decrease is less than that of pregnanediol. In men, dehydroepiandrosterone excretion rises rapidly after puberty, peaks at age 20 years, and then falls rapidly (Gleispach, 1973). The excretion of all oestrogens in women is greatest at about age 30 years, with values about 5 to 10 times greater than those at puberty.

Growth hormone secretion is greater during adult life than in prepubertal children or adolescents.

1.3.1.4. Old age

Significant increases in the plasma concentrations of urea, uric acid, inorganic phosphorus, calcium, cholesterol, total lipids and sodium occur following the menopause in women (Wilding et al., 1972). Alkaline phosphatase activity also increases.

In the elderly, many of the hormonal responses to a specific challenge are reduced. Thus, the growth hormone response to insulin hypoglycaemia is reduced and the marked surges in secretion observed in young adults no longer occur. The plasma TSH concentration is unaffected by ageing but its response to thyrotrophin releasing hormone is reduced, probably due to impairment of its release, as the amount present in the pituitary is unaffected by age. Corticotrophin stimulation produces a smaller increase in the concentration of cortisol in the plasma.

Renal concentration is impaired in the elderly. This is associated with a decreased effective renal plasma flow with a reduced glomerular filtration rate. The creatinine clearance may decrease by as much as 50% between the third and ninth decades. Renal ability to handle an acid load is reduced. The tubular maximum capacity for glucose is also affected (Epstein and Hollenberg, 1976). The secretion rate of renin falls and the plasma renin concentration and renin activity are also reduced. The blood urea concentration rises with age and urinary protein excretion increases. However, vasopressin secretion and the renal response to it are unaffected by age.

The basal metabolic rate and thyroid secretion decrease with age. The degradation of thyroxine is also reduced so that the plasma concentration is not influenced by ageing. The free thyroxine concentration remains constant, although the thyroxine-binding globulin may be increased to a slight extent. In ill elderly patients, the thyroxine-binding globulin is often reduced with a correspondingly reduced T_3 uptake. Triiodothyronine concentration decreases by 25 to 40% in individuals over 50 years of age, possibly as a result of a change in peripheral thyroxine metabolism. The serum triiodothyronine concentration decreases by approximately 50 ng/litre per decade from childhood to old age. There is no decrease in the plasma corticotrophin concentration in the elderly.

The concentration of cortisol in plasma may not be affected by age but the secretion rate of the hormone falls by 30% during adult life. Decreased secretion of cortisol results in a decreased excretion of 17-hydroxycorticosteroids in urine. The urinary excretion of 17-oxosteroids decreases in the elderly of both sexes to values approximately one-half of those in young adults because of lower production by the testes and adrenals (Moncloa et al., 1963). The excretion of dehydroepiandrosterone is decreased to a greater extent than that of the other 17-oxosteroids. The lower production of androgens by the testes and adrenals causes reductions in the plasma concentrations of dehydroepiandrosterone and androsterone to barely detectable values at age 70 years.

The metabolic clearance and secretory rates of aldosterone are decreased in the elderly and its plasma concentration is reduced by about 50% (Flood et al., 1967). Both the plasma aldosterone response to sodium restriction and the urinary excretion of sodium and potassium are reduced in the elderly. At age 70 years, plasma renin activity is only 60% of its concentration in 40-year-old individuals (Crane and Harris, 1976). This is illustrated in Figure 1.3.

Basal insulin secretion is unaffected by ageing but glucose tolerance is reduced. This is probably related to a diminished immediate secretion of insulin. A greater proportion of the insulin secreted in the elderly is proinsulin which is metabolically less active (Duckworth and Kitabchi, 1976). Glucagon secretion and response in the elderly are no different from that in the young.

Falls in the secretion rate and concentration of testosterone occur with age after 50 years in the male. At 80 years, the concentration is reduced to one-half of the value at 50 years. With age, the proportion of protein-bound testosterone increases so that there is an even greater decrease of the free hormone. The concentration of free dihydrotestosterone also decreases. There is no change in the concentration of testosterone in the plasma of women with age.

There is a marked increase in the concentration of pituitary gonadotrophins in blood and urine following the menopause. Oestrogen secretion begins to decrease several years before the menopause. It decreases further between the ages of 50 and 60 years. Oestrone

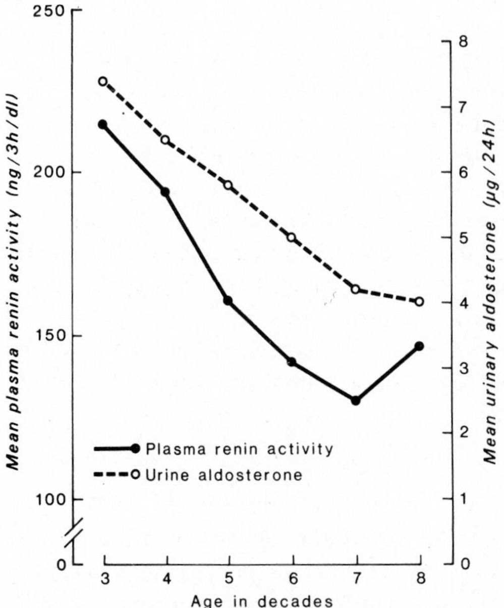

Figure 1.3. Reduction in plasma renin activity and urinary aldosterone excretion with ageing. (Reproduced, by permission, from Crane and Harris, 1976)

is less affected than oestriol and oestradiol. Oestrogen secretion, always at a lower level in men, falls further with age. In men, the free oestradiol actually increases with age (Pirke and Doerr, 1970). The decreased secretion of oestrogens may be partly responsible for the increased secretion of cholesterol that occurs with the menopause, and the increased cholesterol/phospholipid ratio that also occurs. The total lipid concentration increases with the rise in serum cholesterol, but lipoprotein lipase (EC 3.1.1.34) activity declines at the same time. The serum cholesterol concentration in men begins to decline by 0.08 mmol/litre (3 mg/dl) per year after age 60 years, at which time there is no sex difference in the cholesterol concentration. Progesterone secretion is decreased in elderly men and urinary pregnanediol excretion is reduced to one-quarter of that in young adults. The plasma FSH concentration in men aged 70 years is 2 to 4 times that at age 40 years. Plasma dehydroepiandrosterone concentration declines after age 50 years so that the values at 70 years are 20% of those at age 20 years.

Parathyroid hormone concentration in plasma decreases with age. After the menopause, the plasma concentration of calcium increases slightly and urinary excretion is also increased. Plasma phosphate rises and alkaline phosphatase activity in women may increase by 50% from before the menopause to age 70 years. There is considerable reabsorption of calcium from bone after the menopause. Urinary excretion of hydroxyproline declines in the elderly (Saleh and Coenegracht, 1968).

Urinary excretion of epinephrine and norepinephrine does not change with age, although the adrenal medullary response to specific challenges, and hence catecholamine secretion, decreases with age. Ziegler et al. (1976a) reported that the plasma norepinephrine, and its response to stress, is increased in the plasma of the elderly of both sexes, but Weidmann et al. (1975) failed to observe a change. Plasma dopamine-β-hydroxylase activity in the elderly is much less than in young adults (Ogihara et al., 1975).

Liver function tests are generally normal in the elderly although bromosulphthalein retention may be slightly decreased and the serum albumin, which is synthesized in the liver, may be reduced. The serum haptoglobin concentration increases between the ages of 20 and 70 years. In women, the serum uric acid concentration rises when the ovarian secretion of oestrogens is diminished. The activities of lactate dehydrogenase and aspartate aminotransferase increase in the serum of women after the menopause so that the sex difference is eliminated in the elderly. The serum iron concentration is less in the elderly of both sexes. There is also a higher incidence of positive rheumatoid factor and increased concentration of carcinoembryonic antigen in the serum of the elderly.

The blood P_{50} (oxygen tension at 50% oxygen saturation) shows a positive correlation with age (Tweeddale et al., 1976). Plasma zinc concentration decreases by as much as 0.77 μmol/litre (5 μg/dl) per decade (Reinhold, 1975).

1.3.2. Sex

In general, sex differences in laboratory data can be linked to either the influence of sex hormones or the differences in muscle mass between the two sexes. The greatest differences in test values tend to be observed between puberty and the menopause. There is little difference between the concentrations of most constituents of plasma between boys and girls, and the differences that are observed between puberty and the menopause in women and men of a similar age lessen as the hormonal influence on the female values is reduced. The differences are usually sufficiently large that data from the appropriate sex and age group should be used for the correct interpretation of test values.

The activities of alkaline phosphatase, alanine and aspartate aminotransferases, creatine kinase and aldolase are greater in the serum of men than women. After the menopause, the alkaline phosphatase activity of women is greater than men. The total lactate dehydrogenase activity is similar in men and women but LD_1 and LD_3 are higher and LD_2 is lower in young women than men. These differences disappear after the menopause, suggesting an oestrogenic influence (Cohen et al., 1967). α_1-Antitrypsin and α_2-macroglobulin concentrations are higher in women than men (Dawson et al., 1976).

The concentrations of total protein, albumin, calcium and magnesium are higher in men than in women, but the concentration of γ-globulin is less. The concentration of phosphorus may be slightly higher in women, especially at the time of menstruation. With the lower haemoglobin concentration of blood in women, the serum bilirubin is also reduced. The serum iron concentration in women may be low. The plasma ferritin concentration in menstruating women is only one-third of that in healthy men. The plasma zinc concentration is less in women than men. In contrast, the concentration of copper, α-lipoprotein and creatine is higher in the serum of women. Cholesterol is higher in men. Plasma α-amino nitrogen is also higher in men (Feigin, 1969). Dirren et al. (1975) have reported strongly sex-correlated urinary amino acid excretion patterns. Amylase (EC 3.2.1.1) activity may be greater in the serum of women. In keeping with the greater body mass of most men, the concentration of creatinine, urea and uric acid is higher than in women. The plasma concentration and urinary excretion of carnitine is greater in men than women (Cederblad, 1976). The lower gastric output in women has been attributed to their lesser body build (Novis et al., 1973). Indocyanine green disappearance from plasma is greater in women than men (J.F. Martin et al., 1975).

Prolactin concentration is greater in the serum of young women than in young men. While the basal growth hormone concentration is the same in both sexes, or slightly higher in women, a marked rise occurs with activity in women that is not observed in men (Frantz and Rabkin, 1965). The overall secretion of growth hormone may be as much as 50% greater in women than men during a 24-hour period (Merimee et al., 1976).

1.3.3. Race

It is often difficult to separate the influence of race on laboratory data from the effects of socioeconomic conditions. In the United States, for example, many black individuals still belong to the lower economic groups, live in poor environments, and work in jobs requiring much physical activity.

It has long been recognized that the serum total protein concentration is higher in blacks than in whites although the serum albumin is less. α_1-, β- and γ-Globulins may be substantially increased but α_2-globulin is less. γ-Globulin is considerably increased due to IgA as well as IgG. In black men, the serum IgG is as much as 40% higher than in whites and IgA 20% higher. In women the differences are only slightly less, but IgM is reduced in black women (Buckley and Dorsey, 1971). Part of the increase in immunoglobulin concentration may be attributed to a generally increased exposure to infections. The concentration of γ-globulin in blacks and Puerto Ricans living in New York tends to be higher than in the blood of other New Yorkers and appears to be independent of socioeconomic conditions or duration of residence in the city. The concentration of γ-globulin in black Africans decreases when they leave to take up residence in Europe. This is suggestive of an environmental influence. Racially associated dietary taboos may cause nutritional deficiencies which may only become apparent when the individuals move to a different country.

In South Africa, a clear relationship has been demonstrated between an individual's income and his plasma albumin concentration, which may also be correlated with protein intake. There is also a direct correlation between the serum γ-globulin concentration and income, even within a racial group (Bronte-Stewart et al., 1961).

Climatic effects may reveal genetic differences. Thus, Eskimos in summer have higher serum globulins (except for γ-globulin) compared with Caucasian Americans when no such differences exist in winter (Luzzio, 1966). The plasma concentration of potassium is less in blacks in equatorial regions than in individuals living in the temperate zones.

The activity of creatine kinase and lactate dehydrogenase is greater in the serum of blacks than whites. This is probably attributable to the increased manual labouring activities in which the former engage. It is presumed that the increased enzyme activity is of skeletal muscular origin and may be correlated with the increased muscle mass that develops with repeated exercise. The alkaline phosphatase activity of black children at puberty tends to be higher than in white children due to their greater skeletal development. The serum phosphate concentration of blacks may be slightly less than in whites.

Racial differences exist in carbohydrate and lipid metabolism. In general, glucose tolerance is impaired in blacks when compared with matched groups of whites. The plasma glucose in blacks may be as much as 0.84 to 1.40 mol/litre (15 to 25 mg/dl) higher one hour after ingestion of glucose.

The incidence of intestinal lactase (EC 3.2.1.23) deficiency, or lactose intolerance, is only 5 to 15% in Caucasian Gentiles but 70% in Jews and American blacks. In Asians, the incidence is as high as 98% (Rosensweig, 1975). In white men and women, the serum cholesterol is consistently higher than in blacks, especially after age 40 years. This may be related to dietary factors only, as the serum cholesterol is less in Orientals living in Japan than those living in the United States, where no differences can be observed between their values and those of American Caucasians. The serum triglyceride concentration is also less in blacks than in whites (Benedek and Sunder, 1970).

The concentration of uric acid in individuals older than 35 years is more likely to be increased in Orientals than in Caucasians, Mexican Americans or blacks. This again may reflect dietary preferences rather than inherent differences in metabolism. The relative influence of sex, age and race on the serum uric acid concentration is illustrated in Figure 1.4. In Africa the serum urea is consistently less in Africans than Europeans. The urea concentration is known to increase in proportion to the quantity of protein ingested, so that this too is probably a manifestation of different dietary habits. The serum vitamin B_{12} concentration may be as much as 30% higher in European than African women. The serum copper may be as much as 6 μmol/litre (40 μg/dl) less in blacks than in Caucasians or Mexican Americans, but the explanation for this is uncertain. Serum pepsinogen concentrations are higher in male Mexicans than in Caucasians (Kuttner and Mailander, 1965).

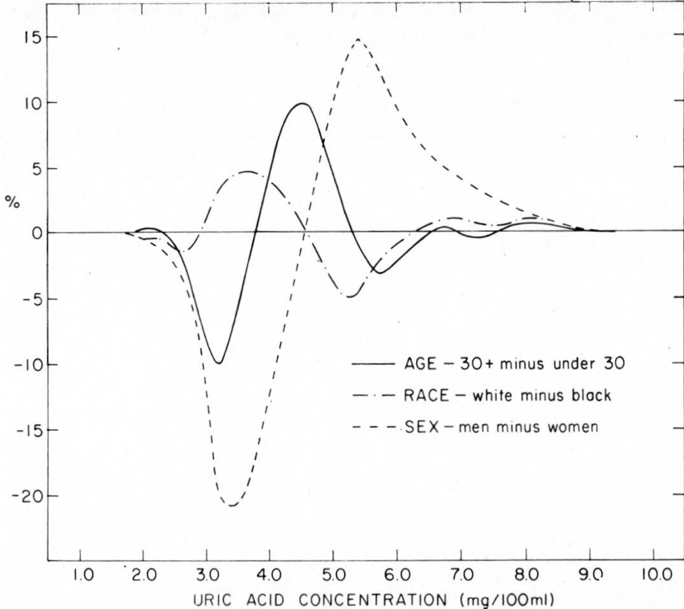

Figure 1.4. Serum uric acid data are plotted from a population of about 80 healthy individuals, who were equally divided according to age, race and sex categories listed. Deviations from the mean value are plotted and demonstrate a preponderance of low values in women, the major influence, and higher values in men. Low values were also observed in the younger age group. In this study more of the low uric acid values were observed in blacks than whites. SI Unit conversion for uric acid, mg/dl × 0.095 = mmol/litre.

Blood haemoglobin concentration may be as much as 10 g/litre higher in whites than blacks (Garn et al., 1975).

There may be some real genetic influences accounting for differences between the erythrocytes of blacks and whites. In erythrocytes from blacks, there is a reduction of potassium content that is compensated for by increased sodium. In blacks, erythrocyte galactose-1-phosphate uridylyltransferase (EC 2.7.7.10) activity is reduced, yet the quantity of cellular water is the same in both racial groups (Munro-Faure et al., 1971). In blacks, erythrocyte pyridoxal kinase (EC 2.7.1.35) may be only 40% of that of Caucasians (Chern and Beutler, 1976). Galactokinase (EC 2.7.1.6) activity is also reduced. The adenosine triphosphate (ATP) content of erythrocytes from blacks is less than in whites. There is growing evidence that enzymes may escape from cells with a reduction of their ATP content. This may provide a partial explanation for the increased activities of certain enzymes in the serum of blacks.

1.3.4. Geographical location

Few studies have been clearly directed to the influence of geographical location on the composition of biological fluids. Most have not differentiated other factors from those of geographical location alone. Many have been short-term studies and have not been continued long enough to determine if adaptation takes place with time.

1.3.4.1. Environmental temperature and climate

Within 30 minutes of an individual's exposure to heat, the blood volume may increase by up to 5%. With hot weather, the blood volume may be increased by up to 27% and the extracellular fluid volume may increase by 6 to 16% over several days. Red cell mass is increased, but not to the extent of the blood volume. Acclimatization to hot weather allows the haemodilution process to occur more rapidly. The blood haemoglobin is decreased by haemodilution but the plasma protein concentration may be unchanged, as the total circulating protein is increased through influx of isotonic cell-free fluid from the interstitial space. There is no general salt and water retention but glomerular filtration and sodium and chloride excretion are reduced. Water and electrolytes are lost by sweating. Some proteins of low molecular mass, for example albumin and α_1-globulin, may be lost to the extravascular space with a corresponding reduction in the plasma protein concentration, but the plasma protein concentration is usually increased with work, with the greatest increase in the β-globulin fraction (Senay et al., 1976). Initially there is no change in the osmolality or plasma sodium concentration, but the plasma potassium concentration may be reduced by as much as 10% as it is taken up by cells.

The early haemodilution is inversely related to the extent of sweating. Heavy sweating causes dehydration and a decrease in the plasma volume. This, in turn, reduces renal plasma flow and glomerular filtration rate with an increased filtered fraction but decreased urinary volume. Sodium and chloride excretion is reduced. With restricted replacement of sodium the secretion of aldosterone is increased, but a negative sodium balance persists with loss of sodium in the sweat. The concentration of sodium chloride in sweat rises in proportion to the rate of secretion. Potassium and nitrogen are also lost in sweat. Urinary potassium excretion is reduced but nitrogen loss is increased. Initially the excretion of 17-oxosteroids and 17-hydroxycorticosteroids is increased, but after three days the excretion of these compounds is reduced to, or below, the baseline values. The plasma glucose concentration is increased and glucose tolerance is impaired. The excretion of uric acid, nitrogen and creatinine in urine is increased for several days.

With contraction of the blood volume, the blood haemoglobin and plasma protein concentrations increase. Venous blood pH is increased. As haemoconcentration develops, the plasma concentration of electrolytes also increases, with an overall increase of the osmolality of perhaps 3%. The plasma cortisol and corticosterone concentrations are increased following exposure of as little as two hours to a high ambient temperature. Urinary catecholamine excretion is reduced with heat exposure.

With acclimatization, which may occur within one week and last for several weeks, salt concentration in sweat and the basal oxygen consumption are reduced (Kirmiz, 1962). An isotonic expansion of the extracellular fluid volume occurs. This and other reactions have been attributed to stimulation of the adrenal cortex.

Exposure to intense cold for a few hours produces little effect on the secretion of TSH; however, secretion is increased by up to 60% with more prolonged exposure. The plasma thyroxine concentration may be slightly decreased. The plasma concentration of growth hormone is unaffected or increased. The secretion and diurnal variation of cortisol are unaffected by cold, although increased plasma concentrations are also reported. Cold provokes a diuresis with increased loss of sodium, magnesium and chloride, initially with a contraction of the plasma volume and increased plasma protein concentration. Interstitial fluid volume is expanded. Glomerular filtration rate and renal plasma flow are unaffected. Short-term exposure to cold increases the urinary excretion of norepinephrine and, to a lesser extent, of epinephrine. Plasma dopamine-β-hydroxylase activity is slightly increased (Frewin et al., 1973). 3-Methoxy-4-hydroxyphenylglycol excretion is increased but the circadian rhythm of its urinary excretion and that of vanillylmandelic acid is abolished (Cymerman and Francesconi, 1975). Plasma tryptophan and tyrosine concentrations are decreased.

1.3.4.2. Other environmental influences

The serum cholesterol concentration has been observed to be higher in individuals who live in areas with hard-water as opposed to soft-water. The serum triglyceride concentration is also higher. The magnesium/potassium ratio is significantly lower in cardiac muscle of individuals who lived in soft-water areas although plasma concentrations are unaffected (Bierenbaum et al., 1973). Trace element concentrations in plasma are affected by the presence of environmental influences. Thus, in individuals living in Billings, Montana and in El Paso, Texas, where there are copper smelters, the serum concentration of copper is higher than elsewhere (Kubota et al., 1968). Blood lead concentration is to a large extent governed by the amount of lead in food but is also related to the concentration of lead in drinking water (Elwood et al., 1976). The lead concentration also tends to be higher in areas of high automobile traffic density compared with more rural areas. The body burden of lead can be correlated with the period for which lead has been added to motor fuel in different countries (Schroeder and Tipton, 1968). Industrial exposure to cadmium may lead to proteinuria, aminoaciduria and a high incidence of renal calculi (Scott et al., 1976). Cadmium may also be released from domestic water pipes by soft acidic water (Schroeder and Nason, 1971), although rarely to the extent that might cause medical problems.

Fluoridation of water has been shown to produce a transient but real decrease in serum alkaline phosphatase activity (Ferguson, 1971).

Carboxyhaemoglobin concentration is higher in urban non-smokers than rural non-smokers, although the rural smoker has a higher concentration than the rural non-smoker. Blood lead concentration is higher in city dwellers than in rural dwellers. The greatest influence is probably from automobile exhaust fumes, but the influence of contamination from lead pipes carrying domestic water cannot be excluded. Automobile driving also increases temporarily the plasma concentrations of catecholamines and 11-hydroxycorticoids (Bellet et al., 1969b).

1.3.5. Body build and obesity

Although digestion is no more efficient in the obese individual than in the lean person, and fat metabolism is similar, there are several differences in laboratory data between the two types of individual. The concentrations of both cholesterol and triglycerides are correlated with body weight, rising with the degree of obesity. These increased concentrations are independent of the influence of ageing. The concentration of the β-lipoproteins in serum also rises in parallel with those of the lipid components, but there is generally no correlation between height, weight or surface area and the concentrations of the serum protein fractions. The total body water increases with the height and mass of an individual and thus is affected by body build (Hume and Weyers, 1971).

The concentration of urate in serum increases in both men and women with increasing body mass. This is most marked in individuals weighing more than 80 kg. With treatment of obesity by means of a restricted diet, there is also a good correlation between the changes in body mass and serum urate concentration. However, starvation or a diet poor in calories leads to an increase in the serum uric acid concentration and a negative nitrogen balance due to the catabolism of tissue, for example skeletal muscle, which is rich in nucleic acids. Competition by oxoacids for renal excretion may also lead to an increase in the serum concentration of urate.

The cortisol secretion rate is correlated with the body cell mass. With obesity the production of cortisol is increased, but its turnover is affected to the same extent, so that the plasma cortisol concentration is unaffected or even may be slightly reduced. The normal circadian variation persists. The increased cortisol secretion causes an increased excretion of 17-hydroxycorticosteroids and 17-oxogenic steroids, especially in women. There is a positive correlation between muscle mass and 17-oxosteroid excretion in young men (Tanner and Gupta, 1968). The concentration of testosterone in the plasma of obese individuals is reduced.

The release of growth hormone by the pituitary gland is reduced in obese individuals (Roth et al., 1963). The fasting plasma growth hormone concentration is less than in people of ideal body weight. The normal increased secretion of growth hormone in response to insulin, arginine, sleep, or exercise is impaired. The normal response to fasting is much impaired, or even absent, in obese individuals, but the response to meals may be exaggerated, especially in women. However, the normal late response of growth hormone secretion to glucose ingestion may be reduced. The plasma growth hormone concentration and its response to different challenges return to normal with loss of weight.

The plasma insulin concentration in obese individuals is generally higher than in non-obese individuals but glucose tolerance is impaired (Nestel and Goldrick, 1976). The binding of insulin to the monocytes or adipocytes of obese individuals is impaired. This decrease is due to a reduction in the number of receptor sites, with possibly some loss of affinity for the binding sites as well (Olefsky, 1976). With restriction of caloric intake, the plasma insulin concentration is decreased and the binding of insulin to cells is improved (Archer et al., 1975). In obese individuals the insulin response to both oral and intravenous glucose, as well as to other stimulants such as tolbutamide, glucagon or aminoacids, is reduced.

Serum triiodothyronine concentration is significantly correlated with body weight and is increased by overeating (Bray et al., 1976). The relationship between body mass and serum concentrations of triiodothyronine and insulin is shown in Figure 1.5. The plasma thyroxine concentration in obese individuals is usually no different from that in individuals of normal body mass.

The fasting plasma pyruvate and lactate concentrations are higher in obese than lean people. The rise of the pyruvate concentration in response to glucose ingestion is both

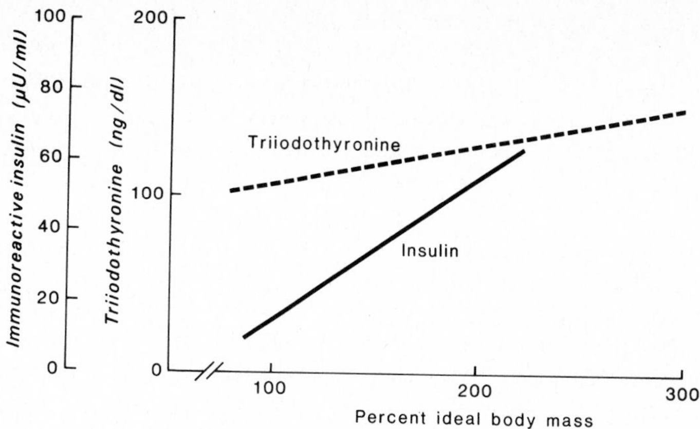

Figure 1.5. Correlation between serum insulin and triiodothyronine concentration and body mass. SI Unit conversion for triiodothyronine, ng/dl × 0.015 = nmol/litre. (Reproduced, by permission, from Bagdade et al., 1976 and Bray et al., 1976)

larger and later in obese individuals. The concentration of both unesterified fatty acids and citrate is higher than in individuals of normal body build; the concentrations fall following glucose ingestion but not to the levels occurring in normal individuals. Unlike his thinner counterpart, the obese individual fails to show an increase in his free fatty acid concentration with enforced reduction in food intake.

Obese individuals generally have higher plasma concentrations of the branched-chain aminoacids and of phenylalanine and tyrosine, but the urinary excretion is not increased. Plasma glycine concentration is usually low. The increased aminoacids probably reflect failure of insulin to control aminoacid uptake and release in skeletal muscles (Scriver and Rosenberg, 1973).

In obese individuals, the activity of creatine kinase in serum is markedly increased in both men and women. With individuals weighing more than 70 kg, there is generally a good correlation between body mass and plasma activities of alanine and aspartate aminotransferases. This is most marked in men. In obese women, especially, there may also be an increased activity of serum alkaline phosphatase (Goldberg and Winfield, 1974).

The basal gastric juice volume and acid output is increased in obese individuals (Vaughan et al., 1975). Peak output of acid is also increased. The bile of obese individuals differs from that of other people in that it is supersaturated with cholesterol (Bennion and Grundy, 1975).

The concentration of iron and the iron-binding capacity of the plasma are often reduced in obese individuals (Seltzer and Mayer, 1963).

1.3.6. Diet

Individuals' total caloric intake, and the relative proportions of protein, carbohydrate and fat in the diet vary throughout the world as a result of available income or food supplies, which determine the quantity and type of food that is ingested. Even within an affluent population, total caloric intake probably changes little from day to day but the variety of food may change quite markedly. Changes in the composition of food, even with the total intake constant, may affect the composition of body fluids within a short period of time so that an understanding of the effects of dietary factors is essential before laboratory data can be correctly interpreted. Both long-term and short-term factors are involved.

1.3.6.1. Habitual diet

The plasma concentrations and urinary excretions of many compounds can be correlated with protein intake. Four days after the change from a normal to a high protein diet, increases of 75% in the plasma urea concentration, 18% in cholesterol, and 10% in phosphate and phosphatide concentrations may occur. Serum osmolality may show a slight increase. In contrast, the plasma glucose concentration may decrease by 8% and plasma insulin by 44%. The changes in urinary composition are also marked. Thus in one study, urea excretion increased by 70% and cyclic AMP excretion doubled, but uric acid excretion decreased by 79% (Astrand, 1967). Urea clearance progressively increases with increased protein intake. Urinary pseudouridine and uracil excretion are similarly affected (Eisen et al., 1962). Urinary alanine, histidine, serine, and tyrosine excretion is greater on a high protein diet but there is little change in plasma concentrations. Much meat in the diet causes a large excretion of carnosine, anserine and 1-methylhistidine (Hill et al., 1976). Uric acid is formed from dietary and endogenous purines or nucleoproteins, as well as from the body nitrogen pool. A high protein diet augments the available supply of precursors and both serum concentration and urinary excretion are high, but a high fat diet depletes the nitrogen pool due to the increased demand for ammonium ions to maintain acid–base homeostasis so that the plasma urate concentration is reduced (Bishop and Talbot, 1953). When a high protein diet is ingested following a normal diet, but with the intake of calcium and phosphate maintained constant, mineral absorption is more efficient. The urinary excretion of calcium increases although its serum concentration is unchanged (Johnson et al., 1970). Activity of ornithine carbamoyltransferase (EC 2.1.3.3) in serum is increased, presumably as a result of induction of urea cycle enzymes in the liver and leakage of the extra enzyme from the cells. The activity in serum increases further when the high protein diet is no longer ingested. Increased activity of the aminotransferases in serum has also been reported (Brohult, 1969). The influence of change in the composition of the diet on the serum ornithine carbamoyltransferase activity and urinary excretion of urea is illustrated in Figure 1.6.

Reduction of dietary fat from 35 to 25% of total calories causes a reduction of serum lactate dehydrogenase activity, with the H type subunits most affected. In men, pyruvate and lactate concentrations in serum are also reduced; the pyruvate concentration is more affected. The increased carbohydrate intake probably increases Krebs cycle activity (Marshall et al., 1976).

Reduction of a normal intake of protein to a much lower amount causes decreased turnover of nitrogen with a sharp reduction in its excretion (Rand et al., 1976). Breakdown of body protein is increased, but this is not completely compensated for by increased synthesis. Endogenous aminoacids are reutilized more efficiently. With a change

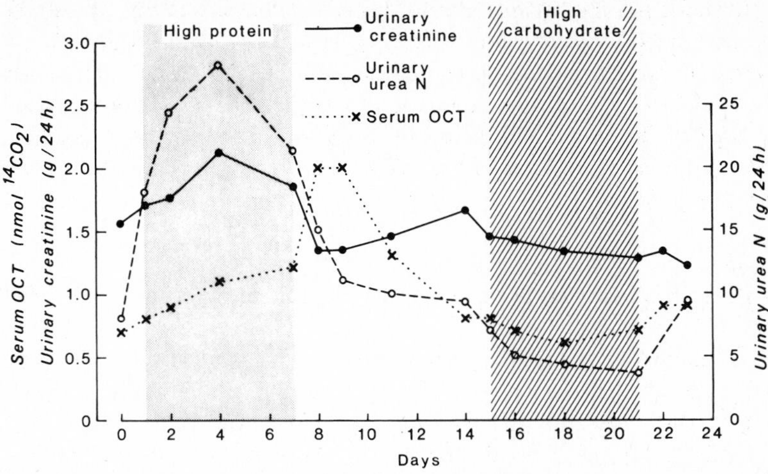

Figure 1.6. Influence of change in composition of diet on plasma ornithine carbamoyl transferase activity and urinary excretion of urea and creatinine. (Reproduced, by permission, from Brohult, 1969)

from a protein-rich to a low protein diet, or vice versa, from 4 to 10 days are required in well-nourished individuals for a new nitrogen equilibrium to be reached.

On diets in which most of the carbohydrate is present as sucrose or starch, the activities of lactate dehydrogenase and alkaline phosphatase in serum are higher in both men and women than when the carbohydrate calories are provided by other sugars (Irwin and Staton, 1969). Aminotransferase activity also varies with the type of carbohydrate ingested. Fructose and sucrose induce intestinal sucrase (EC 3.2.1.26) and maltase (EC 3.2.1.20) activities, although lactase activity is unaffected by lactose intake. Jejunal glycolytic enzymes are also affected by dietary carbohydrates, especially by glucose or fructose, and the changes occur within hours of the sugar ingestion (Rosensweig, 1975). Reduction of sucrose intake tends to reduce plasma triglyceride concentration, and flatter glucose tolerance curves are observed with a bread diet than when an individual ingests a high sucrose diet. High carbohydrate diets cause a lower plasma growth hormone concentration than either a high fat or protein diet (Merimee et al., 1976). A high carbohydrate diet increases the amount of very low density lipoprotein, triglyceride, cholesterol and protein.

The serum cholesterol concentration is generally related to the number of calories derived from fat. Serum cholesterol is also higher in individuals with a low intake of vitamin E. Only fat is able to increase the activity of alkaline phosphatase in serum after it has been reduced by fasting. A change of as much as 50% in the intake of dietary cholesterol may produce a change of only 0.13 or 0.26 mmol/litre (5 or 10 mg/dl) in the plasma cholesterol concentration (Leveille et al., 1962). The hypocholesterolaemic effect of unsaponifiable fat in corn oil is due to sitosterol. The frequency of ingestion of fat, sugar, starch or alcohol is less important than the degree of adiposity in influencing the serum cholesterol and triglyceride concentrations (Nichols et al., 1976). Increased dietary cholesterol, however, does increase the plasma concentrations of cholesterol and phospholipid (Connor et al., 1961). Antonis and Bersohn (1962) have varied the composition of the diets of groups of Caucasians and Bantus in South Africa so that the plasma lipid composition took on the characteristics of the other group. The nature of the habitual diet appears to be largely responsible for the apparent racial difference in plasma lipids.

1.3.6.2. Vegetarianism

Vegetarianism has been most studied in its relationship to lipid metabolism and its treatment of abnormal lipid metabolism.

In vegetarians of long-standing the plasma concentrations of low, very low, and high density lipoproteins are less than in non-vegetarians (Sacks et al., 1975). Total lipid and phospholipid concentrations are also affected. The concentrations of cholesterol and triglycerides may be only two-thirds of that in people on a conventional mixed diet, but the concentration of triglycerides is often less affected. These changes are observed in infants and children as well as in adults. An increase with age in lipid concentrations in serum is observed in vegetarians, as in non-vegetarians, but the changes are slight.

In individuals who have ingested a vegetarian diet for a short time only, the changes in lipid concentration are less marked than in those adhering to a vegetarian diet for a long time. The concentration of lipids is less in individuals who eat only a vegetable diet than in lacto-ovo-vegetarians, but in both groups the lipid concentrations are less than in meat-eaters. In meat-eaters, the serum cholesterol concentration increases in individuals with the frequency of meat ingestion.

The high concentration of lipids in the plasma of non-vegetarians has been correlated with the ingestion of saturated fats. Replacement of saturated fat with polyunsaturated fat has a marked cholesterol-lowering effect. The saturated fats which have most influence on the serum cholesterol concentration contain between 12 and 18 carbon atoms. It has been postulated that polyunsaturated fats cause a shift of cholesterol from the plasma into the tissues. The typical vegetarian diet also contains much fibre which increases faecal bile acid loss and also reduces the serum cholesterol concentration (Antonis and Bersohn, 1962). Cholesterol, when ingested in the form of egg-yolk, produces a significant increase in the serum concentrations of cholesterol and phospholipids. The effect is less marked when purified free cholesterol is substituted.

When individuals, previously on a mixed diet, have their diet replaced by an isocaloric protein-deficient diet, their plasma concentrations of albumin and urea may decrease by as much as 10 and 50%, respectively. However, if long-standing vegetarians and non-vegetarians are compared as groups, there is generally no significant difference between the concentrations of any of the five major protein fractions (Kirkeby, 1966). Generally, the plasma protein concentrations and enzyme activities are not affected (Ellis and Montegriffo, 1970). Following a change from a meat-containing to a meat-free diet, the ratio of concentrations of non-essential to essential aminoacids in plasma gradually increases. In vegetarians there may be some impairment of conversion of creatine into creatinine because urinary excretion of the former is increased whereas that of the latter is reduced.

Urinary pH is usually higher in vegetarians than in meat-eaters due to the reduced intake of precursors of acidic metabolites. This may affect the excretion of urobilinogen and other urine pH-dependent compounds such as certain drugs. Plasma folate concentration is often increased but the plasma concentration of vitamin B_{12} may be reduced to a value suggestive of deficiency (Armstrong et al., 1974). Vegans may have a higher serum bilirubin concentration than meat-eaters, but their urea concentration may be less.

The nocturnal increase in plasma prolactin observed in healthy women is less in individuals ingesting a vegetarian diet. The amplitude of the changes in plasma luteinizing hormone at night is also less (Hill and Wynder, 1976).

1.3.6.3. Synthetic diet

To estimate the contribution of diet to the composition of body fluids, mixtures of pure chemicals containing all known trace elements and vitamins in adequate amounts and sufficient in calories to support normal activities, have been fed to volunteers (Winitz et al., 1970). Urea and cholesterol concentrations are strikingly decreased, and glucose is affected to a lesser extent. The decrease in cholesterol concentration is smaller if dietary sucrose is not completely replaced by glucose. Serum urate and phosphate concentrations are slightly increased. Urinary urea and urate excretions are reduced and the excretion of most electrolytes is affected similarly. Many of the organic compounds normally present in urine of individuals ingesting a typical diet disappear from the urine, or are excreted in greatly reduced amounts, when the synthetic diet is fed (Young et al., 1971). The faecal flora is markedly altered by ingestion of the synthetic diet and the faecal excretions of both acid and neutral steroids are also greatly reduced (Crowther et al., 1973). These studies illustrate the dependency of body fluid composition on the material ingested in the diet. When normal food intake is resumed, the rapid reversion of the composition of the fluids to that found before the synthetic diet was ingested provides further support for the view that day-to-day variations in the composition of the diet may have considerable influence on the concentrations of constituents in body fluids.

1.3.6.4. Malnutrition and protein calorie deficiency

The change in concentrations of constituents in body fluids in response to dietary deficiencies is greatly dependent on the nature of the deficiency, e.g. whether it affects protein only, or protein together with other sources of calories, the age at which the deficiency first occurs, and the geographical location in which an individual resides. Many additional factors are also involved, such as the quality of the protein available, the duration of the deficiency, the individual's prior state of health, and the adequacy of intake of vitamins and trace elements. The biochemical responses listed below will not necessarily be observed in all individuals, and the extent will vary from individual to individual even when they are subject to the same deprivations.

In malnutrition the plasma concentration of total protein is reduced. Albumin is most affected but β-globulin is also reduced and only partly compensated for by an increased γ-globulin. Synthesis and catabolism of most proteins is reduced. However, the concentrations of C4 and immunoglobulins IgA, IgG and IgM are usually unaffected (Olusi et al.,

1975). C3 and transferrin concentrations appear to be most susceptible to malnutrition. The plasma concentrations of cholesterol and triglycerides may be reduced by as much as 50% by severe malnutrition. The lipoprotein concentration is reduced, and phospholipids are similarly affected. Plasma carnitine is also reduced (Khan and Bamji, 1977). The proportion of free cholesterol is greater than normal. Although there is some accumulation of intra- and extra-cellular water, the plasma concentrations of sodium and potassium are unchanged or only slightly reduced. However, total body potassium is reduced (Viteri and Arroyave, 1973). When oedema accompanies protein calorie malnutrition, the plasma sodium and potassium concentrations are reduced. The decrease of plasma glucose is not usually significant. The plasma urea concentration is greatly reduced, because of the reduced protein intake, and is indicative of a negative nitrogen balance. The nitrogen balance remains positive for many months after treatment is commenced. Urinary urea and creatinine concentrations are considerably reduced and creatinine clearance is similarly affected. This is associated with the decrease of muscle tissue and lean body mass.

With protein calorie malnutrition, the plasma cortisol concentration is high and urinary cortisol is also increased. The increases are largely due to a decreased metabolic clearance. Urinary 17-hydroxycorticosteroid excretion is reduced to a greater extent than cortisol production. Plasma corticotrophin concentration is maintained in spite of the increased plasma cortisol. Dexamethasone is less effective in decreasing the plasma cortisol concentration than in a well-nourished individual. Plasma growth hormone concentration is very high in malnourished individuals but falls during refeeding. Plasma insulin concentration is reduced. Somatomedin concentration is also reduced (Lunn et al., 1973). Plasma triiodothyronine concentration may be reduced. The concentration of TSH is affected similarly, and that of thyroxine to an even greater extent. The concentrations of both thyroxine-binding globulin and prealbumin are decreased. Thyroxine-binding prealbumin contains a large proportion of tryptophan and has a rapid turnover, which makes it particularly sensitive to deficiency of the amino acid. Retinol-binding protein is similarly affected (Ingenbleek et al., 1975). There is also believed to be impaired conversion of thyroxine into triiodothyronine. The reduced caeruloplasmin concentration causes a reduction in the serum copper concentration in kwashiorkor, but the copper concentration is normal in marasmus (Reinhold, 1975).

Experimentally induced protein calorie malnutrition has shown that adaptation occurs to improve the conservation of nitrogen. This is associated with a decrease in the release of aminoacids from skeletal muscles which limits gluconeogenesis and thus the loss of nitrogen. Urinary excretion of nitrogen and aminoacids is reduced. However, the excretion of taurine, β-aminoisobutyric acid and ethanolamine may be increased. Reduced excretion of hydroxyproline has been used as a test for marginal malnutrition (Feigin, 1969). In general, the plasma concentrations of essential aminoacids, e.g. methionine and tyrosine, are reduced. The decrease with tyrosine may be much greater and more prolonged than that with phenylalanine; this has been attributed to impaired hydroxylation of the latter (Saunders et al., 1967). The concentrations of threonine, leucine, lysine and valine may be reduced by as much as 50%. The concentration of non-essential aminoacids tends to be variable. Plasma glycine is usually high, both with malnutrition and after refeeding. Glycine concentration appears to be increased in protein deficiency from all causes. Serine also is often increased. In malnutrition, as opposed to experimental starvation, the plasma alanine concentration, like that of other aminoacids, tends to be normal. With refeeding all non-essential aminoacids, except glycine, increase in plasma. The plasma concentrations of the urea cycle aminoacids are much better maintained in malnutrition than in acute starvation. The plasma arteriovenous difference of aminoacids is less in malnutrition than in health, suggesting conservation of aminoacids by skeletal muscles (Smith et al., 1974). The low plasma carnitine may be associated with lysine deficiency (Mikhail and Mansour, 1976). Reductions of the activities of erythrocyte glutathione reductase, glutathione peroxidase (EC 1.11.1.9) and alanine and aspartate aminotransferases occur with protein calorie malnutrition, although vitamin B_6 deficiency may be mainly responsible for the effect on the aminotransferases (Verjee and Behal, 1976).

Erythrocyte and plasma folate concentrations are reduced in protein calorie malnutrition, but the serum vitamin B_{12} concentration is unaffected or slightly increased (Khalil et al., 1973). Plasma iron concentration is maintained but both plasma transferrin and blood haemoglobin concentrations are reduced (Olson, 1975), which may be associated with the reduced demand for oxygen. The plasma concentrations of vitamins A and E are much reduced.

In severe protein calorie malnutrition, renal plasma flow, glomerular filtration rate and tubular function decrease. This may lead to impairment of renal concentrating and acidification abilities. Gastric juice, pancreatic juice and bile production may be reduced, with low to normal enzyme activities and conjugated bile acid concentrations (Viteri and Arroyave, 1973).

Alkaline phosphatase activity is reduced by malnutrition and may fall further when refeeding is initiated before subsequently rising after 2 weeks of therapy. Serum cholinesterase (EC 3.1.1.8) and amylase activities are reduced and also rise with treatment, as do the activities of amylase, lipase (EC 3.1.1.3) and trypsin (EC 3.4.21.4) in the duodenum. While the activities of other enzymes in plasma may be within the normal range during malnutrition, treatment causes increases in their activities.

During dietary therapy for malnutrition, at least 90% of the calories are absorbed. Positive balances for nitrogen, phosphorus and sulphur occur. This is associated with increased protein synthesis, but a negative potassium balance may still occur (Holmes et al., 1956).

1.3.6.5. Fasting and starvation

Enforced reduction of food intake has been used to treat obesity. Withdrawal of most of the nutrients from a previously healthy, but obese, individual may cause important metabolic effects. These change with time so that the immediate and the final responses may be quite different. The responses tend to be different in obese, normal and malnourished individuals. Reduction of food intake which is imposed following surgery, or associated with a severe illness, mimics to some extent the situation of imposed caloric restriction, but the metabolic changes are considerably influenced by the factor precipitating the reduced intake.

From the onset of a period of fasting, the body attempts to conserve protein at the expense of other sources of energy. Fat contributes most of the energy, and body fat is decreased to a greater extent than protein (Yang and Van Itallie, 1976). Initially, the body attempts to maintain glucose production yet the blood glucose may decrease by as much as 1 mmol/litre (18 mg/dl) during the first 3 days after the fast has started. This decrease is usually more marked in women than men (Merimee and Fineberg, 1973). Insulin secretion is reduced, as evidenced by a decrease of immunoreactive insulin concentration in plasma of as much as 70%. A new steady state is normally achieved after three days. Non-suppressible insulin-like activity is also reduced initially in lean individuals, but shows an initial slight increase in obese individuals (Solomon et al., 1968). The plasma glucagon concentration may double with the fall in the insulin concentration (Unger et al., 1963). The increase is usually greater in women than men. The decreased insulin concentration stimulates lipolysis through an increase in the amount of cyclic AMP in adipose tissue, which in turn increases the activities of lipolytic enzymes. Hepatic oxogenesis is stimulated, and oxoacids and fatty acids become the principal sources of energy for muscle. Normal cerebral metabolism is dependent on an adequate supply of glucose. Extracerebral utilization is reduced and gluconeogenesis is maintained by utilization of amino acids and lactate. To a small extent the brain also uses β-hydroxybutyrate and acetoacetate. Bodily fuel reserves are generally small except for protein in muscle and lipid in adipose tissue (Table 1.3).

Starvation induces a considerable increase in the release of aminoacids from skeletal muscle. Lack of food, even for as little as one day, increases the plasma concentration of valine, leucine, isoleucine and α-aminobutyrate by as much as 100% (Adibi and Drash, 1970); these aminoacids are most influenced by insulin secretion. Most of the essential aminoacids are decreased in arterial plasma after several weeks of starvation, but not to the extent normally observed with chronic malnutrition. Glycine and threonine concentrations are usually much increased and methionine slightly increased. Alanine is reduced after one day of fasting and reaches its lowest value in three days. Citrulline, phenylalanine and tyrosine are also reduced. The plasma concentrations of the aminoacids involved in the urea cycle are not well maintained (Saunders et al., 1967). The urinary excretion of 3-methylhistidine, which serves as an indicator of the amount of muscle protein breakdown, decreases with starvation (Young et al., 1973). Starvation for a short period leads to increased excretion of β-aminoisobutyric acid which is derived from the thymine of

TABLE 1.3.

AVAILABLE FUEL RESERVES IN MAN

(Data reproduced, by permission, from Cahill, G.F., Jr. (1976) Clinics in Endocrinology and Metabolism, 5, 397–415)

	Glycogen or glucose		Mobilisable protein		Triglycerides	
	grams	Calories	grams	Calories	grams	Calories
Blood	15	60	0	0	5	45
Liver	100	400	100	400	50	450
Brain	2	8	0	0	0	0
Muscle	300	1200	6000	24000	50	450
Adipose Tissue	20	80	10	40	15000	135000

tissue nucleic acids. Formiminoglutamic acid excretion is reduced with short term calorie restriction (Rosenauerová-Ostrá et al., 1976).

The breakdown of fat leads to a transient increase in body water, but with continued starvation the plasma volume is reduced by an osmotic diuresis. The reduced plasma volume affects the glomerular filtration rate so that the plasma creatinine concentration rises slightly and the creatinine clearance is reduced: this may amount to 15% over four days. Reduction of plasma volume may contribute to impairment of liver function. Increased bromosulphthalein retention may occur and the serum bilirubin concentration increases rapidly in response to fasting. After 24 hours the concentration may rise 1.3 times and after 48 hours by 2.2 times the initial values. These changes have been attributed to decreased clearance from plasma (Barrett, 1971). Increased serum activities of aspartate and alanine aminotransferases and lactate dehydrogenase may be observed, but have been attributed to focal necrosis in the liver rather than to a general circulatory effect.

Immediately after the onset of a fast the plasma renin activity decreases, but it rises to a higher value within a week. The plasma aldosterone concentration is also greatly increased initially (Verdy and de Champlain, 1968). Plasma dopamine concentration and urinary excretion of dopamine are unaffected by three days of fasting whereas urinary epinephrine may increase 2-fold (Christensen et al., 1976).

In spite of the catabolism of tissues, with increased turnover of protein, the concentration of protein in plasma is little changed. However, the increased breakdown of nucleoprotein does result in an increase in the concentration of uric acid in the serum. Contributing to this increase is the reduced glomerular filtration rate and competitive inhibition of tubular secretion by lactate and oxoacids. The concentrations of these constituents also increase in plasma and contribute to the metabolic acidosis (with a reduction of blood pH and pCO_2, with pO_2 often also reduced) that characterizes starvation or semi-starvation. The acidosis is rarely so severe that the individual is incapable of compensating for it.

Urinary loss of vitamins continues during starvation and the plasma concentrations of thiamine, pantothenic acid, riboflavin and pyridoxine may decrease unless supplementation is given. Plasma folate also decreases although vitamin B_{12} is unaffected.

The plasma potassium concentration may be considerably decreased. With the onset of starvation urinary excretion is greatly increased, although it later falls to about 10 mmol/day (Weinsier, 1971). The loss is probably linked to the rate of protein catabolism, and most of it probably originates in skeletal muscle. The pattern of circadian excretion is not affected by fasting (Wesson, 1964). As with potassium, the concentrations of magnesium and calcium in the serum may be reduced, while the urinary excretions of these elements are increased. The normal diurnal excretion pattern of calcium may be abolished. Fasting also reduces the serum alkaline phosphatase activity (Sukumaran and Bloom, 1953). Serum phosphate concentration falls, with an increased urinary excretion initially that steadily decreases with continuation of the fasting. The plasma bicarbonate concentration is decreased with starvation but the concentrations of sodium and chloride show little change. The excretion of sodium increases with the onset of a fast but then declines to about 10 mmol/day (Weinsier, 1971). The increase in sodium excretion is greater than that of chloride, but a negative chloride balance may still occur. The increased sodium excretion occurs largely to compensate for the considerable increase in metabolically produced organic anions. The normal circadian pattern of sodium excretion persists (Wesson, 1964). The starved individual excretes more ammonium ion, and his titratable acidity is also increased, in order to maintain the acid–base balance within physiological limits. The increased excretion of ammonium allows some conservation of sodium. Urinary zinc may be increased 6-fold with fasting. Half of this increase may occur on the first day (McCall et al., 1971). The obligatory water excretion is greatly reduced, because of the marked reduction in urea excretion, to an amount that may be less than that of ammonia. Urine volume may be as low as 200 ml/day. Some of the changes in urine composition that occur with prolonged fasting are illustrated in Figure 1.7.

With increased utilization of fat, and with release and degradation of fatty acids, the concentrations of fatty acids, ketone bodies and glycerol in serum tend to increase (Owen et al., 1969). In the normal individual starvation for one day has little effect on the serum acetoacetate concentration but it rises rapidly with a longer fast. In the obese individual there is a marked and immediate increase. In the lean individual serum glycerol rises almost 3-fold with three days of starvation, but there is little effect in the obese individual. Initially the triglyceride concentration increases, but it ultimately decreases with weight loss. There may be a transient decrease in the serum cholesterol concentration. Urinary carnitine excretion is greatly increased with the lipolysis of fasting (Maebashi et al., 1976).

Fasting may cause the plasma concentration of growth hormone to increase from 2 to 15 times. It peaks on the second day of a fast, and the effect is greater in premenopausal women than men, but the concentration may be reduced to normal after 3 days. Starvation also causes a marked decrease in the serum free triiodothyronine and total triiodo-

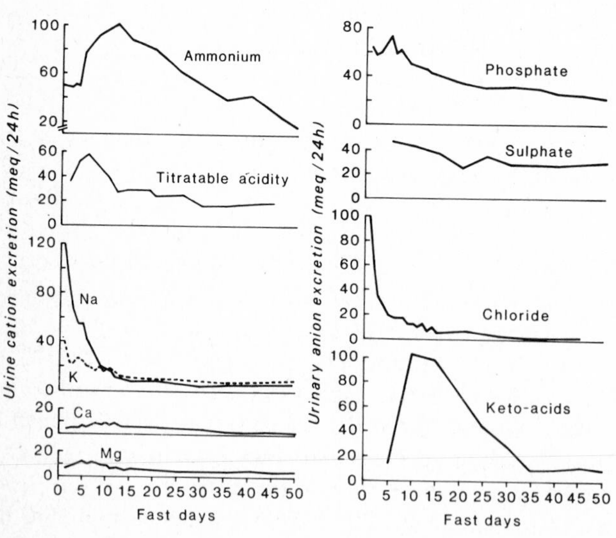

Figure 1.7. Effect of fasting on urinary composition. (Reproduced, by permission, from Bray et al., 1972)

thyronine (by up to 50% in three days) with a slight decrease of the free thyroxine (Portnay et al., 1974; Merimee and Fineberg, 1976). Although slight decreases in the binding capacities of thyroxine-binding globulin and prealbumin have been observed, there is little change in the total thyroxine concentration. Starvation has no effect on TSH or on its response to thyroid releasing hormone. However, peripheral conversion of thyroxine into triiodothyronine is impaired. The concentration of reverse T_3 is increased (Cahill, 1976).

Urinary free cortisol, which serves as an indicator of corticotrophin secretion, changes little in response to fasting but plasma free and total cortisol concentrations increase with a diminution of the day–night variation (Galvão-Teles et al., 1976). However, the plasma concentration of dehydroepiandrosterone increases with fasting and this has been postulated to inhibit the 11β-hydroxylation involved in the synthesis of corticosterone from deoxycorticosterone and the synthesis of cortisol and aldosterone. Increased activity of corticotrophin is masked by inhibition of this enzyme. That the plasma cortisol is maintained in spite of an overall decrease in cortisol secretion is suggested by decreased excretion of 17-hydroxycorticosteroids, 17-oxo- and 17-oxogenic steroids and unconjugated 11-hydroxycorticoids in the urine (Schachner et al., 1965). Pituitary gonadotrophin release is reduced by starvation and testicular function is reduced in men (Cahill, 1976).

With refeeding, urinary excretion of sodium is decreased markedly for some time and weight gain parallels the sodium retention. The urinary chloride excretion parallels that of sodium but potassium excretion decreases less rapidly. The sodium retention is associated with an even greater secretion of aldosterone than during the fasting period. The excretions of ammonium ion and of organic acids are also rapidly reduced as refeeding is initiated. A metabolic alkalosis may supervene with refeeding. The concentrations of the branched chain aminoacids, α-aminobutyrate and growth hormone return rapidly to their normal values. The plasma concentrations of most aminoacids require several weeks to return to normal. Within one day the plasma insulin concentration reverts to normal but a transiently diabetic glucose tolerance curve may be observed as carbohydrate stores are built up. The concentrations of ketones and glycerol decrease promptly with refeeding. A positive nitrogen balance begins early, especially if the non-protein calories are mainly carbohydrate. The cortisol concentration returns rapidly to normal with refeeding. The concentrations of the triiodothyronines rapidly revert to euthyroid values.

1.3.7. Pregnancy

Pregnancy produces many physiological and biochemical changes in a woman (Hytten and Lind, 1973).

The plasma volume may increase by as much as 50% during pregnancy. The total blood volume also increases, but to a lesser extent, due to the almost 15% decrease in haemoglobin concentration and haematocrit. These changes begin about the tenth week of pregnancy. Renal plasma flow increases by about 250 ml/min in pregnancy. Although a decrease at term has been reported, this is probably an artifact due to partial occlusion of the renal veins by the pressure of the uterus. The glomerular filtration rate may be increased by as much as 60% with the increase in the effective renal plasma flow. Creatinine and urea clearances show marked increases, in association with decreased plasma concentrations, so that a creatinine clearance of 200 ml/min may be observed. The plasma urea concentration decreases in early pregnancy and continues to decrease to about three-quarters of the non-pregnant value at term. Plasma renin activity increases by as much as 10 times during pregnancy, but the pregnant woman's response to angiotensin is much reduced. The proportion of inactive to active renin is greatly increased in serum from pregnant women (Leckie et al., 1976).

During pregnancy the plasma concentrations of sodium and potassium decrease by about 2 and 0.2 mmol/litre, respectively. These changes become apparent in the first 8 weeks of pregnancy. In the third trimester the potassium concentration returns to normal. In spite of the decreased plasma sodium concentration, total body sodium is actually increased due to the expansion of the extravascular fluid. The plasma concentration, and urinary excretion, of aldosterone is increased 3-fold during pregnancy. In ambulatory pregnant women the normal diurnal excretory pattern of sodium and water is reversed so that a greater excretion occurs at night than during the day. This is probably attributable to the accumulation of fluid in the limbs in the upright position. There is a reduced response to the excretion of water, especially in late pregnancy. This may contribute, together with haemodilution, to the decrease in osmolality of up to 10 mosmol/kg.

The serum protein concentration begins to fall in the first 3 months of pregnancy, and remains reduced until the end of pregnancy. Most of the change is due to a reduction in the albumin concentration of up to 30%. This is only partly compensated by an increase of about 0.2 g/litre in α-globulin (mainly α_1-antitrypsin and α-lipoproteins) and of about 0.3 g/litre in β-globulin (transferrin and β-lipoproteins). IgG concentration is also reduced, but IgA and IgM are not affected (Song et al., 1970). The plasma colloid osmotic pressure falls in relation to the decrease in the albumin concentration. During pregnancy certain proteins can be detected in serum that are not present in the non-pregnant state. These include an α_2- and β_1-glycoprotein, and α-foetoprotein. Several of the specific hormone-binding globulins are present in increased concentrations in serum. Serum caeruloplasmin and β_{1A}-globulin concentrations are also significantly increased by the last trimester. In contrast, the concentrations of orosomucoid (α_1-acid glycoprotein) and haptoglobin are decreased. Generally, pregnancy has its greatest effects on those proteins that are synthesized in the liver. Increased plasma concentrations are related to increased synthesis, and decreased concentrations to increased catabolism. Bromosulphthalein retention is increased. This is probably an oestrogenic effect and related to delayed excretion or increased binding by plasma proteins (Crawford and Hooi, 1968). The changes in serum concentrations of some of the commonly measured constituents throughout pregnancy are illustrated in Figure 1.8.

The plasma concentrations of calcium and magnesium decrease by 10% at the end of pregnancy, because of a reduction in the plasma albumin concentration. The serum parathyroid hormone concentration has been reported to be both normal and high in the last trimester (Lim et al., 1976). The plasma iron concentration falls by about 35% during pregnancy and the iron-binding capacity increases with the average 50% increase in transferrin concentration. The serum zinc concentration decreases, but that of copper may almost double with the increased synthesis of caeruloplasmin.

Plasma pCO_2 falls from the time of conception until the end of the second trimester. This decrease may be as much as 8 mm Hg (1.1 kPa), and has been attributed to the

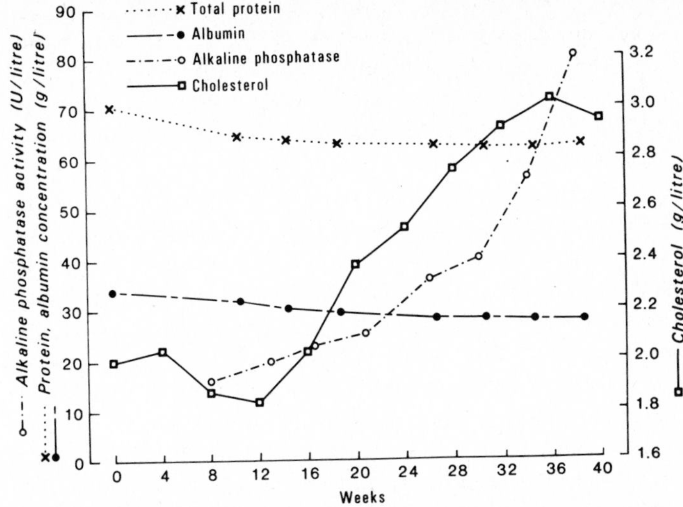

Figure 1.8. Effect of duration of pregnancy on concentration of some commonly measured constituents of serum. SI Unit conversion for cholesterol, g/litre × 2.59 = mmol/litre. (Reproduced, by permission, from Hytten and Lind, 1973)

effect of progesterone on the respiratory centre. The plasma bicarbonate concentration decreases at the same time. Oxygen consumption increases during pregnancy and the blood arteriovenous difference increases from about 33 ml/litre in early pregnancy to the normal value of about 45 ml/litre near term (Palmer and Walker, 1949). The early decrease is due to a relatively greater increase of cardiac output than to change in basal oxygen consumption without a corresponding decrease in the amount of circulating haemoglobin. However, the oxygen consumption greatly increases towards term, with the growth of the foetus and placenta.

In normal pregnancy, there is a slight increase in serum lactate dehydrogenase activity (of the order of 10%) to term. Serum diamine oxidase (histaminase, EC 1.4.3.6) activity begins to rise from the sixth week and it reaches 20 times the non-pregnant value during the third trimester (Elmfors and Tryding, 1976). 17β-Hydroxysteroid oxidoreductase activity, which originates in the placenta and catalyzes the oxidoreduction of oestrone and oestradiol, becomes detectable in serum by the third month and increases to the end of pregnancy. Acid phosphatase (EC 3.1.3.2) and aminopeptidase (EC 3.4.11.1) activities increase during pregnancy with growth of the placenta. Serum creatine kinase activity is reduced during the first half of pregnancy whereas cholinesterase activity declines by up to 30% in the later part. Alkaline phosphatase activity may increase four-fold during pregnancy. The increase is slight to the 20th week and is maximal at term. The increase is largely due to enzyme released from the placenta, which may ultimately comprise 50% of the total. Activity of the heat-stable placental component is detectable after about 25 weeks. Serum lipase activity declines, but amylase activity increases gradually with pregnancy to the 25th week before falling slightly. Although γ-glutamyltransferase is purportedly an indicator of hepatic enzyme induction, which is known to occur in pregnancy, its activity in serum is unchanged by pregnancy (Herzberg et al., 1977). Nevertheless, urinary glucaric acid excretion may increase by 60% from the first to the third trimester.

The concentration of lipids in plasma increases throughout pregnancy. Total lipid concentration at the end of pregnancy may be twice the non-pregnant value. Triglyceride concentration may be 2 to 3 times the non-pregnant value at term and is associated with increased quantities of low density and very low density lipoproteins. After an initial fall in the first trimester the serum cholesterol increases progressively to the last month. The total phospholipid concentration also increases, with the greatest contribution from lecithin or cephalin. These increases are associated with the increased β-lipoprotein concentration. Free fatty acid concentration rises by 50% during pregnancy. The proportion of saturated fatty acids also rises. High density lipoproteins, which are probably affected by increased oestrogen secretion, increase by about 25% in a normal pregnancy.

The concentrations of most aminoacids in plasma decrease during pregnancy although there is usually a rise in the last month. During the first half of pregnancy the aminoacids of the urea cycle are especially low. Tyrosine falls relative to phenylalanine. The kidney's ability to reabsorb sugars and aminoacids is reduced, and this is reflected in large increases in the excretion of threonine, methionine and histidine. The excretion of glycine, serine and alanine is also increased until late pregnancy. The excretion of most other amino acids increases until mid-pregnancy (Armstrong and Yates, 1964). The tubular threshold for glucose is reduced in pregnancy so that glucosuria is quite common. The fasting blood glucose concentration is reduced during pregnancy but glucose tolerance is generally normal. Serum urate concentration decreases early in pregnancy – because its urinary clearance is increased – but it rises towards normal at the end. Plasma folate, ascorbate and vitamins A, B_6 and B_{12} are reduced in pregnancy, and these reductions may be associated with the increased demands of normal pregnancy. Increased activity of hepatic microsomal enzymes, for which folate is a co-factor, may be the cause of the reduced plasma folate (Davis et al., 1973). In contrast to the situation with other vitamins, the concentration of vitamin D is greatly increased in the third trimester of pregnancy. At this time, the concentration of its binding protein may be more than double the non-pregnant value (Haddad and Walgate, 1976). In about one-third of pregnant women, the concentration of 25-hydroxyvitamin D in plasma is reduced below the normal lower limit in the last trimester (Turton et al., 1977).

The plasma progesterone concentration increases to nearly 200 μg/litre at term, from about 20 μg/litre in early pregnancy. Urinary pregnanediol increases 4-fold at the same time. The excretion of oestriol begins to increase at 12 weeks and progressively increases to term. The excretion of other oestrogens, although increased, is much less marked. Chorionic gonadotrophin is detectable in serum within 10 days of ovulation and peaks about the 60th day. A second, but much smaller, peak occurs in the third semester. Slightly higher concentrations occur at term when a female foetus is present. Placental lactogen (choriomammotrophin) is first detectable in serum after six weeks of pregnancy and its concentration increases until just before birth. Serum follicle stimulating hormone concentration decreases as the gonadotrophin concentration increases. The effects of duration of pregnancy on some of these hormones are illustrated in Figure 1.9.

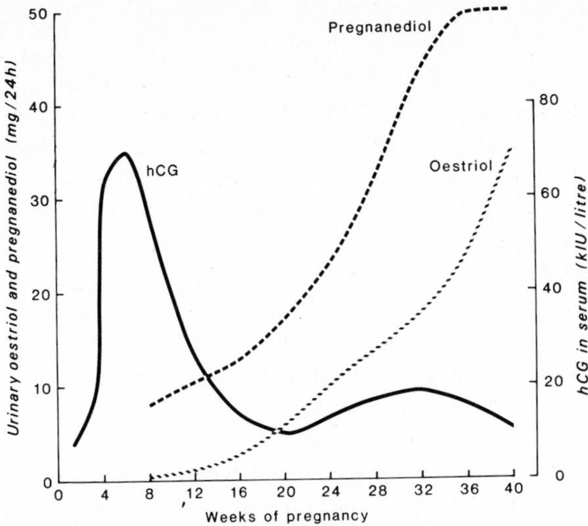

Figure 1.9. Changes in urinary excretion of oestriol and pregnanediol and in plasma chorionic gonadotrophin with duration of pregnancy. (Reproduced, by permission, from Hytten and Lind, 1973)

The concentration of corticotrophin in plasma is greatly reduced in normal pregnancy, whereas that of plasma cortisol increases steadily throughout pregnancy. The increase may be linked, in part, to an increase in the amount of transcortin, which affects the protein-bound portion of the hormone, but free cortisol concentration is also increased. The actual secretion rate of cortisol has been shown to be less in pregnant than non-pregnant women. The plasma concentrations of corticosterone and deoxycorticosterone rise progressively in pregnancy. The concentrations of testosterone and androstenedione increase in the pregnant woman's plasma, but the quantities excreted in urine appear to be unaffected, except in women with a male foetus in whom the excretion of testosterone is greater. The increases in plasma concentration may be due only to the increased concentration of binding protein in the plasma. The excretion of catecholamines is unaffected by pregnancy. Growth hormone secretion is also unaffected by pregnancy. Urinary excretion of cyclic AMP increases by about 70% from the first trimester to its peak about the 34th week (Yuen et al., 1976).

The concentration of melanocyte stimulating hormone in plasma may increase 100-fold during pregnancy. The concentration of prolactin steadily rises throughout pregnancy, especially in the last trimester, and may be twice as high at term as at 6 to 9 weeks (Schenker et al., 1975). TSH concentration is unaffected by pregnancy, but plasma thyroxine may be increased by up to 50%. This is entirely due to an increase in thyroxine-binding globulin, the concentration of which may double, because the concentration of the free hormone remains the same as – or may actually decrease to the lower limit of – the values found in healthy adults. Triiodothyronine concentration rises throughout pregnancy, to a greatly increased value at term, but free T_3 concentration is reduced below normal (Avruskin et al., 1976).

1.3.7.1. Multiple pregnancy

Biochemical changes observed in the mother during a multiple pregnancy are little different from those occurring with a single pregnancy. However, chorionic gonadotrophin secretion is usually increased and the concentration of placental lactogen is significantly increased (Dhant et al., 1976). Testosterone-binding globulin concentration is increased and the concentration of α-foetoprotein in the serum of a mother with a twin pregnancy may be almost twice as high as with a single pregnancy. Bromosulphthalein retention is greater with a multiple pregnancy than with a single pregnancy (Beazley and Tindall, 1966). Activity of alkaline phosphatase is higher in a twin pregnancy than in a single pregnancy. The activities at term of serum cystine aminopeptidase and leucine aminopeptidase may be almost twice as much in a twin pregnancy as in a single pregnancy. The mother's serum folate is substantially reduced in a twin pregnancy.

1.3.7.2. Labour

Fluid lost by sweating and by other routes during labour is usually inadequately replaced so that haemocentration occurs, with an increased concentration of total protein and albumin. The hyperventilation that is caused by the stress of delivery produces respiratory alkalosis that is compensated for by a metabolic acidosis. This results in a reduction of blood pCO_2 and plasma bicarbonate. Plasma sodium concentration decreases during delivery, but the potassium concentration and osmolality show slight but insignificant increases. The plasma urea and uric acid concentrations rise during delivery. This may reflect mild impairment of renal function as well as increased turnover of tissue protein with the stress of the labour. A slight increase of aminotransferase activities in plasma occurs with labour. The free fatty acid concentration rises 2-fold with labour on mobilization from adipose tissue, possibly due to the influence of oxytocin (Burt et al., 1963). Corticotrophin secretion is stimulated. Cortisol secretion is increased two- to three-fold during labour, and the stress of delivery also increases serum dopamine-β-hydroxylase activity and the urinary excretions of epinephrine, norepinephrine and vanillylmandelic acid (Hashimoto et al., 1974). The plasma glucose concentration is increased with or without a change in the insulin concentration. The lactate concentration rises to a high concentration at delivery (Kashyap et al., 1976). The maternal plasma also shows increased concentrations of oestrogens and androgens in response to the stress of labour.

1.3.7.3. Puerperium

Renal plasma flow and glomerular filtration rate return rapidly to normal (Hytten and Lind, 1973). Plasma albumin concentration is least about 36 hours after delivery and does not revert to a normal adult female value until at least a week later. Total protein concentration is restored to normal before the albumin concentration due to increased synthesis of α_2-globulin. The plasma concentrations of sodium, potassium and bicarbonate revert to normal within 3 days. Plasma potassium concentration may be increased early in the puerperium due to the increased tissue breakdown at this time. Tissue breakdown is probably also responsible for the continual increase of the plasma urea concentration during the first week post-partum (MacDonald et al., 1974). During the period of lactation, the higher basal metabolic rate of pregnancy persists, but most changes gradually revert to normal. Urinary excretion of oestrogens remains high until the normal menstrual cycle resumes. The plasma high density lipoprotein concentration remains elevated for up to 6 weeks and the low density lipoprotein concentration also remains high. Plasma renin activity remains high after delivery (Romero and Hoobler, 1970). Serum prolactin concentration is high in post-partum lactating women, but in women who are not breast-feeding a decline begins immediately (Forsyth and Edwards, 1972). At six to eight weeks post-partum a significant decrease below non-pregnant or pregnant values has been observed for the fasting plasma glucagon concentration (Leblanc et al., 1976).

1.3.8. Vasectomy

Vasectomy has been reported to produce conflicting biochemical results. Comparison of a vasectomized population with an unvasectomized population failed to demonstrate differences in plasma concentrations of testosterone and gonadotrophins (Varma et al., 1975). However, significant increases in plasma testosterone and luteinizing hormone, but with reduced oestradiol concentration, have been observed in men studied before and after the operation. Although the plasma concentration of follicle stimulating hormone is initially unaffected, a slight increase occurs by two years. After two years, the oestradiol concentration returns to its baseline value but the concentrations of luteinizing hormone and testosterone remain increased; all changes are small. The measured values do not extend beyond the normal range, although they indicate a statistically significant change (K.D. Smith et al., 1976).

1.3.9. Occupation and social class

Social class has no effect, reportedly, on the plasma concentrations of calcium, phosphate, total bilirubin, total protein and albumin, glucose, lactate dehydrogenase, alkaline phosphatase and urea. Serum urate concentration is associated with drive and achievement; thus the concentration is higher in executives than in labourers, craftsmen or their supervisors (Dunn et al., 1963). The trend can be observed in school children in whom the urate concentration is higher in those with a good academic record. The serum urate concentration can also be correlated with the number of years of schooling.

The activities of aminotransferase enzymes are higher in labourers and farmers than in professional workers. Children of low-income families tend to have lower plasma concentrations of folate than children of other families (Daniel et al., 1975). The serum cholesterol concentration is less in lower socioeconomic groups than in others (Noel and Kilmore, 1971). These effects may be associated with the greater physical activity involved in most labouring jobs, as well as with the poorer quality diet habitually ingested by manual workers. Diet may have the major influence because there is a good correlation between aspartate aminotransferase activities in husbands and wives after middle age, as has also been observed for serum cholesterol concentrations. It is unlikely that occupational influences affecting one spouse could have a significant effect on the other. Similar correlations between husbands and wives have also been observed for albumin and glucose in plasma.

The concentration of blood lead has been found to increase from 1.1 μmol/litre (22 μg/dl) to 2.9 μmol/litre (60 μg/dl) within 3 weeks in new employees of a factory working with lead (Benson et al., 1976). Urinary lead excretion is increased in such people. Long-term occupational exposure to mercury vapour results in increased urinary excretion of mercury, and increased activity of acid lysosomal hydrolases in plasma (Foa et al., 1976). Blood and urinary cadmium concentrations may provide a measure of present or previous exposure to cadmium (Lauwerys et al., 1976).

1.3.10. Season

While circadian variations in the concentrations of blood constituents have received considerable attention, relatively little has been accorded to longer cyclical changes, with the exception of factors associated with the menstrual cycle. Changes that occur over a long period of time are often smaller than those occurring within a day if the observation conditions for the former are standardized. Some of the changes that have been reported may represent artifacts due to the difficulty of assuring reproducibility of analytical methods over a long period of time. On the other hand, this same analytical variability may obscure real changes.

The majority of seasonal changes can be linked to environmental temperature and the different recreational activities that increased temperature allows; to differences in diet that accompany the availability of fresh fruit and vegetables; to changes in overall caloric requirements for the different seasonal activities.

Blood and plasma volumes are significantly increased in hot weather, presumably to compensate for the vasodilatation that hot weather provokes. Changes in composition of blood occur more rapidly in the plasma than in the cells but it still takes several days for the serum protein concentration to adjust to a new set point. In Eskimos in North America, the concentration of protein in serum actually increases during the summer months – a change that has not been observed in Americans. Generally, the total protein concentration increases by 10% from summer to winter (Kawai, 1973). This probably is related to a decreased blood volume as well as to influences of environment and temperature. In summer, α-globulins are low, β-globulins remain constant but γ-globulins may increase by as much as 50%.

Lactate dehydrogenase activity may be increased by as much as 20% in the serum of individuals during the summer, possibly as a result of increased physical activity (Winkelman et al., 1973). Alkaline phosphatase activity may be slightly higher in the autumn than in spring as a result of changes in diet.

Serum cholesterol may be much higher in winter than summer (Thomas et al., 1961): in men, the difference may be almost 1.3 mmol/litre (50 mg/dl) and in women 0.7 mmol/litre (30 mg/dl). This has been attributed to a greater caloric intake in winter, increased activity in summer, and greater exposure to ultraviolet irradiation in summer which may cause oxidation of cholesterol, all of which may effectively reduce the serum concentration in summer. Total lipids have been reported to be decreased in the serum in the late winter months. Serum triglyceride concentration has been reported to decrease from summer to winter, and this has been claimed to occur independently of changes in diet (Fuller et al., 1974). Fahlén et al. (1971) have observed a lower plasma glucose concentration in summer. The plasma insulin concentration is also less, and individuals generally have better glucose tolerance in summer than in winter. Although no changes in plasma concentrations of triiodothyronine, thyroxine and TSH have been reported with change of season, the urinary excretions of triiodothyronine and thyroxine are higher in summer (Rastogi and Sawhney, 1976). Significantly increased plasma triiodothyronine has been found in winter by other observers (Nagata et al., 1976).

Calcium metabolism is considerably altered by changes in the seasons. Sunlight changes 7-dehydrocholecalciferol to cholecalciferol (vitamin D) in the skin. The latter compound undergoes further metabolism in the liver and kidney to produce 1,25-dihydroxycholecalciferol which causes reabsorption of calcium from bone and also enhances its absorption through the gastrointestinal tract. The result is a significant increase in the concentration of calcium in serum, and a rise in its urinary excretion. Typically the excretion is 30% greater in summer than winter (Green, 1974), although a very different pattern has been observed in Alaskan Eskimos, in whom the winter excretion may be up to ten times as much as in summer (Tedeschi, 1973). This presumably also reflects some dietary influence. The plasma concentrations of sodium, potassium and chloride are also slightly higher in summer (Josephson and Dahlberg, 1952), but the urinary excretion of these electrolytes shows no consistent pattern throughout the year.

The urinary excretion of tetrahydrocortisone, metanephrine and normetanephrine, all metabolites of adrenal hormones, tends to be slightly greater in summer than winter, probably reflecting greater physical activity. In northern latitudes, the excretion of 17-oxosteroid and 17-hydroxycorticosteroid is greatest in November and least in May. Excretion of dehydroepiandrosterone is also least in winter. Plasma testosterone concentration in men is higher in summer and autumn than in other seasons (Smals et al., 1976).

Erythrocyte glucose-6-phosphate dehydrogenase (EC 1.1.1.49) activity is greater in winter than in summer, possibly in response to increased thyroxine stimulation (Hilgertová et al., 1972).

In general, day-to-day variability of the concentrations of compounds in serum, and their excretions in urine, is greater in summer than winter, probably reflecting a greater variability in the diet and more physical activity.

1.3.11. Blindness

The secretion and plasma concentration of corticotrophin in normal individuals reach their maxima in the early morning shortly after waking. The plasma concentration of cortisol follows that of corticotrophin, peaking at about 09.00 hours, then rapidly declining in the next hour and, thereafter, gradually declining to reach a minimum about 01.00 hours. In an individual with regular sleep–waking cycles, the diurnal variations in plasma concentrations of corticotrophin and cortisol are remarkably constant. The diurnal variation of cortisol may persist in some blind people, but in others it may be lost. All blind individuals still demonstrate a rise in their plasma cortisol concentration towards the end of sleep, although peak values may not occur at this time. The overall secretion of cortisol in blind individuals may be greater than in sighted people.

Blind individuals often demonstrate features of hypoadrenalism. Thus, the urinary excretion of 17-oxosteroids and 17-hydroxycorticosteroids may be considerably reduced when compared with age- and sex-matched sighted control individuals. Plasma glucose may be significantly reduced in blind individuals. This may be related, in part, to lack of antagonists to insulin, but may also be due to diminished stores of glycogen. Insulin tolerance is often reduced. The night secretion of growth hormone is unaffected.

Plasma concentrations and diurnal variation of FSH, oestradiol, and testosterone are unaffected by blindness in men. Luteinizing hormone concentrations are similar in blind and sighted individuals (Bodenheimer et al., 1973).

Reduced secretion of aldosterone may be responsible for the lowered plasma concentrations of sodium and chloride. The excretion of uric acid is reduced in blind individuals, as is often found in Addison's disease, and the serum concentration is increased as a result. There may be some mild impairment of renal function, as both serum creatinine and urea nitrogen concentrations are increased. The serum calcium concentration may be slightly increased, with a corresponding decrease in the serum phosphate. The reverse pattern occurs in the urine.

A negative nitrogen balance may occur in blind individuals. A reduced plasma protein concentration, may be observed and, typically, the serum cholesterol may be increased, as found in individuals with hypofunctioning adrenals. The serum bilirubin concentration may be increased. The diurnal variation of iron concentration may be lost although the variation of cortisol is unaffected.

1.4. SHORT-TERM PHYSIOLOGICAL INFLUENCES

For the purpose of this review, "short-term" has been considered to be an effect lasting for one month or less. Some of the effects are of very much shorter duration, and it should be recognized that one set of physiological responses may be superimposed on another.

1.4.1. Circadian variation

Many body constituents exhibit variations in concentration in both serum and urine throughout the day. Some of these are regular cyclical variations: others are the result of postural, activity, food or stress effects. Light and darkness, and sleep and wakefulness, may also influence some constituents. Cyclical variations may be quite large, as in the case of serum iron, which may exhibit a variation of more than 50% between 08.00 and 14.00 hours without any variation in the concentration of the protein to which it is bound (Stengle and Schade, 1957). Most hormones are secreted episodically in short bursts. These rapid changes in concentration in plasma are superimposed on the normal cyclical changes and do not replace them. Cyclical patterns which are typical of adults are not present at birth and generally require about three years to become established.

Corticosteroid secretion is subject to a marked circadian influence. This is partly determined by the influence of light and dark, but posture also has an important role. Alteration of the sleep–wake cycle affects the rhythm of corticotrophin secretion to the extent that the 24-hour periodicity of adrenal steroids may be abolished. Corticotrophin secretion increases 3- to 5-fold from its minimum between noon and midnight of 0.14 μmol/litre

(5 μg/dl) to its maximum around waking of 0.41 to 0.69 μmol/litre (15 to 25 μg/dl). Corticotrophin secretion is suppressed by the increased plasma cortisol which reaches its maximum about 06.00 to 08.00 hours, i.e. about the time of, or immediately after, the maximum secretion of corticotrophin. The metabolic clearance of cortisol tends to be greater in the morning than at night. The secretion of cortisol is affected by activity, since a higher concentration is normally observed in the afternoon in an individual when active rather than when inactive. In general, the control of production of cortisol works so efficiently that the concentration of plasma glucocorticoids is appropriate to meet the needs of the body for a particular time of day. The mechanisms involved include not only the activity of the individual, but also the secretion of corticotrophin and its regulation by the plasma cortisol concentration, corticotrophin releasing factor and hypothalamic activity. Actual changes in cortisol output during a 24-hour day appear to be due to differences in frequency and duration of the secretory episodes and not to major changes in the secretory rate. About 15 peaks of cortisol secretion occur in a normal day. The variations in secretion rate, as illustrated by changes in plasma concentrations, are shown for several hormones in Figure 1.10.

The dominant factor affecting aldosterone secretion is upright posture, so that the hormone's secretion and excretion tends to fall with a normal night time sleep schedule, although it may not be primarily affected by light and dark. The postural regulatory mechanism is probably mediated through the pituitary so that corticotrophin secretion ultimately exerts considerable control on the plasma aldosterone concentration (Katz et al., 1975). With restriction of sodium intake, changes in plasma aldosterone are mediated through the renin–angiotensin system, and a close relationship develops between the plasma aldosterone concentration and the plasma renin activity. In a supine man, with

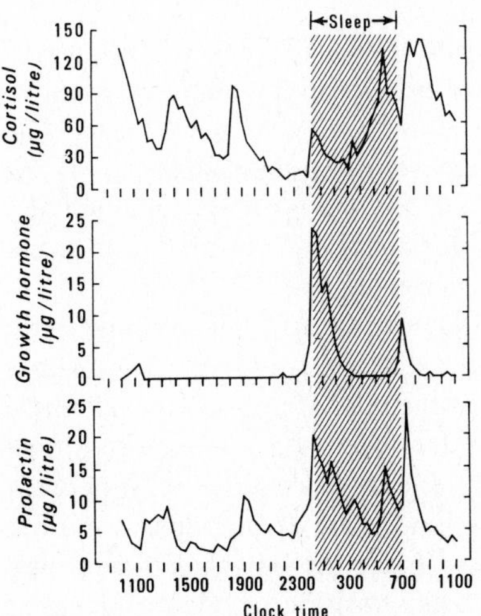

Figure 1.10. Variation in plasma concentration of cortisol, growth hormone and prolactin throughout a normal day. SI Unit conversion for cortisol, mg/litre × 2.76 = nmol/litre. (Reproduced, by permission, from Weitzman, 1976)

normal sodium intake, plasma aldosterone changes more closely parallel those of cortisol than renin activity. During a typical day, the diurnal variation of aldosterone is very like that of cortisol or corticosterone.

Maximum plasma renin activity normally occurs early in the morning during sleep, and its minimum occurs in the late afternoon. It varies reciprocally with the plasma osmolality. A sleep–wake rhythm exists for plasma renin activity, independent of food intake and body posture. Plasma renin substrate concentration is unaffected by sleep. The circadian rhythm of renin–angiotensin–aldosterone may be due to changes in sympathetic or central nervous system factors as well as to haemodynamic factors. Glomerular filtration rate and renal blood flow are minimal at the time of maximal secretion of renin and are approximately 20% greater in mid-afternoon, coinciding with the minimum of plasma renin activity.

The excretion of 17-oxosteroids and 17-hydroxycorticosteroids is low at night and reaches a maximum about midday. Excretion is least during the night. The rhythms of corticosterone and cortisone secretion are parallel, and the excretion of tetrahydrocortisol and tetrahydrocorticosterone vary in parallel in the urine. The cycle of excretion of 17-hydroxycorticosteroids can be altered by modification of the dark–light cycle alone.

No changes related to time of day have been observed in men for the plasma concentrations of LH and FSH, but bursts of secretion of these hormones have been shown to occur with intervals as short as two minutes. There is a nocturnal rise of from 20 to 40% in the plasma testosterone in normal men. This increase is temporally related to the secretion of LH and may be the result of altered metabolic clearance as well as increased production. During the follicular phase of the menstrual cycle in women, there is a transient decrease of plasma LH during sleep. The plasma prolactin concentration may also be markedly increased during sleep (Nokin et al., 1972). Like other hormones, it is secreted in multiple bursts.

There is a significant variation of the plasma concentration of TSH throughout the day. The maximum occurs between 02.00 and 04.00 hours and its minimum between 18.00 and 20.00 hours (Patel et al., 1972); this variation may be related to sleep. The diurnal variation of total plasma thyroxine is probably related to the changes in plasma volume that occur with posture. The concentrations of thyroxine-binding globulin and prealbumin peak between 10.00 and 14.00 hours. Free thyroxine concentration is unaffected by the time of day (De Costre et al., 1971; Johns et al., 1975).

The secretion of growth hormone reaches a maximum shortly after sleep commences, at the time when the secretion of corticotrophin is least. With deprivation of sleep there is no peak secretion of growth hormone. With reversal of the normal day–night cycle there is an immediate adjustment of the time of peak secretion of growth hormone to a time shortly after the start of sleep. Such rapid adjustment does not take place for other hormones. The secretion of growth hormone is normally low during daylight hours. Indeed, its main secretion occurs during the first two hours of sleep in adults, although prepubertal children also secrete the hormone during their awake hours. Plasma glucagon shows little cyclical variation throughout a day. However, the plasma glucagon concentration peaks in response to carbohydrate-rich meals. The insulin response to glucose is greatest in the morning and least about midnight. The basal plasma insulin is higher in the morning than in the afternoon. In response to a glucose tolerance test, the plasma glucose concentration is higher in the afternoon and evening than in the morning. The plasma insulin response is sometimes greater when the tolerance test is performed late in the day, but it is delayed and less effective (Grabner et al., 1975).

Some individuals exhibit a diurnal variation of epinephrine and norepinephrine excretion. Peaks and nadirs of excretion occur at the same time for dopamine, homovanillic acid, 3-methoxy-4-hydroxyphenylglycol, vanillylmandelic acid and total *O*-methylated catecholamines. Excretion is less during the night than during daytime. The activity of dopamine-β-hydroxylase, involved in the conversion of dopamine into norepinephrine, is lowest in plasma about 04.00 hours and highest about 12 hours later (Okada et al., 1974). The concentration of norepinephrine in cerebrospinal fluid is higher at 15.00 hours than at 03.00 hours (Ziegler et al., 1976b). The peak excretion of 5-hydroxyindoleacetic acid occurs in the early morning, with a concentration perhaps 60% higher than during the remainder of the day (Wadsworth et al., 1957).

There may be significant hourly changes in the plasma cholesterol concentration in response to stress, but there generally is an insignificant diurnal variation of cholesterol and phospholipids throughout the day (Kuo and Carson, 1959). Total plasma lipids decrease from 08.00 to 14.00 hours. The concentration of free fatty acids also falls after the first meal of the day: their peak concentration occurs about 17.00 hours but this is followed by a slight fall after the last meal. Their concentration then rises during the early part of the night (Malherbe et al., 1969).

The plasma concentration of aminoacids is lower in the early morning than later in the day. Thus, plasma concentrations of phenylalanine, tyrosine and tryptophan are highest about 10.00 hours and lowest about 02.00 hours. For tyrosine, the 02.00 hours concentration is one-half of that determined later (Wurtman et al., 1968). For most aminoacids, the diurnal variation is between ±30% of the daily mean. The concentrations of methionine, cysteine and isoleucine reveal the biggest cyclical changes. Those aminoacids that are present in serum in highest concentration – glycine, alanine and glutamine – show the smallest diurnal changes. Around the time of peak concentration of aminoacids, the plasma urea concentration falls slightly. Maxima of urinary excretion of aminoacids occur after each meal (Tewksbury and Lohrenz, 1970).

There is a marked change in serum protein concentration throughout the day, with postural haemodilution causing a fall during the night. Total protein concentration may change by 10 to 13 g/litre while albumin may change by 7 g/litre. The proportional change of mucoproteins and γ-globulins is even greater, values of 41% and 28% respectively having been described (Tedeschi, 1973). Total iron-binding capacity, equivalent to transferrin, remains constant throughout the day, and the quantity of bound iron does not change. In contrast to the marked variation of iron during the day, there is no characteristic pattern of variation for serum copper. Serum zinc decreases slightly from 08.00 to 15.00 hours (Hetland and Brubakk, 1973). The changes in iron concentration are directly linked to the turnover of red blood cells. Swings of as much as 40% have been observed to take place within a 30-minute period in children (Werkman et al., 1974). The plasma calcium concentration is least between noon and 20.00 hours. The serum bilirubin concentration parallels that of iron, and both are highest early in the morning when the blood haemoglobin concentration is also highest, although the peak iron concentration has also been reported to occur about 14.00 hours (Wiltink et al., 1973). The plasma inorganic phosphate concentration is least about noon, at which time erythrocyte 2,3-diphosphoglycerate concentration is maximal. Blood P_{50} and pH vary with the 2,3-diphosphoglycerate concentration (Böning et al., 1975). The changes in plasma concentrations of some of the electrolytes are illustrated in Figure 1.11.

There is little diurnal influence on serum enzyme activities although plasma creatine kinase and lactate dehydrogenase activities have been observed to increase in women throughout the day: this has been presumed to be due to muscular activity. The increased serum urate concentration that occurs during the mid-afternoon has also been attributed to increased skeletal muscular activity, with increased turnover of nucleoprotein.

There is a slight circadian influence on the plasma concentrations of bicarbonate, sodium and phosphate, but urinary changes are much greater. On a normal diet, sodium chloride excretion falls spontaneously during the night reaching a minimum at the end of sleep and a maximum about mid-day (Wesson, 1964). The excretions of sodium, potassium, chloride and bicarbonate usually vary together. Variations are linked to changes in urine pH. The rate of electrolyte excretion appears to determine the rate of urine flow. Alkalosis tends to increase the excretion of sodium and potassium (Stanbury and Thomson, 1951). Phosphate excretion is least in the morning and greatest about midnight. Small changes in glomerular filtration rate may contribute to the cyclical pattern of electrolyte excretion, but changes in tubular function are probably of much greater importance. While the peak excretion of sodium and potassium occurs around noon, the peak excretion of calcium and magnesium occurs during the night. The peak excretion of hydroxyproline occurs at the same time suggesting that increased degradation of collagen takes place concomitantly in the bone matrix (Mautalen, 1970).

Urinary volume and creatinine excretion are least during the night, but the relative density and osmolality of the urine rises. Creatinine and inulin clearances may be reduced up to 10% during the night, and night urine contains much more ammonium. Urinary excretion of enzymes is also high (Maruhn et al., 1977). Titratable acidity is lowest and

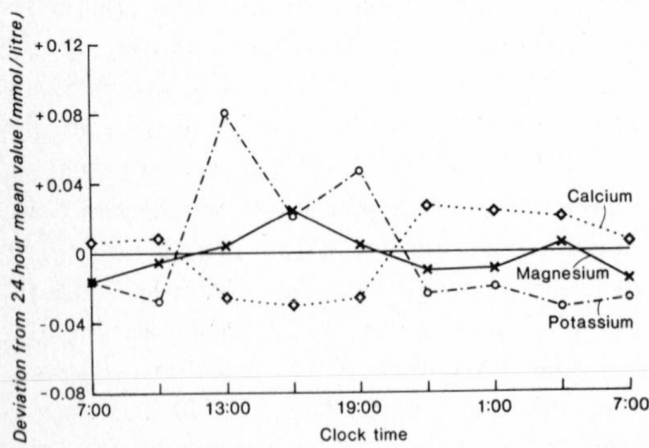

Figure 1.11. Deviation of plasma electrolyte concentration throughout a day from daily mean values. (Reproduced, by permission, from Wesson, 1964)

urine pH highest in the early morning; the opposite occurs during the late hours of sleep. Oxygen consumption and other metabolic activities are generally reduced during the night.

1.4.2. Menstrual cycle

Increases in both plasma renin activity and plasma aldosterone concentration occur from the follicular phase of the menstrual cycle to the luteal phase. The aldosterone concentration may actually double on the pre-ovulatory day compared with the early follicular phase. Its peak plasma concentration occurs in the mid- or late-luteal phase (Michelakis et al., 1975). The rise in plasma aldosterone is caused by increased secretion, and only occurs if ovulation takes place, and its concentration is usually greater in women who retain water prior to menstruation. Urinary aldosterone excretion is also greatest in the luteal phase. The renin activity increases to a peak either just before or at the time of maximum secretion of aldosterone. The change of renin activity is of the order of 1.7 to 3.0 μg/litre from follicular to luteal phase, but renin substrate concentration is unaffected by the menstrual cycle (Katz and Romfh, 1972). The change in progesterone secretion is believed to be the mediator of the increased concentrations of both renin activity and aldosterone.

Fasting plasma growth hormone concentration does not vary during the menstrual cycle, but its response to exercise is greatest at mid-cycle (Hansen and Weeke, 1974). The concentrations of most other hormones are affected by the menstrual cycle. Thus the plasma corticosterone concentration is as much as 50% higher in the luteal phase than in the follicular phase (Schwartz and Abraham, 1975). Plasma androstenedione concentration is highest in the late follicular phase. There is a sharp single peak of luteinizing hormone at mid-cycle. The luteinizing hormone activates adenylate cyclase in the corpus luteum and the urinary excretion of cyclic AMP is increased. Cyclic GMP excretion may also be increased (Lebeau et al., 1975). The plasma FSH concentration also reaches its maximum at the same time. Plasma oestradiol concentration reaches its maximum shortly before the LH peak. Urinary excretion of oestrogens is maximal about ovulation, and minimal 2 to 3 days after the onset of menstruation. Urinary pregnanediol and plasma progesterone concentrations reach their maximum about the mid-point of the luteal phase. Plasma prolactin concentration peaks with the luteinizing hormone peak, being significantly higher in the luteal than in the follicular phase. Plasma testosterone concentration varies throughout the cycle but is usually highest in the mid-third. A slight fall in the plasma thyroxine concentration is observed after menstruation. In contrast, the serum melatonin concentration is highest at the time of menstrual bleeding – 3.8 ng/litre compared with only 0.8 ng/litre at the time of ovulation (Wetterberg et al., 1976). The urinary excretion of 17-hydroxycorticosteroids reaches a peak at mid-cycle. Urinary catecholamine excretion increases at mid-cycle and remains high throughout the luteal phase (Rao and Zuspan, 1970).

The plasma cholesterol is lowest at ovulation, corresponding to the time of maximum oestrogen secretion. Its concentration rises immediately prior to menstruation. The plasma cholesterol ester concentration decreases markedly, and the plasma phospholipid decreases to a lesser extent, so that the cholesterol/phospholipid ratio is also reduced at ovulation. The plasma cholesterol concentration rises in the week immediately following menstruation. The cyclical variation in cholesterol concentration is not observed with anovulatory cycles. Urinary carnitine excretion is also greatest at the time of ovulation (Maebashi et al., 1976).

The total protein and albumin concentrations decrease at mid-cycle, but these are followed by immediate increases. The globulins, with the exception of α_1-globulin, follow a similar variation. Neither α_1-globulin nor its major component, α_1-antitrypsin, are much influenced by the menstrual cycle. The plasma fibrinogen concentration increases markedly with menstruation. The plasma concentrations of several amino acids change with the different phases of the menstrual cycle, with a fall of as much as 50% during the latter part of the cycle (Craft and Peters, 1971).

Serum creatinine and urate concentrations are highest during menstruation and lowest towards the end of the inter-menstrual period. The serum calcium concentration varies slightly, but in parallel with the serum albumin concentration. Serum phosphate concentration is lowest at the time of menstruation. The plasma iron concentration may be greatly reduced at the time of onset of bleeding. The magnesium concentration is highest at this time. Plasma zinc concentration is slightly increased at the time of ovulation. The plasma sodium and chloride concentrations increase up to the onset of menstruation, but a reduction of as much as 2 mmol/litre occurs with the postmenstrual diuresis.

Plasma ascorbic acid concentration is lowest at the time of ovulation, but the concentrations of folate and vitamin B_6 are unaffected by the menstrual cycle. Nevertheless, there may be a functional B_6 deficiency in the preovulatory phase of the menstrual cycle, as the urinary excretions of 3-hydroxykynurenine, xanthurenic acid and anthranilic acid are reduced immediately after menstruation.

Serum creatine kinase activity may be slightly reduced at the time of ovulation, but the activities of other enzymes appear to be unaffected by the menstrual cycle.

In women with the premenstrual syndrome, the serum prolactin concentration is significantly higher throughout the cycle than in other women. Secretion of the hormone increases further premenstrually (Halbreich et al., 1976).

1.4.3. Periodic cyclical variations

Some apparently cyclical variations in the excretions of some compounds have been observed. These are independent of normal diurnal influences or of the menstrual cycle.

In men, an 8 to 10 day cycle of oestrone excretion has been reported. A weekly cycle of 17-oxosteroid excretion has been reported in the same individuals (Exley and Corker, 1966). In another study of one individual over many years a similar cycle was observed. A change in the concentration of plasma testosterone has been observed over a period of 20 to 22 days, but the overall change is no greater than normal diurnal variation (Doering et al., 1975).

The changes observed with these cycles are small and of no apparent clinical significance. Their underlying mechanisms have not yet been elucidated.

1.4.4. Recent food

Although standardization of blood collection procedures might obviate some of the problems caused by different times of specimen collection throughout a day, this is not feasible in hospital or clinic practice: many blood specimens must be drawn at variable times after meals.

Examination of a population one to three hours after lunch, compared with a fasting population, showed little difference in the plasma concentrations of sodium, glucose, calcium and cholesterol. However, after the meal a consistent and statistically significant decrease was observed for serum creatinine, urate, urea, total protein and albumin. A decrease in lipoprotein concentration was also observed, that was greater in women than men. Serum bilirubin concentration increased in both sexes, although the effect of its temporal cyclical variation was not excluded. In men, the concentration of serum inorganic phosphorus was increased, whereas it decreased in women. The biggest change was that of bilirubin which increased approximately 10%, i.e. 2 μmol/litre (0.1 mg/dl). Most of the other changes were less than 5% (Steinmetz et al., 1973). Pyruvate and lactate concentrations in plasma are also increased by meals (Friedemann et al., 1945).

When variability was reduced by settling upon a fixed time after a standard meal, some different findings emerged. Yet this type of regulation would also be difficult to achieve in a hospital. When blood was drawn two hours after a meal of 800 kcal (3.32 MJ), the concentrations in plasma of urea, protein, calcium, sodium and potassium were decreased in both sexes, and the concentration of urate and activity of alkaline phosphatase were decreased in men (Steinmetz et al., 1973). Following the meal, significant increases for glucose and β-lipoprotein concentrations and lactate dehydrogenase activity were observed. Alkaline phosphatase activity decreased by 5 to 10% in women, and urate concentration by more than 10%. The increase of β-lipoproteins exceeded 10% in both sexes and the serum bilirubin increased by a like amount in men. For the other constituents the changes were less than 5%. Some of these changes are illustrated in Figure 1.12.

When the same population was studied both before and 2 hours after a standardized meal, statistically significant increases of serum glucose, phosphorus, bilirubin, urate, calcium, protein, albumin, creatinine, urea and cholesterol concentrations, and activities of lactate dehydrogenase, alkaline phosphatase and aspartate aminotransferase were observed. Alanine aminotransferase activity was increased in men whereas it was decreased in women.

Other observers have noted that a single meal may produce an effect on laboratory data lasting over 12 hours. Thus, a high protein meal taken the previous evening may cause an increase in the concentration of plasma urea, urate and phosphorus that is still apparent the next morning. The increase in urea has been shown to be proportional to the degree of absorption and metabolism of the ingested protein. Nevertheless, the nutritionally induced variability of urea and phosphorus – and for many constituents other than urate – is less than the typical inter-individual variability. The amount of fat in a meal may affect laboratory data both by causing lipaemia, which may make measurement of some of the test constituents less precise, and also by directly affecting the concentration in vivo of some of the serum constituents. Although the concentration of cholesterol is little affected, that of triglycerides is increased immediately following a meal, and peaks

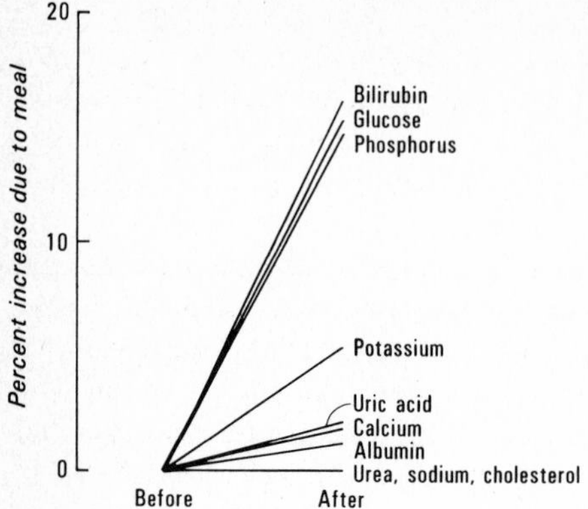

Figure 1.12. Mean change in concentration of some commonly measured serum constituents induced by ingestion of a single standard meal in a group of healthy volunteers. (Reproduced, by permission, from Steinmetz et al., 1973)

after about four hours. The increase is less when the fat is mainly unsaturated, e.g. corn-oil, compared with saturated fats. Serum alkaline phosphatase activity may be particularly stimulated by the ingestion of fats, although other meals may produce the same type of response. The effect is most marked in women and in blood group O secretors. Isoenzyme studies have confirmed that the increase is mainly of the intestinal component, but it should be noted that it occurs only when phenylphosphate, and not the more common *p*-nitrophenylphosphate, is used as substrate (Statland et al., 1973). Lactate dehydrogenase activity is decreased by a high fat diet. The H component of the enzyme shows a relatively greater decrease than the M component. The plasma lactate and pyruvate concentrations are also reduced, with the greatest effect on the pyruvate. Plasma prostaglandin E_1 may increase following food ingestion, probably as a result of the fat present. Carbohydrate ingestion may depress the plasma aldosterone concentration.

The secretion by the stomach of large quantities of acid in response to the ingestion of a meal causes a loss of chloride ions, and the venous blood returning from the stomach contains more bicarbonate than in the resting state. This so-called "alkaline tide" is, in effect, a mild metabolic alkalosis and produces an increase in the pH of both blood and urine, and an increase in blood pCO_2. The metabolic alkalosis is sufficient to reduce the serum ionized calcium by as much as 0.05 mmol/litre (0.1 mEq/litre) 1 hour after a meal. Following a meal the liver becomes the prime site for the metabolism of the ingested substances and its secretory ability may be impaired, which may account for the increased serum bilirubin and impaired excretion of bromosulphthalein that is typically found. After the ingestion of a test meal an increase in the plasma amino acid concentration is found 1 to 2 hours later. The ratio of the different aminoacids varies with the type of meal. A non-protein meal causes a decrease of plasma aminoacids for 8 hours. Ingestion of beef, on the other hand, causes the expected rise in aminoacids and urea, but a reduction in the concentration of glucose (Nasset and Ju, 1969).

The same meal ingested at different times of the day provokes markedly different secretory responses of insulin: it is much greater at breakfast than later in the day. Whether this is due to increased resistance to the action of the hormone or to the involvement of cortisol is uncertain (Malherbe et al., 1969). Protein ingestion stimulates the secretion of glucagon whereas carbohydrate ingestion may cause a slight reduction of its plasma concentration. Aminoacids and protein-rich meals also stimulate growth hormone secretion. This is more marked in children than in adults, and in women than men.

It should be noted that ingestion of one glass of water may significantly affect laboratory data when a blood specimen is drawn 2 hours later (Diot et al., 1974). The plasma concentrations of glucose, insulin, triglycerides, sodium, chloride and urea and the activity of alkaline phosphatase are reduced, but the concentrations of free fatty acids, bilirubin, bicarbonate, protein and calcium are all significantly increased. When 75 grams of glucose are ingested with the water, as might happen with a glucose tolerance test, the concentrations of free fatty acids and bilirubin are also decreased, as is the activity of aspartate aminotransferase. The concentrations of insulin and sodium are increased. It is believed that insulin causes release of sodium from the cells, and the effect on the bilirubin is due to modification of liver metabolism by the massive load of glucose.

1.4.4.1. Coffee

Caffeine, which is present in coffee, tea, cola and various other beverages, and which is to a large extent responsible for the metabolic action of these drinks, has considerable effects on the concentrations of several constituents commonly measured in blood. This is illustrated in Figure 1.13.

Two hundred milligrams of caffeine, or as little as two cups of coffee, have a marked stimulating effect on the adrenal medulla. This causes an increase in the urinary excretion

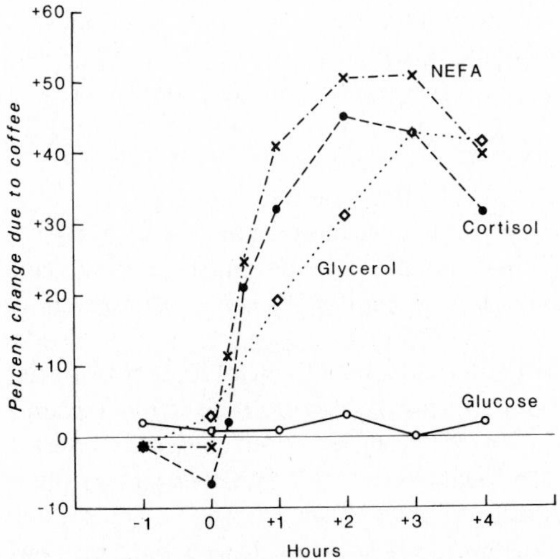

Figure 1.13. Influence of ingestion of coffee on the concentration of several serum constituents. Mean changes for several individuals are illustrated. (Reproduced, by permission, from Avogaro et al., 1973)

of both norepinephrine and epinephrine – the increase being relatively greater for the latter – and a slight increase in the plasma glucose concentration (Bellet et al., 1969a). The plasma insulin concentration is unaffected or reduced. Coffee also causes some impairment of glucose tolerance. The adrenal cortex is also affected. Plasma cortisol concentration is increased and the excretion of 11-hydroxycorticoids and free cortisol is also increased. The normal temporal decrease of the plasma cortisol between 08.00 hours and noon may be prevented by ingestion of coffee with breakfast (Avogaro et al., 1973). The urinary excretion of *N*-acetyltryptophan and 5-hydroxyindoleacetic acid is also increased by coffee.

The most studied effect of coffee is that on lipid metabolism. Plasma free fatty acids may be increased by as much as 30% by two cups of coffee in healthy adults. The effect is less marked in obese than lean adults and in younger than older people. The plasma concentrations of glycerol, total lipids and lipoproteins are also affected. The lipolytic action of coffee is probably mediated through cyclic AMP. Caffeine is a potent inhibitor of phosphodiestérase (EC 3.1.4.17), which breaks down cyclic AMP in adipose tissue, so that the concentration of cyclic AMP rises in tissues. The extent of the response of the serum lipid concentration to caffeine shows a direct correlation with its intake in coronary-prone individuals. Indeed, such individuals show a positive correlation between coffee intake and the serum concentration of cholesterol and lipoproteins. However, Naismith et al. (1970) claim that a slight reduction in serum cholesterol concentration occurs with ingestion of coffee for some weeks, whereas the concentration of triglycerides rises by as much as 16%. That this is a caffeine-related effect is indicated by a quite different response to the ingestion of decaffeinated coffee.

Coffee and caffeine are stimulants for the secretion of gastric juice hydrochloric acid and pepsin, and the serum gastrin concentration may be increased 2- to 5-fold after three cups of coffee. Intermediary metabolism is affected in a manner not as yet understood, and an increased excretion of creatine may be observed. Neither serum nor urinary creatinine nor creatinine clearance are affected by coffee. However, coffee does have an effect on the kidneys. Urine volume may be increased by a direct diuretic effect, but more serious are the other actions which may lead to an increase in the excretion of renal tubular cells and erythrocytes.

1.4.4.2. Specific food effects

Certain foods have specific effects on laboratory findings. Thus bran has been reported to reduce the absorption of certain compounds from the gastrointestinal tract: the substances affected include calcium, cholesterol and triglycerides, the serum concentrations of which are reduced. The concentration of calcium may be reduced by as much as 0.08 mmol/litre (0.15 mEq/litre) and that of triglycerides by up to 20 mg/dl (0.23 mmol/litre) if it were high initially. If initial concentrations are normal, bran has little effect on plasma cholesterol or triglycerides. Pectin ingestion also decreases the serum cholesterol concentration by reduction of apolipoprotein-B (Durrington et al., 1976). Other dietary fibres also reduce the serum cholesterol concentration.

Avocados may contain large quantities of serotonin, as may bananas, eggplant, pineapples, plums and other fruit, so that the excretion of 5-hydroxyindoleacetic acid is increased up to 5 times following their ingestion. Avocados also affect insulin secretion, so that glucose tolerance is impaired (Viktora et al., 1969). Asparagus imparts a characteristic odour to urine, and beets may cause a red urine due to anthocyanins and other pigments. Onions cause a significant decrease of the plasma glucose within four hours of ingestion and a significant decrease in the plasma insulin secretion; they have no effect on the free fatty acid concentration in plasma. Garlic decreases the serum cholesterol concentration and also reduces the plasma concentration of fibrinogen.

With sensitive procedures for the detection of blood in faeces, positive reactions may be obtained after the ingestion of fish or meat. Meat is also a potent stimulant for the secretion of gastrin, histamine and gastric juice hydrochloric acid.

1.4.5. Smoking

Smoking affects several metabolic processes as indicated by alterations of laboratory findings. The extent of alteration appears to be related both to the quantity of cigarettes or cigars smoked and to the extent of inhalation. As far as can be determined, the metabolic effects of smoking are due to nicotine.

Nicotine has a potent effect on the adrenal medulla, and causes a marked increase in the concentration of epinephrine in the plasma and of catecholamines in the urine. The increase of plasma norepinephrine is less than that of epinephrine. The increased catecholamine concentration activates hepatic glycogenolysis. This causes an increase in the concentration of glucose in plasma, which may rise by as much as 0.6 mmol/litre (10 mg/dl) within 10 minutes and remains elevated for 1 hour. The plasma lactate/pyruvate ratio begins to increase within 8 minutes of the start of smoking because of an increase in the lactate and decrease of the pyruvate concentration. The plasma glycerol concentration also increases (Cryer et al., 1976). Plasma insulin concentration is unaffected until one hour after smoking, at which time it shows a slight increase. However, the serum growth hormone concentration may rise by as much as 10-fold within 30 minutes of the onset of smoking. Generally, the fasting plasma glucose concentration is higher in smokers than in non-smokers, and glucose tolerance is mildly impaired (Sandberg et al., 1973). When smokers abandon the habit, the plasma glucose concentration reverts to that found in non-smokers.

Particularly in Caucasians, the plasma cholesterol and β-lipoprotein concentrations tend to be higher in smokers (Boyle et al., 1968). This is presumed to be an adrenal-mediated response, with catecholamines acting on the β-receptors of adipose tissue cells to increase lipid mobilization; this produces the increase in plasma concentration. There is a sustained rise in the plasma triglyceride concentration regardless of whether the smoker inhales or not. The response of free fatty acids to smoking is variable. Thus, there may be no detectable change in concentration if a cigar is smoked or if cigarettes are smoked without inhalation. However, smoking three cigarettes with inhalation has been demonstrated to produce an immediate increase of 30% in the concentration of free fatty acids.

The hormonal responses to smoking are not limited to the adrenal medulla. The concentration of 11-hydroxycorticosteroids in plasma may be increased by 75% following heavy smoking. This is most marked in individuals who are not accustomed to smoking. The plasma cortisol concentration increases by 40% within 15 minutes of the start of smoking (Cryer et al., 1976). The normal diurnal rhythmicity of cortisol is unaffected.

There is usually a difference in the excretion of 17-hydroxycorticosteroids between smokers and non-smokers. The excretion of 5-hydroxyindoleacetic acid is considerably increased in individuals who smoke compared with non-smokers. Tryptophan metabolism may be further affected by smoking, with an increased excretion of 3-hydroxykynurenine and 3-hydroxyanthranilic acid and a reduction in the conversion of 3-hydroxyanthranilic acid into nicotinic acid (Kerr et al., 1965). Nevertheless, the response of a smoker to a tryptophan load is generally the same as that of a non-smoker.

Nicotine exerts an antidiuretic action on the kidneys, which causes some slight alterations in the concentrations of blood constituents. A mild degree of haemodilution occurs, although this is usually masked by the increases in erythrocyte count, haemoglobin concentration and haematocrit that occur to compensate for the lower oxygen carrying capacity of the erythrocytes. In an individual who smokes as many as 40 cigarettes per day, up to 6% of his haemoglobin may be in the form of carboxyhaemoglobin compared with 1% typically found in a non-smoker. The plasma carboxyhaemoglobin concentration is higher when filter cigarettes are smoked than others (Wald et al., 1977). The amount of carboxyhaemoglobin increases throughout the day (Wald and Howard, 1975). The increased haematocrit, at best, allows the smoker the same ability as the non-smoker to transport oxygen. His erythrocyte P_{50} and adenosine triphosphate concentrations are significantly less than in the non-smoker (Sagone et al., 1973). Nevertheless, there is usually a reduction of less than 5 mm Hg (0.65 kPa) in his pO_2 and no significant change in his pCO_2. Smoking several cigarettes within a short time (e.g. 10 minutes) is followed by a significant increase in carboxyhaemoglobin concentration and decrease in pO_2 and oxygen saturation (Dawley et al., 1976). The leucocyte concentration may be as much as 30% more in smokers who inhale than in non-smokers, but this increase does not compensate for the marked decrease in their leucocyte ascorbic acid. Plasma vitamin C concentration is also reduced (Elwood et al., 1970).

The presumed haemodilution which occurs in smokers causes a slight decrease in the plasma concentration of albumin (up to 1 g/litre) and of the globulins, at least in the younger smoker (Dales et al., 1974). However, there is no indication that the plasma calcium concentration is affected nor the activities of any of the enzymes which are commonly measured in plasma or serum. There is usually a slight decrease in the concentration of plasma urate in smokers compared with non-smokers. This may be due more to differences in dietary habits than to metabolic effects, although the latter cannot be excluded. Further support for a possible dietary influence is the slightly lower urea concentration in the plasma of smokers than in non-smokers. The serum creatinine concentration may also be less in smokers than non-smokers. These effects may be manifestations of the antidiuretic action of nicotine with concomitant haemodilution. The impaired excretion of phenolsulphonphthalein observed in smokers is suggestive of a renal-mediated response. Some of the differences observed between a large population of smokers and non-smokers are illustrated in Figure 1.14.

Nicotine is a potent stimulant of the secretion of gastric juice. A marked increase in the volume and in acid secretion can be induced within an hour by four to six cigarettes. Basal acid output is related to the number of cigarettes smoked per day. In contrast, the secretion of pancreatic juice is reduced, especially in heavy smokers, with a fall in both its volume and bicarbonate content.

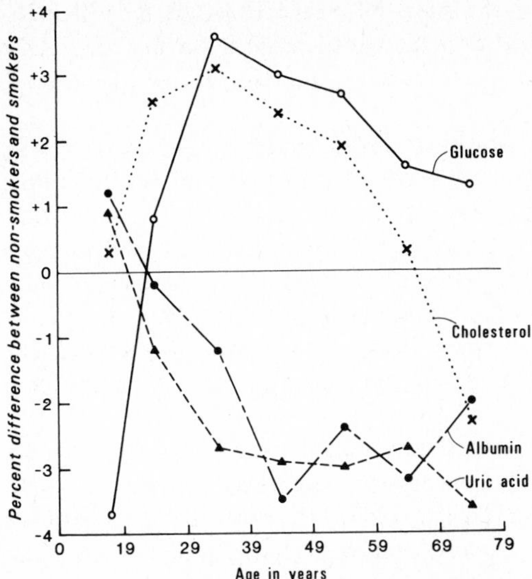

Figure 1.14. Mean differences and changes with age in concentration of several commonly measured serum constituents between smokers and non-smokers. A point above the zero line indicates that the value is higher in smokers. (Reproduced, by permission, from Dales et al., 1974)

Smoking also affects the body's immune response, in a manner that is not yet clearly understood. Typically, smokers show the presence of antinuclear antibodies, weakly positive tests for carcinoembryonic antigen, and the presence of rheumatoid factor in their serum.

The serum vitamin B_{12} concentration of smokers may be markedly reduced, in inverse proportion to the concentration of thiocyanate in their serum. Thiocyanate is derived from the metabolism of cyanide, and its measurement in urine provides a useful screening test for smokers. Cotinine, the major metabolite of nicotine, may be detected in serum for 2 days after cigarettes are smoked.

1.4.6. Posture

When an individual changes from a recumbent to a sitting or standing position, a decrease in the circulating blood volume of about 600 to 700 ml occurs. Concomitantly there is a reduction of both central venous pressure and cardiac output. This is reflected in increased pulse rate and diastolic blood pressure. Fluid moves outwards from capillaries due to the increased hydrostatic pressure at their arterial end that is not balanced by as large a change in the plasma oncotic pressure. Water and small molecules such as the electrolytes and simple organic compounds (including some polypeptides) pass freely through the pores of the capillaries (average size 4.5 nm) and the spaces between the cells (average size 8.0 nm). This causes the reduction in intravascular volume. At the venous end of the capillaries, the plasma hydrostatic pressure is less than the plasma oncotic pressure so that fluid and small molecules return from the interstitial space. However, the gain is less than the loss at the arterial end of the capillaries so that there are actual increases in the concentrations of compounds of large molecular mass, e.g. proteins, and of erythrocytes and other cells.

The opposite effect occurs when an individual lies down after standing or sitting. Hormonal and renal vascular mechanisms prevent overloading of the circulation with fluid returning from the extravascular spaces. Diuresis serves as a protective mechanism. When recumbency continues for a long time, the volume of returning fluid progressively declines. The change from standing to lying causes an increase in the plasma volume of approximately 10%. The cellular volume (haematocrit) is less markedly affected. In healthy individuals, the change in blood volume occurs in less than 30 minutes. The decrease in blood volume that occurs with the change from lying to standing is more rapid, taking up to 10 minutes only.

Postural changes are exaggerated in hypertensives (Eisenberg and Wolf, 1965), and in individuals with a low concentration of plasma proteins, especially albumin, as might occur with malnutrition (Widdowson and McCance, 1951; Eisenberg, 1963). Most of the plasma oncotic pressure is due to albumin, because of its high concentration. α_1-Globulin contributes a large amount to the oncotic pressure per gram, but the protein is normally present at a low concentration. In malnutrition, the plasma albumin concentration is reduced and the postural change in plasma volume may be as large as 20%. Postural changes are less in individuals with abnormally high plasma protein concentration, as in multiple myeloma, due to the increased plasma colloid pressure.

The change from lying to standing stimulates an increased secretion of norepinephrine, aldosterone, angiotensin II, renin and antidiuretic hormone. The plasma concentrations of these hormones respond rapidly to the change, e.g. within 30 minutes for renin in normotensives and even less in hypertensives. Plasma concentrations may rise to at least three times the resting concentration. This is illustrated for plasma renin activity and aldosterone concentration (Figure 1.15). Plasma norepinephrine concentration and dopamine-β-hydroxylase activity are significantly higher within 15 minutes of a change from lying to sitting, but there is no effect on the plasma epinephrine (Moerman et al., 1976). With the change of posture, urinary excretion of aldosterone increases from 0.06 μg/h to 0.4 μg/h. If recumbency continues for as much as one day the normal increase in output that occurs with ambulation will not take place. The excretion of norepinephrine increases with the change from lying to standing but that of epinephrine is not much affected. Contraction of the extracellular fluid volume with standing reduces glomerular filtration rate and it causes a reduction in creatinine clearance and urine flow. Sodium, potassium, and chloride excretion are reduced as a result of the increased hormonal secretion, but the normal circadian variation persists. If any changes in potassium and phosphorus excretion occur, they are small and transient, unless standing is prolonged. Urinary pH decreases and bicarbonate output is reduced as hydrogen ions are exchanged for sodium (Thomas, 1957). The opposite effects occur with lying. The ratio of sodium-to-potassium excretion decreases with standing and increases with lying (Thomas, 1959). In most individuals, the urinary excretion of protein decreases with the reduction in glomerular filtration rate that occurs with standing (Mahurkar et al., 1975).

The change from an upright to a recumbent position affects the concentration not

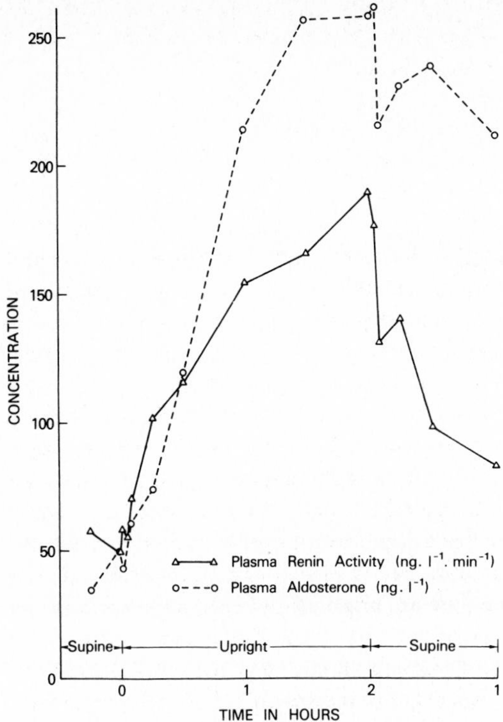

Figure 1.15. Influence of posture on plasma renin activity and aldosterone concentration. SI Unit conversion for aldosterone, ng/dl × 26.5 = pmol/litre. (Reproduced, by permission, from Sassard et al., 1976)

only of plasma proteins but of all those compounds that are bound to, or transported by, them. Thus, after 5 minutes the concentration of cholesterol may fall by 10% and that of triglycerides by 12%, as they are bound to lipoproteins. The activities of enzymes vary with postural changes because of their protein nature. The concentration of thyroxine falls by as much as 8% due to the decreased concentration of thyroxine-binding globulin and prealbumin. Triiodothyronine concentration changes by a similar amount. The concentrations of the protein-bound components of other hormones are affected in the same way, although the concentration of the free component may be unaffected, as, for example, is free thyroxine.

The concentrations of drugs that are transported bound to plasma proteins are also affected by changes in the concentration of the latter. The concentration of calcium and magnesium is changed with alteration of posture only because of changes in the fraction bound to albumin (aboug 40%), without a change in the ionized and complexed fractions, so that the overall change is less than that of cholesterol and triglycerides. Plasma sodium concentration is unaffected by postural changes but a significant increase in potassium concentration occurs with 30 minutes of standing. This has been attributed to release of intracellular potassium from muscle (Sassard et al., 1976). In general, the concentrations of freely diffusible constituents with molecular masses at least as large as that of insulin (5800) are unaffected by postural changes.

The effect of a change from lying to sitting, and vice versa, is approximately two-thirds of that due to the change from lying to standing.

1.4.7. Sleep and wakefulness

Secretion of corticotrophin, growth hormone, prolactin and TSH can be specifically linked to sleep. The secretion of LH in prepubertal children can be similarly associated with sleep, rather than to other influences, although there may be additional factors involved (Daly and Evans, 1974). Shifts in the sleep cycle produce a rapid change in the peak of growth hormone secretion so that the maximum still occurs shortly after the new sleep cycle begins. Adrenocorticosteroid secretion can be completely dissociated from a night-time secretory influence, so that the other factors that are known to affect cortisol secretion must be of greater importance. If the sleep–wakefulness cycle is reversed, the maxima and minima adjust to the new cycle over two weeks. The influence of activity may be quite important in determining the new cycle. Catecholamine excretion is greatly increased during the first week of a change from day to night work. Significant increases in the plasma concentrations of cholesterol, glucose, uric acid and potassium occur at the same time (Theorell and Åkerstedt, 1976).

The diurnal variation in aminoacid concentration in plasma appears to be linked to the sleep–wakefulness cycle (Tedeschi, 1973). Normally blood aminoacid concentration rises during sleep (Feigin, 1969). In night workers the normal diurnal pattern of excretion of sodium and chloride is reversed. The potassium excretion cycle is unaffected. The plasma phosphate and urinary phosphate excretion patterns change with change of the day–night sleep pattern. The highest plasma iron concentration occurs in the evening in night workers.

Deprivation of sleep provokes an increased excretion of epinephrine and norepinephrine in the urine, an increase in the serum thyroxine concentration but a fall in that of serum iron. 17-Hydroxycorticoid excretion is increased after several days. Deprivation for one or two days does not affect cortisol secretion. The plasma cortisol concentration is increased when sleep deprivation is imposed for a few days (Selye, 1976).

1.4.8. Hospitalization and immobilization

Differences in the concentrations of certain plasma constituents have been observed between in-patients and out-patients. These have been attributed to the combined influence of diet, activity and posture, the assumption being made that out-patients generally undertake more activity and spend more time upright. However, the effects of disease should not be ignored, as it is probable that an in-patient's illness is the more severe. Typical differences that have been reported are 0.13 mmol/litre (0.25 mEq/litre) for calcium, 5 g/litre and 3 g/litre for total protein and albumin respectively, and 0.39 to 0.77 mmol/litre (15–30 mg/dl) for cholesterol. In all of these situations the serum concentrations are higher in out-patients. Although the concentration of total serum calcium may not be increased, the ionized concentration is often elevated (Heath et al., 1972). This occurs without any effect on the serum alkaline phosphatase activity. Amador et al. (1967) have observed greater aspartate aminotransferase activity in the serum of outpatients. Creatine kinase activity is affected similarly.

When healthy individuals are confined to bed, the response to change of posture (section 1.4.6.) occurs initially. Subsequently the plasma volume decreases by as much as 5% with one day of bed-rest and 8% after 6 days. This is associated with a reduction of the plasma vasopressin concentration and increased plasma renin activity, possibly related to a decreased inhibition of renin release (Keil and Ellis, 1976). The contraction of blood volume is associated with an increased urine volume. The plasma volume remains contracted until the individual starts to walk again. The change appears to be greatest in physically fit individuals. Concomitant with the decreased blood volume, there is probably a slight decrease in extracellular fluid and total body water (Vogt and Johnson, 1967). Both body mass and serum osmolality show a slight decrease. The small changes in serum calcium concentration are probably manifestations of the reabsorption from bone that occurs with inactivity, because both urinary and faecal excretions are increased. Urinary excretion begins to increase within three days and reaches its maximum of about twice the healthy ambulatory amount in 4 to 5 weeks. The changes in patients with fractures tend to be greater than in healthy volunteers.

Urinary nitrogen excretion begins to increase within a week of immobilization, but faecal excretion is unaffected. Nitrogen excretion is maximal in about 10 days (Deitrick et al., 1948). The excretions of the "fixed" anions, phosphate and sulphate, increase at the same time, but citrate excretion is unaffected. Hydrogen ion excretion decreases, possibly due to decreased production of the normal products of metabolism from muscular activity; the lower basal metabolic rate provides support for this view. Sodium and potassium excretions are also increased but not always accompanied by an increased urinary volume. Creatine and creatinine excretions remain constant, but creatine tolerance is decreased with the decreased muscle mass. There is normally little change in steroid excretion with prolonged bed rest, but a considerable reduction in the serum androgen concentration has been observed in severely ill immobilized male patients compared with ambulatory patients or healthy men. In contrast, the serum corticosteroid concentration is high in immobilized patients (Briggs et al., 1973). The excretion of epinephrine and norepinephrine is decreased to as little as one-third of the quantities excreted when an individual is moderately active. When activity is restricted, but with enforced bed rest, the excretion of the catecholamines is between the extremes observed with bed rest and moderate activity. In spite of the reduced metabolic rate, the serum thyroxine may be slightly increased. This is probably related more to the increased protein concentration following reduction of plasma volume than to the altered metabolic state (Leach et al., 1972). Plasma growth hormone concentration decreases during the first ten days of bed rest but then rises to 1.5 times its basal value at 20 days, before decreasing again. Insulin concentration is high initially but begins to decrease after one month, at the same time as the glucose concentration begins to decrease (Vernikos-Danellis et al., 1976). Inactivity causes decreased glucose tolerance. The plasma cortisol concentration is increased during the first month of bed rest.

When an individual becomes active again after a period of bed rest it takes more than

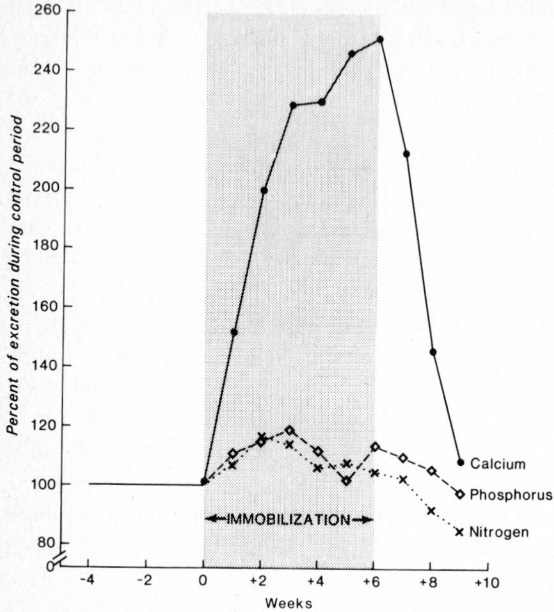

Figure 1.16. Change in excretion of calcium, nitrogen and phosphorus with immobilization and renewed activity. (Reproduced, by permission, from Deitrick et al., 1948)

three weeks for calcium excretion to decrease to normal and another three weeks for the individual to enter positive calcium balance. During the initial period, the serum calcium concentration may increase above the values observed during immobilization. Nitrogen excretion is increased for two weeks after immobilization stops. Thereafter, a period of reduced excretion ensues during which protein stores accumulate. It may take as long as 6 weeks before the habitual nitrogen excretion pattern is regained. This is illustrated in Figure 1.16.

1.4.9. Site of collection of blood

Typically, blood is drawn from a vein in the antecubital fossa of the arm. Occasionally, blood is obtained in the adult by puncturing the earlobe or finger-tip. This capillary (skin puncture) blood has more the characteristics of arterial blood than venous blood, except when the circulation is impaired or venous stasis is present. Capillary blood is more often obtained than venous blood in children. A heel-prick is used to obtain the blood in infants. In all instances in which skin puncture blood is obtained, the extremity must be warmed if arterialized blood is to be obtained. Even with good technique, capillary specimens tend to show more haemolysis than venous blood and some contamination from tissue debris. Trauma to cells during the collection procedure may cause increases in the activities of certain enzymes, e.g. aldolase and lactate dehydrogenase, due to tissue damage. Other constituents that are rich intracellularly, e.g. potassium and inorganic phosphate, show increased plasma concentrations also.

Freely flowing capillary blood is similar to arteriolar blood in composition because of the greater pressure at the arterial than the venous end, so that the bleeding is primarily arterial. Thus there are no measurable differences in pH, pCO_2, pO_2 and oxygen saturation. Plasma carbon dioxide content in capillary blood may be artifactually reduced by exposure to air. There is little difference between the composition of venous and arterial blood in a warm resting extremity, or between capillary pCO_2 in the warmed earlobe and in arterial blood (Maas and Van Heijst, 1961). However, some individuals have reported lower pO_2 values in capillary blood at high pO_2 values. The arteriovenous difference depends on the rate of blood flow and on the metabolism of the tissue drained. The pH of venous blood is up to 0.03 units less than in arterial blood. The pCO_2 is from 6 to 7 mm Hg (0.8–0.9 kPa) higher. Capillary blood, if drawn from a site such as the earlobe in which stasis may be present, has a similar pH to venous blood. Venous blood glucose concentration is less than capillary glucose, by as much as 0.56 mmol/litre (10 mg/dl), due to tissue utilization. Venous serum protein is higher than arterial protein by 2 to 5 g/litre. This may occur as a result of a relative haemoconcentration in the venous side of the circulation. The stasis in the earlobe circulation causes an increase of protein in serum from skin puncture blood when compared with serum from venous blood. Warming of the puncture site improves the circulation and decreases the plasma potassium and protein concentrations when compared with the unwarmed site.

1.4.10. Venous occlusion and blood drawing

With the volume of serum required for analysis being less than 100 μl for most tests, it is rarely necessary to draw more than 10 ml blood for all the tests requested at one time. The fill rate of an evacuated blood tube is approximately 10 ml/min – a rate that can also be achieved with a needle and syringe – so that it is unnecessary to place a tourniquet on an arm for longer than 1 minute in most situations. There should never be a need for a tourniquet to be in place for longer than 3 minutes.

While a tourniquet is used primarily to distend veins, so as to make them easier to locate, it also impedes the venous return to the heart and increases the intravascular pressure and the filtration pressure across capillary walls. This causes loss of fluid and of compounds of low molecular mass to the interstitial fluid. The concentrations of diffusible substances in serum water are unaffected but the concentrations of non-filtrable substances rise.

Slight, and clinically insignificant, changes in the concentration of some serum constituents have been observed with application of a tourniquet for one minute or less. Thus, a 6% increase in serum albumin concentration and a 3% increase in serum calcium have been observed in 40 seconds (Statland et al., 1974). The increase in cholesterol concentration is similar to that of albumin, but the increases for total protein and total lipid are less. A marked increase in serum aspartate aminotransferase activity has been observed, as well as increased creatine kinase activity. These increases may be related to trauma to tissue with aspiration of enzyme into the collected blood, and they may be independent of tourniquet application per se. The anticipated increase of enzyme activity would be only the same as the percentage increase in concentration of other proteins.

The concentration of all protein-bound constituents is increased by tourniquet application, whereas that of freely diffusible compounds is unaffected. Thus the protein-bound moieties of drugs and of ions such as calcium and magnesium are increased, although their free components are unaffected. The magnitudes of the increases will vary with the duration of application of the tourniquet and the magnitude of the cuff-pressure.

The plasma potassium concentration may be increased if opening and closing of the fist is allowed during blood collection. This is unrelated to tourniquet application (Skinner, 1961). Blood lactate may be increased and pH decreased by muscle contractions also.

If considerable stress is exerted on the blood at the time of collection by suction of a syringe, haemolysis will occur with an increase in the plasma haemoglobin and potassium concentrations and lactate dehydrogenase activity. Little haemolysis occurs if the shearing stress on erythrocytes is less than 3000 dynes/cm^2 (300 N m^2) (Nevaril et al., 1968). Haemolysis is generally less with a small bore needle because of the decreased velocity of blood flow (Moss and Staunton, 1970).

Growth hormone secretion is stimulated by venipuncture, especially in children, and an increase is one of the indications that a stress type of response is induced (Helge et al., 1969). Cortisol may be affected likewise (Davis et al., 1967), but in newborn infants the stress of heel-prick causes a decrease in plasma growth hormone concentration (Stubbe and Wolf, 1971). Glucose and glycerol concentrations are increased, presumably as a result of adrenal stimulation. The plasma concentrations of taurine and glutamic acid fall for one hour after venipuncture (Scriver and Rosenberg, 1973).

In young children, movement during blood-drawing and the need for restraining procedures may be sufficient to cause increases in serum creatine kinase and aldolase activities.

1.4.11. Hydration, dehydration and sweating

Although heat stress causes sweating and a reduction of body fluid and electrolytes, an increase in the blood volume occurs within 30 minutes, but it is usually less than 5%, and inversely related to the degree of sweating. The cardiac output is also increased, with a reduction of splanchnic and renal blood flow. The capillary blood flow is augmented. The haemodilution is associated with a decrease in the blood haemoglobin and plasma protein concentration. Most of the decrease in protein is caused by a reduction in the albumin concentration, but about one-quarter of the change can be attributed to lessened concentration of low molecular mass α_1-globulin. The haemodilution is believed to occur by influx of cell-free fluid with reduced protein concentration from the interstitial space into the intravascular space. The increased capillary blood flow is also associated with increased capillary permeability which allows the exchange of fluid. The plasma potassium concentration falls to an extent greater than the haemodilution but no changes in the plasma sodium concentration are usually observed initially.

The plasma volume is reduced within a few hours. The concentration of plasma protein begins to increase within one hour of the initial heat exposure, but it may take as long as 2 weeks for the blood volume and plasma protein concentration to return to normal. Renal plasma flow and glomerular filtration rate are reduced with the reduction in blood volume. This leads to an increase in the filtered fraction but a reduction in the urine volume. Negative nitrogen, potassium and magnesium balances occur early due to diminished dietary intake and increased urinary and sweat loss (Beisel et al., 1968). Urinary sodium and chloride excretion is rapidly diminished, but a negative sodium balance occurs on the day of exposure to heat. On the day of heat exposure urinary creatinine, urea nitrogen, ammonia and α-amino nitrogen excretion are increased, but only the increased excretion of urea nitrogen persists. These changes occur in spite of lack of change in the serum concentrations of urea, creatinine and α-amino nitrogen. Serum urate concentration increases by as much as 0.06 mmol/litre (1.0 mg/dl) on the day of hyperthermia, and persists at the slightly increased concentration. Urinary excretion is reduced initially but then increases above normal. The changes in concentration of some of the serum constituents that are affected by hyperthermia are illustrated in Figure 1.17.

The plasma concentrations of sodium, potassium and chloride may decrease by up to 10% over several days. The decrease in calcium and magnesium concentrations is usually less. The plasma phosphate falls rapidly, possibly related to the respiratory alkalosis that causes an increase in the blood pH of 0.15 units. To conserve phosphate, urinary and sweat excretions are reduced to a very low level. Plasma bicarbonate concentration may be markedly reduced. The fasting blood glucose is increased and glucose tolerance is decreased.

Plasma cortisol and corticosterone concentrations are increased in individuals exposed to a high temperature (Collins and Weiner, 1968; Collins et al., 1969). Urinary 17-hydroxycorticosteroid, 17-oxosteroid and pregnanetriol excretions are increased by hyperthermia. A further indication of increased adrenal secretion is the failure of the plasma

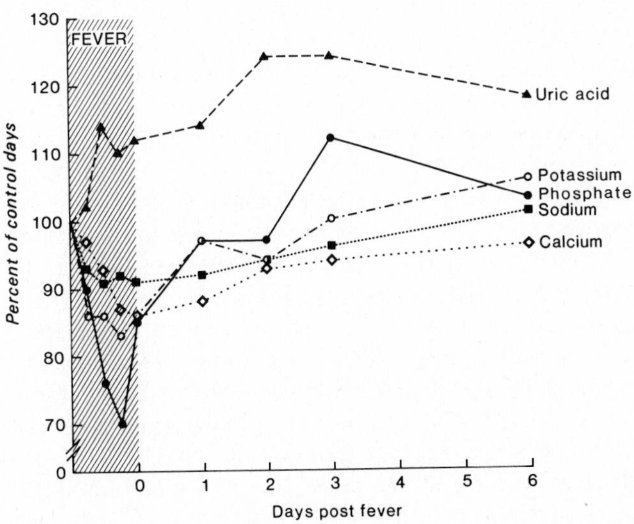

Figure 1.17. Influence of induced fever for one day on concentration of serum constituents. (Reproduced, by permission, from Beisel et al., 1968)

17-hydroxycorticoid concentration to fall in the afternoon. With continued exposure to heat, urinary excretion of 17-hydroxycorticosteroids returns to normal after three days and the excretion of 17-oxosteroids falls below the normal amount. Aldosterone secretion is increased and this effect is responsible for the reduced excretion of sodium. This is most marked when physical exercise accompanies the heat exposure and much sweating occurs. The stimulus to aldosterone secretion is probably related to the decreased plasma or extracellular fluid volume (Streeten et al., 1960).

With hyperthermia for a few hours there is either no change in the plasma growth hormone concentration or a transient slight increase. TSH secretion may be slightly increased, but with a slight fall in the thyroxine concentration. Urinary catecholamine excretion is reduced.

Haemodilution occurs rapidly in a dehydrated individual in response to drinking of water or other fluid.

With rehydration, the initial haemodilution persists and there is a further decrease in the plasma potassium concentration. This can be prevented by exercise. Oral administration of water lowers the concentrations of serum inorganic cations.

1.4.12. Exercise

Unless individuals are confined to bed, activity always plays a role in determining the concentrations of blood constituents. Activity can vary in extent and duration from that incurred during a normal day to that associated with sports, which can range from mild exercise to physical exhaustion. Activity invokes different degrees of stress which may be superimposed on the characteristic exercise response. Frequency of similar activity may modify the individual's response.

With moderate exercise, there is a rise in the plasma glucose concentration due to increased adrenal activity. Even if the exertion is not so marked as to affect the blood glucose, the secretion of growth hormone is increased some hours later. Although the effect is not always observed, the increased blood glucose concentration provokes an increased secretion of insulin. This leads to a slight alteration of the concentration of plasma aminoacids, with a rise in the alanine, glycine and ornithine concentrations but a fall in those of valine, leucine and isoleucine. Prolonged and intense exercise may ultimately produce a mild hypoglycaemia and a reversal in the pattern of change of aminoacids. The decreased plasma glucose is presumably due to increased transport across the muscle cell membrane. The arteriovenous difference of plasma glucose is accentuated through the greater requirements imposed by exercise. Glucose tolerance is improved by severe exercise. Plasma insulin concentration may be decreased even in the absence of a marked change in the glucose concentration (Hartley et al., 1972). A moderate increase in plasma glucagon activity has been reported in the absence of hypoglycaemia. The glucagon response is greater with prolonged exercise, although non-esterified fatty acids increase in response to exercise and inhibit the glucagon response (Galbo et al., 1975). The plasma pyruvate and lactate concentrations increase at the same time but usually return to normal within 1 hour.

The serum urate is increased by mild as well as by severe exercise. Nevertheless, the serum urate in individuals who do not exercise is higher than in those who exercise regularly, especially after middle age. The increased urate arises both from the increased turnover of nucleoprotein and impaired renal excretion of urate through competition for excretion by lactate and oxoacids. Urinary xanthine and hypoxanthine are increased by exercise. Plasma ammonia is also increased (Brodan et al., 1976). Short-term exercise produces no effect on the plasma urea nitrogen concentration but does cause a slight increase in the serum creatinine. Mild exercise does not alter the plasma volume but does produce a slight decrease in the serum cholesterol, although some increase has also been reported.

With more strenuous exercise, there is a reduction in the concentration of plasma proteins. This primarily affects glycoproteins, but plasma albumin is also increased. The change in the haematocrit is somewhat smaller than the change in plasma volume. The reduction in plasma volume is largely caused by a change in the capillary plasma osmotic pressure and not by a change in the hydrostatic pressure. With a short period of intense exercise, there is a small loss of plasma proteins from the capillaries. It has been postulated that this is due to increased capillary permeability which augments exchangable extravascular pools of protein. This process is analogous to the increased permeability of renal glomeruli which allows increased excretion of protein in the urine in response to exertion. With prolonged strenuous exercise, the observed increase in plasma protein concentration probably results from a regain of protein from the extravascular spaces and is not due to increased tissue breakdown or to increased synthesis. The increased plasma protein concentration may be instrumental, in part, for reducing the renal excretion of water by increasing the plasma osmotic pressure. Serum β-globulins show a real decrease with exercise and this may be caused by increased catabolism. The rate of catabolism of albumin is normally less than that of β-globulins so that, even without addition of albumin from extravascular pools, the plasma albumin concentration would increase relative to that of the β-globulins. Exercise of intense, but short, duration, has no effect on IgM, but increases glycoproteins, transferrin and α_2-macroglobulin (Haralambie, 1969). Increased fibrinolytic activity occurs with increases in plasma factors VIII and XII as a result of exercise. The decrease of serum cholesterol that may occur with exercise may be partially influenced by the decreased lipoprotein concentration. The concentration of very low density lipoproteins is significantly reduced during prolonged exercise. The serum cholesterol concentration in people who do not exercise is higher than in those who do. There is a slight fall in the plasma free fatty acid concentration when exercise is begun but this returns to normal within 15 minutes. The proportion of stearic acid is decreased during activity (Carlsten et al., 1962).

With strenuous exercise there is an efflux of enzyme protein from muscle tissue into the blood stream. This occurs with depletion of the cellular ATP which increases the permeability of the cellular membrane (Thomson et al., 1975). Increased ATP can be measured in plasma following muscular exercise. The effect is related to the degree of exhaustion and not to the duration of the exertion. Enzymes most affected include creatine kinase and aldolase. That the increase of serum lactate dehydrogenase activity is of skeletal muscular origin and not of cardiac origin is confirmed by measurements of isoenzyme activity. Following exercise, the increased lactate dehydrogenase activity is almost entirely due to isoenzymes 3, 4 and 5 (Rose et al., 1970). Malate dehydrogenase is also affected. With mild activity, such as that involved in 5 minutes' walking on an ergometer, slight increases in serum activities of aspartate aminotransferase, lactate dehydrogenase, creatine kinase and aldolase have been reported. Serum aminoacid arylpeptidase activity is also increased (Haralambie and Berg, 1976). Alanine aminotransferase activity is generally unaffected. The activities of creatine kinase and aspartate aminotransferase are generally higher immediately after strenuous exercise than during the activity, and the time for the enzyme activities to return to pre-exercise values is related to the magnitude of the physical activity. The maximum increase of ornithine carbamoyltransferase may be delayed for one week after exercise (King et al., 1976). Changes in activity of non-skeletal-muscle enzymes (e.g. γ-glutamyltransferase) with exercise are usually small. Some of the reported changes in serum constituents induced by a short period of exercise are listed in Table 1.4.

Strenuous exercise causes a decrease in hepatic and renal plasma flow and glomerular filtration rate. Urea excretion decreases following moderate to severe exercise, and the decreased glomerular filtration rate also reduces the excretion of creatinine and other non-protein nitrogen. There is an increase in urinary protein as well as an increase in the number of red and white cells and casts. Urine volume is reduced, but its acidity and osmolality are increased (Kachadorian and Johnson, 1971). Associated with the increased acidity, due to accumulation of end-products of metabolism, is an increase in specific gravity. If the ability to concentrate is impaired, a more dilute urine is produced. With moderate exercise, the glomerular filtration rate is unaffected and the urine output is unchanged but the urine is slightly more acid. With mild exercise the glomerular filtration rate is increased, the urine volume is increased and it is more alkaline than at rest. Urinary sodium and chloride excretion may be reduced due to a reduction in the proportion of filtered sodium that is excreted or an increase in the tubular reabsorption of filtered sodium. This effect may persist for more than 30 minutes after exercise is completed.

TABLE 1.4.

EFFECT OF EXERCISE TO EXHAUSTION ON THE CONCENTRATION OF SERUM PROTEINS

(Data reproduced, by permission, from Poortmans (1971), Journal of Applied Physiology, 30, 190–192)

Protein (g/litre)	Concentration prior to exercise	Concentration 2 min after excercise
Total protein	70	76
Albumin	36.5	40.3
α_1-acid glycoprotein	4.05	4.19
Haptoglobin	1.47	1.73
α_2-macroglobulin	3.46	3.62
β-lipoprotein	3.20	3.30
Transferrin	2.35	2.58
β_{1A}-globulin	0.52	0.59
IgA	2.36	2.70
IgM	1.36	1.40
IgG	12.52	14.00

Potassium and phosphate excretion do not correlate well with changes in sodium excretion (Kattus et al., 1949). The normal urinary excretion cycles of calcium and magnesium are reduced by even light exercise. Severe exercise may also cause an increased excretion of haemoglobin and an increase in the clearance of muramidase (lysozyme; EC 3.2.1.17), although that of amylase is unaffected. The degree of proteinuria and haematuria is proportional to the extent of the exercise. The excretion of white blood cells and epithelial cells does not correlate with the activity.

Hard physical work increases the formation of angiotensin and the plasma renin activity is increased. Exercise has no effect on the concentration of TSH, but the concentration of thyroxine rises in proportion to the degree of haemoconcentration (Terjung and Tipton, 1971). However, the concentration of free thyroxine may rise by as much as 30% of its resting values. Strenuous exercise may stimulate cortisol secretion, but with light activity its plasma concentration is either unaffected or may show a slight decrease, probably caused by an increased rate of removal from the circulation (Davies and Few, 1973). Loss of the normal circadian rhythm may occur. A decreased plasma cortisol is sometimes also observed with maximum exercise in untrained individuals (Adlercreutz and Dessypris, 1974). The cortisol-binding affinity of transcortin is decreased with exercise so that the free cortisol concentration is increased. Urinary free cortisol excretion is increased, the extent being related to the severity and duration of the exercise (Bonen, 1976). Plasma prolactin concentration is also raised by exercise, but to a lesser extent than that of growth hormone. The increased growth hormone may occur as a result of the increased demand for oxidizable substrates (Noel et al., 1972).

In the absence of emotional overtones, the urinary excretions of catecholamines and metabolites of cortisol are unaffected. With emotional overtones, urinary steroid excretion is increased and the normal rhythm of excretion of epinephrine is altered. The excretion of norepinephrine is only slightly affected. Plasma norepinephrine concentration is unaffected by mild work but is increased by exercise. Plasma dopamine concentration is increased but urinary output is reduced (Christensen et al., 1976). Plasma epinephrine is little affected initially but also increases with more severe exercise (Moerman et al., 1976). Plasma dopamine-β-hydroxylase activity is slightly increased by exercise in a warm environment (Frewin et al., 1973).

The plasma concentration and urinary excretion of aldosterone are increased both during exercise and in the recovery period. The increase is probably related to decreased metabolism as well as to increased secretion, as the metabolic clearance of aldosterone is correlated with hepatic blood flow. This may be decreased by as much as 80% with severe exercise (Rowell et al., 1964). The increased aldosterone production causes an increase in the excretion of potassium relative to that of sodium. Stimulation of the adrenals is probably also responsible for the increased plasma androstenedione and decreased testosterone concentrations.

While both plasma pyruvate and lactate are increased by vigorous exercise, the latter is more affected and the lactate/pyruvate ratio is increased. Urinary lactate is increased (Miller and Miller, 1949). It is probable that exercise per se, rather than lactate accumulation, serves as the stimulus for growth hormone secretion (Sutton et al., 1976). Plasma alanine is greatly increased by the transamination of pyruvate during exercise. The blood pH, oxygen saturation, and venous bicarbonate concentration are decreased by strenuous exercise (Laurell and Pernow, 1966). Such activity also increases the plasma creatinine and urea concentrations. The increased creatinine concentration rapidly returns to normal with the cessation of exercise, yet the urea concentration may remain elevated. These different responses have been attributed to increased production of creatinine, whereas the urea increase is related to diminished excretion. The plasma sodium, chloride and calcium concentrations are all increased to an extent comparable with the loss of fluid if only water is used as replacement fluid. Activity may cause increased plasma concentrations of potassium, phosphate and bilirubin in plasma (Van Beaumont et al., 1973). The increased bilirubin concentration reflects an increase in breakdown of erythrocytes caused by physical stress. The concentrations of uric acid, phosphate and bilirubin remain increased even when the concentrations of most constituents have reverted to the pre-exercise values. The overall concentration of triglycerides is usually briefly reduced by exercise, but the plasma glycerol is often increased and the concentration of stearic acid is decreased, reflecting an increased removal compared with that of other free fatty acids (Hagenfeldt and Wahren, 1975). Generally, the total free fatty acid concentration is much increased. Extensive mobilization of free fatty acids takes place under the influence of norepinephrine and growth hormone during exercise.

1.4.13. Physical training and conditioning

Physical fitness or condition may have considerable effect on the concentrations of certain plasma constituents, both at rest and in response to activity. In general, body fatness is correlated inversely with the extent of an individual's participation in physical activity.

The activities in plasma of enzymes that have a muscular origin are generally higher in the resting state for athletes than for untrained individuals. This applies, for example, to both the skeletal and cardiac muscular components of lactate dehydrogenase. Plasma creatine kinase activity is also increased. Physical training increases the concentration of ATP in resting muscles and also the activities of malate dehydrogenase (EC 1.1.1.37) and aspartate aminotransferase, although the increases for lactate dehydrogenase and creatine kinase are not significant (Raimondi et al., 1975). Training reduces the creatine kinase response to severe excercise and eliminates that of lactate dehydrogenase (Hunter and Critz, 1971). The increased serum activities of creatine kinase and aspartate aminotransferase in response to submaximal exercise are also reduced. Of those enzymes that are normally thought to have a primarily liver origin, the activity of γ-glutamyltransferase is unaffected by exercise or training whereas the activity of glutamate dehydrogenase (EC 1.4.1.2) is increased in athletes, particularly after the activity. Training also reduces the plasma isocitrate dehydrogenase (EC 1.1.1.41) activity. Muscle succinic oxidase and glycogen synthetase activities are also increased.

In athletes, the concentrations in plasma of urea, urate, creatinine, thyroxine and tryptophan are higher than in comparable control subjects. This may be related to the increased muscle mass and turnover of muscle protein that is likely to occur in athletes. However, it has also been reported that plasma urate is less in athletes who have undertaken a strenuous conditioning program. This is characteristic of the normal stress response (Bosco et al., 1970). Urea clearance may be slightly higher in athletes. In trained athletes, the urinary excretion is little different on days of activity from days of rest (Astrand, 1967).

No significant change in plasma volume occurs with training, and the haemoconcentration that results from exercise is unaffected by training. Plasma protein concentration increases with exercise. Proteins that increase specifically in response to exercise include α_1-antitrypsin, caeruloplasmin and, to a lesser extent, transferrin, which is significantly higher in the serum of athletes than in non-trained individuals. The concentrations of haptoglobin, and many of the glycoproteins and α-macroglobulins are also increased by training. Haralambie (1969) has determined that athletes at rest do not have significantly greater concentrations of bound hexoses than non-athletes. He has further suggested that the increase of α_1-antitrypsin and α_2-macroglobulin – both of which possess antiproteolytic properties – is related to possible increase in serum proteolytic activity after exercise. Poortmans (1973) has demonstrated both increased serum activity and urinary excretion of muramidase after exercise and has postulated that the increased α_1-antitryptic activity is a defence mechanism against the increased proteolytic activity in the plasma. It should be noted that the effect of training on plasma protein concentrations is not long lasting. Some of the differences in concentrations of specific serum proteins between trained and untrained individuals are illustrated in Table 1.5.

Plasma total serum lipids is decreased by physical training. With attention to diet and to a properly planned training programme, serum cholesterol may be decreased by as much as 25%. Several studies have shown a lower serum triglyceride concentration in trained individuals compared with untrained people. The difference is of the order of 20 mg/dl. It is possible that the insulin-like effect of exercise effects a diversion of dietary sugar from lipogenesis in the liver to cause the reduction of plasma triglycerides. Holloszy (1973) has postulated that the increased muscle glycogen observed in muscle after strenuous exercise also contributes to the decreased synthesis of lipids. The free fatty acids in the plasma of fit individuals at rest may be as much as 0.20 mmol/litre higher than in unfit individuals. With exercise, the concentration rises in the fit person but falls in the

TABLE 1.5.

PERCENT CHANGE IN CONCENTRATION OR ACTIVITY OF SERUM COMPONENTS INDUCED BY EXERCISE

(Data reproduced, by permission, from Galteau, M.M. and Siest, G. (1973) In Reference Values in Human Chemistry (Ed. G. Siest) p. 223, Karger, Basel)

Age (years)	Calcium	Cholesterol	Creatinine	Glucose	Magnesium	Phosphate	Urea
20-30	+0.7	+0.9	−0.8	−0.9	+0.5	+6.6	−2.8
40-50	+1.0	+3.5	+2.3	−2.6	+0.5	+10.4	−1.9

Age (years)	Albumin	Alanine amino-transferase	Alkaline phosphatase	Aspartate aminotrans-ferase	Creatine kinase	Total protein
20-30	+2.6	+2.4	+1.3	+1.7	+7.2	+2.4
40-50	+2.7	+2.4	+4.2	+0.3	+7.5	+1.9

unfit. The increase in plasma lactate in trained individuals in response to submaximal exercise is less than in other people, presumably because of the augmented transport of oxygen to muscles. The increased lactate is responsible for the reduction in the free fatty acid concentration (Hartley et al., 1972).

Training improves the maximal oxygen uptake of individuals in response to exercise. Plasma glucose is generally unchanged, or only slightly higher, in trained individuals than others in response to exercise. The plasma insulin concentration is less depressed in fit individuals in response to exercise than in others. Plasma glucagon response to exercise is similar in both fit and unfit people. Although the plasma concentration of growth hormone increases in response to exercise, the rise may be similar in trained and untrained people but the concentration of growth hormone may take longer to return to normal values in the unfit individuals. Growth hormone concentration may increase in an untrained individual with a submaximal exercising that has no effect in a physically fit person. With prolonged exercise to the point of exhaustion, the plasma growth hormone remains high in trained individuals, whereas a marked fall occurs in the untrained individual (Sutton et al., 1969). There is little difference in the response of plasma cortisol to exercise between trained and untrained individuals. Physical conditioning nearly doubles the thyroxine degradation rate but has little effect on the plasma concentrations of either free or total thyroxine; the turnover rate returns to normal with several days rest. The degradation of triiodothyronine is increased by training but the plasma concentration is unaffected (Balsam and Leppo, 1975).

After physical training, there is generally a lesser response of plasma norepinephrine, and lessened urinary excretion of catecholamines, to all degrees of exercise than prior to conditioning.

1.4.14. Altitude

There is little information concerning the effects of long-term exposure to high altitudes. Most have been concerned with an acute change such as occurs with mountain climbing.

There is little or no change in total body water, lean body mass, protoplasmic mass or bone mineral with a change from a moderate to a high altitude over 1 to 2 weeks. There is an overall loss of body protein, with non-muscle protein increasing at the expense of muscle protein. Both this response and the decrease of body fat may be consequences of the physical activity involved in climbing a mountain, which has been involved in the reported studies, but fat intake also tends to be reduced at high altitude with an increase in the carbohydrate intake (Krzywicki et al., 1969). Basal blood glucose concentration is less at high altitudes and utilization of glucose is greater (Picon-Reategui, 1963). Plasma lactate is increased at high altitudes and the lactate/pyruvate ratio is also affected at higher altitudes (Friedemann et al., 1945). Plasma volume is reduced by an increase in insensible water loss and also possibly by a redistribution of fluid within the body. Intracellular space may be markedly increased at the expense of the extracellular space. Albumin synthesis is decreased at high altitude, but plasma oncotic pressure is not usually reduced because of the decreased blood water (Hannon et al., 1969). Globulin forms a relatively greater proportion of the total plasma protein concentration.

The change from a low to a high altitude does not affect overall metabolism as measured by the basal metabolic rate. However, ^{131}I uptake is reduced initially. The degradation of thyroxine is increased, but this reverts to near normal within a few days (Surks et al., 1967). Plasma free and total thyroxine may remain slightly elevated. Urinary 17-oxosteroids and 17-hydroxycorticosteroids are increased by as much as 50% and 300%, respectively, during the first three days of a change from sea-level to an altitude of 4 km. The plasma 17-hydroxycorticosteroid concentration may more than double, reflecting the increased cortisol secretion rate. During the first month of high altitude exposure, plasma and urinary steroid concentrations remain high but revert to normal over 1 year. The extent of the steroid change in response to altitude diminishes with repeated exposure. The urinary excretions of 17-hydroxycorticosteroids and oxosteroids are similar in populations habitually living at sea level or at high altitudes.

Norepinephrine excretion is increased slightly after several days exposure to a high altitude, and urinary vanillylmandelic acid excretion is also increased. These responses suggest increased sympathetic activity. Urinary excretions of epinephrine and metanephrine are unaffected.

Plasma bicarbonate concentration may be reduced by acute exposure to high altitude by as much as 7 mmol/litre. Plasma chloride concentration increases to compensate for this change, with a minor increase in the plasma phosphate. Acidosis is more severe with exercise at high altitude (Moncloa et al., 1970). Sodium and calcium are unaffected, but slight increases of potassium and magnesium occur (Hannon et al., 1971).

Urine volume is decreased markedly with an increased altitude. Sodium intake is decreased but its urinary excretion is also reduced. Urinary potassium is greatly reduced so that the sodium/potassium ratio is increased and the plasma potassium concentration increases. This response is similar to that which would occur with diminished aldosterone secretion, yet some short-term studies at high altitude have demonstrated both decreased aldosterone and renin secretions (Frayser et al., 1975). A negative nitrogen balance may occur at high altitude (Johnson et al., 1969), with a urinary excretion of nitrogen which is greater than the dietary intake; urinary ammonia excretion is reduced to a greater extent. Urate excretion is little affected over the short term. Urinary creatinine excretion has been reported to be decreased immediately following a change to a high altitude, but it has not been established whether this is related to altered renal blood flow or to another cause. The urinary excretions of pregnanediol and pregnanetriol are unchanged by increased altitude. Serum cholesterol concentration may be reduced by altered dietary habits or by the increased secretion of thyroid hormones.

The blood haemoglobin is markedly affected by altitude, and the 2,3-diphosphoglycerate concentration of erythrocytes may be increased by as much as 25% in some individuals who formerly lived at low altitudes (Eaton et al., 1969). The oxygen dissociation curve is shifted to the right. The negative correlation between blood haemoglobin concentration and erythrocyte 2,3-diphosphoglycerate concentration that is observed at sea-level still holds in individuals at a high altitude. The myoglobin concentration in skeletal muscle is also increased by high altitudes (Reynafarje, 1962). The increased number of erythrocytes in the blood leads to an increased turnover of nucleoprotein and excretion of urate. An abrupt change to a high altitude both increases the requirements for iron and reduces its serum concentration.

In individuals who are adapted to a high altitude, the fasting basal growth hormone concentration in plasma is high, but this does not increase much with exercise. In non-adapted individuals, growth hormone concentration is greatly increased by exercise (Sutton et al., 1970).

Increased pressure, as occurs with deep sea diving, causes a significant reduction in the excretion of sodium and calcium, although their serum concentrations are unaffected. Excretion of potassium and magnesium is unaffected. The changes in sodium and calcium can be correlated with the air-pressure. Serum phosphate and potassium concentrations are increased whereas that of albumin is reduced. Substitution of helium for nitrogen reduces the changes. Blood haematocrit and plasma free fatty acids are increased following a dive, but plasma cortisol, complement activity and serum lactate are reduced (Philp et al., 1972). All alterations in urinary excretion or plasma concentration are rapidly restored to normal with decompression (Radomski and Bennett, 1970).

1.4.15. Travel

Travelling long distances by air from east to west or vice versa leads to certain metabolic alterations. The excretion of epinephrine and norepinephrine is increased for 2 days after the flight, while norepinephrine excretion is also increased during the flight. Cortisol concentration remains normal during the travel but is decreased during the following day. It returns to normal within 2 days. The change of time zones has sufficient impact on metabolism that a change of ten hours affects glucocorticoid secretion for five days. An 11-hour time-change initiates alteration of the 17-hydroxycorticoid excretion within 3 days; a complete adjustment to a new diurnal rhythm takes place in 5 days (Lafontaine et al., 1967). Even in a passenger, the serum triglyceride and glucose concentrations increase during a flight, but cholesterol and free fatty acid concentrations are unaffected. Urinary volume is decreased during a flight, resulting in a concentrated urine and reduced excretion of sodium. After 2 days, urine composition returns to normal (Carruthers et al., 1976). Adaptation occurs more rapidly with travel from east to west than vice versa (Aschoff, 1976).

1.4.16. Noise

Exposure to audible noise affects adrenal function. Thus plasma corticosteroids are increased and urinary 11-hydroxycorticosteroids are also affected. In contrast, the excretion of 17-oxosteroids is decreased. The excretions of epinephrine, norepinephrine and vanillylmandelic acid are also increased, as manifested by a smaller reduction in excretion in the afternoon than usually occurs when an individual is not exposed to much extraneous noise. The excretion of gonadotrophins is also increased by noise of certain frequencies. In factory workers exposed to noise and vibration, increased serum activities of aldolase and lactate dehydrogenase have been observed (Gregorczyk et al., 1965). Plasma cholesterol and free fatty acid concentrations may be increased by short-term exposure to high-pitched noise (Ortiz et al., 1974).

1.4.17. Sexual activity

Sexual intercourse has no significant effect on the concentrations of plasma cortisol, follicle stimulating hormone or luteinizing hormone in either sex. Plasma oestradiol and progesterone concentrations are unaffected in women but prolactin concentration may be increased as much as eight times, probably as a result of breast stimulation. The plasma testosterone concentration may be slightly increased in men. Abstinence from sexual activity in men for as long as two months has no effect on the plasma concentrations of the gonadotrophins or testosterone.

Prostatic palpation or catheterization of the ureter may cause a marked increase in serum prostatic acid phosphatase activity (Woodard, 1959).

Masturbation by men increases the plasma concentrations of pregnenolone, dehydroepiandrosterone, androstenedione, testosterone, dihydrotestosterone, oestrone, oestradiol and cortisol. The increases are greatest for pregnenolone and dehydroepiandrosterone (Purvis et al., 1976).

1.4.18. Coughing and muscle massage

Severe coughing may cause doubling of the plasma creatine kinase activity, but the source of the enzyme has not been identified. Muscle massage will produce significant increases in the plasma activity of creatine kinase within one hour and also of alanine aminotransferase, lactate dehydrogenase and myokinase (EC 2.7.4.3) within 8 hours, but none of the changes is large enough to cause confusion in the diagnosis of pathological conditions (Bork et al., 1972).

1.5. DRUG ADMINISTRATION

Although clinical laboratory tests may be insensitive measures of disease, they are useful as indicators of the presence of a disease and as a means of following its progress or treatment. It has been widely accepted that the major cause of changes in laboratory data is disease. This premise is dealt with in the bulk of this book and it is not appropriate for consideration in this section. Disease has widespread effects on laboratory tests – often affecting those that one would not normally associate primarily with a particular disease. Disease may alter some of the normal physiological responses such as diurnal variation, and the changes that occur are usually related to a specific disease.

While drugs are administered primarily to cure a disease, they may exert actions on many organs other than those affected by the disease. Thus disease and its treatment involve a complex series of changes in test values which may be superimposed on the normal physiological changes that have already been discussed in this chapter.

1.5.1. Drug therapy and response

The response of individuals to drug administration depends on many factors. These include the presence or absence of disease and, when disease is present, the nature of the disease and its severity. The bioavailability of the drug, its route of administration, and whether it is administered by itself or in combination with others also may exert substantial effects on the response to its administration. The effect of the drug may be considerably modified by many of the same variables that influence the concentrations of many endogenous constituents.

In general, infants are particularly susceptible to the effects of drugs, and doses should be reduced accordingly; past knowledge and experience are more valuable than rules of thumb in estimating correct dosage regimens. The extent of the effect varies with the type of drug used. In the elderly, responses tend to be less consistent, and the dose calculated to be suitable for an adult may actually be inappropriate. The variable response in the elderly may be related to a combination of factors, amongst which are absorption from the gastrointestinal tract, metabolism and excretion from the body.

Only the concentration of the free component of a drug in plasma is indicative of its effective concentration. For many drugs, the volume of distribution is much greater in obese individuals, and so a bigger dose is required to ensure the same plasma concentration as in a lean individual. Hormonal differences between individuals may significantly affect responses to drug administration: this is especially true of the pregnant woman who may be unusually susceptible to the actions of many drugs.

The time of administration of a drug may affect the response to it. Thus, taken orally in association with a meal, the absorption of a drug is delayed and its peak concentration in plasma is likely to be less. Halberg (1974) has also indicated that the response to certain drugs is affected by the time of day at which they are administered. This is especially true of drugs that affect, or are affected by, adrenal action. The route of administration of a drug has considerable influence on both its plasma concentration, speed of response and duration of action. The route of metabolism or elimination of a drug may be considerably influenced by disease. Thus liver disease may impair the breakdown of certain drugs, and may also affect the conversion of inactive forms into active forms. For a drug that is eliminated from the body wholly or partly through the kidneys, impairment of renal function may lead to prolonged action of the drug; the dose may need to be adjusted to allow for this effect.

Combinations of drugs may produce effects which are different to those when they are administered singly. This may occur, for example, when one drug acts on the liver to induce enzymes that may either accelerate or impair the metabolism of another drug. In the first instance, the dose of the drug required to produce the same effect must be increased, and in the second reduced, to allow for the combination. Considerable danger may result if one drug that affects another's hepatic metabolism is withdrawn, because this may suddenly produce a situation equivalent to that of an overdose in the first case, and a suboptimal blood concentration in the second. Most drugs are transported in plasma bound to plasma proteins, most often to albumin. Two different types of binding sites exist on the albumin molecule, so that acidic and basic substances are bound separately. However, administration of more than one acidic drug, for example, may cause mutual displacement from the binding sites with a transient increase in the circulating free drug, which ultimately adjusts to a lower total concentration but similar free concentration. Thus while the free, and effective, concentration of the drug is unchanged, the total concentration is reduced. This should always be considered when several drugs are administered together and only measurements of total drug concentration are made. It should also be noted that several endogenous compounds such as porphyrins, bile acids and uric acid are also transported bound to the same acidic binding sites on albumin as are most drugs, and that the concentrations of these compounds may also be affected by drug administration.

The many mechanisms involved in changing the requirement for anticoagulant drugs when other drugs are co-administered have been discussed by Williams et al. (1976).

1.5.2. Adaptation to drugs

Individuals may become tolerant to the repeated administration of a drug. The therapeutic effect of the drug may decrease with time so that the administered dose has to be increased, although the plasma concentration of the drug has already achieved what might be considered a therapeutic concentration. Tolerance may occur in one individual to a dose that produces marked effects in others, even when the individual has not previously received the drug. Tolerance may also occur to drugs that are chemically similar to that which produced the tolerance in the first instance. Habituation and addiction are extreme examples of tolerance.

Certain unintended responses to drugs may occur. These include side-effects, the number of which may be so large that a physician has difficulty in remembering all of them and may not attribute unusual effects to a drug that the patient has been receiving. In other instances, a patient may react in an atypical or unusual manner to a drug's administration. Hypersensitivity is a more common abnormal response to drug administration. Drugs act as if they were haptens to produce an allergic response. Such hypersensitivity reactions may take several forms. From the clinical laboratory standpoint, the most important types of response affect the haemopoietic system and liver function. To a lesser extent, the kidneys may also be involved in hypersensitivity reactions. For many drugs, the incidence of this type of reaction has been assessed so that the physician can be alerted to the possibility of problems with those drugs, for which there is a strong indication for their administration. When a drug produces a hypersensitive response, the mechanism of the toxicity is usually fairly characteristic so that there is a typical cholestatic, as opposed to hepatotoxic, response in the liver. Hypersensitivity need not be a characteristic response of one patient to a variety of drugs, nor need it be characteristic of a particular drug, or broad class of drugs, clearly greater for one than for others.

The presence of a disease and its severity may greatly modify the response to a drug's administration. It should also be noted that the effects of a drug may be modified greatly by the duration of its administration. For some drugs considerable time is required for their therapeutic effects to become apparent, and these or other effects may persist long after drug therapy has been stopped.

1.5.3. Self-prescribed drugs

The widespread and often indiscriminate self-administration of certain drugs has resulted in a general attitude of acceptance of the practice to the extent that many are no longer thought of as drugs. Many of these drugs have considerable effects on laboratory tests and yet the physician, as much as the patient, may minimize the importance of these compounds. Drugs that are commonly ingested, and yet are ignored as potential influences on laboratory tests, include iron salts, vitamins, oral contraceptives, hypnotic-sedatives such as barbiturates, and analgesics such as aspirin or paracetamol (acetaminophen). The effects of these and other drugs on laboratory tests have been summarized by Young et al. (1975). Only some of the major effects of a few of the more widely used drugs are discussed here.

1.5.3.1. Oral contraceptives

Throughout the world, a large number of women use steroidal oral contraceptives. Use of "the pill" has a considerable influence on normal metabolism, the extent of which varies with the composition of the drug. In general, an oral contraceptive drug consists of both an oestrogenic and a progestogenic component, each of which may affect specific metabolic processes.

The action of oral contraceptives on serum lipids is dependent on the type and strength of "pill" used. Progestogens (e.g. megestrol) tend to have little effect on the concentration of serum lipids or may cause a decrease of free fatty acids, phospholipids and cholesterol. When administered alone, norgestrol has little effect on the serum triglyceride concentration, but when it is combined with ethinyloestradiol, the triglyceride concentration is increased, together with the low and very low density lipoproteins. The concentrations of phospholipids and cholesterol are also increased but the free fatty acid concentration may, or may not, be increased. There is uncertainty whether the increased lipid concentration is due to impaired removal from the circulation by inhibition of post-heparin lipoprotein lipase and esterase activities, or to increased triglyceride production by the liver. Oestrogens increase the pool size and turnover rate of triglycerides but decrease the free fatty acid pool. The increased circulating insulin observed with oral contraceptive use may also affect lipid metabolism.

Oral contraceptive users usually have a fasting blood glucose higher than normal. Glucose tolerance is also impaired. In addition to an increased circulating insulin concentration, the plasma growth hormone concentration is also increased. Cortisol production is increased and has been implicated in causing altered liver function which affects the blood glucose concentration. The plasma free cortisol may be more than twice as high in contraceptive users as in other women (Durber and Daly, 1976). The plasma pyruvate concentration is usually increased.

The concentrations of many different proteins are affected by steroidal contraceptives, with alterations in the concentrations of compounds which are bound to these proteins. Thus, combined contraceptives cause increased synthesis and plasma concentrations of transferrin, caeruloplasmin, plasminogen, α_2-macroglobulin, C-reactive protein, transcortin (cortisol-binding globulin), sex hormone-binding globulin, thyroxine-binding globulin, vitamin D-binding globulin, α_1-antitrypsin, complement C_3 and several blood-clotting factors. The overall concentration of α_1-, α_2- and β-globulins is slightly increased (Ramcharan et al., 1976). Typically, the increases in plasma concentrations of the binding proteins may be as much as 25% for transferrin, 200% for transcortin, 60% for thyroxine-binding globulin and 190% for caeruloplasmin (Laurell et al., 1967). While other authors have observed less marked increases, the relative amounts of the different proteins are similar. While the serum iron is not necessarily increased, the concentrations of copper and of thyroxine are increased.

The concentrations of the immunoglobulins IgA, IgG and IgM are little affected by oral contraceptive use, but the concentrations of haptoglobin and orosomucoid are usually reduced by as much as 30%. The concentration of albumin may be slightly reduced and this is the probable cause of the decreased serum calcium concentration observed in "pill" users. Plasma zinc, also bound to albumin, is decreased but the serum magnesium concentration may be increased. Most of the changes are oestrogenic effects, except for the alteration of α_2-macroglobulin and transferrin. The effects are greatest on those proteins synthesized in the liver. It should be noted that the oral contraceptive effects are generally less marked than those associated with late pregnancy, but the decreases of orosomucoid and haptoglobin are greater than in pregnancy. The changes in plasma protein concentration are probably due to a steroid influence on the synthesis of protein. The decreased concentrations may be attributable to increased synthesis of proteolytic enzymes, so that the catabolism of these proteins is accelerated. The incidence of serum antibodies, e.g. antinuclear antibodies and rheumatoid factor, is higher in oral contraceptive users than in other women (Kay et al., 1971).

Contraceptive steroids, especially those with a C_{17} α-alkyl-substituted group and an oxygen group at C_3 in the A ring, produce a high dose-related incidence of hepatic dysfunction. The incidence of jaundice, however, is low. Impairment of bromosulphthalein excretion occurs within a few days in up to 40% of the users. Contraceptives produce a bland, reversible, non-inflammatory intrahepatic cholestasis but occasionally, some hepatocellular degeneration and necrosis. Despite continued use of the "pill", most users exhibit a decrease in bromosulphthalein retention after some weeks. The oestrogen component may produce a significant increase in the activities of both alanine aminotransferase and, to a lesser extent, of aspartate aminotransferase. Progestogen-only pills have no effects on aminotransferase activities. The alkaline phosphatase activity in women taking oral contraceptives is generally lower than in other women or men. Serum phosphate concentration is reduced. Serum cholinesterase activity is also reduced but that of γ-glutamyltransferase is unaffected or slightly increased after combined oral contraceptives. Lactate dehydrogenase activity is unaffected (Batt et al., 1974).

Oral contraceptives have considerable influence on the plasma concentrations of hormones, mainly through their effects on the concentrations of binding proteins. The concentration of renin substrate is increased, which leads to increased concentrations of plasma angiotensin II and aldosterone, but renin concentration is reduced. Serum TSH is higher in women receiving oral contraceptives than in normally menstruating women (Weeke and Hansen, 1975). Triiodothyronine and thyroxine concentrations are also higher. Progestogens have no effect on thyroid metabolism and effects are due to the oestrogenic influence on the plasma proteins and thyroid gland. Oral contraceptive steroids cause an increase in the amplitude of the circadian variation of cortisol but do not alter the cycle per se. Prolactin concentration is usually unaffected by oral contraceptives. Generally, urinary excretions of gonadotrophins, pregnanediol, oestrogens and androgen and corticosteroid metabolites are reduced by oral contraceptives. The plasma testosterone concentration is slightly increased, with an increased binding protein concentration, but not in proportion to the decrease in dehydroepiandrosterone and androsterone sulphates (Briggs, 1976). Norepinephrine excretion is increased 3-fold with the ingestion of a combined oral contraceptive (Rao and Zuspan, 1970). The increase is less marked in sequential "pill" users.

Progestogens are believed to be responsible for the decreased plasma concentrations of aminoacids in "pill" users. Urinary excretions of glycine, ornithine and tyrosine are also reduced, but histidine excretion may be increased.

Oral contraceptives cause an increased excretion of kynurenic acid and of xanthurenic acid following a tryptophan load, suggesting either a relative pyridoxine deficiency or increased requirement. Plasma pyridoxal phosphate concentration is reduced. Increased erythrocyte aspartate aminotransferase activity, increased plasma vitamins A, D and E concentrations and falls in erythrocyte folate and plasma carotene concentrations are also observed. Urinary excretion of folate is increased. Steroidal contraceptives also reduce erythrocyte riboflavin concentration and glutathione reductase activity, indicating considerable alteration of nutritional status (Ahmed et al., 1975). These changes become apparent shortly after use of the "pill" begins. Oral contraceptives cause a reduction in the plasma, leucocyte and platelet concentrations of ascorbic acid as well as its urinary excretion. Plasma vitamin B_{12} concentration may be reduced in oral contraceptive users but it is not known whether this is due to an effect on plasma clearance, on renal excretion or on tissue uptake (Anderson et al., 1976).

Contraceptive steroids may impair drug metabolism so that plasma half-lives are prolonged (Carter et al., 1976).

1.5.3.1.1. Contraceptive devices. There is no evidence that intrauterine devices alter normal metabolism. However, devices made of copper produce an inflammatory response with increased serum concentrations of IgG and IgM in consequence (Holub et al., 1971).

1.5.3.2. Vitamins

The diseases due to deficiencies of vitamins are discussed elsewhere in this volume (Chapter 22). Here, we discuss alterations in laboratory data due to the administration of vitamins in conventional doses and also in "megadoses".

Vitamin A has been reported to inhibit ^{131}I uptake and reduce protein-bound iodine by inhibition of the iodination of tyrosine residues. It has also been incriminated as a cause of hypoplastic anaemia, with reductions of the erythrocyte and neutrophil counts.

In large doses, niacin (nicotinic acid) may produce signs of liver damage with increased bromosulphthalein retention and increased serum enzyme activities. It is a potent stimulant of gastric acidity. Serum concentrations of cholesterol, triglycerides, total lipids and phospholipids are decreased by administration of the vitamin. The free fatty acid concentration is markedly reduced and this stimulates the secretion of growth hormone. The plasma glucose concentration is increased, which prompts increased secretion of insulin, which in turn leads to an improvement in glucose tolerance. The serum uric acid concentration may be increased by as much as 0.09 mmol/litre (1.5 mg/dl) with large doses of niacin (Gershon and Fox, 1974); this is largely due to a reduction in its tubular clearance.

Vitamin B_6, especially in the elderly, increases the activity of serum aspartate aminotransferase. This probably only occurs with those individuals who are actually deficient, to some extent, in the vitamin. Vitamin administration allows further activation of the enzyme. Successful treatment of vitamin B_{12}-deficient individuals with the vitamin may cause a mild polycythaemia with increase of both erythrocyte count and haematocrit.

Ascorbic acid administration reduces the serum cholesterol concentration in young adults, but has no effect on the serum concentration in the elderly, even though there is apparently a reduction in the amount of atheroma in their large blood vessels. In atherosclerotic individuals, the serum triglyceride concentration is reduced (Sokoloff et al., 1966). Vitamin D promotes the absorption of calcium from the gastrointestinal tract, so that faecal excretion is reduced; the serum calcium concentration is slightly increased and urinary excretion is augmented. Serum phosphate is reduced initially and urinary phosphate concentration is increased, reflecting the primary action of the vitamin in promoting its mobilization from bone and its urinary excretion. Serum alkaline phosphatase activity may be increased in some individuals. Ultimately, the increased serum calcium concentration caused by secretion of parathyroid hormone is reduced. As a result, urinary excretion of phosphate falls and the serum concentration rises. In middle-aged men, the serum cholesterol concentration may be increased by as much as 0.65 mmol/litre (25 mg/dl).

1.5.3.3. Barbiturates and antiepileptics

Administration of the occasional barbiturate as a sleeping pill probably has little or no effect on the concentrations of commonly measured constituents in body fluids. However, barbiturates and most of the other drugs administered for the treatment of epilepsy are powerful inducers of hepatic microsomal enzymes. This action is exploited in the treatment of the physiological jaundice of newborn infants through the induction of glucuronyltransferase in the liver. The plasma and cerebrospinal fluid concentrations of glutamine and ornithine are also increased, with a reduction in the urea concentration through a presumed effect on the urea cycle in the liver (Perry et al., 1976).

With long-term administration of antiepileptic agents, there may be considerable changes in laboratory data. Thus, serum γ-glutamyltransferase activity may be increased by as much as 200%, and aspartate aminotransferase activity by as much as 40%. Alanine aminotransferase and alkaline phosphatase activities may also be increased by phenobarbitone administration. The alkaline phosphatase is mainly of bone origin. Pheneturide is an even more potent enzyme inducer than phenobarbitone (Latham et al., 1973). Enzyme induction is also manifested in increased urinary excretion of glucaric acid and the diversion of corticosteroid metabolism so that 6β-hydroxycortisol excretion is increased at the expense of 11-hydroxycorticoids. Hepatic synthesis of cholesterol and of bile acids is stimulated by antiepileptic agents. Gastrointestinal absorption of cholesterol is increased through facilitation of micelle formation. Typically, serum cholesterol concentration is increased by 20%, but no consistent change in the triglyceride concentration may be observed. Plasma glucose concentration tends to be higher in treated epileptic individuals than in other individuals. The insulin response to glucose may be reduced and glucose tolerance is impaired. Free triiodothyronine and thyroxine concentrations are reduced in long-term treated epileptic patients, probably as a result of increased metabolism in the liver. TSH concentration is not affected (Liewendahl and Majuri, 1976). Barbiturates may stimulate vasopressin release but this is inhibited by phenytoin (Hays, 1976).

With long-term anticonvulsant therapy, serum 25-hydroxyvitamin D concentration is reduced. Serum calcium concentration is commonly reduced to the lower limit of the normal range, but the concentrations of both constituents tend to be decreased in relation to the duration of treatment. Parathyroid hormone secretion is greatly increased by the decreased serum calcium (Bouillon et al., 1975). There may be no significant change or a reduction in the plasma phosphate concentration. Plasma folate and vitamin B_{12} concentrations are often reduced by phenytoin administration, although the exact mechanism is unknown. Plasma pyridoxal phosphate concentration is reduced by antiepileptic medications (Reinken, 1973). Urinary riboflavin excretion is reduced by phenytoin (Lewis et al., 1975), and this drug also has an immunosuppressive action in reducing the plasma concentrations of immunoglobulins IgA and IgG (Masi et al., 1976). The concentrations of other proteins such as complement C_3 are also reduced.

Antiepileptic agents often stimulate the metabolism of other drugs, thereby reducing their plasma concentrations and half-lives, and therapeutic effectiveness. They may affect drug metabolism in another way also, by displacement of other drugs from their binding sites on albumin.

1.5.3.4. Narcotic drugs

Narcotic drugs may cause spasm of the sphincter of Oddi and, presumably through pressure transmitted back to the liver, cause a release of hepatic alanine and aspartate aminotransferases so as to increase the serum activities of these enzymes. The activities of other enzymes of liver origin are also increased in serum. Amylase and lipase activities are also increased. Many drugs – not only narcotics – which are administered intramuscularly cause increased activities of enzymes of skeletal muscular origin (Greenblatt and Koch-Weser, 1976). The increases tend to be greatest when the drug is administered deeply; when a large volume is injected; when the pH of the drug is very different from the physiological pH; and when the solution that is injected is intrinsically irritating or toxic. Many narcotic drugs administered intramuscularly cause increases in serum creatine kinase, aldolase and lactate dehydrogenase activities. Narcotics may reduce the secretion of norepinephrine and vanillylmandelic acid. Steroid output is reduced through inhibition of corticotrophin and pituitary gonadotrophin release.

In both heroin addicts and methadone-treated patients, a hyperalbuminaemic, hypercatabolic state may be observed (Rothschild et al., 1976). In narcotic addicts, the concentrations of immunoglobulins IgG and IgM in serum are frequently raised. Serum thyroxine concentration is raised in about 25% of addicts. T_3-resin uptake is reduced in a similar number of addicts. Thyroxine-binding globulin capacity is increased, although the protein concentration remains within the normal range. The free thyroxine concentration remains normal (Webster et al., 1973). Many addicts show evidence of abnormal liver function, presumably due to past exposure to hepatitis. Slightly increased concentrations of triiodothyronine and thyroxine may be observed in the serum of methadone-treated addicts.

Heroin addicts have a high incidence of hyperamylasaemia, the enzyme being mainly of non-pancreatic origin (Heffernon et al., 1976). The serum concentrations of corticotrophin, cyclic AMP and cholesterol are reduced in heroin addicts. While plasma cortisol has been reported to be reduced by a single dose of morphine, this is not characteristic of heroin addicts (Ho et al., 1977).

1.5.3.5. Radiographic contrast media

Radiographic contrast agents, particularly when injected intravascularly, may cause release of enzymes from the organ into which the agent is injected. When used for aortography, radiographic contrast agents may reduce glomerular filtration rate and increase the urinary excretion of protein, casts and red cells. Other manifestations of nephrotoxicity include increased concentrations of creatinine and urea in serum. The radiographic contrast media inhibit the excretion of certain compounds such as vanillylmandelic acid and catecholamines so that their urinary excretions are reduced.

1.5.4. Alcohol ingestion

Alcohol (ethanol) may have quite different effects on the composition of the body fluids of a social drinker compared with that of an alcoholic. Even in a normal individual, the amount of alcohol, the time at which it is ingested in relation to meals, and the interval after ingestion at which fluids for analysis are obtained, may affect the data.

With a single moderate dose of ethanol, no effect is observed on the plasma concentrations of glucose or ethanol, but several hours after the ingestion of large quantities of ethanol, the plasma concentrations of urate and glucose may be increased. With ingestion of enough alcohol to produce mild inebriation, a 20 to 50% increase in the blood glucose concentration may occur. Alcohol has a diabetogenic effect and impairs tolerance to both oral and intravenous glucose. Galactose tolerance is reduced by the inhibitory effect of the increased NADH/NAD ratio in the liver on the uridine diphosphate galactose-4-epimerase reaction (Olson, 1973). Large quantities of alcohol reduce insulin secretion and cause an increase in the plasma concentrations of cortisol and 11-hydroxycorticosteroids when the plasma ethanol concentration exceeds 22 mmol/litre (100 mg/dl) (Jenkins and Connolly, 1968). The plasma growth hormone concentration is also increased (Bellet et al., 1971). Ethanol has no effect on the concentration of TSH, but causes an increase in the plasma calcitonin concentration within 15 minutes (Dymling et al., 1976). Large amounts of alcohol cause an increase in plasma renin activity, whereas small amounts have no effect (Linkola, 1975).

Following the ingestion of alcohol, there is a moderate increase in the excretions of epinephrine, norepinephrine, dopamine and metanephrine in the urine. This is associated with a marked decrease of vanillylmandelic acid in the urine but a compensatory increase of 3-methoxy-4-hydroxyphenylglycol, reflecting a shift from oxidative to reductive metabolism (Davis et al., 1967). Tryptophan metabolism is also affected, as indicated by an increased excretion of 5-hydroxytryptophol and reduced formation of 5-hydroxytryptamine (serotonin). The causes of these changes are uncertain, but they are probably associated with competitive inhibition by acetaldehyde of the conversion of 5-hydroxyindoleacetaldehyde into 5-hydroxyindoleacetic acid. The availability of hepatic NAD is important in the regulation of the oxidation of ethanol and the conversion of acetaldehyde into acetylcoenzyme A.

After a single dose of alcohol there is a prompt diuresis with increased excretion of 17-hydroxysteroids and a reduction of the plasma steroid concentration within 2 hours. The plasma concentration returns to normal after 4 hours but urinary excretion falls and remains low for 12 hours. Urinary oxogenic steroid excretion is not affected by alcohol ingestion. Alcohol ingestion may increase the urinary excretion of urate and urea nitrogen (McDonald and Margen, 1976). The plasma zinc concentration is decreased but urinary zinc excretion is increased in chronic alcoholics, either with or without cirrhosis. With abstension by the latter group of individuals, the zinc excretion reverts to normal (McCall et al., 1971).

Alcohol ingestion causes a marked increase in the concentrations of triglycerides and free fatty acids in plasma. There is increased mobilization of free fatty acids from adipose tissue. The increase in the serum concentration of triglycerides may be related both to inhibition of lipoprotein lipase and to increase in the NADH/NAD ratio which enhances the supply of fatty acids for triglyceride synthesis. If intoxication develops, the concentration of triglycerides in plasma decreases, possibly due to reduced release from the liver.

In large quantities, ethanol causes a decrease in the plasma concentrations of potassium, magnesium and phosphate. A syndrome with low osmolar concentrations in plasma and urine has been reported in beer drinkers (Hilden and Svendsen, 1975). Small quantities are sufficient to cause an increase in the serum γ-glutamyltransferase activity. The ability of alcohol to induce hepatic microsomal enzymes enhances the rate of metabolism of certain drugs such as meprobamate, phenytoin, warfarin and tolbutamide (Lieber, 1976). Serum aminotransferase activities may be increased with a comparable reduction in the hepatic enzyme activities. Freer and Statland (1977) have observed increases of 26% in creatine kinase activity 5 hours after ingestion of a single dose of ethanol, and of 18% for aspartate aminotransferase and 14% for lactate dehydrogenase after one hour. They also noted a decrease of alanine aminotransferase activity. They speculated that the increased enzyme activity is derived from skeletal muscle.

Alcohol may occasionally cause a severe and profound hypoglycaemia in previously malnourished individuals with lactic acidosis. This syndrome is associated with a low plasma insulin concentration, a metabolic acidosis and normal or low plasma pyruvate concentration. The alcoholic hypoglycaemia is associated with impaired hepatic gluconeogenesis, and enhanced formation of α-glycerophosphate from glucose (Marks, 1975).

Alcohol in the duodenum causes spasm of the sphincter of Oddi with increased secretin output occurring within a few minutes of its ingestion (Straus et al., 1975). The serum gastrin concentration is unaffected. Alcohol may reduce the absorption of vitamins.

When administered to men at a dose of 3 g/kg body mass per day, alcohol causes, within a few days, reductions in the mean plasma concentration of testosterone and its production rate. The metabolic clearance of testosterone is increased and may be associated with reduced protein binding and increased testosterone A-ring reductase activity. Ethanol has no consistent effect on plasma LH or FSH concentrations (Gordon et al., 1976).

1.5.4.1. Alcoholism

Overall there is no difference between the body composition of alcoholics and non-alcoholics. However, the alcoholic may have impaired hepatic function. Typically, the aspartate aminotransferase activity increases in serum after ingestion of alcohol. Occasionally, increased activities of alkaline phosphatase and alanine aminotransferase may occur. Ornithine carbamoyl transferase activity may also be increased in heavy drinkers.

Other conventional liver function tests are unaffected, with the exception of γ-glutamyltransferase activity which may greatly exceed the upper limit of normal: with withdrawal of alcohol the plasma enzyme activity decreases. With liver damage, secretion of triglycerides by the liver is impaired and the plasma triglyceride concentration is reduced. Serum creatine kinase activity may be increased in the serum of alcoholics; it is derived from skeletal muscle (Song and Rubin, 1972). This may be the tissue origin of other enzymes with increased plasma activities. Alcoholics tend to have reduced tissue stores of most vitamins.

The plasma phosphate concentration is often reduced in chronic alcoholism. The increase in plasma glucose concentration which is observed in non-alcoholics in response to alcohol fails to occur. Plasma cortisol has been reported to be decreased in fasted chronic alcoholics but a positive correlation between the plasma concentrations of alcohol and cortisol has also been reported and attributed to impaired metabolism of cortisol in the liver or to a pituitary-mediated response. Cortisol concentration is high in alcoholics early in the withdrawal period. The highest plasma cortisol is observed in individuals with gastrointestinal symptoms.

Alcoholics excrete large quantities of catecholamines in their urine when allowed to ingest alcohol; epinephrine excretion is most affected. Plasma sodium concentration may be increased and urinary excretion reduced in the alcoholic. Low doses of alcohol – average plasma alcohol concentration 22 mmol/litre (100 mg/dl) – have been reported to increase aldosterone secretion, but with continued ingestion over several days, aldosterone secretion was reduced although the blood ethanol continued to increase.

TABLE 1.6.

CONCENTRATION OF SERUM CONSTITUENTS IN ALCOHOLICS BEFORE AND AFTER WITHDRAWAL OF ALCOHOL

Mean concentrations of 75 male alcoholics are shown. SI Unit conversions: bilirubin, mg/litre × 1.7 = μmol/litre; cholesterol, g/litre × 2.59 = mmol/litre; creatinine, mg/litre × 8.84 = μmol/litre; phosphate, mg/litre × 0.32 = mmol/litre; uric acid, mg/litre × 0.006 = mmol/litre. (Data reproduced, by permission, from Gellens, H.K., Gottheil, E., Arayata, L. and Alterman, A.I. (1976) British Journal of Addiction, 71, 103–108)

Constituent	Normal range	Before	After
Albumin (g/litre)	35–50	42	43
Alkaline Phosphatase (U/litre)	30–85	67	54
Aspartate Aminotransferase (U/litre)	10–50	59	38
Bilirubin, Total (mg/litre)	1.5–10	6.5	5.4
Calcium (mmol/litre)	2.1–2.6	2.5	2.4
Cholesterol (g/litre)	1.5–3.0	2.1	2.2
Creatinine (mg/litre)	0–10	11	10
Lactate Dehydrogenase (U/litre)	80–200	178	150
Inorganic Phosphate (mg/litre)	25–45	36	39
Protein, Total (g/litre)	60–80	72	70
Uric Acid (mg/litre)	25–80	59	61

In alcoholic cirrhotic men, the plasma concentration, production rate and metabolic clearance of testosterone are reduced, but testosterone binding to proteins is increased. Androstenedione production rate and plasma concentration are increased. A higher production rate and plasma concentration of oestradiol is observed. The plasma concentration of oestrone is increased but that of the gonadotrophins is variable (Gordon et al., 1976). A 2-fold increase in plasma prolactin concentration may be observed in chronic alcoholics (Van Thiel et al., 1975).

With withdrawal of alcohol, serum γ-glutamyltransferase activity decreases. The activities of other enzymes revert to normal even more rapidly. Hypomagnesaemia is very common in alcoholics. Respiratory alkalosis may be caused by hyperventilation. Blood pH, which is unaffected by drinking, has been reported to increase within eight hours of alcohol withdrawal. This was associated with a fall in the plasma bicarbonate concentration. It has been claimed that the α-amino-n-butyrate/leucine ratio is higher in the plasma of alcoholics than in other individuals (Shaw et al., 1976). Both acute alcohol intoxication and chronic alcohol administration lead to increased formiminoglutamate excretion (Rosenauerová-Ostrá et al., 1976). The effect of withdrawal of alcohol from alcoholics is illustrated in Table 1.6.

The concentration of homovanillic acid in spinal fluid is decreased in alcoholics (Roos and Silfverskiöld, 1973).

1.6. GENERAL PHYSIOLOGICAL RESPONSES

There are several syndromes that are characteristic of disease states in general. These syndromes persist regardless of the specific disease, but may be modified by features characteristic of a particular disease. Indeed, the features associated with a specific disease may predominate.

1.6.1. Fever

The biochemical reaction to fever is a general response on which effects of specific diseases may be superimposed. Much of our knowledge of the metabolic response to infection is due to the experimental studies of Beisel and his colleagues on the induction of fever in healthy individuals (1967, 1975).

The early response to fever causes a slight hyperglycaemia with impaired glucose tolerance (Rayfield et al., 1973); hypoglycaemia may occur later. Although the concentration of glucose is increased initially, that of insulin is also increased. The anticipated decrease of glucose due to increased insulin secretion is negated by the slightly increased secretion of both glucagon and growth hormone. Growth hormone secretion is increased within one hour of induction of an artificial fever (Baylis et al., 1968). The augmented hormonal secretion activates adenylate cyclase which increases the formation of cyclic AMP. Glycogenolysis occurs, with a negative nitrogen balance that is mainly due to the wastage of skeletal muscle, but also arises from the decreased intake of food, and increased urinary and sweat losses as well. Faecal excretion of nitrogen is unaffected. The urinary excretion of creatinine varies in parallel with the extent of the fever. The excretions of urea,

α-amino nitrogen and ammonium ions peak 1 or 2 days after the fever reaches its maximum. The excretion of urate may also be augmented by an infection or fever with the resulting considerable tissue catabolism. Vitamin metabolism is little affected by fever. Only the excretion of riboflavin is enhanced, and this may be correlated with the negative nitrogen balance (Beisel et al., 1972).

Fever generally causes a slight increase in plasma volume (Bass and Henschel, 1956) and there is also an increase in the concentrations of uric acid, creatinine, and non-protein nitrogen in serum. Increased bromosulphthalein retention may occur as result of increased reflux of the dye from liver to plasma. Fever also causes increased synthesis of protein in the liver. Activities of hepatic tyrosine aminotransferase (EC 2.6.1.5) and tryptophan oxygenase (EC 1.13.11.11) are increased. The production of acute phase reactants and glycoproteins in the liver is accelerated, and this is manifested by increased quantities of haptoglobin, α_1-antitrypsin, C-reactive protein, fibrinogen, caeruloplasmin and orosomucoid and an increase in the γ-globulin fraction in plasma. While a transient increase in C-reactive protein concentration is normally observed after an operation, the increase is sustained if infection occurs (Fischer et al., 1976). Increased protein turnover, mainly from skeletal muscle, results in an increase in the concentration of phenylalanine in the plasma but a decrease in the concentrations of all other amino acids. An increased plasma phenylalanine/tyrosine ratio is characteristic of most fevers (Wannemacher et al., 1976). Changes in amino acid concentration may occur before clinical changes are apparent. Hyperamino-acidaemia may occur before fever becomes apparent, but with its onset the plasma concentration decreases, with an increased liver uptake of the amino acids. Increased urinary excretion occurs and the negative nitrogen balance may persist well into the recovery period.

There is a marked adrenal response to infection. In response to increased corticotrophin secretion, the plasma cortisol concentration increases to a value slightly greater than the usual morning peak concentration. The normal circadian variation, with its progressive fall throughout the day, may be lost so that the plasma cortisol concentration in the afternoon or evening is very high in comparison with the usual state. Hyperthermia also increases the urinary excretion of free cortisol, 17-hydroxycorticosteroids and 17-oxosteroids. Pregnanetriol secretion is also enhanced. These hormonal responses are all mediated through the anterior pituitary via corticotrophin. As recovery occurs, the hormonal secretion reverts to normal. This may even happen when the fever changes from an acute to a subacute or chronic state.

With the onset of infection the secretion of thyroxine may be reduced, possibly due to increased secretion of glucocorticoids. Thyroxine bound to prealbumin is frequently decreased, but the free thyroxine concentration is increased. Triiodothyronine turnover is increased by fever (Gregerman and Solomon, 1967). The concentration of reverse T_3 (3,3′,5′-triiodothyronine) is increased with less peripheral conversion of thyroxine into triiodothyronine. The concentration of active thyroid hormones is reduced in acute illnesses even without fever (Burger, 1976).

Increased metabolism of lipids occurs with infection, so that the serum concentrations of cholesterol, non-esterified fatty acids and other lipids may decrease. Within a few days, the plasma free fatty acid concentration may greatly increase above normal (Rayfield et al., 1973). With an individual's recovery from infection, the lipid concentration returns to normal. The lipid response occurs regardless of dietary intake and is associated to a greater extent with the infection itself than with fever. Lipid concentrations have been shown to vary inversely with the white cell count.

The plasma phosphate concentration commonly decreases with fever due to the respiratory alkalosis that often occurs (Beisel et al., 1968). Urinary phosphate excretion increases, as does that of magnesium and potassium. Increased losses of these ions occur in sweat also. Initially, there is also a loss of sodium and chloride, but this falls off rapidly and the subsequently decreased excretion may persist for several days following recovery from an infection due to the increased secretion of aldosterone. Plasma iron and zinc concentrations fall during infections, whereas the copper concentration rises. Pekarek and Beisel (1971) have attributed the effects on iron and zinc to the release of a hormone-like protein that transfers these elements from the plasma to the liver. The apparently anomalous response of copper is due to the increased concentration of caeruloplasmin. The percentage of saturation of transferrin by iron is decreased by fever, but the serum ferritin concentration rises rapidly and is sustained for several days even when a single injection of aetiocholanolone is used to produce an artificial fever (Elin et al., 1977).

1.6.2. Shock and trauma

The physiological and biochemical response to trauma is a combination of the responses to the precipitating cause and to the general stress. The extent of response is largely governed by the extent of tissue damage and the state of health of the individual at the time of the injury.

Increased secretion of corticotrophin occurs immediately following an injury. This, in turn, leads to increased secretion of cortisol, causing a 3- to 5-fold increase in the plasma concentration. Impaired liver metabolism and delayed removal from the circulation may contribute to the increased plasma concentration (Johnston, 1972). Anaesthesia and surgery decrease binding of cortisol to albumin but do not affect transcortin binding. The urinary excretion of 17-hydroxycorticosteroids may be increased by up to 6 times over the 4 days following a severe injury, but the output of 17-oxosteroids and metabolites of adrenal androgens is barely affected or actually reduced. Aldosterone secretion is increased in response to the increase in corticotrophin and to stimulation of the renin–angiotensin system. Plasma renin activity may be greatly increased following operations, burns or blood loss. The increased plasma renin and angiotensin II may persist for many days. The liberation of 5-hydroxytryptamine that occurs following injury may also stimulate aldosterone secretion. The decreased plasma volume and increased concentration of electrolytes following an injury are suggestive of increased secretion of vasopressin. Plasma vasopressin concentration is frequently increased following surgery. Growth hormone, glucagon and insulin secretions are also increased. Trauma decreases the secretion of gonadotrophic and gonadal hormones in both sexes.

Trauma, such as surgery, has been shown to affect catecholamine metabolism, and increased quantities of metanephrine, normetanephrine, *N*-methylmetanephrine and 3-methoxytyramine are excreted in the urine. These changes probably reflect increased secretion of epinephrine and increased activity of the sympathetic nervous system. While the urinary excretions of norepinephrine and epinephrine are increased after surgery, their plasma concentrations are not necessarily affected by trauma. Some of the changes may be attributable to the anaesthesia rather than to the surgery.

Within the first 24 hours following an injury, the blood vessels become more permeable in the general area of the injury. This may lead to a decreased blood volume and even impairment of the circulation. If the circulation is affected, glomerular filtration decreases and, in its most severe form, acute renal failure ensues. Diminished renal function leads to an increase in the plasma concentration of urea and other end-products of nitrogen metabolism. The circulatory impairment may also affect deamination of aminoacids so that the plasma concentrations of both essential and non-essential aminoacids may increase. More usually, immediately following an injury there may be an actual decrease in the plasma concentration with an increased excretion of both aminoacids and peptides. The plasma concentrations of urea cycle aminoacids usually decrease progressively with severity of shock (Feigin, 1969). A negative nitrogen balance may persist for some time following an injury.

The general metabolic response to trauma causes mobilization of free fatty acids and, to a lesser extent, of cholesterol, neutral fat and phospholipids. The triglyceride concentration is often unaffected. Invariably the plasma glucose concentration increases following a severe injury and the change is inversely related to the change in the plasma aminoacid concentration. Aerobic metabolism of glucose is affected to a greater extent than anaerobic metabolism. The tricarboxylic acid cycle is also affected by injury, and liver tissue contains reduced quantities of citrate, glutamate and aspartate but an increased quantity of pyruvate. Glycogenolysis and glycolysis are increased in proportion to the degree of injury. Glucose tolerance is reduced by trauma. The plasma insulin does not increase in response to the hyperglycaemia of trauma (Stoner and Heath, 1973).

The plasma sodium concentration is considerably reduced after extensive burns. In previously well-nourished individuals there may be no change, or a slight decrease, in the urinary excretion of sodium. With tissue catabolism there are increased excretions of nitrogen, sulphate, phosphate, magnesium, zinc and creatine; the loss of potassium is greater than can be accounted for by the damaged tissue alone. The plasma potassium concentration also increases. Urinary calcium excretion is affected in the same manner as the excretion of sodium. The increased tissue catabolism creates a demand for increased oxygen consumption and also leads to the production of acid metabolites. If tissue anoxia arises, and respiratory and renal function are also impaired, metabolic acidosis ensues.

Total body protein may decrease by as much as 12% within 10 days of severe physical injury (Cuthbertson, 1964). Any major injury may cause the plasma albumin concentration to decrease, often by as much as 8 g/litre. The largest decreases occur in burned patients, and the turnover of protein is also greatest in these individuals. Albumin is lost through the damaged tissue, and its peak loss occurs simultaneously with the maximum loss of nitrogen. The concentrations of both α_1- and α_2-globulins increase following surgery. The concentrations of caeruloplasmin and many other proteins are similarly affected. Diminished activity of testosterone, manifested by a decreased plasma concentration, may contribute to the protein catabolism following an injury. While its concentration remains increased for 2 weeks, that of haptoglobin peaks in 4 days and is increased for only 1 week. An α_2-glycoprotein, not normally detectable in plasma, becomes detectable within 18 hours of injury and remains measurable for over a week.

The concentration of transferrin in plasma decreases after surgery, generally varying with the albumin concentration. Following haemorrhage, plasma transferrin concentration increases for 10 to 20 days.

γ-Globulin concentration increases after burn injuries and may also increase following surgery. Plasma fibrinogen concentration may double two to eight days after surgery. The concentrations of mucoproteins and protein-bound carbohydrates rise with stress. Plasma protein changes are generally attributable to increased synthesis for those constituents whose concentrations are increased, and augmented catabolism for those whose concentration is decreased. Both catabolism and anabolism of protein are increased following injury.

The increased adrenal activity that occurs with an injury is associated with increased gastric acidity and pepsin secretion, as well as with increased urinary uropepsin (Cuthbertson and Tilstone, 1969).

1.6.3. Stress

There is a single biochemical response to stress, which may be modified according to the precipitating cause. Despite the many different precipitating causes of a stress reaction, which may include exercise, thermal responses – both to heat and cold – trauma, surgery, electroconvulsive therapy or mental stress such as pain, fear or anxiety, the reaction is hormonally mediated and similar in character from one situation to another.

It is presumed that the stress reaction is centrally mediated through the hypothalamus or pituitary gland, which in turn acts on the adrenal and other glands. The plasma corticotrophin concentration is increased up to ten times the normal value during the immediate stress of surgery and remains elevated for several hours; it does not fall to normal values for 24 hours. Both psychological stress and tissue necrosis produce similar effects. Stress influences can overrule control of corticotrophin secretion by diurnal rhythm and feedback control. Cortisol secretion increases in response to the outpouring of corticotrophin and reaches its maximum at the height of the stress. Even in the absence of an acute stress situation, individuals subjected to repeated stresses show higher plasma concentrations of 17-hydroxycorticosteroids. The urinary excretions of these steroids and of 17-oxo- and 17-oxogenic-steroids are increased. Aldosterone secretion is increased at the same time.

The secretion of TSH is decreased in many forms of stress but has also been reported to be unaffected by surgery. Thyroxine turnover is often reduced immediately after a stress but in general there is an increased turnover of thyroxine and triiodothyronine with increased free thyroxine in plasma. The plasma triiodothyronine falls continually for 24 hours after stress such as surgery (Brandt et al., 1976), and an acute rise in the concentration of reverse T_3 occurs.

Plasma growth hormone concentration is increased by physical stress, and may also be increased by psychic stress. The release of the hormone closely parallels the increased secretion of corticotrophin. Schalch (1967) has calculated that as much as 20% of the typical daily output of growth hormone may be released in response to a single stress situation.

The effect of stress on the adrenal medulla may be quite marked. Thus, there is increased secretion of epinephrine, norepinephrine and their metabolites, 3-methyl-4-hydroxy-phenylglycol and vanillylmandelic acid, with the increase of epinephrine occurring earliest. The normal circadian rhythm of these compounds is abolished by stress. Apprehension increases renin release (Romero and Hoobler, 1970). Plasma dopamine-β-hydroxylase activity is not consistently affected by stress (Goodwin et al., 1975). While mobilization of lipids and an increased concentration of glucose usually follow increased adrenal medullary activity, these responses are not necessarily apparent if exercise has provoked the stress reaction, as these compounds are used as metabolic fuels. The plasma phosphate concentration falls immediately after surgery. The free fatty acid concentration is usually increased by most forms of stress. The response is rapid, rising by as much as 0.13 mmol/litre within 5 minutes (Cardon and Gordon, 1959). This is probably related to an increased rate of release of the non-esterified fatty acids from adipose tissue. The plasma glucagon is often increased by stress and this, more than increased catecholamine secretion, may be responsible for the increased concentration of free fatty acids in plasma because of its greater lipolytic activity than that of the catecholamines. The increased epinephrine secretion may be responsible for the reduction of plasma insulin concentration. In spite of the reduced plasma insulin concentration the blood glucose concentration may also be reduced by emotional stress. Serum hexosamine concentration is increased by stress (Boas et al., 1955). The plasma zinc concentration decreases rapidly in response to an acute stress, whereas the copper and nickel concentrations increase (Reinhold, 1975).

Stress causes a reduction in the plasma concentrations of testosterone and luteinizing hormone. Prolactin secretion is stimulated. Gastric hydrochloric acid and pepsin secretions are stimulated, with an increase in the urinary uropepsin as a result (Gray et al., 1953).

The stress of examinations has been shown to increase the serum cholesterol concentration by as much as 1.8 mmol/litre (70 mg/dl) in healthy students. The same stress has caused a reduction in the plasma glucose concentration. Similar effects have been observed in professional individuals in response to stressful work situations, with a rapid reversal when the provocative situation is removed.

With both cold-water stress and heat stress associated with physical exercise, urinary urate is increased in relation to the creatinine excretion. Other studies have demonstrated an increased serum urate concentration in individuals faced with a stimulating challenge, but a fall in the urate concentration during periods of anxiety. The acute heat stress of a sauna causes increases in the plasma renin activity, and in angiotensin II and aldosterone concentrations (Kosunen et al., 1976). With hypothermia there are usually increased plasma activities of creatine kinase, hydroxybutyrate dehydrogenase and aspartate aminotransferase (Maclean et al., 1974). These changes are probably related to alterations of the acid–base status.

Urinary ascorbic acid excretion is increased following stress situations, presumably indicating reduction of adrenal reserves. Urinary vasopressin excretion may be markedly increased by different types of stress. The urinary excretion of amino acids may also be increased.

Casey (1973) has demonstrated a significant correlation between states of anxiety or neurosis and the concentrations of albumin and urea. Serum albumin is increased whereas urea is decreased. The cause of these changes is unknown. Plasma fibrinogen concentration is also increased by anxiety and stress.

In contrast to the increase that occurs with stress, the plasma cortisol concentration is significantly reduced by transcendental meditation, although it is not affected by relaxation in normal healthy adults. The plasma prolactin concentration is similarly affected. Unusually low production of cortisol and 17-hydroxycorticoid excretion is observed with hypnosis (Sachar et al., 1966).

1.6.4. Pain

Pain is characterized by the typical biochemical features of the stress response. These include increased secretion and urinary excretion of vasopressin which causes a reduced output of urine. Catecholamine secretion is increased, but the plasma glucose concentration is reduced. If the pain is severe, the basal metabolic rate is increased.

1.6.5. Transfusion

Immediately following an injury, there is dilution of the blood with protein-poor fluid which is subsequently replaced with a fluid similar in composition to plasma. Replacement of lost blood by plasma or whole blood may increase the plasma protein concentration by up to 5 g/litre. The nitrogen released by the breakdown of red cells is not excreted but is re-used by the body. With adequate replacement of lost blood, the usual retention of sodium, chloride and water is reduced. Nitrogen excretion is also reduced in transfused individuals compared with untransfused injured people. Serum iron and iron-binding capacity (transferrin) are reduced following major trauma, but extensive blood transfusion can lead to siderosis with an increased serum iron concentration.

Infusion of saline solutions of glucose causes a reduction of the plasma phosphate which may be severe enough to reduce the red cell glycolytic rate (Guillou et al., 1976).

1.7. IN VITRO EFFECTS

Regardless of the nature of the disease from which a patient may be suffering, the concentrations of constituents in body fluids may be modified by factors outside the patient, so that the measured concentrations are not representative of the in vivo situation. In spite of careful in vivo control of the patient, in vitro factors outside the patient can invalidate the results obtained in the clinical laboratory. Lack of knowledge of the in vitro factors affecting the specimen can lead to misinterpretations of data and inappropriate clinical action.

1.7.1. Lipaemia

Lipaemia affects analytical methods for most constituents which are measured in plasma or serum unless a serum blank is included with each test. As well as colorimetric measurements, light-scattering and kinetic techniques may be affected.

1.7.2. Haemolysis

Haemolysis is, in effect, the leakage of components from red cells into the plasma. Thus measurements of those constituents that are present in large amounts in erythrocytes will be affected most by haemolysis. The most sensitive measure of haemolysis is the plasma haemoglobin concentration. Other constituents that are readily affected are the plasma lactate dehydrogenase activity and potassium concentration. Unless a specific substrate for the prostatic component is used, serum acid phosphatase activity is increased by haemolysis. Serum arginase activity and creatine concentration are markedly affected even by slight haemolysis because of the large gradient between cells and plasma. Slightly increased concentrations of magnesium, phosphate and protein may be observed. Alanine and aspartate aminotransferase activities are only slightly increased by haemolysis. Aldolase, isocitrate dehydrogenase and argininosuccinate lyase (EC 4.3.2.1) activities are also affected. Haemolysis may cause a reduction in the apparent albumin and bilirubin concentrations, and in lipase activity, due to interference with the analytical procedures. The background absorbance of haemoglobin may cause inaccurate results with many procedures unless appropriate corrections are made.

Constituents of haemolyzed erythrocytes can degrade insulin so that non-haemolyzed specimens are required for this assay.

1.7.3. Icterus

Icterus is due to an increased concentration of bilirubin in plasma. This causes problems in determining accurately the concentrations of various constituents by increasing the background absorbance in the yellow region of the spectrum. Bilirubin may also affect other determinations because its binding to albumin may reduce the number of available binding sites for coloured dyes, thereby decreasing the apparent concentration of the protein.

1.7.4. Anticoagulants and preservatives

If allowance is made for the increased volume of specimen occupied by the fibrinogen from plasma, very few tests are influenced by the choice of plasma over serum. Serum is generally preferred in most laboratories (especially when narrow-bore tubing is used in mechanized analyzers) because of potential problems from accumulation of fibrin, but plasma could equally well be used. However, plasma is preferable for electrolyte determinations because of the possible release of potassium from cells during the clotting process. Even in healthy individuals, serum potassium is about 0.2 mmol/litre higher than plasma potassium. In individuals who have abnormal blood cells, as, for example, in leukaemia, the serum potassium may be as much as 1.6 mmol/litre higher than the plasma values. Those constituents that are present in large amounts in the cells also tend to leak out, so that higher activities of enzymes such as acid phosphatase and lactate dehydrogenase are observed in serum than plasma even in healthy individuals. The plasma amino nitrogen concentration may be as much as 40% less than the serum concentration. The absence of fibrinogen in serum means that a serum total protein value will be less than the plasma value by the amount of fibrinogen. However, the concentration of calcium is higher in plasma than serum (Lester and Varghese, 1977).

Antiglycolytic agents are required to ensure that the concentration of glucose remains constant in blood specimens. Fluoride, by inhibiting glycolysis by cells in whole blood, effectively maintains the glucose concentration constant. However, by doing this, it affects the integrity of the cell membranes so that intracellular constituents leak out with accompanying haemolysis. Thus, specimens to which fluoride are added cannot be used for other determinations. The presence of added fluoride may also inhibit some reagent enzymes, such as urease, which are used in the measurement of constituents of body fluids.

Preservatives must be added to urine to ensure that the concentration of many constituents is maintained. Alterations are likely to occur from bacterial metabolism of carbohydrate or protein, but certain other constituents, for example urate and calcium in the form of phosphate salts, may be precipitated out of solution by inappropriate pH.

1.7.5. Handling of blood

Certain constituents of plasma are sufficiently unstable or reactive that specimens of whole blood must be handled specially to prevent changes in their concentrations. Such constituents are plasma glucose, gastrin and renin activities, vitamin D, pyruvate, ammonia and blood pH and pCO_2. All laboratories should have developed a standard code of practice for handling specimens for these determinations, so that maximum stability of the test constituents is assured.

In all institutions, delay between collection of a specimen and its transport to the laboratory should be kept to a minimum to avoid deterioration. In some institutions, pneumatic tube systems have been used to ensure rapid delivery of specimens but unless the blood tubes are carefully wrapped, and are filled with blood, haemolysis may result due to the agitation of the specimen.

Care must be taken to ensure that the specimens are not contaminated by the container. Cork stoppers may contain calcium, and siliconized stoppers cadmium, so that the tests for these elements may be invalidated. The stoppers of evacuated blood tubes may also affect the accurate measurement of some therapeutic drugs, e.g. meperidine, propranolol and quinidine (Cotham and Shand, 1976).

1.7.6. Storage of specimens

Stability of constituents also determines the procedure that should be used for storage of the separated plasma or serum specimens prior to analysis. Thus, most constituents are more stable when stored at –20°C than in a 4°C refrigerator or at ambient temperature. Yet for some, e.g. lactate dehydrogenase, the activity is greater when the specimen has been stored at ambient temperature rather than in a refrigerator or freezer. Amino-acid concentrations fall unless the specimens are stored at –80°C. While long-term storage of serum specimens at –20°C has no effect on their calcium concentration, calcium concentrations in plasma show a progressive decline (Lester and Varghese, 1977). At –5°C, prorenin is gradually converted into renin at the normal blood pH, although this does not occur at –20°C or at pH 5.0 at –5°C (Sealey et al., 1976).

1.8. ANALYTICAL METHODOLOGY

The analytical methods in use in the clinical laboratory are the final determinants of the concentrations of constituents in body fluids. The analytical method must be considered in conjunction with the equipment and reagents used for the analysis, the standards for calibrating the system and the means of calculation. The laboratory must pay considerable attention to all these facets of the analytical determination to ensure that the results are optimal. The method that is used should be specific and sensitive, as well as simple and cheap, so that if necessary many results can be produced each day. The method should be sufficiently accurate and precise that the analytical variability is always very small compared with the biological variability. This should be assured even when different drugs that might affect the method through lack of specificity are administered to the patient, or when the patient is studied under standardized conditions that might minimize biological variability. Inappropriate analytical methods may well mask the precision of physiological regulation of the concentrations of blood constituents.

Ultimately all analytical methods should be capable of reference back to procedures that have been validated against definitive analytical methods such as isotope dilution–mass spectrometry. Only by this approach will it be possible to ensure that a method used in one centre is comparable with those used elsewhere, so that the analytical data are truly interchangeable.

REFERENCES

Acharya, P.T. and Payne, W.W. (1965) Blood chemistry of normal full-term infants in the first 48 hours of life. Archives of Disease in Childhood, 40, 430–435.

Adibi, S.A. and Drash, A.L. (1970) Hormone and amino acid levels in altered nutritional states. Journal of Laboratory and Clinical Metabolism, 76, 772–732.

Adlercreutz, H. and Dessypris, A. (1974) Effect of exertion on hormone secretion. British Medical Journal, 2, 726.

Ahmed, F., Bamji, M.S. and Iyengar, L. (1975) Effect of oral contraceptive agents on vitamin nutrition status. American Journal of Clinical Nutrition, 28, 606–615.

Amador, E., Massod, M.F. and Franey, R.J. (1967) Characterization of the normal serum glutamic-oxaloacetic transaminase activity of healthy adults. American Journal of Clinical Pathology, 47, 3–8.

Anderson, K.E., Bodansky, O. and Kappas, A. (1976) Effects of oral contraceptives on vitamin metabolism. Advances in Clinical Chemistry, 18, 247–287.

Antonis, A. and Bersohn, I. (1962) The influence of diet on serum lipids in South African white and Bantu prisoners. American Journal of Clinical Nutrition, 10, 484–499.

Archer, J.A., Gordon, P. and Roth, J. (1975) Defect in insulin binding to receptors in obese man. Journal of Clinical Investigation, 55, 166–174.

Armstrong, B.K., Davis, R.E., Nicol, D.J., van Merwyk, A.J. and Larwood, C.J. (1974) Hematological, vitamin B_{12}, and folate studies on Seventh-day Adventist vegetarians. American Journal of Clinical Nutrition, 27, 712–718.

Armstrong, M.D. and Stave, U. (1973) A study of plasma free amino acid levels. III. Variations during growth and aging. Metabolism: Clinical and Experimental, 22, 571–578.

Armstrong, M.D. and Yates, K.N. (1964) Amino acid excretion during pregnancy. American Journal of Obstetrics and Gynecology, 88, 381–390.

Aschoff, J. (1976) Circadian systems in man and their implications. Hospital Practice, 11, 51–57.

Astrand, P.-O. (1967) Diet and athletic performance. Federation Proceedings, 26, 1772–1777.

Avogaro, P., Capri, C., Pais, M. and Cazzolato, G. (1973) Plasma and urine cortisol behavior and fat mobilization in man after coffee ingestion. Israel Journal of Medical Sciences, 9, 114–119.

Avruskin, T.W., Mitsuma, T., Shenkman, L., Sau, K. and Hollander, C.S. (1976) Measurement of free and total serum T_3 and T_4 in pregnant subjects and in neonates. American Journal of Medical Sciences, 271, 309–315.

Bagdade, J.D., Bierman, E.L. and Porte, D., Jr., (1967) The significance of basal insulin levels in the evaluation of the insulin response to glucose in diabetic and nondiabetic subjects. Journal of Clinical Investigation, 46, 1549–1557.

Balsam, A. and Leppo, L.E. (1975) Effect of physical training on the metabolism of thyroid hormones in man. Journal of Applied Physiology, 38, 212–215.

Banerjee, B. and Saha, N. (1969) Interrelation of serum cholesterols, ABO-Rh blood groups and body fat. Medical Journal of Malaysia, 24, 41–44.

Barrett, P.V.D. (1971) Hyperbilirubinemia of fasting. Journal of the American Medical Association, 217, 1349–1353.

Bass, D.E. and Henschel, A. (1956) Responses of body fluid compartments to heat and cold. Physiological Reviews, 36, 128–144.

Batt, A.M., Siest, G., Loppinet, V., Guerin, P., Gueguen, R. and Floch, A.Y. (1974) Médicaments et valeurs de référence en biologie. 1. Contraceptifs oraux. Annales de Biologie Clinique, 32, 245–256.

Baylis, E.M., Greenwood, F., James, V., Jenkins, J., Landon, J., Marks, V. and Samols, E. (1968) An examination of the control mechanisms postulated to control growth hormone secretion in man. In Growth Hormone International Congress Series No. 158 (Eds. A. Pecile and E.E. Muller) Excerpta Medica, Amsterdam.

Beazley, J.M. and Tindall, V.R. (1966) Changes in liver function during multiple pregnancy – using a modified bromsulphthalein test. Journal of Obstetrics and Gynaecology. British Commonwealth, 73, 658–661.

Beisel, W.R. (1975) Metabolic response to infection. Annual Review of Medicine, 26, 9–20.

Beisel, W.R., Goldman, R.F. and Joy, R.J.T. (1968) Metabolic balance studies during induced hyperthermia in man. Journal of Applied Physiology, 24, 1–10.

Beisel, W.R., Herman, Y.F., Sauberlich, H.E., Herman, R.H., Bartelloni, P.J. and Canham, J.E. (1972) Experimentally induced sandfly fever and vitamin metabolism in man. American Journal of Clinical Nutrition, 25, 1165–1173.

Beisel, W.R., Sawyer, W.D., Ryll, E.D. and Crozier, D. (1967) Metabolic effects of intracellular infections in man. Annals of Internal Medicine, 67, 744–779.

Bellet, S., Roman, L., De Castro, O., Kim, K.E. and Kershbaum, A. (1969a) Effect of coffee ingestion on catecholamine release. Metabolism: Clinical and Experimental, 18, 288–291.

Bellet, S., Roman, L. and Kostus, J. (1969b) The effect of automobile driving on catecholamine and adrenocortical excretion. American Journal of Cardiology, 24, 365–368.

Bellet, S., Yoshimine, N., De Castro, O.A.P., Roman, L., Parmar, S.S. and Sandberg, S. (1971) Effects of alcohol ingestion on growth hormone levels: their relation to 11-hydroxycorticoid levels and serum FFA. Metabolism: Clinical and Experimental, 20, 762–769.

Benedek, T.G. and Sunder, J.H. (1970) Comparisons of serum lipid and uric acid content in white and Negro men. American Journal of Medical Science, 260, 331–340.

Bennion, L.J. and Grundy, S.M. (1975) Effects of obesity and caloric intake on biliary lipid metabolism in man, Journal of Clinical Investigation, 56, 996–1011.

Benson, G.I., George, W.H.S., Litchfield, M.H. and Seaborn, D.J. (1976) Biochemical changes during the initial stages of industrial lead exposure. British Journal of Industrial Medicine, 33, 29–35.

Berg, K., Hames, C., Dahlen, G., Frick, M.H. and Krishan, I. (1976) Genetic lipoprotein variation and lipid levels in man. Clinical Genetics, 10, 97–103.

Bierenbaum, M.L., Fleischman, A.I., Dunn, J.P., Hayton, T., Pattison, D.C. and Watson, P.B. (1973) Serum parameters in hard and soft-water communities. American Journal of Public Health, 63, 169–173.

Bishop, C. and Talbot, J.H. (1953) Uric acid: its role in biological processes and the influence upon it of physiological, pathological, and pharmacological agents. Pharmacological Reviews, 5, 231–273.

Biss, K., Ho, K.-J., Mikkelson, B., Lewis, L. and Taylor, C.B. (1971) Some unique biologic characteristics of the Masai of East Africa. New England Journal of Medicine, 284, 694–699.

Boas, N.F., Bollet, A.J. and Bunim, J.J. (1955) Effect of acute clinical stress on the levels of hexosamine in serum and its excretion in urine. Journal of Clinical Investigation, 34, 782–789.

Bodenheimer, S., Winter, J.S.D. and Faiman, C. (1973) Diurnal rhythms of serum gonadotropins, testosterone, estradiol and cortisol in blind men. Journal of Clinical Endocrinology and Metabolism, 37, 472–475.

Bonen, A. (1976) Effects of exercise on excretion rates of urinary free cortisol. Journal of Applied Physiology, 40, 155–158.

Böning, D., Meier, U., Schweigart, U. and Kunze, M. (1975) Diurnal changes of the 2,3-diphosphoglycerate concentration in human red cells and the influence of posture. European Journal of Applied Physiology, 34, 11–17.

Bork, K., Korting, G.W. and Faust, G. (1972) The increase of some serum enzyme levels (GOT, LDH, CPK, MK) after body massage and its significance in dermatomyositis. Klinische Wochenschrift, 50, 332–333.

Bosco, J.S., Greenleaf, J.E., Kaye, R.L. and Averkin, E.G. (1970) Reduction of serum uric acid in young men during physical training. American Journal of Cardiology, 25, 46–52.

Bouillon, R., Reynaert, J., Claes, J.H., Lissens, W. and De Moor, P. (1975) The effect of anticonvulsant therapy on serum levels of 25-hydroxyvitamin D, calcium and parathyroid hormone. Journal of Clinical Endocrinology and Metabolism, 41, 1130–1135.

Boyle, E. Jr., Morales, I.B., Nichaman, M.Z., Talbert, C.R. Jr. and Watkins, R.S. (1968) Serum beta lipoproteins and cholesterol in adult men. Geriatrics, 23, 102–111.

Brandt, M.R., Kehlet, H., Skovsted, L. and Hansen, J.M. (1976) Rapid decrease in plasma-triiodothyronine during surgery and epidural analgesia independent of afferent neurogenic stimuli and of cortisol. Lancet, II, 1333–1336.

Bray, G.A., Davidson, M.B. and Drenick, E.J. (1972) Obesity: a serious symptom. Annals of Internal Medicine, 77, 779–795.

Bray, G.A., Fisher, D.A. and Chopra, I.J. (1976) Relation of thyroid hormones to body-weight. Lancet, I, 1206–1208.

Briggs, M. (1976) Biochemical effects of oral contraceptives. Advances in Steroid Biochemistry and Pharmacology, 5, 65–160.

Briggs, M.H., Garcia-Webb, P. and Cheung, T. (1973) Androgens and exercise. British Medical Journal, 3, 49–50.

Brodan, V., Kuhn, E., Pechar, J. and Tomkova, D. (1976) Changes of free amino acids in plasma of healthy subjects induced by physical exercise. European Journal of Applied Physiology, 35, 69–77.

Brohult, J. (1969) Effects of high protein and low protein diets on ornithine carbamoyl transferase activity in human serum (S-OCT). Acta Medica Scandinavica, 185, 357–362.

Bronte-Stewart, B., Antonis, A., Rose-Innes, C. and Moodie, A.D. (1961) An interracial study on the serum protein pattern of adult men in Southern Africa. American Journal of Clinical Nutrition, 9, 596–605.

Buckley, C.E. and Dorsey, F.C. (1971) Serum immunoglobulin levels throughout the life-span of healthy men. Annals of Internal Medicine, 75, 673–682.

Burger, A. (1976) Reduced active thyroid-hormone levels in acute illness. Lancet, II, 97.

Burt, R.L., Leake, N.H. and Dannenburg, N.N. (1963) Effect of synthetic oxytocin on plasma nonesterified fatty acids, triglycerides and blood glucose. Obstetrics and Gynecology, 21, 708–712.

Butenandt, O., Eder, R., Wohlfarth, K., Bidlingmaier, F. and Knorr, D. (1976) Mean 24-hour growth hormone and testosterone concentrations in relation to pubertal growth spurt in boys with normal or delayed puberty. European Journal of Pediatrics, 122, 85–92.

Cacciari, E., Cicognani, A., Pirazoli, P., Dallacasa, P., Mazzaracchio, M.A., Tassoni, P., Bernardi, F., Salardi, S. and Zappulla, F. (1976) GH, ACTH, LH and FSH behaviour in the first seven days of life. Acta Paediatrica Scandinavica, 65, 337–341.

Cahill, G.F. Jr. (1976) Starvation in man. New England Journal of Medicine, 282, 668–675.

Cardon, P.V. Jr. and Gordon, R.S. Jr. (1959) Rapid increase of plasma unesterified fatty acids in man during fear. Journal of Psychosomatic Research, 4, 5–9.

Carlsten, A., Hallgren, B., Jagenburg, R., Svanborg, A. and Werkö, L. (1962) Arterial concentrations of free fatty acids and free amino acids in healthy human individuals at rest and at different work loads. Scandinavian Journal of Clinical and Laboratory Investigation, 14, 185–191.

Carruthers, M., Arguelles, A.E. and Mosovich, A. (1976) Man in transit: biochemical and physiological changes during intercontinental flights. Lancet, I, 977–981.

Carter, D.E., Bressler, R., Hughes, M.R., Haussler, M.R., Christian, C.D. and Heine, M.W. (1976) Effect of oral contraceptives on plasma clearance. Clinical Pharmacology and Therapeutics, 18, 700–707.

Casey, A.E. (1973) Serum chemistry in the anxiety states: albumin and urea changes. Journal of the American Medical Association, 224, 1532.

Cederblad, G. (1976) Plasma carnitine and body composition. Clinica Chimica Acta, 67, 207–212.

Cheek, D.B. (1968) Human Growth, Energy and Intelligence. Lea and Febiger, Philadelphia, Pa.

Chern, C.J. and Beutler, E. (1976) Biochemical and electrophoretic studies of erythrocyte pyridoxine kinase in white and black Americans. American Journal of Human Genetics, 28, 9–17.

Christensen, N.J., Mathias, C.J. and Frankel, H.L. (1976) Plasma and urinary dopamine; studies during fasting and exercise and in tetraplegic man. European Journal of Clinical Investigation, 6, 403–409.

Christian, J.C., Cheung, S.W., Kang, K., Harmath, F.P., Huntzinger, D.J. and Powell, R.C. (1976) Variance of plasma free and esterified cholesterol in adult twins. American Journal of Human Genetics, 28, 174–178.

Cohen, L., Block, J. and Djordjevich, J. (1967) Sex related differences in isoenzymes of serum lactic dehydrogenase (LDH). Proceedings of the Society for Experimental Biology and Medicine, 126, 55–60.

Cohn, S.H., Vaswani, A., Zanzi, I., Aloia, J.F., Roginsky, M.S. and Ellis, K.J. (1976a) Changes in body chemical composition with age measured by total body neutron activation. Metabolism, 25, 85–95.

Cohn, S.H., Vaswani, A., Zanzi, I. and Ellis, K.J. (1976b) Effect of aging on bone mass in adult women. American Journal of Physiology, 230, 143–148.

Collins, K.J., Few, J.D., Forward, T.J. and Giec, L.A. (1969) Stimulation of adrenal glucocorticoid secretion in man by raising the body temperature. Journal of Physiology (London), 202, 645–660.

Collins, K.J. and Weiner, J.S. (1968) Endocrinological aspects of exposure to high environmental temperatures. Physiological Reviews, 48, 785–839.

Connor, W.E., Hodges, R.E. and Bleiler, R.E. (1961) The serum lipids in men receiving high cholesterol-free diets. Journal of Clinical Investigation, 40, 894–901.

Cotham, R.H. and Shand, D.G. (1976) Spuriously low plasma propranolol concentrations resulting from blood collection methods. Clinical Pharmacology and Therapeutics, 18, 535–538.

Craft, I.L. and Peters, T.J. (1971) Quantitative changes in plasma amino acids induced by oral contraceptives. Clinical Science, 41, 301–307.

Crane, M.G. and Harris, J.J. (1976) Effect of aging on renin activity and aldosterone excretion. Journal of Laboratory and Clinical Medicine, 87, 947–959.

Crawford, J.S. and Hooi, H.W.Y. (1968) Binding of bromsulphthalein by serum albumin from pregnant women, neonates and subjects on oral contraceptives. British Journal of Anaesthesia, 40, 723–729.

Crowther, J.S., Drasar, B.S., Boddard, P., Hill, M.J. and Johnson, K. (1973) The effect of a chemically defined diet on the faecal flora and faecal steroid concentration. Gut, 14, 790–793.

Cryer, P.E., Haymond, M.W., Santiago, J.V. and Shah, S.D. (1976) Norepinephrine and epinephrine release and adrenergic mediation of smoking-associated hemodynamic and metabolic events. New England Journal of Medicine, 295, 573–577.

Cuthbertson, D.P. (1964) Physical injury and its effect on protein metabolism. In Mammalian Protein Metabolism (H.N. Munro and J.B. Allison Eds.) Academic Press, New York, pp. 373–414.

Cuthbertson, D.P. and Tilstone, W.J. (1969) Metabolism during the postinjury period. Advances in Clinical Chemistry, 12, 1–55.

Cymerman, A. and Francesconi, R.F. (1975) Alteration of circadian rhythmicities of urinary 3-methoxy-4-hydroxyphenylglycol (MHPG) and vanilmandelic acid (VMA) in man during cold exposure. Life Sciences, 16, 225–236.

Dales, L.G., Friedman, G.D., Siegelaub, A.B. and Seltzer, C.C. (1974) Cigarette smoking and serum chemistry tests. Journal of Chronic Diseases, 27, 293–307.

Daly, J.R. and Evans, J.I. (1974) Daily rhythms of steroid and associated pituitary hormones in man and their relationship to sleep. Advances in Steroid Biochemistry and Pharmacology, 4, 61–110.

Daniel, W.A. Jr., Gaines, E.G. and Bennett, D.L. (1975) Dietary intakes and plasma concentrations of folate in healthy adolescents. American Journal of Clinical Nutrition, 28, 363–370.

Davies, C.T.M. and Few, J.D. (1973) Effects of exercise on adrenocortical function. Journal of Applied Physiology, 35, 887–891.

Davis, J., Morrill, R., Fawcett, J., Upton, V., Bondy, P.K. and Spiro, H.M. (1962) Apprehension and elevated serum cortisol levels. Journal of Psychosomatic Research, 6, 83–86.

Davis, M., Simmons, C.J., Dordoni, B., Maxwell, J.D. and Williams, R. (1973) Induction of hepatic enzymes during normal pregnancy. Journal of Obstetrics and Gynaecology. British Commonwealth, 80, 690–694.

Davis, V.E., Cashaw, J.L., Huff, J.A., Brown, H. and Nicholas, N.L. (1967) Alteration of endogenous catecholamine metabolism by ethanol ingestion. Proceedings of the Society for Experimental Biology and Medicine, 125, 1140–1143.

Dawley, H.H. Jr., Ellithorpe, D.B. and Tretola, R. (1976) Aversive smoking: carboxyhemoglobin levels before and after rapid smoking. Journal of Behavioural Therapeutics and Experimental Psychiatrics, 7, 13–15.

Dawson, A., Allardyce, M., Allan, T.M., Ogston, D., Kerridge, D.F. and Lewis, H.B.M. (1976) Interrelations between ABO blood group, plasminogen, α_1-antitrypsin, α_2-macroglobulin and the platelet count in blood donors. Acta Haematologica (Basle), 56, 19–26.

De Costre, P., Buhler, U., De Groot, L.J. and Refetoff, S. (1971) Diurnal rhythm in total serum thyroxine levels. Metabolism, 20, 782–791.

Deitrick, J.E., Whedon, G.D. and Shorr, E. (1948) Effects of immobilization upon various metabolic and physiologic functions of normal men. American Journal of Medicine, 4, 3–36.

Dhant, M., Thiery, M. and Vandekerckhove, D. (1976) Hormonal screening for detection of twin pregnancies. Lancet, II, 861.

Diot, M.-N., Claude, J.-R., Eschwege, E., Warnet, J.-M., Mollaret, C., Rosselin, E.-G. and Richard, J.-L. (1974) Variations de 16 paramètres biologiques plasmatiques sous l'influence d'une charge orale en glucose ou en eau chez 116 sujets normaux. Annales de Biologie Clinique, 32, 493–498.

Dirren, H., Robinson, A.B. and Pauling, L. (1975) Sex-related patterns in profiles of human urinary amino acids. Clinical Chemistry, 21, 1970–1975.

Doering, C.H., Kraemer, H.C., Brodie, H.K.H. and Hamburg, D.A. (1975) A cycle of plasma testosterone in the human male. Journal of Clinical Endocrinology and Metabolism, 40, 492–500.

Duckworth, W.C. and Kitabchi, A.E. (1976) The effect of age on plasma proinsulin-like material after oral glucose. Journal of Laboratory and Clinical Medicine, 88, 359–367.

Dunn, J.P., Brooks, G.W., Mausner, J., Rodnan, G.P. and Cobb, S. (1963) Social class gradient of serum uric acid levels in males. Journal of the American Medical Association, 185, 431–436.

Durber, S.M. and Daly, J.R. (1976) A simple method for the determination of free cortisol in plasma, with normal levels in men and women, including women taking low oestrogen contraceptives. Clinica Chimica Acta, 68, 43–48.

Durrington, P.N., Manning, A.P., Bolton, C.H. and Hartog, M. (1976) Effect of pectin on serum lipids and lipoproteins, whole-gut transit-time, and stool weight. Lancet, II, 394–396.

Dybkaer, R. and Gräsbeck, R. (1973) Theory of reference values. Scandinavian Journal of Clinical and Laboratory Investigation, 32, 1–7.

Dymling, J.F., Ljungberg, O., Hillyard, C.J., Greenberg, P.B., Evans, I.M.A. and MacIntyre, I. (1976) Whisky: a new provocative test for calcitonin secretion. Acta Endocrinologica, 82, 500–509.

Eaton, J.W., Brewer, G.J. and Grover, R.F. (1969) Role of red cell 2,3-diphosphoglycerate in the adaptation of man to altitude. Journal of Laboratory and Clinical Medicine, 73, 603–609.

Eisen, A.Z., Weissman, S. and Karon, M. (1962) Pseudouridine metabolism. I. Isolation and the effect of diet on urinary excretion. Journal of Laboratory and Clinical Medicine, 59, 620–629.

Eisenberg, S. (1963) Postural changes in plasma volume in hypoalbuminemia. Archives of Internal Medicine, 112, 544–549.

Eisenberg, S. and Wolf, P.C. (1965) Plasma volume after posture change in hypertensive subjects. Archives of Internal Medicine, 115, 17–22.

Elin, R.J., Wolff, S.M. and Finch, C.A. (1977) Effect of induced fever on serum iron and ferritin concentrations in man. Blood, 49, 147–153.

Ellis, F.R. and Montegriffo, V.M.E. (1970) Veganism, clinical findings and investigations. American Journal of Clinical Nutrition, 23, 249–255.

Ellis, K.J., Vaswani, A., Zanzi, I. and Cohn, S.H. (1976) Total body sodium and chlorine in normal adults. Metabolism, 25, 645–654.

Elmfors, B. and Tryding, N. (1976) Date of confinement prediction from serum diamine oxidase determination in early pregnancy. British Journal of Obstetrics and Gynaecology, 83, 6–10.

Elwood, P.C., Hughes, R.E. and Hurley, R.J. (1970) Ascorbic acid and serum cholesterol. Lancet, II, 1197.

Elwood, P.C., St. Leger, A.S. and Morton, M. (1976) Dependence of blood lead on domestic water lead. Lancet, I, 1295.

Epstein, M. and Hollenberg, N.K. (1976) Age as a determinant of renal sodium conservation in normal man. Journal of Laboratory and Clinical Medicine, 87, 411–417.

Exley, D. and Corker, C.S. (1966) The human male cycle of urinary oestrone and 17-oxosteroids. Journal of Endocrinology, 35, 83–99.

Fahlén, M., Odén, A., Björntorp, P. and Tibblin, G. (1971) Seasonal influence on insulin secretion in man. Clinical Science, 41, 453–458.

Feigin, R.D. (1969) Blood and urine amino acid aberrations. American Journal of Diseases of Children, 117, 24–47.

Ferguson, D.B. (1971) Effects of low doses of fluoride on serum proteins and a serum enzyme in man. Nature, New Biology, 231, 159–160.

Fischer, C.L., Gill, C., Forrester, M.G. and Nakamura, R. (1976) Quantitation of "acute-phase proteins" postoperatively. American Journal of Clinical Pathology, 66, 840–846.

Fisher, D.A., Dussault, J.H., Hobel, C.J. and Lam, R. (1973) Serum and thyroid gland triiodothyronine in the human fetus. Journal of Clinical Endocrinology, 36, 397–400.

Flood, C., Gherondache, C., Pincus, G., Tait, J.F., Tait, S.A.S. and Willoughby, S. (1967) The metabolism and secretion of aldosterone in elderly subjects. Journal of Clinical Investigation, 46, 960–966.

Foa, V., Caimi, L., Amante, L., Antonini, C., Gattinoni, A., Tettamanti, G., Lombardo, A. and Giuliani, A. (1976) Patterns of some lysosomal enzymes in the plasma and of proteins in urine of workers exposed to inorganic mercury. International Archives of Occupational and Environmental Health, 37, 115–124.

Forbes, G.B. (1976) The adult decline in lean body mass. Human Biology, 48, 161–173.

Forsyth, I.A. and Edwards, C.R.W. (1972) Human prolactin, its isolation, assay and clinical applications. Clinical Endocrinology, 1, 293–314.

Frantz, A.G. and Rabkin, M.T. (1965) Effects of estrogen and sex difference on secretion of human growth hormone. Journal of Clinical Endocrinology and Metabolism, 25, 1470–1480.

Frayser, R., Rennie, I.D., Gray, G.W. and Houston, C.S. (1975) Hormonal and electrolyte response to exposure to 17500 feet. Journal of Applied Physiology, 38, 636–642.

Freer, D.E. and Statland, B.E. (1977) The effects of ethanol (0.75 g/kg body weight) on the activities of selected enzymes in sera of healthy young adults: 1. Intermediate-term effects. Clinical Chemistry, 23, 830–834.

Frewin, D.B., Downey, J.A. and Levitt, M. (1973) The effect of heat, cold, and exercise on plasma dopamine-β-hydroxylase activity in man. Canadian Journal of Physiology and Pharmacology, 51, 986–989.

Friedemann, T.E., Haugen, G.E. and Kmieciak, T.C. (1945) Pyruvic acid: III. The level of pyruvic and lactic acids, and the lactic-pyruvic ratio, in the blood of human subjects, the effect of food, light muscular activity, and anoxia at high altitude. Journal of Biological Chemistry, 157, 673–689.

Friedman, G. and Goldberg, S.J. (1975) Concurrent and subsequent serum cholesterols of breast- and formula-fed infants. American Journal of Clinical Nutrition, 28, 42–45.

Fuller, J.H., Grainger, S.L., Jarrett, R.J. and Keen, H. (1974) Possible seasonal variation of plasma lipids in a healthy population. Clinica Chimica Acta, 52, 305–310.

Gairdner, D., Marks, J., Roscoe, J.D. and Brettell, R.O. (1958) The fluid shift from the vascular compartment immediately after birth. Archives of Disease in Childhood, 33, 489–498.

Galbo, H., Holst, J.J. and Christensen, N.J. (1975) Glucagon and plasma catecholamine responses to graded and prolonged exercise in man. Journal of Applied Physiology, 38, 70–76.

Galvão-Teles, A., Graves, L., Burke, C.W., Fotherby, K. and Fraser, R. (1976) Free cortisol in obesity: effect of fasting. Acta Endocrinologica, 81, 321–329.

Garn, S.M., Smith, N.J. and Clark. D.C. (1975) The magnitude and the implications of apparent race differences in hemoglobin values. American Journal of Clinical Nutrition, 28, 563–568.

Gershon, S.L. and Fox, I.H. (1974) Pharmacologic effects of nicotinic acid on human purine metabolism. Journal of Laboratory and Clinical Medicine, 84, 179–186.

Gleispach, H. (1973) Excretion of androgens, pregnanes and oestrogens depending on age and sex. In Reference Values in Human Chemistry (Ed. G. Siest) Karger, Basel.

Goldberg, D.M. (1976) Demographic and analytic factors affecting the normal range of serum enzyme activities. Clinical Biochemistry, 9, 168–172.

Goldberg, D.M. and Winfield, D.A. (1974) Relationship of serum enzyme activities to demographic variables in a healthy population. Clinica Chimica Acta, 54, 357–368.

Goodwin, P.M., Harrop, J. and Marks, V. (1975) Dopamine-beta-hydroxylase and sympatho-adrenal activity. Lancet, I, 170–171.

Gordon, G.G., Altman, K., Southren, A.L., Rubin, E. and Lieber, C.S. (1976) Effect of alcohol (ethanol) administration on sex-hormone metabolism in normal men. New England Journal of Medicine, 295, 793–797.

Grabner, W., Matzkies, F., Prestele, H., Rose, A., Daniel, U., Phillip, J. and Fischer, K. (1975) Diurnal variation of glucose tolerance and insulin secretion in man. Klinische Wochenschrift, 53, 773–778.

Gray, S.J., Ramsey, C., Reifenstein, R.W. and Benson, J.A., Jr. (1953) The significance of hormonal factors in the pathogenesis of peptic ulcer. Gastroenterology, 25, 156–172.

Green, A.G. (1974) Circannual excretory patterns in man. Journal of Clinical Pathology, 27, 932.

Greenblatt, D.J. and Koch-Weser, J. (1976) Intramuscular injection of drugs. New England Journal of Medicine, 295, 542–546.

Gregerman, R.I. and Solomon, N. (1967) Acceleration of thyroxine and triiodothyronine turnover during bacterial pulmonary infections and fever; implications for the functional state of the thyroid during stress and in senescence. Journal of Clinical Endocrinology and Metabolism, 27, 93–105.

Gregorczyk, J., Lewandowska-Tokarz, A., Stanosek, J. and Hepa, J. (1965) The effects of physical work and work under conditions of noise and vibration on the human body. I. Behaviour of serum alkaline phosphatase, aldolase and lactic dehydrogenase activities. Acta Physiologica Polanska, 16, 701–708.

Guillou, P.J., Morgan, D.B. and Hill, G.L. (1976) Hypophosphataemia: a complication of "innocuous dextrose-saline". Lancet, II, 710–712.

Haddad, J.G., Jr. and Walgate, J. (1976) Radioimmunoassay of the binding protein for vitamin D and its metabolites in human serum. Journal of Clinical Investigation, 58, 1217–1222.

Hagenfeldt, L. and Wahren, J. (1975) Turnover of plasma free stearic and oleic acids in resting and exercising human subjects. Metabolism, 24, 1299–1304.

Halberg, F. (1974) Protection by timing treatment according to bodily rhythms - an analogy to protection by scrubbing before surgery. Chronobiologia 1, Suppl. 1, 27–68.

Halbreich, U., Assael, M., Ben-David, M. and Bornstein, R. (1976) Serum prolactin in women with premenstrual syndrome. Lancet, II, 654–655.

Hannon, J.P., Chinn, K.S.K. and Shields, J.L. (1971) Alterations in serum and extracellular electrolytes during high-altitude exposure. Journal of Applied Physiology, 31, 266–273.

Hannon, J.P., Shields, J.L. and Harris, C.W. (1969) Effects of altitude acclimatization on blood composition of women. Journal of Applied Physiology, 26, 540–547.

Hansen, A.A.P. and Weeke, J. (1974) Fasting serum growth hormone levels and growth hormone responses to exercise during normal menstrual cycles and cycles of oral contraceptives. Scandinavian Journal of Clinical and Laboratory Investigation, 34, 199–205.

Haralambie, G. (1969) Serum glycoproteins and physical exercise. Clinica Chimica Acta, 26, 287–291.

Haralambie, G. and Berg, A. (1976) Resting muscle levels and the influence of exercise on serum amino acid-arylpeptidase activity in man. Clinica Chimica Acta, 69, 433–439.

Hartley, L.H., Mason, J.W., Hogan, R.P., Jones, L.G., Kotchen, T.A., Mougey, E.H., Wherry, F.E., Pennington, L.L. and Ricketts, P.T. (1972) Multiple hormonal responses to graded exercise in relation to physical training. Journal of Applied Physiology, 33, 602–606.

Hashimoto, Y., Kurobe, Y. and Hirota, K. (1974) Effect of delivery on serum dopamine-beta-hydroxylase activity and urinary vanillylmandelic acid excretion of normal pregnant subjects. Biochemical Pharmacology, 23, 2185–2187.

Havlik, R., Garrison, R., Fabsitz, R. and Feinleib, M. (1977) Genetic variability of clinical chemical values. Clinical Chemistry, 23, 659–662.

Hays, R.M. (1976) Antidiuretic hormone. New England Journal of Medicine, 295, 659–665.

Heath, H., III, Earll, J.M., Schaff, M., Piechocki, J.T. and Li, T.-K. (1972) Serum ionized calcium during bed rest in fracture patients and normal men. Metabolism, 21, 633–640.

Heffernon, J.J., Smith, W.R., Berk, J.E., Fridhandler, L., Glauser, F.L. and Montgomery, K.A. (1976) Hyperamylasemia in heroin addicts. American Journal of Gastroenterology, 66, 17–22.

Helge, H., Weber, B. and Quabbe, H.J. (1969) Growth hormone release and venepuncture, Lancet, I, 204.

Herzberg, M., Penebaum, E., Fishel, B. and Wiener, M.H. (1977) D-Glucaric acid and gamma-glutamyltransferase as indices of hepatic enzyme induction in pregnancy. Clinical Chemistry, 23, 596–598.

Hetland, O. and Brubakk, E. (1973) Diurnal variation in serum zinc concentration. Scandinavian Journal of Clinical and Laboratory Investigation, 32, 225–226.

Hilden, T. and Svendsen, T.L. (1975) Electrolyte disturbances in beer drinkers. Lancet, II, 245–246.

Hilgertová, J., Straková, M., Vrbová, H., Gregorová, I., Sónka, J. and Josifko, M. (1972) Seasonal variations of human erythrocyte glucose 6-phosphate dehydrogenase activity in relation to temperature and dehydroepiandrosterone excretion. Clinica Chimica Acta, 36, 511–515.

Hill, A., Casey, R. and Zaleski, W.A. (1976) Difficulties and pitfalls in the interpretation of screening tests for the detection of inborn errors of metabolism. Clinica Chimica Acta, 72, 1–15.

Hill, P. and Wynder, F. (1976) Diet and prolactin release. Lancet, II, 806–807.

Ho, W.K.K., Wen, H.L., Fung, K.P., Ng, Y.H., Au, K.K. and Ma, L. (1977) Comparison of plasma hormonal levels between heroin-addicted and normal subjects. Clinica Chimica Acta, 75, 415–419.

Hodgson, P.A., Ellefson, R.D., Elveback, L.R., Harris, L.E., Nelson, R.A. and Weidman, W.H. (1976) Comparison of serum cholesterol in children fed high, moderate, or low cholesterol milk diets during neonatal period. Metabolism, 25, 739–746.

Hoffman, R.G. and Waid, M.E. (1965) The "average of normals" method of quality control. American Journal of Clinical Pathology, 43, 134–141.

Holloszy, J.O. (1973) Cellular adaptations to exercise. In Reference Values in Human Chemistry (Ed. G. Siest) pp. 216–222, Karger, Basel.

Holmes, E.G., Jones, E.R., Lyle, M.D. and Stanier, M.W. (1956) Malnutrition in African Adults. 3. Effect of diet on body composition. British Journal of Nutrition, 10, 198–219.

Holub, W.R., Reyner, F.C. and Forman, G.H. (1971) Increased levels of serum immunoglobulin G and M in women using intrauterine contraceptive devices. American Journal of Obstetrics and Gynecology, 110, 362–365.

Honour, J.W., Valman, H.B. and Shackleton, C.H.L. (1977) Aldosterone and sodium homeostasis in preterm infants. Acta Paediatrica Scandinavica, 66, 103–109.

Hume, R. and Weyers, E. (1971) Relationship between total body water and surface area in normal and obese subjects. Journal of Clinical Pathology, 24, 234–238.

Hunter, J.B. and Critz, J.B. (1971) Effect of training on plasma enzyme levels in man. Journal of Applied Physiology, 31, 20–23.

Hytten, F.E. and Lind, T. (1973) Diagnostic Indices in Pregnancy. Ciba-Geigy. Basel.

Ingenbleek, Y., Van Den Schrieck, H.-G., De Nayer, P. and De Visscher, M. (1975) Albumin, transferrin and the thyroxine-binding pre-albumin/retinol-binding protein (TBPA-RBP) complex in assessment of malnutrition. Clinica Chimica Acta, 63, 61–67.

Irwin, M.I. and Staton, A.J. (1969) Dietary wheat starch and sucrose. Effect on levels of five enzymes in blood serum of young adults. American Journal of Clinical Nutrition, 22, 701–709.

Jenkins, J.S. and Connolly, J. (1968) Adrenocortical response to ethanol in man. British Medical Journal, 2, 804–805.

Jensen, J., Blankenhorn, D.H., Chin, H.P., Sturgeon, P. and Ware, A.G. (1965) Serum lipids and serum uric acid in human twins. Journal of Lipid Research, 6, 193–204.

Johns, M.W., Masterton, J.P., Paddle-Ledinek, J.E., Patel, Y.C., Winikoff, D. and Malinek, M. (1975) Variations in thyroid function and sleep in healthy young men. Clinical Science and Molecular Medicine, 49, 629–632.

Johnson, H.L., Consolazio, C.F., Matoush, L.O. and Kryzwicki, H.J. (1969) Nitrogen and mineral metabolism at altitude. Federation Proceedings, 28, 1195–1198.

Johnson, N.E., Alcantara, E.N. and Linkswiler, H. (1970) Effect of level of protein intake on urinary and fecal calcium and calcium retention of young adult males. Journal of Nutrition, 100, 1425–1430.

Johnston, I.D.A. (1972) Endocrine response to trauma. Advances in Clinical Chemistry, 15, 255–285.

Jones, C.R., Bergman, M.W., Kittner, P.J. and Pigman, W.W. (1964) Urinary hydroxyproline excretion in normal children and adolescents. Proceedings of the Society for Experimental Biology and Medicine, 115, 85–87.

Josephson, B. and Dahlberg, G. (1952) Variations in the cell-content and chemical composition of the human blood due to age, sex and season. Scandinavian Journal of Clinical and Laboratory Investigation, 4, 216–236.

Josephson, B., Dahlberg, G. and Tötterman, G. (1952) On the effect of nutrition upon the blood count and chemical composition of the blood. Scandinavian Journal of Clinical and Laboratory Investigation, 4, 237–241.

Kachadorian, W.A. and Johnson, R.E. (1971) The effect of exercise on some clinical measures of renal function. American Heart Journal, 82, 278–280.

Kang, K.W., Christian, J.C., Hedges, B., Corey, L.A. and Powell, R. (1976) Fatty acid variability of plasma lipids and cholesteryl esters in adult male twins and their brothers. Lipids, 11, 722–726.

Kashyap, M.L., Sivasamboo, R., Sothy, S.P., Cheah, J.S. and Gartside, P.A. (1976) Carbohydrate and lipid metabolism during human labor: free fatty acids, glucose, insulin, and lactic acid metabolism during normal and oxytocin-induced labor for post-maturity, Metabolism, 25, 865–875.

Kattus, A.A., Sinclair-Smith, B., Genest, J. and Newman, E.V. (1949) The effect of exercise on the renal mechanism of electrolyte excretion in normal subjects. Bulletin of the Johns Hopkins Hospital, 84, 344–368.

Katz, F.H. and Romfh, P. (1972) Plasma aldosterone and renin activity during the menstrual cycle. Journal of Clinical Endocrinology and Metabolism, 34, 819–821.

Katz, F.H., Romfh, P. and Smith, J.A. (1975) Diurnal variation of plasma aldosterone, cortisol and renin activity in supine man. Journal of Clinical Endocrinology and Metabolism, 40, 125–134.

Kawai, T. (1973) Clinical Aspects of the Plasma Proteins. Lippincott, Philadelphia, Pa.

Kay. D.R., Bole, G.G. Jr. and Ledger, W.J. (1971) Antinuclear antibodies, rheumatoid factor and C-reactive protein in serum of normal women using oral contraceptives. Arthritis and Rheumatism, 14, 239–248.

Keil, L.C. and Ellis, S. (1976) Plasma vasopressin and renin activity in women exposed to bed rest and $+G_z$ acceleration. Journal of Applied Physiology, 40, 911–914.

Kerr, W.K., Barkin, M., Levers, P.E., Woo, S.K.-C. and Menczyk, Z. (1965) The effect of cigarette smoking on bladder carcinogens in man. Canadian Medical Association Journal, 93, 1–7.

Keys, A. (1955) Atherosclerosis; mode of life and prevalence of coronary heart disease. Minnesota Medicine, 38, 578–766.

Khalil, M., Tanios, A., Moghazy, M., Aref, M.K., Mahmoud, S. and El Lozy, M. (1973) Serum and red cell folates, and serum vitamin B_{12} in protein calorie malnutrition. Archives of Disease in Childhood, 48, 366–369.

Khan, L. and Bamji, M.S. (1977) Plasma carnitine levels in children with protein-calorie malnutrition before and after rehabilitation. Clinica Chimica Acta, 75, 163–166.

King, S.W., Statland, B.E. and Savory, J. (1976) The effect of a short burst of exercise on activity values of enzymes in sera of healthy young men. Clinica Chimica Acta, 72, 211–218.

Kirkeby, K. (1966) Blood lipids, lipoproteins and proteins in vegetarians. Acta Medica Scandinavica, 179, Suppl. 443, 1–84.

Kirmiz, J.P. (1962) Adaptation to Desert Environment. Butterworths, London.

Kosunen, K.J., Pakarinen, A.J., Kuoppasalmi, K. and Adlercreutz, H. (1976) Plasma renin activity, angiotensin II, and aldosterone during intense heat stress. Journal of Applied Physiology, 41, 323–327.

Krovetz, L.J. (1965) The physiologic significance of body surface area. Journal of Pediatrics, 67, 841–862.

Krzywicki, H.J., Consolazio, C.F., Matoush, L.O. and Johnson, H.L. (1968) Metabolic aspects of acute starvation; body composition changes. American Journal of Clinical Nutrition, 21, 87–97.

Krzywicki, H.J., Consolazio, C.F., Matoush, L.O., Johnson, H.L. and Barnhart, R.A. (1969) Body composition changes during exposure to altitude. Federation Proceedings, 28, 1190–1194.

Kubota, J., Lazar, V.A. and Losee, F. (1968) Copper, zinc, cadmium, and lead in human blood from 19 locations in the United States. Archives of Environmental Health, 16, 788–793.

Kuo, P.T. and Carson, J.C. (1959) Dietary fats and the diurnal serum triglyceride levels in man. Journal of Clinical Investigation, 38, 1384–1393.

Kuttner, R.E. and Mailander, J.C. (1965) Serum pepsinogen in migrant Mexicans and stressed Caucasians. Journal of the National Medical Association, 57, 109–111.

Lafontaine, E., Lavernhe, J., Courillon, J., Medvedeff, M. and Ghata, J. (1967) Influence of air travel east-west and vice versa on circadian rhythms of urinary elimination of potassium and 17-hydroxycorticosteroids. Aerospace Medicine, 38, 944–947.

Latham, A.N., Millbank, L., Richens, A. and Rowe, D.J.F. (1973) Liver enzyme induction by anticonvulsant drugs, and its relationship to disturbed calcium and folic acid metabolism. Journal of Clinical Pharmacology, 13, 337–342.

Laurell, C.-B., Kullander, S. and Thorell, J. (1967) Effect of administration of a combined estrogen-progestin contraceptive on the level of individual plasma proteins. Scandinavian Journal of Clinical and Laboratory Investigation, 21, 337–343.

Laurell, H. and Pernow, B. (1966) Effect of exercise on plasma potassium in man. Acta Physiologica Scandinavica, 66, 241–242.

Lauwerys, R.R., Buchet, J.P. and Roels, H. (1976) The relationship between cadmium exposure or body burden and the concentration of cadmium in blood and urine in man. International Archives of Occupational and Environmental Health, 36, 275–285.

Leach, C.S., Johnson, P.C. and Driscoll, T.B. (1972) Effects of bed rest and centrifugation of humans on serum thyroid function tests. Aerospace Medicine, 43, 400–402.

Lebeau, M., Dumont, J.E. and Golstein, J. (1975) Urinary cyclic AMP and cyclic GMP excretion during the menstrual cycle. Hormone and Metabolic Research, 7, 190–194.

Leblanc, H., Anderson, J.R. and Yen, S.S.C. (1976) Glucagon secretion in late pregnancy and the puerperium. American Journal of Obstetrics and Gynecology, 125, 708–710.

Leckie, B., Brown, J.J., Lever, A.F., McConnell, A., Morton, J.J., Robertson, J.I.S. and Tree, M. (1976) Inactive renin in human plasma. Lancet, II, 748–749.

Lee, P.A., Xenakis, T., Winer, J. and Matsenbaugh, S. (1976) Puberty in girls: correlation of serum levels of gonadotropins, prolactin, androgens, estrogens, and progestins with physical changes. Journal of Clinical Endocrinology and Metabolism, 43, 775–783.

Lester, E. and Varghese, Z. (1977) Differences in the calcium concentration of serum and plasma initially and after storage. Annals of Clinical Biochemistry, 14, 39–44.

Leveille, G.A., Sauberlich, H.E., Powell, R.C. and Nunes, W.T. (1962) The influence of dietary protein on plasma lipids in human subjects. Journal of Clinical Investigation, 41, 1007–1011.

Lewis, J.S., Baer, M.T. and Lauffer, M.A. (1975) Urinary riboflavin and creatinine excretion in children treated with anticonvulsant drugs. American Journal of Diseases of Children, 129, 394.

Lieber, C.S. (1976) The metabolism of alcohol. Scientific American, 234, 25–33.

Lie-Injo, L.E., Ng, T. and Balakrishnan, S. (1974) Red cell enzymes in cord blood and plasma bilirubin levels in the first week of life. Clinica Chimica Acta, 50, 77–83.

Liewendahl, K. and Majuri, H. (1976) Thyroxine, triiodothyronine, and thyrotropin in serum during long-term diphenylhydantoin therapy. Scandinavian Journal of Clinical and Laboratory Investigation, 36, 141–144.

Lim, V.S., Katz, A.I. and Lindheimer, M.D. (1976) Acid-base regulation in pregnancy. American Journal of Physiology, 231, 1764–1770.

Linkola, J. (1975) Natriuresis after diluted ethanol solutions. Lancet, II, 1157.

Lunn, P.G., Whitehead, R.G., Hay, R.W. and Baker, B.A. (1973) Progressive changes in serum cortisol, insulin and growth hormone concentrations and their relationship to the distorted amino acid pattern during the development of kwashiorkor. British Journal of Nutrition, 29, 399–422.

Luzzio, A.J. (1966) Comparison of serum proteins in Americans and Eskimos. Journal of Applied Physiology, 21, 685–688.

Maas, A.H.J. and Van Heijst, A.N.P. (1961) The accuracy of the microdetermination of the pCO_2 of blood from the ear-lobe. Clinica Chimica Acta, 6, 34–37.

MacDonald, H.N., Good, W. and Stone, J. (1974) Changes in common plasma solute levels during labour and the puerperium. Journal of Obstetrics and Gynaecology of the British Commonwealth, 81, 888–894.

Maclean, D., Murison, J. and Griffiths, P.D. (1974) Serum enzyme activities in accidental hypothermia and hypothermic myxoedema. Clinica Chimica Acta, 52, 197–201.

Maebashi, M., Kawamura, N., Sato, M., Yoshinaga, K. and Suzuki, M. (1976) Urinary excretion of carnitine in man. Journal of Laboratory and Clinical Medicine, 87, 760–766.

Mahurkar, S.D., Dunea, G., Pillay, V.K.G., Levine, H. and Gandhi, V. (1975) Relationship of posture and age to urinary protein excretion. British Medical Journal, 1, 712–714.

Malherbe, C., De Gasparo, M., De Hertogh, R. and Hoet, J.J. (1969) Circadian variations of blood sugar and plasma insulin levels in man. Diabetologia, 5, 397–404.

Marks, V. (1975) Alcohol and changes in body constituents: glucose and hormones. Proceedings of the Society of Experimental Biology and Medicine, 68, 377–380.

Marshall, M.W., Iacono, J.M., Wheeler, M.A., Mackin, J.F. and Canary, J.J. (1976) Changes in lactate dehydrogenase, LDH isoenzymes, lactate, and pyruvate as a result of feeding low fat diets to healthy men and women. Metabolism, 25, 169–178.

Martin, H.F., Gudzinowicz, B.J. and Fanger, H. (1975) Normal Values in Clinical Chemistry: A Guide to Statistical Analysis of Laboratory Data. Dekker, New York.

Martin, J.F., Mikulecky, M., Blaschke, T.F., Waggoner, J.G., Vergalla, J. and Berk, P.D. (1975) Differences between the plasma indocyanine green disappearance rates of normal men and women. Proceedings of the Society of Experimental Biology and Medicine, 150, 612–617.

Maruhn, D., Strozyk, K., Gielow, L. and Bock, K.D. (1977) Diurnal variations of urinary enzyme excretion. Clinica Chimica Acta, 75, 427–433.

Masi, M., Paolucci, P., Perocco, P. and Franceschi, C. (1976) Immunosuppression by phenytoin. Lancet, I, 860.

Mautalen, C.A. (1970) Circadian rhythm of urinary total and free hydroxyproline excretion and its relation to creatinine excretion. Journal of Laboratory and Clinical Medicine, 75, 11–18.

McCall, J.T., Goldstein, N.P. and Smith, L.H. (1971) Implications of trace metals in human disease. Federation Proceedings, 30, 1011–1015.

McDonald, J.T. and Margen, S. (1976) Wine versus ethanol in human nutrition. 1. Nitrogen and calorie balance. American Journal of Clinical Nutrition, 29, 1093–1103.

Merimee, T.J. and Fineberg, E.S. (1973) Homeostasis during fasting. II. Hormone substrate differences between men and women. Journal of Clinical Endocrinology and Metabolism, 37, 698–702.

Merimee, T.J. and Fineberg, E.S. (1976) Starvation-induced alterations of circulating thyroid hormone concentrations in man. Metabolism, 25, 79–83.

Merimee, T.J., Pulkkinen, A.J. and Burton, C.E. (1976) Diet-induced alterations of hGH secretion in man. Journal of Clinical Endocrinology and Metabolism, 42, 931–937.

Meyer, K. (1962) Serum cholesterol and heredity: a twin study. Acta Medica Scandinavica, 172, 401–404.

Michelakis, A.M., Yoshida, H. and Dormois, J.C. (1975) Plasma renin activity and plasma aldosterone during the normal menstrual cycle. American Journal of Obstetrics and Gynecology, 123, 724–726.

Mikhail, M.M. and Mansour, M.M. (1976) The relationship between serum carnitine levels and the nutritional status of patients with schistosomiasis. Clinica Chimica Acta, 71, 207–214.

Miller, A.T., Jr. and Miller, J.O., Jr. (1949) Renal excretion of lactic acid in exercise. Journal of Applied Physiology, 1, 614–618.

Moerman, E.J., Bogaert, M.G. and de Schaepdryver, A.F. (1976) Estimation of plasma catecholamines in man. Clinica Chimica Acta, 72, 89–96.

Moncloa, F., Carcelen, A. and Beteta, L. (1970) Physical exercise, acid-base balance, and adrenal function in newcomers to high altitude. Journal of Applied Physiology, 28, 151–155.

Moncloa, F., Gomez, R. and Pretell, E. (1963) Response to corticotrophin and correlation between excretion of creatinine and urinary steroids and between the clearance of creatinine and urinary steroids in aging. Steroids, 1, 437–444.

Moss, G. and Staunton, C. (1970) Blood flow, needle size and hemolysis – examining an old wives tale. New England Journal of Medicine, 282, 967.

Munro-Faure, A.D., Hill, D.M. and Anderson, J. (1971) Ethnic differences in human blood cell sodium concentration. Nature, 231, 457–458.

Nagata, H., Izumiyama, T., Kamata, K., Kono, S., Yukimura, Y., Tawata, M., Aizawa, T. and Yamada, T. (1976) An increase of plasma triiodothyronine concentration in man in a cold environment. Journal of Clinical Endocrinology and Metabolism, 43, 1153–1156.

Naismith, D.J., Akinyanju, P.A., Szanto, S. and Yudkin, J. (1970) The effect in volunteers of coffee and decaffeinated coffee on blood glucose, insulin, plasma lipids and some factors involved in blood clotting. Nutrition and Metabolism, 12, 144–151.

Nasset, E.S. and Ju, J.S. (1969) Amino acids and glucose in human blood plasma after beef and non-protein meals. Proceedings of the Society of Experimental Biology and Medicine, 132, 1077–1080.

Nestel, P. and Goldrick, B. (1976) Obesity: changes in lipid metabolism and the role of insulin. Clinics in Endocrinology and Metabolism, 5, 313–335.

Nevaril, C.G., Lynch, E.C., Alfrey, C.P. Jr. and Hellums, J.D. (1968) Erythrocyte damage and destruction induced by shearing stress. Journal of Laboratory and Clinical Medicine, 71, 784–790.

Nichols, A.B., Ravenscroft, C., Lamphiear, D.E. and Ostrander, L.D., Jr. (1976) Independence of serum lipid levels and dietary habits: The Tecumseh study. Journal of the American Medical Association, 236, 1948–1953.

Noel, G.L., Suh, H.K., Stone, J.G. and Frantz, A.G. (1972) Human prolactin and growth hormone release during surgery and other conditions of stress. Journal of Clinical Endocrinology and Metabolism, 35, 840–851.

Noel, W.K. and Kilmore, M.A. (1971) Socioeconomic status and blood chemistry, Journal of the American Osteopathic Association, 70, 1103–1107.

Nokin, J., Vekemans, M., L'Hermite, M. and Robyn, C. (1972) Circadian periodicity of serum prolactin concentration in man. British Medical Journal, 2, 561–562.

Novis, B.H., Marks, I.N., Bank, S. and Sloan, A.W. (1973) The relation between gastric acid secretion and body habitus, blood groups, smoking and the subsequent development of dyspepsia and duodenal ulcer. Gut, 14, 107–112.

Ogihara, T., Nugent, C.A., Shen, S.-W. and Goldfein, S. (1975) Serum dopamine-β-hydroxylase activity in parents and children. Journal of Laboratory and Clinical Medicine, 85, 566–573.

Okada, T., Fujita, T., Ohta, T., Kato, T., Ikuta, K. and Nagatsu, T. (1974) A 24-hour rhythm in human serum dopamine-β-hydroxylase activity. Experientia, 30, 605–607.

Olefsky, J.M. (1976) Decreased insulin binding to adipocytes and circulating monocytes from obese subjects. Journal of Clinical Investigation, 57, 1165–1172.

Oliver, T.K. Jr., Demis, J.A. and Bates, G.D. (1961) Serial bloodgas tensions and acid-base balance during the first hour of life in human infants. Acta Paediatrica, 50, 346–360.

Olson, R.E. (1973) Nutrition and alcoholism. In Modern Nutrition in Health and Disease (Eds. R.S. Goodhart and M.E. Shils), 5th edition, Lea and Febiger, Philadelphia, Pa.

Olson, R.E. (1975) Introductory remarks: nutrient, hormone, enzyme interactions. American Journal of Clinical Nutrition, 28, 626–637.

Olusi, S.O. and McFarlane, H. (1976) Effects of early protein-calorie malnutrition on the immune response. Pediatric Research, 10, 707–712.

Olusi, S.O., McFarlane, H., Osunkoya, B.O. and Adesina, H. (1975) Specific protein assays in protein-calorie malnutrition. Clinica Chimica Acta, 62, 107–116.

Ortiz, G.A., Argüelles, A.E., Crespin, H.A., Sposari, G. and Villafañe, C.T. (1974) Modifications of epinephrine, norepinephrine, blood lipid fractions and the cardiovascular system produced by noise in an industrial medium. Hormone Research, 5, 57–64.

Owen, O.E., Felig, P., Morgan, A.P., Wahren, J. and Cahill, G.F. Jr. (1969) Liver and kidney metabolism during prolonged starvation, Journal of Clinical Investigation, 48, 574–583.

Palmer, A.J. and Walker, A.H.C. (1949) The maternal circulation in normal pregnancy. Journal of Obstetrics and Gynaecology of the British Empire, 56, 537–547.

Passmore, R. and Draper, M.H. (1970) Nutritional disorders. In Biochemical Disorders in Human Disease (Eds. R.H.S. Thomson and I.D.P. Wootton) 3rd ed., pp. 15–33, Academic Press, New York.

Patel, Y.C., Alford, F.P. and Burger, H.G. (1972) The 24-hour plasma thyrotrophin profile. Clinical Science, 43, 71–77.

Pekarek, R.S. and Beisel, W.R. (1971) Characterization of the endogenous mediator(s) of serum zinc and iron depression during infections and other stresses. Proceedings of the Society of Experimental Biology and Medicine, 138, 728–732.

Perry, T.L., Hansen, S. and Maclean, J. (1976) Cerebrospinal fluid and plasma glutamine elevation by anticonvulsant drugs: a potential diagnostic and therapeutic trap. Clinica Chimica Acta, 69, 441–445.

Philp, R.B., Ackles, K.N., Inwood, M.J., Livingstone, S.D., Achimastos, A., Binns-Smith, M. and Radomski, M.W. (1972) Changes in the hemostatic system and in blood and urine chemistry of human subjects following decompression from a hyperbaric environment. Aerospace Medicine, 43, 498–505.

Picon-Reategui, E. (1963) Intravenous glucose tolerance test at sea level and at high altitudes. Journal of Clinical Endocrinology and Metabolism, 23, 1256–1261.

Pierson, M., Grignon, G., Malaprade, D. and Hartemann, P. (1976) L'activité somatomédine du sérum au cours de l'enfance chez le sujet normal et dans les retards de croissance. Annales de Biologie Clinique, 34, 11–18.

Pincus, J.B., Gittleman, I.F., Saito, M. and Sobel, A.E. (1956) A study of plasma values of sodium, potassium, chloride, carbon dioxide, carbon dioxide tension, sugar, urea and the protein base - binding power, pH and hematocrit in prematures on the first day of life. Pediatrics, 18, 39–49.

Pirke, K.M. and Doerr, P. (1970) Age related changes in free plasma testosterone, dihydrotestosterone and oestradiol. Acta Endocrinologica, 80, 171–178.

Poortmans, J.R. (1973) Body fluids fluctuations induced by physical activities. In Reference Values in Human Chemistry (Ed. G. Siest) pp. 255–263. Karger, Basle.

Portnay, G.I., O'Brian, J.T., Bush, J., Vagenakis, A.G., Azizi, F., Arky, R.A., Ingbar, S.H. and Braverman, L.E. (1974) The effect of starvation on the concentration and binding of thyroxine and triiodothyronine in serum and on the response to TRH. Journal of Clinical Endocrinology and Metabolism, 39, 191–194.

Purvis, K., Landgren, B.-M., Cekan, Z. and Diczfalusy, E. (1976) Endocrine effects of masturbation in men. Journal of Endocrinology, 70, 439–444.

Radomski, M.W. and Bennett, P.B. (1970) Metabolic changes in man during short exposure to high pressure. Aerospace Medicine, 41, 309–313.

Raimondi, G.A., Puy, R.J.M., Raimondi, A.C., Schwarz, E.R. and Rosenberg, M. (1975) Effects of physical training on enzymatic activity of human skeletal muscle. Biomedicine, 22, 496–501.

Ramcharan, S., Sponzilli, E.E. and Wingerd, J.C. (1976) Serum protein fractions: effects of oral contraceptives and pregnancy. Obstetrics and Gynecology, 48, 211–215.

Rand, W.M., Young, V.R. and Scrimshaw, N.S. (1976) Change of urinary nitrogen excretion in response to low-protein diets in adults. American Journal of Clinical Nutrition, 29, 639–644.

Rao, P.N. and Zuspan, F.P. (1970) Urinary catecholamine excretion and basal body temperature alterations with oral contraceptives. Surgical Forum, 21, 412–413.

Rastogi, G.K. and Sawhney, R.C. (1976) Thyroid function in changing weather in a subtropical region. Metabolism, 25, 903–908.

Rayfield, E.J., Curnow, R.T., George, D.T. and Beisel, W.R. (1973) Impaired carbohydrate metabolism during a mild viral illness. New England Journal of Medicine, 289, 618–621.

Reinhold, J.G. (1975) Trace elements – a selective survey. Clinical Chemistry, 21, 476–500.

Reinken, L. (1973) Die Wirkung von Hydantoin und Succinimid aus den Vitamin B_6-Stoffwechsel. Clinica Chimica Acta, 48, 435–436.

Reiter, E.O. and Root, A.W. (1975) Hormonal changes of adolescence, Medical Clinics of North America, 59, 1289–1304.

Reynafarje, B. (1962) Myoglobin content and enzymatic activity of muscle and altitude adaptation. Journal of Applied Physiology, 17, 301–305.

Romero, J.C. and Hoobler, S.W. (1970) The renin-angiotensin system in clinical medicine. American Heart Journal, 80, 701–708.

Roos, B.-E. and Silfverskiöld, B.P. (1973) Homovanillic acid in cerebrospinal fluid of alcoholics. New England Journal of Medicine, 288, 1358.

Rose, L.I., Bousser, J.E. and Cooper, K.H. (1970) Serum enzymes after marathon running. Journal of Applied Physiology, 29, 355–357.

Rosenauerová-Ostrá, A., Hilgertová, J. and Sonka, J. (1976) Urinary formiminoglutamate in man. Clinica Chimica Acta, 73, 39–43.

Rosensweig, N.S. (1975) Diet and intestinal adaptation: implications for gastrointestinal disorders. American Journal of Clinical Nutrition, 28, 648–655.

Roth, J., Glick, S.M., Yalow, R.S. and Berson, S.A. (1963) Secretion of human growth hormone: physiologic and experimental modification. Metabolism, 12, 577–579.

Rothschild, M.A., Kreek, M.J., Oratz, M., Schreiber, S.S. and Mongelli, J.G. (1976) The stimulation of albumin synthesis by methadone. Gastroenterology, 71, 214–220.

Rowe, D.S., Crabbé, P.A. and Turner, M.W. (1968) Immunoglobulin D in serum, body fluids and lymphoid tissues. Clinical and Experimental Immunology, 3, 477–490.

Rowell, L.B., Blackmon, J.R. and Bruce, R.A. (1964) Indocyanine green clearance and estimated hepatic blood flow during mild to maximal exercise in upright man. Journal of Clinical Investigation, 43. 1677–1690.

Sachar, E.J., Cobb, J.C. and Shor, R.E. (1966) Plasma cortisol changes during hypnotic trance. Relation to depth of hypnosis. Archives of General Psychiatry, 14, 482–490.

Sack, J., Fisher, D.A. and Wang, C.C. (1976) Serum thyrotropin, prolactin, and growth hormone levels during the early neonatal period in the human infant. Journal of Pediatrics, 89, 298–300.

Sacks, F.M., Castelli, W.P., Donner, A. and Kass, E.H. (1975) Plasma lipids and lipoproteins in vegetarians and controls. New England Journal of Medicine, 292, 1148–1151.

Sagone, A.L., Jr., Lawrence, A. and Balcerzak, S.P. (1973) Effect of smoking on tissue oxygen supply. Blood, 41, 845–851.

Saleh, A.E. and Coenegracht, J.M. (1968) The influence of age and weight on the urinary excretion of hydroxyproline and calcium. Clinica Chimica Acta, 21, 445–452.

Sandberg, H., Roman, L., Zavodnick, J. and Kupers, N. (1973) The effect of smoking on serum somatotropin, immunoreactive insulin and blood glucose levels of young adult males. Journal of Pharmacology and Experimental Therapeutics, 184, 787–791.

Sassard, J., Vincent, M., Annat, G. and Bizollon, C.A. (1976) A kinetic study of plasma renin and aldosterone during changes of posture in man. Journal of Clinical Endocrinology and Metabolism, 42, 20–27.

Saunders, S.J., Truswell, A.S., Barbezat, G.O., Wittman, W. and Hansen, J.D.L. (1967) Plasma free amino acid pattern in protein-calorie malnutrition. Reappraisal of its diagnostic value. Lancet, II, 795–797.

Savage, D.C.L., Forsyth, C.C., McCafferty, E. and Cameron, J. (1975) The excretion of individual adrenocortical steroids during normal childhood and adolescence. Acta Endocrinologica, 79, 551–567.

Schachner, S.H., Wieland, R.G., Maynard, D.E., Kruger, F.A. and Hamwi, G.J. (1965) Alterations in adrenal cortical function in fasting obese subjects. Metabolism, 14, 1051–1058.

Schalch, D.S. (1967) The influence of physical stress and exercise on growth hormone and insulin secretion in man. Journal of Laboratory and Clinical Medicine, 69, 256–269.

Schenker, J.G., Ben-David, M. and Polishuk, W.Z. (1975) Prolactin in normal pregnancy: relationship of maternal, fetal, and amniotic fluid levels. American Journal of Obstetrics and Gynecology, 123, 834–838.

Schroeder, H.A. and Nason, A.P. (1971) Trace element analysis in clinical chemistry. Clinical Chemistry, 17, 461–473.

Schroeder, H.A. and Tipton, I.H. (1968) The human body burden of lead. Archives of Environmental Health, 17, 965–978.

Schwartz, U.D. and Abraham, G.E. (1975) Corticosterone and aldosterone levels during the menstrual cycle. Obstetrics and Gynecology, 45, 339–342.

Scott, R., Paterson, P.J., Mills, E.A., McKirdy, A., Fell, G.S., Ottoway, J.M., Husain, F.E.R., Fitzgerald-Finch, O.P., Yates, A.J., Lamont, A. and Roxburgh, S. (1976) Clinical and biochemical abnormalities in coppersmiths exposed to cadmium. Lancet, II, 396–398.

Scriver, C.R. and Rosenberg, L.E. (1973) Amino Acid Metabolism and its Disorders. Saunders, Philadelphia, Pa.

Sealey, J.E., Moon, C., Laragh, J.H. and Alderman, M. (1976) Plasma prorenin: Cryoactivation and relationship to renin substrate in normal subjects. American Journal of Medicine, 61, 731–738.

Seltzer, C.C. and Mayer, J. (1963) Serum iron and iron-binding capacity in adolescents. II. Comparison of obese and nonobese subjects. American Journal of Clinical Nutrition, 13, 354–361.

Selye, H. (1976) Stress in Health and Disease. Butterworth, Boston, Mass.

Senay, L.C., Mitchell, D. and Wyndham, C.H. (1976) Acclimatization in a hot, humid environment: body fluid adjustments. Journal of Applied Physiology, 40, 786–796.

Shaw, S., Stimmel, B. and Lieber, C.S. (1976) Plasma alpha-amino-*n*-butyric acid to leucine ratio: an empirical biochemical marker of alcoholism. Science, 194, 1057–1058.

Skinner, S.L. (1961) A cause of erroneous potassium levels. Lancet, I, 478–480.

Smals, A.G.H., Kloppenborg, P.W.C. and Benraad, T.J. (1976) Circannual cycle in plasma testosterone levels in man. Journal of Clinical Endocrinology and Metabolism, 42, 979–982.

Smith, J.C., Jr., Zeller, J.A., Brown, E.D. and Ong, S.C. (1976) Elevated plasma zinc: a heritable anomaly. Science, 193, 496–498.

Smith, K.D., Tcholakian, R.K., Chowdhury, M. and Steinberger, E. (1976) An investigation of plasma hormone levels before and after vasectomy. Fertility and Sterility, 27, 145–151.

Smith, S.R., Posefsky, T. and Chhetri, M.K. (1974) Nitrogen and amino acid metabolism in adults with protein-calorie malnutrition. Metabolism, 23, 603–618.

Sokoloff, B., Hori, M., Saelhol, C.C., Wrzolek, T. and Imai, T. (1966) Aging, atherosclerosis and ascorbic acid metabolism. Journal of the American Geriatric Society, 14, 1239–1260.

Sollberger, A. (1975) Rhythmic changes in clinical laboratory values. CRC Critical Reviews in Clinical Laboratory Sciences, 6, 247–285.

Solomon, S.S., Ensinck, J.W. and Williams, R.H. (1968) Effects of starvation on plasma immunoreactive insulin and non-suppressible insulin-like activity in normal and obese humans. Metabolism, 17, 528–534.

Song, C.S., Merkatz, I.R., Rifkind, A.B., Gillette, P.N. and Kappas, A. (1970) The influence of pregnancy and oral contraceptive steroids on the concentration of plasma proteins. American Journal of Obstetrics and Gynecology, 108, 227–231.

Song, S.K. and Rubin, E. (1972) Ethanol produces muscle damage in human volunteers. Science, 175, 327–328.

Stanbury, S.W. and Thomson, A.E. (1951) Diurnal variations in electrolyte excretion. Clinical Science, 10, 267–293.

Statland, B.E., Bokelund, H. and Winkel, P. (1974) Factors contributing to intra-individual variation of serum constituents. 4. Effects of posture and tourniquet application on variation of serum constituents in healthy subjects. Clinical Chemistry, 20, 1513–1519.

Statland, B.E., Winkel, P. and Bokelund, H. (1973) Serum alkaline phosphatase after fatty meals: the effect of substrate on the assay procedure. Clinica Chimica Acta, 49, 299–300.

Steinmetz, J., Panek, E., Sourieau, F. and Siest, G. (1973) Influence of food intake on biological parameters. In Reference Values in Human Chemistry. (Ed. G. Siest) p. 193, Karger, Basel.

Stengle, J.M. and Schade, A.L. (1957) Diurnal-nocturnal variations of certain blood constituents in normal human subjects. British Journal of Haematology, 3, 117–124.

Stoner, H.B. and Heath, D.F. (1973) The effects of trauma on carbohydrate metabolism. British Journal of Anaesthesia, 45, 244–251.

Straus, E., Urbach, H.J. and Yalow, R.S. (1975) Alcohol-stimulated secretion of immunoreactive secretion. New England Journal of Medicine, 293, 1031–1032.

Streeten, D.H.P., Conn, J.W., Louis, L.H., Fajans, S.S., Seltzer, H.S., Johnson, R.D., Gittler, R.D. and Dube, A.H. (1960) Secondary aldosteronism: metabolic and adrenocortical responses of normal men to high environmental temperatures. Metabolism, 9, 1071–1092.

Stubbe, P. and Wolf, H. (1971) The effect of stress on growth hormone, glucose and glycerol in newborn infants. Hormone and Metabolic Research, 3, 175–179.

Sukumaran, M. and Bloom, W.L. (1953) Influence of diet on serum alkaline phosphatase in rats and men. Proceedings of the Society of Experimental Biology and Medicine, 84, 631–634.

Surks, M.I., Beckwitt, H.J. and Chidsey, C.A. (1967) Changes in plasma thyroxine concentration and metabolism, catecholamine excretion and basal oxygen consumption in men during acute exposure to high altitude. Journal of Clinical Endocrinology and Metabolism, 27, 789–799.

Sutton, J.R., Jones, N.L. and Toews, C.J. (1976) Growth hormone secretion in acid-base alterations at rest and during exercise. Clinical Science and Molecular Medicine, 50, 241–247.

Sutton, J.R., Young, J.D., Lazarus, L., Hickie, J.B. and Maksyvtis, J. (1969) The hormonal response to physical exercise. Australasian Annals of Medicine, 18, 84–90.

Sutton, J.R., Young, J.D., Lazarus, L., Hickie, J.B., Garmendia, F. and Velasquez, T. (1970) Hormonal response to altitude. Lancet, II, 1194.

Tanner, J.M. and Gupta, D. (1968) A longitudinal study of urinary excretion of individual steroids in children from 8 to 12 years old. Journal of Endocrinology, 41, 139–156.

Tedeschi, C.G. (1973) Circadian challenges in "quality control". Human Pathology, 4, 281–287.

Terjung, R.L. and Tipton, C.M. (1971) Plasma thyroxine and thyroid-stimulating hormone levels during submaximal exercise in humans. American Journal of Physiology, 220, 1840–1845.

Tewksbury, D.A. and Lohrenz, F.N. (1970) Circadian rhythm of human urinary amino acid excretion in fed and fasted states. Metabolism, 19, 363–371.

Theorell, T. and Åkerstedt, T. (1976) Day and night work: changes in cholesterol, uric acid, glucose and potassium in serum and in circadian patterns of urinary catecholamine excretion. Acta Medica Scandinavica, 200, 47–53.

Thomas, C.B., Holljes, H.W.D. and Eisenberg, F.F. (1961) Observations on seasonal variations in total serum cholesterol level among healthy young prisoners. Annals of Internal Medicine, 54, 413–430.

Thomas, S. (1957) Some effects of change of posture on water and electrolyte excretion by the human kidney. Journal of Physiology (London), 139, 337–352.

Thomas, S. (1959) Effects of change of posture on the diurnal renal excretory rhythm. Journal of Physiology (London), 148, 489–506.

Thomson, W.H.S., Sweetin, J.C. and Hamilton, I.J.D. (1975) ATP and muscle enzyme efflux after physical exertion. Clinica Chimica Acta, 59, 241–245.

Turton, C.W.G., Stanley, P., Stamp, T.C.B. and Maxwell, J.D. (1977) Altered vitamin-D metabolism in pregnancy. Lancet, I, 222–225.

Tweeddale, P.M., Leggett, R.J.E. and Flenley, D.C. (1976) Effect of age on oxygen-binding in normal human subjects. Clinical Science and Molecular Medicine, 51, 185–188.

Unger, R.H., Eisentraut, A.M. and Madison, L.L. (1963) The effects of total starvation upon the levels of circulating glucagon and insulin in man. Journal of Clinical Investigation, 42, 1031–1039.

Van Beaumont, W., Strand, J.C., Petrofsky, J.S., Hipskind, S.G. and Greenleaf, J.E. (1973) Changes in total plasma content of electrolytes and proteins with maximal exercise, Journal of Applied Physiology, 34, 102–106.

Van Thiel, D.H., Gavaler, J.S., Lester, R., Loriaux, D.L. and Braunstein, G.D. (1975) Plasma estrone, prolactin, neurophysin and sex steroid binding globulin in chronic alcoholic men. Metabolism, 24, 1015–1019.

Varma, M.M., Varma, R.R., Johanson, A.J., Kowarski, A. and Migeon, C.J. (1975) Long-term effects of vasectomy on pituitary-gonadal function in man. Journal of Clinical Endocrinology and Metabolism, 40, 868–871.

Vaughan, R.W., Bauer, S. and Wise, L. (1975) Volume and pH of gastric juice in obese patients. Anesthesiology, 43, 686–689.

Verdy, M. and de Champlain, J. (1968) Fasting in obese females: II. Plasma renin activity and urinary aldosterone. Canadian Medical Association Journal, 98, 1034–1037.

Verjee, Z.H. and Behal, R. (1976) Protein-calorie malnutrition: a study of red blood cell and serum enzymes during and after crisis. Clinica Chimica Acta, 70, 139–147.

Vernikos-Danellis, J., Leach, C.S., Winget, C.M., Goodwin, A.L. and Rambaut, P.C. (1976) Changes in glucose, insulin, and growth hormone levels associated with bed rest. Aviation, Space and Environmental Medicine, 47, 583–587.

Viktora, J.K., Johnson, B.F., Penhos, J.C., Rosenberg, C.A. and Wolff, F.W. (1969) Effect of ingested mannoheptulose in animals and man. Metabolism, 18, 87–102.

Viteri, F.E. and Arroyave, G. (1973) Protein calorie malnutrition. In Modern Nutrition in Health and Disease. (Eds. R.S. Goodhart and M.E. Shils) 5th edition, Lea and Febiger, Philadelphia. Pa.

Vogt, F.B. and Johnson, P.C. (1967) Plasma volume and extracellular fluid volume change associated with 10 days bed recumbency. Aerospace Medicine, 38, 21–25.

von Berger, L., Henrichs, I., Raptis, S., Heinze, E., Jonatha, W., Teller, W.M. and Pfeiffer, E.F. (1976) Gastrin concentration in plasma of the neonate at birth and after the first feeding. Pediatrics, 58, 264–267.

Wadsworth, G.L., Halberg, F., Albrecht, P. and Skaff, G. (1957) Peak urinary excretion of 5-hydroxyindoleacetic acid following arousal in human beings. Physiologist, 1, 86.

Wald, N. and Howard, S. (1975) Variations in carboxyhaemoglobin levels in smokers. British Medical Journal, I, 393.

Wald, N., Idle, M. and Smith, P.G. (1977) Carboxyhaemoglobin levels in smokers of filter and plain cigarettes. Lancet, I, 110–112.

Wannemacher, R.W., Jr., Klainer, A.S., Dinterman, R.E. and Beisel, W.R. (1976) The significance and mechanism of an increased serum phenylalanine-tyrosine ratio during infection. American Journal of Clinical Nutrition, 29, 997–1006.

Webster, J.B., Coupal, J.J. and Cushman, P., Jr. (1973) Increased serum thyroxine levels in euthyroid narcotic addicts. Journal of Clinical Endocrinology, 37, 928–934.

Weeke, J. and Hansen, A.P. (1975) Serum TSH and serum T_3 levels during normal menstrual cycles and during cycles on oral contraceptives. Acta Endocrinologica, 79, 431–438.

Weidmann, P., De Myttenaere-Bursztein, S., Maxwell, M.H. and de Lima, J. (1975) Effect of aging on plasma renin and aldosterone in normal man. Kidney International, 8, 325–333.

Weinshilboum, R.M., Raymond, F.A., Elveback, L.R. and Weidman, W.H. (1974) Correlation of erythrocyte catechol-*O*-methyl-transferase activity between siblings. Nature, 252, 490–491.

Weinsier, R.L. (1971) Fasting – a review with emphasis on the electrolytes. American Journal of Medicine, 50, 233–240.

Weitzman, E.D. (1976) Circadian rhythms and episodic hormone secretion. Annual Review of Medicine, 27, 225–243.

Werkman, H.P.T., Trijbels, J.M.F. and Schretlen, E.D.A.M. (1974) The short-term iron rhythm. Clinica Chimica Acta, 53, 65–68.

Wesson, L.G., Jr. (1964) Electrolyte excretion in relation to diurnal cycles of renal function. Medicine, 43, 547–592.

Westgren, U., Burger, A., Ingemansson, S., Melander, A., Tibblin, S. and Wahlin, E. (1976) Blood levels of 3,5,3′-triiodothyronine and thyroxine: differences between children, adults and elderly subjects. Acta Medica Scandinavica, 200, 493–495.

Wetterberg, L., Arendt, J., Paunier, L., Sizonenko, P.C., Van Donselaar, W. and Heyden, T. (1976) Human serum melatonin changes during the menstrual cycle. Journal of Clinical Endocrinology and Metabolism, 42, 185–188.

Widdowson, E.M. and McCance, R.A. (1951) The effect of undernutrition and of posture on the volume and composition of the body fluids. Special Reports Series, Medical Research Council, London, 275, 165–174.

Wilding, P., Rollason, J.G. and Robinson, D. (1972) Patterns of change for various biochemical constituents detected in well population screening. Clinica Chimica Acta, 41, 375–387.

Williams, G.Z. (1967) Individuality of clinical biochemical patterns in preventive health maintenance. Journal of Occupational Medicine, 9, 567–570.

Williams, J.R.B., Griffin, J.P. and Parkins, A. (1976) Effect of concomitantly administered drugs on the control of long term anticoagulant therapy. Quarterly Journal of Medicine, 45, 63–76.

Williams, R.J. (1956) Biochemical Individuality. Wiley, New York.

Wiltink, W.F., Kruithof, J., Mol, C., Bos, G. and Van Eijk, H.G. (1973) Diurnal and nocturnal variations of the serum iron in normal subjects. Clinica Chimica Acta, 49, 99–104.

Winitz, M., Seedman, D.A. and Graff, J. (1970) Studies in metabolic nutrition employing chemically defined diets. I. Extended feeding of normal human adult males. American Journal of Clinical Nutrition, 23, 525–545.

Winkelman, J.W., Cannon, D.C., Pileggi, V.J. and Reed, A.H. (1973) Estimation of norms from a controlled sample survey. II. Influence of body habitus, oral contraceptives, and other factors on values for the normal range derived from the SMA 12/60 screening group of tests. Clinical Chemistry, 19, 488–491.

Woodard, H.Q. (1959) The clinical significance of serum acid phosphatase. American Journal of Medicine, 27, 902–910.

Wurtman, R.J., Rose, C.M., Chou, C. and Larin, F.F. (1968) Daily rhythms in the concentrations of various amino acids in human plasma.New England Journal of Medicine, 279, 171–175.

Yang, M.-U. and Van Itallie, T.B. (1976) Composition of weight lost during short-term weight reduction. Journal of Clinical Investigation, 58, 722–730.

Young, D.S., Epley, J.A. and Goldman, P. (1971) Influence of a chemically defined diet on the composition of serum and urine. Clinical Chemistry, 17, 765–773.

Young, D.S., Pestaner, L.C. and Gibberman, V. (1975) Effects of drugs on clinical laboratory tests. Clinical Chemistry, 21, 1D-432D.

Young, V.R., Haverberg, L.N., Bilmazes, C. and Munro, H.N. (1973) Potential use of 3-methylhistidine excretion as an index of progressive reduction in muscle protein catabolism during starvation. Metabolism, 22, 1429–1436.

Yuen, B.H., Wittman, B. and Staley, K. (1976) Cyclic adenosine 3′,5′-monophosphate (cAMP) in pregnancy body fluids during normal and abnormal pregnancy. American Journal of Obstetrics and Gynecology, 125, 597–602.

Ziegler, M.G., Lake, C.R. and Kopin, I.J. (1976a) Plasma noradrenaline increases with age. Nature, 261, 333–335.

Ziegler, M.G., Lake, C.R., Wood, J.H. and Ebert, M.H. (1976b) Circadian rhythm in cerebrospinal fluid noradrenaline of man and monkey. Nature, 264, 656–658.

Zonana, J. and Rimoin, D.L. (1976) Inheritance of diabetes mellitus. New England Journal of Medicine, 295, 607.

FURTHER READING

Albrink, M.J. (1974) Overnutrition and the fat cell. In Duncan's Diseases of Metabolism. (Eds. P.K. Bondy and L.E. Rosenberg) seventh ed., p. 417, Saunders, Philadelphia, Pa.

Beisel, W.R. (1975) Metabolic response to infection. Annual Reviews of Medicine, 26, 9–20.

Briggs, M. (1976) Biochemical effects of oral contraceptives. Advances in Steroid Biochemistry and Pharmacology, 5. 65–160.

Cahill, G.F., Jr. (1976) Starvation in man. Clinics in Endocrinology and Metabolism, 5, 397–415.
Cuthbertson, D.P. (1964) Physical injury and its effect on protein metabolism. In Mammalian Protein Metabolism (Eds. H.N. Munro and J.B. Allison) pp. 373–414, Academic Press, New York.
Cuthbertson, D.P. and Tilstone, W.J. (1969) Metabolism during the postinjury period. Advances in Clinical Chemistry, 12, 1–55.
De Groot, L.J. and Stanbury, J.B. (1975) The Thyroid and Its Disorders, 4th edition, Wiley, New York, N.Y.
Feigin, R.D. (1969) Blood and urine amino acid aberrations. American Journal of Diseases of Children, 117, 24–47.
Fessel, W.J. (1972) Hyperuricemia in health and disease. Seminars in Arthritis and Rheumatism, 1, 275–299.
Johns, M.W., Masterton, J.P., Paddle-Ledinek, J.E., Patel, Y.C., Winikoff, D. and Malinek, M. (1975) Variations in thyroid function and sleep in healthy young men. Clinical Science and Molecular Medicine, 49, 629–632.
Johnson, W.R. (1960) Science and Medicine of Exercise and Sports. Harper, New York.
Kawai, T. (1973) Clinical Aspects of the Plasma Proteins. Lippincott, Philadelphia, Pa.
Krzywicki, H.J., Consolazio, C.F., Matoush, L.O. and Johnson, H.L. (1968) Metabolic aspects of acute starvation; body composition changes. American Journal of Clinical Nutrition, 21, 87–97.
Lie-Injo, L.E., Ng, T. and Balakrishnan, S. (1974) Red cell enzymes in cord blood and plasma bilirubin levels in the first week of life. Clinica Chimica Acta, 50, 77–83.
Martin, H.F., Gudzinowicz, B.J. and Fanger, H. (1975) Normal Values in Clinical Chemistry: A Guide to Statistical Analysis of Laboratory Data. Dekker, New York.
Mendelson, J.H. (1970) Biologic concomitants of alcoholism. New England Journal of Medicine, 283, 24–32 and 71–81.
Olson, R.E. (1973) Nutrition and Alcoholism. In Modern Nutrition in Health and Disease (Eds. R.S. Goodhart and M.E. Shils), 5th edition, Lea and Febiger, Philadelphia, Pa.
Saudek, C.D. and Felig, P. (1976) The metabolic events of starvation. American Journal of Medicine, 60, 117–126.
Scriver, C.R. and Rosenberg, L.E. (1973) Amino Acid Metabolism and its Disorders. Saunders, Philadelphia, Pa.
Selye, H. (1976) Stress in Health and Disease. Butterworth, Boston, Mass.
Statland, B.E. and Winkel, P. (1977) Effects of preanalytical factors on the intraindividual variation of analytes in the blood of healthy subjects: consideration of preparation of the subject and time of venipuncture. CRC Critical Reviews in Clinical Laboratory Science, 8, 105–144.
Wesson, L.G., Jr. (1964) Electrolyte excretion in relation to diurnal cycles of renal function. Medicine, 43, 547–592.
Williams, R.H. (1974) Textbook of Endocrinology, 5th edition, Saunders, Philadelphia, Pa.
Williams, R.J. (1965) Biochemical Individuality, Wiley, New York.

Chapter 2

Chemical analysis of body fluids other than blood

William Z. Borer

National Institutes of Health, Clinical Chemistry Service, Clinical Pathology Department, Bethesda, MD 20014, U.S.A.

CONTENTS

2.1. INTRODUCTION

Few individuals are admitted to a hospital, or examined by a specialist physician, without having some chemical tests performed on their blood or urine. Generally these tests yield

Chemical diagnosis of disease, edited by S.S. Brown, F.L. Mitchell and D.S. Young

quantitative data, but in some instances only qualitative determinations are possible. Laboratory tests are sometimes used to establish the diagnosis of a disease, but are used more often to confirm a physician's clinical impressions. They may also be used to gauge the severity of a disease, or to monitor its progress. Assessment of a patient's response to treatment and the monitoring of drug concentrations are additional uses of laboratory determinations.

At best, the measurement of the concentrations of compounds in body fluids provides an indirect indication of the metabolic processes within the body. The non-cellular part of the blood (plasma or serum) is the most commonly examined fluid. However, this is primarily a transport medium that conveys nutrients to the actively metabolizing cells and removes their metabolites for further processing or excretion. The plasma is also involved in the regulation of physiological processes. Its composition and volume influence the actions of other organ systems which, in turn, maintain the metabolic homoeostasis of the entire body.

Besides plasma or serum, a number of other body fluids may be submitted for analysis, depending on the clinical circumstances. In this chapter, the chemical analysis of body fluids other than blood, plasma or serum is addressed, with particular emphasis on tests which provide the most useful clinical information. In addition there is discussion of several tests which have shown diagnostic potential, but which have not yet gained widespread clinical acceptance. Many of these chemical determinations provide data which are interpreted together with the results of microbial culture, cell counts, and cytology so as to reach the appropriate clinical decision.

2.2. FLUIDS OF THE CENTRAL NERVOUS SYSTEM AND SPECIAL SENSES

2.2.1. Cerebrospinal fluid (CSF)

Cerebrospinal fluid is analyzed by the laboratory less commonly than is blood or urine. The findings, however, may be of importance in the diagnosis of disorders of the central nervous system, such as infection or haemorrhage. CSF production is closely regulated by the choroid plexus lying within the lateral ventricles, which are fluid-filled spaces deep within the brain substance (Milhorat, 1976). From the ventricles, the CSF follows a tortuous route, flowing through tiny canals and openings to the cisterns surrounding the cerebellum. It then passes upward over the outer surface of the cerebrum in the subarachnoid space where it is reabsorbed by the arachnoid villi. That portion of the CSF that flows downward in the spinal canal is thought to be reabsorbed via the capillaries and lymphatics which supply the spinal nerves.

There is little doubt that one of the major functions of the CSF is protective; the central nervous system is, in effect, cushioned by the fluid which surrounds it. The delicate nervous tissues are thus protected from the effects of sudden external shocks to the skull and spine. A second, but less clearly defined, function of the CSF involves the maintenance of a precise hydrostatic and chemical milieu surrounding the central nervous system. The circular flow suggests a lymphatic role for CSF by which both soluble and particulate debris may be removed from metabolically active tissue. Recent observations point to a possible neuroendocrine role for the CSF, in which it functions as a transport system for biogenic amines affecting pituitary function (Milhorat, 1975).

In the normal adult, the total volume of CSF bathing the central nervous system is about 150 ml. In a single day, 800 to 900 ml are produced and reabsorbed. The rate of absorption varies directly with the CSF pressure, which normally lies between 5 and 14 torr (0.67 and 1.86 kPa). The production of CSF is thought to be a resultant of the processes of ultrafiltration and active transport. A key role in chemical homoeostasis is held by the choroid plexus which mediates complex ionic exchanges between blood and CSF. Homeostasis is further enforced by the so-called blood–brain and blood–CSF barriers (Guyton et al., 1975). These barriers prevent the passage of ionic species and large molecules, but are permeable to lipid-soluble substances such as carbon dioxide, alcohol, and anaesthetic agents.

The CSF specimen is usually obtained on the medical or surgical ward by lumbar puncture. This procedure involves the insertion of a narrow gauge spinal needle into the lumbar subarachnoid space, under local anaesthesia and with aseptic technique (Blount et al., 1974). Ventricular or cisternal fluid may be obtained during a specialized radiological or neurosurgical procedure. The fresh CSF is then transported to the laboratory, usually in three tubes kept separate for differential cell counts, cultures, and chemical analyses.

A CSF specimen which is sent for glucose analysis must either be preserved with fluoride or analyzed immediately. A separate fluoride-preserved blood specimen drawn at the time of lumbar puncture should also be sent for glucose determination, because glucose enters the CSF from the blood via a carrier transport system which is dependent upon the glucose concentration in the plasma. For example, bacterial meningitis is often associated with a decreased CSF glucose concentration. If, however, a patient has both hyperglycaemia and meningitis, the CSF glucose concentration may appear to be normal unless it is compared with the concomitant plasma glucose concentration (Thompson et al., 1975). The CSF glucose concentration is normally about 60 to 80% of the plasma glucose concentration (Greenawald et al., 1973). This proportion decreases with worsening hyperglycaemia, i.e. a plasma glucose concentration above 16.7 mmol/litre (300 mg/dl). The CSF glucose concentration follows the plasma glucose concentration with a lag period of about 1 or 2 hours; this becomes important if the plasma glucose is changing rapidly. Under these circumstances a low CSF glucose could be a reflection of earlier hypoglycaemia (Calabrese, 1976). Low CSF glucose concentration is often – but not always – seen with the bacterial meningitides, especially tuberculosis. Other possible causes include central nervous system sarcoidosis, meningeal carcinomatosis, and subarachnoid haemorrhage.

The composition of the CSF reflects the balance of multiple physiological processes. This is illustrated by variability in protein concentration: because of the barriers to the passage of protein, its concentration in the CSF is less than 1% of the concentration in serum. The specific CSF protein concentration depends upon the sampling site. Lower protein concentrations are found in ventricular and cisternal fluid than in lumbar fluid. Knowledge of the source of the CSF sample is, therefore, mandatory for the correct interpretation of protein concentration. Very high CSF protein concentrations are seen with tuberculous meningitis and with Guillain–Barré syndrome. Moderate increases are characteristic of bacterial meningitis, while viral illness may produce only a small increase. Subarachnoid haemorrhage and tissue trauma occurring at the time of lumbar puncture may also increase the CSF protein concentration, as a result of the spillage of plasma proteins into the CSF.

If tumour, demyelinating disease or syphilis of the central nervous system is suspected, the physician is likely to request that protein fractionation studies be done on the CSF. The collodial gold test of Lange has now been supplanted by quantitative immunoglobulin determinations and, in some cases, by protein electrophoresis on polyacrylamide gel. Tumours of the central nervous system, whether benign or malignant, usually produce an elevation in total protein concentration with increased α_1- and γ-globulins (Bartko et al., 1970). Demyelinating diseases, such as multiple sclerosis, may produce changes in CSF γ-globulin with little or no increase in total protein. These changes are most pronounced in those patients whose disease is the most debilitating (Laterre et al., 1970). Unfortunately, this means that during the earliest stages of the disease – when diagnosis is most difficult – the CSF γ-globulin may be normal. Conversely, an elevated γ-globulin concentration is not specific for multiple sclerosis, but if the γ_3 and γ_4 fractions are increased on polyacrylamide gel electrophoresis, this strongly suggests that multiple sclerosis is the correct diagnosis (Clausen et al., 1969).

CSF enzymology has found minimal clinical application, mainly because of its limited diagnostic specificity. Plasma enzymes do not pass into the CSF: therefore, increased CSF enzyme activities are the result of tissue destruction, tumour growth, or infection. This is discussed in several reviews (Gilland, 1971). CSF aldolase activity is reported to be elevated in cases of tuberculous and bacterial meningitis, but not in cases of viral infections of the central nervous system (Sherlin, 1969). Carcinoma which has metastasized to the central nervous system may produce increases in lactate dehydrogenase and aspartate aminotransferase activities. Increased activities of these enzymes have not been found in the CSF of patients with benign primary intracranial tumours (Davies-Jones, 1969).

Biogenic amine metabolites such as 5-hydroxyindoleacetic acid and homovanillic acid (Chapter 24) have been studied in the CSF of both animals and man (Moir et al., 1970). While it is likely that the CSF concentrations of these substances can give information about brain metabolism, conclusions must be drawn with caution because of the complex relationship between cerebral metabolism and CSF transport. CSF concentrations of monoamine metabolites have been measured in a number of neurologic and psychiatric diseases including schizophrenia, depression, Parkinson's and Alzheimer's diseases (Gilland, 1971). The pituitary hormones, corticotrophin, growth hormone, thyrotrophin, prolactin, luteinizing hormone and follicle stimulating hormone have been measured in the CSF of patients with pituitary tumours. The concentration of one or more of these hormones is increased in 95% of those patients who had extension of the tumour above the diaphragma sellae. In addition, the investigators found that serial measurement of the hormones is of value in monitoring patients' response to therapy (Jordon et al., 1976).

Electrolyte concentrations and acid–base balance in the CSF play crucial roles in the maintenance of homeostasis, not only of the central nervous system, but of the entire body, and tables of normal values for these substances have been compiled (Shapiro,

1975; Krieg, 1974). For practical reasons, CSF electrolyte concentrations are rarely determined in clinical practice. CSF chloride may still be measured occasionally in suspected cases of meningitis, but lack of diagnostic specificity limits the usefulness of this test. Potassium, sodium and calcium concentrations affect the excitability of nervous tissue and modulate such vital functions as respiration and hydration. In most clinical circumstances, however, the plasma concentration adequately serves to monitor these electrolytes.

The acid–base composition of the CSF is at least as critical as the concentrations of the electrolytes. The bicarbonate concentration in the CSF is about the same as that of arterial whole blood, but the hydrogen ion concentration and the pCO_2 are both slightly higher (Shapiro, 1975). Because of the low protein concentration and the absence of erythrocytes, the CSF is rather poorly buffered in comparison with whole blood. This leads to technical problems in the accurate measurement of CSF pH and pCO_2. Nonetheless, several meticulous investigators have made acid–base measurements in the CSF of patients with metabolic or respiratory disorders (Campkin et al., 1974; Plum and Siesjo, 1975). These studies demonstrated a lower pH in lumbar fluid than in cisternal fluid in nearly all cases. It must be remembered (Chapter 3) that carbon dioxide is lipid soluble, and therefore it easily penetrates the blood–brain barrier (Manheim et al., 1975). This means that changes in blood pCO_2 will result in rapid changes in the pCO_2 of CSF. Changes in CSF bicarbonate concentration may require several hours to reach a new equilibrium state. The mechanisms involved in the acid–base homeostasis of CSF continue to provide a challenge for the innovative and skilled investigator (Blayo et al., 1975; Forster et al., 1975).

2.2.2. Aqueous humour and vitreous humour

The aqueous humour is located in both the anterior chamber and the posterior chamber of the eye. It is formed at a rate of 3 to 5 μl/min from the surface of the highly vascular ciliary body. Although the mode of its secretion is not completely understood, it appears that processes of both active transport and ultrafiltration are involved (Green and Pederson, 1973; Bill, 1973). Aqueous humour flows from the site of its formation in the posterior chamber, past the periphery of the lens, through the pupil and into the anterior chamber where it is absorbed by a lattice work of trabeculae lying in the angle between the cornea and the iris. The intraocular pressure, which averages about 15 torr (2.0 kPa) in the normal eye, is maintained by the balance between formation and reabsorption of the aqueous humour (Guyton et al., 1975).

Because of the small total volume (about 300 μl in each eye) and because of technical problems in sampling, the chemical analysis of aqueous humour has remained primarily a tool of the investigator rather than of the clinician. Tables of the chemical composition of the intraocular fluids have been compiled from a number of sources (Altman and Dittmer, 1961; Maren, 1974). The electrolytes sodium, chloride, and bicarbonate have been of particular research interest because of their role in the formation of aqueous humour. Methods for the automated determination of electrolytes and total protein concentration in human aqueous humour have been described (Bessière et al., 1973). Ascorbic acid also has attracted the attention of physiologists. Ascorbate concentrations are

15 to 20 times higher in aqueous humour than in blood. The reason for the active transport of this vitamin into the intraocular fluids is unknown. There is, however, speculation that ascorbate may be an essential nutrient for normal lens metabolism, at least in some species (Cole, 1970). Wide variability in aqueous humour ascorbate concentration occurs among the various types of glaucoma. Metabolites of glycolysis have been studied in the aqueous humour in a group of patients with senile cataracts (Laursen and Lorentzen, 1974). Specimens of 70 to 200 μl were obtained at the time of surgery and the concentrations of glucose, pyruvate and citrate were measured. The investigators demonstrated a positive correlation between cataract density and concentration of citrate in aqueous humour.

Aminoacids are among the low molecular mass substances that have been measured in aqueous humour. Specimens for analysis were obtained from patients after the induction of general anaesthesia at the time of surgery. Fluid was withdrawn using a fine gauge micro-paracentesis needle. Statistically significant increases in the concentrations of six aminoacids (threonine, glutamine, proline, alanine, ornithine and lysine) were found in the aqueous humour of patients with intraocular malignant melanoma. Striking elevations in both proline and glycine concentrations were noted in those patients with uveitis (Durham et al., 1971).

The protein constituents of aqueous humour have been studied on the basis of their electrophoretic mobility (Praus, 1961). The technique involved labeling of the proteins with ^{131}I followed by paper electrophoresis. The albumin and globulin fractions were then quantitated by direct radioactive counting or by photometric scanning of an autoradiogram. An immunoelectrophoretic technique in agarose gel has been used to determine caeruloplasmin and transferrin concentrations in human aqueous humour (Zirm et al., 1975). With a similar technique, others have shown that the only lipoprotein which is detectable in aqueous humour is the α subfraction (Schmut and Zirm, 1974). This is because the large size of the lipoprotein molecule precludes its passage from the blood into the aqueous humour. The presence of complement components C1, C3, and C4 has been demonstrated by haemolytic assay, and immunoglobulin concentrations have been determined in a small number of patients with ocular disease (Chandler, 1974). As noted by these authors, the source and function of these proteins have not yet been determined.

The assay of lactate dehydrogenase (Chapter 7) in aqueous humour has some potential for clinical application. Increased serum lactate dehydrogenase activity in patients with cancer (Chapter 25) has prompted a number of investigators to measure this enzyme in the aqueous humour of patients with various intraocular tumours. One such study demonstrated a marked increase in lactate dehydrogenase of aqueous humour in eyes containing a retinoblastoma (Swartz et al., 1974). Another series showed no increase in activity in the aqueous humour of patients with intraocular malignant melanoma (Porter and Skillen, 1972). Isoenzymes of lactate dehydrogenase have also been studied in retinoblastoma (Kabak and Romano, 1975). The LD_5/LD_1 ratio is greater than 5 in the aqueous humour of affected eyes.

The vitreous humour (or vitreous body) occupies the major portion of the eye lying behind the iris. It is a gelatinous semi-solid matrix of water, collagen, and hydrated mucopolysaccharide. The vitreous fluid can be studied only after a surgical procedure or at necropsy. Tables of values for the concentrations of a number of biochemical constituents have been compiled (Altman and Dittmer, 1961; Cole, 1974). Chemical determinations on vitreous humour have found application in forensic pathology. The concentrations of many chemical constituents in blood change dramatically at the time of death and for the first few hours thereafter. The eye, however, is well isolated and anatomically protected. As a result, chemical analyses done on vitreous humour obtained postmortem have been found to be helpful in determining the cause and time of death (Coe, 1972).

2.2.3. Endolymph and perilymph

Detailed biochemical studies of the inner ear fluids, endolymph and perilymph, have been hampered by the extreme inaccessibility and the small total volume of these fluids. The perilymph is contained within the bony labyrinth in the temporal bone. The perilymph is connected with CSF through the cochlear aqueduct and maintains a biochemical composition which is nearly the same as CSF except that the protein concentration is 5 to 10 times higher in perilymph. There is, however, no evidence of fluid flow or free exchange between the CSF and perilymph (Maren, 1974).

The endolymph is contained within the membranous labyrinth which is cushioned by the perilymph within the bony labyrinth. The endolymph is in intimate contact with the highly specialized organs responsible for the perception of sound and the maintenance of equilibrium and posture. The total volume of the endolymph is about 3 μl. It differs markedly from the perilymph, especially in its electrolyte composition. The sodium and potassium concentrations of endolymph approximate to those of cytosol, with the potassium concentration ranging from 140 to 160 mmol/litre and the sodium concentration from 13 to 16 mmol/litre (Doutremepuich, 1975). The chloride content of the endolymph is about 110 mmol/litre. The high activity of carbonic anhydrase in the endolymphatic sac suggests that bicarbonate plays an important role in endolymph formation.

Perilymph composition has been studied in a number of disease states, both pre- and postmortem. Up to 350 μl may be obtained from a cadaver after removal of overlying bone. The fluid thus obtained has been used to measure ethanol, γ-globulin, and α_1-antitrypsin concentrations, and blood group antigens (Trela, 1975). Perilymph has also been obtained at the time of surgery by inserting a fine glass capillary through the oval window followed by withdrawal of up to 20 μl of fluid (Schindler and Schneider, 1966). A modification of this technique has been used to show that there is markedly increased protein concentration in the perilymph of patients with acoustic neurinoma (Silverstein, 1972). Oxygen tension has been measured in vivo using a polarographic micro-electrode with a tip having a diameter of less than 100 μm (Fisch et al., 1976).

2.3. EFFUSION

An effusion is a pathological collection of fluid in any of the potential spaces of the body, which include the pericardial sac, the pleural space, the peritoneal space, the bursae, and the joint spaces. A small amount of fluid is normally present in each of these spaces. This fluid, which is rich in mucin, acts as a lubricant which permits free movement of the viscera or articular surfaces of the joints within each of the potential spaces. A complex system of fluid dynamics prevents the collection of effusion under normal circumstances. The factors involved include colloid osmotic pressure of the plasma, capillary pressure and permeability, and lymphatic drainage (Guyton et al., 1975). An imbalance affecting any one of these factors may result in the development of an effusion. For example, infection or other inflammation may increase vascular permeability, or tumour may result in lymphatic obstruction. A specimen of the effusion is usually obtained by paracentesis. This involves the use of local anaesthesia and sterile technique to withdraw a fluid sample through a needle or catheter inserted into the effusion (Lowell, 1977; McCoy and Wolma, 1971).

2.3.1. Pleural effusion

The pleural space has been the subject of more physiologic studies than any other potential space. The normal pleural space contains a few millilitres of fluid with a protein concentration of 10 to 20 g/litre. Normal pleural fluid is almost impossible to obtain, hence extensive reference ranges have not been compiled. Water and solutes equilibrate rapidly across the membranes which line the potential spaces. As a result, the composition of normal pleural fluid is probably similar to that of interstitial fluid (Agostoni, 1972).

Microscopic examination of the cellular elements in a pleural effusion should always be a part of the laboratory analysis, especially when the diagnosis remains in doubt. A leucocyte count of greater than 1000 cells/mm^3 strongly suggests an infectious aetiology, but tumour is not ruled out. Polymorphonuclear leucocytes predominate in pyogenic infections, whereas large numbers of lymphocytes suggest that the effusion may be due to tuberculosis or lymphoma (Lowell, 1977). Cytologic examination of the pleural fluid reveals malignant cells in 60% of the cases in which the effusion is secondary to neoplasm. This is increased to 80% when the metastases are from carcinoma of the breast (Dines et al., 1975). If grossly blood-stained pleural fluid is obtained from a patient who has not experienced chest trauma, the chances are about two to one that he has a malignancy involving the pleura (Lowell, 1977).

The determination of total protein has replaced that of specific gravity in determining whether an effusion is an exudate or transudate. These two classes of effusion are fundamentally distinguished on a pathophysiologic basis. A transudate occurs with increased plasma osmotic pressure or increased capillary hydrostatic pressure. An exudate is the result of a disease which causes inflammation or irritation of the pleura leading to increased capillary permeability. Traditionally, a pleural fluid protein concentration of greater than 30 g/litre indicates an exudate and one of less than 30 g/litre, a transudate. Problems with misclassification have prompted others to classify as exudates those fluids with (a) a fluid/serum protein concentration ratio greater than 0.5; or (b) a fluid lactate dehydrogenase activity greater than 200 U/litre; or (c) a fluid/serum lactate dehydrogenase activity ratio greater than 0.6 (Light et al., 1972). This kind of distinction does not make a diagnosis, but it does add to the sum of clinical information which the physician may use to arrive at a diagnosis and to manage the patient.

Inflammatory diseases such as pneumonia, tuberculosis and rheumatoid arthritis, tend to produce pleural effusions with high total protein concentrations. This is also true for effusions caused by pulmonary infarction and by malignant neoplasm which has metastasized to the pleura. Uraemic pleural effusion may show increased total protein concentration and increased lactate dehydrogenase activity in the absence of infection or malignancy (Berger et al., 1975). Multiple myeloma involving the pleura has been reported to show increased total protein in the pleural fluid and a sharp spike in the γ-globulin region on protein electrophoresis (Safa and Van Ordstrand, 1973). Quantitative immunoglobulin and rheumatoid factor determinations have been of little value in detecting the cause of pleural effusions (Levine et al., 1968; Shallenberger and Daniel, 1972).

Clinical studies of pleural fluid enzymes have concentrated mainly on lactate dehydrogenase and amylase. Early reports suggested that increased total lactate dehydrogenase activity was an indicator of a malignant pleural effusion. Subsequent studies have demonstrated that this enzyme may help to distinguish exudate from transudate, but that it is of little value in determining the cause of the effusion (Chandrasekhar et al., 1969). Evaluation of the lactate dehydrogenase isoenzymes may, however, be of value in detecting a pleural effusion secondary to metastatic malignancy. Of 28 malignant pleural effusions studied, 14 showed LD_2 to be greater than 35%, or LD_5 to be less than 12%. This pattern was found in only one of 48 benign exudates. Total lactate dehydrogenase activity and isoenzyme patterns were essentially unchanged by the presence of intact erythrocytes in the pleural fluid (Light and Ball, 1973a).

Pleural effusion is associated with 5 to 10% of cases of pancreatitis. This effusion is usually left-sided, but may be bilateral (Miridjanian et al., 1969). It is nearly always characterized by a strikingly high amylase activity. Amylase is thought to enter the pleural space via the transdiaphragmatic lymphatic channels (Kaye, 1968). Among the other diseases which may be associated with increased amylase activity in pleural fluid are pancreatic pseudocyst, carcinoma of the pancreas and carcinomas of other organs (Light and Ball, 1973b). Rupture of the oesophagus with pleural effusion has also been reported (Bellman and Rajaratnam, 1974). In this case, the high amylase activity found in the pleural fluid is the result of salivary amylase which leaks into the pleural space through the perforation (Sherr et al., 1972).

Glucose concentration (Chapter 4), like protein concentration, may be helpful but not diagnostic in determining the cause of a pleural effusion. The glucose content of pleural fluid changes in response to fluctuations in plasma glucose concentration, again demonstrating the rapid equilibration which occurs between blood and pleural fluid (Russakoff et al., 1962). This means that the most appropriate specimen for measurement of glucose in pleural fluid is one which is obtained after an overnight fast. A glucose concentration greater than 5.3 mmol/litre (95 mg/dl) is nearly always associated with a transudate. The glucose concentration found in an exudate, however, is highly variable, depending to some degree on the disease process (Light and Ball, 1973b). Empyema, pneumonia, and malignancy all may be associated with a pleural fluid glucose concentration which is less than 3.3 mmol/litre (60 mg/dl) (Berger and Maher, 1971). A glucose concentration of less than 1.7 mmol/litre (30 mg/dl) is not uncommon in cases of pleural effusion caused by tuberculosis or rheumatoid arthritis (Lowell, 1977). In one series, 42% of the cases of rheumatoid pleural effusion were associated with a glucose content of less than 0.6 mmol/litre (10 mg/dl) (Lillington et al., 1971). It must be remembered, however, that there is much overlap in the glucose concentrations of fluids associated with various diseases. The clinician must always pursue a suspicious result with appropriate cultures, cytology and, if necessary, a pleural biopsy.

The pH of pleural fluid may be measured using the same technique as for arterial acid–base status. The specimen must be drawn anaerobically and it must be analyzed promptly. The pH range for pleural fluid is wide, but low values may be of diagnostic importance. For example, leakage of gastric fluid through a perforated oesophagus into the pleural space produces an effusion with a pH of less than 6 (Dye and Laforet, 1974). The pH of fluid from an empyema or parapneumonic effusion is commonly between 6 and 7 (Lowell, 1977). Pleural effusion is not likely to be associated with malignancy if the pH is less than 7.3; a pH greater than 7.4 militates against a diagnosis of tuberculosis (Light et al., 1973). Low pH (7.0 to 7.2) and high pCO_2 (60 to 70 mm Hg) are seen in pleural effusions associated with rheumatoid arthritis (Funahashi et al., 1971). A high lactate concentration may also be seen in rheumatoid effusions (Feagler et al., 1971).

Chylothorax refers to the presence of pleural fluid which is composed of lymph containing lipid droplets (chylomicrons, Chapter 5). This gives the fluid a milky or creamy appearance. Chylothorax is the result of lymphatic obstruction or laceration of the thoracic duct. This can occur in cases of mediastinal tumour or with chest trauma or surgery (Nix et al., 1957). Spontaneous chylothorax may also occur in the neonatal period. Congenital anomalies in the lymphatic system have been implicated as the cause (Peitersen and Jacobsen 1977). Cholesterol (pseudochylous) effusion may occur rarely in association with tumour or tuberculosis (Coe and Aikawa, 1961). The presence of cholesterol crystals imparts a satin sheen or opalescence to the fluid. The pathophysiology of the production of the fluid and of cholesterol is unknown.

The analysis of pleural fluid lipids has been used to distinguish chylothorax from cholesterol effusion. The creamy fluid of chylothorax can be cleared with an ether extraction, or the chylomicrons can be stained with Sudan III. A cholesterol effusion does not clear with ether, and characteristic cholesterol crystals are seen microscopically (Chandrasekhar and Buehler, 1974). The concentration of cholesterol in pleural fluid may range from 2.6 to 116 mmol/litre (100 to 4500 mg/dl). A few cases have been reported in which no cholesterol crystals are seen in the fluid and yet the cholesterol concentration is high (Matsuura et al., 1971). Lipoprotein electrophoresis has been used to confirm chylothorax. A heavy chylomicron band is seen at the origin of the electrophoretic pattern of fluid from a chylothorax; this is not present in pleural fluid originating from other causes (Seriff et al., 1977).

The concentration of orosomucoid (α_1-acid glycoprotein) has been studied in effusions of various aetiologies using a radial immunodiffusion technique (Rudman et al., 1974). The lowest concentrations are found in transudates; intermediate concentrations are associated with inflammatory exudates; and the highest concentrations are found in malignant exudates. Others have been able to detect no significant difference in orosomucoid concentration between malignant and inflammatory exudates (Agostoni and Marasini, 1977). Correlations between orosomucoid and β_2-microglobulin concentrations have been observed. The highest concentration of β_2-microglobulin is seen in effusions associated with lymphoma or autoimmune disorders (Vladutiu, 1976). It is possible that diagnostic discrimination might be improved if the concentrations of both proteins were determined on the same fluid.

Copper, zinc and iron concentrations in pleural fluid have been determined with the hope of finding a method of differentiating benign from malignant effusions. Pleural fluid copper shows correlations with pleural fluid protein and with serum copper. Unfortunately, the data are too widely scattered to provide any diagnostic information regarding the underlying disease in the individual patient (Dines et al., 1974).

2.3.2. Ascites

Ascites (peritoneal effusion) has much in common with pleural effusion. The aetiologies and underlying pathophysiology of formation of the effusions are similar. The clinical usefulness of the distinction between transudate and exudate is impaired when this is based upon the total protein concetration, which does not reliably discriminate between the two types of effusions. Again, it must be emphasized that the classification does not establish a diagnosis, but it may provide a clue as to the nature of the underlying disease process.

The protein concentration in ascites fluid has been evaluated in the study of several diseases. Ascites is commonly associated with hepatic cirrhosis. The total protein concentration in cirrhotic ascites varies widely; higher concentrations are seen in early cirrhosis and lower concentrations are characteristic of advanced cirrhosis (Witte et al., 1969). Protein concentrations ranging from 1 to 43 g/litre have been encountered in cirrhotic ascites (Sampliner and Iber, 1974). Tuberculous peritonitis almost always produces ascitic fluid with a protein concentration greater than 25 g/litre (Borhanmanesh et al., 1972). Consequently, fluids with high protein concentrations should always be examined and cultured for tubercle bacilli. Bacterial peritonitis may occur spontaneously with cirrhosis and ascites. The protein concentration in ascitic fluid is usually lower in bacterial peritonitis than in tuberculous peritonitis: the mean value in bacterial peritonitis is around 18 g/litre (Conn and Fessel, 1971). Cell counts and cultures of the fluid establish the diagnosis.

The removal of large quantities of fluid from patients with cirrhotic ascites is dangerous because shock or hyponatraemia may result. However, this is not a problem when the ascites is secondary to ovarian carcinoma, in which case paracentesis provides symptomatic relief. A study of both ascites fluid and serum showed that neither total protein nor albumin were significantly decreased even after multiple paracenteses (Cruikshank and Buchsbaum, 1973; Lifshitz and Buchsbaum, 1976). The protein concentration is very low (less than 7 g/litre) in the ascites fluid of a small proportion of patients with intra-abdominal malignancy: the portal venous system of these patients has been shown at surgery or necropsy to be obstructed by tumour mass (Witte et al., 1972).

Ascites occasionally occurs in patients with pancreatitis or following trauma to the pancreas. Total protein concentration in the fluid is greater than 30 g/litre in 70% of cases of pancreatic ascites. The amylase activity of the fluid is nearly always high, occasionally exceeding 20,000 Somogyi units (Donowitz et al., 1974). Other diseases in which the peritoneal fluid shows increased amylase activity are perforated duodenal ulcer and strangulated small bowel (Mansberger, 1964). The measurement of methaemalbumin in serum and ascites fluid may be helpful in distinguishing haemorrhagic from acute oedematous pancreatitis. This provides useful information regarding the prognosis of the disease, and it may alter the management of these cases (Geokas et al., 1974).

Ascites may occur in patients who are undergoing haemodialysis for treatment of chronic renal insufficiency, and the ascites fluid contained a protein concentration ranging from 33 to 54 g/litre in one series (Gutch et al., 1974). In many cases, the onset of ascites follows the use of peritoneal dialysis (Craig et al., 1974). Some patients show complete resolution of ascites following renal transplantation or even after exploratory laparotomy (Rodriguez et al., 1974). The pathogenesis of nephrogenic ascites awaits further elucidation.

Determination of the glucose concentration in ascites fluid may provide some diagnostic information. Tuberculous peritonitis – like tuberculous pleuritis – is frequently associated with a low glucose concentration in the fluid. This is occasionally found to be less than 1.7 mmol/litre (30 mg/dl) (Brown and Dac An, 1976). Others have examined larger series' of patients with ascites of varying aetiologies by measuring both plasma glucose and ascitic fluid glucose concentrations. The highest glucose concentrations were found in transudates associated with cirrhosis or congestive heart failure. The lowest glucose concentrations were found in exudates associated with diseases such as peritoneal carcinomatosis and tuberculous peritonitis. Considerable overlap was seen, but it is evident that disease processes which involve the peritoneum produce ascites fluid which contains lower glucose concentrations (Polak and Torres da Costa, 1973).

Chylous ascites occurs relatively rarely. The presence of chylomicrons, which cause the creamy appearance of the fluid, may be confirmed by microscopic or biochemical methods (section 2.3.1). The pathophysiology involves the leakage or transudation of chyle from the lymphatic channels into the peritoneal space. A number of diseases may be associated with chylous ascites, including infection, malignancy, trauma and congenital anomalies of the lymphatic system (Nix et al., 1957; Tsuchiya et al., 1973). The origin of the lipids in the chylous ascites of patients with hepatic cirrhosis has been studied in detail (Malagelada et al., 1974). These patients appear to develop increased pressure in the intestinal lymphatic system, which results in abnormal permeability or rupture of the lymphatic ducts into the peritoneal cavity.

Extravasation of urine into the peritoneal cavity presents rarely as ascites. In the adult it may occur after trauma or surgery (Bourdeau et al., 1974). The diagnosis must be strongly entertained if the urea and creatinine concentrations in the fluid are higher than those in the serum (Singh et al., 1973). Passage of urine into the peritoneal cavity may occur in the neonate either spontaneously or following a difficult delivery (Gregory et al., 1975). Spontaneous bile duct perforation has also been reported in the neonate followed by the accumulation of bile-stained ascites (Howard et al., 1976). Another rare cause of ascites is the accumulation of cerebrospinal fluid in the peritoneal space after the placement of a ventriculoperitoneal shunt for treatment of hydrocephalus (Weidmann, 1975).

Recent advances in the surgical technique of peritoneoscopy have permitted the sampling of normal peritoneal fluid (Maathuis et al., 1973). The procedure is more complicated than simple paracentesis, and it is usually undertaken for exploratory purposes or for sterilization. Others have employed culdocentesis to obtain fluid specimens for chemical analysis (McGowan et al., 1973). These techniques have permitted the compilation of reference ranges for a number of biochemical constituents found in peritoneal fluid. Thus, cholesterol concentration was found to be markedly increased in the ascites fluid of patients with active ovarian carcinoma. Multifactorial analysis of peritoneal fluid has also been of value in the detection of recurrence of mesothelioma involving the peritoneum (McGowan et al., 1975). Realization of the full diagnostic potential of this approach awaits further study.

2.3.3. Pericardial effusion

Pericardial effusion may result in cardiac tamponade. This potentially fatal complication arises when the fluid accumulates very rapidly within the pericardial sac. Haemorrhage into the pericardium secondary to trauma or anticoagulant therapy is the most common cause of cardiac tamponade. Malignant neoplasm, autoimmune disease and infective pericarditis may, however, cause an effusion which accumulates rapidly enough to produce tamponade. Under these circumstances, aspiration of as little as 25 ml of fluid from the pericardium may be life saving (Fowler, 1976). After relief of the tamponade the cause of the effusion must then be established so that appropriate follow-up therapy may be instituted.

Not all pericardial effusions cause pericardial tamponade. Most effusions either resolve completely (e.g. idiopathic pericarditis) or accumulate slowly allowing expansion of the pericardial sac to accommodate the increasing volume. Few clinicians request the chemical analysis of pericardial fluid. Most biochemical tests are quite non-specific as indicators of the underlying disease process, but an exception is provided by data obtained from the study of pericardial effusion associated with autoimmune disorders.

Pericarditis with or without effusion occurs in 30 to 50% of patients with rheumatoid arthritis. The chemical composition of pericardial fluid obtained from patients with rheumatoid pericarditis is quite similar to that obtained from pleural and synovial effusions associated with rheumatoid arthritis (sections 2.3.1 and 2.3.4). A low glucose concentration – often less than 1.7 mmol/litre (30 mg/dl) – and a high total protein concentration are common to these fluids. Another feature of the fluid produced by rheumatoid pericarditis is the markedly elevated lactate dehydrogenase activity (Franco et al., 1972). γ-Globulin complexes have also been demonstrated in rheumatoid pericardial fluid (Ball et al., 1975). Low or absent haemolytic complement activity is found in the pericardial fluid associated with both rheumatoid disease and systemic lupus erythematosus (Franco et al., 1972; Goldenberg et al., 1975).

Chylopericardium and cholesterol pericarditis are rare conditions which may be associated with any one of a number of diseases. Cholesterol pericarditis is the term which has been applied to chronic pericardial effusions which contain high concentrations of cholesterol. It may be associated with hypothyroidism, tuberculosis, malignancy or rheumatoid arthritis (Brawley et al., 1966). Some cases arise spontaneously in patients who appear to be otherwise in good health. Lipid analysis of the fluid has been reported in only a few isolated cases. Analytical difficulties undoubtedly arise due to the turbidity of the fluid. A dense chylomicron band has been reported on lipoprotein electrophoresis of fluid from chylopericardium (Csanády and Kovács, 1973). Cholesterol concentration may be markedly increased – over 18.2 mmol/litre (700 mg/dl) – in the fluid associated with cholesterol pericarditis (Eisalo and Konttinen, 1972). However, cholesterol concentrations ranging from 2.6 to 5.2 mmol/litre (100 to 200 mg/dl) are more commonly seen in either chylopericardium or cholesterol pericarditis (Brawley et al., 1966; Lee et al., 1974).

2.3.4. Synovial effusion

The synovium lacks a distinct membrane of the type found in the pleural, peritoneal and pericardial spaces. The synovial lining is formed instead of loosely bound connective tissue cells which permit free exchange of water, ions and small molecules between the joint space and the blood (Guyton et al., 1975). Normal synovial fluid, which is present in small amounts in all of the joints, is essentially a dialysate of plasma. The synovial lining secretes hyaluronic acid which imparts a high viscosity and lubricating properties to the synovial fluid (Swann et al., 1974). The fluid specimen is obtained by needle aspiration of the joint space using local anaesthesia and careful aseptic technique (Scott, 1975). The knee is the joint which is aspirated most frequently. One reason for this may be that an effusion here is the most readily accessible.

As with the other effusions, the chemical analysis of synovial fluid is employed in conjuction with the appearance of the fluid, cell counts, microbial cultures and clinical information to provide diagnostic clues as to the nature of the underlying disorder (Rodnan, 1973). Inflammatory arthropathy is often associated with sufficient capillary permeability to permit the exudation of fibrinogen and other clotting factors into the effusion. Upon aspiration, this may result in the spontaneous formation of a clot the size of which is roughly proportional to the severity of the inflammation (Teloh, 1975). For this reason fluid which is to be examined for cell counts and crystals should be placed in a tube containing an anticoagulant such as EDTA or heparin. Potassium oxalate should be avoided for this purpose because oxalate crystals may produce a confusing microscopic artifact (Cracchiolo, 1971).

The clinical usefulness of both quantitative and qualitative chemical tests has been demonstrated in differentiating the various causes of a joint effusion. One of the favourite qualitative tests of the rheumatologist is the assessment of "mucin clot" formation. To perform this test, one part of synovial fluid is mixed with four parts of 2% acetic acid. The suspension is mixed rapidly with a glass rod and the results are interpreted promptly. Formation of a tight ropey mass in a clear solution is described as "good mucin clot" whereas a "poor mucin clot" shows fragmentation, causing the solution to become turbid (Cohen et al., 1975). This test depends upon the interaction of protein and hyaluronate in acid. The quality of the mucin clot may be assessed using as little as 0.5 μl of synovial fluid (Goldenberg et al., 1973). The viscosity of the fluid may be estimated by noting whether a "string" will form when a drop of fluid is expressed from a syringe or stretched between the thumb and forefinger. High quality normal hyaluronate results in the formation of a long (5 cm or more) string. If the molecular size is smaller, the fluid will be thin and watery, showing no tendency to form a string (Cracchiolo, 1971). Low viscosity fluid associated with poor mucin clot formation is characteristic of inflammatory joint diseases such as rheumatoid arthritis, septic arthritis and gout (Percy and Russell, 1975).

The determination of glucose concentration in joint fluid is often useful, and for this purpose specimens should be preserved with sodium oxalate and potassium fluoride. As with other effusions, glucose in the joint fluid equilibrates with that in blood. A lag period can be demonstrated between the two compartments if the blood glucose concentration is changing rapidly (Teloh, 1975). As a result, it is preferable, but not imperative, to aspirate the synovial fluid for glucose determination after an overnight fast. In any case, a concomitant blood specimen should be drawn so that plasma glucose may be determined for comparison (Cohen et al., 1975). A glucose concentration in synovial fluid which is nearly equal to that of plasma is characteristic of normal fluid or of non-inflammatory effusion such as that seen with degenerative joint disease. Inflammatory diseases such as rheumatoid arthritis may lower the glucose concentration to about 60% of that in plasma. The lowest levels (30 to 40% of the plasma concentration) are seen with the septic arthritides (Rodnan, 1973).

Microscopic examination of a wet smear of synovial fluid for crystals and sediment may make the diagnosis. The demonstration (Chapter 21) of needle-like monosodium urate crystals, engulfed by leucocytes, in the fluid from an acutely inflamed joint establishes the diagnosis of gout. Identification of calcium pyrophosphate dihydrate crystals is the most important criterion for the diagnosis of pseudogout (Rodnan, 1973). These crystals are recognized by their appearance and by their properties of birefringence when viewed using a polarizing microscope equipped with a first order red compensator (Phelps et al., 1968). An adequate polarizing microscope may be fabricated by fitting an ordinary light microscope with two inexpensive polarizing filters and a colour compensator constructed from cellophane tape (Fagan and Lidsky, 1974; Wild and Zvaifler, 1975). Cholesterol crystals or crystals of corticosteroid which have been previously injected into the joint capsule may also be seen; these, however, are quite different in appearance from urate or calcium pyrophosphate dihydrate crystals (Kitridou, 1972; Yehia and Duncan, 1975).

Other diagnostic clues may be found in the non-crystalline sediment in synovial fluid. Dark fragments floating in the specimen are suggestive of ochronosis (Schumacher and Holdsworth, 1977). Masses of tangled microscopic fibrils are often seen in fluid associated with the arthropathy of hypothyroidism. These fibrils, which are thought to contain collagen, show weak birefringence when viewed through a polarizing microscope (Dorwart and Schumacher, 1975). Amyloid arthropathy is a well-documented complication of multiple myeloma. The synovial fluid from these patients often shows fragments of amyloid which exhibit a green birefringence by polarizing light microscopy (Gordon et al., 1973); the diagnosis may be confirmed by staining with Congo red. Haemochromatosis is suggested if the phagocytic synovial fluid cells show a positive iron stain with Prussian blue (Schumacher, 1975).

McCarty (1974) and McCarty and Silcox (1973) have proposed the term "crystal deposition disease" to embrace both classic gout (monosodium urate deposition) and pseudogout or chondrocalcinosis (calcium pyrophosphate dihydrate deposition). This permits precise distinction between the two disorders based upon a final common biochemical pathway (Chapter 21). As a result, interest has been stimulated in the physical chemistry of calcium pyrophosphate crystallization (Brown and Gregory, 1976). Others have studied the concentration of inorganic pyrophosphate in patients with various arthritic conditions (Silcox and McCarty, 1974). As expected, the highest concentrations of pyrophosphate are found in the synovial fluid of patients with pseudogout. Moderately increased concentrations are associated with degenerative joint disease and gout, while near normal concentrations are characteristic of the synovial effusions produced by rheumatoid arthritis. Other diseases in which intra-articular deposition of calcium pyrophosphate dihydrate has been identified are neuroarthropathy (Jacobelli et al., 1973), haemochromatosis, ochronosis, acromegaly, Wilson's disease, hypothyroidism and hyperparathyroidism (Schumacher, 1975). The pyrophosphate assays are long and difficult procedures; thus, for most clinical applications, polarizing light microscopy provides an adequate method of crystal identification. If the diagnosis of gout remains in question after microscopic examination for crystals, knowledge of the uric acid concentration of the synovial fluid may be of considerable value. Many patients with gout have a synovial fluid uric acid concentration which is higher than the serum uric acid concentration, and this is considered by some authors to be diagnostic of gout (Reeves, 1965).

The calcium concentration ranges from 1.3 to 1.5 mmol/litre (2.5 to 3 mEq/litre) in the synovial fluids associated with a number of arthropathies (Altman et al., 1973). Unfortunately, no diagnostic discrimination is provided by this measurement alone. The phosphorus/calcium ratio of particles obtained from joint fluid may provide another method for crystal identification. The technique requires the use of an electron microscope equipped with an energy-dispersive microanalytical system. Using this method, crystals of calcium hydroxyapatite have been identified in the synovial fluid of patients with degenerative joint disease, and this may represent a third type of crystal deposition disease (Dieppe et al., 1976).

The determination of protein concentration in synovial fluid is of limited diagnostic value. Differences can be demonstrated between groups of patients, but overlap between the groups precludes sufficient diagnostic specificity for the individual case. A concentration of total protein greater than 25 g/litre strongly suggests that the synovial fluid is abnormal. When the concentration is greater than 45 g/litre, a severe inflammatory process is likely to be present (Cohen et al., 1975). The fluid/serum concentration ratio for all proteins has been shown to be higher in a group of patients with rheumatoid arthritis than in a second group with degenerative joint disease. This is explained by the exudation of plasma proteins through the capillaries of the inflamed synovium (Pruzanski et al., 1973). Others have shown that the protein concentration is directly related to the severity of the inflammation (Collins and Cosh, 1970). The latter, however, is more reliably assessed on clinical grounds than by laboratory tests.

The immunoglobulins present in the synovial fluid of rheumatoid patients are in higher concentrations than expected when compared to the fluid/serum ratios for the other proteins. This suggests that the immunoglobulins are produced within the synovial space, in addition to their exudation across the capillaries (Pruzanski et al., 1973). Pathological paraproteins ("M components") have been demonstrated in the joint fluid of patients with amyloid arthritis secondary to multiple myeloma. In two cases, these were identified as κ light chains by immunoelectrophoresis (Gordon et al., 1973). Both α_1-antitrypsin and β_2-microglobulin have been found in increased concentrations in the synovial fluid of patients with rheumatoid arthritis (Swedlund et al., 1974; Talal et al., 1975). Determination of total haemolytic complement in synovial fluid has been proposed as a diagnostic aid in inflammatory joint disease. When compared to total protein, the complement concentration is low in about 60 to 70% of joint effusions secondary to rheumatoid arthritis, systemic lupus erythematosis, or septic arthritis (Bunch et al., 1974). Increased concentrations of IgG and IgM anti-γ-globulins (rheumatoid factors) are associated with decreased total complement in rheumatoid synovial effusions (Panush et al., 1971). Unfortunately, the demonstration of rheumatoid factor in the joint fluid is of little diagnostic value because it may be associated with a number of different forms of synovitis (Scott, 1975).

Increased activities of several enzymes have been demonstrated in the synovial effusions associated with inflammatory joint disease, but these studies have been generally unrewarding from a diagnostic standpoint (Teloh, 1975). Lysozyme and collagenase have been investigated because these enzymes have been postulated to play a role in the pathogenesis of the disease (Cohen et al., 1975). Lysozyme activity measured simultaneously with lactoferrin concentration in synovial fluid has been suggested as a potentially useful index of both joint inflammation and cartilage destruction (Bennett and Skosey, 1977). Widespread clinical use of such tests is limited by low specificity and relatively high cost for the amount of information gained.

Lipid analysis of synovial fluid is of little diagnostic value except to confirm the presence of a cholesterol or chylous effusion. If necessary, cholesterol and triglyceride determinations on specimens of fluid may be done with the same techniques as for serum lipid measurements (Cohen et al., 1975). Chylous effusions have been reported to be associated with both rheumatoid arthritis (Newcombe and Cohen, 1965) and with systemic lupus erythematosus (Ryan et al., 1973). Cholesterol effusion is an infrequent complication of rheumatoid arthritis. Cholesterol-rich synovial fluid may be very similar in appearance to a purulent effusion (Meyers and Watermeyer, 1976). The distinction is made by the results of the culture and by microscopic identification of the cholesterol crystals. These crystals may occur in the form of either needles or rhomboid plates (Nye et al., 1968).

2.3.5. Middle ear effusion

The accumulation of middle ear effusion has long been recognized as a complication of infection, inflammation and trauma involving the middle ear. Yet until recently very little was known about the epidemiology, pathophysiology and natural history of this condition (Paradise, 1976). Classification of the middle ear fluids has been largely based upon their appearance and the clinical course surrounding their accumulation. The four basic types are serous, mucoid, bloody and purulent. These may occur individually or in any combination (Paparella, 1976). The biochemical characteristics of middle ear fluid have been studied primarily for the purposes of elucidating pathophysiology, with the diagnosis being made on clinical grounds (Juhn and Huff, 1976).

Studies of the protein fractions in middle ear effusion suggest that the fluid is an exudate resulting from mucosal reaction (Pahor et al., 1976). The total protein concentration, which ranges from 60 to 90 g/litre, is usually higher in the effusion than in serum (Mogi and Honjo, 1972). Most of the proteins appear to arise from the serum. An important exception is the immunoglobulins. High concentrations of IgE and secretory IgA are characteristic of the effusion fluids (Bernstein et al., 1974; Phillips et al., 1974). These data suggest that immunoglobulins are produced by a distinct local immune system within the middle ear. High lysozyme activity, which is also characteristic of middle ear fluids, may act in concert with the immunoglobulins to provide an effective antimicrobial system (Veltri and Sprinkle, 1973).

2.4. FLUIDS OF THE GENITOURINARY SYSTEM

2.4.1. Urine

Urine was the first of the body fluids to be examined for diagnostic clues. Hippocrates noted that foam persisting on the surface of urine – evidence of proteinuria – was associated with renal disease. By the early nineteenth century, chemists had developed qualitative tests for sugar, protein, urea and bilirubin. Modern techniques of urine analysis still employ some of the principles of these early tests.

The primary functional unit which is responsible for the formation of urine is the nephron of the kidney. In addition to the elimination of metabolic waste products, the kidney has an equally inportant role in the maintenance of homeostasis i.e. regulation of the volume and composition of body fluid. These aspects of renal function are reviewed in Chapter 9 and described in detail in a number of monographs (Pitts, 1974; Bauman and Chinard, 1975; Deetjen et al., 1975).

Few patients undergo a complete medical examination without providing a urine specimen for routine analysis. This should be a cleanly voided midstream sample so that it is free of contaminating bacteria and epithelial cells from the external genitalia. Special cleansing procedures are necessary if a bacterial culture is to be made or if vaginal discharge or haemorrhage is present. Examination of the specimen within 30 minutes of voiding is crucial if the results are to be meaningful. Microbial growth may alter pH, falsely increase the bacterial count, and cause lysis of cells or distort their morphology. Glucose and bilirubin concentrations may decrease on standing. The first morning specimen is usually the most concentrated and is, therefore, preferable for determination of the specific gravity or osmolality and the nature of the sediment. If the urine sample is used to assess the control of diabetes, a second specimen is collected either when the patient is fasting or 2 to 3 hours after a meal. The collection of a 24 hour specimen for clearance and excretion studies requires a larger container, refrigeration, an appropriate preservative and careful instruction to the patient about the collection procedure (Free and Free, 1975).

Clues to the chemical and cellular constituents of a urine specimen may be given by its physical appearance (Kark et al., 1963). A red colour suggests the presence of haem pigments or vegetable dyes. A deep golden colour may be due to the presence of bilirubin or riboflavin. Turbidity can be caused by a fine precipitate of urates or phosphates, or by a suspension of lipid droplets or cells. The presence of red blood cells has been described as imparting a smoky appearance to a urine specimen.

The chemistry of urine analysis has been simplified by the introduction of the immersible reagent strip. The technique uses a plastic-coated strip with dry reagents impregnated on a porous substrate. After dipping the reagent strip into a urine specimen, the colours which develop are compared with those on a chart to provide semi-quantitative estimates of pH, and of the presence of protein, glucose, ketones, haemoglobin and bilirubin. Some of these tests are subject to interference by drugs, but if good technique is used, the reagent strip provides an adequate screening procedure for routine analysis (Hall et al., 1976). The chemical methods used on the reagent strips are, of course, subject to change by the manufacturer.

Estimation of urinary pH provides an indication of acid–base balance and of the ability of the renal tubules to eliminate the hydrogen ions released by fixed acids such as sulphate and phosphate. Urinary pH may be estimated to within 0.5 pH units by the reagent strip method: electrometric measurements are necessary for the more specialized tests of hydrogen ion excretion which are described in Chapter 9. Normal kidneys produce urine with a pH which may vary from 4.4 to 8.0. A freshly voided urine specimen from a healthy adult is usually mildly acidic, but the specimen obtained after a meal may be slightly alkaline. Urine which is persistently alkaline should suggest a systemic alkalosis or infection of the urine with a urea-splitting organism. Urine may become alkaline when the specimen is allowed to stand for too long before analysis (Kark et al., 1963).

The healthy adult may excrete up to 150 mg of protein in the urine in 24 hours. Immunodiffusion techniques have been used to identify in normal urine about 30 different proteins that are also present in plasma (Berggard, 1970). Other proteins may originate from within the renal parenchyma (Tamm–Horsfall glycoprotein) or from the prostate and seminal vesicles in the male. A benign form of postural or orthostatic proteinuria occurs in about 5% of adolescents and young adults. Persistent or constant proteinuria is nearly always pathological and in most cases is related to the increased passage of plasma proteins across the glomerular membrane. Bence Jones protein – produced by myeloma, lymphoma, or leukaemia cells (Chapter 6.3.3.4) – is of sufficiently low molecular mass to cross the glomerular barrier whenever excessive quantities appear in the blood (Rennie, 1971).

The usual reagent strip method for proteinuria employs the protein error of a pH indicator, bromphenol blue, which is held at pH 3 with a citrate buffer; change in colour from yellow to blue-green indicates the presence of protein, and the extent of the colour change affords a rough quantitative estimate. The sensitivity of the reagent strip method corresponds to approximately 0.30 g of albumin per litre and the test is less sensitive for globulins and Bence Jones protein than for albumin. A visual turbidimetric method using hot acetic or sulfosalicylic acid will detect any protein in concentrations as low as 0.15 g/litre. False positive turbidity tests may occur due to the presence of radiographic contrast material and a number of drugs (Hall et al., 1976). Persistent proteinuria should be quantified by a 24-hour collection. Bence Jones proteinuria may be confirmed and the protein identified, when necessary, by immunoelectrophoresis.

Glycosuria may occur in hyperglycaemic states (e.g. diabetes mellitus) or in renal disease (e.g. nephrotic syndrome). Glucose is detected on the reagent strip by a fairly specific glucose oxidase method. Sensitivity corresponds to about 0.6 mmol of glucose per litre (10 mg/dl), but quantitation is poor. False negative reactions may occur due to ascorbic acid, but a separate reagent strip can be used to screen for the presence of ascorbic acid in urine. Copper reduction methods such as Benedict's Test and Clinitest (Ames Division, Miles Laboratories, Elkhart, Indiana) are much less sensitive for glucose. They are also non-specific in that they respond to a wide variety of reducing substances

(Wilson, 1975), but this can be advantageous if one of the less common melliturias is suspected. Thin layer chromatography may then be used to identify the specific sugar.

Ketone bodies are produced as a result of incomplete lipid metabolism (Chapter 4). This can occur in diabetic ketoacidosis or even in a healthy individual after a 24-hour fast (Kerr, 1973). The usual reagent strip method is based on the nitroprusside reaction and is most sensitive for acetoacetate. False positive reactions may occur with bromosulphthalein, or with large amounts of phenylketones or metabolites of L-DOPA.

Haematuria is detected by microscopic examination or by a reagent strip method which is based on the catalase activity of haemoglobin. This test is most sensitive for free haemoglobin, and can detect concentrations as low as 150 μg/litre. There is less sensitivity to intact erythrocytes and to myoglobin. In one series, only 54% of patients with microscopic haematuria also had positive reagent strip tests for blood (Wilson, 1975). Ascorbic acid may cause a false negative reaction. High bacterial counts may cause false positive reactions due to the presence of bacterial peroxidases (Hall et al., 1976). Accurate detection of haematuria is of great clinical importance, and for this reason it is essential to examine the sediment for erythrocytes before the reagent strip test for blood is interpreted.

Urine tests for bile pigments (bilirubin and urobilinogen) may provide early diagnostic information in cases of inflammatory or toxic liver disease. The absence of bilirubin from the urine in the presence of increased urine urobilinogen suggests that jaundice is the result of a haemolytic state (Kerr, 1973). Bilirubin is detected on the usual reagent strip by a diazotization reaction. The tablet form of this test (Ictotest, Ames Division, Miles Laboratories, Elkhart, Indiana) is about twice as sensitive as the reagent strip, but both are subject to interferences by drugs such as chlorpromazine and pyridium (Hall et al., 1976). The presence of urobilinogen is best determined using Ehrlich's reagent followed by a solvent extraction (Kark et al., 1963). Details of the interpretation of these tests are given in Chapter 10, and urine tests for porphyrias are discussed in Chapter 20.

The measurement of specific gravity gives a rough indication of the solute concentration of urine and is usually included in a routine analysis. The refractometer provides a convenient estimate of specific gravity and avoids many of the problems associated with the hydrometer (urinometer) which are referred to in Chapter 9. Knowledge of whether urine is concentrated or dilute is useful in the interpretation of other analytical tests on urine. For example, cells lyse more readily in dilute urine and, therefore, microscopic haematuria might be missed in a dilute specimen. In particular, tests for proteinuria should always be interpreted with a knowledge of urine concentration. A low concentration of protein in a dilute specimen may be of greater concern than the same concentration in a less dilute specimen. Because of the precision required to measure the concentrating ability of the distal tubule (Chapter 9), osmolality must be determined. This is usually done by measurement of the depression of the freezing point (Hall et al., 1976), but this technique includes the contribution to osmolality of volatile compounds such as ethanol. It is important to note here that the vapour pressure osmometer does *not* detect the contribution of organic volatiles to the osmolality of the sample (Barlow, 1976). Clearly, both the chemist and the clinician should be aware of the capabilities and limitations of the instrumentation used.

Microscopic examination of the urinary sediment is still considered by nephrologists and urologists to be of key importance in routine analysis of urine. Yet the value of this simple test is all too frequently lost amongst the more complex testing procedures of modern medicine (Winkel et al., 1974). Improper collection technique, faulty handling of the specimen and an inadequately trained analyst often act in concert to provide a result which is worthless, and which may actually mislead the physician. Proper identification of the formed elements in urinary sediment necessitates the examination of a freshly voided specimen. As a result, many meticulous physicians prefer to examine the sediment themselves. Unless gross blood or pus is present, the urine sediment is concentrated by centrifugation and examined microscopically (Kark et al., 1963).

The four general classes of formed elements in the urinary sediment are cells, casts, crystals, and micro-organisms. A thick film of suspended sediment should be scanned under the microscope using low power for casts and crystals. A thin film is then examined, so that cells and bacteria may be identified. Several excellent atlases of the components of urinary sediment have been compiled (Lippman, 1957; Brody et al., 1971; Spencer and Pedersen, 1971). Quantitative (Addis) counts of the urinary formed elements are now rarely done, because they are laborious and because the yield of new clinical information is low.

Cells appearing in the urinary sediment consist of erythrocytes, leucocytes and epithelial cells. All of these may appear in small quantities in the normal urine specimen. The mechanism of extravasation of blood cells into the normal urinary tract is unclear, and numerous causes of haematuria have been outlined by Kark et al. (1963). During the menses, increased numbers of red blood cells appear in the urine of females. Numerous cornified epithelial cells in the urine indicate contamination with vaginal discharge. Large numbers of leucocytes in the sediment are suggestive of acute infection, but non-infectious inflammatory disease of the kidney, bladder or urethra may also result in increased numbers of urinary leucocytes. Hypotonic alkaline urine results in rapid lysis of leucocytes, again emphasizing the importance of prompt examination of the sediment (Wilson, 1975).

Casts are cylindrically shaped mouldings of the renal tubules and collecting ducts. They are composed of precipitated protein, agglutinated cells and debris. Formation of casts is favoured by decreased urine flow rate and increased urine osmolality and acidity. Casts may be classified on the basis of their content and appearance (Levinsky, 1967). A few hyaline casts are seen in the normal urine specimen. They consist of precipitated Tamm–Horsfall protein which has a refractive index close to that of urine. Granular casts in the absence of fever or recent vigorous exercise nearly always indicate renal disease with proteinuria.

Haematuria (i.e. free-floating erythrocytes) may be the result of blood loss from any part of the urinary tract, but red cell casts are diagnostic of damage to the capillary vessels of the renal parenchyma. Autoimmune diseases such as acute post-streptococcal glomerulonephritis and systemic lupus erythematosus are known to cause sufficient glomerular bleeding for the formation of red cell casts. Leucocyte casts are characteristic of acute pyelonephritis, whereas renal epithelial cell casts occur with acute tubular damage or in the active stage of glomerulonephritis. The size of a cast is also important clinically. Broad granular or waxy casts originate in the larger ducts of the renal collecting system. This implies malfunction of entire segments of the kidney and usually accompanies end-stage renal failure. Fatty casts and oval fat bodies display a typical Maltese cross pattern under polarized light. Lipiduria – the presence of fat in the urine – may occur with the nephrotic syndrome and diabetic glomerulosclerosis (Brody et al., 1971). Severe, rapidly progressive glomerular or vascular disease results in a so-called "telescoped urine sediment". This simply means that a mixture of elements such as red cell casts, granular casts, fat bodies and broad waxy casts are all seen in the same specimen.

Most crystals seen in urine are of minimal clinical significance. They may appear in the urine of a normal subject or in a wide variety of disease states. Amorphous urates and phosphates may precipitate as a freshly voided urine specimen cools to room temperature. These often complicate the examination of the urinary sediment. The formation of most crystals in urine is pH dependent; thus the refractile hexagonal crystals of cystine appear in the urine of patients with cystinosis when the pH of the specimen is slightly acid. Crystals which form in the urine of patients with renal lithiasis may be of clinical interest (Chapter 9.3.7), but only if pH and temperature are controlled at the time of examination of the urine.

Proper diagnosis and treatment of urinary tract infections requires detection, identification and quantitation of bacteriuria. Bacteria are detected by urine microscopy, but they may be obscured in a centrifuged sediment by masses of leucocytes. A bacterial culture of the urine then serves to identify and quantitate the organism. A Gram stain of unspun urine sediment, when carefully examined under an oil-immersion objective, shows good correlation with urine culture results (Wilson, 1975). A chemical test for bacteriuria has been recently revived, having been discovered nearly one hundred years ago. When significant numbers of bacteria are present in the urine, naturally excreted nitrate is reduced to nitrite, which can be detected by a diazotization reaction on a reagent strip. When done in triplicate on separate morning specimens (Kunin, 1974), the test gave no false positives, but had a 10% false negative rate.

Specialized stains may also be used to assist in the identification of components of the sediment. Occasionally, lipid which is non-refractile may appear in the urine, and this can be detected with a specific fat stain such as Sudan III. Papanicolaou stains of urinary sediment can be used by an experienced cytologist to detect malignant cells and inclusion bodies which are found in some viral diseases such as rubeola and cytomegalic inclusion disease (Kark et al., 1963). Differential staining of the elements of urinary sediment may be done easily with a mixture of crystal violet and safranin: this stain was originally developed to differentiate leucocytes according to their origin within the urinary tract (Sternheimer and Malbin, 1951). Unfortunately, the staining characteristics of leucocytes have not proved to be entirely reliable. This, however, does not detract from the usefulness of the stain to help delineate and identify the various components of urinary sediment. Another test has recently been reported which shows a high degree of specificity in the localization of urinary tract infections (Thomas et al., 1974). This test uses a simple immunofluorescent staining technique to detect antibody-coated bacteria which originate from infection within the kidney.

Several optical methods have been developed to help distinguish and differentiate the elements of urinary sediment. Most microscopes used in hospital laboratories employ bright-field illumination, whereby the specimen is evaluated using transmitted light. Phase-contrast microscopy is based on subtle differences in refractive index between sediment particles and the surrounding medium, and this permits better delineation of certain formed elements. Polarizing filters assist in the identification of birefringent crystals and lipids. In combination, these three types of illumination provide a powerful tool for examination of urinary sediment (Spencer and Pedersen, 1971).

2.4.2. Semen

Seminal plasma, the fluid elaborated by the male reproductive system, acts as a vehicle and a nutrient support medium for the spermatozoa. The volume of the ejaculate is normally from 3 to 3.5 ml. A semen volume of less than 1 ml or greater than 4 ml is associated with an increased prevalence of infertility (Milne, 1976). Well over 50% of the total volume of semen is produced by the seminal vesicles, and 10 to 20% is of prostatic origin. Secretions from the epididymides, vasa deferentia, bulbourethral and urethral glands comprise the remainder. The sperm count is normally higher in the first half of the ejaculate than in the remainder (Tresidder, 1975).

Immediately upon ejaculation, semen appears as an off-white viscous gel or coagulum with a distinct odour due to the presence of polyamines. The substrate for coagulation is a fibrin-like protein produced by the seminal vesicles. Within 20 minutes, liquefaction of the coagulum occurs, catalyzed by the powerful fibrinolytic and proteolytic enzymes of prostatic origin. When the seminal vesicles and vasa deferentia are congenitally absent, semen fails to coagulate (Amelar, 1962). Semen analysis should be delayed until liquefaction occurs, because spermatozoa attain full motility only after this process is complete, but delays longer than 2 or 3 hours must be avoided. A qualitative estimate of semen viscosity may be made during pipetting steps for other analytical procedures. Semen which demonstrates impaired liquefaction may be associated with infertility (Syner et al., 1975).

Prostatic fluid is slightly acidic, but the pH of normal seminal plasma is about 7.6 due to the alkaline secretions from the seminal vesicles. Patients whose ejaculate mainly consists of prostatic secretions have not only a low semen volume but also a semen pH which is below 7.0 (Raboch and Skachova, 1965). The alkaline pH of normal semen serves to buffer metabolites such as lactate and to protect the spermatozoa from the lethal acidic environment of the vagina.

The semen specimen is best collected by masturbation in a clean, detergent-free glass or polystyrene container. Ideally, it should be provided at the physician's laboratory so that coagulation and liquefaction may be observed. If the specimen is obtained in the patient's home, it must be collected in a pre-warmed container and then kept near body temperature at least until liquefaction has occurred. Failure to do so may result in a significant decrease in sperm motility referred to as "cold shock" (Watson and Robertson, 1966). A 3-day period of abstinence from sexual activity is requested of the patient. If the patient is unable to produce a specimen by masturbation, a plastic condom may be used. Rubber condoms are to be avoided because of potential for contamination of the specimen with talcum powder or lubricants.

Semen analysis has become an integral part of the evaluation of the infertile couple. In 35% or more of such cases, the male is solely responsible. In addition, semen analysis is relatively simple compared with the detailed investigation of female infertility. Much excellent work has been done to elucidate the biochemistry of semen (Mann, 1964), but relatively little of this knowledge has been applied to the routine solution of clinical problems. In most centres, semen analysis involves a semi-quantitative estimate of sperm count, motility, and morphology. The details, expected ranges, and drawbacks of microscopic semen analysis are discussed in a number of reviews (MacLeod, 1965; Glover, 1974; Sobrero and Rehan, 1975).

Seminal plasma contains several carbohydrates which are unique to mammalian fluids; some of these are present in unusually high concentrations. For example, the fructose concentration is of the order of 14 mmol/litre (2.5 g/litre) making this the principal monosaccharide found in normal human semen. Several studies have demonstrated a relationship between the fructose concentration of semen and fertility (Schirren, 1963; Phadke et al., 1973, 1975). The metabolism of fructose depends upon the presence of normal spermatozoa. Indeed, the data of Schirren (1963) and Phadke et al. (1973) clearly show an inverse relationship between fructose concentration and sperm count. Seminal fructose content has also been shown to decline with advancing age. In addition, a group of infertile men has been identified whose sperm appear normal but whose semen shows an abnormally low fructose concentration. This group of patients with post-pubescent interstitial cell deficiency has responded well to treatment with methyltestosterone (Schirren, 1963). The secretory activity of the seminal vesicles under the influence of testosterone is responsible for the fructose concentration in human semen. Thus, conditions in which there is a low endogenous androgen level (e.g. Klinefelter's syndrome) or seminal vesicle insufficiency (e.g. congenital aplasia of the seminal vesicles) may be the cause of low or zero fructose concentration (Mauss et al., 1974).

The citrate concentration in human seminal plasma ranges from 5 to 50 mmol/litre (1 to 10 g/litre). Because citrate is produced by the prostate gland, it may be used as an indicator of prostatic function in relation to possible causes of infertility. For example, semen which has a low pH and a very high citric acid concentration, but little or no fructose, suggests that the seminal plasma is composed of prostatic secretions only, without contribution from the seminal vesicles (Marberger et al., 1962).

Trace element analysis is gaining ever wider attention as an indicator of deficiency syndromes and toxicity states (Chapter 19). Magnesium and zinc are both secreted by the prostate, so that their concentrations in semen are much higher than those in serum. Complex dynamics inter-relate zinc uptake by cells (spermatozoa and leucocytes) to zinc concentration in prostatic or seminal plasma (Stankova et al., 1976). Measurement of zinc concentration in whole human semen has demonstrated no difference between groups of normal volunteers and post-vasectomy patients. However, patients with prostatitis show a definite decrease in semen zinc concentration which increases 2-fold on supplementation with oral zinc sulphate (Marmar et al., 1975). This may prove to be of therapeutic importance, because a positive correlation has been found between the concentration of zinc and the antibacterial activity of seminal fluid (Colleen et al., 1975). Another group of oligospermic men with low semen zinc content showed increased sperm count, improved sperm motility and morphology, and increased semen zinc concentration following oral zinc therapy (Marmar et al., 1975). Unfortunately, the diagnostic value of zinc and magnesium determinations is limited because of the wide ranges of concentrations which are found in both normal and abnormal semen.

Detailed studies of the effects of fluids from the prostate and seminal vesicles on spermatozoa have been performed (Eliasson, 1976). These have shown that the zinc and magnesium concentrations are 5 to 10 times higher in the first fractions of an ejaculate than in the last fractions. This is not surprising because the prostatic fluid is ejaculated first. Paradoxically, however, the zinc content of the spermatozoa is almost 4 times higher in the *last* fraction than in the first fraction of the ejaculate. Infertile males with prostatic dysfunction may have a zinc concentration in spermatozoa which is twice as high as that of fertile males, and a higher percentage of spermatozoa which are morphologically abnormal. The data support the hypothesis that the zinc uptake of spermatozoa depends upon the ratio of free to bound zinc, or upon the presence or absence of seminal plasma factors.

The measurement of hormones in seminal plasma is a logical extension of the radioimmunoassay techniques used to measure these compounds in blood plasma. Studies of six unconjugated steroids in human semen have shown that azoospermic men have lower concentrations of pregnenolone and dihydrotestosterone than do normal or oligospermic men (Purvis et al., 1975). A similar study has demonstrated a marked decrease in semen concentration of dihydrotestosterone associated with less striking decreases in dehydroepiandrosterone and androstenedione in men who had undergone vasectomy (Purvis et al., 1976a). To obtain reliable results, it was necessary to control the liquefaction period prior to steroid assays. Incubation periods longer than 30 minutes produced false elevations in a number of the unconjugated steroids in seminal plasma. This is the result of the action of enzymes such as sulphatases and glucuronidases which are present in semen and which hydrolyze the conjugated steroids (Purvis et al., 1976b). The pituitary hormones prolactin (Sheth et al., 1975) and luteinizing hormone (Sheth et al., 1976) have been found in human semen in concentrations which are several-fold higher than those in serum. The concentrations of both of these hormones are significantly lower in the seminal plasma of azoospermic men than in that of normal men.

In addition to the glucoproteins, semen contains a number of proteins which resemble those found in blood plasma. The total protein concentration in semen (50 to 60 g/litre) is slightly lower than that of blood plasma. Albumin represents about one-third of the total, with a pre-albumin fraction and the globulins comprising the remainder (Mann, 1975). A number of plasma proteins have been examined in human split ejaculates in an attempt to determine which of the accessory glands is responsible for their secretion (Tauber et al., 1975; Nishimura et al., 1977). Protein electrophoresis of seminal plasma on cellulose acetate has been suggested as another method for the assessment of the functional state of the prostate and seminal vesicles (Lewin et al., 1974). Beta-trace protein has been associated with renal disease and disorders of the central nervous system, and one study showed a positive correlation between sperm count and beta-trace protein concentration in human semen (Olsson, 1975).

Enzyme activities in semen have provided information about secretory activities of the accessory organs, and correlations have been made with specific causes of infertility. Acid phosphatase, well known as a secretory product of the prostate, shows highest activity in the first fraction of the ejaculate. This enzyme has been measured, together with the concentrations of zinc and citrate, as an index of prostatic function (Glover, 1974). Prostatitis usually results in decreased acid phosphatase activity in seminal plasma. Conversely, lactate dehydrogenase activity has been observed to increase in the semen of patients with prostatic dysfunction. Determination of lactate dehydrogenase isoenzymes by agar-gel electrophoresis revealed a sixth isoenzyme (designated LD_x) in semen which migrated between the third and fourth fractions. LD_x appeared to be closely associated with the spermatozoa in that there was a positive correlation between sperm count and LD_x activity (Eliasson, 1968).

The presence of polyamines, particularly spermine, in human semen has been well documented (Mann, 1974). Recent studies of the enzymes involved in spermine metabolism have shown some degree of correlation with sperm count (Thakur et al., 1974) and with sperm motility (Fair et al., 1972). Diamine oxidase is intimately associated with the spermatozoa, yet both diamine oxidase and spermine appear to be derived from the prostate gland. Oxidation products of the polyamines are known to immobilize spermatozoa; thus it is possible that polyamines in the presence of oxidative enzymes may have a direct effect on the activity and fertilizing capacity of the spermatozoa (Pulkkinen et al., 1975). Diamine oxidase activity has recently been shown to be inversely related to sperm motility. Conversely, fumarase activity in semen shows a positive correlation with sperm motility suggesting that enzyme assays might well serve as replacements for semi-quantitative motility studies (Crabbe, 1976).

Prostaglandins are a group of unsaturated fatty acids which are characterized by a cyclopentanone ring system. At least 13 of these compounds have been identified in human semen (Mann, 1975). The prostaglandins are a secretory product of the seminal vesicles and their production is highly androgen dependent. Early experiments demonstrated a stimulatory effect of these compounds upon smooth muscle. They are known to be rapidly absorbed through the vaginal mucosa. The major prostaglandin components of human semen have been identified as 19-hydroxyprostaglandin E_1 and 19-hydroxyprostaglandin E_2 (Kelly et al., 1976).

The prostaglandin concentration in semen has been measured in both fertile and infertile males (Bygdeman et al., 1970). About 40% of a group of infertile men had low prostaglandin E levels in their semen. No other abnormality could be found in these men which would account for their infertility. Attempts to correct the infertility and to increase the semen prostaglandin concentration have been unsuccessful (Collier et al., 1975).

2.4.3. Amniotic fluid

During the past 20 years, the analysis of amniotic fluid has become increasingly important in the diagnosis of foetal distress, foetal maturity and in the prenatal diagnosis of genetic disorders. The specimen is usually obtained by transabdominal amniocentesis. This procedure is done under sterile conditions using a long, narrow gauge spinal needle to penetrate the amniotic cavity through the maternal abdominal wall. Care is taken to determine the location of the foetus and placenta so that injury to these structures may be avoided. Amniocentesis may be performed at any time from the twelfth week of gestation to the termination of the pregnancy, but the actual timing of the procedure is dependent upon the condition being evaluated (Alpern, 1974). When bilirubin is to be determined, the aspirate should be placed in an opaque container to avoid photodecomposition. If the amniotic fluid is contaminated with blood, it should be centrifuged as soon as possible. A bloody tap should always be noted in the record.

The production and reabsorption of amniotic fluid is a complicated process, the details of which have not been entirely elucidated. Early in pregnancy, the amniotic fluid may be thought of as an extension of the extracellular fluid. The low protein concentration suggests that the source is transudation through the foetal membranes, and perhaps across the umbilical cord (Seeds, 1974). Transfer of water may also occur across the foetal skin and through the tracheobronchial tree. At term, the foetus swallows about 500 ml of fluid daily and produces about the same volume of hypotonic urine. As a result, the osmolality of the amniotic fluid drops to around 260 mosmol/litre and the concentrations of creatinine, urea and uric acid increase toward the end of pregnancy (Pitkin, 1974).

The amniotic fluid serves to cushion the developing foetus against external shock. It also provides lubrication between the foetus and the amnion, thereby allowing movement within the amniotic cavity. About 2 weeks before term, the amniotic fluid reaches maximum volume, averaging around one litre with a range from 0.2 to 1.5 litres. At this time, the normal fluid turnover rate is about 500 ml/hour with total replacement occurring once every 3 hours. These rates of exchange are altered by the presence of specific foetal congenital defects, or by pathological states of pregnancy (Ostergard, 1974).

Analysis of bilirubin in the amniotic fluid provided the first step toward successful management of erythroblastosis foetalis, or haemolytic disease of the newborn. This is a pathologic state of pregnancy which results when maternal antibodies to foetal red cell antigens cross the placenta and cause destruction of the foetal erythrocytes. The classic example is that of rhesus isoimmunization where Rh-positive foetal cells stimulate antibody production in the Rh-negative mother. The involvement of the foetus is classified according to the severity of the anaemia and the estimated chances for survival of the infant (Misenhimer, 1974). Prediction of the magnitude of foetal involvement was woefully inaccurate until the advent of amniocentesis and of spectrophotometric measurement of bile pigment concentration in amniotic fluid. This led to the development of an appropriate plan of management based on the severity of foetal involvement as related to gestational age.

The bilirubin-like pigments in amniotic fluid decrease in concentration throughout the term of a normal pregnancy. When the foetus becomes affected by haemolysis secondary to isoimmunization, the bile pigment concentration does not show its normal decrease and indeed may increase with the severity of foetal involvement. This permits the construction of prediction charts which allow assessment of foetal distress based upon measurement of bile pigments in the amniotic fluid (Fairweather et al., 1976). It is now generally agreed that unconjugated bilirubin is the major component of these pigments (Willis and Faulkner, 1965).

Measurement of the apparent absorbance at 450 nm provides an adequate estimation of bile pigment concentration in most cases. A spectrum of the clear amniotic fluid from 340 nm to 600 nm is obtained, and a baseline drawn to connect the minima at 365 nm and 550 nm. The difference in absorbance between this baseline and the 450 nm spectrum is a measure of the bile pigments (Liley, 1961). If the specimen is contaminated with blood, an oxyhaemoglobin peak at 415 nm is seen. The method is not reliable with grossly blood stained samples unless the contribution made by oxyhaemoglobin is determined at another wavelength (Dubin, 1974). Others have demonstrated that a solvent extraction method for the determination of bilirubin eliminates most of the interference from haem pigments (Simkins and Worth, 1976). A prediction diagram which uses the amniotic fluid bilirubin concentration to estimate foetal prognosis has been constructed (Bock et al., 1976).

Assessment of foetal pulmonary maturity is of greatest importance when early delivery of the infant is anticipated. The premature foetus – before the 35th week of gestation – has not yet developed the biochemical apparatus to produce the surface-active phospholipids (principally lecithin) which are necessary to prevent pulmonary alveolar collapse and progressive atelectasis in the neonatal period. These infants are at high risk for the development of the respiratory distress syndrome (Forman, 1974). A dramatic 3–4-fold increase in amniotic fluid lecithin concentration occurs between the 34th and 36th gestational week. Many methods for the assessment of foetal pulmonary maturity, based upon amniotic fluid phospholipid concentration have now been published.

Determination of the lecithin/sphingomyelin (L/S) ratio was one of the first methods reported (Gluck et al., 1971). It continues, with some modification, to be the principal method in use today. The procedure involves solvent extraction followed by thin layer chromatography and densitometric quantitation of the lipid fractions. Much of the recent literature suggests that an L/S ratio of 2 or greater indicates pulmonary maturity in the foetus, and that these infants may be delivered with essentially no risk of respiratory distress syndrome (Aubry et al., 1976). Unfortunately the earlier methods did not report the conditions used for initial centrifugation of the specimens. This is of key importance because increasing centrifugal force and centrifugation time causes sedimentation of the phospholipids, and leads to an apparent decrease in the L/S ratio (Wilkinson et al., 1977). A carefully detailed method has been presented by Olson et al. (1975). These data support an L/S ratio of 3.5 (rather than 2) or greater as the indicator of foetal pulmonary maturity.

Other investigators have indicated a preference for the determination of the amniotic fluid lecithin concentration only (Bhagwanani et al., 1972; Falconer et al., 1973). This procedure is much more laborious but it does avoid problems resulting from the lack of standardization of the L/S ratio (Gebhardt and Dubbeldam, 1973). No matter which method is used, care must be taken to remove the cellular debris and either analyze the fluid or freeze it immediately to prevent degradation of the lecithin by phosphodiesterase which is present in amniotic fluid. Fluids stained with meconium present problems with lipid extraction. Contamination of the amniotic fluid with maternal blood causes an absolute increase in the concentration of both lecithin and sphingomyelin, but the L/S ratio is falsely decreased (Gibbons et al., 1974).

The clinical utility of measurement of hormone concentrations in amniotic fluid has become apparent as the sensitivity and accuracy of analytical methods have improved. A review of the steroids present in amniotic fluid suggested early on that the concentrations of some of these hormones are related to foetal well-being (Klopper, 1970). Amniotic fluid cortisol concentrations appear to correlate well with the corresponding values in cord serum but not in maternal serum. An abrupt rise in cortisol concentration occurs in the 2-week period prior to delivery (Murphy et al., 1975). This pattern has been confirmed by others although absolute values differ with methodology. The rise in amniotic fluid cortisol concentration at the end of pregnancy may be associated with the onset of foetal lung maturity and has been proposed as a marker of this process (Fencl and Tulchinsky, 1975). A good correlation between amniotic fluid cortisol and the L/S ratio has been demonstrated (Tan et al., 1976). It is noteworthy that the palmitic acid concentration, which reflects the amniotic fluid lecithin concentration, correlates poorly with the cortisol concentration. Again differences in methodology or a host of biologic variables may be responsible (Sharpe-Cageorge et al., 1977).

During pregnancy, the maternal excretion of oestrogens increases by 2 or 3 orders of magnitude. The foetus and placenta acting in concert are responsible for this dramatic rise in production. Amniotic fluid oestriol, 95% of which is conjugated, reflects the foetal rather than the maternal serum pattern. Abnormally low oestriol levels have been associated with severely affected erythroblastotic foetuses (Scommegna, 1974), but management of these cases is still based primarily upon the amniotic fluid bile pigment concentration.

Progesterone is involved in the regulation of uterine muscle activity. The amniotic fluid concentration of this hormone decreases while maternal blood concentration increases as gestation progresses. The dynamics of these changes are not well understood. A sudden paradoxical increase in progesterone concentration has been observed in the amniotic fluid of patients undergoing elective prostaglandin-induced abortion at 15 to 20 weeks of gestation. Alterations in uterine blood flow and intrauterine pressure are thought to be responsible for this phenomenon (Koren et al., 1976). Amniotic fluid testosterone has been used to successfully predict the sex of the foetus prior to 20 weeks of gestation (Giles et al., 1974). A retrospective study of amniotic fluid 17α-hydroxyprogesterone has shown that an increased concentration may have predictive value in the prenatal diagnosis of congenital adrenal hyperplasia secondary to 21-hydroxylase deficiency (Frasier et al., 1975).

Studies of the thyroid hormones and thyrotrophin (Chapter 13) in amniotic fluid have been directed toward prenatal assessment of foetal thyroid status (Chopra and Crandall, 1975). Total T_4 (thyroxine) concentration in amniotic fluid is 1/20th to 1/30th of that in either cord blood or maternal serum. The concentration of T_3 (3,3′,5-triiodothyronine) is also very low. Conversely, the concentration of reverse T_3 (3,3′,5′-triiodothyronine) is much higher in amniotic fluid than in maternal serum during the mid-trimester of pregnancy. Near term, reverse T_3 decreases so that concentrations in amniotic fluid and maternal serum are equal, but cord blood taken at delivery still shows a high concentration of reverse T_3 (Burman et al., 1976). Thyrotrophin is undetectable in amniotic fluid, and thyroxine binding globulin is present in much lower concentration than in either foetal or maternal serum. The interpretation of these values is difficult because the physiologic dynamics are not well understood. Further study is needed to clarify the role of amniotic fluid hormone assays in prenatal diagnosis of foetal thyroid disease (Fisher, 1975).

The amniotic fluid concentrations of many different proteins have been investigated. The most promising of these from a clinical standpoint is α-foetoprotein. This is the principal foetal protein during the first few weeks following conception. It is synthesized first in the yolk sac, then in the foetal liver, appearing in foetal serum by the sixth week of gestation (Brock, 1976). Foetal urine appears to be the major source of α-foetoprotein in the amniotic fluid of the normal pregnancy. Transudation of the protein from foetal serum via a highly vascular organ into the amniotic cavity is thought to be the mechanism by which α-foetoprotein becomes elevated in defective pregnancies (Weiss et al., 1976b). It is also now clear that the α-foetoprotein concentration decreases as the normal pregnancy progresses (Ainbender and Hirschhorn, 1976). Some investigators feel that the ratio of amniotic fluid to maternal serum α-foetoprotein shows a better correlation with gestational age (Buffe et al., 1976), and that the maternal serum concentration provides an adequate screen for an increased amniotic fluid concentration.

Quantitation of α-foetoprotein has been of greatest value in the prenatal diagnosis of open neural tube defects such as anencephaly and spina bifida. Very high concentrations are most often seen with this type of defect (Weiss et al., 1976a). Other pathological foetal conditions have also been detected by elevated α-foetoprotein concentrations, including foetal death, omphalocoele, Turner syndrome, Meckel syndrome, oesophageal atresia and congenital nephrosis (Brock, 1976). Unfortunately, minor congenital defects such as pilonidal sinus, which is easily treatable, may also be associated with an elevated α-foetoprotein concentration (Jandial et al., 1976).

Because of the gravity of the decision as to whether or not to terminate a suspected defective pregnancy, the user of this test must be well acquainted with its limitations. Closed neural tube defects frequently escape detection. Fortunately, this represents a small proportion of the total. The test is most reliable if done prior to the 26th week of pregnancy. After this time, the α-foetoprotein level may become normal as the defective foetus approaches term (Weiss et al., 1976a). In a large series, the false positive rate was approximately 1%, based upon *normal* foetuses aborted because of increased amniotic fluid α-foetoprotein concentration (Milunsky and Alpert, 1976). A fluid contaminated with foetal blood is the most likely source of a false positive. The foetal serum concentration of α-foetoprotein is about 150 times higher than that in the amniotic fluid (Brock, 1976). Detection of foetal haemoglobin is suggestive of, but is *not* conclusive of, iatrogenic contamination of the amniotic fluid with foetal blood (Milunsky, 1976). Standardization of the assay has become a major problem. In much of the original work very little was mentioned about the source and purity of the standards (Keyser et al., 1976), and comparison between laboratories, methods and commercial kits has been poor (Watson and Pow, 1976). For these reasons it is crucial that each laboratory establish a firm reference range related to gestational age before accepting any specimens for diagnostic determinations.

The activities of a number of enzymes have been measured in the amniotic fluid. Some of these are related to gestational age. All of the phosphatases (i.e. acid, alkaline, heat-labile and placental) show peak activities in the last 8 weeks before delivery. The heat-labile fraction shows an additional peak of activity about the 15th week of gestation (Sutcliffe et al., 1972). Amniotic fluid amylase (DeCastro et al., 1973) and peroxidase (Armstrong et al., 1976) show a similar abrupt rise in activity after the 36th gestational week. These enzymes may be detected as early as the 16th or 17th week of gestation. The increase in activity near term is thought to be related to the maturation of the salivary glands and pancreas (Wolf and Taussig, 1973). A study of lactate dehydrogenase isoenzymes revealed no significant differences between normal pregnancies and those in which Rh haemolytic disease was present (Miotti et al., 1973).

During the last trimester, α_1-antitrypsin concentration in amniotic fluid normally shows a decrease associated with gestational age. This parallels the decrease in total protein (Guibaud et al., 1975). The amniotic fluid α_1-antitrypsin is elevated in about 40% of cases in which the infants develop respiratory distress syndrome. Interestingly, over 80% of the infants who have some degree of respiratory difficulty also have low α_1-antitrypsin concentrations (less than 0.2 g/dl) in their cord blood (Singer et al., 1976).

The total protein concentration in amniotic fluid reaches a peak of 6 to 7 g/litre by the 25th week of gestation. A gradual decline then occurs, so that the concentration at delivery is about 2.5 g/litre. A table of the proteins studied in amniotic fluid, including the analytical methods, has been compiled (Warshaw and Pesce, 1974). It appears that most of these proteins are maternal in origin, a notable exception being α-foetoprotein. Attempts to use amniotic fluid total protein concentration as a diagnostic indicator have been generally discouraging (Jonasson, 1973).

An extensive analysis of the chemical composition of amniotic fluid in early pregnancy has been done (Weisberg, 1974), and generally there was agreement with the data reported by others. Non-protein nitrogenous compounds have engendered interest as possible measures of foetal maturity. The concentrations of these substances in amniotic fluid increase with gestational age until a plateau is reached at the 36th week. Weiss et al. (1974) have shown that a uric acid concentration of 0.6 mmol/litre (10 mg/dl) or more, combined with creatinine of 190 μmol/litre (2.2 mg/dl) or more, is absolutely predictive of foetal maturity. Results should be interpreted with caution in cases of pre-eclampsia or during maternal diuretic therapy (McAllister et al., 1973). A decline with gestational age in osmolality and sodium and chloride concentrations in amniotic fluid is characteristic of a normal pregnancy. An increasing solute concentration near term is associated frequently with foetal distress (Cassady and Barnett, 1968; Bailey et al., 1976).

The infant of a diabetic mother is at risk of incurring a number of serious complications including foetal distress, neonatal hypoglycaemia and perinatal death. Identification of infants at high risk by amniotic fluid analysis has recently been investigated. A study of glucose concentration showed marked hypoglycaemia in a group of 6 out of 15 infants whose amniotic fluid glucose concentration was greater than 1.7 mmol/litre (30 mg/dl) shortly before delivery. The mothers of all six of these infants were known to have diabetes mellitus (Wood and Sherline, 1975). Others have suggested that the insulin concentration in the amniotic fluid may provide another prognostic indicator of foetal compromise in the diabetic mother (Newman and Tutera, 1976).

The bladder and uterus are in close anatomic proximity. As a result, the need occasionally arises to differentiate maternal urine from amniotic fluid. Reagent strips may be used to test for glucose and protein; both are present in measurable quantities in amniotic fluid, but are essentially absent in normal urine (Pirani et al., 1976). This test is not reliable when the case is complicated by maternal glycosuria or renal disease. As an alternative, urea and potassium may be measured to provide the differential identification (Guibaud et al., 1976).

Much attention has recently been given to the prenatal diagnosis of genetic disorders based upon the analysis of amniotic fluid or cells, but this type of testing is of benefit only when there is a high index of suspicion for a specific genetic defect. The information derived is then made available through genetic counselling to the couple at risk (Tegenkamp and Tegenkamp, 1974). Chromosomal disorders such as trisomy 21 (Down's syndrome) may be identified by determining the foetal karyotype. Groups at risk are pregnant patients over 40 years of age, and known carriers of chromosomal abnormalities (Gerbie and Simpson, 1976). Intricate methodology is evolving for the detection of enzyme deficiencies which are responsible for a number of inborn errors of metabolism (Seegmiller, 1974; Milunsky, 1976). The details of these disorders are reviewed in Chapter 18.8. Estimation of the specific enzyme activities in amniotic fluid per se has been disappointing from the diagnostic standpoint. Enzyme analysis conducted on cultured amniotic fluid cells shows considerably more promise. Numerous variables such as gestational age, stage of cell growth in culture and culture technique, must be rigorously accounted for and controlled (Ressler, 1974). As a result, most of the techniques remain confined to specialist laboratories.

Disadvantages of the cell culture methods are the long cultivation period (4 to 8 weeks) and the limited number of cells obtainable. To circumvent these problems, an elegant microanalytic procedure has been developed. Cells are cultured on plastic film for 1 to 2 weeks: they are then lyophilized, counted, and separated into groups of a few hundred using a microdissection technique. Next the cells are incubated with a few microlitres of substrate, and a micro-spectrofluorometer is used to measure the fluorescent or chromogenic product (Galjaard et al., 1975). Much remains to be learned about the diagnostic accuracy of such techniques before they can be reliably employed in the diagnosis and prevention of genetic disorders.

2.4.4. Cervical mucus

Investigations of the biochemical and biophysical properties of human cervical mucus have recently increased in both number and depth (Moghissi, 1973). This interest has been stimulated by the recognition of the importance of cervical mucus in fertility and contraception. The quantity, quality, and chemical composition of cervical mucus changes with the phases of the menstrual cycle under the influence of the ovarian steroid hormones. The secretory activity of the endocervical mucosal crypts is maximal during the period of oestrogen stimulation near the time of ovulation. The daily volume of mucus production is approximately 0.7 ml during the mid-cycle ovulatory phase. Less than 0.1 ml/day is produced during the luteal (post-ovulatory) phase of the cycle which is under progestogen influence (Moghissi, 1972).

Sampling techniques depend upon the visco-elastic state of the mucus. A non-lubricated vaginal speculum is used to visualize the cervix which is wiped dry with a cotton pledget. Mucus is then aspirated from the endocervix into a small syringe or plastic catheter. The latter method is particularly useful for fractional analysis of contents of the cervical canal. Very viscous or tenacious mucus may be removed using a specially designed mucus forceps. Evaporation is minimized by immediate transfer of the specimen to a small pre-weighed vial which is promptly sealed, re-weighed, and appropriately refrigerated according to the type of analysis to be performed. Rheological and sperm penetration studies should not be done on specimens which have been frozen and thawed because alterations may occur in the biophysical characteristics of the mucin (Elstein et al., 1973).

The uterine cervix with its secretions has been likened to a biological valve which allows entry of sperm only during the period of maximum fertility. The mucus at mid-cycle is alkaline (pH 7 to 8.5), thereby protecting the sperm from the acidic environment of the vagina. Healthy, motile sperm are protected from phagocytosis while non-motile or abnormal sperm are selected out and removed. Cervical mucus provides a reservoir for sperm storage with subsequent slow release into the uterine cavity. Supplemental energy requirements are provided, while the sperm migrate along mucus strands toward the site of fertilization (Elstein et al., 1973).

Several qualitative microscopic tests of sperm penetration into cervical mucus have found some clinical application (Lemert and Mastroianni, 1974). The usefulness of these tests is limited by lack of adequate standardization (Linford, 1974). Some investigators have found that meticulous examination of post-coital cervical mucus may provide important information for the diagnosis and management of infertility (Moghissi, 1976). This type of test permits microscopic observation of sperm motility in the context of the support provided by the cervical mucus. Results, which must be read with care, are most reliable when interpreted by an experienced observer (Makler, 1976).

The principal constituent of cervical mucus is mucin, a glycoprotein which contains more than 40% carbohydrate in numerous branched side chains (Masson, 1972). Mucin is primarily responsible for the unique rheological properties of cervical mucus – its properties of flow, elasticity and deformability. Cervical mucus is not a true Newtonian fluid, but a heterogenous mixture of components with high and low viscosities (Elstein et al., 1973). It is almost impossible for sperm to penetrate the tacky, viscous, tenacious mucus of the luteal and early follicular phases of the cycle. A marked decrease in viscosity occurs a few days before ovulation, and it is this mucus which is most favourable for sperm transport.

"Spinnbarkeit" is a characteristic of mid-cycle low viscosity mucus which refers to its fibrosity, or its ability to be drawn into threads. This property is easy to measure but it is less reliable than viscosity or crystallization studies. "Arborization" or "ferning" is a phenomenon of electrolyte crystallization modified by the presence of proteins. It occurs only where the concentration of each is optimal. It is a sensitive indicator of changes in the concentration of sex hormones, and it is widely used for the detection of ovulation. The extent of crystallization also bears a direct relationship to sperm receptivity (Kesserii, 1972). A detailed study of the rheological characteristics of human cervical mucus in all phases of the menstrual cycle has recently been published (Wolf et al., 1977).

Changes in the chemical composition are responsible for the altered rheological properties which are seen at mid-cycle. Cervical mucus contains about 92 to 95% water during the luteal and early follicular phases, but at ovulation the water content rises to about 98% with a corresponding decrease in protein concentration. A technique for the detection of increased water content has been developed and has shown potential for detection of the fertile period (Polishuk and Ron, 1976). Inorganic solutes comprise about 1% of the weight of cervical mucus, and the salt present in highest concentration (120 mmol/litre) is sodium chloride.

The concentration of chloride remains fairly constant throughout the menstrual cycle; however, the increased mucus secretion at mid-cycle produces a larger total quantity of chloride. This observation has been proposed as the basis for a semi-quantitative spot test for the detection of ovulation (France and Boyer, 1975). Unfortunately, the test has the disadvantage of wide variability not only between subjects but between cycles of the same subject. It is possible that improvement in the methodology for quantitation of chloride in cervical mucus would provide a reliable test for the detection of the fertile period.

The soluble organic compounds which are present in cervical mucus include free sugars such as glucose, maltose, and mannose. Glucose concentration may play a role in sperm viability at the time of ovulation. Normally, there is an increase in glucose concentration up to 8 or 11 mmol/litre (150 or 200 mg/dl) at mid-cycle. Low concentrations of glucose occur in the cervical mucus of some infertile women (Kellerman and Weed, 1970). Attempts to detect ovulation by testing for glucose in cervical mucus have not met with success (France and Boyer, 1975).

Soluble proteins comprise about 30% of the high molecular weight non-dialyzable compounds in cervical mucus. These include a variety of serum proteins, secretory proteins and enzymes. In general, the concentration of cervical mucus protein decreases under oestrogen stimulation at mid-cycle and increases with progestogen stimulation during the luteal phase. Quantitative analysis of the protein is hampered by the small volume of specimen and by its high viscosity and tacky nature, but micro-immunoelectrophoresis and micro-radial-diffusion have proved to be useful techniques (Schumacher, 1972). The latter method has demonstrated that the lowest concentrations of proteinase inhibitors and of immunoglobulins G and A coincide with ovulation and maximum sperm receptivity. Secretory IgA and IgG are produced by human cervical tissue in culture, suggesting that a localized immune response may occur in response to specific inciting antigens such as those found in semen (Behrman and Lieberman, 1973).

Several enzymes contained in normal human cervical mucus have been studied in relationship to the menstrual cycle. Methodological differences and sampling difficulties have led to conflicting results. Alkaline phosphatase activity has been reported to rise markedly during the fertile period (Sobrero et al., 1973). A more recent study, however, has demonstrated a significant *decrease* in alkaline phosphatase activity before, and an increase after, ovulation (Moghissi et al., 1976). Amylase activity in cervical mucus appears to be related to hormonal cycles, with highest values during the progestational phase and lowest during the fertile period under oestrogen stimulation. Conversely, lysozyme (muramidase) activity has been reported to be markedly increased during the ovulatory and luteal phases (Musacchio et al., 1972).

Lipid concentrations in cervical mucus undergo cyclic changes, as do most of the other chemical constituents (Singh, 1975a). Total lipid concentration shows a 3-fold decrease at mid-cycle. Cholesterol and triglyceride concentrations parallel this pattern but the magnitude of the mid-cycle decrease is less. The administration of oral contraceptives causes an increase in the concentrations of total lipids, cholesterol and triglyceride and it abolishes the cyclic variation.

Interest in the trace elements in cervical mucus has centred mainly around copper and zinc (Elstein and Daunter, 1972). Copper and zinc manifest a reciprocal type of relationship such that an excess of one may result in a deficiency of the other. Metallic copper has proven to be an effective intrauterine contraceptive material which prevents the implantation of the fertilized ovum. In addition, metallic copper has an inhibitory effect upon alkaline phosphatase and carbonic anhydrase, both of which require zinc as a cofactor (Oster, 1972). The presence of a copper intrauterine device produces a 2- to 4-fold increase in the copper concentration in cervical mucus (Hagenfeldt, 1972; Singh, 1975b). It is possible that this is a part of the mechanism by which copper exerts its contraceptive effect.

2.4.5. Follicular, oviductal and vaginal fluids

Follicular fluid is produced within the graafian follicles as they develop on the surface of the ovary with each new menstrual cycle. The fluid is composed of both transudates from the plasma and secretions from the follicle. The developing oocyte is contained within the follicle and it is the follicular fluid which provides protection, transport and nourishment especially near the time of ovulation. Human follicular fluid may be obtained only during a surgical procedure such as laparoscopy or laporatomy during which the ovaries are visualized. As a result, the biochemical information which has been compiled has found little clinical application. A review of the chemical composition and function of follicular fluid from both human and animal sources has been published (Edwards, 1974).

Synthesis of steroid hormones is a major endocrine function of the ovary. Cyclic variations of these hormones in follicular fluid have now been documented. At mid-cycle, a very high concentration of oestradiol in follicular fluid is closely associated with a high concentration of oestradiol in the venous plasma which drains the corresponding ovary. These data suggest that a graafian follicle may be assumed to be functionally active when the concentration of oestradiol in the fluid exceeds 3.5 mmol/litre (Baird and Fraser, 1975). Other investigators have studied the concentrations of androgens in follicular fluid throughout the phases of the menstrual cycle (McNatty et al., 1976). This is of interest in relation to the high concentration of androstenedione found in the fluid of patients with polycystic ovaries (Stein-Leventhal syndrome) (Edwards, 1974).

Oviductal fluid provides the milieu in which spermatozoa and ova unite and development of the conceptus begins. Unfortunately, human oviductal fluid is even less accessible than is follicular fluid. Nonetheless, a few investigators have succeeded in cannulating the oviduct at the time of surgery. This procedure has provided enough fluid for a cursory study of the chemical composition (Brackett and Mastroianni, 1974); however, the clinical utility of such studies has yet to be demonstrated.

Vaginal secretions contain a number of volatile aliphatic acids containing from two to five carbon atoms. Some of these have been identified as pheromones, or sex attractants, in other primate species (Sokolov et al., 1976). Human vaginal secretions have been collected using tampons, and chromatographic analysis of the volatile constituents revealed that the secretion rate of the low molecular mass fatty acids is highest during the fertile period at mid-cycle. Additionally, the use of oral contraceptives was shown to lower the secretory rate and to obliterate the mid-cycle increase in volatile compounds (Michael et al., 1974). Elucidation of an active human pheromonal system awaits further investigation.

2.5. SALIVA, FAECES AND MECONIUM

The chemical analysis of the contents of the gastrointestinal tract is an important part of the diagnosis of many disorders. Specialized collection procedures permit sampling of specific fluids such as saliva, gastric contents and pancreatic secretions. The chemical pathology of many of these fluids is discussed in other chapters: the metabolism of bile is detailed in Chapter 10, section 10.2; tests of intestinal and pancreatic function are covered in Chapter 12, sections 12.4 and 12.5; saliva and gastric analysis is discussed in Chapter 11, sections 11.1, 11.2 and 11.3. In this section recent developments in the chemical analysis of saliva and faeces are summarized which have found clinical utility in the evaluation or management of diseases involving not only the gastrointestinal tract but other organ systems as well.

2.5.1. Saliva

The physiology of salivary secretion and measurement of salivary flow rate are outlined in Chapter 11, section 11.1, but they are also considered in this section since they bear so directly on the concentrations of the various chemical constituents.

Saliva is secreted mainly by three pairs of glands – the parotid, the submaxillary and the sublingual glands. The principal stimulus for salivary secretion appears to be neuronal with both sympathetic and parasympathetic contributions. Several physiological studies support the hypothesis that a hydrostatic pressure differential across the secretory epithelium is a major salivary secretory mechanism (Shannon et al., 1974). The parotid glands, located at the side of the face, are the largest, weighing from 20 to 30 grams each. Numerous other small glands located in mucus membranes of the mouth also contribute secretions to the mixed salivary fluid. About 0.8 to 1.2 litres of saliva are produced daily, with highest secretions occurring at meal-times. Saliva has lubricant and cleansing actions and the digestion process begins as salivary amylase initiates the breakdown of dietary carbohydrates into maltose and glucose. Salivary glands also function as excretory organs for a number of chemical substances and micro-organisms (Hightower and Janowitz, 1973).

Collection of saliva samples has been facilitated by a number of devices which fit over the openings of the various salivary ducts (Stephen and Speirs, 1976). A plastic suction cup may be used to collect parotid saliva. Submandibular and sublingual saliva is collected by triangular plastic appliances or trays which, if necessary, may be individually fitted to each subject. Mixed saliva, collected by gravity drainage or by suction, can be stimulated by the chewing of wax, gum base, or rubber bands. The investigator must, however, be familiar with changes in the composition which may occur with each of the various methods used to induce salivary flow. Lipophilic drugs are absorbed by paraffin containing materials chewed to stimulate salivary flow. Losses from saliva of up to 40% have been reported for chlorpromazine and butaperazine when Parafilm (3M Company, St. Paul, Minnesota) is used as a masticatory stimulant (Chang and Chiou, 1976).

The chemical composition of saliva is affected by a number of physiological variables such as diet, age, endocrine status, circadian rhythms, flow rate, type of stimulus and proximity of collection time to meal-time. Composition and flow-rate may also be altered by a variety of drugs (Mason and Chisholm, 1975). Collection of resting saliva may be hampered by the stimulatory effect of cannulation of the duct or application of a suction device (Benedek-Spät, 1973a). The salivary flow rate varies from near zero to as high as 3 or 4 ml/min under maximal stimulation. In order to compile reference data relating chemical composition to flow rate, a number of authors have studied the effects of varying degrees of salivary stimulation on the concentrations of the electrolytes and many other metabolites (Kreusser et al., 1972; Benedek-Spät, 1973b; Dawes, 1974a). Even though the data show some degree of variability between individuals, they still provide the investigator with correlative information regarding solute concentration and flow rate. A reference table for human parotid saliva collected at varying degrees of exogenous stimulation has been published (Shannon, 1973; Shannon et al., 1974).

Circadian variations in parotid saliva flow rate and composition can be fitted to curves derived from a combination of a fundamental sine wave of 24-hour period and its first harmonic. Similar, but not identical, circadian rhythms were demonstrated for both resting and stimulated saliva (Ferguson et al., 1973; Ferguson and Fort, 1974). The curves are reproducible with a given individual, but considerable variation occurs between subjects. Many investigators collect saliva between 07.30 and 10.00 hours when most of the constituents are subject to maximum rates of variation. The studies cited above demonstrate that the minimum rate of change in composition occurs during mid-afternoon, indicating that the optimal collection time is between 14.00 and 16.00 hours. Dawes (1974b) has reviewed the salient features of rhythms in salivary flow rate and composition.

Despite difficulties with biological variability, a growing body of literature has begun to document the value of salivary secretions as a potential source of important chemical information (Wotman and Mandel, 1973). Among the first studies relating salivary composition to systemic disease were those which examined changes in the saliva electrolyte composition in aldosteronism (Lauler et al., 1962). Sodium/potassium ratios in saliva increased following surgical removal of the aldosterone-producing adrenal adenoma (Wotman et al., 1969). In a similar study, the salivary potassium concentration was higher in a group of patients with primary hyperaldosteronism (Conn's syndrome) than in a group of patients with adrenal hyperplasia (Wotman et al., 1970). Limitations in the use of sodium/potassium ratios as a diagnostic screen for aldosteronism have, however, been reported (Wilson et al., 1971).

Others have examined salivary electrolytes throughout the menstrual cycle. Sodium and calcium concentrations decrease whereas that of potassium increases during the ovulatory period at mid-cycle (Puskulian, 1972). A study of the endocrine effects of pregnancy on salivary secretions has shown an antepartum decrease in sodium and calcium concentrations, with an increase in potassium concentration (Marder et al., 1972). This work demonstrates the responsiveness of the salivary glands to endocrine hormones. Because saliva is the most accessible of the body fluids, it has been suggested that it could provide the basis of a simple self-administered test to detect the fertile pre-ovulatory period of the menstrual cycle (France and Boyer, 1975). Changes in the salivary concentration of both glucose (Davis and Balin, 1973) and phosphate (Ben-Aryeh et al., 1976) have been suggested as indicators of ovulation. The submandibular saliva of patients with cystic fibrosis contains a higher concentration of calcium, sodium and chloride than that of normal controls (Blomfield et al., 1973). A method has been developed for the collection of stimulated secretions from the small salivary glands of the lip. Saliva obtained by this method from patients with cystic fibrosis contains a sodium concentration which is 2- to 4-fold higher than that of normal controls (Wiesmann et al., 1972). The wide variability of electrolyte concentrations in parotid saliva precludes their use in the diagnosis of cystic fibrosis (Blomfield et al., 1976). Trisomy 21 (Down's syndrome) may be associated with physiological and biochemical anomalies which are manifest by changes in the composition of saliva (Cutress, 1972; Winer and Feller, 1972). However, the relationship between the observed changes and the possible causes remains obscure.

The chemical analysis of saliva has been proposed as an adjunct to the diagnosis of chronic pancreatic disorders (Kakizaki et al., 1976). The test measures salivary output, bicarbonate concentration and amylase activity of parotid saliva. Pilocarpine hydrochloride is given intramuscularly to stimulate salivary secretion, and consecutive 5-minute samples are collected for a total of 25 minutes, so that the maximum for each of the three secretory parameters may be determined. The reference range for each of the three is determined by testing normal volunteers. The saliva test appears to have a diagnostic accuracy greater than that of the secretin–pancreozymin test which is usually used to assess pancreatic function (Chapter 12, section 12.5), and is much simpler to perform.

The determination of potassium and calcium concentrations in saliva has shown clinical potential for the detection of digitalis intoxication (Wotman et al., 1971). The product of the potassium and calcium concentrations is generally higher in patients with a toxic serum concentration of digoxin, than in those whose digoxin concentration is in the therapeutic range. Unfortunately, some investigators have been unable to confirm these findings (Gould et al., 1973). One of the variables which clearly affects salivary electrolyte excretion is the severity of renal insufficiency. Patients whose urine output is less than 1 litre/day have high potassium and calcium concentrations in their saliva whether or not they are taking digoxin (Swanson et al., 1973). Other problem areas have been defined, such as techniques for the collection of saliva and standardization of analytical methods (Wotman and Bigger, 1974).

A number of trace elements have been measured in saliva, including toxic metals such as lead (Fung et al., 1975), mercury (Windeler, 1973) and selenium (Hadjimarkos and Shearer, 1971). Correlations between the concentration of these elements in saliva and blood await further definition. Zinc is normally secreted by the salivary glands in a concentration of about 50 mg/litre. Studies (Henkin et al., 1975a) of a group of patients with hypogeusia (loss of taste acuity) showed that their saliva has an abnormally low zinc concentration (about 10 mg/litre). In addition, a unique zinc-containing metalloprotein which appears to be associated with the taste process has been isolated from saliva (Henkin et al., 1975b).

Among the anions which have been studied in saliva are the halides and their congeners, pertechnetate and thiocyanate (Stephen et al., 1973). Most iodinated radiographic contrast media are rapidly excreted by the kidneys, but in patients with renal insufficiency, there is evidence for in vivo deiodination of these compounds with subsequent elimination of inorganic iodide via the salivary glands (Talner et al., 1973). Pertechnetate and thiocyanate are handled in much the same way as iodide. One study has shown that smokers secrete salivary thiocyanate in a concentration which is twice as high as that of non-smokers. Conversely, the iodide concentration in the saliva of smokers is significantly lower than that of non-smokers (Tenovuo and Mäkinen, 1976). Pertechnetate has been used in the study of thyroid and salivary concentrating mechanisms (Mason and Chisholm, 1975). Nitrate is secreted normally in saliva in concentrations ranging from 15 to 40 mg/litre. Micro-organisms in the oral cavity then convert a variable percentage of the nitrate to nitrite. This process has attracted attention because of the carcinogenic nitrosoamines which may be formed from nitrite and amines in the acid environment of the stomach or by the action of bacteria in the mouth (Tannenbaum et al., 1974).

The concentrations of calcium and phosphate in the oral fluids have become a topic of interest in the dental literature because of the involvement of these ions in the remineralization of enamel and the formation of dental calculus (Gron, 1973). Depending upon pH, saliva may become supersaturated with respect to calcium and phosphate, resulting in the formation of crystalline deposits within the matrix of the dental plaque (Leach, 1974). Salivary proteins and oral bacteria provide a nidus for the formation of the precipitate. There is strong positive correlation between the amount of calcium found in dental calculus and that found in spontaneous precipitates from whole saliva (McGaughey et al., 1975). High concentrations of calcium and phosphorus occur in the saliva of patients with cystic fibrosis. In these and other patients with heavy calculus formation, it appears that the crystalline nature and composition of the calcium phosphate deposits change as plaque formation progresses (Tannenbaum et al., 1976).

The salivary concentration of fluoride has been studied because of the importance of this ion in the prevention of dental caries. In parotid saliva, the fluoride concentration is independent of flow rate. Oral administration of sodium fluoride results in an increased secretion of fluoride by the parotid gland (Shannon et al., 1976). Gastroinstestinal absorption of fluoride may be inhibited by the presence of aluminium which occurs in the normal diet as well as in a number of antacids (Brudevold et al., 1973).

The protein concentration in human mixed saliva normally ranges from 1 to 3 g/litre. Because of problems with contamination of mixed saliva by bacterial proteins and food debris, most investigators prefer to work with isolated secretions from individual salivary glands (Bonilla, 1972). Higher concentrations of albumin are found in mixed (whole) saliva than in individual glandular secretions. The albumin concentration increases even more with gingival stimulation. These data suggest that protein enters the oral fluids with the exudation of serum proteins across the gingival epithelium (Oppenheim and Hay, 1972). This hypothesis is further supported by the detection of increased concentrations of IgA and IgG in the mixed saliva of patients with periodontal diseases (Lindstrom and Folke, 1973).

Electrophoresis of salivary proteins has been explored as a potential predictive or diagnostic technique for a number of disease states. Parotid saliva has been subjected to polyacrylamide gel electrophoresis in an attempt to identify patterns which distinguish individuals who are caries-susceptible from those who are caries-resistant. Patients with active caries showed significantly higher concentrations of anionic proteins at pH 9, which were predominantly isoamylases, than did subjects who were caries-resistant (Balekjian et al., 1975). Conversely, the caries-resistant group had higher salivary concentrations of cationic proteins at pH 9.

Electrophoretic fractionation of the proteins found in the saliva of patients with diabetes mellitus has shown a densely staining band in the γ-globulin region. This abnormality was seen in 85% of the diabetic patients surveyed (Finestone et al., 1973). Isoelectric focussing has demonstrated the presence of additional anionic proteins in the saliva of patients with rheumatoid arthritis and Sjögren's syndrome (Chisholm et al., 1973). Patients with these diseases have an increased salivary concentration of β_2-microglobulin which decreases concurrently with a clinical response to treatment (Talal et al., 1975). A detailed quantitative study of the submandibular salivary proteins in patients with cystic fibrosis has demonstrated a significant increase in three specific fractions. These include two fractions with amylase and acid phosphatase activities, but the protein comprising the third fraction remains unidentified (Mayo et al., 1976).

A small group of parotid proteins has recently been the subject of study by human geneticists. These are proteins of low molecular mass with a high percentage of basic residues such as proline and glycine (Hay and Oppenheim, 1974). They chemically resemble both collagen and enamel protein and have a marked affinity for hydroxyapatite. The most interesting aspect of these proteins is the high frequency of genetic polymorphism occurring in various populations (Azen and Oppenheim, 1973). The concordance between parotid salivary protein patterns is highest for monozygotic twins, followed by dizygotic twins and non-twin siblings; unrelated subjects show the lowest concordance (Smith et al., 1976). This type of polymorphism is potentially useful in genetic research and in the establishment of linkage.

One of the most publicized applications of the analysis of saliva has been in the area of therapeutic drug monitoring. The concentration of a drug which is secreted in saliva correlates well with the concentration of free (non-protein bound) drug circulating in the plasma. It is the free drug which is pharmocologically active and which produces toxicity when present in concentrations above the therapeutic range. A review of the saliva-to-plasma ratio of a number of drugs in relation to the proportion of free circulating drug has been published (Horning et al., 1977).

It is important that both the chemist and the attending physician be aware of potential problems when whole mixed saliva is collected for drug analysis. There may be absorption of lipophilic drugs onto paraffin-containing masticatory stimulants (Chang and Chiou, 1976). It is also important to know the form in which the dose of drug was administered. If the drug was given as an uncoated tablet or in an aqueous suspension, enough drug may remain in the oral cavity to give a falsely elevated concentration in whole saliva (Chiou et al., 1976). This problem may be avoided by giving an oral dosage which is sealed in a capsule or in a coated tablet. Another alternative is to collect the saliva produced by a single gland using a suction cup collecting device.

A study of the plasma and saliva levels of phenytoin has demonstrated the value of the latter in patients with epilepsy and chronic renal insufficiency (Reynolds et al., 1976). In these patients, the concentration of total phenytoin in plasma is unreliable as an indicator of the free drug concentration. Better correlation has been demonstrated between drug concentration in saliva and the free drug concentration in plasma. Using a radioimmunoassay technique, it has been demonstrated that phenytoin concentrations are similar in parotid and submandibular saliva, and that they are independent of the volume of saliva produced (Paxton et al., 1976, 1977).

Lithium carbonate is used to treat manic depressive illness. Lithium is secreted in the saliva in a concentration which may be as high as 4 times the plasma concentration although the usual saliva-to-plasma ratio for this drug is about 2.3. The relationship of saliva lithium concentration to flow rate has not yet been completely elucidated (Lazarus et al., 1973). There is some evidence that variation in the capacity of the salivary glands to concentrate lithium may be related to the duration of administration. Caution must also be exercised when interpreting results if the patient is also taking a psychotropic agent, such as phenothiazine, which has atropine-like effects and which may lead to inhibition of salivary secretion of both water and solute, thereby altering salivary drug concentrations (Neu and DiMascio, 1977).

Pharmacokinetic studies of theophylline show an excellent linear correlation between drug concentrations in plasma and saliva: the concentrations in plasma are about twice as high as those in saliva (Koysooko et al., 1974). Successful clinical application of saliva theophylline measurements has been published in the paediatric literature. Specimens can be obtained non-invasively in children and the results give a good indication of compliance – whether or not the patient is taking the drug. This permits a more accurate assessment of therapeutic response (Eney and Goldstein, 1976).

2.5.2. Faeces and meconium

The colon of the normal adult presents from 100 to 200 grams of faeces daily to the rectum for elimination. The mass may be higher if the diet contains a high proportion of vegetable fibre. About 75% of the total faecal mass is water. The solids are comprised of bacteria (30 to 40%), fat (10 to 20%), inorganic salts (10 to 20%), undigested roughage (about 30%), and protein (2 to 3%) (Guyton, 1976). The characteristic brown colour of faeces is due to bile pigments.

Meconium is the substance passed per rectum by the neonate during the first 2 to 3 days of extrauterine life. It is a viscous greenish-brown material which contains desquamated epithelial cells and hair which were swallowed along with amniotic fluid. Meconium contains no bacteria until colonization of the colon begins a few hours after birth (Davidson, 1972).

The collection and laboratory manipulation of faecal specimens are unpleasant tasks. As a result, different methods for handling faeces have been suggested. One of these uses plastic bags for collection, with secondary containment in a sealable plastic pail or paint-can (Hoffman et al., 1973). Another uses a deep-freeze toilet for the collection of the total specimen. The frozen faeces is then weighed and homogenized in a garbage-disposal unit. After a sample is removed for analysis, the remainder of the faecal specimen is flushed away (Ghoos and Vantrappen, 1977). Of more fundamental importance than the aesthetics of the handling procedures is the assurance of a complete collection when a timed specimen is required and of complete homogenization of the specimen prior to sampling. This is especially true for tests such as the quantitative faecal fat determination which is performed on a 72-hour collection.

Testing of the faeces for the presence of occult blood involves the use of a qualitative chemical test and requires only a small random faecal specimen. The importance of a simple screening test for gastrointestinal bleeding cannot be over-emphasized, because it is such a test which may alert the physician to a clinically silent peptic ulcer or a cancer of the stomach or colon. Normal gastrointestinal blood loss amounts to about 1 to 2 ml of blood daily (O'Neill et al., 1973). Alteration of the haemoglobin by partial digestion occurs, especially when the blood originates in the oesophagus, stomach or duodenum (Burton et al., 1976).

The commonly employed screening tests for occult blood in faeces depend upon detection of the peroxidase activity of haemoglobin. This activity decreases as the haemoglobin is degraded to haematin. False-positive reactions may occur in the presence of myoglobin and haemoglobin contained in dietary meat. Plant and bacterial peroxidases also contribute to the false-positive rate. False-negative results may occur if the blood is not uniformly mixed with the stool or if the patient is ingesting ascorbic acid (Jaffe et al., 1975). In addition, there are large differences in the sensitivities of the various chromogens which are commonly used for detection. All of these shortcomings have led some authors to conclude that there is no diagnostic value in the screening of faeces for occult blood by employing the peroxidase activity of haem (Ford-Jones and Cogswell, 1975; Lauridsen and Bohn, 1976).

It is unlikely, however, that the experienced clinician will abandon a simple test which he believes has served him and his patients well. Indeed, there is support for his steadfastness, provided that he uses the test rationally and is aware of its shortcomings (Winawer, 1976). A commercial modification of the guaiac method (Hemoccult, Smith-Kline Diagnostics, Sunnyvale, California) has emerged as a clinically useful indicator of gastrointestinal bleeding (Morris et al., 1976; Stroehlein et al., 1976). The Hemoccult slide test was compared with guaiac and with orthotolidine reagents while actual gastrointestinal blood loss was quantitated using a radioactive tracer technique. The false-positive rate for the Hemoccult method ranged from 7 to 12% while the other two methods yielded over 70% false-positive reactions. The sensitivity of the Hemoccult slides is less, but this problem is minimized by testing three or more separate faecal samples to reduce the false-negative rate.

Analyses of the water and electrolyte composition of faeces have found more application in studies of gastrointestinal physiology than in clinical medicine. Situations may occasionally arise, however, when it is helpful to estimate faecal electrolyte losses. For example, patients with chronic hormonally mediated diarrhoeas may lose up to 7 litres of fluid daily, accompanied by the loss of several hundred millimol of sodium and potassium (Graham et al., 1975; Spiro, 1977). In these circumstances, the physician may wish to have an approximate idea of the daily faecal electrolyte losses so that the appropriate replacement therapy may be instituted. Acid–base balance may also be assessed from the faecal concentrations of sodium, potassium and chloride. Faecal pH and bicarbonate measurements are unreliable because of alterations produced by bacterial metabolism (Fordtran, 1973).

Profuse diarrhoea produces fluid faeces which contain greater than 90% water. A well mixed 24-hour specimen should be submitted for optimal assessment of electrolyte losses. An aliquot is either centrifuged or filtered, to remove particulate matter and the supernatant or filtrate is analyzed to provide a reasonable estimate of faecal electrolyte concentrations. In vitro and in vivo dialysis methods have also been used to obtain specimens for faecal fluid analysis. The in vivo dialysis technique, however, provides fluid which differs in composition from that obtained by centrifugation (Tarlow and Thom, 1974; Owens and Padovan, 1976).

Faecal analysis may also be helpful in the diagnosis of diarrhoea which is due to chronic laxative abuse. Patients who ingest excessive amounts of Epsom salts or Glauber's salt often excrete an increased quantity of sulphate. The faecal sulphate concentration is usually less than 2.3 mmol/litre (4.5 mEq/litre) when the diarrhoea is of a hormonal aetiology. The magnesium content of faeces varies with diet and physical activity. Consequently its measurement is of less value than that of the urinary magnesium excretion, which may be greatly increased if the patient is ingesting Epsom salts. Alkalinization of faeces or urine has been employed to detect the red colour of phenolphthalein which is a commonly used laxative (Cummings, 1974).

An increased albumin concentration has been found in the meconium of infants with cystic fibrosis (Bull et al., 1974). This discovery has subsequently led to the development of a commercial reagent strip test (Boehringer-Mannheim Corporation) for the detection of albumin in meconium (Bruns et al., 1977). Evaluations of the test as a screening procedure indicate that it has a specificity of 99 to 99.5% (Kollberg and Hellsing, 1975; Stephan et al., 1975). False-positive results may be seen with various neonatal gastrointestinal disorders such as atresia, malabsorption, and melaena. The use of glycerine suppositories has also caused false-positive results (Berger et al., 1977). The sensitivity of the test ranges from 50 to 80% depending on the size and design of the study. At least a portion of the false-negative results may be attributed to normal pancreatic function in perhaps 15 to 20% of infants with cystic fibrosis. This has raised questions as to the value of the test as a screening procedure (Ryley et al., 1976). In any case, the parents of an infant at high risk for cystic fibrosis should not be counselled solely on the basis of a meconium test. Such an infant must have the sweat electrolyte test (section 2.6.3.) and must be followed carefully for clinical manifestations of the disease.

The study of immunoglobulins in faeces has been hampered by the digestion and reabsorption of proteins in the gastrointestinal tract. Nonetheless several serum proteins including immunoglobulins have now been detected in the faeces of infants and children. A higher IgA concentration is present in the faeces of infants receiving human milk than those fed on cow's milk (Haneberg, 1974). The use of radioisotopes for the quantitation of protein loss in exudative enteropathy is discussed in Chapter 12, section 12.1. A variation of this technique using [^{131}I]albumin and [^{125}I]immunoglobulin G has been used for topographic diagnosis (localization) of chronic inflammatory bowel disease (Jarnum and Jensen, 1975).

Carcinoembryonic antigen (CEA) has been detected in the sera of patients with colorectal carcinoma (Chapter 25, section 25.5.). This antigen is present in detectable concentrations in the faeces of normal adults as well as those with cancer (Freed and Taylor, 1972). It has been postulated that the high faecal concentrations of CEA originate from the surface of the epithelial cells of the normal, as well as the diseased, gastrointestinal tract (Elias et al., 1974). CEA is also produced in the foetal gastrointestinal tract and, therefore, subsequently appears in the meconium. Foetal hypoxia is associated with meconium staining of the amniotic fluid. As a result, measurement of CEA concentrations in amniotic fluid has been suggested as an indicator of the severity of foetal distress (Goldenberg et al., 1972).

The chemical pathology of the bile acids in serum is discussed in Chapter 10, section 10.2. Measurement of bile acids in faeces or in serum is a complicated and time consuming procedure. Comparison is poor between isotopic turnover studies and faecal bile acid excretion as measured by gas chromatography–mass spectrometry (Subbiah et al., 1976). The study of faecal bile acids is further complicated by bacterial alteration of these compounds in the colon. Patterns of bile acid excretion change with age; the proportion of secondary bile acids excreted in the faeces increases as the infant grows into adulthood (Huang et al., 1976). High dietary intake of certain types of vegetable fibre also results in increased faecal bile acid excretion (Walters et al., 1975; Baird et al., 1977).

The quantity of bile acids excreted in the faeces is increased in certain diseases and following surgical resection of segments of the bowel. For example, some patients who undergo surgical resection of the ileum develop watery diarrhoea associated with the excretion of excessive amounts of bile acids. It appears that chenodeoxycholic acid entering the colon is an important factor in subsequent water and electrolyte loss (Mitchell et al., 1973). Similar increases in the faecal excretion of secondary bile acids have been implicated in the pathogenesis of post-vagotomy diarrhoea (Gerskowitch et al., 1973). A group of patients with cancer of the large bowel has been shown to have an increased concentration of bile acids in their faeces. There is growing concern that these compounds may be involved in colon carcinogenesis (Hill et al., 1975).

The laboratory investigation of malabsorption syndromes is reviewed in Chapter 12, section 12.4. Steatorrhoea is diagnosed by quantitation of the daily faecal fat excretion. This involves saponification followed by either titration or spectrophotometric measurement of the liberated free fatty acids. The latter method has the advantage of good recovery of the medium-chain as well as the long-chain fatty acids (Massion and McNeely, 1973). Attention must be paid to the dietary fat intake if results are to be interpreted correctly (Walker et al., 1973; Losowsky et al., 1974). Microbial hydroxylation of fatty acids in the colon may be excessive in certain pathological states such as small bowel disease and pancreatic insufficiency. In some cases, the increased excretion of hydroxylated fatty acids has been associated with diarrhoea or steatorrhoea, or both (Soong et al., 1972). Measurement of faecal hydroxystearic acid has been suggested as a diagnostic test for ileal disease and small bowel stasis (Wiggins et al., 1974).

Patterns of excretion of cholesterol and its metabolites in faeces are dependent upon the age of the subject (Huang et al., 1976) and upon the fat and fibre content of the diet (Nestel et al., 1975; Walters et al., 1975). Patients with familial polyposis coli excrete a greater amount of cholesterol in their faeces than do normal controls (Watne and Core, 1975). Others have confirmed these data and suggested that the analysis of faeces for cholesterol and its metabolites could be used as a screening test for the disease in patients at high risk (Reddy et al., 1976). The interaction of intestinal bacterial flora with dietary substances and digestive secretions has been postulated as a factor in colon carcinogenesis. Population studies have demonstrated differences in faecal steroid excretion which are associated with diet. Americans and Western Europeans have a higher incidence of colon cancer than do Africans and Asians. This is strongly associated with increased faecal bile acid and neutral sterol excretion resulting from the Western-type diet which is high in animal protein and fat (Hill and Aries, 1971; Reddy and Wynder, 1973).

2.6. SPECIALIZED GLANDULAR SECRETIONS

2.6.1. Mucus

Mucus-secreting glands and mucous membranes produce fluids which are necessary for lubricating and cleansing functions throughout the body. Mucus is produced in the gastro-intestinal tract, the genitourinary system (section 2.4.4.) and in the respiratory tract. Bronchial mucus (sputum) may be obtained by expectoration or by the technique of broncho-alveolar lavage. Nonetheless, technical problems associated with the collection of normal sputum specimens have precluded the compilation of reliable reference ranges for the chemical constituents (Boat and Matthews, 1973). The biochemical composition of the lung washings has been shown to reflect the nature of certain underlying disease processes (Ramirez et al., 1971). The cellular and protein content of broncho-alveolar lavage fluid has been analyzed to explore the diagnostic, therapeutic and investigative worth of this technique in evaluating patients with various types of fibrotic pulmonary disease (Reynolds et al., 1977).

Most of the recent studies which employ the chemical analysis of bronchial washings have focussed on the concentrations of specific proteins as markers of the underlying disease. Bronchogenic carcinoma is associated with an increased amount of IgG and IgA in pulmonary lavage fluids (Mandel et al., 1976). Because the dilution factor of the washings is unknown, the ratio of immunoglobulin concentration to potassium concentration is calculated. The washings from the patient's "normal" lung provide a reference value against which the washings from the diseased lung are compared. Inflammatory disease does not produce the increased immunoglobulin concentrations which are seen with malignant disease. Other immunoreactive proteins which have been detected in the bronchial washings of patients with bronchogenic carcinoma are carcinoembryonic antigen and a high molecular mass adrenocorticotrophic hormone ("big" ACTH) (Blair and Goldenberg, 1974; Ayvazian et al., 1975).

2.6.2. Milk

The chemical analysis of human milk has been employed primarily to investigate problems of a nutritional or toxicological nature. The biochemical differences between human milk and proprietary infant formulae have been critically assessed from a nutritional standpoint (Hambraeus, 1977). Others have demonstrated that breast milk undergoes a change in nutritional composition while the infant is feeding (Hall, 1975). This change in composition may be functionally important as an appetite control mechanism in the breast-fed infant. This mechanism would be lost with synthetic formulae of constant composition and flavour. Immunoglobulins, especially IgA, occur in human milk but may be entirely lacking from proprietary milks. There is evidence that these proteins serve a protective function for the infant. The immunoglobulin concentration in milk is highest in the immediate post-natal period (Peitersen et al., 1975).

Several studies reflect growing concern over the appearance of drugs and toxic substances in human milk. The transport of these compounds from plasma to milk is dependent upon a number of factors including blood flow, glandular transport mechanisms and lipid concentration in the milk. Also important are the plasma concentration of the substance and its solubility in lipids and in water (Catz and Giacoia, 1972). Most drugs appear in milk in amounts which are less than 1% of the daily dose ingested by the mother. Certain lipophilic drugs, such as phenytoin and phenobarbital, may appear in slightly higher concentrations (Vorherr, 1974). Some drugs, such as the sex steroids found in oral contraceptive preparations, may interfere with hepatic metabolism or cause development of secondary sex characteristics in the nursing infant. Breast feeding should be discontinued when the mother is receiving radioisotopes, steroids, anticoagulants or antineoplastic agents (Knowles, 1974).

Halogenated hydrocarbon pesticides are among the lipophilic substances which readily accumulate in human tissues (Bakken and Seip, 1976). DDT has been found in human milk in a concentration which is over 100 times greater than the maximum concentration permitted by the World Health Organization (Winter et al., 1976; Woodard et al., 1976). Heavy accidental exposures to polyhalogenated biphenyls (PCB and PBB) have resulted in high concentrations of these compounds in human milk (Miller, 1977). This was associated with obvious toxic manifestations in nursing infants. Identification of the problem of exposure to environmental toxins requires alertness on the part of the physician and the ability to characterize the toxic materials in human fluids and tissues when necessary (Finberg, 1977).

2.6.3. Sweat

The only widely accepted test done on sweat is the determination of sodium and chloride concentrations for the diagnosis of cystic fibrosis. Increased concentrations of these two ions in sweat is the most constant and clearly defined abnormality associated with the disease (Lobeck, 1972). This finding is most helpful in children, and is present at the time of birth, provided adequate sweat can be obtained for analysis. In healthy subjects, the concentrations of sodium and chloride in sweat increase with age, but even in adults, the test may be useful if cystic fibrosis is suspected on clinical grounds. Sodium and chloride concentrations increase with an increase in the rate of sweat production. Other disorders such as Addison's disease may be associated with an abnormally high sweat electrolyte concentration, but these are easily distinguished on the basis of other clinical information (Lobeck, 1972).

Sweat may be safely and painlessly collected by the technique of pilocarpine iontophoresis, which involves the use of an electric current to introduce pilocarpine into the skin and stimulate localized sweating. This continues for about 30 minutes, allowing adequate time for collection. From 150 to 1500 mg of sweat may be obtained by this method (Gibson and Cooke, 1959). Others have used thermal stimulation in an environmental chamber to collect whole body sweat for research purposes (Cohen et al., 1976). Sodium and potassium concentrations in whole body sweat correlate well with those found in sweat stimulated by pilocarpine iontophoresis. The use of ion-specific electrodes for the measurement of sodium and chloride in sweat is appealing because of its simplicity (Grice et al., 1975). These electrodes may be used to measure the electrolytes in situ, thereby avoiding the necessity of collecting the sweat and transporting it to the laboratory for analysis (Steinrud et al., 1974).

ACKNOWLEDGEMENTS

I wish to express my gratitude to Marilyn White for assisting with the preparation of the bibliography, to Barbara Young for secretarial assistance, and to Dr. E. Arthur Robertson for his critique of the manuscript.

REFERENCES

Section 2.2. Fluids of the central nervous system and special senses

Altman, P.L. and Dittmer, D.S. (Eds.) (1961) Blood and Other Body Fluids. Federation of American Societies for Experimental Biology, Washington, D.C.

Bartko, D., Danisova, J. and Wagnerova, M. (1970) Protein spectrum changes in brain tumors with special regard to quantitative analysis of cerebrospinal fluid protein. Ceskoslovenska Neurologie, 33, 83–88.

Bessière, E., Crockett, R., Le Rebeller, M.J., Maurain, C. and Grenie, D. (1973) Méthodes chimiques de dosage de l'humeur aquese normal. Albrecht von Graefes Archiv für Klinische und Experimentelle Ophthalmologie, 187, 273–288.

Bill, A. (1973) The role of ciliary blood flow and ultra filtration in aqueous humor formation. Experimental Eye Research, 16, 287–298.

Blayo, M.C., Coudert, J. and Pocidalo, J.J. (1975) Comparison of cisternal and lumbar cerebrospinal fluid pH in high altitude natives. Pflügers Archiv; European Journal of Physiology, 356, 159–167.

Blount, M., Kinney, A.B. and Donohoe, K.M. (1974) Obtaining and analyzing cerebrospinal fluid. Nursing Clinics of North America, 9, 593–609.

Calabrese, V.P. (1976) The interpretation of routine CSF tests. Virginia Medical Monthly, 103, 207–209.

Campkin, T.V., Barker, R.G., Pabari, M. and Grove, L.H. (1974) Acid-base changes in arterial blood and cerebrospinal fluid during craniotomy and hyperventilation. British Journal of Anaesthesia, 46, 263–267.

Chandler, J.W. (1974) Quantitative determinations of complement components and immunoglobulins in tears and aqueous humor. Investigative Ophthalmology, 13, 151–153.

Clausen, J., Fog, T. and Roboz-Einstein, E. (1969) The clinical value of assaying proteins in the CSF: a comparative study in methods. Acta Neurologica Scandinavica, 45, 513–528.

Coe, J.I. (1972) Use of clinical determinations on vitreous humor in forensic pathology. Journal of Forensic Sciences, 17, 541–546.

Cole, D.F. (1970) Aqueous and ciliary body. In Biochemistry of the Eye (Ed. C.N. Graymore), Academic Press, London.

Cole, D.F. (1974) Comparative aspects of the intraocular fluids. In The Eye, (Eds. H. Davson and L.T. Graham), Academic Press, New York.

Davies-Jones, G.A.B. (1969) LDH and GOT of the CSF in tumors of the CNS. Journal of Neurology, Neurosurgery and Psychiatry, 32, 324–327.

Doutremepuich, C. (1975) Biochimie des liquides de l'oreille interne. Revue de Laryngologie Otologie-Rhinologie, 96, 535–548.

Durham, D.G., Dickinson, J.C. and Hamilton, P.B. (1971) Ion-exchange chromatography of free amino acids in human intraocular fluids. Clinical Chemistry, 17, 285–289.

Fisch, U., Murata, K. and Hossli, G. (1976) Measurement of oxygen tension in human perilymph. Acta Oto-laryngologica, 81, 278–282.

Forster, H.V., Dempsey, J.A. and Chosy, L.W. (1975) Incomplete compensation of CSF [H^+] in man during acclimatization to high altitude. Journal of Applied Physiology, 38, 1067–1072.

Gilland, O. (1971) Cerebrospinal fluid. Progress in Neurology and Psychiatry, 26, 329–361.

Green, K. and Pederson, J.E. (1973) Aqueous humor formation. Experimental Eye Research, 16, 273–286.

Greenawald, K.A., Speicher, C.E., Evers, W. and Henry, J.B. (1973) Glucose content in cerebrospinal fluid. American Journal of Clinical Pathology, 59, 518–520.

Guyton, A.C., Taylor, A.E. and Granger, H.J. (1975) Special fluid systems: eye, brain, liver, intestines, muscle, and bone. In Circulatory Physiology II: Dynamics and control of the body fluids (Eds. A.C. Guyton, A.E. Taylor and H.J. Granger) pp. 206–224, W.B. Saunders, Philadelphia.

Jordon, R.M., Kendall, J.W. and Seaich, J.L. (1976) CSF hormone concentration in the evaluation of pituitary tumors. Annals of Internal Medicine, 85, 49–55.

Kabak, J. and Romano, P.E. (1975) Aqueous humour lactic dehydrogenase isoenzymes in retinoblastoma. British Journal of Ophthalmology, 59, 268–269.

Krieg, A.F. (1974) Cerebrospinal fluid and other fluids. In Clinical Diagnosis by Laboratory Methods, (Eds. I. Davidsohn and J.B. Henry) pp. 1254–1279, W.B. Saunders, Philadelphia.

Laterre, E.C., Callewaert, A., Heremans, J.F. and Sfaello, Z. (1970) Electrophoretic morphology of gamma globulins in CSF of multiple sclerosis and other diseases of the nervous system. Neurology, 20, 982–989.

Laursen, A.B. and Lorentzen, S.E. (1974) Glucose, pyruvate and citrate concentrations in the aqueous humour of human cataractous eyes. Acta Ophthalmologica, 52, 477–489.

Manheim, A., Perez, R.E., Jr. and Soyangco, A. (1975) CSF pH and pCO_2. Virginia Medical Monthly, 102, 625–626.

Maren, T.H. (1974) The cerebrospinal fluid with notes on aqueous humor and endolymph. In Medical Physiology, Vol. II, (Ed. V.B. Mountcastle) pp. 1116–1141, C.V. Mosby, Saint Louis.

Milhorat, T.H. (1975) The third circulation revisited. Journal of Neurosurgery, 42, 628–645.

Milhorat, T.H. (1976) Structure and function of the choroid plexus and other sites of cerebrospinal fluid formation. International Review of Cytology, 47, 225–288.

Moir, A.T.B., Ashcroft, G.W., Crawford, T.B.B., Eccleston, D. and Guldberg, H.C. (1970) Cerebral metabolites in cerebrospinal fluid as a biochemical approach to the brain. Brain, 93, 357–368.

Plum, F. and Siesjo, B.K. (1975) Recent advances in cerebrospinal fluid physiology. Anesthesiology, 42, 708.

Porter, R. and Skillen, A.W. (1972) Lactic dehydrogenase activity in the aqueous humour of eyes containing malignant melanomas. British Journal of Ophthalmology, 56, 709–710.

Praus, R. (1961) Paper electrophoresis of aqueous humor proteins labelled with radioactive I^{131}. Experimental Eye Research, 1, 67–73.

Schindler, K. and Schneider, E.A. (1966) Perilymph in patients with otosclerosis. Archives of Otolaryngology, 84, 373–394.

Schmut, O. and Zirm, M. (1974) Immunologische bestimmung von lipoproteinen im kammerwasser. Albrecht von Graefes Archiv für Klinische und Experimentelle Ophthalmologie, 191, 19–23.

Shapiro, H.M. (1975) CSF . . . neural urine or more? Anesthesiology, 42, 647–650.

Sherlin, L.G. (1969) Clinical diagnostic significance of cerebrospinal fluid aldolase in acute neuroinfections. Zhurnal Nevropatologü i Psikhiatrü imeni S.S. Korsakova, 69, 643–647.

Silverstein, H. (1972) A rapid protein test for acoustic neurinoma. Archives of Otolaryngology, 95, 202–203.

Swartz, M., Herbst, R.W. and Goldberg, M.F. (1974) Aqueous humor lactic acid dehydrogenase in retinoblastoma. American Journal of Ophthalmology, 78, 612–617.

Thompson, E.J., Norman, P.M. and Macdermot, J. (1975) The analysis of cerebrospinal fluid. British Journal of Hospital Medicine, 14, 645–652.

Trela, F.M. (1975) Die Bedeutung der Innenohrflussigkeit für die gerichtliche Medizin. Zeitschrift für Rechtsmedizin, 77, 17–23.

Zirm, M., Petek, W., Schmut, V., Hofmann, H. and Holasek, A. (1975) Quantitative Bestimmung von Kammerwasserproteinen durch die Elektroimmundiffusion in einem antiserumhaltigen Agarosegel. Albrecht von Graefes Archiv für Klinische und Experimentelle Ophthalmologie, 196, 127–132.

Section 2.3. Effusion

Agostoni, E. (1972) Mechanics of the pleural space. Physiological Reviews, 52, 57–128.

Agostoni, A. and Marasini, B. (1977) Orosomucoid contents of pleural and peritoneal effusion of various etiologies. American Journal of Clinical Pathology, 67, 146–148.

Altman, R.D., Muniz, O.E., Pita, J.C. and Howell, D.S. (1973) Articular chondrocalcinosis. Microanalysis of pyrophosphate (PPi) in synovial fluid and plasma. Arthritis and Rheumatism, 16, 171–178.

Ball, G.V., Schrohenloher, R. and Hester, R. (1975) Gamma globulin complexes in rheumatoid pericardial fluid. American Journal of Medicine, 58, 123.

Bellman, M.H. and Rajaratnam, H.N. (1974) Perforation of the oesophagus with amylase rich pleural effusion. British Journal of Diseases of the Chest, 68, 197–201.

Bennett, R.M. and Skosey, J.L. (1977) Lactoferrin and lysozyme levels in synovial fluid: differential indices of articular inflammation and degradation. Arthritis and Rheumatism, 20, 84–90.

Berger, H.W. and Maher, G. (1971) Decreased glucose concentration in malignant pleural effusions. American Review of Respiratory Disease, 103, 427–429.

Berger, H.W., Rammohan, G., Neff, M.S. and Buhain, W.J. (1975) Uremic pleural effusion. A study in 14 patients on chronic dialysis. Annals of Internal Medicine, 82, 362–364.

Bernstein, J.M., Tomasi, T.B. Jr and Ogra, P. (1974) The immunochemistry of middle ear effusions. Archives of Otolaryngology, 99, 320–326.

Borhanmanesh, F., Hekmat, K., Vaezzadeh, K. and Rezai, H.R. (1972) Tuberculous peritonitis. Prospective study of 32 cases in Iran. Annals of Internal Medicine, 76, 567–572.

Bourdeau, G.V., Jindal, S.L., Gillies, R.R. and Berry, J.V. (1974) Urinary ascites secondary to ureteroperitoneal fistula. Urology, 4, 209–211.

Brawley, R.K., Vasco, J.S. and Morrow, A.G. (1966) Cholesterol pericarditis. American Journal of Medicine. 41, 235–248.

Brown, J.D. and Dac An, N. (1976) Tuberculous peritonitis. Low ascitic fluid glucose concentration as a diagnostic aid. American Journal of Gastroenterology, 66, 277–282.

Brown, W.E. and Gregory, T.M. (1976) Calcium pyrophosphate crystal chemistry. Arthritis and Rheumatism 19, Suppl. 3, 446–462.

Bunch, T.W., Hunder, G.G., McDuffie, F.C., O'Brien, P.C. and Markowitz, H. (1974) Synovial fluid complement determination as a diagnostic aid in inflammatory joint disease. Mayo Clinic Proceedings 49, 715–720.

Chandrasekhar, A.J. and Buehler, J.H. (1974) Diagnostic evaluation of pleural effusion. Geriatrics, 29, 116–119.

Chandrasekhar, A.J., Palatao, A., Dubin, A. and Levine, H. (1969) Pleural fluid lactic acid dehydrogenase activity and protein content. Archives of Internal Medicine, 123, 48–50.

Coe, J.E. and Aikawa, J.K. (1961) Cholesterol pleural effusion. Archives of Internal Medicine, 108, 763–774.

Cohen, A.S., Brandt, K.D. and Krey, P.R. (1975) Synovial fluid. In Laboratory Diagnostic Procedures in the Rheumatic Diseases, 2nd edn., (Ed. A.S. Cohen) pp. 1–62, Little, Brown and Co., Boston.

Collins, A.J. and Cosh, J.A. (1970) Temperature and biochemical studies of joint inflammation. A preliminary investigation. Annals of the Rheumatic Diseases, 29, 386–392.

Conn, H.O. and Fessel, J.M. (1971) Spontaneous bacterial peritonitis in cirrhosis. Medicine, 50, 161–197.

Cracchiolo, A., III (1971) Joint fluid analysis. American Family Physician, 4, 87–94 (November).

Craig, R., Sparberg, M., Ivanovich, P., Rice, L. and Dordal, E. (1974) Nephrogenic ascites. Archives of Internal Medicine, 134, 276–279.

Cruikshank, D.P. and Buchsbaum, H.J. (1973) Effects of rapid paracentesis. Cardiovascular dynamics and body fluid composition. Journal of the American Medical Association, 225, 1361–1362.

Csanády, M. and Kovács, G.S. (1973) Isolated massive chylopericardium. Annals of Thoracic Surgery, 15, 427–433.

Dieppe, P.A., Crocker, P., Huskisson, E.C. and Willoughby, D.A. (1976) Apatite deposition disease. A new arthropathy. Lancet, I, 266–269.

Dines, D.E., Elveback, L.R. and McCall, J.T. (1974) Zinc, copper, and iron contents of pleural fluid in benign and neoplastic disease. Mayo Clinic Proceedings, 49, 102–106.

Dines, D.E., Pierre, R.V. and Franzen, S.J. (1975) The value of cells in the pleural fluid in the differential diagnosis. Mayo Clinic Proceedings, 50, 571–572.

Donowitz, M., Kerstein, M.D. and Spiro, H.M. (1974) Pancreatic ascites. Medicine, 53, 183–195.

Dorwart, B.B. and Schumacher, H.R. (1975) Joint effusions, chondrocalcinosis and other rheumatic manifestations in hypothyroidism. A clinicopathologic study. American Journal of Medicine, 59, 780–790.

Dye, R.A. and Laforet, E.G. (1974) Esophageal rupture: diagnosis by pleural fluid pH. Chest, 66, 454–456.

Eisalo, A. and Konttinen, A. (1972) Composition of pericardial fluid in cholesterol pericarditis. Acta Medica Scandinavica, 191, 125–128.

Fagan, T.J. and Lidsky, M.D. (1974) Compensated polarized light microscopy using cellophane adhesive tape. Arthritis and Rheumatism, 17, 256–262.

Feagler, J.R., Sorenson, G.D., Rosenfeld, M.G. and Osterland, C.K. (1971) Rheumatoid pleural effusion. Archives of Pathology, 92, 257–266.

Fowler, N.O. (1976) Pericardial disease. In Cardiac Diagnosis and Treatment, 2nd edn., pp. 858–888, Harper and Row, Hagerstown.

Franco, A.E., Levine, H.D. and Hall, A.P. (1972) Rheumatoid pericarditis. Report of 17 cases diagnosed clinically. Annals of Internal Medicine, 77, 837–844.

Funahashi, A., Sarkar, T.K. and Kory, R.C. (1971) pO_2, pCO_2, and pH in pleural effusion. Journal of Laboratory and Clinical Medicine, 78, 1006.

Geokas, M.C., Rinderknecht, H., Walberg, C.B. and Weissman, R. (1974) Methemalbumin in the diagnosis of acute hemorrhagic pancreatitis. Annals of Internal Medicine, 81, 483–486.

Goldenberg, D.L., Brandt, K.D., Cohen, A.S. (1973) Rapid, simple detection of trace amounts of synovial fluid. Arthritis and Rheumatism, 16, 487–490.

Goldenberg, D.L., Leff, G. and Grayzel, A.I. (1975) Pericardial tamponade in systemic lupus erythematosus; with absent hemolytic complement activity in pericardial fluid. New York State Journal of Medicine, 75, 910–912.

Gordon, D.A., Pruzanski, W., Ogryzlo, M.A. and Little, H.A. (1973) Amyloid arthritis simulating rheumatoid disease in five patients with multiple myeloma. American Journal of Medicine, 55, 142–154.

Gregory, J.G., Schoenberg, H.W., Sana, U. and Thompson, J. (1975) Neonatal urinary ascites. Urology, 85, 394–396.

Gutch, C.F., Mahony, J.F., Pingerra, W., Holmes, J.H., Ramirez, G. and Ogden, D.A. (1974) Refractory ascites in chronic dialysis patients. Clinical Nephrology, 2, 59–62.

Guyton, A.C., Taylor, A.E. and Granger, H.J. (1975) Fluid dynamics of the potential spaces. In Circulatory Physiology II: Dynamics and Control of the Body Fluids, pp. 194–205, W.B. Saunders, Philadelphia.

Howard, E.R., Johnson, D.I. and Mowat, A.P. (1976) Spontaneous perforation of common bile duct in infants. Archieves of Disease in Childhood, 51, 883–886.

Jacobelli, S., McCarty, D.J., Silcox, D.C. and Mall, J.C. (1973) Calcium pyrophosphate dihydrate crystal deposition in neuropathic joints. Four cases of polyarticular involvement. Annals of Internal Medicine, 79, 340–347.

Juhn, S.K. and Huff, J.S. (1976) Biochemical characteristics of middle ear effusions. Annals of Otology, Rhinology and Laryngology (Suppl.) 85, 110–116.

Kaye, M.D. (1968) Pleuropulmonary complications of pancreatitis. Thorax, 23, 297–306.

Kitridou, R.C. (1972) Synovianalysis. American Family Physician 5, 101–107.

Lee, C.Y., Di Loreto, P.C. and Kim, S. (1974) Isolated primary chylopericardium in pregnancy. Obstetrics and Gynecology, 43, 586–591.

Levine, H., Szanto, M., Grieble, H.G., Bach, G.L. and Anderson, T.O. (1968) Rheumatoid factor in non-rheumatoid pleural effusions. Annals of Internal Medicine, 69, 487–492.

Lifshitz, S. and Buchsbaum, H.J. (1976) The effect of paracentesis on serum proteins. Gynecologic Oncology, 4, 347–353.

Light, R.W. and Ball, W.C. Jr. (1973a) Lactic dehydrogenase isoenzymes in pleural effusions. American Review of Respiratory Disease, 108, 660–664.

Light, R.W. and Ball, W.C. Jr. (1973b) Glucose and amylase in pleural effusions. Journal of the American Medical Association, 225, 257–259.

Light, R.W., MacGregor, M.I., Ball, W.C. Jr. and Luchsinger, P.C. (1973) Diagnostic significance of pleural fluid pH and pCO_2. Chest, 64, 591–596.

Light, R.W., MacGregor, M.I., Luchsinger, P.C. and Ball, W.C. Jr. (1972) Pleural effusions: the diagnostic separation of transudates and exudates. Annals of Internal Medicine, 77, 507–513.

Lillington, G.A., Carr, D.T. and Mayne, J.G. (1971) Rheumatoid pleurisy with effusion. Archives of Internal Medicine, 128, 764–768.

Lowell, J.R. (1977) Diagnosis: fluid and tissue examination. In Pleural Effusions, pp. 45–73, University Park Press, Baltimore.

McCarty, D.J. (1974) Crystal deposition joint disease. Annual Review of Medicine, 25, 279–288.

McCarty, D.J. Jr. and Silcox, D.C. (1973) Gout and pseudogout. Geriatrics, 28, 110–120.

McCoy, J. and Wolma, F.J. (1971) Abdominal tap: indication, technic, and results. American Journal of Surgery, 122, 693–695.

McGowan, L., Bunnag, B. and Arias, L.F. (1975) Mesothelioma of the abdomen in women. Monitoring of therapy by peritoneal fluid study. Gynecologic Oncology, 3, 10–14.

McGowan, L., Davis, R.H. and Bunnag, B. (1973) The biochemical diagnosis of ovarian cancer. American Journal of Obstetrics and Gynecology, 116, 760–768.

Maathuis, J.B., Houx, P.C., Bastiaans, L.A. and Mastboom, J.L. (1973) Proceedings: some properties of peritoneal fluid obtained by laparoscopy from fertile and infertile women. Journal of Reproduction and Fertility, 35, 630–632.

Malagelada, J.R., Iber, F.L. and Linscheer, W.G. (1974) Origin of fat in chylous ascites of patients with liver cirrhosis. Gastroenterology, 67, 878–886.

Mansberger, A.R. Jr. (1964) The diagnostic value of abdominal paracentesis. American Journal of Gastroenterology, 42, 150–164.

Matsuura, C., Murakami, T. and Kajiyama, G. (1971) A case of cholesterol pleurisy with special reference to lipid analysis of the serum and pleural fluid. Hiroshima Journal of Medical Sciences, 20, 195–206.

Meyers, O.L. and Watermeyer, G.S. (1976) Cholesterol-rich synovial effusions. South African Medical Journal, 50, 973–975.

Miridjanian, O., Ambruoso, U.N., Derby, B.M. and Tice, D.A. (1969) Massive bilateral hemorrhagic pleural effusions in chronic relapsing pancreatitis. Archives of Surgery, 98, 62–66.

Mogi, G. and Honjo, S. (1972) Middle ear effusion. Analysis of protein components. Annals of Otology, Rhinology and Laryngology, 81, 99–105.

Newcombe, D.S. and Cohen, A.S. (1965) Chylous synovial effusion in rheumatoid arthritis. American Journal of Medicine, 38, 156–164.

Nix, J.T., Albert, M. and Dugal, J.E. (1957) Chylothorax and chylous ascites: a study of 302 selected cases. American Journal of Gastroenterology, 28, 40–53.

Nye, W.R., Terry, R. and Rosenbaum, D.L. (1968) Two forms of crystalline lipid in cholesterol effusions. American Journal of Clinical Pathology, 49, 718–728.

Pahor, A.L., Sözen, N., Beetham, R. and Raine, D.N. (1976) Immunoelectrophoretic study of proteins in middle ear effusion. A study of secretory otitis media in children. Journal of Laryngology and Otology, 90, 1033–1040.

Panush, R.S., Bianco, N.E. and Schur, P.H. (1971) Serum and synovial fluid IgG, IgA and IgM anti-gammaglobulins in rheumatoid arthritis. Arthritis and Rheumatism, 14, 737–747.

Paparella, M.M. (1976) Middle ear effusions. Annals of Otology, Rhinology and Laryngology (Suppl.), 85, 8–11.

Paradise, J.L. (1976) Pediatrician's view of middle ear effusions. Annals of Otology, Rhinology and Laryngology (Suppl.), 85, 20–24.

Peitersen, B. and Jacobsen, B. (1977) Medium chain triglycerides for treatment of spontaneous, neonatal chylothorax. Lipid analysis of the chyle. Acta Paediatrica Scandinavia, 66, 121–125.

Percy, J.S. and Russell, A.S. (1975) Laboratory diagnosis and monitoring of rheumatologic diseases. Canadian Medical Association Journal, 112, 1320–1328.

Phelps, P., Steele, A.D. and McCarty, D.J. (1968) Compensated polarized light microscopy. Journal of the American Medical Association, 203, 508–512.

Phillips, M.J., Knight, N.J., Manning, H., Abbott, A.L. and Tripp, W.G. (1974) IgE and secretory otitis media. Lancet, II, 1176–1178.

Polak, M. and Torres da Costa, A.C. (1973) Diagnostic value of the estimation of glucose in ascitic fluid, Digestion, 8, 347–352.

Pruzanski, W., Russell, M.L., Gordon, D.A. and Ogryzlo, M.A. (1973) Serum and synovial fluid proteins in rheumatoid arthritis and degenerative joint deseases. American Journal of the Medical Sciences, 265, 483–490.

Reeves, B. (1965) Significance of joint fluid uric acid levels in gout. Annals of the Rheumatic Diseases, 24, 569–571.

Rodnan, G.P. (ed.) (1973) Primer on the rheumatic diseases. Journal of the American Medical Association 224, 661–812.

Rodriguez, H.J., Walls, J., Slatopolsky, E. and Klahr, S. (1974) Recurrent ascites following peritoneal dialysis. Archives of Internal Medicine, 134, 283–287.

Rudman, D., Chawla, R.K., Del Rio, A.E., Hollins, B.M., Hall, E.C. and Conn, J.M. (1974) Orosomucoid content of pleural and peritoneal effusions. Journal of Clinical Investigation, 54, 147–155.

Russakoff, A.H., LeMaistre, C.A. and Dewlett, H.J. (1962) An evaluation of the pleural fluid glucose determination. American Review of Respiratory Disease, 85, 220–223.

Ryan, W.E., Ellefson, R.D. and Ward, L.E. (1973) Clinical conference: lipid synovial effusion. Unique occurrence in systemic lupus erythematosus. Arthritis and Rheumatism, 16, 759–764.

Safa, A.M. and Van Ordstrand, H.S. (1973) Pleural effusion due to multiple myeloma. Chest, 64, 246–248.

Sampliner, R.E. and Iber, F.L. (1974) High protein ascites in patients with uncomplicated hepatic cirrhosis. American Journal of the Medical Sciences, 267, 275–289.

Schumacher, H.R. Jr. (1975) Laboratory diagnosis of degenerative joint disease. Annals of Clinical and Laboratory Science, 5, 242–247.

Schumacher, H.R. and Holdsworth, D.E. (1977) Ochronotic Arthropathy. I. Clinicopathologic studies. Seminars in Arthritis and Rheumatism, 6, 207–246.

Scott, J.T. (1975) The analysis of joint fluids. British Journal of Hospital Medicine, 14, 653–658.

Seriff, N.S., Cohen, M.L., Samuel, P. and Schulster, P.L. (1977) Chylothorax: diagnosis by lipoprotein electrophoresis of serum and pleural fluid, Thorax, 32, 98–100.

Shallenberger, D.W. and Daniel, T.M. (1972) Quantitative determination of several pleural fluid proteins. American Review of Respiratory Disease, 106, 121–122.

Sherr, H.P., Light, R.W., Merson, M.H., Wolf, R.O., Taylor, L.L. and Hendrix, T.R. (1972) Origin of pleural fluid amylase in oesophageal rupture. Annals of Internal Medicine, 76, 985–986.

Silcox, D.C. and McCarty, D.J. Jr. (1974) Elevated inorganic pyrophosphate concentrations in synovial fluids in osteoarthritis and pseudogout. Journal of Laboratory and Clinical Medicine, 83, 518–531.

Singh, S., Aoki, S., Mitra, S. and Berman, L.B. (1973) Ascites. An unusual manifestation of urinary leak in a renal allograft recipient. Journal of the American Medical Association, 226, 777–778.
Swann, D.A., Radin, E.L., Nazimiec, M., Weisser, P.A., Curran, N. and Lewinnek, G. (1974) Role of hyaluronic acid in joint lubrication. Annals of the Rheumatic Diseases, 33, 318–326.
Swedlund, H.A., Hunder, G.G. and Gleich, G.J. (1974) Alpha 1-antitrypsin in serum and synovial fluid in rheumatoid arthritis. Annals of the Rheumatic Diseases, 33, 162–164.
Talal, N., Grey, H.M., Zvaifler, N., Michalski, J.P. and Daniels, T.E. (1975) Elevated salivary and synovial fluid beta 2-microglobulin in Sjogren's syndrome and rheumatoid arthritis. Science, 187, 1196–1198.
Teloh, H.A. (1975) Clinical pathology of synovial fluid. Annals of Clinical and Laboratory Science, 5, 282–287.
Tsuchiya, M., Okazaki, I., Maruyama, K., Asakura, H. and Morita, A. (1973) Chylous ascites formation and a review of 84 cases. Angiology, 24, 576–584.
Veltri, R.W. and Sprinkle, P.M. (1973) Serous otitis media. Immunoglobulin and lysozyme levels in middle ear fluids and serum. Annals of Otology, Rhinology and Laryngology, 82, 297–301.
Vladutiu, A.O. (1976) Beta 2-microglobulin in pleural fluids. New England Journal of Medicine, 294, 903.
Weidmann, M.J. (1975) Ascites from a ventriculoperitoneal shunt. Journal of Neurosurgery 43, 233–235.
Wild, J.H. and Zvaifler, N.J. (1975) An office technique for identifying crystals in synovial fluid. American Family Physician 12, 72–81 (July).
Witte, C.L., Witte, M.H., Cole, W.R., Chung, Y.C., Bleiseh, V.R. and DuMont, A.E. (1969) Dual origin of ascites in hepatic cirrhosis. Surgery, Gynecology and Obstetrics, 129, 1027–1033.
Witte, M.H., Witte, C.L., Davis, W.M., Cole, W.R. and DuMont, A.E. (1972) Peritoneal transudate. A diagnostic clue to portal system obstruction in patients with intra-abdominal neoplasms or peritonitis. Journal of the American Medical Association 221, 1380–1383.
Yehia, S.R. and Duncan, H. (1975) Synovial fluid analysis. Clinical Orthopaedics and Related Research, 107, 11–24.

Section 2.4. Fluids of the genitourinary system

Ainbender, E. and Hirschhorn, K. (1976) Routine alpha-fetoprotein studies in amniotic fluid. Lancet, I, 597–598.
Amelar, R.D. (1962) Coagulation, liquefaction, and viscosity of human semen. Journal of Urology, 87, 187–190.
Alpern, W.M. (1974) Techniques of amniocentesis. In Amniotic Fluid (Eds. S. Natelson, A. Scommegna and M.B. Epstein) pp. 201–204, John Wiley and Sons, New York.
Armstrong, D., Van Wormer, D.E., Dimmell, S., May, P. and Gideon, W.P. (1976) The determination of peroxidase in amniotic fluid. Obstetrics and Gynecology, 47, 593–598.
Aubry, R.H., Rourke, J.E., Almanza, R., Cantor, R.M. and Van Doren, J.E. (1976) The lecithin/sphingomyelin ratio in high risk obstetric population. Obstetrics and Gynecology, 47, 21–27.
Bailey, P., Blake, M., Younger, B., Hinkley, C. and Cassady, G. (1976) Amniotic fluid osmolality in pregnancies complicated by diabetes. American Journal of Obstetrics and Gynecology, 124, 257–262.
Baird, D.T. and Fraser, I.S. (1975) Concentration of oestrone and oestradiol in follicular fluid and ovarian venous blood of women. Clinical Endocrinology (Oxford), 4, 259–266.
Barlow, W.K. (1976) Volatiles and osmometry. Clinical Chemistry, 22, 1230–1232.
Bauman, J.W. and Chinard, F.P. (1975) Renal Function: Physiological and Medical Aspects, C.V. Mosby, St. Louis.
Behrman, S.J. and Lieberman, M.E. (1973) Biosynthesis of immunoglobulins by the human cervix. In The Biology of the Cervix, (Eds. R.J. Blandau and K. Moghissi) pp. 235–249, University of Chicago Press, Chicago.

Berggard, I. (1970) Plasma proteins in normal human urine. In Proteins in Normal and Pathological Urine, (Eds. Y. Manuel, J.P. Revillard and H. Betnel), pp. 7–19, University Park Press, Baltimore.

Bhagwanani, S.G., Fahmy, D. and Turnbull, A.C. (1972) Lecithin in amniotic fluid. Lancet, I, 159–162.

Bock, J.E., Nørgaard-Pedersen, E. and Trolle, D. (1976) Amniotic fluid bilirubin as a prognostic indicator in Rhesus isoimmunization. Acta Obstetrica et Gynecologica Scandinavica, 53, 3–6.

Brackett, B.G. and Mastroianni, L. (1974) Composition of oviductal fluid. In The Oviduct and Its Functions (Eds. A.D. Johnson and C.W. Foley) pp. 133–159, Academic Press, New York.

Brock, D.J.H. (1976) Prenatal diagnosis – chemical methods. British Medical Bulletin, 32, 16–20.

Brody, L.H., Salladay, J.R. and Armbruster, K. (1971) Urinalysis and the urinary sediment. Medical Clinics of North America, 55, 243–266.

Buffe, D., Rimbaut, C., Henrion, R., Boue, J. and Boue, A. (1976) Alpha fetoprotein in amniotic fluid and maternal serum. New England Journal of Medicine, 295, 51.

Burman, K., Read, J., Dimond, R.C., Strum, D., Wright, F.D., Patow, W., Earll, J.M. and Wartofsky, L. (1976) Measurements of 3,3′,5′-triiodothyronine, (reverse T_3), 3,3′-L-duodothyronine, T_3 and T_4 in human amniotic fluid and in cord and maternal urine. Journal of Clinical Endocrinology and Metabolism, 43, 1351–1359.

Bygdeman, M., Fredricsson, B., Svanborg, K. and Samuelsson, B. (1970) The relationship between fertility and prostaglandin content of seminal fluid in man. Fertility and Sterility, 21, 622–629.

Cassady, G. and Barnett, R. (1968) Amniotic fluid electrolytes and perinatal outcome. Biologia Neonatorum 13, 155–174.

Chopra, I.J. and Crandall, B.F. (1975) Thyroid hormones and thyrotropin in amniotic fluid. New England Journal of Medicine, 293, 740–743.

Colleen, S., Mardh, P.-A. and Schytz, A. (1975) Magnesium and zinc in seminal fluid of healthy males and patients with non-acute prostatitis with and without gonorrhoea. Scandinavian Journal of Urology and Nephrology, 9, 192–197.

Collier, J.G., Flower, R.J. and Stanton, S.L. (1975) Seminal prostaglandin in infertile man. Fertility and Sterility, 26, 868–871.

Crabbe, M.J.C. (1976) Enzyme assay for sperm motility. Lancet, II, 1295.

DeCastro, A.F., Ustalegui-Gomez, M. and Spellacy, W.N. (1973) Amniotic fluid amylase. American Journal of Obstetrics and Gynecology, 116, 931–936.

Deetjen, P., Boylan, J.W. and Kramer, K. (1975) Physiology of the Kidney and of Water Balance, Springer-Verlag, New York.

Dubin, A. (1974) Application of multiwavelength spectroscopy to analysis of amniotic fluid bilirubin. In Amniotic Fluid, (Eds. S. Natelson, A. Scommegna and M.B. Epstein) pp. 191–197, John Wiley and Sons, New York.

Edwards, R.G. (1974) Follicular fluid. Journal of Reproduction and Fertility, 37, 189–219.

Eliasson, R. (1968) Biochemical analysis of human semen in the study of the physiology and pathophysiology of the male accessory genital glands. Fertility and Sterility, 19, 344–350.

Eliasson, R. (1976) Accessory glands and seminal plasma with special reference to infertility as a model for studies on induction of sterility in the male. Journal of Reproduction and Fertility (Suppl.), 24, 163–174.

Elstein, M. and Daunter, B. (1972) Trace elements in cervical mucus. In Cervical Mucus in Human Reproduction, (Eds. M. Elstein, K.S. Moghissi and R. Borth) pp. 122–127, Scriptor, Copenhagen.

Elstein, M., Moghissi, K.S. and Borth, R. (Eds.) (1973) Cervical mucus: present state of knowledge. In Cervical Mucus in Human Reproduction (Eds. M. Elstein, K.S. Moghissi and R. Borth) pp. 11–23, Scriptor, Copenhagen.

Fair, W.R., Clark, R.B. and Wehner, N. (1972) A correlation of seminal polyamine levels and semen analysis in the human. Fertility and Sterility, 23, 38–42.

Fairweather, D.V.I., Whyley, G.A. and Millar, M.D. (1976) Six years' experience of the prediction of severity in Rhesus haemolytic disease. British Journal of Obstetrics and Gynecology, 83, 698–706.

Falconer, G.F., Hodge, J.S. and Gadd, R.L. (1973) Influence of amniotic fluid volume on lecithin estimation in prediction of respiratory distress. British Medical Journal, 2, 689–691.

Fencl, M. DeM. and Tulchinsky, D. (1975) Total cortisol in amniotic fluid and fetal lung maturation. New England Journal of Medicine, 292, 133–136.

Fisher, D.A. (1975) Reverse tri-iodothyronine and fetal thyroid status. New England Journal of Medicine, 293, 770–772.

Forman, D.T. (1974) The lecithin to sphingomyelin ratio in amniotic fluid and its predictive value for fetal lung immaturity (respiratory distress syndrome). In Amniotic Fluid, (Eds. S. Natelson, A. Scommegna and M.B. Epstein) pp. 247–258, John Wiley and Sons, New York.

France, J.T. and Boyer, K.G. (1975) The detection of ovulation in humans and its application in contraception. Journal of Reproduction and Fertility (Suppl.), 22, 107–120.

Frasier, S.D., Thorneycroft, I.H., Weiss, B.A. and Horton, R. (1975) Elevated amniotic fluid concentration of 17 α-hydroxyprogesterone in congenital adrenal hyperplasia. Journal of Pediatrics, 86, 310–311.

Free, A.H. and Free, H.M. (1975) Urinalysis in Clinical Laboratory Practice, CRC Press, Cleveland.

Galjaard, H., Sacks, E.S., Kleijer, W.J. and Niermeijer, M.F. (1975) Prenatal diagnosis of genetic diseases. In Early Diagnosis and Prevention of Genetic Diseases (Eds. L.N. Went and A.G.J.M. Van der Linden) pp. 82–91, Leiden University Press, Leiden.

Gebhardt, D.O.E. and Dubbeldam, A. (1973) Relationship between lecithin/sphingomyelin ratios of amniotic fluid and method of determination, Lancet, I, 726.

Gerbie, A.B. and Simpson, J.L. (1976) Antenatal detection of genetic disorders. Postgraduate Medicine, 59, 129–136.

Gibbons, J.M., Huntley, T.E. and Corral, A.G. (1974) Effect of maternal blood contamination on amniotic fluid analysis, Obstetrics and Gynecology, 44, 657–660.

Giles, H.R., Lox, C.D., Heine, M.W. and Christian, C.D. (1974) Intrauterine fetal sex determination by radioimmunoassay of amniotic fluid testosterone. Gynecologic Investigation, 5, 317–323.

Glover, T.D. (1974) Recent progress in the study of male reproductive physiology: testis stimulation, sperm formation, transport and maturation (epididymal physiology), semen analysis, storage and artificial insemination. In Reproductive Physiology, Vol. 8, Physiology Series I (Ed. R.O. Greep) pp. 221–277, University Park Press, Baltimore.

Gluck, G., Kulovich, M.V., Borer, R.C., Brenner, P.H., Anderson, G.G. and Spellacy, W.N. (1971) Diagnosis of the respiratory distress syndrome by amniocentesis. American Journal of Obstetrics and Gynecology, 109, 440–445.

Guibaud, S., Bonnet, M., Dury, A., Thoulon, J.M. and Dumont, M. (1976) Amniotic fluid or maternal urine? Lancet, I, 746.

Guibaud, S., Bonnet, M., Thoulon, J.M. and Dumont, M. (1975) Alpha-1-antitrypsin in amniotic fluid. Obstetrics and Gynecology, 45, 34–38.

Hagenfeldt, K. (1972) Intrauterine contraception with the copper-T device. Contraception, 6, 37–54.

Hall, P.M., Schuman, M. and Vidt, D.G. (1976) Laboratory tests of renal function. CRC Critical Reviews in Clinical Laboratory Sciences, 7, 33–47.

Jandial, V., Thom, H. and Gibson, J. (1976) Raised α-fetoprotein levels associated with minor congenital defect. British Medical Journal, 2, 22.

Jonasson, L.E. (1973) The clinical value of amniotic fluid analysis in pregnancies complicated by Rh-isoimmunization or hepatosis. Acta Obstetrica et Gynaecologica Scandinavica, 52, 113–130.

Kark, R.M., Lawrence, J.R., Pollack, V.E., Pirani, C.L., Muehrcke, R.C. and Silva, H. (1963) A Primer of Urinalysis, 2nd edn., Hoeber Medical Division, Harper and Row, New York.

Kellerman, A.S. and Weed, J.C. (1970) Sperm motility and survival in relation to glucose concentration: an in vitro study. Fertility and Sterility, 21, 802–805.

Kelly, R.W., Taylor, P.L., Hearn, J.P. and Short, R.V. (1976) 19-Hydroxyprostaglandin E as major component of the semen of primates. Nature, 260, 544–545.

Kerr, D.N.S. (1973) A critic looks at urine studies. In Urinalysis in the '70's (Ed. G.E. Schreiner) pp. 54–57, Medcom, New York.

Kesserii, E. (1972) Assessment of the rheology of cervical mucus. In Cervical Mucus in Human Reproduction (Eds. M. Elstein, K.S. Moghissi and R. Borth) pp. 45–57, Scriptor, Copenhagen.

Keyser, J.W., Kohn, J. and Ward, A.M. (1976) Standardization of alpha-fetoprotein assays. Lancet, I, 1015.

Klopper, A. (1970) Steroids in amniotic fluid. Annals of Clinical Research, 2, 289–299.

Koren, Z., Schulman, H., Lev-Gur, M., Gatz, M., Thysen, B. and Bloch, E. (1976) Progesterone levels in amniotic fluid and maternal plasma in prostaglandin $F_2\alpha$-induced midtrimester abortion. Obstetrics and Gynecology, 48, 472–474.

Kunin, C.M. (1974) Detection, Prevention, and Management of Urinary Tract Infections, 2nd edn., Lea and Febiger, Philadelphia.

Lemert, M. and Mastroianni, L. (1974) Cervical factors in infertility. Clinical Obstetrics and Gynecology, 17, 29–43.

Levinsky, N.G. (1967) The interpretation of proteinuria and the urinary sediment. Disease-a-Month, 3, 3–40.

Lewin, L.M., Beer, R. and Glezerman, M. (1974) Electrophoretic separation of proteins on cellulose acetate: a technique for the study of prostatic and vesicular contributions in human seminal fluid. Fertility and Sterility, 25, 416–423.

Liley, A.W. (1961) Liquor amnii analysis in the management of the pregnancy complicated by rhesus sensitization. American Journal of Obstetrics and Gynecology, 82, 1359–1370.

Linford, E. (1974) Cervical mucus: an agent or a barrier to conception? Journal of Reproduction and Fertility, 37, 239–250.

Lippman, R.W. (1957) Urine and the Urinary Sediment, Charles C. Thomas, Springfield.

MacLeod, J. (1965) The semen examination. Clinical Obstetrics and Gynecology, 8, 115–127.

McAllister, C.J., Stull, C.G. and Churey, N.G. (1973) Amniotic fluid levels of uric acid and creatinine in toxemic patients; possible relation to diuretic use. American Journal of Obstetrics and Gynecology, 115, 560–563.

McNatty, K.P., Baird, D.T., Bolton, A., Chambers, P., Corker, C.S. and McLean, H. (1976) Concentration of oestrogens and androgens in human ovarian venous plasma and follicular fluid throughout the menstrual cycle. Journal of Endocrinology, 71, 77–85.

Makler, A. (1976) A new method for evaluating cervical penetrability using daily aspirated and stored cervical mucus. Fertility and Sterility, 27, 533–540.

Mann, T. (1964) Biochemistry of Semen and of the Male Reproductive Tract, John Wiley and Sons, New York.

Mann, T. (1974) Secretory function of the prostate, seminal vesicle and other male accessory organs of reproduction. Journal of Reproduction and Fertility, 37, 179–188.

Mann, T. (1975) Biochemistry of semen. In Handbook of Physiology, Vol. 5 (Eds. R.O. Greep and E.B. Astwood) pp. 461–471, Williams and Wilkins, Baltimore.

Marberger, H., Marberger, E., Mann, T. and Lutwak-Mann, C. (1962) Citric acid in human prostatic secretion and metastasizing cancer of prostate gland. British Medical Journal, 1, 835–836.

Marmar, J.L., Katz, S., Praiss, D.T. and DeBenedictes, T.J. (1975) Semen zinc levels in infertile and postvasectomy patients and patients with prostatitis. Fertility and Sterility, 26, 1057–1063.

Masson, P.L. (1972) Carbohydrate content of cervical mucus. In Cervical Mucus in Human Reproduction (Eds. M. Elstein, K.S. Moghissi and R. Borth) pp. 82–91, Scriptor, Copenhagen.

Mauss, J., Börsch, G. and Torok, L. (1974) Differential diagnosis of low or absent seminal fructose in man. Fertility and Sterility, 25, 411–415.

Michael, R.P., Bonsall, R.W. and Warner, P. (1974) Human vaginal secretions: volatile fatty acid content. Science, 186, 1217–1219.

Milne, J.A. (1976) The investigation of infertility. Scottish Medical Journal, 21, 218–227.

Milunsky, A. (1976) Prenatal diagnosis of genetic disorders. New England Journal of Medicine, 295, 377–380.

Milunsky, A. and Alpert, E. (1976) Routine testing for α-fetoprotein in amniotic fluid. Lancet, I, 1015.

Miotti, A.B., Alter, A.A., Moltz, A. and Sabb, F. (1973) Serum and amniotic fluid lactic dehydrogenase in pregnant women. American Journal of Obstetrics and Gynecology, 117, 1129–1136.

Misenhimer, R.H. (1974) Role of amniotic fluid studies (ΔA_{450}) in the management of Rh immunization. In Amniotic Fluid (Eds. S. Natelson, A. Scommegna and M.B. Epstein) pp. 171–178, John Wiley and Sons, New York.

Moghissi, K.S. (1972) The function of cervix in fertility. Fertility and Sterility, 23, 295–305.

Moghissi, K.S. (1973) Composition and function of cervical secretion. In Handbook of Physiology, Vol. 2 (Eds. R.O. Greep and E.B. Astwood) pp. 25–48, American Physiological Society, Washington.

Moghissi, K.S. (1976) Postcoital test: physiological basis, technique and interpretation. Fertility and Sterility, 27, 117–129.

Moghissi, K.S., Syner, F.N. and Borin, B. (1976) Cyclic changes of cervical mucus enzymes related to the time of ovulation. American Journal of Obstetrics and Gynecology, 125, 1044–1048.

Murphy, B.E.P., Patrick, J. and Denton, R.L. (1975) Cortisol in amniotic fluid during human gestation. Journal of Clinical Endocrinology and Metabolism, 40, 164–167.

Musacchio, I., Epstein, J.A. and Sobrero, A.J. (1972) Enzymes in normal human cervical mucus. In Cervical Mucus in Human Reproduction (Eds. M. Elstein, K.S. Moghissi and R. Borth) pp. 114–121, Scriptor, Copenhagen.

Newman, R.L. and Tutera, G. (1976) The glucose–insulin ratio in amniotic fluid. Obstetrics and Gynecology, 47, 599–601.

Nishimura, T., Mobley, D.F. and Carlton, C.E. (1977) Clinical use of immunoelectrophoresis of split ejaculates. I. Variation of patterns due to antisera. Urology, 9, 39–41.

Olson, E.B., Graven, S.N. and Zachman, R.D. (1975) Amniotic fluid lecithin to sphingomyelin ratio of 3.5 and fetal pulmonary maturity. Pediatric Research, 9, 65–69.

Olsson, J.E. (1975) Correlation between concentration of β-trace protein and the number of spermatozoa in human semen. Journal of Reproduction and Fertility, 42, 149–151.

Oster, G. (1972) Chemical reactions of the copper intrauterine device. Fertility and Sterility, 23, 18–22.

Ostergard, D.R. (1974) The physiology and clinical importance of amniotic fluid. In Amniotic Fluid (Eds. S. Natelson, A. Scommegna and M.B. Epstein) pp. 213–220, John Wiley and Sons, New York.

Phadke, A.M., Samant, N.R. and Deval, S.D. (1973) Significance of seminal fructose studies in male infertility. Fertility and Sterility, 24, 894–903.

Phadke, A.M., Samant, N.R. and Deval, S.D. (1975) Seminal fructose content in necrospermia. Fertility and Sterility, 26, 1021–1023.

Pirani, B.B., Doran, T.A. and Benrie, R.J. (1976) Amniotic fluid or maternal urine? Lancet, I, 303.

Pitkin, R.M. (1974) Changes in osmolality, nonprotein nitrogen, and bilirubin in amniotic fluid during the course of pregnancy. In Amniotic Fluid (Eds. S. Natelson, A. Scommegna and M.B. Epstein) pp. 81–94, John Wiley and Sons, New York.

Pitts, R.F. (1974) Physiology of the Kidney and Body Fluids, 3rd edn., Year Book Medical Publishers, Chicago.

Polishuk, W.Z. and Ron, M. (1976) Detection of ovulation by water content of vaginal mucus. Israel Journal of Medical Sciences, 12, 1207–1208.

Pulkkinen, P., Kanerva, S., Elfving, K. and Janne, J. (1975) Association of spermine and diamine oxidase activity with human spermatozoa. Journal of Reproduction and Fertility, 43, 49–55.

Purvis, K., Landgren, B.-M., Cekan, Z. and Diczfalusy, E. (1975) Indices of gonadal function in the human male. II. Seminal plasma levels of steroids in normal and pathological conditions. Clinical Endocrinology (Oxford), 4, 247–258.

Purvis, K., Saksena, S.K., Cekan, Z., Diczfalusy, E. and Giner, J. (1976a) Endocrine effects of vasectomy. Clinical Endocrinology (Oxford), 5, 263–272.

Purvis, K., Saksena, S.K., Landgren, B.-M., Cekan, S.Z. and Diczfalusy, E.R. (1976b) Importance of controlled liquefaction periods for valid steroid assays in human seminal plasma. Fertility and Sterility, 27, 929–932.

Raboch, J. and Skachova, J. (1965) The pH of human ejaculate. Fertility and Sterility, 16, 252–256.

Rennie, I.D. (1971) Proteinuria. Medical Clinics of North America, 55, 213–230.

Ressler, N. (1974) Enzymes and principles of their assay in the prenatal diagnosis of inherited diseases. In Amniotic Fluid (Eds. S. Natelson, A. Scommegna and M.B. Epstein) pp. 317–326, John Wiley and Sons, New York.

Schirren, C. (1963) Relation between fructose content of semen and fertility in man. Journal of Reproduction and Fertility, 5, 347–358.

Schumacher, G.F.B. (1972) Soluble proteins of human cervical mucus. In Cervical Mucus in Human Reproduction (Eds. M. Elstein, K.S. Moghissi and R. Borth) pp. 93–113, Scriptor, Copenhagen.

Scommegna, A. (1974) Concentration of steroids and other hormones in amniotic fluid: changes in estrogen concentrations and their interpretation. In Amniotic Fluid (Eds. S. Natelson, A. Scommegna and M.B. Epstein) pp. 259–272, John Wiley and Sons, New York.

Seeds, A.E. (1974) Dynamics of amniotic fluid. In Amniotic Fluid (Eds. S. Natelson, A. Scommegna and M.B. Epstein) pp. 23–36, John Wiley and Sons, New York.

Seegmiller, J.E. (1974) Amniotic fluid and cells in the diagnosis of genetic disorders. In Amniotic Fluid, (Eds. S. Natelson, A. Scommegna and M.B. Epstein) pp. 291–316, John Wiley and Sons, New York.

Sharp-Cageorge, S.M., Blicher, B.M., Gordon, E.R. and Murphy, B.E.P. (1977) Amniotic fluid cortisol and human fetal lung maturation. New England Journal of Medicine, 296, 89–92.

Sheth, A.R., Mugatwala, P.P., Shah, G.U. and Rao, S.S. (1975) Occurrence of prolactin in human semen. Fertility and Sterility, 26, 905–907.

Sheth, A.R., Shah, G.U. and Mugatwala, P.P. (1976) Levels of luteinizing hormone in semen of fertile and infertile men and possible significance of luteinizing hormone in sperm metabolism. Fertility and Sterility, 27, 933–936.

Simkins, A. and Worth, H.G.J. (1976) Determination of bilirubin in amniotic fluid: a comparison of some current methods. Annals of Clinical Biochemistry, 13, 510–515.

Singer, A.D., Thibeault, D.W., Hobel, C.J. and Heiner, D.C. (1976) $Alpha_1$-antitrypsin in amniotic fluid and cord blood of preterm infants with the respiratory distress syndrome. Journal of Pediatrics, 88, 87–93.

Singh, E.J. (1975a) Oral contraceptives and human cervical mucus lipids. American Journal of Obstetrics and Gynecology, 123, 128–132.

Singh, E.J. (1975b) Effect of oral contraceptives and IUD's on the copper in human cervical mucus. Obstetrics and Gynecology, 45, 328–330.

Sobrero, A.J. and Rehan, N.-E. (1975) The semen of fertile men. II. Semen characteristics of 100 fertile men. Fertility and Sterility, 26, 1048–1056.

Sobrero, A.J., Szlachter-Aisemberg, B.N., Musacchio, I. and Epstein, J.A. (1973) Cyclic changes in sialic acid and alkaline phosphatase levels from normal and infected cervices. In The Biology of the Cervix (Eds. R.J. Blandau and K. Moghissi) pp. 357–366, University of Chicago Press, Chicago.

Sokolov, B.A., Harris, R.T. and Hecker, M.R. (1976) Isolation of substances from human vaginal secretions previously shown to be sex attractant pheromones in higher primates. Archives of Sexual Behavior, 5, 269–274.

Spencer, E.S. and Pedersen, I. (1971) Hand Atlas of the Urinary Sediment, University Park Press, Baltimore.

Stankova, L., Drach, G.W., Hicks, T., Zukoski, C.F. and Chvapil, M. (1976) Regulation of some functions of granulocytes by zinc of the prostatic fluid and prostate tissue. Journal of Laboratory and Clinical Medicine, 88, 640–648.

Sternheimer, R. and Malbin, B. (1951) Clinical recognition of pyelonephritis, with a new stain for urinary sediments. American Journal of Medicine, 11, 312.

Sutcliffe, R.G., Brock, D.J.H., Robertson, J.G., Scrimgeour, J.B. and Monaghan, J.M. (1972) Enzymes in amniotic fluid: a study of specific activity patterns during pregnancy. Journal of Obstetrics and Gynaecology of the British Commonwealth, 79, 895–901.

Syner, F.N., Moghissi, K.S. and Yanez, J. (1975) Isolation of a factor from normal human semen that accelerates dissolution of abnormally liquefying semen. Fertility and Sterility, 26, 1064–1069.

Tan, S.Y., Gewolb, I.H. and Hobbins, J.C. (1976) Unconjugated cortisol in human amniotic fluid: relationship to lecithin/sphingomyelin ratio. Journal of Clinical Endocrinology and Metabolism, 43, 412–418.

Tauber, P.F., Zaneveld, L.J.D., Propping, D. and Schumacher, G.F.B. (1975) Components of human split ejaculates. I. Spermatozoa, fructose, immunoglobulins, albumin, lactoferrin, transferrin and other plasma proteins. Journal of Reproduction and Fertility, 43, 249–267.

Tegenkamp, T.R. and Tegenkamp, I.E. (1974) Cytogenetic studies of amniotic fluid as a basis for genetic counseling. In Amniotic Fluid (Eds. S. Natelson, A. Scommegna and M.B. Epstein) pp. 281–290, John Wiley and Sons, New York.

Thakur, A.N., Sheth, A.R. and Rao, S.S. (1974) Polyamines in human semen: presence of S-adenosyl-L-methionine decarboxylase. Clinica Chimica Acta 55, 377–381.

Thomas, V., Shelokov, A. and Forland, M. (1974) Antibody-coated bacteria in the urine and the site of urinary tract infection. New England Journal of Medicine, 290, 588–590.

Tresidder, G.C. (1975) Male fertility. Proceedings of the Royal Society of Medicine, 68, 291–298.

Warshaw, M.M. and Pesce, A.J. (1974) Electrophoretic and immunologic analysis of amniotic fluid proteins. In Amniotic Fluid (Eds. S. Natelson, A. Scommegna and M.B. Epstein) pp. 125–144, John Wiley and Sons, New York.

Watson, D. and Pow, M. (1976) Diagnostic reagents for α-fetoprotein. Lancet I, 1015–1016.

Watson, A.A. and Robertson, C.M.G. (1966) Male infertility: a reappraisal of semen analysis. Journal of Medical Laboratory Technology, 23, 1–10.

Weisberg, H.F. (1974) Clinical chemical analyses of 62 amniotic fluids from women in early pregnancy. In Amniotic Fluid (Eds. S. Natelson, A. Scommegna and M.B. Epstein) pp. 47–72, John Wiley and Sons, New York.

Weiss, R.R., Duchin, S., Evans, M.I., Finkelstein, F. and Mann, L.I. (1974) Amniotic fluid uric acid and creatinine as measures of fetal maturity. Obstetrics and Gynecology, 44, 208–214.

Weiss, R.R., Elligers, K., Princler, G.L., McIntire, K.R. and Waldeman, T.A. (1976a) Amniotic fluid α-fetoprotein as a marker in prenatal diagnosis of neural tube defects. Obstetrics and Gynecology, 47, 148–151.

Weiss, R.R., Macri, J.N. and Elligers, K.W. (1976b) Origin of amniotic fluid alpha-fetoprotein in normal and defective pregnancies. Obstetrics and Gynecology, 47, 697–700.

Wilkinson, E.J., Cherayil, G.D. and Borkowf, H.I. (1977) L/S ratio and the G-force factor. New England Journal of Medicine, 296, 286–287.

Willis, C.E. and Faulkner, W.R. (1965) Nature of the yellow pigment in amniotic fluid of mothers with Rh sensitization. Clinical Chemistry 11, 814.

Wilson, D.M. (1975) Urinalysis and other tests of renal function. Minnesota Medicine 58, 9–17.

Winkel, P., Statland, B.E. and Jørgensen, K. (1974) Urine microscopy, an ill-defined method, examined by a multifactorial technique. Clinical Chemistry 20, 436–439.

Wolf, D.P., Blasco, L., Khan, M., Litt, M. and Sokoloski, J. (1977) Human cervial mucus. Fertility and Sterility, 28, 41–58.

Wolf, R.O. and Taussig, L.M. (1973) Human amniotic fluid isoamylases. Obstetrics and Gynecology, 41, 337–342.

Wood, G.P. and Sherline, D.M. (1975) Amniotic fluid glucose: a maternal, fetal, and neonatal correlation. American Journal of Obstetrics and Gynecology, 122, 151–154.

Section 2.5. Saliva, faeces and meconium

Azen, E.A. and Oppenheim, F.G. (1973) Genetic polymorphism of proline-rich human salivary proteins. Science, 180, 1067–1069.

Baird, I.M., Walters, R.L., Davies, P.S., Hill, M.J., Drasar, B.S. and Southgate, D.A. (1977) The effects of two dietary fiber supplements on gastrointestinal transit, stool weight and frequency, and bacterial flora, and fecal bile acids in normal subjects. Metabolism, 26, 117–128.

Balekjian, A.Y., Meyer, T.S., Montague, M.E. and Longton, R.W. (1975) Electrophoretic patterns of parotid fluid proteins from caries-resistant and caries-susceptible individuals. Journal of Dental Research, 54, 850–856.

Ben-Aryeh, H., Filmar, S., Gutman, D., Szargel, R. and Paldi, E. (1976) Salivary phosphate as an indicator of ovulation. American Journal of Obstetrics and Gynecology, 125, 871–878.

Benedek-Spät, E. (1973a) The composition of unstimulated human parotid saliva. Archives of Oral Biology, 18, 39–47.

Benedek-Spät, E. (1973b) The composition of stimulated human parotid saliva. Archives of Oral Biology, 18, 1091–1097.

Berger, H.M., Reynolds, S.J. and Lee, K.H. (1977) False positive meconium screen. Lancet, I. 458.

Blomfield, J., Rush, A.R., Allars, H.M. and Brown, J.M. (1976) Parotid gland function in children with cystic fibrosis and child control subjects. Pediatric Research, 6, 574–578.

Blomfield, J., Warton, K.L. and Brown, J.M. (1973) Flow rate and inorganic components of submandibular saliva in cystic fibrosis. Archives of Disease in Childhood, 48, 267–274.

Bonilla, C.A. (1972) Human mixed saliva protein concentration. Journal of Dental Research, 51, 664.

Brudevold, F., Bakhos, Y. and Gron, P. (1973) Fluoride in human saliva after ingestion of aluminium chloride and sodium fluoride or sodium monofluorophosphate. Archives of Oral Biology, 18, 699–706.

Bruns, W.T., Connell, T.R., Lacey, J.A. and Whisler, K.E. (1977) Test strip meconium screening for cystic fibrosis. American Journal of Diseases in Children, 131, 71–73.

Bull, F.E., Gladwin, D.E. and Griffiths, A.D. (1974) Immunochemical method for detection of albumin in human meconium. Archives of Disease in Childhood, 49, 602–605.

Burton, R.M., Landreth, K.S., Barrows, G.H., Jarrett, D.D. and Songster, C.L. (1976) Appearance, properties, and origin of altered human hemoglobin in feces. Laboratory Investigation, 35, 111–115.

Chang, K. and Chiou, W.L. (1976) Interactions between drugs and saliva-stimulating parafilm and their implications in measurements of saliva drug levels. Research Communications in Chemical Pathology and Pharmacology, 13, 357–360.

Chiou, W.L., Chang, K. and Peng, G.W. (1976) Precaution in the monitoring of drug levels in saliva: abnormal salicylate levels after oral dosing. Journal of Clinical Pharmacology, 16, 158–160.

Chisholm, D.M., Beely, J.A. and Mason, D.K. (1973) Salivary proteins in Sjögren's syndrome: separation by isoelectric focusing in acrylamide gels. Oral Surgery, Oral Medicine and Oral Pathology, 35, 620–630.

Cummings, J.H. (1974) Progress report: laxative abuse. Gut, 15, 758–766.

Cutress, T.W. (1972) Composition, flow-rate and pH of mixed and parotid salivas from trisomic 21 and other mentally retarded subjects. Archives of Oral Biology, 17, 1081–1094.

Davidson, M. (1972) The gastrointestinal tract. In Pediatrics, 15th edn. (Eds. H.L. Barnett and A.H. Einhorn) pp. 1565–1572, Meredith Corp., New York.

Davis, R.H. and Balin, H. (1973) Saliva glucose: a useful criterion for determining the time of fertility in women. American Journal of Obstetrics and Gynecology, 115, 287–288.

Dawes, C. (1974a) The effects of flow rate and duration of stimulation on the concentrations of protein and the main electrolytes in human submandibular saliva. Archives of Oral Biology, 19, 887–895.

Dawes, C. (1974b) Rhythms in salivary flow rate and composition. International Journal of Chronobiology, 2, 253–279.

Elias, E.G., Holyoke, E.D. and Chu, T.M. (1974) Carcinoembryonic antigen (CEA) in feces and plasma of normal subjects and patients with colorectal carcinoma. Diseases of the Colon and Rectum, 17, 38–41.

Eney, R.D. and Goldstein, E.O. (1976) Compliance of chronic asthmatics with oral administration of theophylline as measured by serum and salivary levels. Pediatrics, 57, 513–517.

Ferguson, D.B. and Fort, A. (1974) Circadian variations in human resting submandibular saliva flow rate and composition. Archives of Oral Biology, 19, 47–55.

Ferguson, D.B., Fort, A., Elliott, A.L. and Potts, A.J. (1973) Circadian rhythms in human parotid saliva flow rate and composition. Archives of Oral Biology, 18, 1155–1173.

Finestone, A.J., Schacterle, G.R. and Pollack, R.L. (1973) The comparative analysis of diabetic and non-diabetic saliva, study 1; protein separation by disc gel electrophoresis. Journal of Periodontology, 44, 175–176.

Ford-Jones, A.E. and Cogswell, J.J. (1975) Tests for occult blood in stools of children. Archives of Disease in Childhood, 50, 238–240.

Fordtran, J.S. (1973) Diarrhea. In Gastrointestinal Disease (Eds. M.H. Sleisenger and J.S. Fordtran) pp. 291–319, W.B. Saunders, Philadelphia.

France, J.T. and Boyer, K.G. (1975) The detection of ovulation in humans and its application in contraception. Journal of Reproduction and Fertility (Suppl.), 22, 107–120.

Freed, D.L. and Taylor, G. (1972) Carcinoembryonic antigen in faeces. British Medical Journal, 1, 85–87.

Fung, H.L., Yaffe, S.J., Mattar, M.E. and Lanighan, M.C. (1975) Blood and salivary lead levels in children. Clinica Chimica Acta, 61, 423–424.

Gerskowitch, V.P., Allan, J.G., Russell, R.I. and Blumgart, L.H. (1973) Increased faecal excretion of bile-acids in post-vagotomy diarrhoea. British Journal of Surgery, 60, 912 (abstract).

Ghoos, Y. and Vantrappen, G. (1977) Clean collection and manipulation of stools. Lancet, I, 884–885.

Goldenberg, D.M., Tchilinguirian, N.G., Hansen, H.J. and Vandevoorde, J.P. (1972) Carcinoembryonic antigen present in meconium: the basis of a possible new diagnostic test of fetal distress. American Journal of Obstetrics and Gynecology, 113, 66–69.

Gould, L., Reddy, C.V., Pfeiffer, N., Marini, J., Marcus, M. and Gomprecht, R.F. (1973) Evaluation of digitalis toxicity by salivary electrolytes. Angiology, 24, 528–532.

Graham, D.Y., Johnson, C.D., Bentlif, P.S. and Kelsey, J.R. (1975) Islet cell carcinoma, pancreatic cholera and vasoactive intestinal peptide. Annals of Internal Medicine, 83, 782–785.

Gron, P. (1973) Saturation of human saliva with calcium phosphates. Archives of Oral Biology, 18, 1385–1392.

Guyton, A.C. (1976) Textbook of Medical Physiology, 5th edn., W.B. Saunders Company, Philadelphia.

Hadjimarkos, D.M. and Shearer, T.R. (1971) Selenium concentration in human saliva. American Journal of Clinical Nutrition, 24, 1210–1211.

Haneberg, B. (1974) Immunoglobulins in feces from infants fed human or bovine milk. Scandinavian Journal of Immunology, 3, 191–197.

Hay, D.I. and Oppenheim, F.G. (1974) The isolation from human parotid saliva of a further group of proline-rich proteins. Archives of Oral Biology, 19, 627–632.

Henkin, R.I., Mueller, C.W. and Wolf, R.O. (1975a) Estimation of zinc concentration of parotid saliva by flameless atomic absorption spectrophotometry in normal subjects and in patients with idiopathic hypogeusia. Journal of Laboratory and Clinical Medicine, 86, 175–180.

Henkin, R.I., Lippoldt, R.E., Bilstad, J. and Edelhoch, H. (1975b) A zinc protein isolated from human parotid saliva. Proceedings of the National Academy of Sciences of the U.S.A., 72, 488–492.

Hightower, N.C. and Janowitz, H.D. (1973) Salivary secretion. In Physiological Basis of Medical Practice, 9th edn. (Ed. J.R. Brocheck) pp. 217–230, Williams and Wilkins, Baltimore.

Hill, M.J. and Aries, V.C. (1971) Faecal steroid composition and its relationship to cancer of the large bowel. Journal of Pathology, 104, 129–139.

Hill, M.J., Drasar, B.S., Williams, R.E., Meade, T.W., Cox, A.G., Simpson, J.E. and Morson, B.C. (1975) Faecal bile-acids and clostridia in patients with cancer of the large bowel. Lancet, I, 535–539.

Hoffman, N.E., LaRusso, N.F. and Hofmann, A.F. (1973) An improved method for faecal collection: the faecal field-kit. Lancet, I, 1422–1433.

Horning, M.G., Brown, L., Nowlin, J., Lertratanangkoon, K., Kellaway, P. and Zion, T.E. (1977) Use of saliva in therapeutic drug monitoring. Clinical Chemistry, 23, 157–164.

Huang, C.T., Rodriguez, J.T., Woodward, W.E. and Nichols, B.L. (1976) Comparison of patterns of fecal bile acid and neutral sterol between children and adults. American Journal of Clinical Nutrition, 29, 1196–1203.

Jaffe, R.M., Kasten, B., Young, D.S. and McLowry, J.D. (1975) False-negative stool occult blood tests caused by ingestion of ascorbic acid (vitamin C). Annals of Internal Medicine, 83, 824–826.

Jarnum, S. and Jensen, K.N. (1975) Fecal radioiodide excretion following intravenous injection of 131-I-albumin and 125-I-immunoglobulin G in chronic inflammatory bowel disease: an aid to topographic diagnosis. Gastroenterology, 68, 1433–1444.

Kakizaki, G., Saito, T., Soeno, T., Sasahara, M. and Fujiwara, Y. (1976) A new diagnostic test for pancreatic disorders by examination of parotid saliva. American Journal of Gastroenterology, 65, 437–445.

Kollberg, H. and Hellsing, K. (1975) Screening for cystic fibrosis by analysis of albulin in meconium. Acta Paediatrica Scandinavica, 64, 477–482.

Koysooko, R., Ellis, E.F. and Levy, G. (1974) Relationship between theophylline concentration in plasma and saliva of man. Clinical Pharmacology and Therapeutics, 15, 454–460.

Kreusser, W., Heidland, A., Hennemann, H., Wigand, M.E. and Knauf, H. (1972) Mono- and divalent electrolyte patterns, pCO_2 and pH in relation to flow rate in normal human parotid saliva. European Journal of Clinical Investigation, 2, 398–406.

Lauler, D.P., Hickler, R.B. and Thorn, G.W. (1962) The salivary sodium-potassium ratio. New England Journal of Medicine, 267, 1136–1137.

Lauridsen, L.H. and Bohn, L. (1976) Testing of feces for occult blood: a review. Danish Medical Bulletin, 23, 230–235.

Lazarus, J.H., Fell, G.S., Robertson, J.W., Millar, W.T. and Bennie, E.H. (1973) Secretion of lithium in human parotid saliva in manic depressive patients treated with lithium carbonate. Archives of Oral Biology, 18, 329–335.

Leach, S.A. (1974) Salivary products in plaque and saliva. Journal of Dental Research, 53, 310–313.

Lindstrom, F.D. and Folke, L.E. (1973) Salivary IgA in periodontal disease. Acta Odontologica Scandinavica, 31, 31–34.

Losowsky, M.S., Walker, B.E. and Kelleher, J. (1974) Assessment of fat absorption. In Malabsorption in Clinical Practice, pp. 74–104, Churchill Livingstone, London and Edinburgh.

McGaughey, C., Campbell, J.E., Pazo, C. and Stowell, E.C. (1975) Relations between early dental calculus production and calcium and phosphate parameters of salivary fractions. Journal of Periodontology, 46, 681–684.

Marder, M.Z., Wotman, S. and Mandel, I.D. (1972) Salivary electrolyte changes during pregnancy. I. Normal pregnancy. American Journal of Gynecology, 112, 233–236.

Mason, D.K. and Chisholm, D.M. (1975) Salivary Glands in Health and Disease, W.B. Saunders, London.

Massion, C.G. and McNeely, M.D. (1973) Accurate micromethod for estimation of both medium- and long-chain fatty acids and triglycerides in fecal fat. Clinical Chemistry, 19, 499–505.

Mayo, J.W., Wallace, W.M., Matthews, L.W. and Carlson, D.M. (1976) Quantitation of submandibular proteins resolved from normal individuals and children with cystic fibrosis. Archives of Biochemistry and Biophysics, 175, 507–513.

Mitchell, W.D., Findlay, J.M., Prescott, R.J., Eastwood, M.A. and Horn, D.B. (1973) Bile acids in the diarrhoea of ileal resection. Gut, 14, 348–353.

Morris, D.W., Hansell, J.R., Ostrow, J.D. and Lee, C.S. (1976) Reliability of chemical tests for fecal occult blood in hospitalized patients. American Journal of Digestive Diseases, 21, 845–852.

Nestel, P.J., Havenstein, N., Homma, Y., Scott, T.W. and Cook, L.J. (1975) Increased sterol excretion with polyunsaturated-fat high-cholesterol diets. Metabolism, 24, 189–198.

Neu, C. and DiMascio, A. (1977) Saliva lithium levels: clinical applications. Psychopharmacology Bulletin, 13, 55–57.

O'Neill, B.J., Shum, H.Y. and Streeter, A.M. (1973) Normal faecal blood loss after injection of 51-Cr-labelled red cells. Lancet I, 262.

Oppenheim, F.G. and Hay, D.I. (1972) Further studies of human serum albumin in oral fluid. Helvetica Odontologica Acta, 16, 22–26.

Owens, C.W. and Padovan, W. (1976) Limitations of ultracentrifugation and in vivo dialysis as methods of stool analysis. Gut, 17, 68–74.

Paxton, J.W., Rowell, F., Ratcliffe, J.G., Lambie, D.G., Nanda, R., Melville, I.D. and Johnson, R.H. (1977) Salivary phenytoin radioimmunoassay. A simple method of the assessment of non-protein bound drug concentrations. European Journal of Clinical Pharmacology, 11, 71–74.

Paxton, J.W., Whiting, B., Rowell, F.J., Ratcliffe, J.G. and Stephen, K.W. (1976) Salivary concentrations of antiepileptic drugs. Lancet, II, 639–640.

Puskulian, L. (1972) Salivary electrolyte changes during the normal menstrual cycle. Journal of Dental Research, 51, 1212–1216.

Reddy, B.S., Mastromarino, A., Gustafson, C., Lipkin, M. and Wynder, E.L. (1976) Fecal bile acids and neutral sterols in patients with familial polyposis. Cancer, 38, 1694–1698.

Reddy, B.S. and Wynder, E.L. (1973) Large-bowel carcinogenesis: fecal constituents of populations with diverse incidence rates of colon cancer. Journal of the National Cancer Institute, 50, 1437–1442.

Reynolds, F., Ziroyanis, P.N., Jones, N.F. and Smith, S.E. (1976) Salivary phenytoin concentration in epilepsy and in chronic renal failure. Lancet, II, 384–386.

Ryley, H.C., Neale, L.M. and Bray, P.T. (1976) False-negative meconium tests for cystic fibrosis. Lancet, II, 365–366.

Shannon, I.L. (1973) Reference table for human parotid saliva collected at varying levels of exogenous stimulation. Journal of Dental Research, 52, 1157.

Shannon, I.L., Feller, R.P. and Chauncey, H.H. (1976) Fluoride in human parotid saliva. Journal of Dental Research, 55, 506–509.

Shannon, I.L., Suddick, R.P. and Dowd, F.J., Jr. (1974) Saliva: composition and secretion. Monographs in Oral Science, 2, 1–103.

Smith, Q.T., Shapiro, B.L. and Hamilton, M.J. (1976) Polyacrylamide gel electrophoresis of twin and nontwin parotid salivary proteins. Proceedings of the Society for Experimental Biology and Medicine, 151, 535–538.

Soong, C.S., Thompson, J.B., Poley, J.R. and Hess, D.R. (1972) Hydroxy fatty acids in human diarrhea. Gastroenterology, 63, 748–757.

Spiro, H.M. (1977) Clinical Gastroenterology, 2nd edn., p. 365, MacMillan, New York.

Stephan, U., Busch, E.W., Kollberg, H. and Hellsing, K. (1975) Cystic fibrosis detection by means of a test-strip. Pediatrics, 55, 35–38.

Stephen, K.W., Robertson, J.W., Harden, R.M. and Chisholm, D.M. (1973) Concentration of iodide, pertechnetate, thiocyanate, and bromide in saliva from parotid, submandibular, and minor salivary glands in man. Journal of Laboratory and Clinical Medicine, 81, 219–229.

Stephen, K.W. and Speirs, C.F. (1976) Methods for collecting individual components of mixed saliva: the relevance to clinical pharmacology. British Journal of Clinical Pharmacology, 3, 315–319.

Stroehlein, J.R., Fairbanks, V.F., McGill, D.B. and Go, V.L. (1976) Hemoccult detection of fecal occult blood quantitated by radioassay. American Journal of Digestive Diseases, 21, 841–844.

Subbiah, M.T., Tyler, N.E., Buscaglia, M.D. and Marai, L. (1976) Estimation of bile acid excretion in man: comparison of isotopic turnover and fecal excretion methods. Journal of Lipid Research 17, 78–84.

Swanson, M., Cacace, L., Chun, G. and Itano, M. (1973) Saliva calcium and potassium concentrations of digitalis toxicity. Circulation, 47, 736–743.

Talal, N., Grey, H.M., Zvaifler, N., Michalski, J.P. and Daniels, T.E. (1975) Elevated salivary and synovial fluid beta-2-microglobulin in Sjögren's syndrome and rheumatoid arthritis. Science, 187, 1196–1198.

Talner, L.B., Coel, M.N. and Lang, J.H. (1973) Salivary secretion of iodine after urography. Further evidence for in vivo deiodination and salivary secretion of contrast media. Radiology, 106, 263–268.

Tannenbaum, P.J., Posner, A.S. and Mandel, I.D. (1976) Formation of calcium phosphates in saliva and dental plaque. Journal of Dental Research, 55, 997–1000.

Tannenbaum, S.R., Sinskey, A.J., Weisman, M. and Bishop, W. (1974) Nitrite in human saliva. Its possible relationship to nitrosamine formation. Journal of the National Cancer Institute, 53, 79–84.

Tarlow, M.J. and Thom, H. (1974) A comparison of stool fluid and stool dialysate obtained in vivo. Gut, 15, 608–613.

Tenovuo, J. and Mäkinen, K.K. (1976) Concentration of thiocyanate and ionizable iodine in saliva of smokers and nonsmokers. Journal of Dental Research, 55, 661–663.

Walker, B.E., Kelleher, J., Davies, T., Smith, C.L. and Losowsky, M.S. (1973) Influence of dietary fat on fecal fat. Gastroenterology, 64, 233–239.

Walters, R.L., Baird, I.M., Davies, P.S., Hill, M.J., Drasar, B.S., Southgate, D.A., Green, J. and Morgan, B. (1975) Effects of two types of dietary fibre on faecal steroid and lipid excretion. British Medical Journal 2, 536–538.

Watne, A.L. and Core, S.K. (1975) Fecal steroids in polyposis coli and ileorectostomy patients. Journal of Surgical Research, 19, 157–161.

Wiesmann, U.N., Boat, T.F. and Di Sant'Agnese, P.A. (1972) Flow-rates and electrolytes in minor-salivary-gland saliva in normal subjects and patients with cystic fibrosis. Lancet, II, 510–512.

Wiggins, H.S., Pearson, J.R., Walker, J.G., Russell, R.I. and Kellock, T.D. (1974) Incidence and significance of faecal hydroxystearic acid in alimentary disease. Gut, 15, 614–621.

Wilson, D.R., Laidlaw, J.C. and Ruse, J.L. (1971) Fecal and salivary electrolytes in the diagnosis of primary aldosteronism. Canadian Medical Association Journal, 105, 1300–1305.

Winawer, S.J. (1976) Fecal occult blood testing. American Journal of Digestive Diseases, 21, 885–888.

Windeler, A.S., Jr. (1973) Determination of mercury in parotid fluid. Journal of Dental Research, 52, 19–22.

Winer, R.A. and Feller, R.P. (1972) Composition of parotid and submandibular saliva and serum in Down's syndrome. Journal of Dental Research, 51, 449–454.

Wotman, S. and Bigger, J.T., Jr. (1974) Salivary electrolytes and digitalis toxicity. Journal of the American Medical Association, 228, 696–697.

Wotman, S., Bigger, J.T., Jr., Mandel, I.D. and Bartelstone, H.J. (1971) Salivary electrolytes in the detection of digitalis toxicity. New England Journal of Medicine, 285, 871–876.

Wotman, S., Baer, L., Mandel, I.D. and Laragh, J.H. (1970) Submaxillary potassium concentration in true and pseudoprimary aldosteronism. Archives of Internal Medicine, 126, 248–251.

Wotman, S., Goodwin, F.J., Mandel, I.D. and Laragh, J.H. (1969) Changes in salivary electrolytes following treatment of primary aldosteronism. Archives of Internal Medicine, 124, 477–480.

Wotman, S. and Mandel, I.D. (1973) Salivary indicators of systemic disease. Postgraduate Medicine, 53, 73–78.

Section 2.6. Specialized glandular secretions

Ayvazian, L.F., Schneider, B., Gewirtz, G. and Yalow, R.S. (1975) Ectopic production of big ACTH in carcinoma of the lung. Its clinical usefulness as a biologic marker. American Review of Respiratory Disease, 111, 279–287.

Bakken, A.F. and Seip, M. (1976) Insecticides in human breast milk. Acta Paediatrica Scandinavica, 65, 535–539.

Blair, O.M. and Goldenberg, D.M. (1974) A correlative study of bronchial cytology, bronchial washing carcinoembryonic antigen, and plasma carcinoembryonic antigen in the diagnosis of bronchogenic cancer. Acta Cytologica, 18, 510–514.

Boat, T.F. and Matthews, L.W. (1973) Chemical composition of human tracheo-bronchial secretions. In Sputum: Fundamentals and Clinical Pathology (Ed. M.J. Dulfano) pp. 243–274, Charles C. Thomas, Springfield.

Catz, C.S. and Giacoia, G.P. (1972) Drugs and breast milk. Pediatric Clinics of North America, 19, 151–166.

Cohen, L.F., Farrell, P.M., Lundgren, D.W. and di Sant' Agnese, P.A. (1976) Electrolyte values of sweat obtained by local and whole body collection methods in cystic fibrosis patients. Journal of Pediatrics, 89, 430–433.

Finberg, L. (1977) Pollutants in breast milk: PBBs: the ladies' milk is not for burning. Journal of Pediatrics, 90, 511–512.

Gibson, L.E. and Cooke, R.E. (1959) A test for concentration of electrolytes in sweat in cystic fibrosis of the pancreas utilizing pilocarpine iontophoresis. Pediatrics, 23, 545–549.

Grice, K., Sattar, H., Casey, T. and Baker, H. (1975) An evaluation of Na^+, Cl^- and pH ion-specific electrodes in the study of the electrolyte contents of epidermal transudate and sweat. British Journal of Dermatology, 92, 511–518.

Hall, B. (1975) Changing composition of human milk and early development of an appetite control. Lancet, I, 779–781.

Hambraeus, L. (1977) Proprietary milk versus human breast milk in infant feeding. A critical appraisal from the nutritional point of view. Pediatric Clinics of North America, 24, 17–36.

Knowles, J.A. (1974) Breast milk: a source of more than nutrition for the neonate. Clinical Toxicology, 7, 69–82.

Lobeck, C.C. (1972) Cystic fibrosis. In The Metabolic Basis of Inherited Disease, 3rd edn. (Eds. J.B. Stanbury, J.B. Wyngaarden and D.S. Fredrickson) pp. 1605–1626, McGraw-Hill, New York.

Mandel, M.A., Dvorak, K.J., Worman, L.W. and DeCosse, J.J. (1976) Immunoglobulin content in the bronchial washings of patients with benign and malignant pulmonary disease. New England Journal of Medicine, 295, 694–698.

Miller, R.W. (1977) Pollutants in breast milk: PCB's and cola-colored babies. Journal of Pediatrics, 90, 510–511.

Peitersen, B., Bohn, L. and Andersen, H. (1975) Quantitative determination of immunoglobulins, lysozyme, and certain electrolytes in breast milk during the entire period of lactation, during a 24-hour period, and in milk from the individual mammary gland. Acta Paediatrica Scandinavica 64, 709–717.

Ramirez, R.J., Schwartz, B., Dowell, A.R. and Lee, S.D. (1971) Biochemical composition of human pulmonary washings. Archives of Internal Medicine, 127, 395–400.

Reynolds, H.Y., Fulmer, J.D., Kazmierowski, J.A., Roberts, W.C., Frank, M.M. and Crystal, R.G. (1977) Analysis of cellular and protein content of broncho-alveolar lavage fluid from patients with idiopathic pulmonary fibrosis and chronic hypersensitivity pneumonitis. Journal of Clinical Investigation, 59, 165–175.

Steinrud, J., Winkel, S. and Flensborg, E.W. (1974) Screening for cystic fibrosis with chloride. An investigation of sweat chloride with chloride electrode orion 417 in normal persons and in patients with cystic fibrosis. Danish Medical Bulletin, 21, 251–255.

Vorherr, H. (1974) Drug excretion in breast milk. Postgraduate Medicine, 56, 97–104.

Winter, M., Thomas, M., Wernick, S., Levin, S. and Farvar, M.T. (1976) Analysis of pesticide residues in 290 samples of Guatemalan mother's milk. Bulletin of Environmental Contamination and Toxicology, 16, 652–657.

Woodard, B.T., Ferguson, B.B. and Wilson, D.J. (1976) DDT levels in milk of rural indigent blacks. American Journal of Diseases in Children, 130, 400–403.

FURTHER READING

Fluids of the central nervous system and special senses

Calabrese, V.P. (1976) The interpretation of routine CSF tests. Virginia Medical Monthly, 103, 207–209.

Thompson, E.J., Norman, P.M. and Macdermot, J. (1975) The analysis of cerebrospinal fluid. British Journal of Hospital Medicine, 14, 645–652.

Effusion

Cohen, A.S., Brandt, K.D. and Krey, P.R. (1975) Synovial fluid. In Laboratory Diagnostic Procedures in the Rheumatic Diseases, 2nd edn., (Ed. A.S. Cohen) pp. 1–62, Little, Brown and Co., Boston.

Donowitz, M., Kerstein, M.D. and Spiro, H.M. (1974) Pancreatic ascites. Medicine, 53, 183–195.

Lowell, J.R. (1977) Diagnosis: fluid and tissue examination. In Pleural Effusions, pp. 45–73, University Park Press, Baltimore.

Mansberger, A.R. Jr. (1964) The diagnostic value of abdominal paracentesis. American Journal of Gastroenterology, 42, 150–164.

Scott, J.T. (1975) The analysis of joint fluids. British Journal of Hospital Medicine, 14, 653–658.

Fluids of the genitourinary system

Brock, D.J.H. (1976) Prenatal diagnosis – chemical methods. British Medical Bulletin, 32, 16–20.

Fairweather, D.V.I., Whyley, G.A. and Millar, M.D. (1976) Six years' experience of the prediction of severity in Rhesus haemolytic disease. British Journal of Obstetrics and Gynaecology, 83, 698–706.

Forman, D.T. (1974) The lecithin to sphingomyelin ratio in amniotic fluid and its predictive value for fetal lung immaturity (respiratory distress syndrome). In Amniotic Fluid (Eds. S. Natelson, A. Scommegna and M.B. Epstein) pp. 247–258, John Wiley and Sons, New York.

Hall, P.M., Schuman, M. and Vidt, D.G. (1976) Laboratory tests of renal function. CRC Critical Reviews in Clinical Laboratory Sciences, 7, 33–47.

Kark, R.M., Lawrence, J.R., Pollack, V.E., Pirani, C.L., Muehrcke, R.C. and Silva, H. (1963) A Primer of Urinalysis, 2nd edn., Hoeber Medical Division, Harper and Row, New York.

Wilson, D.M. (1975) Urinalysis and other tests of renal function. Minnesota Medicine, 58, 9–17.

Saliva, faeces and meconium

Horning, M.G., Brown, L., Nowlin, J., Lertratanangkoon, K., Kellaway, P. and Zion, T.E. (1977) Use of saliva in therapeutic drug monitoring. Clinical Chemistry, 23, 157–164.

Morris, D.W., Hansell, J.R., Ostrow, J.D. and Lee, C.S. (1976) Reliability of chemical tests for fecal occult blood in hospitalized patients. American Journal of Digestive Diseases, 21, 845–852.

Winawer, S.J. (1976) Fecal occult blood testing. American Journal of Digestive Diseases, 21, 885–888.

Wotman, S. and Mandel, I.D. (1973) Salivary indicators of systemic disease. Postgraduate Medicine, 53, 73–78.

Specialized glandular secretions

Bakken, A.F. and Seip, M. (1976) Insecticides in human breast milk. Acta Paediatrica Scandinavica, 65, 535–539.

Hambraeus, L. (1977) Proprietary milk versus human breast milk in infant feeding. A critical appraisal from the nutritional point of view. Pediatric Clinics of North America, 24, 17–36.

Lobeck, C.C. (1972) Cystic fibrosis. In The Metabolic Basis of Inherited Disease, 3rd edn. (Eds. J.B. Stanbury, J.B. Wyngaarden and D.S. Fredrickson) pp. 1605–1626, McGraw-Hill, New York.

Chapter 3

Hydrogen ions and blood gases

Ole Siggaard-Andersen

Københavns Amts Sygehus i Herlev, Department of Clinical Chemistry, Herlev Ringvej, 2730 Herlev, Denmark

CONTENTS

Chemical diagnosis of disease, edited by
S.S. Brown, F.L. Mitchell and D.S. Young

3.1. INTRODUCTION

This Chapter deals with three important components in the blood: hydrogen ion, carbon dioxide, and oxygen. Each component can be described by: (a) a quantity related to the chemical potential or the activity of the component in blood or plasma; or (b) a quantity related to the stoichiometric amount of the component in blood or plasma. The Chapter contains a systematic description of the following quantities.

Concentration of free hydrogen ion in arterial plasma.
Concentration of titratable hydrogen ion in plasma, blood, or extracellular fluid.

Partial pressure of carbon dioxide in arterial blood.
Concentrations of total carbon dioxide and of bicarbonate in plasma.
Partial pressure of oxygen in arterial and mixed venous blood.
Partial pressure of oxygen at half saturation.
Saturation of oxygen in haemoglobin in arterial blood.

The systematic clinical chemical description employed here differs from most other accounts of pH and blood gases. For more detailed descriptions of the various clinical or aetiological entities, the reader is referred to textbooks of internal medicine (e.g. Schwartz, 1975). The elementary principles of acid–base chemistry, biochemistry, and physiology are described in appropriate textbooks (Masoro and Siegel, 1971; Bates, 1973; Campbell, 1974; Davenport, 1974; Siggaard-Andersen, 1974; Rooth, 1974; Weisberg, 1975; Natelson and Natelson, 1975). For more detailed accounts of analytical methods, reference should be made to textbooks of clinical chemistry techniques (Henry et al., 1974; Tietz, 1976) and to the various original publications.

Each description of the foregoing quantities includes the following sections.

(1) *Introduction,* with comments on the most important clinical applications or indications for measurements.

(2) *Chemistry,* including a discussion of terminology, symbols, and units of measurement.

(3) *Reference values,* giving reference intervals, and commenting on the extreme pathological range.

(4) *Causes of change,* describing the pathophysiological causes of change in the quantity, i.e. the various aetiologies of disturbances.

(5) *Effects of change,* dealing with the changes in the body which can be considered secondary to a change in the given quantity, i.e. the signs and symptoms related to a change in the quantity.

(6) *Therapy,* containing a brief comment on some therapeutic measures in cases where these are directly aimed at normalizing the given quantity.

(7) *Analysis,* summarizing the most important analytical principles.

Sections 4 and 5 above together give a description of the physiological regulation of the quantity, i.e. the negative feed-back mechanisms which are illustrated by means of cybernetic diagrams (Schemes 3.1–3.4). With regard to the layout of these diagrams, the following principles apply. The *variables,* i.e. the different measurable quantities, are indicated by rounded boxes. Each variable may be considered as a function of several other variables and each *function* or mechanism is represented by a rectangular box. Each function expresses a *dependent variable* as a function of several *independent variables.* The arrow leading from an independent variable to a given function may be closed (black) or open (white) indicating, respectively, a positive or a negative correlation between the independent and the dependent variables. When a feed-back loop contains an uneven number of open arrows, it is a negative feed-back loop – a regulatory mechanism. When the loop contains an even number of open arrows, it is a positive feed-back loop – a vicious circle. The reader is referred to Ashby (1973) for a more detailed account of the principles of cybernetics.

3.1.1. Quantities, symbols and abbreviations

A quantity is a measurable property of a stated physical or chemical system: the name of the quantity requires a specification of the property (e.g. volume, mass, amount of substance, temperature, etc.) and a sufficiently detailed characterization of the component and system (Dybkaer, 1970).

Concerning symbols for quantities, the following principles are applied. The symbol for the property is a single letter (Latin or Greek) which is printed in italics (International Organization for Standardization, 1974). The symbols for the component and system are written in Roman type immediately following the symbol for the property. Thus:

concentration of free hydrogen ion in plasma = $c\mathrm{fH}^+ \subset \mathrm{P}$.

Alternatively the symbol might be written $c(\mathrm{fH}^+ \subset \mathrm{P})$, but in the author's opinion the parentheses are unnecessary. Tables 3.1 and 3.2 give a list of symbols and abbreviations employed in this Chapter. The system (plasma = P) is a set of elements (molecules), and the set of component molecules (free hydrogen ion = fH^+) is a subset of the system: $\mathrm{fH}^+ \subset \mathrm{P}$. The measurement equation is the equation which expresses the quantity as a numerical value times the appropriate unit, where the multiplication sign is generally omitted. Thus:

$c\mathrm{fH}^+ \subset \mathrm{P}$ = 40 nmol/litre.

TABLE 3.1

LIST OF QUANTITIES, WITH THE SYMBOLS IN ALPHABETICAL ORDER, THE LATIN ALPHABET PRECEDING THE GREEK

Symbol	Name	Primary unit
a	(relative) activity	1
c	(substance) concentration	mol/litre
F	Faraday constant = 96485	C/mol
m	mass	kg
$\acute{m}$	molality	mol/kg
n	amount of substance	mol
$\dot{n}$	substance flux	mol/min
p	(partial) pressure	Pa
R	gas constant = 8.314	$\mathrm{J} \times \mathrm{K}^{-1} \times \mathrm{mol}^{-1}$
s	saturation fraction	1
T	(absolute) temperature	K
V	volume	litre
$\dot{V}$	volume flux	litre/min
x	substance fraction	mol/mol = 1
α	solubility coefficient	mol/J
γ	activity coefficient	1
μ	(standard) chemical potential	J/mol
ρ	mass concentration	kg/litre

TABLE 3.2

LIST OF SYSTEMS AND COMPONENTS, WITH SYMBOLS IN ALPHABETICAL ORDER

A	alveolar air
a	arterial (used as prefix)
B	blood
Csf	cerebrospinal fluid
E	erythrocyte
Ecf	extracellular fluid
f	free (used as prefix)
Hb	haemoglobin (Fe)
I	humidified inspired air
P	plasma
Pt	patient or whole body
t	total (used as prefix)
U	urine
V	venous (used as prefix)

A quantity may change with time, in which case a dot above the symbol for the property indicates the rate of change. Thus:

rate of change in the amount of oxygen in the patient = $\dot{n}O_2 \subset Pt$.

Unless otherwise specified, this refers to the net change, i.e. the sum or balance of changes due to various processes. The rate of change in the amount of oxygen in the patient due to uptake of oxygen in the lungs [= $\dot{n}O_2 \subset Pt$ (uptake in lungs) $\approx +12.5$ mmol/min] is numerically equal to the rate of change in the amount of oxygen in the patient due to oxidative metabolism in the tissues [= $\dot{n}O_2 \subset Pt$ (metabolism) ≈ -12.5 mmol/min]; in the steady state $\dot{n}O_2 \subset Pt$ (net) = 0. In other words, the process which causes the change is indicated in parenthesis.

When a composite symbol appears in the text or in the Figures, *it is essential to translate and read each symbol in the sequence* as if the quantity name were written in full. Only a few of the symbols, notably pH, pCO_2 and pO_2, have become so familiar that they are meaningful without translation.

3.2. CONCENTRATION OF FREE HYDROGEN ION IN ARTERIAL PLASMA

The concentration of free hydrogen ion (cfH^+) in arterial plasma (or the plasma pH) is an indicator of the acidity of the extracellular milieu: its measurement is indicated on suspicion of a respiratory or metabolic acidosis or alkalosis. Usually the pCO_2 and the concentration of titratable hydrogen ion or of bicarbonate are measured simultaneously. This set of quantities is designated the acid–base status of the blood.

3.2.1. Chemistry

The chemical potential of H^+ in a solution, commonly termed the acidity of the solution, is usually expressed in terms of the pH value, the activity of H^+, or the concentration of "free" H^+.

The absolute chemical potential (μ^*) is defined as the partial molar internal energy (E) with respect to amount of substance (n) of added H^+:

$$\mu^*H^+ = \partial E/\partial nH^+ \text{, by definition .} \quad [1]$$

Absolute chemical potentials cannot be determined – only the difference between two systems (Moore, 1972). Hence *the (standard) chemical potential* of H^+ in a given solution (S) is defined as the absolute chemical potential of H^+ in the solution minus the absolute chemical potential of H^+ in an arbitrary reference solution (S^θ):

$$\mu H^+ \subset S = \mu^*H^+ \subset S - \mu^*H^+ \subset S^\theta \text{, by definition .} \quad [2]$$

In other words, the chemical potential is the energy liberated by reversible transfer of a differential amount of component from the given test solution to a given reference solution, expressing the energy liberated per unit amount of substance. The conventional reference is an ideal aqueous solution with a molality of HCl of 1 mol/kg – "ideal" indicating that inter-molecular and inter-ionic forces between solute molecules are absent.

The (relative) activity of H^+ is defined on the basis of the chemical potential:

$$aH^+ = \exp(\mu H^+/R \times T) \text{, by definition} \quad [3]$$

where R is the gas constant and T is the absolute temperature. The negative logarithm of the activity is conventionally called pH (p = –log) *:

$$-\log aH^+ = \text{p}\, aH^+ = \text{pH} \text{, by definition .} \quad [4]$$

It follows from these equations that the chemical potentials of H^+ and pH are proportional:

$$\mu H^+ = -R \times T \times \ln 10 \times \text{pH}$$
$$= -5.938 \times \text{pH kJ/mol} \Leftarrow T = 310.15 \text{ K.} \quad [5]$$

The concentration of free H^+ in the plasma or other body fluids is derived from:

$$cfH^+ = (aH^+ \times \rho H_2O)/(\gamma H^+ \times \text{kg} \times \text{mol}^{-1}) \quad [6]$$

which approximates to cfH^+ in nmol/litre $\approx aH^+ \times 10^9 = \text{antilog}(9 - \text{pH})$ [7]

* In the present text log signifies decadic logarithm.

For normal plasma, the activity coefficient (γ) of H^+ is about 0.8, while the mass concentration (ρ) of water is 0.94 kg/litre (Maas et al., 1971). The free hydrogen ions are actually bound to H_2O and exist mainly as hydroxonium ions (H_3O^+).

The relationship between paH^+ and $paOH^-$ is:

$$paH^+ + paOH^- - paH_2O = pKH_2O \ , \qquad [8]$$

where paH_2O in dilute aqueous solution approaches the value (zero by convention) for pure water and $pKH_2O = 13.622$ for $T = 310.15$ K.

Although the chemical potential of H^+ in plasma is the most relevant quantity, the more familiar pH and hydrogen ion concentration are used in the following treatment.

3.2.2. Reference values

The reference intervals (95%) for the concentration of free hydrogen ions and the pH of arterial plasma from healthy resting individuals and the approximate extreme pathological ranges are tabulated:

Quantity	Reference interval	Extremes of range
cfH^+ (nmol/litre)	35 – 43	16 – 160
pH	7.45 – 7.37	7.8 – 6.8

The pH values tend to be slightly higher for women than for men (0.01 units). There is no pronounced variation with age although the pH value tends to fall slightly (0.02 units) in old age. Newborn infants often have a respiratory acidosis immediately after birth (pH as low as 7.2) with values approaching the reference interval in the course of a few hours.

Capillary blood may often be used as a substitute for arterial blood except in cases where the peripheral circulation is markedly decreased, as in cases of shock.

In *venous plasma,* the pH value is 0.01 to 0.03 lower than in arterial plasma. However, prolonged venous stasis or muscular pumping may cause a considerably greater arterio-venous difference (up to 0.1 units lower in the vein).

The extremes of range refer to acute disturbances, e.g. hyperventilation or severe muscular exercise. In chronic diseases, cfH^+ rarely exceeds the range 25 to 63 nmol/litre (≈pH 7.6 to 7.2).

Decreased plasma pH has been designated hyperhydrionaemia, hyperprotonaemia, or *acidaemia.* Increased plasma pH is similarly designated hypohydrionaemia, hypoprotonaemia, or *alkalaemia* (Winters, 1966).

3.2.3. Causes of change in cfH^+ and pH in the arterial plasma

The causes of change in the hydrogen ion concentration of the arterial plasma are classified as metabolic or respiratory disturbances. Temperature variation is another cause which will be described separately.

3.2.3.1. Metabolic and respiratory acid–base disturbances

The concentration of free H^+ in plasma is a function of two independent variables.

(a) The concentration of titratable H^+ (ctH^+) in the extracellular fluid, which is primarily dependent on the previous balance of H^+ in the organism. This variable is also designated the metabolic or non-respiratory factor.

(b) The pCO_2 of the arterial blood, which is primarily dependent on the alveolar ventilation. This variable is designated the respiratory factor.

In the intact organism, a primary change in one of these variables, by way of a change in plasma pH, causes a secondary or compensatory change in the other, which tends to reduce the primary change in pH. The causes of change in the free hydrogen ion concentration in the plasma and the negative feed-back mechanisms (regulatory mechanisms) are illustrated in the cybernetic flow diagram (Scheme 3.1). The quantitative relationships between the variables are illustrated in the Cartesian diagram (Figure 3.1) in which the bivariate reference areas for the various types of acid–base disturbances are shown (Siggaard-Andersen, 1971).

In considering the *cybernetics* of the regulation of the concentration of free hydrogen ions in the arterial plasma, renal and respiratory mechanisms must be distinguished.

The renal mechanism involves an increase in $cfH^+ \subset aP$ which tends to enhance the rate of excretion of titratable H^+ in the urine ($\dot{n}tH^+ \subset U$) via an increase in cfH^+ in the tubule cells and thus in the secretion of H^+ in the kidney tubules. However, the H^+ excretion in the urine is affected by several other variables: the concentration of carbonic anhydrase in the kidneys ($cCA \subset Ren$); the concentration of glutaminase in the kidneys ($cGA \subset Ren$); the concentration of aldosterone in plasma ($cAldost \subset P$); the concentration of parathyroid hormone in plasma ($cPTH \subset P$); and the concentration of potassium in plasma ($cK^+ \subset P$). Furthermore, the filtration of titratable H^+ in the glomeruli is dependent on $ctH^+ \subset Ecf$.

An increase in $\dot{n}tH^+ \subset U$ tends to cause a decrease in the amount of titratable H^+ in the patient ($ntH^+ \subset Pt$), provided that the rate of change in the amount of H^+ in the patient due to other processes is constant. Such processes are: production of lactic acid or keto-acids, oral intake or loss of acid or base, intravenous infusion of acid or base, or loss of base in stools. In Scheme 3.1, the rate of change in titratable H^+ in the patient due to a given process, e.g. oral intake or loss, is symbolized: $\dot{n}H^+ \subset Pt$ (p.o.).

Due to the law of electro-neutrality, a loss of H^+ from the body (metabolic alkalosis) must be accompanied by an equivalent accumulation of other cations (e.g. Na^+ or K^+, often termed "accumulation of base"), or by an equivalent loss of anion (e.g. Cl^-, often termed "loss of acid"). Disturbances involving H^+ therefore always involve disturbances in several other electrolytes as well.

A fall in $ntH^+ \subset Pt$ tends to cause a decrease in the amount of H^+ in the extracellular fluid ($ntH^+ \subset Ecf$), but the distribution of H^+ between the extracellular and intracellular fluids is dependent on the distribution of K^+. The buffering properties of bone tissue are dependent on parathyroid function.

A decrease in $ntH^+ \subset Ecf$ causes a decrease in $ctH^+ \subset Ecf$ depending upon the volume of extracellular fluid in the patient ($VEcf \subset Pt$). A fall in $ctH^+ \subset Ecf$ tends to cause a fall in $ctH^+ \subset P$, although the distribution of H^+ between erythrocytes, plasma, and interstitial fluid is slightly dependent upon the pCO_2. A fall in $ctH^+ \subset aP$ gives a fall in $cfH^+ \subset aP$ and

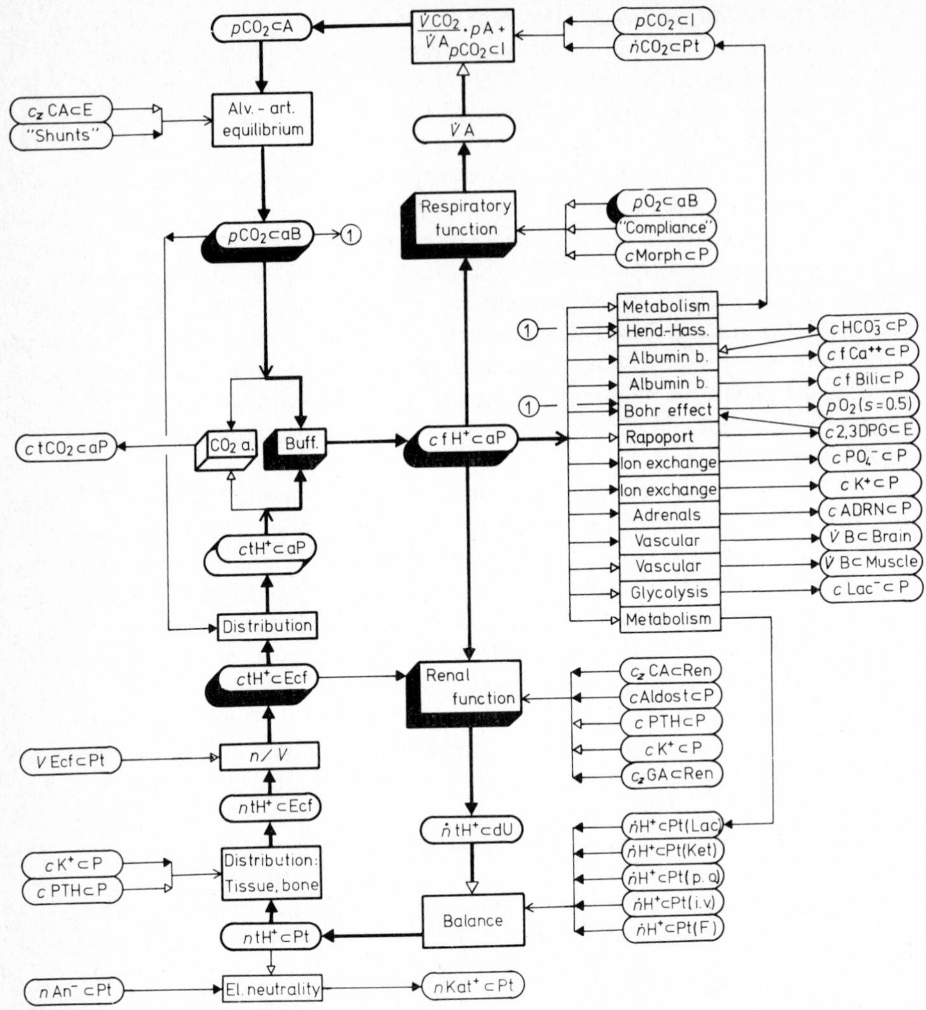

Scheme 3.1. Cybernetic diagram of the regulation of the concentration of free hydrogen ions in the arterial plasma. Descriptions of the different parts of the diagram are given in sections 3.2.3, 3.2.4, 3.3.3, 3.3.4, 3.4.3 and 3.4.4. Symbols and abbreviations are explained in section 3.1 and in Tables 3.1 and 3.2. The most important *variables* (rounded boxes) are emphasized – the concentration of free hydrogen ion in the arterial plasma ($cfH^+ \subset aP$). which is a function of the concentration of titratable H^+ in the extracellular fluid ($ctH^+ \subset Ecf$) and the partial pressure of CO_2 in the arterial blood ($pCO_2 \subset aB$). The most important *functions* or mechanisms (rectangular boxes) are also emphasized – the buffer function of plasma, renal function and respiratory function. The circled number (1) indicates that a change in pCO_2 has a specific effect on the relevant mechanism, apart from the effect of cfH^+.

hence there is negative feed-back, or a regulation of the initial rise in $cfH^+ \subset aP$.

The respiratory mechanism involves an increase in $cfH^+ \subset aP$ which tends to cause an increase in the alveolar ventilation ($\dot{V}A$ = volume flux of alveolar air). However, $\dot{V}A$ is also dependent on several other variables: the partial pressure of O_2 in the arterial blood

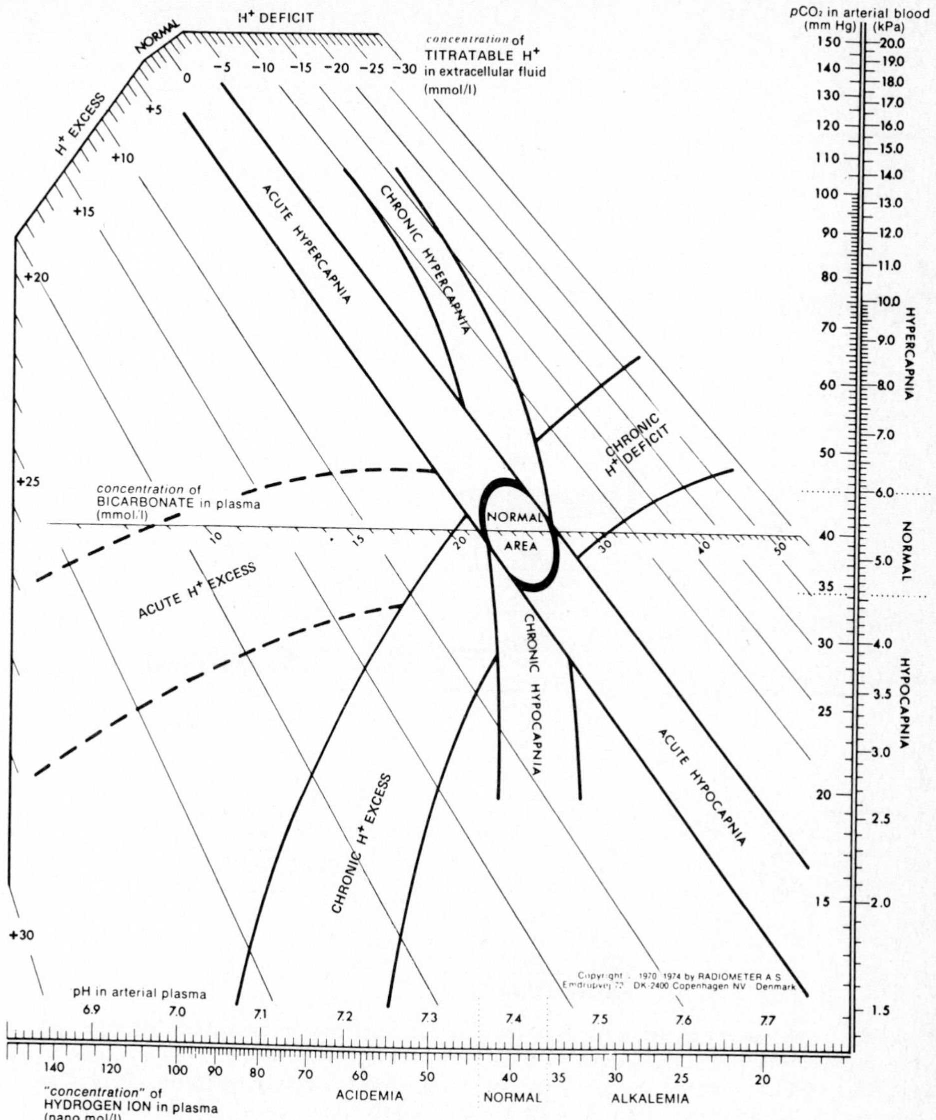

Figure 3.1. Cartesian diagram of the regulation of the concentration of free hydrogen ion in the arterial plasma. A description of the diagram is given in section 3.2.3.1.

($pO_2 \subset aB$), lung compliance, and the concentrations of respiratory depressants such as morphine or stimulants. The respiratory mechanism is further expanded in Scheme 3.2.

The rise in $\dot{V}A$ tends to cause a fall in the pCO_2 of the alveolar air ($pCO_2 \subset A$), but the latter is also dependent on pCO_2 of the inspired air ($pCO_2 \subset I$) and the rate of CO_2 production in the patient ($\dot{n}CO_2 \subset Pt$). The quantitative relationships between these variables are considered in section 3.4.3.

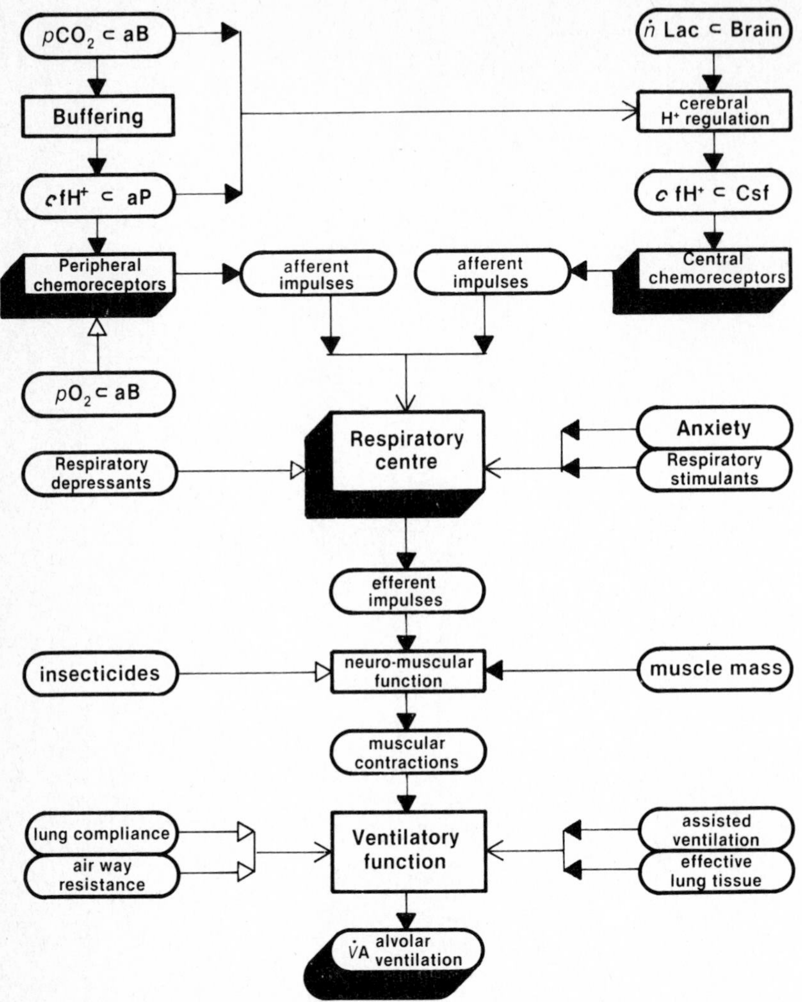

Scheme 3.2. Cybernetic diagram of the causes of a change in the alveolar ventilation, $\dot{V}$A. Descriptions of the various mechanisms are given in section 3.4.3.3. Symbols and abbreviations are explained in section 3.1. and in Tables 3.1 and 3.2. The effects of a change in alveolar ventilation, i.e. changes in $p\text{CO}_2$ and $p\text{O}_2$ of the arterial blood, are illustrated in Schemes 3.1 and 3.3, respectively.

The values of $p\text{CO}_2 \subset$ A and $p\text{CO}_2 \subset$ aB are almost equal provided that the concentration of carbonic anhydrase in the erythrocytes (cCA ⊂ E) is normal.

A fall in $p\text{CO}_2 \subset$ aB causes a fall in $c\text{fH}^+ \subset$ P, thus providing a negative feed-back regulation of the original increase in $c\text{fH}^+ \subset$ P.

A more detailed description of the many other effects of a change in $c\text{fH}^+ \subset$ P, such as effects on the vasculature system, on intermediary metabolism and albumin binding, is given in section 3.2.4.

In considering the Cartesian diagram (Figure 3.1) it is appropriate to discuss the significance of both the coordinates and the marked areas.

(a) The concentration of free hydrogen ion and the pH of the arterial plasma are both indicated on the abscissa.

(b) The pCO_2 is indicated on the ordinate in kilopascals (kPa) and in mm Hg.

(c) The concentration of titratable H^+ in the extracellular fluid ($ctH^+ \subset$ Ecf) is indicated on the scale to the upper left. Projections to this scale should be made along the slanting lines of the diagram. These lines of constant $ctH^+ \subset$ Ecf represent so-called in vivo CO_2 titration lines.

(d) The concentration of bicarbonate in the plasma is indicated on the horizontal scale in the middle of the diagram. Projections to the bicarbonate scale should be made at an angle of $-45°$; for this reason, divisions on the scale are slanting with slope -1.

With regard to the areas which are marked in the figure:

(a) The normal area for resting adults is shown near the centre of the diagram.

(b) Acute hypercapnia (acute respiratory acidosis) indicates the values which are obtained in normal individuals following an acute rise in pCO_2 (e.g. CO_2 breathing) before any renal compensation occurs.

(c) Chronic hypercapnia (chronic respiratory acidosis) indicates the values which are obtained in patients with a chronic respiratory insufficiency in the steady state, and with a normal renal function and maximal renal compensation. Following an acute rise in pCO_2, the maximal renal compensation is achieved in the course of 2 to 3 days.

(d) Acute hypocapnia (acute respiratory alkalosis) indicates values which are obtained in normal individuals immediately following hyperventilation, and before lactic acid production or renal compensation modify the results.

(e) Chronic hypocapnia (chronic respiratory alkalosis) indicates the values which are obtained in normal individuals at high altitude after acclimatization. Maximal renal compensation requires 2 to 3 days.

(f) Acute hydrogen ion excess (acute metabolic acidosis) indicates the values which are obtained after an acute accumulation of H^+ in the body, e.g. due to lactic acid production in the context of severe anaerobic muscular exercise. The rise in cfH^+ in the arterial plasma stimulates the peripheral chemoreceptors, so causing a moderate hyperventilation, with a slight fall in pCO_2.

(g) Chronic hydrogen ion excess (metabolic acidosis) indicates the values which are obtained in states with a chronic H^+ excess and with a maximal respiratory compensation, which require equilibrium of H^+ across the blood–brain barrier and stimulation of the central chemoreceptors. To achieve this equilibrium requires 4 to 6 hours after an acute accumulation of H^+ in the extracellular fluid.

(h) Chronic hydrogen ion deficit (metabolic alkalosis) indicates the values which are obtained in patients with a chronic H^+ deficit and with a maximal respiratory compensation.

It should be noted that a point falling within the reference area of acute hypercapnia does not necessarily indicate that the patient belongs to the reference population in question (viz. that there is an acute respiratory acidosis). The patient may very well have a chronic respiratory acidosis complicated with a metabolic acidosis. In statistics, this is called an error of the second kind. Similarly, the point for a patient with an acute respiratory acidosis may very well fall just outside the reference area – about 10% do fall outside. In statistics, this is called error of the first kind. The interpretation of reference intervals or reference areas therefore requires a statistical approach.

The designation "*fully compensated*" is sometimes used when pCO_2 of the arterial blood and ctH^+ of the extracellular fluid are both abnormal but balancing each other, so that the plasma pH is within the normal range. However, this designation can be misleading because fully compensated in a physiological sense would indicate values within the reference areas of chronic respiratory or non-respiratory disturbances, not necessarily associated with a normal pH.

3.2.3.2. Variation of the hydrogen ion concentration with temperature

In pure water, the variation of pH with temperature is $\partial pH/\partial T = -0.015\ K^{-1}$. With plasma or whole blood in a closed system in vitro, the temperature effects are $-0.012\ K^{-1}$ and $-0.015\ K^{-1}$, respectively. These coefficients vary slightly with the haemoglobin concentration, the plasma protein concentration and the pCO_2, but for most practical purposes this variation can be ignored (Siggaard-Andersen, 1974).

Among different homeothermic species, a correlation between the arterial plasma pH and body temperature has been demonstrated: $\Delta pH/\Delta T = +0.03\ K^{-1}$ (Chapot et al., 1972). In hibernating animals, a correlation between pH of the arterial plasma and body temperature when awake and during hibernation has been found: $\Delta pH/\Delta T = -0.010\ K^{-1}$ (Malan et al., 1973). In poikilothermic animals, the relationship between pH and body temperature is the same as found for pure water in vitro: $\partial pH/\partial T = -0.015\ K^{-1}$ (Truchot, 1973; Rahn, 1974).

For therapeutic hypothermia of the human body, very little is known about the optimal arterial plasma pH value as a function of body temperature. The general practice is to try to maintain pH = 7.40 as measured at the actual body temperature. This can be achieved by breathing CO_2 so that the pCO_2 remains about 5.3 kPa, irrespective of temperature.

3.2.4. Effects of change in cfH^+ and pH in the arterial plasma

The principal effects of changes in the hydrogen ion concentration of arterial plasma should be considered in relation to the cybernetic diagram (Scheme 3.1).

3.2.4.1. Renal function

A high cfH^+ causes an increased excretion of H^+ in the kidney tubules, probably due to a rise in cfH^+ in the cytoplasm of the tubule cells, so causing an increased secretion of H^+ in exchange for Na^+ and K^+. A low $cfH^+ \subset P$ has the opposite effect.

3.2.4.2. Respiratory function

A rise in $cfH^+ \subset aP$ provides a direct stimulus to the peripheral chemoreceptors, resulting in hyperventilation (Sørensen, 1971). A primary rise in cfH^+, after distribution of H^+ across the blood–brain barrier, also eventually causes a rise in $cfH^+ \subset Csf$. This causes stimulation of the central chemoreceptors on the surface of medulla oblongata and a further stimulation of ventilation (Mitchell et al., 1963). A fall in $cfH^+ \subset aP$ has the opposite effect, resulting in hypoventilation.

3.2.4.3. Cardiovascular effects

The local effect of H^+ on the vessels seems to be a vasodilatation as cfH^+ rises, and a vasoconstriction as cfH^+ falls. These effects are the predominant ones in brain, skin, and myocardium. In respiratory as well as metabolic acidosis, cerebral vasodilatation with increased intracranial pressure may be the cause of coma.

The sympathetic nervous system is stimulated by a rise in cfH^+ resulting in a markedly increased concentration of adrenaline and noradrenaline in the plasma (Nahas, 1974). At the same time, however, the sensitivity of the tissues to catecholamines decreases. The overall effect on the muscular, pulmonary, and splanchnic vessels is a vasocontriction as cfH^+ rises, and a dilatation as cfH^+ falls.

The cardiac output, the total peripheral resistance, and the blood pressure tend to increase slightly as cfH^+ increases, and the opposite effects are caused by a cfH^+ fall.

3.2.4.4. Intermediary metabolism

Oxygen consumption and CO_2 production (both associated with energy production) are negatively correlated to $cfH^+ \subset P$ (Albers, 1974). The same applies to the rate of glycolysis, probably because the catalytic effect of phosphofructokinase (EC 2.7.1.11) increases with increasing pH. Hence the lactate concentration in the plasma tends to rise significantly as $cfH^+ \subset P$ falls. Both effects tend to cause a negative feed-back regulation of $cfH^+ \subset P$, as shown in Scheme 3.1, but these mechanisms are not nearly as effective as the renal and the respiratory mechanisms. The effect of cfH^+ on the rate of glycolysis is also shown with blood in vitro. The rise in blood lactate when $cfH^+ \subset P$ falls in the whole organism is in part due to the increased rate of glycolysis in the blood, and in part to a release of hepatic lactate probably due to vasoconstriction in the liver resulting in local tissue hypoxia.

The intracellular concentration of organic phosphates increases when cfH^+ falls and decreases when cfH^+ rises. This is especially marked for the concentration of 2,3-diphosphoglycerate in erythrocytes. This explains why the concentration of inorganic phosphate in plasma is positively correlated to $cfH^+ \subset P$.

3.2.4.5. Potassium distribution

The concentration of K^+ in the plasma is closely correlated to the plasma pH during acute changes in pH: $\Delta cK^+/\Delta pH = -1$ to -3 mmol/litre. This is probably due to an ion-exchange mechanism, with H^+ entering the cells in exchange for K^+ and vice versa (Kilburn, 1966). Conversely, K^+ depletion seems to cause a loss of intracellular K^+ in exchange for H^+, so causing a rise in intracellular cfH^+ and a fall in extracellular cfH^+ (hypokalaemic alkalosis with intracellular acidosis).

3.2.4.6. Binding of Ca^{2+} and bilirubin to albumin

The albumin binding of Ca^{2+} increases with decreasing cfH^+ and consequently the concentration of free Ca^{2+} falls: $\partial \log cfCa^{2+}/\partial\, pH \approx -0.24$ (Pedersen, 1971). This may explain the tendency to twisting paresthaesias, muscular fibrillation, and tetany in alkalaemic patients.

The binding of bilirubin to albumin is also dependent on H^+, and concentration of free bilirubin increases with increasing cfH^+. A high $cfH^+ \subset P$ therefore accentuates the danger of hyperbilirubinaemia in the newborn infant. The binding of various drugs to albumin is probably also H^+-dependent, and the toxicities of various drugs may very well be accentuated in the presence of a high cfH^+.

3.2.4.7. Oxygen affinity of haemoglobin

The direct effect of changes in pH on the oxygen affinity of haemoglobin (the Bohr effect) is described in section 3.7.3.2. An indirect and opposite effect of pH on the oxygen affinity is due to the change, mentioned above, in the concentration of 2,3-diphosphoglycerate in the erythrocytes (the Rapoport effect, section 3.7.3.4.).

3.2.5. Therapy

The therapeutic measures to be adopted in a patient with abnormal hydrogen ion concentration depend entirely upon the aetiology. In a case of acidaemia, symptomatic therapy is aimed at either decreasing ctH^+ (e.g. by infusion of sodium bicarbonate) or decreasing pCO_2 (by artificial ventilation). In a case of alkalaemia, symptomatic therapy is aimed at either increasing ctH^+ (e.g. by infusion of NH_4Cl, or enchancing the renal reabsorption of H^+ by infusion of NaCl and KCl), or increasing pCO_2 (e.g. by increasing pCO_2 of the inspired air, as in rebreathing).

3.2.6. Analysis

3.2.6.1. Blood collection

Arterial blood is obtained from the radial or femoral artery. In newborn infants, a catheter is usually inserted in the umbilical artery. The blood is collected in a heparinized syringe, the dead space of which is filled with a neutral solution of heparin. (Heparin preparations may be acid, and the effect of the heparin on the pH of a 7.4 phosphate buffer should be checked before use). Special syringes are available with a vent for the escape of air so that the syringe fills directly, without suction, by the arterial pressure (Jacobsen and Rosen, 1975). The blood and heparin should be gently but thoroughly mixed by rotating the syringe between the hands.

Exposure to air causes a loss of CO_2 and hence a fall in cfH^+. However, a small air bubble in the syringe is of little significance. If the volume of air amounts to 10% of the blood volume, the pH would rise only about 0.01 to 0.02 units. The site of arterial puncture should be firmly compressed for at least 3 minutes after blood sampling.

Capillary blood is obtained from the ear lobe or the finger tip, or in newborns from the edge of the heel. Capillary blood may also be obtained from the scalp of the foetus during labour (Saling, 1966). The site of puncture may be arterialized mechanically by rubbing with vaseline, chemically with tetrahydrofurfuryl nicotinate or a similar vasodilator or by heating with a lamp or wet towel. The scalp of the foetus may be arterialized by means of ethylene chloride spray.

Insufficient arterialization of the site of cutaneous puncture may cause an erroneously low pH, but the effect of admixture of venous blood is usually of minor importance for the plasma pH.

A puncture – never a cut – 3 to 5 mm deep is made with a sharp, sterile, disposable lancet, with the blade following the lines of the skin. A few drops of blood are wiped off, and the freely flowing blood is collected in heparinized glass capillary tubes, each containing a small magnetic follower.

Freely flowing cutaneous blood originates from the arterioles and therefore corresponds to arterial blood in composition.

Severe haemolysis causes an erroneously low pH but moderate haemolysis is of little significance.

3.2.6.2. Storage of blood

The blood should be stored for as short a time as possible, preferably at 2 to 4 °C, and for not more than 2 hours. Capillary tubes should be stored horizontally to avoid the sedimentation of erythrocytes in one end, which would render subsequent mixing difficult.

Glycolysis causes a fall in plasma pH of about 0.06 units per hour when blood is kept at 37 °C. At 2 to 4 °C, the fall is only about 0.003 units/h except in cases of leucocytosis where the fall may be as high as 0.01 units/h. Sodium fluoride cannot be recommended to inhibit glycolysis; the requisite concentration of fluoride significantly affects the ionic strength, and also causes an undesirable exchange of H^+ between plasma and erythrocytes.

Inadequate mixing of blood prior to pH measurement can cause a considerable error. If, when the measuring temperature is higher than the temperature of storage, a disproportionate amount of plasma is aspirated into the electrode, too high pH values will be obtained; if a disproportionate amount of erythrocytes is aspirated too low pH values will be obtained. These effects are due to the different pH-temperature coefficients for plasma and for whole blood, together with the suspension effect of erythrocytes on the liquid junction potential.

3.2.6.3. pH measurement

pH is measured by means of a H^+-selective electrode, usually of glass, the electromotive force (E) of the following cell being measured:

Inner reference electrode	Inner reference solution	Glass membrane	Solution X	Saturated KCl solution	Outer reference electrode
glass electrode				liquid junction	calomel electrode

Calibration is established by means of two buffer solutions (S_1 and S_2), each with defined or known pH (Bates, 1973), and preferably bracketing the pH of the samples to be measured. The pH of a sample, pH(X), is then calculated from:

$$\mathrm{pH(X)} = \mathrm{pH(S_1)} + \frac{\mathrm{pH(S_2)} - \mathrm{pH(S_1)}}{E(\mathrm{S_2}) - E(\mathrm{S_1})} \times (E(\mathrm{X}) - E(\mathrm{S_1})) \qquad [9]$$

The theoretical slope of the calibration function is the Nernst factor (N):

$$N = \frac{R \times T \times \ln 10}{F} = -\frac{E(\mathrm{S_2}) - E(\mathrm{S_1})}{\mathrm{pH(S_2)} - \mathrm{pH(S_1)}} \qquad [10]$$

$T = 310.15\ \mathrm{K} \Rightarrow N = 61.5\ \mathrm{mV}$.

Malfunction of the glass electrode generally results in an abnormally low slope on calibrating or an abnormally long response time. A slow response, or a memory effect, may be due to a protein coating on the glass membrane which may be removed by means of a suitable detergent or enzyme preparation.

Incorrect temperature of the cell reveals itself by an inconsistency among the pH values of the different calibration buffers because the temperature coefficients of the latter vary considerably, from $-0.0020\ K^{-1}$ for the phosphate buffers to $-0.0264\ K^{-1}$ for the Tris buffer. The temperature of the electrode should be accurate within 0.1 K, and the temperature of the liquid junction should be the same as the temperature of the glass electrode. If the temperature of the patient deviates from the temperature of measurement, the pH value referring at the patient's temperature may be calculated using a pH-temperature coefficient of $-0.015\ K^{-1}$.

Erroneous composition of the standard solutions may be revealed by checking for consistency among the pH values of several different calibration buffers.

An abnormal liquid junction potential may arise if the saturated KCl solution becomes diluted or contaminated. The presence of erythrocytes at the liquid junction causes a junction potential of about 0.6 mV so that the pH $\subset$ P measured in whole blood is about 0.01 units lower than the pH measured in the corresponding plasma. With increasing volume fraction of erythrocytes in blood, the error may increase towards +0.04 units.

3.2.6.4. Precision and accuracy

The pH of plasma can be estimated from measurements on whole blood with an analytical standard deviation of 0.005 units or better. Accuracy depends on several factors, primarily the inaccuracy of the calibration buffers which should be of the order of ±0.005 units. The accuracy of pH measurements on whole blood is further reduced by the uncertainty concerning the liquid junction potential, so that the overall inaccuracy is about −0.04 to +0.005 units.

3.3. CONCENTRATION OF TITRATABLE HYDROGEN ION IN PLASMA, BLOOD, OR EXTRACELLULAR FLUID

The concentration of titratable hydrogen ion (ctH^+) indicates the stoichiometric concentration of total added or removed H^+. A positive value indicates a net gain of H^+; a negative value indicates a net loss of H^+. The concentration of titratable H^+ in the total extracellular fluid is the most explicit measure of a metabolic (non-respiratory) acid–base disturbance. This quantity is generally determined in connection with measurements of the plasma pH and pCO_2.

3.3.1. Chemistry

The concentration of titratable H^+ in plasma or whole blood is defined operationally by titrating plasma or whole blood with strong acid or base to an endpoint in the plasma phase of pH = 7.40 at pCO_2 = 5.3 kPa and T = 37 °C. Truly representative extracellular fluid is not accessible for sampling, but a specimen of arterial blood diluted with its own plasma to a haemoglobin concentration of about 3.6 mmol/litre can be used as a model of total extracellular fluid (including erythrocytes), and ctH^+ can be estimated for this model (section 3.3.6.4.). Titratable H^+ may also be called titratable acid or with opposite sign, *titratable base* or "*base excess*" (BE) (Siggaard-Andersen and Engel, 1960).

This quantity may also be defined as the concentration of total H^+ in the original system minus the concentration of total H^+ in the titrated system, i.e. after addition or removal of H^+ (together with an indifferent anion) in an open system (i.e. CO_2 equilibrium with a gas phase) until pH = 7.40 and pCO_2 = 5.33 kPa in the titrated system (T = 37 °C). The symbol would then be ΔctH^+ and a negative value would not be a contradiction. A more detailed discussion of the concept "stoichiometric concentration" is given elsewhere (Siggaard-Andersen, 1977a).

Several other quantities have been proposed as stoichiometric indicators of accumulated H^+. Thus Van Slyke proposed to standardize the pH ⊂ P to 7.40 by CO_2 equilibration and then measure the concentration of bicarbonate. With opposite sign, the Van Slyke "corrected bicarbonate" is equal to the concentration of titratable H^+ when titrating to pH ⊂ P = 7.40 at pCO_2 = 0. Singer and Hastings (1948) proposed that the concentrations of bicarbonate and protein anion, be summed to give *the concentration of buffer base.* With opposite sign, the concentration of buffer base is equal to the concentration of titratable H^+ when titrating to a pH equal to the overall iso-ionic pH of the proteins at pCO_2 = 0.

Several others have proposed to standardize the pCO_2 to 5.3 kPa by equilibration with CO_2 and then measure the concentration of bicarbonate in the plasma. Although this "*standard bicarbonate*" reflects an accumulation or loss of H^+ (a fall in standard bicarbonate indicating an accumulation of H^+), there is no stoichiometric relationship between accumulation or loss of H^+ and standard bicarbonate.

Many others have proposed that the *actual bicarbonate concentration* in the plasma (or the concentration of total carbon dioxide) be used as a measure of a metabolic acid–base disturbance (Peters and Van Slyke, 1946; Schwartz and Relman, 1963; Rispens, 1970). However, the actual bicarbonate concentration is not a stoichiometric indicator of accumulation or loss of H^+, and furthermore, it varies with the pCO_2 at a constant concentration of titratable H^+.

3.3.2. Reference values

The reference intervals (95%) for the concentrations of titratable H^+ in the arterial blood, plasma, or total extracellular fluid from healthy resting individuals, and the approximate extreme of the pathological range are tabulated.

Quantity (titratable H^+)	Men	Women	Children (0–3 years)	Extremes of range
ctH^+ (mmol/litre)	–3.0 to +1.5	–2.0 to +3.0	–2.0 to +4.0	–30 to +30

Towards the end of pregnancy, the value rises to a mean of about +5 mmol/litre. After acclimatization to high altitude, the values are higher by about 1.6 mmol/litre per km above sea level.

The extreme range refers to acute disturbances. In chronic states the values rarely fall outside the range –20 to +15 mmol/litre.

Capillary blood is equivalent to arterial blood.

Venous blood has lower values (by about 1.5 mmol/litre) due to the binding of H^+ to deoxyhaemoglobin.

An increased value of ctH^+ in blood or extracellular fluid may be termed hydrogen ion excess or *metabolic* (non-respiratory) *acidosis*; a decreased (negative) value is termed hydrogen ion deficit or *metabolic alkalosis.* Some authors prefer to restrict the designations metabolic acidosis or alkalosis to a primary hydrogen ion excess or deficit, i.e. a H^+ accumulation or loss which is not secondary or compensatory to a primary change in pCO_2 (Nahas, 1966; Winters, 1966).

3.3.3. Causes of change in ctH^+ in blood and extracellular fluid

The most important cause of change in the concentration of titratable H^+ in blood, plasma, or total extracellular fluid is accumulation or loss of H^+ in the respective phases due to an abnormal H^+ balance in the body. However, an abnormal distribution of H^+ within the body is another mechanism; thus a change in pCO_2 alters the distribution of H^+ within the extracellular fluid so that ctH^+ of whole blood and plasma change in opposite directions. The various causes of change in ctH^+ are illustrated in the cybernetic diagram (Scheme 3.1).

3.3.3.1. Abnormal H^+ balance

Altered renal elimination of acid or base with a change of pH in the arterial plasma, due to a primary change in pCO_2 (primary respiratory acidaemia or alkalaemia), causes a change in the excretion of H^+ in the urine. The resulting change in ctH^+ in the extracellular fluid is termed secondary or compensatory; it represents the metabolic compensation of a primary respiratory disturbance.

Insufficient excretion of H^+, resulting in a rise in ctH^+ (metabolic acidosis), may be caused by a pathologic condition, for example chronic pyelonephritis, renal tubular acidosis, or implantation of the ureters in the intestine. Renal acidosis may also be due to a bicarbonate-losing pyelonephritis, or caused by carbonic anhydrase inhibitors which inhibit the reabsorption of bicarbonate in the kidney tubules. Increased bicarbonate excretion with a moderate metabolic acidosis is also seen in primary hyperparathyroidism, and is caused by a direct effect of parathyroid hormone on reabsorption of bicarbonate in the kidney tubules.

Enhanced excretion of acid – or inhibited excretion of base – leading to a fall in ctH^+ (renal metabolic alkalosis) may be caused by diuretics such as mercurials, ethacrynic acid, thiazides, furosemide. The effect may be secondary to depletion of sodium and chloride with a secondary hyperaldosteronism. Potassium depletion also enhances the H^+ excretion in the kidneys, perhaps due to an increase in the cfH^+ in the renal tubule cells.

Increased intake or administration of non-carbonic acid or base, with an increased intake of acid (e.g. NH_4Cl) or base (e.g. $NaHCO_3$) generally leads to a moderate change in cH$^+$ because the kidneys are able to excrete large amounts of acid as well as base. Increasing the daily intake of acid or of base, by 100 mmol in an adult, only causes a rise, or fall, respectively, in cH$^+$ in the blood of about 3 mmol/litre. However, prolonged use of antacids (e.g. aluminium or barium preparations) may produce a significant metabolic alkalosis (milk alkali syndrome).

Infusion of NH_4Cl or $NaHCO_3$ for therapeutic purposes causes a change in cH$^+$ which depends on the time allowed for distribution in the body. The initial volume of distribution for H^+ equals the volume of extracellular fluid, which is approximately 20% of the body volume. In the course of 3 to 4 hours, the apparent volume of distribution has doubled, i.e. the initial change in cH$^+$ in the extracellular fluid is halved. In the course of days, the apparent volume of distribution expands even further due to the participation of bone tissues in the buffering mechanism.

Extra-renal loss of base or non-carbonic acid may give rise to severe metabolic acidosis or alkalosis. Gastrointestinal loss of base may be due to alkaline diarrhoeas in cases of severe gastroenteritis, cholera, gall- or pancreatic-fistulas and vomiting in patients with achylia.

Loss of non-carbonic acid with a fall in cH$^+$ may be due to vomiting, as in pyloric stenosis, or to continual stomach drainage with loss of HCl, as in unconscious patients. A transient fall in cH$^+$ is seen after a heavy meal due to the secretion of gastric juice – the post-prandial alkali tide.

Organic acidosis, reflecting the accumulation of organic acids which are normally metabolized to CO_2 and H_2O, is an important cause of metabolic acidosis. The accumulation may be due to an increased rate of production or a decreased rate of oxidation of the respective acids, or to both effects. Accumulation of lactate can be due to anaerobic muscular exercise, shock, phenformin poisoning, or it may be of unknown aetiology (Cohen and Woods, 1976).

Accumulation of β-hydroxybutyrate and acetoacetate (ketonaemia or ketosis) can be due to diabetes mellitus, chronic alcoholism, or starvation. Formate accumulates in methanol poisoning.

An abnormal accumulation of base from intermediary metabolism (e.g. NH_3) does not lead to metabolic alkalosis.

Dilution and concentration may give rise, respectively, to acidosis or alkalosis. Dilution acidosis, i.e. dilution of the extracellular fluid with a rise in cH$^+$, is of limited clinical significance. However, it should be recalled that, according to the definition, the concentration of titratable H^+ of water or physiological saline is about +25 mmol/litre, i.e. 25 mmol of strong base must be added per litre to obtain pH = 7.40 at pCO$_2$ = 5.3 kPa.

Concentration alkalosis is caused by dehydration, i.e. by loss of water which effectively represents a loss of titratable H^+ (Kildeberg and Engel, 1971).

3.3.3.2. Abnormal H^+ distribution

Potassium depletion presumably leads to a loss of K^+ from the cells in exchange for Na^+ as well as H^+. The net result therefore tends to be a rise in the intracellular cfH$^+$ (normally pH = 6.8 for muscle cells) and a fall in extracellular cfH$^+$ and cH$^+$ (hypokalaemic alkalosis).

The *Hamburger shift* is a change in the distribution of H^+ between the erythrocytes and the plasma and interstitial fluid, due to a change in pCO_2. The immediate effects of an acute rise in pCO_2 (e.g. CO_2 inhalation) are a rise in ctH^+ in erythrocytes and in whole blood, with a fall in ctH^+ in plasma and interstitial fluid, while ctH^+ in the total extracellular fluid remains unaltered. An acute fall in pCO_2 (e.g. hyperventilation) has the opposite effects (section 3.4.4.3.).

3.3.3.3. The Haldane effect

Changes in oxygen saturation cause a slight change in ctH^+ in the blood in vitro (Haldane effect). Oxygenation of 1 mmol of haemoglobin causes the liberation of about 0.47 mmol of H^+. The liberated H^+ is not distributed equally between plasma and erythrocytes, so that the rise in $ctH^+ \subset B$ is therefore only 0.31 mmol/litre when the rise in the concentration of oxyhemoglobin is 1 mmol/litre.

3.3.3.4. Temperature

Change in temperature does not affect the concentration of titratable H^+ in blood or plasma, and it has not been possible to demonstrate any change in the distribution of H^+ between plasma and erythrocytes upon cooling.

3.3.4. Effects of change in ctH^+ in blood, plasma or total extracellular fluid

3.3.4.1. Effects on cfH^+ in plasma and other body fluids

Most effects are secondary to the change in the concentration of free H^+ (Scheme 3.1). The relationship between ctH^+ in the extracellular fluid and cfH^+ in the arterial plasma in metabolic acidosis or alkalosis is illustrated in Figure 3.1. The effect of cfH^+ on the chemoreceptors causes the respiratory compensation of a primary change in ctH^+, and the degree of compensatory change in pCO_2 is illustrated in the figure. H^+ is distributed rather slowly between the body phases, compared with the rate of distribution of CO_2. Following intravenous infusion of HCl or $NaHCO_3$ in experimental animals, the average intracellular pH therefore changes very slowly, in contrast to the rapid changes caused by CO_2.

3.3.4.2. Effect on the glomerular filtration of titratable H^+

The renal excretion of H^+ is dependent on the glomerular filtration of titratable H^+ as well as on the tubular secretion of titratable H^+. The former is directly proportional to ctH^+ in the plasma, whereas the latter is dependent on the concentration of free H^+ in the tubule cells. In chronic respiratory acidosis, the compensatory fall in ctH^+ causes a decreased filtration of titratable H^+ while the rise in cfH^+ in the plasma causes an increased secretion of titratable H^+. The maximal renal compensation is achieved when these two mechanisms balance each other.

3.3.4.3. Associated changes in the concentrations of other electrolytes

According to the law of electro-neutrality, H^+ must be transported in association with an anion (accumulation of acid) or exchanged for another cation (loss of base). Accumulation of non-carbonic acid involves an accumulation of an accompanying anion such as chloride (hyperchloraemic acidosis), sulphate, lactate or β-hydroxybutyrate. Loss of non-carbonic acid usually involves a fall in the concentration of chloride. Accumulation or loss of base involves an increase, or fall respectively, in the concentration of the cation which exchanged for H^+, which is primarily Na^+.

A change in ctH^+ is always associated with an equivalent change in the *sum* of the concentrations of the various buffer bases – mainly HCO_3^- – but also net protein anion and inorganic phosphate. For this reason, the concentration of HCO_3^- is often used as a non-stoichiometric indicator of an accumulation or loss of H^+.

3.3.5. Therapy

Therapy is primarily aimed towards the pathophysiological process which caused the change in ctH^+. The dangers of an abnormal ctH^+ are closely associated with an accompanying change in cfH^+, cNa^+, or cK^+ in plasma. Therapeutic measures are therefore generally directed towards normalizing cfH^+ rather than ctH^+, and formulae for calculating the required amount of titrant for normalizing ctH^+ cannot be recommended.

When a direct titration of the body fluids is necessary, the common therapeutic agents are NH_4Cl (for acidification) and $NaHCO_3$ (for alkalinization). The efficacy of NH_4^+ depends upon normal liver function forming urea, with liberation of H^+. In case of hepatic failure with severe metabolic alkalosis, infusion of hydrochloric acid into a large vein may therefore be necessary. Sodium lactate is sometimes employed as a base; it also must be metabolized in the liver to CO_2 and H_2O, in order to bind H^+ and function as a base. Tris-hydroxymethylaminomethane (Tris) has also been used as a base, especially in cases where the administration of Na^+ is undesirable (Nahas, 1963).

3.3.6. Analysis

3.3.6.1. Blood collection and storage

Arterial or capillary blood is collected as described previously (section 3.2.6.1.). Glycolysis during storage causes a rise in the concentration of titratable hydrogen ion in the blood of about +0.5 mmol/litre per hour at room temperature; this is reduced to +0.1 mmol/litre per hour at 0 to 4 °C, but the rise is higher when the leucocyte concentration is elevated.

3.3.6.2. Titration of ctH^+ in plasma or whole blood

Several methods have been described for titration of H^+ in plasma or serum by the addition of an excess of H^+, elimination of the liberated CO_2, and back titration with strong base to pH = 7.40 at $pCO_2 = 0$ and $T = 37$ °C (Maas, 1970). The concentration of titratable H^+, defined by titrating to pH = 7.40 at $pCO_2 = 5.3$ kPa and $T = 37$ °C, is obtained by adding 24.4 mmol/litre, i.e. the concentration of bicarbonate in plasma with pH = 7.40 and $pCO_2 = 5.3$ kPa.

A method has also been described for titrating whole blood directly to an end point of pH ⊂ P = 7.40 at $pCO_2 = 5.3$ kPa (Agostoni et al., 1972).

3.3.6.3. *Calculation of ctH^+ by means of the Van Slyke equation*

A set of equations is formed on the basis of approximating the CO_2 equilibration curves for plasma or whole blood as straight lines in a coordinate system with pH on the abscissa and $cHCO_3^-$ in plasma on the ordinate (often called the Davenport diagram). $cHCO_3^- \subset P$ is first calculated from pH ⊂ P and $pCO_2 \subset B$ (section 3.5.1, Eqn. 9). ctH^+ is then calculated from $cHCO_3^- \subset P$ and pH ⊂ P by means of the following equations (Siggaard-Andersen, 1977a) where $cHb \subset B$ is the haemoglobin concentration in the blood.

$$ctH^+ \subset B = \zeta \times (\Delta cHCO_3^- \subset P + \beta \times \Delta pH \subset P) \quad [1]$$

$$\Delta cHCO_3^- \subset P = cHCO_3^- \subset P - 24.4 \text{ mmol/litre} \quad [2]$$

$$\Delta pH \subset P = pH \subset P - 7.40 \quad [3]$$

$$\beta = 2.30 \times cHb \subset B + 7.7 \text{ mmol/litre} \quad [4]$$

$$\zeta = 1 - 0.023 \times cHb \subset B/(\text{mmol/litre}) \quad [5]$$

The concentration of HCO_3^- is 24.4 mmol/litre in normal plasma when pH = 7.40, pCO_2 = 5.3 kPa, and T = 37 °C. β is a measure of the buffer value of non-bicarbonate buffers; for normal plasma, the buffer value is 7.7 mmol/litre – mainly due to the plasma proteins. ζ is a distribution coefficient which takes into account the difference between $cHCO_3^-$ in plasma and erythrocytes. When calculating ctH^+ for plasma, $cHb \subset B = 0$ should be employed. When calculating ctH^+ for the total extracellular fluid, $cHb \subset Ecf$ = 3.6 mmol/litre can be used. The haemoglobin concentration of the total extracellular fluid can be calculated from:

$$cHb \subset Ecf = \frac{cHb \subset B \times VB}{VEcf}$$

Inserting $cHb \subset B$ = 9.1 mmol/litre, $VB/VBody$ = 0.08, and $VEcf/VBody$ = 0.20, gives $cHb \subset Ecf$ = 3.6 mmol/litre. Calculating ctH^+ on the basis of this haemoglobin concentration therefore provides an estimate of ctH^+ in the total extracellular fluid. The biological variation in $cHb \subset Ecf$ due to polycythaemia, dehydration or overhydration can be ignored for practical clinical purposes.

3.3.6.4. *Nomograms*

The alignment nomograms of Singer and Hastings (1948) and Siggaard-Andersen (1963) are based on approximating the CO_2 equilibration curves for plasma or whole blood as straight lines in a coordinate system with pH on the abscissa and log pCO_2 on the ordinate. Again ctH^+ is calculated from the measured plasma pH and pCO_2, using $cHb \subset Ecf$ = 3.6 mmol/litre for estimating $ctH^+ \subset Ecf$.

The Cartesian coordinate system shown in Figure 3.1 allows calculation of $ctH^+ \subset Ecf$ by plotting the point which represents the pH ⊂ P and pCO_2 measured in the arterial blood, and then projecting the point to the ctH^+ scale along the oblique lines of the chart. These lines represent in vivo CO_2 titration curves, or CO_2 equilibration curves of total extracellular fluid, or CO_2 equilibration curves of diluted whole blood with a haemoglobin concentration of 3.6 mmol/litre.

3.3.6.5. Precision and accuracy

The precision of the calculated ctH^+ is dependent on the precision with which pH, pCO_2 and cHb are measured; generally the analytical standard deviation is about 0.4 mmol/litre. The accuracy depends on the accuracy of the pH, pCO_2 and cHb measurements, as well as on the approximations made in the derivation of the Van Slyke equation and the nomogram. The Van Slyke equation tends to give slightly lower values (about 0 to 3 mmol/litre) than the nomogram when calculating $ctH^+ \subset$ Ecf. A rough estimate of the inaccuracy for values inside the normal reference area (Figure 3.1) is ±1 mmol/litre. For values outside the normal reference area, the inaccuracy may amount to ±3 mmol/litre.

3.4. PARTIAL PRESSURE OF CARBON DIOXIDE IN ARTERIAL BLOOD

The partial pressure of carbon dioxide (pCO_2) in arterial blood is important for evaluation of the alveolar ventilation, and its measurement is indicated on suspicion of a respiratory disturbance. The pO_2 and the plasma pH are generally measured simultaneously.

3.4.1. Chemistry

The *partial pressure* of CO_2 in a gas phase ($pCO_2 \subset G$) equals the substance fraction of CO_2 in the gas phase ($xCO_2 \subset G$) times the total pressure of the gas (pG):

$$pCO_2 \subset G = xCO_2 \subset G \times pG \text{, by definition} \quad [1]$$

The traditional unit is mm Hg while the SI unit is the pascal (Pa = N/m^2 = J/m^3). The proportionality factor is 0.133 kPa/mm Hg. An interconversion scale for mm Hg and kPa is included on the ordinate in Figure 3.1.

The partial pressure of CO_2 in the plasma (or actually in an hypothetical gas phase in the plasma) is closely related to the concentration of free dissolved CO_2 in the plasma (including the small amount of hydrated CO_2):

$$cdCO_2 \subset P = \alpha CO_2 \subset P \times pCO_2 \subset P \,. \quad [2]$$

αCO_2 is the *solubility coefficient* for carbon dioxide. For normal plasma at $T = 37$ °C the value is $\alpha CO_2 = 0.230$ mmol/J, with a biological standard deviation of 0.002 mmol/J (corresponding to 0.0306 ± 0.0003 mmol $\times$ litre^{-1} $\times$ mm Hg^{-1}). The value increases with increasing lipid concentration and falls with increasing protein concentration.

The chemical potential of CO_2 is directly proportional to $\log pCO_2$:

$$\mu CO_2 = R \times T \times \ln 10 \times \log(pCO_2/4051 \text{ kPa}) \quad [3]$$

where 4051 kPa is the pCO_2 which provides a molality of dissolved CO_2 in pure water of 1 mol/kg; in other words, the (standard) chemical potential of CO_2 is arbitrarily taken to be zero for a pure aqueous solution with a molality of dissolved CO_2 of 1 mol/kg.

3.4.2. Reference values

The reference intervals (95%) for the pCO_2 of the arterial blood from resting healthy subjets in the recumbent position, and the approximate extremes of the pathological range are tabulated.

Quantity	Men	Women and children	Umbilical artery	Extremes of range
pCO_2 (kPa)	4.7 – 6.0	4.3 – 5.7	4.1 – 8.9	1.3 – 32
pCO_2 (mm Hg)	35 – 45	32 – 43	31 – 67	10 – 240

In the last trimester of pregnancy, the mean value falls for unknown reasons to about 3.7 kPa (= 28 mm Hg). Sitting and standing, the pCO_2 is about 0.4 kPa lower than in the recumbent position. High altitude results in a fall in pCO_2 of about 0.4 kPa/km above sea level after acclimatization. Anxiety during blood sampling may cause a significant change in pCO_2 due to hyperventilation or holding of breath.

Venous blood from the right atrium shows a pCO_2 value that is 0.8 to 0.9 kPa higher than the arterial. Values for venous blood from a peripheral vein vary considerably, depending upon the temperature and the muscular activity of the extremity. Venous blood may be arterialized in vivo by warming the hand at 45 °C for 10 minutes.

The extreme range refers to acute experimental disturbances (hyperventilation and apnoeic oxygenation). In chronic disease states, the value rarely falls outside the range 2.7 to 10.6 kPa.

An increased arterial pCO_2 value is called *hypercapnia,* and decreased pCO_2 *hypocapnia*: the designations hypercarbia and hypocarbia have been used. A primary increase in pCO_2 which is not due to a rise in plasma pH is designated *respiratory acidosis,* while a primary fall in pCO_2 is designated *respiratory alkalosis.*

3.4.3. Causes of change in pCO_2 in the arterial blood

The principal mechanisms are illustrated in the cybernetic diagram (Scheme 3.1). In the steady state, the rate of CO_2 production in the tissues is balanced by the rate of CO_2 elimination in the lungs, and the latter ($\dot{n}CO_2$) is proportional to the alveolar ventilation (expired) times the pCO_2 of the alveolar air, minus the alveolar ventilation (inspired) times the pCO_2 of the humidified inspired air (I):

$$\dot{n}CO_2 = \frac{pCO_2 \subset A \times \dot{V}A(ex.) - pCO_2 \subset I \times \dot{V}A(in.)}{pA \times V_mCO_2} \qquad [4]$$

where V_mCO_2 is the molar volume of CO_2 at the temperature and pressure of the alveolar air (pA). Assuming that the respiratory quotient (RQ) is about one, then $\dot{V}A(ex.) = \dot{V}A(in.) = \dot{V}A$. Rearrangement of equation (4) then gives the pCO_2 of the alveolar air as a function of the alveolar ventilation, the rate of CO_2 production, and the pCO_2 of the humidified inspired air:

$$pCO_2 \subset A = \frac{\dot{n}CO_2}{\dot{V}A} \times pA \times V_mCO_2 + pCO_2 \subset I \qquad [5]$$

For a normal resting adult, representative values are:

$\dot{n}CO_2 = 10$ mmol/min, $\dot{V}A = 5$ litres/min, $pA = 101.3$ kPa,

$V_mCO_2 = 22.26 \times \frac{310.15}{273.15}$ litres/mol $= 25.28$ litres/mol, $pCO_2 \subset I = 0 \Rightarrow$

$pCO_2 \subset A = 5.1$ kPa .

Carbon dioxide normally diffuses very rapidly across the alveolar membrane, so that the pCO_2 of the arterial blood almost equals the pCO_2 of the alveolar air. However, disturbances of this equilibrium may influence the blood pCO_2. Finally, changes in temperature influence the pCO_2.

3.4.3.1. Increased pCO_2 in the inspired air

An increase in pCO_2 in the inspired air gives a proportional increase in the pCO_2 of the alveolar air according to equation [5]. In the whole body, however, due to the stimulation of ventilation, the increase in pCO_2 is much smaller. For example, if the pCO_2 of the inspired air is 5.3 kPa, the rise in pCO_2 in the arterial blood will be only 1.3 kPa due to the increase in ventilation by a factor of about 3.6. This value, however, is subject to great individual variation.

3.4.3.2. Change in the rate of production of CO_2

Doubling the rate of production of CO_2 tends to give a doubling of the alveolar pCO_2, according to equation [5]. In the whole body, however, due to the stimulation of ventilation, the pCO_2 only rises by about 10%.

3.4.3.3. Changes in the alveolar ventilation

The major causes of change in alveolar ventilation are illustrated in the cybernetic diagram (Scheme 3.2; Cunningham and Lloyd, 1963). The diagram represents a subdivision of the box designated "respiratory function" in Scheme 3.1.

The alveolar ventilation ($\dot{V}A$) is the result of contractions of the intercostal muscles and the diaphragm, but several variables modulate the result: increase in thoracic compliance (stiffness of the thoracic skeleton, kyphoscoliosis), severe trauma of the thorax, pneumothorax, increase in airway resistance (suffocation, foreign body in trachea, larynx oedema, aspiration of fluid in the lungs, submersion, status asthmaticus), diminution of effective lung tissue (severe pulmonary oedema, hyaline membrane disease of the newborn, chronic bronchitis, cystic fibrosis, silicosis, advanced pulmonary tuberculosis) – all tend to decrease the alveolar ventilation.

Muscular contractions are the result of efferent impulses from the respiratory centre, but the neuromuscular transmission may be blocked (as in poliomyelitis, or by certain insecticides) or the muscles may be atrophic or injured, resulting in decreased alveolar ventilation.

The efferent impulses from the respiratory centre in the medulla oblongata are due to afferent impulses from the peripheral and central chemoreceptors, but various drugs may either stimulate (salicylate, nikethamide) or depress (morphine, barbiturates) the function of the respiratory centre.

The central chemoreceptors located at the antero-lateral surface of the medulla oblongata are stimulated by an increase in the hydrogen ion concentration in the cerebrospinal fluid and in brain extracellular fluid. Local accumulation of H^+ in the brain due to lactate formation – cerebral trauma – may cause an isolated stimulation of the central chemoreceptors. The peripheral chemoreceptors located in the aortic and carotid bodies are stimulated by an increase in cfH^+ of arterial plasma and also by a decrease in pO_2 in the arterial blood. Rapid accumulation of H^+ in the extracellular fluid (e.g. muscular exercise with production of lactic acid) may cause an isolated stimulation of the peripheral chemoreceptors because H^+ only slowly equilibrates across the blood–brain barrier and the choroid plexus. A rise in pCO_2, however, rapidly causes a stimulation of peripheral as well as central chemoreceptors because of the rapid diffusion of CO_2 across biological membranes.

In some cases, the stimulus for increased ventilation is unknown, e.g. during pregnancy or in hepatic cirrhosis. A few cases have been reported where, for unknown reasons, the respiratory centre apparently maintains an abnormally high pCO_2.

The stimulation or inhibition of the respiratory centre caused by a primary change in cfH^+ of arterial plasma is the cause of the respiratory compensation of a metabolic acidosis or alkalosis.

Several of the conditions mentioned above as causes of decreased alveolar ventilation also involve an arterio-alveolar block and/or disturbance in the perfusion–ventilation relationship (lung oedema, status asthmaticus); these effects cause a hypoxia, with stimulation of the respiratory centre, which outweighs the tendency to decreased alveolar ventilation.

Total apnoea – cessation of breathing – and cardiac arrest are extreme situations where CO_2 cannot be elimінted. The pCO_2 therefore continues to rise at a rate which is proportional to the rate of CO_2 production. The rate of CO_2 production per unit of body mass may be about 0.13 mmol kg^{-1} min^{-1}, and the rate of rise in the concentration of total CO_2 in the plasma may be about 0.11 mmol $litre^{-1}$ min^{-1}; in a closed system this causes a rise in pCO_2 of about 0.5 to 0.8 kPa/min.

An anaesthetized and curarized person can be kept in total apnoea for about 40 minutes without any serious fall in arterial pO_2 provided that the subject has been breathing pure O_2 for 40 minutes in advance (de-nitrogenation), and provided that O_2 is supplied through a catheter leading to the tracheal bifurcation; the pCO_2 thereby rises to as much as 30 kPa. This procedure is called apnoeic oxygenation (Frumin et al., 1959; Ichiyanagi et al. 1969).

3.4.3.4. Arterioalveolar block

Equality of the pCO_2 in arterial blood and in alveolar air is dependent on the activity of carbonic anhydrase (EC 4.2.1.1) in the erythrocytes, which accelerates the dehydration of

H_2CO_3 to CO_2 and H_2O. Complete inhibition of carbonic anhydrase by means of acetazolamide results in an arterioalveolar pCO_2 gradient of about 2.0 to 2.7 kPa (Maren, 1967). The pCO_2 of the arterial blood therefore rises slightly, whereas the pCO_2 of the alveolar air falls significantly due to stimulation of respiration.

Carbon dioxide diffuses very easily across biological membranes and therefore conditions (e.g. pulmonary oedema) which impede the diffusion of CO_2 from the lung capillary to the alveole have to be very severe before an arterio-alveolar pCO_2 difference arises. Oxygen, however, diffuses less easily and therefore an arterio-alveolar O_2 block can develop quite quickly.

Shunting of blood from the venous to the arterial side (as in congenital cyanotic heart disease) only causes a minor arterio-alveolar pCO_2 difference, because of the relatively small arteriovenous pCO_2 difference.

3.4.3.5. Binding or liberation of CO_2 in a closed system

Carbon dioxide is liberated from bicarbonate by addition of strong acid, and in a closed system this would cause a rise in pCO_2. Addition of a CO_2-free base (e.g. NaOH or Tris) would similarly cause a fall in pCO_2. However, the body is an open system in equilibrium with a gas phase (the alveolar air), so that liberated CO_2 will disappear, and the pCO_2 therefore returns to the original value even if ventilation remains constant.

3.4.3.6. Variation of pCO_2 with temperature

In a pure solution of CO_2-HCO_3^-, the change in pCO_2 with temperature can be expressed as $\partial \log pCO_2/\partial T = 0.0096\ K^{-1}$. In normal plasma and whole blood, the coefficients are $+0.019\ K^{-1}$ and $+0.021\ K^{-1}$, respectively. The latter coefficients vary with the plasma protein concentration, the haemoglobin concentration, and the pCO_2 (Siggaard-Andersen, 1974).

Among different homeothermic species, a correlation has been demonstrated between body temperature and pCO_2 of the arterial blood: $\Delta \log pCO_2/\Delta T = 0.03\ K^{-1}$. This means that ventilation increases relatively more than CO_2 production as temperature rises (Chapot et al., 1972). In hibernating animals, the correlation between pCO_2 and temperature is: $\Delta \log pCO_2/\Delta T = +0.008\ K^{-1}$. This means that CO_2 production falls relatively more than the alveolar ventilation when temperature falls (Malan et al., 1973). In poikilothermic animals, the relationship is: $\partial \log pCO_2/\partial T = +0.021\ K^{-1}$, i.e. similar to the coefficient for blood in vitro (Howell et al., 1970).

For therapeutic hypothermia of the human body, attempts are usually made to maintain an arterial plasma pH of 7.40 as measured at body temperature. This can be achieved by breathing CO_2 so that the pCO_2 remains about 5.3 kPa at all temperatures (see also section 3.2.3.2).

3.4.4. Effects of change in pCO_2 in the arterial blood

3.4.4.1. Effect on cfH^+ in plasma and other body fluids

Most effects of a change in pCO_2 are secondary to the effect on the concentration of free H^+ (Scheme 3.1). The relationships between pCO_2 and cfH^+ in the arterial plasma in acute and chronic respiratory acidosis and alkalosis are illustrated in Figure 3.1. The pH effect on the kidneys causes the renal compensation of a primary respiratory acid–base disturbance. The pH effect on the chemoreceptors causes a respiratory compensation in those cases where the primary respiratory disturbance is not a disturbance of the respiratory centre. The pH effects on the cardiovascular system, particularly the cerebral vessels, are especially pronounced in acute respiratory acid–base disturbances because of the rapid diffusion of CO_2 through biological membranes.

3.4.4.2. Binding of CO_2 – effect on the oxygen affinity of haemoglobin

A few effects of a change in pCO_2 are observed even if cfH^+ is maintained constant. These are due to the binding of CO_2 in the form of HCO_3^- and carbamate ($Pr\text{-}NHCOO^-$). The preferential binding of CO_2 to deoxyhaemoglobin causes a fall in the oxygen affinity of haemoglobin at high pCO_2, as described in section 3.7.3.3.

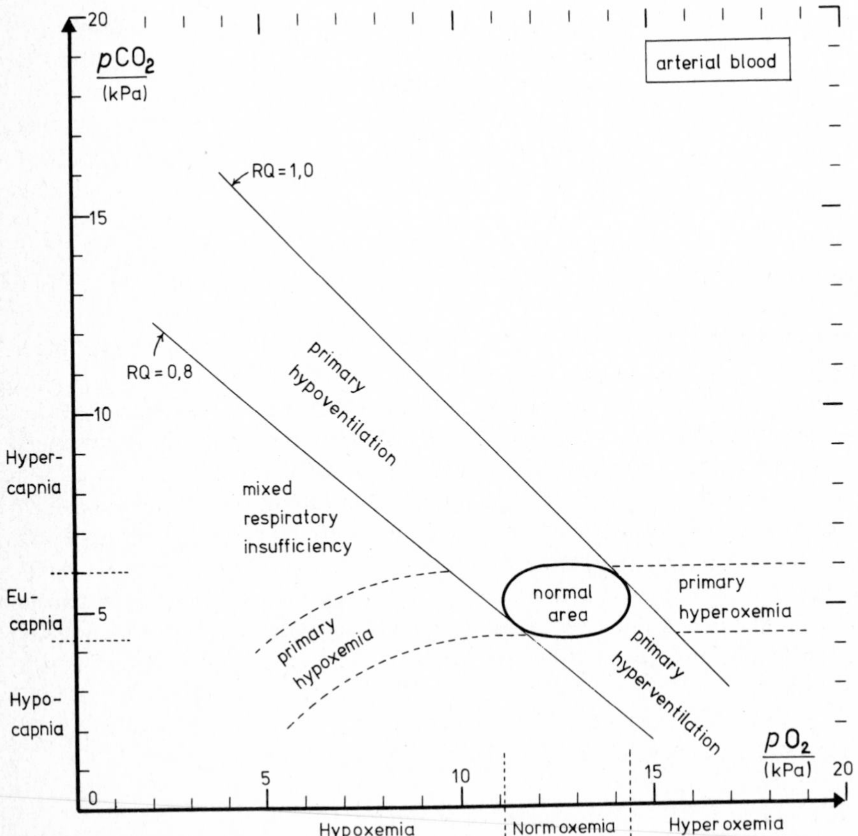

Figure 3.2. Cartesian diagram of the relationship between pO_2 and pCO_2 in arterial blood. A description of this diagram is given in section 3.6.3.1.

3.4.4.3. The Hamburger shift

The ionic equilibrium between the body fluids is disturbed by changes in the pCO_2. A rise in pCO_2 causes the chemical reaction: $CO_2 + H_2O \rightarrow H_2CO_3 \rightarrow H^+ + HCO_3^-$, the extent of which is more pronounced in well buffered body fluids (e.g. erythrocyte fluid) than in weakly buffered fluids (e.g. interstitial fluid), because of a buffering of the H^+ liberated in the reaction. cfH^+ therefore tends to rise less and $cHCO_3^-$ tends to rise more in the erythrocytes than in plasma and interstitial fluid. In effect therefore, H^+ rapidly diffuses into the erythrocytes together with Cl^- (and HCO_3^- diffuses out), whereas transfer of H^+ from interstitial fluid into the general intracellular fluid apparently is so slow as to be negligible. Hamburger (1902) studied this phenomenon in whole blood in vitro, and Shaw and Messer (1932) described the same phenomenon during inhalation of CO_2 in vivo.

The immediate effects of an acute rise in pCO_2 therefore are an unaltered ctH^+ in the total extracellular fluid (including erythrocytes), but a rise in ctH^+ in the erythrocytes and in whole blood with a fall in ctH^+ in plasma and interstitial fluid. An acute fall in pCO_2 gives rise to the opposite effects.

3.4.4.4. The alveolar air equation

In breathing atmospheric air, there is a reciprocal relationship between the pCO_2 and the pO_2 of the alveolar air when the alveolar ventilation is varied. The mathematical expression of this relationship is called the alveolar air equation (section 3.6.3.1 and Figure 3.2). Hypoventilation is therefore associated with hypercapnia as well as with hypoxia, and the latter is generally the more dangerous.

3.4.5. Therapy

Therapeutic measures are directed towards normalizing the pO_2 and pH rather than the pCO_2.

In the acute hyperventilation syndrome, rebreathing in a plastic bag causes a return of pCO_2 and pH towards normal, followed by a dilatation of the previously contracted cerebral vessels which probably brings about the normalization of ventilation.

Addition of CO_2 to the anaesthetic gas mixture has been used in connection with therapeutic hypothermia (sections 3.2.3.2 and 3.4.3.6) in order to maintain a pCO_2 of about 5.3 kPa and pH around 7.40 at all temperatures.

A decrease in pCO_2 is achieved by mechanical hyperventilation. The pCO_2 should be decreased slowly and not too much, so as to avoid cerebral vasoconstriction and convulsions. Decreasing the CO_2 production therapeutically by means of thiouracil has been attempted for the reduction of pCO_2 in chronic hypercapnia, but without significant success. Respiratory stimulants (e.g. nikethamide) are of little value in the treatment of chronic respiratory insufficiency.

3.4.6. Analysis

3.4.6.1. Blood collection

The blood should be collected anaerobically as previously described (section 3.2.6.1).

Arterialized capillary blood can often be used as an adequate substitute for arterial blood. Insufficient arterialization of the site of capillary puncture may cause an increase in the pCO_2, but a small admixture of venous blood is usually of minor importance because of the relatively small arterio-venous pCO_2 difference.

Exposure to air causes a loss of CO_2 and hence a fall in pCO_2. However, a small air bubble in the syringe is of little significance: a volume of air amounting to 10% of the blood volume would cause a fall in pCO_2 of only 0.2 to 0.3 kPa.

Glycolysis with lactic acid formation during storage causes a rise in pCO_2 of about 0.7 kPa/h at 37 °C. At 2 to 4 °C this rate is reduced to about 0.1 to 0.2 kPa/h. Therefore, specimens which cannot be analyzed immediately should be stored in ice water, but for no longer than 2 hours.

Insufficient mixing of the blood prior to pCO_2 measurement can cause a significant error because the pCO_2–temperature coefficient is lower for plasma than for whole blood (cf. section 3.2.6.2).

3.4.6.2. The pCO_2 electrode

The pCO_2 electrode consists of a pH electrode which measures the pH in a thin layer of a stationary sodium bicarbonate solution (5 mmol/litre) separated from the test solution or test gas by a CO_2-permeable membrane (polytetrafluorethylene or silastic). The pH of the bicarbonate solution is a simple function of the pCO_2, as obtained by rearranging the Henderson–Hasselbalch equation:

$$\mathrm{pH} = -\log pCO_2 - \log \alpha + \mathrm{p}K' + \log c\mathrm{HCO_3^-} \qquad [6]$$

where α is the solubility coefficient of CO_2 in the bicarbonate solution and K' is the apparent overall first dissociation constant of carbonic acid (Stow et al., 1957; Severinghaus and Bradley, 1958).

The calibration function is established by measuring the electromotive force (E) of the cell with two different standard gas mixtures with known pCO_2, or with two aqueous solutions in equilibrium with the standard gases. If possible, the pCO_2 of the samples to be tested should be bracketed by the standards. The measurement function is:

$$\log pCO_2 \subset \mathrm{X} = \log pCO_2 \subset \mathrm{S}_1 + \frac{\log pCO_2 \subset \mathrm{S}_2 - \log pCO_2 \subset \mathrm{S}_1}{E\mathrm{S}_2 - E\mathrm{S}_1} \times (E\mathrm{X} - E\mathrm{S}_1) \qquad [7]$$

and the theoretical slope of the calibration function is:

$$\frac{\mathrm{d}\,E}{\mathrm{d}(\log pCO_2)} = N\ (= 61.5\ \mathrm{mV\ for}\ T = 310.15\ \mathrm{K}), \qquad [8]$$

where N is the Nernst factor. In terms of the pH of the bicarbonate solution the theoretical slope is:

$$\frac{\mathrm{d\,pH}}{\mathrm{d}(\log pCO_2)} = -1.0\,. \qquad [9]$$

The substance fraction of CO_2 in the calibration gases should be carefully measured by a standard gasometric method (e.g. Haldane apparatus or Scholander apparatus). If tonometered aqueous solutions are used for calibration, the accuracy of tonometry should be carefully checked.

pCO_2 values measured at 37 °C may be corrected to the actual temperature of the patient by means of the temperature coefficient for whole blood in vitro: $d(\log pCO_2)/dT = +0.021\ K^{-1}$.

pCO_2 can be measured with an analytical coefficient of variation, within a series, of about 2%. The inaccuracy may be kept as low as the inaccuracy of the pCO_2 of the standard gas mixtures.

3.4.6.3. The CO_2 equilibration method

pCO_2 may be calculated from the measured pH by interpolation on the CO_2 equilibration curve. The calibration function is established for each individual sample by tonometry with two standard gas mixtures with different (but known) pCO_2 values. The measurement function is:

$$\log pCO_2 \subset B = \log pCO_2 \subset B_1 + \frac{\log pCO_2 \subset B_2 - \log pCO_2 \subset B_1}{pH \subset P_2 - pH \subset P_1} \times (pH \subset P - pH \subset P_1) \quad [10]$$

where B_1 and B_2 represent the blood sample after equilibration with the two different gas mixtures and P_1 and P_2 represent the corresponding plasmas. The theoretical slope of the measurement function $(\partial(\log pCO_2 \subset B)/\partial pH \subset P)$ is about −1.57 for normal whole blood, varying slightly with the pH value, decreasing (i.e. becoming more negative) with increasing pH. For this reason, the unknown pCO_2 should be bracketed by the pCO_2 values of the standard gas mixtures and the bracketing interval should not be too great.

Oxygenation of haemoglobin causes a liberation of H^+. The Haldane coefficient, which expresses the liberation of H^+ in mols of H^+ formed per mol of oxyhaemoglobin is normally about 0.3 as described in section 3.7.3.2. Correction for this H^+ formation is most simply performed by means of a nomogram (Siggaard-Andersen, 1974).

The analytical coefficient of variation within one series of measurements is about 2%. Certain inaccuracies are introduced by assuming a linear pH–log pCO_2 relationship (irrespective of the slight pH variation of the slope) and by making a fixed correction for oxygenation of haemoglobin during tonometry. Due to these factors, the relative inaccuracy is about ±3%.

3.4.6.4. Calculation of pCO_2 by means of the Henderson–Hasselbalch equation

The pCO_2 can be calculated from the following equation which is obtained by rearranging the Henderson–Hasselbalch equation:

$$pCO_2 = \frac{ctCO_2}{\alpha \times (\text{antilog}(pH - pK') + 1)} \quad [11]$$

The pH of arterial plasma is measured as previously described. The concentration of total CO_2 in the arterial plasma, $ctCO_2$, is measured as described in section 3.5.5.2. α is the solubility coefficient of CO_2 in plasma (section 3.4.1). pK' is the first apparent overall dissociation exponent for carbonic acid in plasma; for normal plasma, this value is 6.10 with a 95% interval of about 6.08 to 6.11. The range is mainly due to variations in ionic strength of the plasma, and the value also changes slightly with pH (decreasing to about 6.08 at pH = 7.6, and increasing to about 6.11 at pH = 7.0).

The analytical coefficient of variation is generally about 3%, depending upon the precision of the pH and $ctCO_2$ measurements. An inaccuracy is introduced by using standard values for α and pK' irrespective of the composition of the plasma. Inaccuracy may also be due to inaccuracy of the pH measurement or the total CO_2 measurement. Routine measurements of total CO_2, e.g. by means of the AutoAnalyzer, are generally too inaccurate for calculation of pCO_2 due to insufficient precautions being taken against loss of CO_2 from the specimen.

3.4.6.5. Other methods for measuring pCO_2

The pCO_2 can also be measured by gasometric analysis of a small air bubble in equilibrium with the blood or by mass spectrometric analysis (Brantigan et al., 1970). However, the former method is too complicated for routine use and the latter is too specialized for most laboratories.

3.5. CONCENTRATIONS OF TOTAL CARBON DIOXIDE AND BICARBONATE IN PLASMA

The concentrations of total CO_2 ($ctCO_2$) and bicarbonate ($cHCO_3^-$), formerly termed the alkali reserve, are both used as indicators of a metabolic acid–base disturbance, i.e. as indicators of an accumulation or loss of H^+. The quantities are used as substitutes for the concentration of titratable H^+ in the blood or extracellular fluid because they are easier to measure directly, often with automated multichannel equipment. The bicarbonate concentration is often determined simultaneously with the other major electrolytes: Na^+, K^+, and Cl^-, and is employed together with them for the calculation of the concentration of undetermined anions (the "anion gap").

In routine clinical work the concentration of total CO_2 (or bicarbonate) in venous plasma is generally the initial acid–base quantity which is measured. Only when an abnormal value indicates the presence of an acid–base disturbance or where a respiratory disturbance is suspected is the analysis supplemented by measurement of pH, pCO_2, and pO_2 of the arterial blood.

3.5.1. Chemistry

The total CO_2 or bicarbonate concentration may refer to the plasma phase of an anaerobically drawn blood specimen, i.e. the so-called *actual total CO_2 or bicarbonate concentration.* Alternatively, the bicarbonate concentration may refer to the plasma of a blood sample equilibrated at 37 °C with a standard gas mixture having pCO_2 = 5.33 kPa and pO_2 > 13 kPa, i.e. the so-called *standard bicarbonate concentration.* Finally, the total CO_2 concentration may refer to plasma or serum separated from erythrocytes under anaerobic conditions and then equilibrated with a standard gas mixture having pCO_2 = 5.33 kPa, i.e. the so-called *CO_2 combining power* of the plasma.

In early literature, the "total CO_2" was often expressed in "volumes per cent", i.e. ml of total CO_2 per 100 ml of plasma. This is calculated as $ctCO_2 \times V_mCO_2$, where V_mCO_2 (= 22.26 litre/mol) is the molar volume of CO_2 at p = 101.3 kPa and T = 0 °C.

Total CO_2 designates all CO_2, both free and bound, that can be liberated with H^+ by causing a displacement to the left of the following chemical reactions (equilibrium constants refer to 37 °C):

$$CO_2 + H_2O \xrightleftharpoons{K_a=10^{-2.64}} H_2CO_3 \xrightleftharpoons{K_a=10^{-3.69}} H^+ + HCO_3^-$$

$$HCO_3^- \xrightleftharpoons{K_a=10^{-10.20}} H^+ + CO_3^{2-} \qquad [1]$$

$$CO_2 + \text{Pr-NH}_2 \xrightleftharpoons{K_a=10^{0.7}} \text{Pr-NHCOOH} \xrightleftharpoons{K_a=10^{-5.2}} H^+ + \text{Pr-NHCOO}^- \qquad [2]$$

where Pr-NH_2 symbolizes the N-terminal amino groups of proteins, which react with CO_2 at physiological pH to form carbamate (Pr-$NHCOO^-$). The concentration of total CO_2 therefore represents the following sum:

$$ctCO_2 = cfCO_2 + cH_2CO_3 + cHCO_3^- + cCO_3^{2-} + c\text{Pr-NHCOO}^- \qquad [3]$$

where

$$cfCO_2 + cH_2CO_3 = \alpha CO_2 \times pCO_2 = cdCO_2 \qquad [4]$$

The bicarbonate concentration is usually determined as

$$cHCO_3^- = ctCO_2 - cdCO_2\,, \qquad [5]$$

and it then includes the small concentrations of carbamate and carbonate.

Often the two first CO_2 equilibrium constants are combined:

$$K_1 = \frac{aH^+ \times aHCO_3^-}{aCO_2 \times aH_2O} = 10^{-6.33} (T = 37\ °C) \qquad [6]$$

The activity of water, aH_2O, is approximately 1.00 for dilute aqueous solutions (about 0.994 for plasma), and the activity of CO_2 in aqueous solutions at 37 °C is related to the pCO_2 as follows: $aCO_2 = pCO_2/4051$ kPa. The activity of bicarbonate can therefore be derived from aH^+ and pCO_2 as follows:

$$aHCO_3^- = 115.5 \times 10^{-12} \times \frac{pCO_2/\text{kPa}}{aH^+} \qquad [7]$$

The concentration of bicarbonate in the plasma is related to the activity as follows:

$$\frac{cHCO_3^- \subset P}{(\text{mol/litre})} \doteq aHCO_3^- \subset P \times \frac{\rho H_2O \subset P/(\text{kg/litre})}{\gamma HCO_3^- \subset P} \qquad [8]$$

where the mass concentration of water in plasma is $\rho H_2O \subset P \approx 0.94$ kg/litre, and the activity coefficient for bicarbonate in plasma is $\gamma HCO_3^- \subset P \approx 0.6$, which varies with the ionic strength ($\log \gamma = -0.5 \times \sqrt{I/(\text{mol/kg})}$). The equation for calculating the concentration of bicarbonate therefore is:

$$\frac{cHCO_3^- \subset P}{(\text{mol/litre})} = 180.9 \times \frac{pCO_2 \subset P/\text{kPa}}{aH^+ \subset P \times 10^9} = 180.9 \times \frac{pCO_2 \subset P/\text{kPa}}{\text{antilog}(9 - \text{pH})} \qquad [9]$$

where the factor 180.9 varies with the ionic strength of the plasma.

The ionic strength (I) is defined as:

$$I = 0.5 \times \sum_i ((zI_i)^2 \times \acute{m}I_i)\,, \qquad [10]$$

where zI_i is the charge number of the ion I_i, and $\acute{m}I_i$ is the molality of the ion. This equation only ápplies to small ions, however, and the contribution of macromolecular zwitter ions is unknown. For normal plasma, the ionic strength is estimated to be about 0.17 mol/kg (Siggaard-Andersen, 1974).

The relationship between aH^+ (or pH), pCO_2, and the concentration of bicarbonate is traditionally expressed in logarithmic form in the Henderson–Hasselbalch equation (sections 3.4.1 and 3.4.6.4):

$$\text{pH} = \text{p}K' + \log \frac{cHCO_3^-}{\alpha \times pCO_2} \qquad [11]$$

where $\text{p}K' = 6.10$ for plasma (varying with ionic strength) and $\alpha = 0.23$ mmol/J (varying with the mass concentration of water).

The concentration of bicarbonate derived from Eqn. [9] or Eqn. [11] is actually the relative activity of bicarbonate ion (compare concentration of free hydrogen ion or concentration of free calcium ion).

3.5.2. Reference values

The concentration of total CO_2 ($ctCO_2 = 26.4$ mmol/litre) equals the sum of the concentrations of the following components, for which the mean values in normal arterial plasma are:

Bicarbonate	(HCO_3^-)	25.0 mmol/litre
Carbon dioxide	(CO_2)	1.2 mmol/litre
Carbamate	(Pr-$NHCOO^-$)	0.2 mmol/litre
Carbonic acid	(H_2CO_3)	0.004 mmol/litre
Carbonate	(CO_3^{2-})	0.001 mmol/litre

The 95% reference intervals for arterial plasma from resting adult individuals, and the extreme pathological ranges, are tabulated

Quantity	Men	Women	Extremes of range
$ctCO_2$ (mmol/litre)	24.6–28.6	22.7–28.5	1–60
$cHCO_3^-$ (mmol/litre)	23.6–27.2	21.8–27.2	1–55
Standard $cHCO_3^-$ (mmol/litre)	22.5–26.9	21.8–26.2	5–55

The values for venous plasma from a resting extremity are higher by about +2.2 mmol/litre for $ctCO_2$ and about +2.0 mmol/litre for $cHCO_3^-$. For standard bicarbonate, the same values are obtained for venous and arterial blood because both refer to the plasma phase of completely oxygenated blood.

The low extremes are encountered in patients with severe metabolic acidosis (e.g. diabetic acidosis) and the high extremes in patients with severe metabolic alkalosis (e.g. prolonged gastric aspiration with potassium depletion and dehydration).

3.5.3. Causes of change in $ctCO_2$ and $cHCO_3^-$ in the plasma

The concentrations of total CO_2 and bicarbonate in plasma are both functions of the two independent variables: the pCO_2 and the concentration of titratable H^+. The various causes of change are therefore described in connection with these quantities.

3.5.3.1. Primary changes in ctH^+

Metabolic disturbances cause the greatest change in $ctCO_2$ or $cHCO_3^-$. With opposite sign, the change in $ctCO_2$ or $cHCO_3^-$ from the normal mean is a reasonably good estimate of ctH^+ in plasma, although they are slightly less numerically, depending upon the concomitant change in pCO_2.

3.5.3.2. Primary changes in pCO_2

Acute changes in pCO_2, as in acute respiratory acid–base disturbances, cause minor changes in $ctCO_2$ or $cHCO_3^-$. An acute rise in pCO_2 from 5.3 to 10.6 kPa causes a rise of only 4.5 mmol/litre for $ctCO_2$ and about 3.0 mmol/litre for $cHCO_3^-$. The standard bicarbonate concentration, however, changes in the opposite direction and *falls* about 3 mmol/litre. This is due to the rise in ctH^+ in the blood caused by the Hamburger shift, as described in section 3.4.4.3.

Chronic respiratory acid–base disturbances are associated with a compensatory change of ctH^+ in plasma, which is the main cause of change in $ctCO_2$ and $cHCO_3^-$ in chronic respiratory acidosis or alkalosis.

The variation in $cHCO_3^-$ with different acid–base disturbances is illustrated in Fig. 3.1, where the (actual) bicarbonate concentration for any point can be read by projecting at an angle of –45° to the bicarbonate scale.

3.5.4. Effects of change in $ctCO_2$ and $cHCO_3^-$

Nearly all effects of a change in $ctCO_2$ or $cHCO_3^-$ are secondary to the effects of the underlying change in ctH^+ or pCO_2 and are described in connection with these quantities. Few effects can be specifically ascribed to the bicarbonate ion; one example, however, is the binding of Ca^{2+}, which is quantitatively of minor importance ($CaHCO_3^+ \rightleftharpoons Ca^{2+} + HCO_3^-$, $K_c \approx 0.10$ mmol/litre, Schaer, 1974), another being the effect on carbohydrate and lipid metabolism (Nahas and Schaefer, 1974).

3.5.5. Analysis

3.5.5.1. Blood collection

Loss of CO_2 from the blood specimen is a source of error in the determination of $ctCO_2$ as well as $cHCO_3^-$. The blood is therefore best collected in a heparinized syringe (section 3.2.6.1) and the collection tube should be as nearly full as possible and half closed during centrifugation. The use of paraffin oil to prevent loss of CO_2 is not to be recommended due to the solubility of CO_2 in the oil. Plasma or serum ought to be separated from the cells at 37 °C, but the effect of temperature on the distribution of CO_2 between erythrocytes and plasma is insignificant.

The major advantage of determining the standard bicarbonate concentration is that blood can be collected without careful precautions to prevent loss of CO_2, because of subsequent equilibration with a standard gas mixture before measurement (Jørgensen and Astrup, 1957).

Glycolysis during storage does not appreciably affect the concentration of total CO_2 or bicarbonate, but causes a fall in standard bicarbonate proportional to the rise in the concentration of titratable H^+ in the blood.

3.5.5.2. Gasometric measurement of total CO_2

The wide variety of analytical methods which is available for measuring total CO_2 has been reviewed by Gill and Brown (1977). In the classical methods, CO_2 is liberated from the sample by vacuum after addition of an excess of acid, and the gas phase is then analyzed manometrically or volumetrically by absorption of the CO_2 into strong alkali (Van Slyke and Neil, 1924; Natelson, 1951). These methods have been considered as the reference methods (Reiner, 1953). The analytical coefficient of variation may be less than 2%; the accuracy mainly depends on correct calibration of the volumetric or manometric device. However, some inaccuracy may be caused by reabsorption of CO_2 into the sample after vacuum extraction.

In the AutoAnalyzer methods, the CO_2 diffuses through a silastic membrane into an alkaline buffer, the pH of which is measured colorimetrically (Skeggs, 1960). The CO_2 may also be absorbed in a buffer and determined by titration, as in the Cediometer of Rispens et al., 1969. Alternatively, the gas phase may be analyzed by gas chromatography (Ortega, 1969), infrared spectrometry (Rabinow et al., 1977), or mass spectrometry (Lotz et al., 1970).

3.5.5.3. Other methods

Measurement of the concentration of total CO_2 by means of the pCO_2 electrode is based upon the liberation of CO_2 by addition of acid and measurement of the resulting pCO_2 in the solution. This method does not require transfer of CO_2 into a gas phase, but it necessitates establishment of a calibration function by means of several standard solutions (Severinghaus, 1960; Cameron, 1971).

Enzymatic measurement of the total CO_2 concentration utilizes phosphoenolpyruvate carboxylase (EC 4.1.1.38) for the binding of CO_2, with formation of oxaloacetate which is measured colorimetrically or enzymatically with an NADH-linked reaction (Forrester et al., 1976).

Titrimetric determination of the concentration of bicarbonate is based on addition of excess acid, elimination of the liberated CO_2 into a gas phase, and back titration of the sample to the original pH (corrected for the effect of dilution). The result ought to be corrected for carbamate and carbonate, which are included by the titration, but generally this correction amounts to less than 0.2 mmol/litre (Maas, 1970).

3.5.5.4. Calculation from pH and pCO_2

The bicarbonate concentration may be calculated from pH and pCO_2 by means of equation 9 (section 3.5.1). Some inaccuracy is introduced by using a constant factor irrespective of the ionic strength of the sample, but this is generally of minor importance compared with the inaccuracies of the measured pH and pCO_2 values. The calculation is performed electronically in several commercial instruments which are equipped with combined pH, pCO_2 and pO_2 electrodes.

3.6. PARTIAL PRESSURE OF OXYGEN IN ARTERIAL AND MIXED VENOUS BLOOD

A detailed description of oxygen in blood (the oxygen status of the blood) comprises the following:

(a) pO_2 as a measure of the activity of oxygen or the concentration of free O_2 in the blood;

(b) concentration of total oxygen, which is often stated implicitly in the form of the oxygen saturation and the haemoglobin concentration (which on multiplication gives the concentration of bound O_2);

(c) relationship between pO_2 and concentration of total O_2 (or oxygen saturation), i.e. the oxygen dissociation curve, the position of which is indicated by means of the pO_2 at half saturation.

In special cases, measurement of the oxygen status of arterial as well as mixed venous blood is necessary for accurate evaluation of the arteriovenous differences and hence the oxygen supply to the tissues.

For routine evaluation of the degree of arterial hypoxia or hyperoxia, determination of the arterial pO_2 alone will be sufficient, for example for the evaluation of the degree of respiratory insufficiency or during oxygen therapy where it is essential to avoid the toxic effects of hyperoxia. However, for evaluation of the degree of hypoxia in cardiac diseases with right to left shunting, measurement of the oxygen saturation is sometimes preferred because it indicates the size of the shunt more directly than the pO_2 value.

3.6.1. Chemistry

The *partial pressure* of oxygen in the arterial blood refers to a hypothetical gas phase in equilibrium with blood (cf. section 3.4.1).

The *concentration of free dissolved* O_2 in a solution is closely related to the pO_2:

$$cfO_2 = \alpha O_2 \times pO_2 \qquad [1]$$

where αO_2 is *the solubility coefficient* for O_2. For pure water at $T = 37\ ^\circ C$ the value is 10.504 μmol/J. The value decreases with increasing ionic strength and increasing protein concentration, but increases with increasing lipid concentration. For normal plasma and whole blood, the mean values are 9.453 μmol/J and 10.203 μmol/J, respectively.

The chemical potential of O_2 in arterial blood is directly proportional to log pO_2:

$$\mu O_2 = R \times T \times \ln 10 \times \log(pO_2/95.21\ \text{MPa}) \qquad [2]$$

where 95.21 MPa is the pO_2 corresponding to a molality of dissolved O_2 in pure water of 1 mol/kg; in other words, μO_2 is arbitrarily taken to be zero for a pure aqueous solution with a molality of dissolved O_2 of 1 mol/kg.

3.6.2. Reference values

The reference intervals (95%) for the pO_2 of the arterial blood from resting healthy subjects in the recumbent position, and the approximate extreme pathological ranges are:

Quantity	Age <40 years	Age >40 years	Extremes of range
pO_2 (kPa)	11.1–14.4	9.6–13.7	4.0–400
pO_2 (mm Hg)	83–108	72–104	30–3000

The relationship between the normal mean $pO_2 \subset aB$ and age (a, years) of the patient (tPt) can be approximated as follows:

$$pO_2 \subset aB/\text{kPa} = 13.7–0.0360 \times tPt/a \qquad [3]$$

This expression refers to subjects at sea level. No significant sex difference has been demonstrated for pO_2, unlike that for pCO_2. *Venous blood* from the right atrium shows a pO_2 of about 4.8 to 5.9 kPa. For peripheral venous blood, the pO_2 varies greatly with skin temperature, duration of venous stasis, and muscular pumping.

The lowest values compatible with life are about 4.0 kPa for arterial blood and about 2.7 kPa for mixed venous blood. The highest values which have been produced by hyperbaric oxygenation are about 400 kPa.

Decreased and increased arterial pO_2 are called *hypoxaemia* and *hyperoxaemia*, respectively. Decreased and increased mixed venous pO_2 indicate general tissue hypoxia and tissue hyperoxia, respectively.

3.6.3. Causes of change in pO_2 in arterial blood

The principal mechanisms are illustrated in the cybernetic diagram (Scheme 3.3).

In the steady state, the rate of O_2 consumption in the tissues equals the rate of O_2 uptake in the lungs, and the latter ($\dot{n}O_2$) is proportional to the alveolar ventilation (inspired) times the pO_2 of the humidified inspired air (I) minus the alveolar ventilation (expired) times the pO_2 of the alveolar air:

$$\dot{n}O_2 = \frac{pO_2 \subset I \times \dot{V}A(in) - pO_2 \subset A \times \dot{V}A(ex)}{pA \times V_mO_2}, \qquad [4]$$

where V_mO_2 is the molar volume of O_2 at the temperature and pressure of the alveolar air (pA). Assuming that the respiratory quotient (RQ) is about one, then $\dot{V}A(ex) = \dot{V}A(in) = \dot{V}A$. Rearrangment of equation [4] gives the pO_2 of the alveolar air as a function of the alveolar ventilation, the rate of O_2 consumption, and the pO_2 of the humidified inspired air:

$$pO_2 \subset A = pO_2 \subset I - \frac{\dot{n}O_2}{\dot{V}A} \times V_mO_2 \times pA\,. \qquad [5]$$

Representative values for a normal resting adult are:

$\dot{n}O_2 = 12.5$ mmol/min; $\dot{V}A = 5$ litre/min; $pA = 101.3$ kPa;

$V_mO_2 = 22.38 \times 310.15/273.15$ litre/mol $= 25.43$ litre/mol; $pO_2 \subset I =$

$20.0 \text{ kPa} \Rightarrow pO_2 \subset A = 13.6$ kPa .

Oxygen normally diffuses rapidly across the alveolar membrane so that the pO_2 of the arterial blood almost equals the pO_2 of the alveolar air. However, disturbances of this equilibrium may influence the blood pO_2.

Finally, the temperature influences the pO_2.

3.6.3.1. Changes in the alveolar ventilation

The major causes of change in the alveolar ventilation are illustrated in the cybernetic diagram (Scheme 3.2) and are described in connection with causes of change in pCO_2 (section 3.4.3.3).

A change in alveolar ventilation causes a change in both pO_2 and pCO_2 (equations 4 and 5, sections 3.4.3 and 3.6.3). Assuming that pCO_2 in the inspired air is zero, these equations can be combined so as to eliminate the alveolar ventilation. The resulting equation is called *the alveolar air equation*:

$$pO_2 \subset A = pO_2 \subset I - pCO_2 \subset A \times (1 - xO_2 \subset I \times (1 - RQ))/RQ \qquad [6]$$

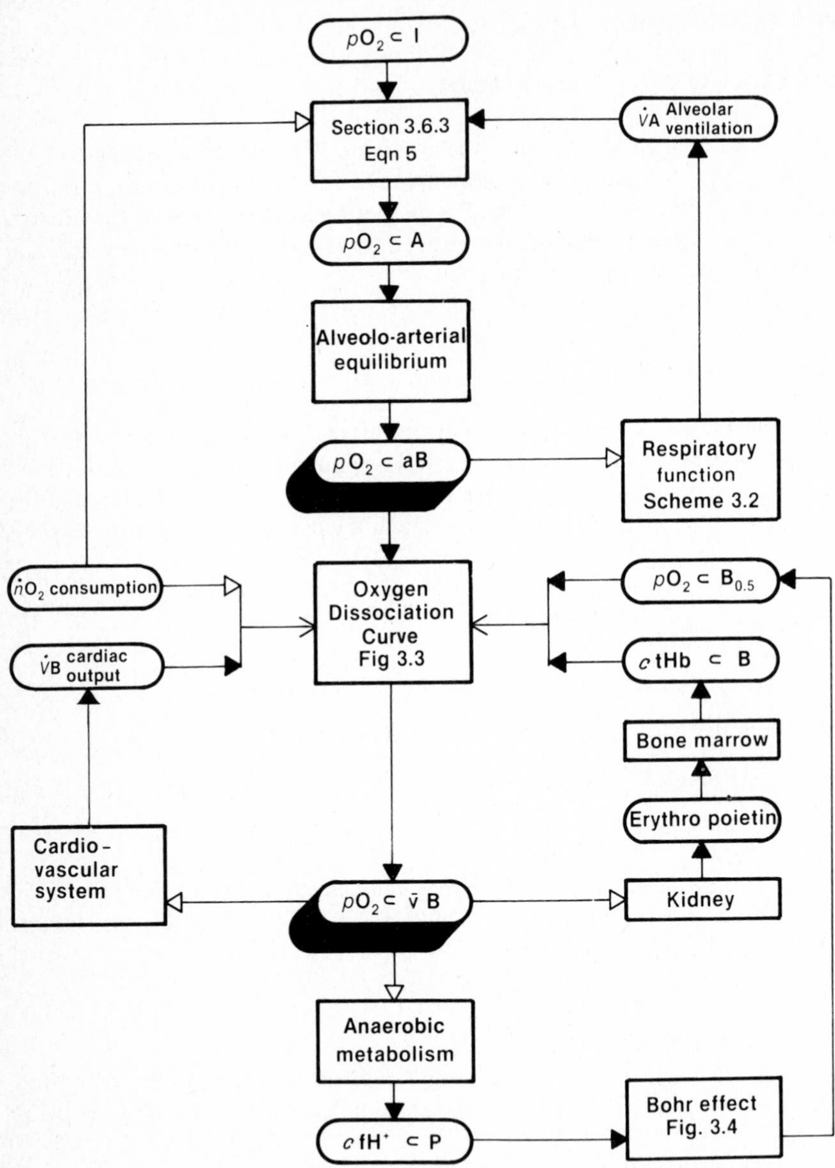

Scheme 3.3. Cybernetic diagram of the regulation of the partial pressure of oxygen in arterial and mixed venous blood ($pO_2 \subset$ aB and $pO_2 \subset \bar{v}$B, respectively). Descriptions of the various mechanisms are given in sections 3.6.3.1 and 3.6.4.1. The symbols are explained in section 3.1 and in Table 3.1. Tracing the arrow backwards from $pO_2 \subset$ aB reveals the *causes* of a change in the arterial pO_2, while the *effects* of such a change are revealed by following the arrows emerging from $pO_2 \subset$ aB.

where $xO_2 \subset I$ is the substance fraction of O_2 in the humidified inspired air (19.7%) and RQ is the ventilatory quotient: $RQ = \dot{n}CO_2(ex)/\dot{n}O_2(in)$. This equation gives the correlation between pO_2 and pCO_2 in the alveolar air when the alveolar ventilation varies. On a diet of carbohydrate, RQ approaches 1 and then: $pO_2 \subset A = pO_2 \subset I - pCO_2 \subset A$, i.e. $pCO_2 \subset A = 5.3$ kPa $\Rightarrow pO_2 \subset A = 14.7$ kPa. On a usual diet, $RQ \approx 0.8$ and then $pO_2 \subset A = pO_2 \subset I - 1.20 \times pCO_2 \subset A$, i.e. $pCO_2 \subset A = 5.3$ kPa $\Rightarrow pO_2 \subset A = 13.6$ kPa.

The correlation between pO_2 and pCO_2 is illustrated in Fig. 3.2 (Rahn and Fenn, 1955). The areas designated primary hypoventilation and hyperventilation indicate the relationship between pCO_2 and pO_2 when the alveolar ventilation is altered with a normal composition of the inspired air.

A respiratory disturbance with a primary hypoventilation, e.g. depression of the respiratory centre with morphine, is sometimes designated respiratory insufficiency type II. A primary hypoxemia causes a stimulation of ventilation and hence a fall in pCO_2. A respiratory disturbance with a primary hypoxaemia, e.g. pulmonary disease with alveolar-arterial block, is sometimes called respiratory insufficiency type I.

A rise in pO_2 does not cause a rise in pCO_2 unless the pO_2 was initially decreased, as indicated by the arrow designated O_2-breathing.

3.6.3.2. *Change in pO_2 of the inspired air*

At high altitude, the pO_2 of the inspired air falls in proportion to the fall in ambient pressure: approximately −11% per km above sea level. A low pO_2 is also encountered in wells and mines because of oxygen deficiency in stagnant air.

3.6.3.3. *Change in the rate of O_2 consumption*

Doubling the rate of O_2 consumption tends to reduce the pO_2 of the alveolar air by about 50% according to equation 5 above. In the whole body, however, CO_2 production simultaneously rises, producing a rise in pCO_2 with stimulation of ventilation, so that the resulting fall in pO_2 would be only about 4%.

3.6.3.4. *Arterioalveolar block and venoarterial shunts*

Diffusion of O_2 across the alveolar membrane is much slower than that of CO_2. A thickening of the alveolar membrane by interstitial or alveolar oedema, therefore, rapidly causes a significant alveoloarterial pO_2 difference. An alveoloarterial pO_2 difference also arises when the perfusion–ventilation relationship in the lungs is abnormal, i.e. when certain sections of the lungs are less well ventilated than others, or when blood is shunted through the lungs without passing functioning alveoli. Finally, an alveoloarterial pO_2 difference arises in congenital heart diseases with venoarterial shunts.

The extent of shunting can be assessed by measuring the pO_2 after breathing pure oxygen for some minutes. Normally the pO_2 should increase to >10 kPa; smaller values indicate venoarterial shunting.

3.6.3.5. *Variations of pO_2 with temperature*

With simple aqueous solutions, a change in pO_2 with temperature can be expressed as $\partial(\log pO_2)/\partial T = +0.005\ \mathrm{K}^{-1}$. The rise in pO_2 with increasing temperature is due to a fall in the solubility of oxygen.

With whole blood in vitro, two other mechanisms contribute to the change in pO_2 with temperature: (a) the binding of O_2 to haemoglobin decreases with increasing temperature: $\partial(\log pO_2 \subset B_{0.5})/\partial T = +0.024\ K^{-1}$ (for constant pH); (b) the binding of O_2 to haemoglobin decreases with decreasing pH, and since pH decreases with increasing temperature, the overall effect is: $d(\log pO_2 \subset B_{0.5})/dT = 0.031\ K^{-1}$. The expression $pO_2 \subset B_{0.5}$ refers to the pO_2 at half saturation of haemoglobin (see section 3.7). At a low pO_2, a rise in temperature causes a liberation of O_2 from oxyhaemoglobin, but the saturation of oxygen only falls slightly (less than 1%) and the change in pO_2 with temperature is therefore almost the same as the displacement of the oxygen dissociation curve, i.e. $d(\log pO_2)/dT = 0.030\ K^{-1}$. At a high pO_2, where the saturation of O_2 in haemoglobin is 1.0 irrespective of temperature, the solubility change is the dominating effect and the temperature coefficient therefore is $d(\log pO_2)/dT = +0.005\ K^{-1}$. The overall relationship between pO_2 and temperature for normal blood is worked out in the form of a convenient slide rule (Severinghaus, 1966).

3.6.4. Effects of change in pO_2 in arterial blood

3.6.4.1. Stimulation of the peripheral chemoreceptors

A fall in pO_2 of the arterial blood causes a stimulation of the peripheral chemoreceptors in the aortic and carotic bodies (Scheme 3.3). This leads to hyperventilation, but the effect is not pronounced until the arterial pO_2 falls below about 8 kPa.

A rise in pO_2 above normal does not cause a decrease in ventilation unless the pO_2 was originally decreased. This is illustrated in Fig. 3.2 which shows that the pCO_2 falls slightly when the pO_2 is decreased below normal, whereas an increase in pO_2 above normal does not cause a rise in pCO_2.

3.6.4.2. Changes in the saturation of oxygen in haemoglobin – the oxygen dissociation curve

The relationship between the pO_2 of the blood and the saturation of oxygen in haemoglobin is illustrated by the classical oxygen absorption curve (Figure 3.3) or the Hill plot (Figure 3.4; see below). Figure 3.3 shows the oxygen absorption curve with the concentration of total oxygen in the blood ($ctO_2 \subset B$) on the ordinate; ctO_2 is the sum of the concentrations of oxyhaemoglobin and dissolved oxygen.

3.6.4.3. Effects on tissue oxygenation and the mixed venous pO_2

The mixed venous pO_2 is determined by the ctO_2 in the mixed venous blood, which in turn is determined by the arteriovenous ctO_2 difference, and by the ctO_2 in the arterial blood. The arteriovenous oxygen difference (ΔctO_2) is determined by the oxygen uptake in the tissues ($\dot{n}O_2$) and the blood flow ($\dot{V}B$): $\Delta ctO_2 = \dot{n}O_2/\dot{V}B$.

An increased oxygen supply to the tissues can be provided in two different ways: by increasing the blood flow ($\dot{V}B$), or by increasing the arteriovenous oxygen difference. This implies increasing either the length or the width of the $\dot{n}O_2$ rectangle in Figure 3.3. The latter can be achieved in several ways (Scheme 3.3).

(a) Increasing the pO_2 at half saturation causes a parallel displacement of the oxygen absorption curve to the right. With unaltered pO_2 of arterial and mixed venous blood, the

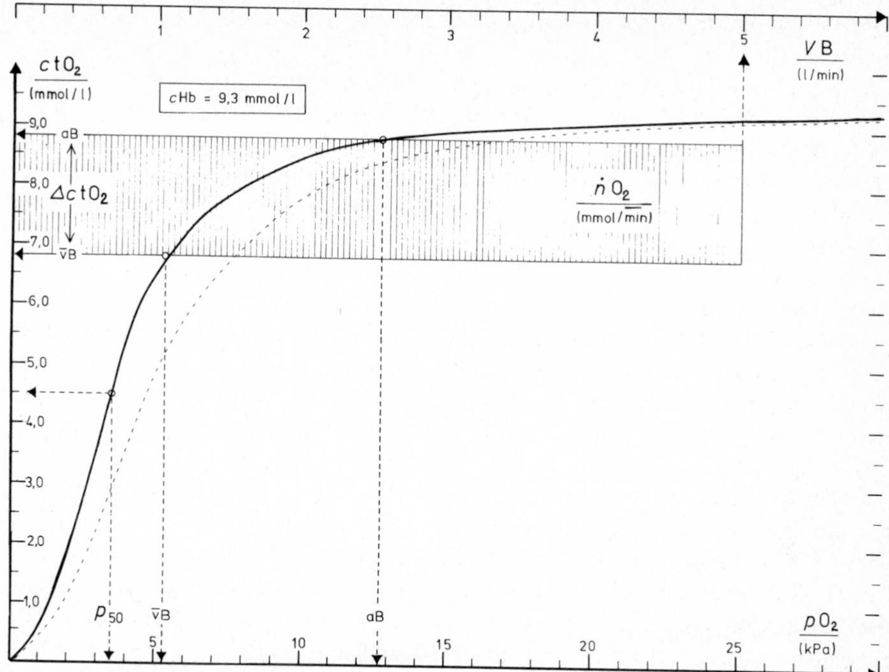

Figure 3.3. The oxygen absorption curve for human blood and the oxygen uptake function (Metcalfe and Dhindsa, 1972). The normal mean values for arterial and mixed venous pO_2 are indicated on the abscissa. The ordinate shows the concentration of total O_2 in arterial and mixed venous blood, and the sigmoid curve is the O_2 absorption curve. The upper abscissa indicates the blood flow ($\dot{V}B$), and the area of the shaded rectangle indicates the rate of oxygen uptake ($\dot{n}O_2 = \dot{V}B \times \Delta ctO_2$).

ctO_2 of mixed venous blood falls a good deal more than ctO_2 of the arterial blood, i.e. the arteriovenous difference increases. This happens as a result of an increase in the concentration of free H^+ in the blood, or a rise in temperature.

(b) Increasing the haemoglobin concentration causes an expansion of the ordinate (Figure 3.3) and hence increases the arteriovenous difference. This is the ultimate regulating mechanism which is brought about by an increased production of erythropoietin in the kidneys.

(c) Increasing the arterial pO_2, and thereby increasing the concentration of total oxygen in arterial blood, has very little effect unless the pO_2 is initially decreased (see Figure 3.3).

(d) Decreasing the mixed venous pO_2, and hence the mixed venous ctO_2, implies decreasing the pO_2 at the mitochondrial level. In the brain, a fall in mixed venous pO_2 below 2.7 kPa is accompanied by anaerobic metabolism. This is what the organism tries to prevent by every means, i.e. by all the foregoing mechanisms of regulation.

Anaerobic metabolism causes accumulation of lactic acid with a rise in the concentration of lactate and of titratable H^+, and free H^+ in the plasma. Concomitant effects are increases in the concentrations of inorganic phosphate, urate and hypoxanthine in the plasma (Saugstad, 1975).

The *clinical symptoms* in severe acute hypoxaemia are at first euphoria and confusion, later unconsciousness. The brain suffers irreversible damage if the oxygen supply is interrupted for more than 3 minutes. However, hypothermia delays the onset of irreversible damage. In chronic hypoxaemia the clinical symptoms are cyanosis, erythrocytosis and swelling of the fingertips (drumstick fingers) caused by hypertrophy of the arteriovenous anastomoses.

3.6.4.4. Oxygen toxicity

Oxygen toxicity is especially pronounced in the newborn, where oxygen treatment causes fibrosis in the eye with blindness (retrolental fibroplasia). Therefore it is essential to control the pO_2 in the newborn during oxygen therapy to avoid values higher than 15 kPa for unnecessarily long periods. In the adult, exposure to pure oxygen at atmospheric pressure is tolerated for 4 days at the most, and causes substernal pain, cough, and progressive deterioration of pulmonary function. Oxygen at high partial pressures damages the pulmonary capillaries causing a fibrinous exudate. However, at reduced pressure (30 kPa), pure oxygen is well tolerated. Hyperbaric oxygen causes vasoconstriction, and eventually convulsions. The sources of the oxygen toxicity are thought to be the unstable intermediates of oxygen reduction, e.g. superoxide anion ($O_2^{-}\cdot$), hydroxyl radicals ($\cdot OH$), oxygen singlets (O_2^*), and hydrogen peroxide (H_2O_2) (Clark, 1974).

When all the oxygen required for metabolism is transported in the form of dissolved O_2, as in hyperbaric oxygenation, no deoxyhaemoglobin is formed in the blood. Since deoxyhaemoglobin is the major vehicle for the transport of CO_2 in the form of carbamate ($R{-}NHCOO^-$), tissue pCO_2 would tend to rise slightly, but this effect is probably of minor importance.

3.6.5. Therapy

The treatment of hypoxaemia depends on the aetiology. In the case of pulmonary insufficiency, the pO_2 of arterial blood can sometimes be increased by increasing the pO_2 of the inspired air, if necessary together with artificial ventilation. When hypoxaemia is due to venoarterial shunting of blood, as in congenital cyanotic heart disease, oxygen breathing is ineffective.

3.6.6. Analysis

3.6.6.1. Blood collection and storage

The blood should be collected anaerobically as previously described (section 3.2.6.1). Arterialized capillary blood can sometimes be used as a substitute for arterial blood, but true arterial blood is always to be preferred for measurement of pO_2.

Insufficient arterialization of the site of capillary puncture with admixture of blood from the venules causes an erroneously low pO_2. The error is especially pronounced in the following situations – (a) in shocked patients in whom the arterial pressure is low, the venous pressure high and the arteriovenous pO_2 difference large; (b) in newborn infants in the first hours, or even days, after birth; (c) in newborn infants with respiratory distress syndrome; (d) in patients receiving oxygen therapy.

Capillary blood is not suitable for estimation of high pO_2 values; even a slight admixture of venous blood, which causes a fall in oxygen saturation of only a few per cent, causes a very marked fall in pO_2 owing to the shallow profile of the oxygen dissociation curve (Figure 3.3) at high pO_2 values. *Exposure to air* can cause either an increase or decrease in the pO_2 depending on the original value.

Glycolysis with lactic acid formation during storage tends to cause a liberation of O_2 from oxyhaemoglobin and an increase in pO_2, while *oxygen consumption* causes a fall in pO_2. The combined effect is a fall in pO_2 of about 0.4 to 1.6 kPa/h at 37 °C if the pO_2 is in the normal range. At high pO_2 values, the rate is greater: at $pO_2 > 50$ kPa the fall is 0.3 kPa/min. At 2 to 4 °C, the rates are reduced by a factor of about 10. The blood should therefore be chilled in ice water if measurement is delayed. Leucocytes, thrombocytes and reticulocytes account for virtually all of the oxidative metabolism. Erythrocytes lack mitochondria with the necessary enzymes of the tricarboxylic acid cycle, but they do contain glucose-6-phosphate dehydrogenase (EC 1.1.1.49) and are able to oxidize some glucose to CO_2 via the pentose phosphate pathway.

Insufficient mixing of the blood prior to pO_2 measurement can cause a significant error because of the effect on plasma pH (section 3.2.6.1). An erroneous pH would change the position of the oxygen dissociation curve and hence affect the pO_2 value.

3.6.6.2. The pO_2 electrode

The most widely used analytical principle (Clark, 1956) is amperometric measurement of the reduction of oxygen at a platinum cathode maintained at –0.6 volts with respect to a non-polarized anode (e.g. Ag/AgCl). The cathode is separated from the sample by an oxygen-permeable membrane which prevents reduction at the cathode of non-diffusible substances such as disulphide groups of proteins. Ionic connection between the cathode and anode is provided by an inner electrolyte solution.

In the absence of oxygen in the sample, the electric current is almost zero because the cathode is polarized, i.e. converted into a hydrogen electrode which generates a counter electromotive force (cathode process: $2H^+ + 2e^- \rightleftharpoons H_2$). A significant zero current may indicate contamination of the inner electrolyte by micro-organisms.

In the presence of oxygen, an electric current (I) flows due to a diffusion of O_2 from the sample through the membrane to the cathode, where it is reduced:

$$O_2 + 2\,H_2O + 4\,e^- \rightleftharpoons 4\,OH^- .$$

The anode process is:

$$Ag \rightleftharpoons Ag^+ + e^- ,$$

where Ag^+ precipitates as AgCl. The current is thus determined by the amount of oxygen which diffuses to the cathode. At the cathode surface, the pO_2 is zero due to the continual reduction of O_2. The amount of O_2 diffusing to the cathode is therefore determined by the pO_2 gradient, i.e. the pO_2 of the sample and the diffusion coefficient of oxygen in the vicinity of the cathode. The dependence on the diffusion coefficient of O_2

in the sample may be reduced by stirring the sample, or better by using a micro-cathode and a membrane with limited oxygen permeability (e.g. polypropylene) so that the diffusion zone is limited to the thin membrane without extending significantly into the sample.

The response time of the electrode is dependent on: (a) the size of the cathode, increasing with increasing area of the cathode; (b) the membrane characteristics, being proportional to l^2/D where l is the membrane thickness and D the diffusion coefficient of O_2 in the membrane material. During use, the area of the cathode tends to increase due to a gradual deposition of Ag on it, which can, if necessary, be removed by nitric acid. A slow or erratic response may be due to a poorly mounted membrane, leaving too much or too little electrolyte between the membrane and the cathode, or to actual leaks through it.

The specificity for O_2 is not absolute. Other diffusible substances may be reduced at the cathode potential of –0.6 volts. One of particular interest is the anaesthetic gas halothane; it has been recommended that the polarizing voltage should be changed to –0.5 volts in order to avoid this reaction.

The calibration function ($I = F(pO_2)$) is established by using two gases (or solutions) with known pO_2. In general, one of these has a pO_2 of zero (pure nitrogen or argon) while the other is atmospheric air or pure oxygen. A solution with pO_2 zero can also be prepared chemically. *The calibration function* is generally linear from $pO_2 = 0$ to about 70 kPa. With commercial micro-electrodes, the slope dI/dpO_2 is usually about 150 fA/Pa, depending upon the size of the cathode and the type of membrane. This corresponds to an oxygen reduction of about 5 fmol/s at a pO_2 of 13 kPa. This O_2 consumption leads to a small downwards drift of the reading. The pO_2 of the test sample (X) is derived from *the calculation function*:

$$pO_2 \subset X = pO_2 \subset S_1 + \frac{pO_2 \subset S_2 - pO_2 \subset S_1}{IS_2 - IS_1} \times (IX - IS_1) \times r \qquad [7]$$

where r is a factor which takes into account differences in the diffusion coefficient for O_2 in the test sample (X) and in the calibration samples (S_1 and S_2). When the calibration is performed with gases, and the test sample is blood, r is generally about 1.05.

The temperature of the electrode should be accurate within ±0.1 K. The pO_2 of blood rises 7% for a temperature rise of 1 K. The electrode adds 3% due to increasing current with increasing temperature, so that the total error amounts to +10% per K. Values for pO_2 measured at 37 °C should be corrected to the actual temperature of the patient by means of the Severinghaus (1966) slide rule (cf. section 3.6.3.5).

Precision and accuracy. The analytical coefficient of variation in measuring pO_2 repeatedly on the same blood specimen is about 2%. The relative inaccuracy due to variations in the diffusion coefficient for O_2 between samples probably amounts to about ±2%. Larger systematic errors may be due to errors in the pO_2 of the calibration samples, unduly large extrapolations from the calibration function (as in measurement of high pO_2 values), or erroneous temperature of the electrode.

Attempts have been made to estimate arterial pO_2 by transcutaneous measurement. The electrode is mounted in a small heating unit which keeps the skin temperature at about 44 °C and vasodilates the underlying skin (Huch et al., 1973). In general, the values so found correlate well with simultaneously measured arterial pO_2 values, but identity can not be expected due to the difficulty in obtaining complete arterialization and due to the influence of temperature on the blood pO_2.

3.6.6.3. Other methods of measuring pO_2

A variety of other methods is available (Payne and Hill, 1975). The blood pO_2 can be measured by gasometric analysis of a small gas bubble aspirated into a syringe with a large volume of blood, but this technique has proved too complicated for routine application. Mass spectrometry has also been employed (Wolding et al., 1966).

Blood pO_2 can also be calculated from the oxygen saturation, pH, and temperature by means of the standard oxygen dissociation curve. Several nomograms and a slide rule have been constructed for this purpose (Severinghaus, 1966). However, the calculation is only an approximation, due to the significant effect of CO_2, as well as that of 2,3-diphosphoglycerate (DPG), on the oxygen dissociation curve (section 3.7.3).

3.7. PARTIAL PRESSURE OF OXYGEN IN BLOOD AT HALF SATURATION OF OXYGEN IN HAEMOGLOBIN

The pO_2 at half saturation ($p_{0.5}$) is a measure of the affinity of oxygen binding to haemoglobin, or in other words a measure of the position of the oxygen dissociation curve. A decreased value, i.e. leftward displacement of the oxygen dissociation curve, indicates an increased oxygen affinity of haemoglobin and hence an inhibition of oxygen supply to the tissues. On the other hand, an increased $p_{0.5}$ value, i.e. displacement of the oxygen dissociation curve to the right, indicates a decreased oxygen affinity, which facilitates O_2 delivery to the tissues.

The pO_2 value at half saturation is part of a detailed description of the oxygen status of the blood and is necessary for a detailed description of the oxygen supply to the tissues (see section 3.6, pO_2 of arterial blood). Measurement of $p_{0.5}$ is also indicated in rare cases where the presence of an abnormal haemoglobin with deviant oxygen affinity is suspected. However, for routine clinical evaluation of states of hypoxia or hyperoxia the $p_{0.5}$ value is rarely determined (Cook, 1976).

3.7.1. Chemistry

The relationship between the saturation of oxygen in haemoglobin and the pO_2 is illustrated by the haemoglobin–oxygen dissociation curve, the Hill plot (Figure 3.4).

The pO_2 of the blood at half saturation of haemoglobin $pO_2 \subset B_{0.5}$ (or $p_{0.5}$ or P_{50}), is a measure of the affinity of oxygen binding to haemoglobin. A low value signifies a high affinity and vice versa. The binding affinity of a ligand at half saturation is defined quite generally as the negative chemical potential of the ligand at half saturation. The normal mean value for the binding affinity of O_2 to haemoglobin at half saturation therefore is: $-\mu O_2 \subset Hb_{0.5} = -R \times T \times \ln 10 \times \log(pO_2 \subset B_{0.5}/95.21\ \mathrm{MPa}) = 26.3\ \mathrm{kJ/mol}$.

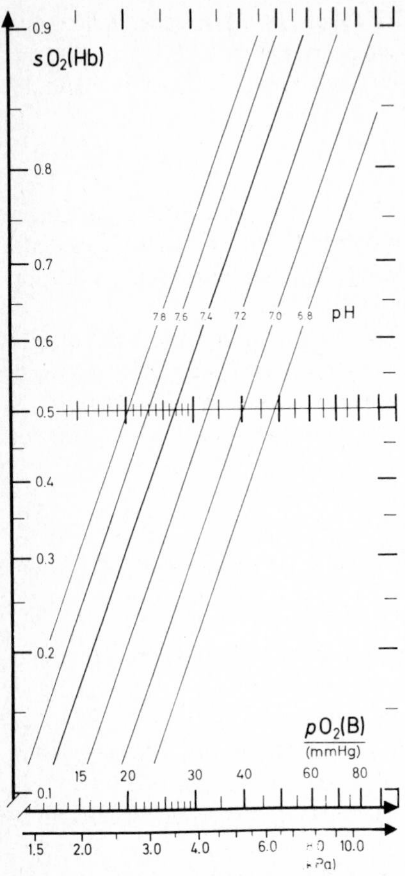

Figure 3.4. Oxygen dissociation curves illustrating the relationship between the pO_2 of the blood and the saturation of oxygen in haemoglobin for human blood with different plasma pH but with constant pCO_2 (=5.33 kPa) normal concentration of 2,3-diphosphoglycerate in the erythrocytes (=4.8 mmol/litre), and temperature (37 °C). The plot is a so-called Hill plot, with pO_2 on a logarithmic scale and sO_2 on a logit scale (logit sO_2 = log(sO_2/(1 – sO_2)). The scale in the middle of the chart indicates the pO_2 at half saturation (pO_2 ⊂ $B_{0.5}$ or $p_{0.5}$). The slope of the lines is about 2.7, but it can be shown that the slope must approach unity at very high as well as very low sO_2 values. The displacement of the lines with changing pH is called the Bohr effect (section 3.7.3.2) but it is not uniform over the range, falling off at high pH as well as low pH values; the maximum effect is at pH ⊂ P = 7.1.

3.7.2. Reference values

The reference intervals (95%) for the partial pressure of O_2 in the blood at half saturation of O_2 in haemoglobin, and the extremes of the pathological range are tabulated.

	Adults	Newborn infants	Extremes of the range
$p_{0.5}$ (kPa)	3.3–3.7	2.4–3.2	1.6–6.7
$p_{0.5}$ (mm Hg)	25–28	18–24	12–50

3.7.3. Causes of change in $p_{0.5}$

The principal causes of change in $p_{0.5}$ are shown in Scheme 3.4. The affinity of haemoglobin for O_2 is primarily dependent on the type of haemoglobin, and secondly on various so-called allosteric effectors (Rørth and Astrup, 1972).

3.7.3.1. Type of haemoglobin

Several abnormal haemoglobins are known with abnormal oxygen affinity (Chapter 17, section 17.2.4). Hb Seattle and Hb Kansas both have low oxygen affinity, while Hb Yakima, Malmø, Rainier and others have a high oxygen affinity.

Foetal haemoglobin, HbF, has a high oxygen affinity so that newborn infants have a low $p_{0.5}$. However, in pure haemoglobin solutions, HbA and HbF show the same $p_{0.5}$, the difference only appearing in the presence of 2,3-diphosphoglycerate which binds more strongly to HbA than to HbF and therefore decreases the oxygen affinity of HbA to a greater extent than that of HbF.

3.7.3.2. Changes with the hydrogen ion concentration

The effect of H^+ on the oxygen binding of haemoglobin is called the Bohr effect (Figure 3.4). The binding sites of the oxygen-linked hydrogen ions (Bohr protons) have been mapped as a result of extensive studies involving X-ray crystallography as well as chemical modifications of the haemoglobin molecule (Perutz, 1970; Kilmartin, 1972). The

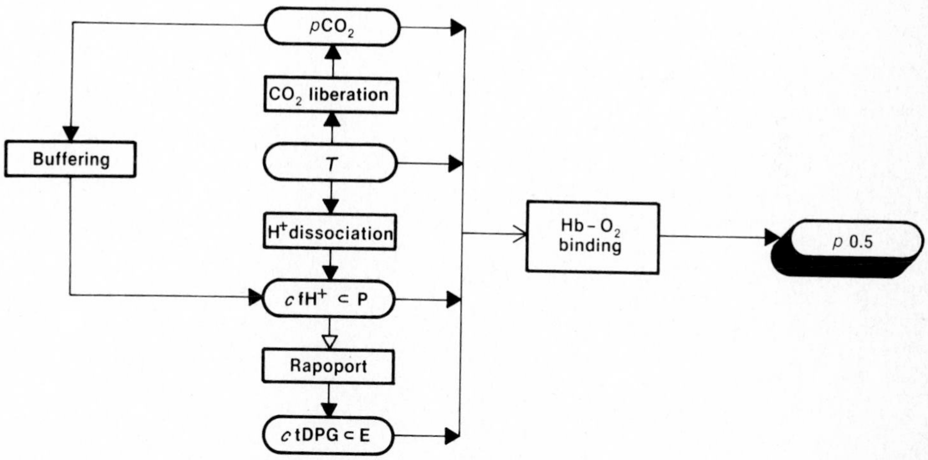

Scheme 3.4. Cybernetic diagram of the causes of change in the pO_2 at half saturation of oxygen in haemoglobin ($p_{0.5}$, section 3.7). A rise in $cfH^+ \subset P$, in $pCO_2 \subset B$, in concentration of total 2,3-diphosphoglycerate in the erythrocytes (ctDPG), and in temperature, all cause a rise in $p_{0.5}$, i.e. a fall in the affinity of oxygen binding to haemoglobin. However, the effect of a rise in pCO_2 is primarily due to the concomitant rise in cfH^+ (the Bohr effect), whereas the effect at constant cfH^+ is much smaller. The effect of a change in temperature is also enhanced by the concomitant changes in cfH^+ and pCO_2. On the other hand, a rise in cfH^+ *gradually* causes a fall in the concentration of DPG in the erythrocytes (Rapoport, 1968) which counteracts the direct effect of cfH^+ on the $p_{0.5}$ value.

groups involved are the imino groups of the C-terminal histidines of the two β-chains (HC3(146)β), the amino groups of the N-terminal valines of the two α-chains (NA1(1)α), and possibly also the imino groups of one of the histidines of the two α-chains (H5(122)α). In deoxyhaemoglobin, these groups participate in the formation of salt bridges, and the pK values are thereby increased. In oxyhaemoglobin the salt bridges rupture and the pK values fall. The events at the oxygen binding sites, i.e. the ferrous ions of the haem groups, which trigger the rupturing of the salt bridges, have also been clarified in detail. These interactions have been reviewed by Antonini and Brunori (1971), Rørth (1972) and Siggaard-Andersen and Garby (1973).

The change in pO_2 at half saturation with a change in pH is the Bohr coefficient:

$$\left(\frac{\partial \log pO_2}{\partial \text{ pH} \subset \text{P}}\right)_{sO_2, pCO_2, ct\text{DPG}, T} = -0.38 \qquad [1]$$

where the value refers to normal blood. The value varies with pH, pCO_2, and concentration of total DPG in the erythrocytes (ctDPG ⊂ E) as shown in Figure 3.5. The Bohr coefficient applies to conditions in which the pCO_2 is constant and changes in pH ⊂ P

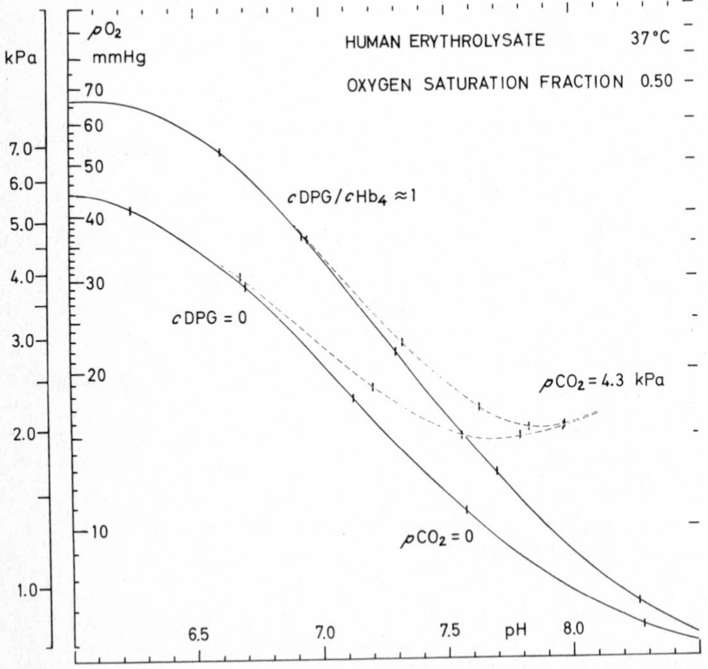

Figure 3.5. The pO_2 of blood at half saturation of oxygen in haemoglobin ($p_{0.5}$) as a function of pH in the presence and absence of CO_2 and 2,3-diphosphoglycerate (section 3.7.3.2). The slope of the curves ($\partial \log p_{0.5}/\partial$ pH) is the Bohr coefficient. The figure indicates a variation in the Bohr coefficient with pH as well as with pCO_2 and concentration of 2,3-diphosphoglycerate in the erythrocytes (ctDPG ⊂ E). (Reproduced, by permission, from Siggaard-Anderson et al., 1972)

are caused by changes in the concentration of titratable H^+. If, however, the concentration of titratable H^+ is constant and pH changes are being caused by changes in pCO_2, the coefficient includes the pH and the pCO_2 effects and its absolute value is therefore higher:

$$\left(\frac{\partial \log pO_2}{\partial \text{pH} \subset \text{P}}\right)_{sO_2, ctH^+ \subset \text{B}, ct\text{DPG} \subset \text{E}, T} = -0.53 \qquad [2]$$

It should be emphasized that coefficients (1) and (2) both refer to whole blood but the pH values refer to the plasma phase. The actual values of the two coefficients change with the different variables, so that any calculations based on them are therefore only approximate.

3.7.3.3. Changes with the pCO_2

The effect of CO_2 on the oxygen binding of haemoglobin is due to its binding as carbamino–CO_2 (R–$NHCOO^-$) to the terminal amino groups of the four peptide chains of the haemoglobin molecule. Carbon dioxide binds preferentially to the N-terminal valine moieties of the two β-chains in deoxyhaemoglobin and thereby stabilizes the deoxy-conformation, so that the oxygen affinity falls even at constant pH. Another consequence of this binding is that the pH effect on the oxygen affinity diminishes; thus at a pCO_2 of 27 kPa and pH = 7.6, the Bohr effect completely vanishes, and at even higher pCO_2 values the Bohr effect is reversed. The effect of CO_2 can be expressed as:

$$\left(\frac{\partial \log pO_2}{\partial \log pCO_2}\right)_{sO_2, \text{pH}, ct\text{DPG}, T} = +0.11 \qquad [3]$$

The value refers to half saturation in normal blood with a normal pH and ctDPG. The effect of CO_2 when pH varies but ctH^+ is constant is much greater, because the effect of H^+ is included. The value of the coefficient is then estimated to be about +0.83 for normal blood.

3.7.3.4. Changes with ctDPG

The effect of DPG on the oxygen binding of haemoglobin is due to its binding in the so-called central cavity between the two β-chains of deoxyhaemoglobin, where it stabilizes the deoxy-conformation (Chapter 17, section 17.2.5) In oxyhaemoglobin, the central cavity narrows and DPG is expelled. The effect of DPG can be expressed as:

$$\left(\frac{\partial \log pO_2}{\partial \, ct\text{DPG}/ct\text{Hb}}\right)_{sO_2, \text{pH}, pCO_2, T} = +0.44 \qquad [4]$$

In other words, a rise in the concentration of total DPG relative to the concentration of total haemoglobin causes an increase in pO_2 at half saturation.

The binding of DPG to deoxyhaemoglobin presumably causes an increase in the concentration of total DPG when the average concentration of deoxyhaemoglobin in the total volume of erythrocytes in the circulation is increased, i.e. when the average oxygen saturation of haemoglobin is decreased (Bellingham and Grimes, 1973). However, it has not been possible to demonstrate this effect in vitro (Rørth, 1972). The general effect of DPG is that of counteracting the effect of H^+ on the oxygen binding: an increase in cfH^+ causes an increase in $p_{0.5}$ but also gradually causes a fall in the concentration of DPG in the erythrocytes which leads to a return of $p_{0.5}$ to normal.

The effect of H^+ on the ctDPG is probably due to the pH dependence of the phosphofructokinase (EC 2.7.1.11) activity. A rise in pH causes a rise in phosphofructokinase activity, resulting in an increased rate of glycolysis and increased formation of DPG from 1,3-diphosphoglycerate (Rapoport and Luebering, 1950). Other enzymes which influence the DPG concentration are hexokinase (EC 2.7.1.1), deficiency of which leads to a low DPG concentration, and pyruvate kinase (EC 2.7.1.40), deficiency of which leads to a rise in DPG concentration.

3.6.3.5. Changes with temperature

The effect of temperature on the oxygen binding can be expressed as:

$$\left(\frac{\partial \log pO_2}{\partial T}\right)_{sO_2,\mathrm{pH},pCO_2} = +0.24\ \mathrm{K}^{-1} \qquad [5]$$

If pH and pCO_2 vary but $ctCO_2$ and ctH^+ are constant, i.e. the temperature changes in a closed system, the temperature effect is greater because the effects of a change in pH and pCO_2 are included, so that the effect is then about $0.32\ \mathrm{K}^{-1}$.

3.7.3.6. Other ligands

Adenosine triphosphate (ATP) has a similar effect to DPG. However, the concentration of ATP in erythrocytes is much lower than that of DPG. Inorganic phosphate and many other anions slightly inhibit the binding of oxygen to haemoglobin.

Carbon monoxide causes a significant increase in oxygen affinity of the remaining haem groups – the Haldane–Smith effect – and methaemoglobin has a similar effect (Hlastala et al., 1976).

3.7.4. Effects of change in $p_{0.5}$

The $p_{0.5}$ value and the arterial pO_2 together determine the arterial oxygen saturation of haemoglobin and, with the concentration of haemoglobin, these variables determine the concentration of total O_2 in arterial blood. On the venous side, however, the $p_{0.5}$ value and the concentration of total O_2 remaining after O_2 uptake in the tissues, together determine the mixed venous pO_2. A high oxygen affinity (low $p_{0.5}$) tends to cause a low mixed venous pO_2 and a low tissue pO_2. Usually the body compensates by increasing the blood flow or, given sufficient time, by increasing the DPG concentration in the erythrocytes; eventually there is an increase in haemoglobin concentration (Scheme 3.3). Stored bank blood depleted in DPG and with a low $p_{0.5}$ value is therefore not ideal for oxygen transport until 12 to 24 hours after infusion by which time new DPG has been synthesized in the erythrocytes.

Due to the variability of the $p_{0.5}$ value, calculation of the oxygen saturation from the

pO_2 or vice versa by means of the so-called standard oxygen dissociation curve, taking the pH and temperature into account, can be considerably biased, especially when the DPG concentration deviates from the normal.

3.7.5. Therapy

At present, no methods are available for therapeutic alteration of the $p_{0.5}$ value. It can be speculated, however, that it will be possible, in future, to synthesize substances which will bind selectively to the central cavity of deoxyhaemoglobin, thereby increasing the $p_{0.5}$ value. In shocked patients, it might be beneficial to give such a drug in order to facilitate the dissociation of O_2 in the tissues so that the oxygen supply to the tissues would be maintained in spite of a low cardiac output.

3.7.6. Analysis

The simplest means of estimating $p_{0.5}$ consists of measuring both the pO_2 (with a Clark electrode) and the oxygen saturation (by a spectrophotometric method) on a venous blood sample drawn anaerobically in a heparinized syringe. Another technique consists of establishing a known pO_2 by equilibrating blood with a gas mixture of known pO_2 and measuring the resulting oxygen saturation. Alternatively, a known oxygen saturation can be established by mixing equal volumes of fully oxygenated and fully deoxygenated blood and measuring the resulting pO_2. In all three methods, the plasma pH and pCO_2 should be measured simultaneously. The pO_2 at half saturation is then calculated from the measured pO_2 and oxygen saturation by means of the following equation:

$$\log p_{0.5}/\text{kPa} = \log pO_2/\text{kPa} - \frac{1}{2.7} \times \text{logit } sO_2 \qquad [6]$$

where 2.7 is the Hill slope, which is assumed to be independent of the other variables. Alternatively, two points of the oxygen dissociation curve may be determined, preferably with sO_2 above and below 0.5; the $p_{0.5}$ value is then determined by interpolation on a Hill plot.

Methods are also available by which the pO_2 is measured continually while the blood is titrated with oxygen, so that the oxygen saturation gradually increases from zero to one. The oxygen saturation may also be measured by continuous spectrophotometric monitoring during the titration (Clerbaux, 1976).

The value for $p_{0.5}$ can be corrected to the desired temperature, pH, and pCO_2 using the foregoing coefficients, but large corrections are subject to considerable error due to changes in the coefficients with all the variables. It is essential to specify whether the $p_{0.5}$ value which is reported pertains to the actual pH and pCO_2 of the venous or arterial blood, or whether it has been corrected to pH = 7.40 and pCO_2 = 5.3 kPa. The latter value is mainly an indicator of the concentration of DPG in the erythrocytes, or it may reveal the presence of an abnormal haemoglobin.

3.8. SATURATION OF OXYGEN IN HAEMOGLOBIN IN ARTERIAL BLOOD

The haemoglobin oxygen saturation ($sO_2 \subset Hb$) is part of a complete description of the oxygen status of the blood comprising: pO_2, oxygen saturation, concentration of total oxygen, and pO_2 at half saturation (see section 3.6, pO_2 of arterial blood). Multiplication of oxygen saturation and haemoglobin concentration gives the concentration of bound O_2 in the blood, which approximately equals the concentration of total oxygen except at elevated pO_2 values.

For routine clinical evaluation of states of hypoxia or hyperoxia the arterial pO_2 is generally employed. Occasionally, however, the oxygen saturation is preferred as indicator of the degree of hypoxia, e.g. in cardiac diseases with cyanosis due to right to left shunting, because the oxygen saturation value more directly than the pO_2 value indicates the size of the shunt.

3.8.1. Chemistry

The saturation of oxygen in haemoglobin ($sO_2 \subset Hb$) is defined as the substance amount of O_2 bound to haemoglobin ($nO_2 \subset Hb$) divided by the substance amount of O_2 bound when the haemoglobin is saturated with O_2:

$$sO_2 \subset Hb = \frac{nO_2 \subset Hb}{nO_2 \subset Hb_{sat}}, \text{ by definition} \qquad [1]$$

which can be expressed as:

$$sO_2 \subset Hb = \frac{cHbO_2}{cHbO_2 + cHb}, \qquad [2]$$

where $cHbO_2$ is the concentration of oxyhaemoglobin and cHb is the concentration of deoxyhaemoglobin in the blood. The sum of the concentrations of HbO_2 and Hb is the concentration of "active" haemoglobin which is often called the "oxygen capacity"; it equals the concentration of total haemoglobin ($ctHb$) minus the concentration of "inactive haemoglobins" (i.e. carboxyhaemoglobin, methaemoglobin, and sulphaemoglobin). Usually the fraction of inactive haemoglobin amounts to about 4% of the total haemoglobin. The oxygen saturation is often determined as the concentration of total O_2 in blood (the so-called "oxygen content") divided by the "oxygen capacity". However, the concentration of total O_2 in the blood ($ctO_2 \subset B$) includes the low concentration of physically dissolved O_2.

3.8.2. Reference values

The reference intervals (95%) for the saturation of O_2 in haemoglobin in the arterial blood from healthy resting adults, and the extremes of the pathological range are tabulated.

Quantity	Reference interval	Extremes of range
$sO_2 \subset Hb$	0.919–0.985	0.5–1.0

For mixed venous blood, the value is about 0.73. The lowest values are seen in patients with severe respiratory insufficiency. Values of 1.0 may be obtained by hyperbaric oxygenation.

3.8.3. Causes of change in $sO_2 \subset Hb$

The oxygen saturation of the arterial blood is a function of the pO_2 of the arterial blood and the pO_2 at half saturation (i.e. the position of the oxygen dissociation curve); causes of change are described in connection with these quantities and shown graphically in Figure 3.4.

3.8.4. Effects of change in $sO_2 \subset Hb$

The effects of an abnormal sO_2 are mostly secondary to the associated change in pO_2. One effect which is unrelated to the pO_2 is the cyanotic appearance which is related to a low sO_2 but also dependent upon the haemoglobin concentration, the blood flow and oxygen consumption in the skin. For example, cyanosis becomes apparent sooner (i.e. at a higher sO_2) when the patient has a high haemoglobin concentration than when the patient is anaemic. The presence of methaemoglobin or sulphaemoglobin also causes cyanosis.

A low sO_2 in mixed venous blood, with a concentration of deoxyhaemoglobin of about 2 mmol/litre, causes a binding of H^+ of about 0.6 mmol/litre (the Haldane effect) as well as a binding of CO_2 of about 0.4 mmol/litre (as carbamino–CO_2). Both effects have been considered to be important for the regulation of neutrality and the transport of CO_2 but the physiological significance has probably been exaggerated: during hyperbaric oxygenation, where sO_2 of the mixed venous blood remains high, no adverse effects can be ascribed to the absence of the Haldane effect or the carbamino transport of CO_2.

3.8.5. Analysis

3.8.5.1. Measurement of the saturation of oxygen in haemoglobin

Spectrometric measurement of the oxygen saturation by transmission spectrometry is based on the Beer–Lambert law according to which the total absorbance at any wavelength is the sum of the contribution from each individual pigment:

$$a_\lambda = l \cdot \Sigma_i \epsilon_\lambda C_i \cdot cC_i \qquad [3]$$

where a_λ is the absorbance at wavelength λ, l is the pathlength, $\epsilon_\lambda C_i$ is the molar absorption coefficient at wavelength λ for component C_i, and cC_i is the concentration of component C_i.

The oxygen saturation is determined by the ratio of the concentrations of deoxyhaemoglobin and oxyhaemoglobin. Measurement of the ratio of the absorbances at two different wavelengths in a haemolysate is therefore sufficient for determination of the oxygen saturation, provided that the contribution of other pigments (e.g. carboxyhaemoglobin, methaemoglobin, sulphaemoglobin, bilirubin) is negligible (Siggaard-Andersen et al., 1972). In the instrument (OSM2) manufactured by Radiometer (Denmark), the blood is haemolysed directly inside the cuvette by means of ultrasound (Siggaard-Andersen, 1977c). By measuring at three different wavelengths, it is possible to calculate the saturation of oxygen in haemoglobin as well as the fraction of carboxyhaemoglobin; this is the principle employed in the CO-oximeter manufactured by Instrumentation Laboratory (U.S.A.).

The precision of spectrometric methods can be very high (standard deviation 0.002), but the accuracy is less certain due to interferences from other pigments or to turbidity.

Transcutanous measurement of the oxygen saturation has also been described. The Hewlett Packard (U.S.A.) ear oximeter measures the transmission through the ear lobe (41 °C) at eight different wavelengths; a computer program calculates the oxygen saturation after correction for skin pigments and inactive haemoglobin.

Reflection spectrometry has also been applied to in vitro as well as in vivo transcutanous measurement (Zijlstra, 1958).

3.8.5.2. Measurement of the concentration of total O_2 in the blood

Classical gasometric methods are based upon the liberation of all bound O_2 by oxidation of haemoglobin to methaemoglobin using potassium ferricyanide, and manometric or volumetric measurement of the liberated gaseous O_2 by absorption in alkaline pyrogallol using the Van Slyke apparatus or the Natelson micro-gasometer. Another technique consists of converting O_2 into CO_2 by combustion, followed by titrimetric determination of CO_2 (Dijkhuizen et al., 1976).

Amperometric measurement is based on liberation of the bound O_2 by means of ferricyanide or carbon monoxide, and measurement of the resulting pO_2 with a pO_2 electrode. Coulometric measurement is based on using a very large oxygen electrode in which essentially all the O_2 of the blood is consumed by the cathode reaction (Lexington Instrument Company, U.S.A.). Gas chromatographic methods have also been described and instruments specially designed for gas chromatographic measurement of the concentrations of total oxygen and total carbon dioxide in blood are available.

3.9. CASE HISTORIES

3.9.1. Acute respiratory acidosis

The patient, a premature newborn infant (birth weight 1700 grams), developed signs of respiratory distress syndrome shortly after birth: cyanosis, intercostal retractions, expiratory grunt. Catheters were inserted in the umbilical artery and vein; the first arterial blood specimen 1 hour after birth, while the infant was breathing pure oxygen, showed the following values: pH = 7.14, pCO_2 = 10.4 kPa, pO_2 = 9.5 kPa. The laboratory diagnoses therefore are: acidaemia, hypercapnia, and relative hypoxaemia. The pH and pCO_2 values fall within the reference area of acute hypercapnia (Figure 3.1), i.e. there is no indication of a metabolic or non-respiratory component of the acidaemia, and the estimated concentration of titratable H^+ in the extracellular fluid (+3 mmol/litre) is within the limits of the reference interval. However, the calculated concentration of titratable H^+ in the blood is +8 mmol/litre (base excess = –8 mmol/litre), and the standard bicarbonate concentration is low (18 mmol/litre) both indicating accumulation of titratable H^+ *in the blood,* but this is merely due to the Hamburger shift within the extracellular phase caused by the rise in pCO_2 and does not indicate a metabolic acidosis. Sodium bicarbonate (2 mmol) was given intravenously, and 2 hours later the values were: pH = 7.10, pCO_2 = 13.5 kPa, titratable H^+ of extracellular fluid –1 mmol/litre (of blood +7 mmol/litre), pO_2 = 8.5 kPa. The infant was then intubated and ventilated with a respirator: 30 minutes later the values were: pH = 7.38, pCO_2 = 5.8 kPa, titratable H^+ of extracellular fluid +1 mmol/litre (of blood 0.0 mmol/litre), pO_2 = 20 kPa. The change in titratable H^+ in the blood from +7 to zero mmol/litre accompanying the change in pCO_2 is due to a reversal of the Hamburger shift.

After 6 days of respirator treatment, breathing was spontaneous and the infant eventually recovered successfully. Other treatment worth mentioning is blood transfusion twice during the first 2 weeks due to blood sampling!

3.9.2. Chronic respiratory insufficiency

The patient, a 65-year-old woman with chronic bronchitis and emphysema, was admitted to hospital restless and confused, with acute exacerbation, severely dyspnoeic, and with pronounced cyanosis. Analysis of the arterial blood revealed a severe hypoxaemia (pO_2 = 4.1 kPa), severe hypercapnia (pCO_2 = 10.4 kPa), renal compensation with a fall in the extracellular concentration of titratable H^+ (–19 mmol/litre), and a normal pH (7.39). The pH and pCO_2 values fall outside the area of simple chronic hypercapnia (Figure 3.1) indicating that the patient might have a superimposed metabolic alkalosis. This could be due to prolonged treatment with a diuretic drug (thiazide), with depletion of Na^+ and K^+ leading to hypokalaemic alkalosis (plasma K^+ = 2.9 mmol/litre).

The pCO_2 and pO_2 values fall outside the area of simple hypoventilation (Figure 3.2) indicating a mixed respiratory insufficiency probably due to hypoventilation complicated by bronchial obstructions with atelectases.

Oxygen breathing caused a moderate rise in pO_2 and simultaneously the pCO_2 rose. After 1 hour, the values were: pH = 7.28, pCO_2 = 13.8 kPa, pO_2 = 7.7 kPa. The patient was therefore intubated and ventilated with a respirator. After 4 days on the respirator and with antibiotic treatment of the bronchial infection, the patient was extubated and breathed spontaneously: pH = 7.34, pCO_2 = 10.5 kPa, pO_2 = 8.4 kPa. The pH and pCO_2 values now fall inside the area of chronic hypercapnia (Figure 3.1), and the pCO_2 and pO_2 values fall in the area of simple hypoventilation (Figure 3.2) indicating that the component of hypoxaemia due to bronchial obstruction had been eliminated.

3.9.3. Diabetic ketoacidosis

A 58-year-old man with diabetes mellitus was admitted in deep coma, dehydrated, with ketonuria, and a blood glucose concentration of 36.5 mmol/litre. The arterial blood values were pH = 6.73, pCO_2 = 2.0 kPa, and pO_2 = 18.6 kPa. This was considered a unique case of survival after such a low pH until the value was corrected to the actual temperature of the patient which was 29.2 °C. The values were then: pH = 6.85, pCO_2 = 1.4 kPa, pO_2 = 17.0 kPa, and the concentration of titratable H^+ in the extracellular fluid +30 mmol/litre. The pH and pCO_2 values fall in the area between acute and chronic H^+ excess (Figure 3.1). X-ray revealed a left pulmonary infiltration which probably precipitated the ketoacidosis. The severe hyperventilation threatened to exhaust the patient and artificial ventilation with a respirator was therefore instituted. The patient was given insulin (low dose intramuscular, 6 IU/h), antibiotics, potassium chloride, and sodium bicarbonate in an amount of 75 mmol/h for the first 4 hours. The expected fall in the concentration of titratable H^+ in the extracellular fluid due to the bicarbonate infusion was 10 mmol/litre (body weight 75 kg, volume of distribution of bicarbonate assumed to be 40% of body volume). After 4 hours the values were: pH = 7.15, pCO_2 = 3.6 kPa, ctH^+ = +18 mmol/litre, and after 11 hours the values were: pH = 7.45, pCO_2 = 4.3 kPa, ctH^+ = +1.0 mmol/litre. The patient recovered successfully.

3.9.4. Chronic metabolic alkalosis

A 32-year-old man was admitted to hospital for observation for encephalitis because of progressive confusion and, finally, general seizures after 4 days of vomiting. On admission the patient was slow cerebrated, disoriented, and dehydrated. An arterial puncture revealed a very severe metabolic alkalosis with pH = 7.63, pCO_2 = 7.6 kPa, extracellular titratable H^+ = –40 mmol/litre, actual bicarbonate concentration 59 mmol/litre and pO_2 = 10.5 kPa. Plasma sodium and potassium concentrations were 127 and 2.4 mmol/litre, respectively. The pH and pCO_2 values fall in the area of chronic H^+ deficit (Figure 3.1).

The patient was treated by infusion of Na^+, K^+, and Cl^- and the next day he was able to tell his story. He had had symptoms of duodenal ulcer for 15 years and had treated himself with large amounts of sodium bicarbonate (600 to 1200 mmol/day) and milk (3 to 4 litres/day).

The aetiology of the metabolic alkalosis is mixed: (a) loss of H^+ due to vomiting; (b) excessive intake of base ($NaHCO_3$); (c) dehydration with contraction alkalosis. The convulsions were due to a low concentration of free calcium ion (1.09 mmol/litre, with reference values of 1.17 to 1.33 mmol/litre) in spite of elevated total calcium (3.05 mmol/litre, with reference values of 2.20 to 2.70 mmol/litre). Even after 10 days, a significant metabolic alkalosis persisted, with pH = 7.55, pCO_2 = 5.9 kPa, and ctH^+ = –14 mmol/litre. At this point the patient got impatient and it was impossible to persuade him to continue the medical treatment.

The causes of the persistence of the alkalosis may be as follows: (a) sodium and potassium depletion would render the kidneys unable to excrete sodium and potassium bicarbonate; however, the patient received ample amounts of sodium and potassium chloride and plasma sodium and potassium rose to 139 and 4.2 mmol/litre, respectively; (b) the plasma creatinine was persistently elevated, indicating a chronic renal insufficiency, which would contribute to the inability to reabsorb H^+ in the distal tubules even in the presence of Na^+ and K^+; (c) the patient had a secondary hypoparathyroidism (concentration of parathyroid hormone in the plasma below the limit of detection) due to the large intake of milk (calcium and vitamin D). One of the effects of parathyroid hormone is to enhance the excretion of phosphate and bicarbonate in the kidneys, so that lack of parathyroid hormone might be contributing to the inability of the kidneys to excrete bicarbonate. The clinical picture is consistent with a typical milk–alkali syndrome which may lead to chronic renal insufficiency, osteosclerosis, and keratopathia.

REFERENCES

Agostoni, A.; Luzzana, M., Raffaele, I., Stella, G. and Rossi-Bernardi, L. (1972) A new technique for the evaluation of base excess (Abstract). Scandinavian Journal of Clinical and Laboratory Investigation, 29, Suppl. 126, 30.16.

Albers, C. (1974) Carbon dioxide and the utilization of oxygen. In Carbon Dioxide and Metabolic Regulations (Ed. G.G. Nahas and K.E. Schaefer) pp. 144–149, Springer-Verlag, New York.

Antonini, E. and Brunori, M. (1971) Hemoglobin and Myoglobin in their Reaction with Ligands. pp. 1–436, North Holland-Publishing Co., Amsterdam.

Ashby, W.R. (1973) An Introduction to Cybernetics. Chapman and Hall Ltd., London.

Bates, R.G. (1973) Determination of pH. Theory and Practice, 3rd. edn. John Wiley and Sons, New York.

Bellingham, A.J. and Grimes, A.J. (1973) Red cell 2,3-diphosphoglycerate (Annotation). British Journal of Haematology, 25, 555–562.

Brantigan, J.W., Gott, V.L., Vestal, M.L., Fergusson, G.J. and Johnston, W.H. (1970) A non-thrombogenic diffusion membrane for continous in vivo measurement of blood gases by mass spectroscopy. Journal of Applied Physiology, 28, 375–377.

Cameron, J.N. (1971) Rapid method for determination of total carbon dioxide in small blood samples. Journal of Applied Physiology, 31, 632–634.

Campbell, E.J.M. (1974) Hydrogen ion (acid–base) regulation. In Clinical Physiology, 4th edn. (Eds. E.J.M. Campbell, C.J. Dickinson and J.D.M. Slater) Chap. 5, Blackwell Scientific Publications, Oxford.

Chapot, G., Barrault, N., Müller, M. and Dargnat (1972) Comparative study of Pa_{CO_2} in several homeothermic species. American Journal of Physiology, 223, 1354–1357.

Clark, J.C. Jr. (1956) Monitor and control of blood and tissue oxygen tension. Transactions of the American Society of Artificial Internal Organs, 2, 41–48.

Clark, J.M. (1974) The toxicity of oxygen. American Review of Respiratory Disease, 110, 40–50.

Clerbaux, Th. (1976) Methodes pour déterminer la courbe de dissociation de l'hémoglobine (Revue). Bulletin Europeénnes de Physiopathologie Respiratoire, 12, 487–505.

Cohen, R.D. and Woods, H.F. (1976) Clinical and Metabolic Aspects of Lactic Acidosis. Blackwell Scientific Publications, Oxford.

Cook, D.A. (1976) A practical and theoretical appraisal of the significance of P_{50} and 2,3-diphosphoglycerate determinations in the routine chemical pathology department. Medical Laboratory Sciences, 33, 287–297.

Cunningham, D.J.C. and Lloyd, B.B. (1963) The Regulation of Human Respiration. Blackwell Scientific Publications, Oxford.

Davenport, H.W. (1974) The ABC of Acid–Base Chemistry. The Elements of Physiological Blood-Gas Chemistry for Medical Students and Physicians, 6th edn. pp. 124, University of Chicago Press, Chicago.

Dijkhuizen, P., Kwant, G. and Zijlstra, W.G. (1976) A new reference method for the determination of the oxygen content of blood. Clinica Chimica Acta, 68, 79–85.

Dybkaer, R. (1970) Nomenclature for quantities and units. Standard Methods of Clinical Chemistry, 6, 223–244.

Forrester, R.L., Wataji, L.J., Silverman, D.A. and Pierre, K.J. (1976) Enzymatic method for determination of carbon dioxide in serum. Clinical Chemistry, 22, 243–245.

Frumin, M.U., Epstein, R.M. and Cohen, G. (1959) Apneic oxygenation in man. Anesthesiology, 20, 789–798.

Gill, P.E. and Brown, S.S. (1977) Measurement of carbon dioxide in blood. CRC Critical Reviews in Clinical Laboratory Sciences, pp. 99–120.

Hamburger, H.J. (1902) Osmotischer Druck und Ionenlehre, 1st edn. pp. 1–539, J.F. Bergman, Wiesbaden.

Henry, R.J., Cannon, D.C. and Winkelman, J.W. (1974) Clinical Chemistry, Principles and Technics, 2nd edn. Harper and Row, Hagerstown, Maryland.

Hlastala, M.P., McKenna, H.P., Franada, R.L. and Detter, J.C. (1976) Influence of carbon monoxide on hemoglobin–oxygen binding. Journal of Applied Physiology, 41, 893–899.

Howell, B.J., Baumgardner, F.W., Bondi, K. and Rahn, H. (1970) Acid–base balance in cold-blooded vetebrates as a function of body temperature. American Journal of Physiology, 218, 600–606.

Huch, A., Huch, R., Arner, B. and Rooth, G. (1973) Continous transcutaneous oxygen tension measured with a heated electrode. Scandinavian Journal of Clinical and Laboratory Investigation, 31, 269–275.

Ichiyanagi, K., Masuko, K., Nishisaka, N., Matsuki, M., Horikawa, H. and Watanabee, R. (1969) Acid–base changes of arterial plasma during exogenous and endogenous hypercapnia in man. Respiration Physiology, 7, 310–325.

International Organization for Standardization (1974) General Principles Concerning Quantities, Units and Symbols. International Standard ISO, 31/0, 1–14.

Jacobsen, E. and Rosen, J. (1975) Improved syringe for arterial blood sampling. Anaesthesiology, 42, 112.

Jørgensen, K. and Astrup, P. (1957) Standard bicarbonate, its clinical significance, and a new method for its determination. Scandinavian Journal of Clinical and Laboratory Investigation, 9, 122–132.

Kilburn, K.H. (1966) Movements of potassium during acute respiratory acidosis and recovery. Journal of Applied Physiology, 21, 679–684.

Kildeberg, P. and Engel, K. (1971) Metabolic alkalosis in infants: Role of water depletion and changes in composition of stool. Acta Paediatrica Scandinavica, 60, 637–641.

Kilmartin, J.V. (1972) Molecular mechanisms of the Bohr effect. Alfred Benzon Symposium (Copenhagen), 4, 93–100.

Lotz, P., Dahners, N. and Pichotka, J.P. (1970) Massenspektrometrische Bestimnung des O_2 und CO_2 Gehaltes von Blut. Pfluegers Archiv Gesammelte Physiologie Menschen und Tiere, 315, 86–92.

Maas, A.H.J. (1970) A titrimetric method for the determination of actual bicarbonate in cerebrospinal fluid and plasma or serum. Clinica Chimica Acta, 29, 567–574.

Maas, A.H.J., van Heijst, A.N.P. and Visser, B.F. (1971) The determination of the true equilibrium constant ($p\bar{K}_{1g}$) and the practical equilibrium coefficient ($p\widetilde{K}_{1g}$) for the first ionization of carbonic acid in solutions of sodium bicarbonate, cerebrospinal fluid, plasma, and serum at 25 °C and 38 °C. Clinica Chimica Acta, 33, 325–343.

Malan, A., Arens, H. and Waechter, A. (1973) Pulmonary respiration and acid–base state in hibernating marmots and hamsters. Respiration Physiology, 17, 45–61.

Maren, T.H. (1967) Carbonic anhydrase: chemistry, physiology and inhibition. Physiological Reviews, 47, 595–78.

Masoro, E.J. and Siegel, P.D. (1971) Acid–Base Regulation: Its Physiology and Pathophysiology. W.B. Saunders Company, Philadelphia, London, Toronto.

Metcalfe, J. and Dhindsa, D. (1972) The physiological effects of displacements of the oxygen dissociation curve. Alfred Benzon Symposium (Copenhagen) 4, 613–628.

Mitchell, R.A., Loeschcke, H.H., Massion, W. and Severinghaus, J.W. (1963) Respiratory responses mediated through superficial chemosensitive areas on the medulla. Journal of Applied Physiology, 18, 523–533.

Moore, W.J. (1972) Physical Chemistry, 5th edn. Longman Group Ltd., London.

Nahas, G.G. (1963) The clinical pharmacology of THAM (Tris(hydroxymethyl)-aminomethane). Clinical Pharmacology and Therapeutics, 4, 784–803.

Nahas, G.G. (Ed.) (1966) Current Concepts of Acid–Base Measurement (Symposium). Annals of the New York Academy of Science, 133, 1–274.

Nahas, G.G. (1974) Mechanisms of carbon dioxide and pH effects on metabolism. In Carbon Dioxide and Metabolic Regulations (Eds. G.G. Nahas and K.E. Schaefer) pp. 107–117, Springer-Verlag, New York.

Nahas, G.G. and Schaefer, K.E. (Eds.) (1974) Carbon Dioxide and Metabolic Regulations (Symposium). Springer-Verlag, New York.

Natelson, S. (1951) Routine use of ultramicro methods in the clinical laboratory. A practical micro gasometer for estimation of carbon dioxide. American Journal of Clinical Pathology, 21, 1153–1172.

Natelson, S. and Natelson, E.A. (1975) Principles of Applied Clinical Chemistry, I. Maintenance of Fluid and Electrolyte Balance, pp. 393, Plenum Publishing Corp., New York.

Ortega, F.G. (1969) Clinical Blood Gas Analysis. Comparison and Evaluation of Some Methods, Particularly Gas Chromatography (Thesis), 1st edn. pp. 1–163, VRG Off-set Drukkerij, Groningen, The Netherlands.

Payne, J.P. and Hill, D.W. (Eds.) (1975) Oxygen Measurements in Biology and Medicine (Symposium). pp. 1–415, Butterworths, London.

Pedersen, K.O. (1971) The effect of bicarbonate, pCO_2, and pH on serum calcium fractions. Scandinavian Journal of Clinical and Laboratory Investigation, 27, 145–150.

Perutz, M.F. (1970) Stereochemistry of cooperative effects in haemoglobin. Haem–haem interaction and the problem of allostery. The Bohr effect and combination with organic phosphates. Nature (London), 228, 726–739.

Peters, J.P. and Van Slyke, D.D. (1946) Quantitative Clinical Chemistry. I. Interpretations, 2nd edn. Williams and Wilkins, Baltimore.

Rabinow, B.E., Geisel, A., Webb, L.E. and Natelson, S. (1977) Automated system for infrared spectrometric analysis for total CO_2 of plasma contained in capillary tubes. Clinical Chemistry, 23, 180–185.

Rahn, H. (1974) P_{CO_2}, pH and body temperature. In Carbon Dioxide and Metabolic Regulations (Eds. G.G. Nahas and K.E. Schaefer) pp. 152–160, Springer-Verlag, New York.

Rahn, H. and Fenn, W.O. (1955) Graphical Analysis of the Respiratory Gas Exchange. American Physiological Society, Washington.

Rapoport, S. and Luebering, J. (1950) The formation of 2,3-diphosphoglycerate in rabbit erythrocytes. The existence of a diphosphoglyceratemutase. Journal of Biological Chemistry, 183, 507–516.

Rapoport, S. (1968) The regulation of glycolysis in mammalian erythrocytes. In Essays in Biochemistry, Vol. 4 (Eds. P.N. Campbell and G.D. Greville) p. 69, Academic Press, New York, London.

Reiner, M. (1953) Carbon dioxide determination by the Van Slyke volumetric and manometric apparatus. Standard Methods of Clinical Chemistry, 1, 23–36.

Rispens, P., Brunsting, J.R., Zijlstra, W.G. and Van Kampen, E.J. (1969) Determination of total carbon dioxide in blood and plasma by means of the cediometer: theory and experimental verification. Clinica Chimica Acta, 22, 261–270.

Rispens, P. (1970) Significance of Plasma Bicarbonate for the Evaluation of H^+ Homeostasis. Van Gorcum, Assen, The Netherlands.

Rooth, G. (1974) Acid–Base and Electrolyte Balance, pp. 118, Studentlitteratur Publication, Year Book Medical Publishers Inc., Chicago.

Rørth, M. (1972) Hemoglobin interactions and red cell metabolism. Series Haematologica, 5, 1–104.

Rørth, M. and Astrup, P. (Eds.) (1972) Oxygen affinity of hemoglobin and red cell acid base status, Alfred Benzon Symposium IV. Munksgaard, Copenhagen and Academic Press, New York.

Saling, E. (1966) Das Kind im Bereich der Geburtshilfe. pp. 219, Thieme, Stutgart.

Saugstad, O.D. (1975) Hypoxanthine as a measurement of hypoxia. Pediatric Research 9, 158–161.

Schaer, H. (1974) Decrease in ionized calcium by bicarbonate in physiological solutions. Pfluegers Archives, 347, 249–254.

Schwartz, W.B. and Relman, S.A. (1963) A critique of the parameters used in the evaluation of acid–base disorders. New England Journal of Medicine, 268, 1382–1388.

Schwartz, W.B. (1975) Disorders of fluid, electrolyte, and acid–base balance. In Textbook of Medicine, 14th edn. (Eds. P.B. Beeson and W. McDermott) pp. 1579–1599, W.B. Saunders Co., Philidelphia.

Severinghaus, J.W. (1960) Methods of measurement of blood and gas carbon dioxide during anesthesia. Anesthesiology, 27, 717–726.

Severinghaus, J.W. (1966) Blood gas calculator, Journal of Applied Physiology, 21, 1108–1116.

Severinghaus, J.W. and Bradley, A.F. (1958) Electrodes for blood pO_2 and pCO_2 determination. Journal of Applied Physiology, 13, 515–520.

Shaw, L.A. and Messer, A.C. (1932) The transfer of bicarbonate between the blood and tissues caused by alterations of carbon dioxide concentration in the lungs. American Journal of Physiology, 100, 122–136.

Siggaard–Andersen, O. (1963) Blood acid–base alignment nomogram. Scales for pH, pCO_2, base excess of whole blood of different hemoglobin concentrations, plasma bicarbonate, and plasma total CO_2. Scandinavian Journal of Clinical and Laboratory Investigation, 15, 211–217.

Siggaard-Andersen, O. (1971) An acid–base chart for arterial blood with normal and pathophysiological reference areas. Scandinavian Journal of Clinical and Laboratory Investigation, 27, 239–245.

Siggaard-Andersen, O. (1974) The Acid–Base Status of the Blood, 4th edn. Munksgaard, Copenhagen and William and Wilkins, Baltimore.

Siggaard-Andersen, O. (1977a) Stoichiometric concentration and chemical potential. Scandinavian Journal of Clinical and Laboratory Investigation, 37, Suppl. 146, 7–13.

Siggaard-Andersen, O. (1977b) The Van Slyke equation. Scandinavian Journal of Clinical and Laboratory Investigation, 37, Suppl. 146, 15–20.

Siggaard-Andersen, O. (1977c) Experiences with a new direct reading oxygen saturation photometer using ultrasound for hemolyzing the blood. Scandinavian Journal of Clinical and Laboratory Investigation, 37, Suppl. 146, 45–50.

Siggaard-Andersen, O. and Engel, K. (1960) A new acid–base nomogram. An improved method for calculation of the relevant acid–base data. Scandinavian Journal of Clinical and Laboratory Investigation, 12, 177–186.

Siggaard-Andersen, O. and Garby, L. (1973) The Bohr effect and the Haldane effect (Editorial). Scandinavian Journal of Clinical and Laboratory Investigation, 31, 1–8.

Siggaard-Andersen, O., Nørgaard-Pedersen, B. and Rem, J. (1972) Hemoglobin pigments. I. Spectrophotometric determination of oxy-, carboxy-, met-, and sulfhemoglobin in capillary blood. Clinica Chimica Acta, 42, 85–100.

Siggaard-Andersen, O., Salling, N., Nørgaard-Pedersen, B. and Rørth, M. (1972) Oxygen-linked hydrogen ion binding of human hemoglobin. Effects of carbon dioxide and 2,3-diphosphoglycerate. III. Comparison of the Bohr effect and the Haldane effect. Scandinavian Journal of Clinical and Laboratory Investigation, 29, 185–193.

Singer, R.B. and Hastings, A.B. (1948) An improved method for the estimation of disturbances of the acid–base balance of human blood. Medicine (Baltimore), 27, 223–242.

Skeggs, L.T. (1960) An automatic method for the determination of carbon dioxide in blood plasma. American Journal of Clinical Pathology, 33, 181–185.

Sørensen, S.C. (1971) The chemical control of ventilation (Thesis). Acta Physiologica Scandinavica, Suppl. 361, 1–72.

Stow, R.W., Baer, R.F. and Randall, B.F. (1957) Rapid measurement of the tension of carbon dioxide in the blood. Archives of Physical and Medical Rehabilitation, 38, 646–650.

Tietz, N.W. (Ed.) (1976) Fundamentals of Clinical Chemistry, 2nd edn. W.B. Saunders Co., Philidelphia.

Truchot, J.P. (1973) Temperature and acid–base regulation in the shore crab *Carcinus maenas* (L.). Respiration Physiology, 17, 11–20.

Van Slyke, D.D. and Neil, J.M. (1924) The determination of gases in blood and other solutions by vacuum extraction and manometric measurement. Journal of Biological Chemistry, 61, 523–575.

Weisberg, H.F. (1975) Water, Electrolyte, and Acid–Base Balance; Normal and Pathologic Physiology as a Basis for Therapy, 3rd edn. William and Wilkins Co., Baltimore.

Winters, R.W. (1966) Terminology of acid–base disorders. Annals of the New York Academy of Science, 133, 211–224.

Wolding, S., Owens, G. and Woolford, D. (1966) Blood gases: continous in vivo recording of partial pressures by mass spectrography. Science, 153, 885–887.

Zijlstra, W.G. (1958) A Manual of Reflection Oximetry. Van Gorcum, Assen, The Netherlands.

FURTHER READING

Antonini, E. and Brunori, M. (1971) Hemoglobin and Myoglobin in their Reaction with Ligands. North-Holland Publishing Co., Amsterdam.

Bates, R.G. (1973) Determination of pH. Theory and Practice, 3rd edn. John Wiley and Sons, New York.

Campbell, E.J.M. (1974) Hydrogen ion (acid–base) regulation. In Clinical Physiology, 4th edn. (Eds. E.J.M. Campbell, C.J. Dickinson and J.D.M. Slater), Chap. 5, Blackwell Scientific Publications, Oxford.

Cohen, R.D. and Woods, H.F. (1976) Clinical and Metabolic Aspects of Lactic Acidosis. Blackwell Scientific Publications, Oxford.

Cunningham, D.J.C. and Lloyd, B.B. (1963) The Regulation of Human Respiration. Blackwell Scientific Publications, Oxford.

Davenport, H.W. (1974) The ABC of Acid–Base Chemistry. The Elements of Physiological Blood-Gas Chemistry for Medical Students and Physicians, 6th edn. University of Chicago Press, Chicago.

Dybkaer, R. (1970) Nomenclature for quantities and units. Standard Methods of Clinical Chemistry, 6, 223–244.

Gill, P.E. and Brown, S.S. (1976) Measurement of carbon dioxide in blood. CRC Critical Reviews in Clinical Laboratory Sciences, 7, 99–120.

International Organization for Standardization (1974) General Principles Concerning Quantities, Units and Symbols. International Standard ISO, 31/0, 1–14.

Nahas, G.G. (Ed.) (1966) Current Concepts of Acid–Base Measurement (Symposium). Annals of the New York Academy of Science, 133, 1–274.

Natelson, S. and Natelson, E.A. (1975) Principles of Applied Clinical Chemistry. I. Maintenance of Fluid and Electrolyte Balance. Plenum Publishing Corp., New York.

Peters, J.P. and Van Slyke, D.D. (1946) Quantitative Clinical Chemistry. I. Interpretations, 2nd edn. William and Wilkins, Baltimore.

Rispens, P. (1970) Significance of Plasma Bicarbonate for the Evaluation of H^+ Homeostasis. Van Gorcum, Assen, The Netherlands.

Rooth, G. (1974) Acid–Base and Electrolyte Balance, Studentlitteratur Publication, Year Book Medical Publishers Inc., Chicago.

Rørth, M. (1972) Hemoglobin interactions and red cell metabolism. Series Haematologica, 5, 1–104.

Schwartz, W.B. (1975) Disorders of fluid, electrolyte, and acid–base balance. In Textbook of Medicine, 14th edn. (Eds. P.B. Beeson and W. McDermott) pp. 1579–1599, W.B. Saunders Co., Philidelphia.

Siggaard-Andersen, O. (1974) The Acid–Base Status of the Blood, 4th edn. Munksgaard, Copenhagen and William and Wilkins, Baltimore.

Chapter 4

Glucose metabolism

C. Nicholas Hales and Robert D.G. Milner

Department of Biochemistry, Addenbrooke's Hospital, Hills Road, Cambridge CB2 2QR and Department of Paediatrics, Children's Hospital, Sheffield S10 2TH, England

CONTENTS

Chemical diagnosis of disease, edited by S.S. Brown, F.L. Mitchell and D.S. Young

4.1. INTRODUCTION

A comprehensive account of all the many clinical situations in which the metabolism of glucose is altered is clearly impossible, even within the well-defined objectives of this volume. Indeed, there are a number of subsections of the topic which have been the subject of entire monographs, some of which we have recommended for further reading. We have, therefore, been highly selective in this presentation. Inevitably our selection has been biased by our own particular interests within the subject. However, we hope that our attempts to concentrate on the areas of major clinical importance have been at least partially successful. Equally, we are aware of a need to cut corners by the use of dogmatic statements on matters over which there is still room for debate. We justify this on the grounds of brevity and as a result of the editors' instructions that we are to avoid a review format which attempts to mention everybody and decide nothing. We are very grateful to our many colleagues who have provided guidance and helpful discussion: they shall not be named for fear of involving them in the shortcomings of our effort.

4.2. NORMAL GLUCOSE METABOLISM IN MAN

The oral glucose tolerance test remains the most widely used diagnostic procedure in the investigation of glucose metabolism in man. Therefore, in attempting to provide a brief review of the mechanisms responsible for the maintenance of normal glucose homeostatis, we have chosen to concentrate on those mechanisms likely to be involved in the oral glucose tolerance test. This test can be regarded essentially as a slow switch that converts carbohydrate, lipid and protein metabolism from the pattern characteristic of the overnight fasting state into that of the carbohydrate-fed state. In the mildest form of diabetes, the main demonstrable abnormality is the increased time taken for this complex mechanism to operate. Viewed in this light, there are three elements in the description of normal glucose metabolism: the relatively steady metabolic state that is the normal sequel of an overnight fast; the qualitative changes in this state which are produced by the uptake of glucose from the gut; and finally, a quantitative description of the rate and amount of change occurring in the transition between the two metabolic states.

The complex series of metabolic alterations which glucose induces is due both to the increase in circulating glucose concentration and to the associated changes in hormone concentrations. In order to simplify the discussion of these changes, the effects of glucose on a number of endocrine systems are described first. This is followed by an account of the state of glucose metabolism after an overnight fast. Finally, the endocrine mechanisms which act to regulate metabolism during the absorption and utilization of oral glucose are described. Wherever possible, quantitative estimates of glucose utilization are given in order to illustrate the relative importance of the metabolic pathways.

4.2.1. Neurological and endocrine effects of glucose

4.2.1.1. Autonomic nervous system

The autonomic nervous system has been shown to affect insulin secretion, both basal and glucose-stimulated, in a number of preparations. Relatively little is known of how important such mechanisms may be in maintaining glucose tolerance. Nevertheless, since changes which occur in pathological states, such as severe stress or trauma, may be related to the effects of the autonomic nervous system, a brief summary of these observations is included here.

Cholinergic compounds and stimulation of the vagus nerve are capable of eliciting insulin secretion, and the latter effect is blocked by atropine. It is possible that such a mechanism is involved during the oral glucose tolerance test, and even more likely that neurogenic stimulation may play a part in insulin release during normal nutrition.

Adrenaline and noradrenaline inhibit insulin secretion – an effect which appears to be mediated via an adrenergic α-receptor of the β-cell itself. Under conditions in which this α-receptor is blocked, evidence has been obtained for a β-mediated adrenaline stimulation of insulin secretion. In man, basal insulin secretion appears to be modulated by adrenergic activity, since infusion of phentolamine (an α-blocker) in the fasting state raises basal insulin concentrations, whereas propranalol (a β-blocker) lowers them (Robertson and Porte, 1973). It is not known whether the administration of glucose affects this proposed tonic control of basal insulin secretion.

4.2.1.2. Gut hormones

In man, the intraduodenal infusion of glucose results in higher peripheral plasma insulin concentrations than are observed if the same blood glucose concentrations are produced by an intravenous glucose infusion (McIntyre et al., 1964). One possible explanation of this effect is that there is stimulation of the secretion of a gut hormone which in turn potentiates the action of glucose on the β-cell. A number of gut factors have been investigated with this possibility in mind, including secretin, gastrin, gut glucagon-like immunoreactive substances, cholecystokinin–pancreozymin and gastric inhibitory polypeptide (see review by Brown, 1974). While it is not yet clear whether the effects of any one of these compounds can explain the difference between the responses to oral and intravenous glucose, gastric inhibitory peptide has many of the necessary characteristics.

4.2.1.3. Insulin

Glucose acts directly on the β-cell to stimulate insulin release and biosynthesis. These effects are most marked over the range of concentrations observed in plasma during an oral glucose tolerance test. Although a number of other compounds of nutritional, diagnostic or therapeutic importance, such as amino acids (e.g. leucine and arginine) and the sulphonylureas, stimulate insulin secretion, glucose is so far the only physiologically important compound which has been shown to have a stimulatory effect on insulin synthesis.

Our understanding of the pathway of insulin synthesis and storage has advanced greatly in the last few years, thanks to the discovery of the insulin precursor proinsulin (Steiner et al., 1972). Since a knowledge of this pathway has important implications for the investigation and treatment of abnormalities of insulin secretion, the major facts will be summarized.

Proinsulin is a single chain disulphide-bridged molecule with a molecular weight of approximately 9000 which is converted into insulin by the removal of the C-peptide and four basic amino acids (Figure 4.1). The enzýmes responsible for this cleavage have not been isolated but the process appears to take place during the production of the insulin-storage granule. As a result, insulin is "co-packaged" and secreted with equimolar amounts of C-peptide. Under normal conditions, the stimulation of insulin secretion leads to very little release of proinsulin. However, insulin, proinsulin and C-peptide – together with other ill-characterized compounds of still higher molecular weight containing insulin-like immunological activity – may be extracted from normal animal or human pancreas. One important consequence of this, as will become obvious later, is the inclusion of these, often highly antigenic, compounds in many therapeutic preparations of insulin.

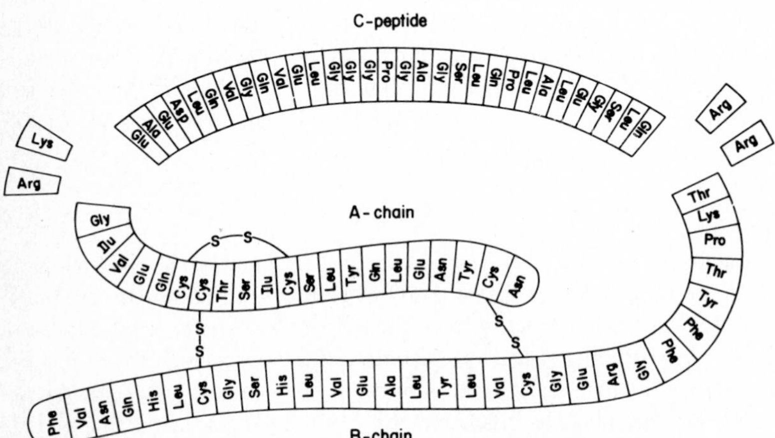

Fig. 4.1. Structure of human proinsulin and its cleavage to insulin and C-peptide. The four basic aminoacids released during cleavage are shown slightly displaced from the sequence; it is assumed that these aminoacids are identical to those which have been shown to be in these positions in both porcine and bovine proinsulin (drawn after the fashion of Steiner et al., 1972).

Although there are only slight differences between the amino acid sequence of human insulin and those which are used therapeutically (porcine and bovine insulin), there are much greater differences in the sequences of the respective C-peptides (Table 4.1). Thus,

TABLE 4.1.

COMPARISON OF THE SEQUENCES OF C-PEPTIDES FROM PROINSULINS OF VARIOUS SPECIES

Note that in some species deletions (–) have occurred and the aminoacids have been placed to show the maximum homology (from the data in Snell and Smythe, 1975).

	C1	2	3	4	5	6	7	8	9	10	11
Human	Glu	Ala	Glu	Asp	Leu	Gln	Val	Gly	Gln	Val	Glu
Monkey	Glu	Ala	Glu	Asp	Pro	Gln	Val	Gly	Gln	Val	Glu
Pig	Glu	Ala	Glu	Asn	Pro	Gln	Ala	Gly	Ala	Val	Glu
Ox, sheep	Glu	Val	Glu	Gly	Pro	Gln	Val	Gly	Ala	Leu	Glu
Guinea pig	Glu	Leu	Glu	Asp	Pro	Gln	Val	Glu	Gln	Thr	Glu
Chinchilla	Glu	Leu	Glu	Asp	Pro	Gln	Val	Gly	Gln	Ala	Asp
Rat I	Glu	Val	Glu	Asp	Pro	Gln	Val	Pro	Gln	Leu	Glu
Rat II	Glu	Val	Glu	Asp	Pro	Gln	Val	Ala	Gln	Leu	Glu
Horse	Glu	Ala	Glu	Asp	Pro	Gln	Val	Gly	Glu	Val	Glu
Dog									Asp	Val	Glu

	12	13	14	15	16	17	18	19	20	21	22
Human	Leu	Gly	Gly	Gly	Pro	Gly	Ala	Gly	Ser	Leu	Gln
Monkey	Leu	Gly	Gly	Gly	Pro	Gly	Ala	Gly	Ser	Leu	Gln
Pig	Leu	Gly	Gly	Gly	Leu	–	–	Gly	Gly	Leu	Gln
Ox, sheep	Leu	Ala	Gly	Gly	Pro	Gly	Ala	Gly	Gly	Leu	–
Guinea pig	Leu	Gly	Met	Gly	Leu	Gly	Ala	Gly	Gly	Leu	Gln
Chinchilla	Pro	Gly	Val	Val	Pro	Glu	Ala	Gly	Arg	Leu	Gln
Rat I	Leu	Gly	Gly	Gly	Pro	Glu	Ala	Gly	Asp	Leu	Gln
Rat II	Leu	Gly	Gly	Gly	Pro	Gly	Ala	Gly	Asp	Leu	Gln
Horse	Leu	Gly	Gly	Gly	Pro	Gly	Leu	Gly	Gly	Leu	Gln
Dog	Leu	Ala	Gly	Ala	Pro	Gly	Glu	Gly	Gly	Leu	Gln

	23	24	25	26	27	28	29	30	31
Human	Pro	Leu	Ala	Leu	Glu	Gly	Ser	Leu	Gln
Monkey	Pro	Leu	Ala	Leu	Glu	Gly	Ser	Leu	Gln
Pig	Ala	Leu	Ala	Leu	Glu	Gly	Pro	Pro	Gln
Ox, sheep	–	–	–	–	Glu	Gly	Pro	Pro	Gln
Guinea pig	Pro	Leu	–	–	Gln	Gly	Ala	Leu	Gln
Chinchilla	Pro	Leu	Ala	Leu	Glu	Met	Thr	Leu	Gln
Rat I	Thr	Leu	Ala	Leu	Glu	Val	Ala	Arg	Gln
Rat II	Thr	Leu	Ala	Leu	Glu	Val	Ala	Arg	Gln
Horse	Pro	Leu	Ala	Leu	Ala	Gly	Pro	Gln	Gln
Dog	Pro	Leu	Ala	Leu	Glu	Gly	Ala	Leu	Gln

whilst antibodies prepared against one of these three insulins frequently cross-react with the other two, this is not the case for antibodies against the C-peptides.

The release of insulin in response to glucose is subject to adaptation over a period of days according to the carbohydrate intake. A severe reduction in the carbohydrate content of the diet (in man, to less than 50 g/day) causes a reduced and delayed rise in plasma insulin concentration following oral glucose. Experiments in animals have shown that after 48 hours' restriction of carbohydrate intake, the reduced insulin release is not explained by a reduction in the insulin content of the pancreas. There is some evidence in animals that an unusually high carbohydrate intake may be accompanied by an adaptive change in the opposite direction.

4.2.1.4. Glucagon

A rise in the blood glucose concentration reduces the release of glucagon from the A_2-cells of the islets of Langerhans. This effect occurs over the physiological range of blood glucose concentration and requires the presence of insulin (Unger, 1974). Glucagon secretion is also affected by the sympathetic system, being stimulated by catecholamines and by stimulation of the sympathetic nerves. To what extent basal and glucose-depressed glucagon secretion are modulated through the release of catecholamines is not known. The hyperglucagonaemia of shock may be mediated via adrenergic and cortisol stimulation of the A_2-cells (Unger, 1974).

There appears to be a number of immunologically glucagon-like polypeptides in the gut, which may interfere with the immunoassay of pancreatic glucagon in plasma. Their physiological role is, at present, undefined. It is also uncertain whether an endocrine link operates to suppress glucagon secretion by the A_2-cells; such a link would be analogous – but reciprocal to – that mediating the effect of glucose in the gut to stimulate insulin secretion.

Unger (1974) has emphasized the importance of considering insulin and glucagon together in the regulation of glucose metabolism. Glucose, presumably because of its significance as a source of energy for the brain, provides the dominating regulatory factor in man, but its actions are modulated by the autonomic nervous system and by hormones produced by the intestine and the adrenal gland. An important implication of this relationship between insulin and glucagon is that henceforth increasing emphasis will be placed on changes in glucagon concentration, in considering the aetiology and treatment of disorders of glucose metabolism. Agents such as somatostatin have clearly demonstrated the dramatic effects which reduction of glucagon release can have on glucose metabolism.

4.2.1.5. Growth hormone

The concentration of growth hormone in plasma falls after the administration of oral glucose. There is a marked rebound rise in concentration 2 to 5 hours later. The mechanism of the latter phenomenon is not known but may be associated with relative hypoglycaemia. Insulin-induced hypoglycaemia is a potent means of stimulating the release of growth hormone.

4.2.2. Glucose metabolism after an overnight fast

In this relatively steady state, glucose is produced predominantly by the liver as a result of gluconeogenesis and glycogenolysis; the rate of production equals the consumption by peripheral tissues. Not more than 20% of the glucose so produced is contributed by the kidneys. This proportion, however, rises considerably during prolonged starvation or in acidosis. The contribution of total glucose oxidation to the energy requirements of the body in starvation is quite small, since lipid oxidation is responsible for the provision of over 80% of energy.

4.2.2.1. Gluconeogenic pathways

Gluconeogenesis may be conceived as a segment of two different types of inter-tissue metabolic pathway. In the first (Figure 4.2), non-carbohydrate substances – mainly aminoacids and glycerol – are converted into glucose for complete oxidation in tissues where glucose oxidation is essential in the fasting state. The second type of pathway is cyclic and involves no net synthesis or oxidation of glucose: the best known example is the glucose–lactate (Cori) cycle, but it has recently been proposed that a glucose–

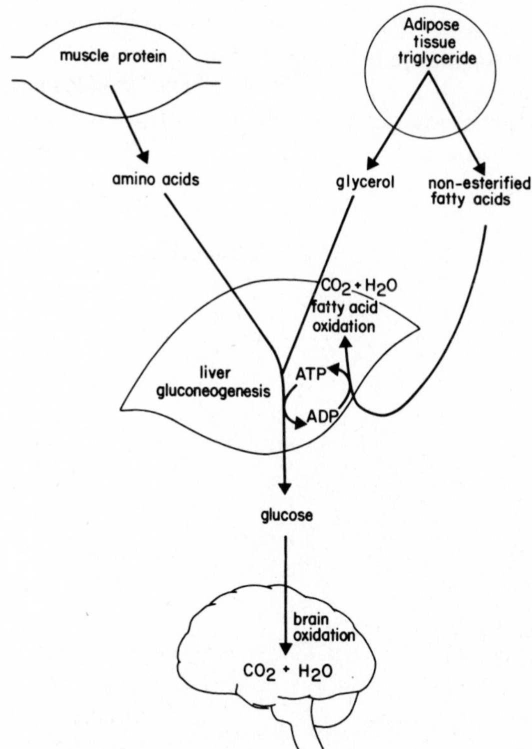

Fig. 4.2. Inter-tissue pathway for the conversion of amino acids and glycerol from muscle and adipose tissue to glucose for complete oxidation by brain.

alanine cycle (Figure 4.3) is of similar importance (Felig, 1973). Quantitative estimates of the components show that there is an hepatic output of approximately 10 g glucose per hour, after an overnight fast. Approximately 7% comes from the conversion of non-carbohydrates into glucose, and of this fraction one-third is derived from adipose tissue triglyceride glycerol. The Cori cycle, in which should be included lactate produced by blood cells, accounts for 10 to 15% of the total glucose production, and the alanine cycle 5 to 10%. Therefore, about 70% comes from glycogenolysis. Details of the relevant hepatic intracellular metabolic reactions are provided in a review by Exton (1972).

The Cori and glucose–alanine cycles function on an inter-tissue basis in a fashion analogous to the cycles between enzyme pathways which are mediated by co-factors such as ATP (Campbell and Hales, 1976). In essence, glucose produced by the liver carries energy derived from fatty acid oxidation by the liver (Figure 4.3) mainly to muscle and red cells, and pyruvate carries back amino groups in the form of alanine. The ability to carry amino groups in this apparently innocuous fashion is clearly of considerable importance. The precise fate of the carbon skeletons released from the other amino acids during deamination is uncertain. Aminoacids such as leucine, isoleucine and valine are very readily oxidized by muscle, but a quantitative balance sheet of this pathway in comparison with those for metabolism in the liver and elsewhere has yet to be worked out.

It may be seen from Figure 4.3 that lactate does not – contrary to some statements – carry reducing equivalents back to the liver since, in the redox sense, it is equivalent to glucose. Lactate is better considered in the Cori cycle as being analogous to ADP since, by conversion into glucose, it is available to carry some of the free energy from fatty acid oxidation to muscle and red cells.

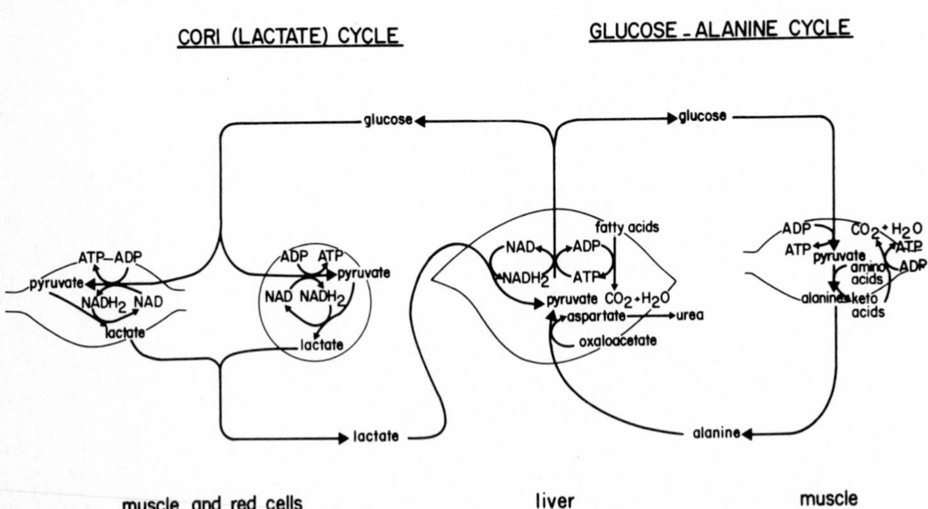

Fig. 4.3. Cori and glucose–alanine cycles showing the role of gluconeogenesis in pathways which do not involve net glucose oxidation, but may act as carriers of the free energy of oxidation of fatty acids by liver.

4.2.2.2. Gluconeogenic regulation

The rates of hepatic uptake and utilization of gluconeogenic precursors are affected by the type and quantity of the precursor presented. Thus a prime point of regulation is the output of aminoacids, lactate and pyruvate by peripheral tissues. There is a close correlation between the circulating concentrations of these substances in the basal state, presumably due to the fact that the rates of pyruvate production and utilization by muscle are most important determinants of their rates of release by this tissue. The rates of amino acid oxidation and output by muscle are regulated by the action of insulin so as to inhibit proteolysis and stimulate protein synthesis (Figure 4.4). The fall in plasma insulin concentration consequent upon fasting could account for the subsequent negative nitrogen balance exhibited by muscle. At the same time, increased oxidation of the carbon skeletons of valine, leucine and isoleucine, and of fatty acids and ketone bodies, serves to inhibit oxidation of pyruvate, thereby increasing its availability for transamination to alanine.

The role of the other hormones in regulating protein metabolism and aminoacid release by muscle is less well understood. Glucocorticoids increase protein breakdown in vivo, but the concentration range in man over which this occurs, and its significance in the resting state after an overnight fast, are not clear. Glucagon has an important stimulatory effect on gluconeogenesis and on the maintenance of blood glucose concentration, but whether this is mediated partially by direct effects on muscle after a shorter fast is uncertain.

Hepatic gluconeogenesis is regulated both by substrate supply and by hormones. High concentrations of long chain fatty acids stimulate gluconeogenesis, but the concentrations which are found in plasma after an overnight fast may be too low to be important under these conditions. Glucagon stimulates aminoacid uptake by the liver and gluconeogenesis, and this process is dependent on the normal availability of glucocorticoids. Insulin opposes the process. Thus, after an overnight fast, a key factor regulating hepatic gluconeogenesis is likely to be the insulin/glucagon ratio in portal blood.

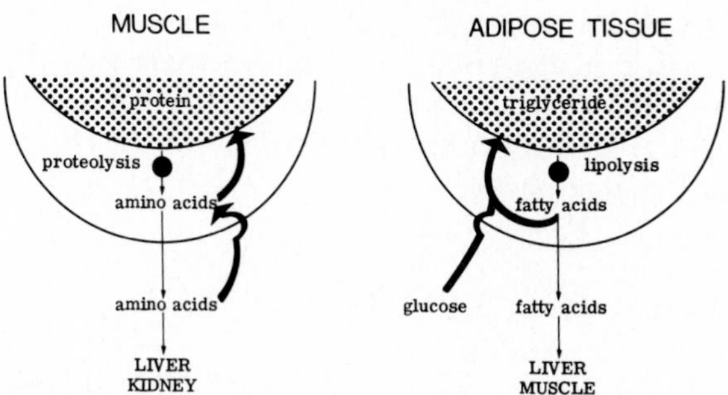

Fig. 4.4. Some actions of insulin which may mediate the effect of carbohydrate intake to inhibit breakdown of protein and triglyceride. (→, stimulation; -●- , inhibition, [transport symbol], transport).

4.2.2.3. *Glycogenolysis*

Although the amount of glycogen in a normal liver is too small to sustain more than a short period of total starvation, it would seem that in man it is quantitatively the most important source of glucose during the usual intervals between meals. Thus, at such times, 70 to 80% of hepatic glucose output may be attributed to hepatic glycogenolysis. The regulation of this process in vivo appears to be mediated by the blood glucose concentration (high levels inhibiting glycogenolysis and stimulating glycogen synthesis) and by the insulin/glucagon ratio in the blood of the portal vein. A fall in this ratio, such as occurs after an overnight fast, serves to activate glycogenolysis.

The amount of glycogen in muscle falls little after an overnight fast, and the main role of this source of carbohydrate is to sustain anaerobic contraction of muscle.

4.2.2.4. *Glucose utilization*

Approximately 60% of the glucose produced by the liver during a short-term fast is completely oxidized by the brain. Most of the remainder of the hepatic output is used by blood cells and muscle. The amount and fate of glucose taken up by muscle is influenced by the availability of other substrates which are available for oxidation as well as by the fall in insulin concentration. The most important alternative substrates are free fatty acids. The plasma concentrations of free fatty acids and of ketone bodies are raised in the fasting state. The fall in concentration of insulin, during fasting, decreases transport of glucose into muscle and glycogen synthesis by this tissue. Glucose uptake may also be reduced during the oxidation of free fatty acids and ketone bodies. A second important effect of the oxidation of the non-glucose substrates is to inhibit oxidation of pyruvate. The result is that the reduced amount of glucose taken up by muscle in the fasting state is only oxidized as far as pyruvate. The pyruvate is then converted into lactate and alanine, so that pyruvate, lactate and alanine are released to be recycled to glucose by the liver. Thus, there is very little complete oxidation of glucose by muscle in the fasting state.

The uptake and utilization of glucose by adipose tissue are insulin dependent and hence greatly reduced during fasting. An important consequence of the reduction of plasma insulin concentration and of glucose uptake by adipose tissue is an enhanced rate of release of free fatty acid by this tissue (Figure 4.4). This in turn increases the circulating concentration of free fatty acids. Fatty acid uptake by tissues such as liver and muscle appears to be mainly regulated by the plasma fatty acid concentration. Hence increased fatty acid oxidation by liver and muscle in the fasting state may be explained. The increased oxidation of fatty acid by the liver appears to be linked to increased ketone body production, since in the fasting state there is a close correlation between the plasma concentrations of free fatty acids and of ketone bodies.

4.3. INVESTIGATION OF GLUCOSE METABOLISM

The measurement of the concentration of glucose in blood poses several technical problems which have been extensively reviewed (Marks, 1969). Authoritative texts on the diagnosis of diabetes continue to reveal a wide range of reference values, and in view of the potential for variation derived from different methods of sampling and assay, and the continuing uncertainty as to the significance of minor changes in glucose tolerance, it is not worthwhile to add another set of arbitrary values to the literature. It is proposed therefore to review some of the more common tests of carbohydrate metabolism, in relation to the diagnostic information which they provide. The role and value of more or less elaborate means of testing carbohydrate metabolism must be viewed in the light of our continued ignorance of the long-term significance of minor changes in the oral glucose test, which has been the standard diagnostic tool for many years. If it is true that we cannot interpret moderate degrees of intolerance to oral glucose in the context of age so as to afford an acceptable prognosis and optimum treatment, little additional value is to be expected from a more controlled test (e.g. intravenous glucose tolerance) or a more physiological test (e.g. oral starch), or one involving the administration of drugs, be they ancient or modern.

4.3.1. Provocative diagnostic tests

4.3.1.1. Oral glucose tolerance test

The fact that the oral glucose test is not highly reproducible is well recognized; nevertheless, it uses the physiological route of carbohydrate absorption and remains the reference test for all other investigations of carbohydrate metabolism. With careful attention to standardization of the procedure, it is certainly adequate to demonstrate degrees of abnormality which warrant treatment. Indeed, in view of the current uncertainties as to the long-term significance of minor – or even moderate – degrees of deviation of oral glucose tolerance test from the norm, and also the controversy surrounding the methods and advantages of treatment, it is only realistic to accept that the standard diagnostic procedures are attended by uncertainties of interpretation. Certain procedures, the results of which are presented as single numbers, may induce an unjustified confidence of interpretation in the unwary observer.

Glucose tolerance deteriorates with age, and in subjects over the age of 60 as many as 20% may have a "diabetic" oral glucose tolerance. Again it has to be recognized that the prognostic significance of such a result is obscure. Undoubtedly, in the present state of knowledge, when treating minor degrees of carbohydrate intolerance in the elderly, due regard should be paid to the impact of treatment on the quality of life of the individual.

The importance of various aspects of preparation of the subject before the test, such as the preceding diet and the length of fast or rest, are matters for debate, but it is clear that they should be standardized as far as possible. The antecedant level of carbohydrate intake can influence glucose tolerance unless the carbohydrate intake is less than 100 g/day; unless there is reason to believe that such a diet may be in use, it is usual to accept the patient's normal intake as adequate preparation for the test. It is sometimes recommended that a diet containing 300 g of carbohydrate be taken for each of three days before the test. However, this is likely to be in excess of the normal intake, and since it is known that a high intake will improve glucose tolerance, there is little point in seeking to relate the results of such a procedure to the patient's usual metabolic pattern. One potential and well recognized difficulty in preparation concerns the patient who has been found to have glucosuria on testing in general practice. Patients are often sufficiently aware of the implications of this finding to reduce their carbohydrate intake spontaneously. This is well known to improve glucose tolerance in mild and moderate diabetics, so that the results of subsequent urine testing may be very misleading.

Glucose tolerance varies according to the time of day, being worse in the afternoon. It is doubtful if this variation reflects a genuine change during normal nutrition, since subjects on standardized meals tend to show lower rather than higher glucose concentrations during mid-day and evening meals (Figure 4.5). This finding, however, does indicate that the results of oral glucose tolerance tests carried out at different times of the day may not be comparable; therefore it is very important to standardize this aspect of the procedure. Chronobiological aspects of glucose metabolism are of considerable interest but have been relatively little studied (see review by Simpson, 1976).

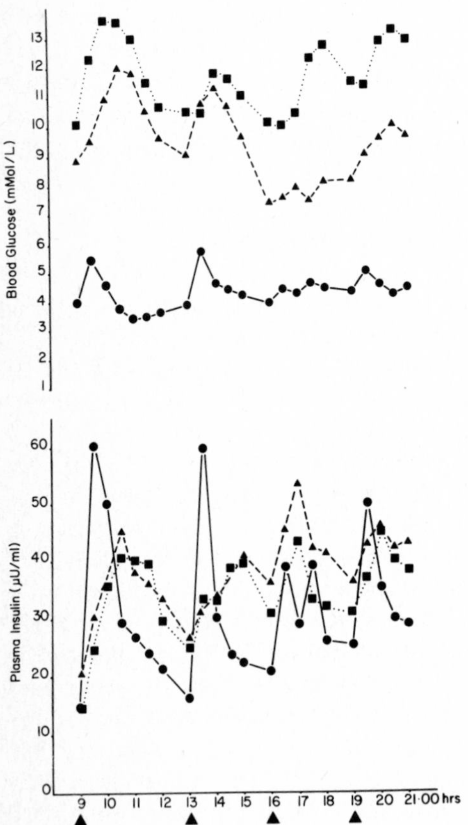

Fig. 4.5. Variations of blood glucose and plasma insulin concentrations in normal subjects and in two groups of diabetic patients (with differing degrees of glucose tolerance) throughout a day in which they were fed four meals each containing the same total calories and carbohydrate, at the times shown ▲. Normal subjects, ●———●; diabetics, ▲- - - - - -▲ and ■· · · · · ·■ (data kindly provided by Dr. D.R. Owens).

The amount of glucose administered in the oral test varies from 50 to 100 g, or may be given as a weight-related dose. In practice, although the plasma insulin concentrations which are achieved may be considerably altered by the amount of glucose given, the concentrations of blood glucose are less affected. The problems of giving a weight-related dose to an obese subject and of the nausea produced by large amounts of glucose have led to the 50 g test being most commonly used, at least in Great Britain. It is usually carried out over a 2-hour period, although periods of 3 to 6 hours are used in the investigation of reactive hypoglycaemia and of growth hormone release.

Variations in oral glucose tolerance due to gastrointestinal factors have been reviewed by Holdsworth (1969), but in spite of these influences, long established use and ease of performance of the test justify its continued application to the diagnosis of diabetes mellitus.

4.3.1.2. Intravenous glucose tolerance test

The advantages claimed for this test are that it avoids the variability associated with gastrointestinal absorption, and that the data it yields may be manipulated to yield a single number which represents glucose tolerance. In the present authors' opinion, these factors are outweighed by the following considerations: there is a much greater wealth of information about the results of the oral test and a better consensus of opinion on the levels of normality, even though these are arbitrary; the oral test is simpler and more acceptable to patients; the representation of the results of an intravenous test by a single number gives an even more arbitrary and disputed index of abnormality, together with a misleading sense of precision; the oral test uses the physiological route.

4.3.1.3. Steroid-augmented glucose tolerance tests

The rationale behind the introduction of these tests was that, by their effect in decreasing glucose tolerance, the use of steroids might afford information about early stages of abnormal carbohydrate metabolism which were not revealed by the administration of glucose alone. Current evaluation of the tests, however, suggests that they merely displace the results of the standard oral glucose tolerance test by an approximately constant factor. Hence they do not provide information which cannot be obtained by careful examination of the results of a standardized test. To put the situation another way, if somewhat arbitrary concentrations of glucose are accepted as indicative of "chemical diabetes", steroid treatment may push certain individuals into this range; they may then be considered in need of careful follow-up. In practice, examination of the results of such an individual's standard oral test, will also show that the glucose concentrations were already higher than those achieved by a comparable subject not made "diabetic" by administration of a steroid.

4.3.1.4. Other tests

As interest has focussed on one or another aspect of the pathology of diabetes or its treatment, so various procedures have been investigated for their effect in modifying metabolism in the disease. Accordingly, many of these procedures have been proposed as "tests" for diabetes, but the diagnosis of clinical diabetes is not a problem: at present, the major uncertainties relate to the long-term effects of subclinical decreases in glucose tolerance, and the effects of treatment. In the absence of definitive long-term studies of these crucial questions, it is hard to see the merit of newer procedures such as the tolbutamide and the steroid–tolbutamide tests.

4.3.2. Measurement of glucose in urine

If a sufficiently sensitive assay is used, glucose can be detected in the urine of most, if not all, normal subjects. Ordinarily, however, the detection of "true" glucose in urine by the usual, less sensitive, screening procedures in the fasting state almost always indicates diabetes mellitus. Renal glucosuria is a rare cause of fasting glucosuria (section 4.6.1.2.) and the possibility of its presence should be eliminated by a glucose tolerance test; it is probably a benign condition, although this interpretation is not universally accepted. The absence of glucose from the urine by no means precludes the diagnosis of diabetes. The significance of glucosuria during a "normal" glucose tolerance test is much more uncertain. The commonest cause is the so-called "lag storage" effect, in which blood glucose concentrations early in the oral glucose tolerance test exceed the renal threshold. There is evidence that such individuals may subsequently develop diabetes.

4.3.3. Measurement of glucose in cerebrospinal fluid

It is an unfortunate fact that the binding of a low glucose concentration in cerebrospinal fluid continues to be the first indication of hypoglycaemia as a cause of unconsciousness in a small proportion of patients (Marks, 1974). It is therefore important to consider hypoglycaemia in the differential diagnosis of the unconscious patient, along with commoner conditions such as poisoning or bacterial meningitis.

In the presence of large numbers of cells and bacteria, the glucose concentration in the cerebrospinal fluid may be reduced. The true cause of such a reduction should be obvious from other investigations and it is doubtful whether, under these circumstances, the estimation of glucose provides useful information.

4.4. INVESTIGATION OF INSULIN METABOLISM

The measurement of insulin in plasma or serum using a radioimmunoassay technique is a relatively straightforward procedure. Although this assay was the first radioimmunoassay method to be introduced, its clinical – as opposed to research – applications remain very limited. Peripheral blood is collected for the assay of insulin, and it has been claimed that the concentration varies according to whether plasma or serum is used. This difference seems to be due to a failure to appreciate that anticoagulants may affect the assay. It is necessary, therefore, to check the effect of anticoagulants, at the appropriate concentrations, on the standard curve since it is not possible to predict whether there will be interference for a particular antiserum. Since insulin is relatively stable in blood at 4 °C, it may be more convenient to assay insulin in serum, thereby eliminating potential variation due to the addition of anticoagulants. Most radioimmunoassays are subject to non-specific effects from proteins which, according to the separation procedure employed, may spuriously elevate or depress the apparent insulin concentration. Such effects are reduced, but not eliminated, by the use of assay and instrument calibrators made up in human serum. As a result, the reference ranges for fasting plasma insulin concentrations vary considerably from laboratory to laboratory. In the past, nearly all patients who had been treated with exogenous insulin for three months or more possessed circulating antibodies to insulin. These antibodies interfered with the radioimmunoassay of insulin, so that invalid results were obtained. More recently, purer preparations of therapeutic insulin have become available and such preparations may not give rise to antibody production. Nevertheless, extreme care must be taken to exclude interference by insulin antibodies in serum when measuring insulin concentration, even if insulin administration has been discontinued for months or even years. Haemolysis also interferes with the assay of insulin, probably because of the release of proteolytic enzymes. It is, therefore, unwise to assay insulin in a plasma or serum specimen which has visible haemolysis.

Insulin is, of course, secreted into the portal circulation, and approximately 50% is thought to be removed during a single passage through the liver. The interpretation of insulin concentrations as measured in peripheral plasma therefore suffers from uncertainty as to the amount and variation of insulin uptake by the liver. Insulin may be measured in portal blood obtained by means of cannulation of the umbilical vein, but this procedure has only been used for research purposes. Proinsulin may be released together with insulin, the ratio of the two varying with the degree of stimulation of insulin secretion. Most antisera to insulin cross-react strongly with proinsulin. This substance has a longer half-life than insulin and so perhaps forms a higher proportion of the apparent insulin content of serum from fasting subjects. Approximately 20% of the insulin determined by immunoassay under these conditions is generally considered to be due to proinsulin. Since this proportion diminishes under stimulation of insulin secretion, interference by proinsulin in the assay is not normally significant.

Insulin-secreting tumours, on the other hand, may release relatively large amounts of proinsulin, and in these circumstances the estimated concentration of insulin in plasma may be seriously in error. A rare cause of an elevated concentration of plasma proinsulin is an apparent defect in the conversion of proinsulin into insulin. This defect has in the past been considered to be a possible cause of diabetes. If a consequence of the defect were a slow uncontrolled steady conversion of proinsulin into insulin peripherally, the apparently surprising feature of hypo- rather than hyper-glycaemia due to sustained insulin action may be explained.

The half-life of insulin in the circulation is approximately 5 minutes, but the mechanisms responsible for insulin removal and destruction are still poorly understood. An hepatic enzyme system capable of splitting the disulphide bonds of insulin has been described, but no good evidence exists that this system is physiologically important. An alternative mechanism which envisages insulin being destroyed while bound to its plasma membrane receptor has been proposed, but also lacks definitive support at present. There is also no well-defined pathological situation resulting from changes in the rate of insulin destruction.

The investigation of insulin metabolism, therefore, includes a number of aspects whose clinical value remains to be fully evaluated. The scope and limitations of the principal assays are now summarized.

4.4.1. Plasma insulin

It is now well established that many diabetics show abnormal patterns of plasma insulin concentration following a number of procedures designed to stimulate secretion of insulin. Unfortunately, there is no good evidence that knowledge of these changes is of value in determining the aetiology or treatment of the condition. Measurement of plasma insulin concentrations after an overnight fast, on at least three separate occasions, and with a knowledge of the blood glucose concentrations, is probably one of the most useful tests in the diagnosis of an insulin-secreting tumour.

4.4.2. Serum proinsulin

Raised concentrations of serum proinsulin in the fasting state are frequently encountered in patients with insulin-secreting tumours. Unfortunately, the assay is technically demanding and it has not been clearly demonstrated that the information so derived is superior to evaluation of the concentrations of plasma insulin and blood glucose.

4.4.3. Serum C-peptide

The assay of C-peptide is also difficult due to the scarcity of reagents and to problems created by cross-reactivity of antisera to human C-peptide with proinsulin. At present, the main value of the technique is in research studies of β-cell function in insulin-treated diabetics, who, as indicated above, may have circulating antibodies to insulin which interfere with the immunoassay of insulin. C-peptide is secreted in equimolar amounts to insulin and is highly species-specific. It is possible, therefore, to assess β-cell function by determination of changes in the peripheral concentration of C-peptide in patients who have insulin antibodies and who may be receiving heterologous C-peptide as a contaminant of therapeutic insulin. Human proinsulin is capable of binding to circulating insulin antibodies and therefore it may still react with antibodies to human C-peptides. Thus, in order to assay the latter specifically, it is necessary to remove antibody-bound or free proinsulin.

4.4.4. Insulin antibodies

A number of procedures have been described for the measurement both of insulin antibodies and of free insulin in the presence of insulin antibodies. It has been claimed that insulin antibodies cause insulin resistance and that labile (or "brittle") diabetes in patients on insulin treatment can be related to the concentration of insulin antibodies (Dixon et al., 1975). Whether or not such a correlation is confirmed, it has to be admitted that a knowledge of the concentration of insulin antibodies in the circulation does not determine the treatment to be followed. Estimation of free insulin in the presence of insulin antibodies is made difficult by the need to separate free from bound insulin. The procedures which are used necessarily alter the equilibrium between free and bound insulin, and hence negate any extrapolation to the situation in vivo. Current studies of residual β-cell function in insulin-treated diabetics, by the measurement of C-peptides, show that in the ten years after the start of treatment, a surprisingly high proportion of patients are still producing insulin. It appears that the stability of control of diabetes is closely related to the residual ability to produce endogenous insulin.

With most radioimmunoassay procedures, the presence of endogenous insulin antibodies in diabetics results in apparently high concentrations of "insulin". From time to time, samples of plasma are submitted for the assay of insulin without it being specified or known that the patient has previously received exogenous insulin, either with therapeutic control or by self-administration. The present authors know of one patient who was subjected to a partial pancreatectomy because of this artefact. Suspicion may be aroused by the discovery of considerably raised and unvarying "insulin" concentrations in patients who were not hypoglycaemic when the samples were taken for insulin assay. This possibility serves to re-emphasize the major importance of hypoglycaemia in the diagnosis of insulin-secreting tumours.

4.4.5. Urinary insulin

It has been shown that a relatively constant proportion of circulating insulin is cleared in the urine, so that in theory it is possible to obtain an index of the daily production of insulin by the determination of the amount excreted in urine. In practice, however, urinary insulin determinations have not been shown to provide useful diagnostic information.

4.4.6. Provocative diagnostic tests

Procedures designed to stimulate insulin secretion, such as the administration of glucose, leucine, tolbutamide or glucagon, have been proposed for the diagnosis of insulin-secreting tumours (Marks, 1974) and some details of the performance of these tests are given in section 4.6.3.3. High plasma insulin concentrations following such tests are often difficult to interpret because of normal individual variation and the effects of obesity. Excessive insulin output following the administration of leucine in adults who have not been treated with sulphonylureas is virtually diagnostic of an insulinoma. Unfortunately, a normal result is inconclusive, as only about one-third of patients exhibit this phenomenon. It is very doubtful whether other tests are helpful in cases in which repeated samples of plasma taken after an overnight or prolonged fast yield equivocal results.

Production of hypoglycaemia by alcohol or by the administration of fish insulin, which is not detected by radioimmunoassays for mammalian insulin, may allow the demonstration of inappropriate elevation of the concentration of endogenous insulin. At present, there is insufficient experience of these procedures for them to be evaluated with confidence in the diagnosis of insulin-secreting tumours.

The rate and characteristics of insulin degradation have been studied by the administration of iodine-labelled or non-labelled exogenous insulin (Symposium on Insulin Metabolism, 1973). Changes in the rate of removal of insulin from blood have been described in diabetes, but the clinical significance of such findings is not clear, and there is as yet no diagnostic indication for the use of such procedures. Similarly, the administration of insulin as a test of insulin sensitivity is used as a diagnostic test of pituitary and adrenal function, rather than to determine the effect on glucose metabolism. The procedure is therefore considered in detail in Chapter 14.4.1.

4.5. INVESTIGATION OF GLUCAGON METABOLISM

The estimation of glucagon in serum has posed particular technical problems due to the presence in serum of material of gut origin which cross-reacts with many antisera raised against pancreatic glucagon. This material appears to cross-react mainly with antisera which are directed against the N- rather than C-terminal part of the glucagon molecule. It is therefore possible to produce radioimmunoassays which are relatively specific for pancreatic glucagon, by selecting antisera which react with the C-terminal end of the hormone.

Serum glucagon concentrations are considerably elevated in a variety of illnesses involving severe stress, including infections, trauma, burns and following surgery (Unger, 1974). Insulin and glucagon concentrations are often reciprocally related, and therefore the need to interpret the two together has been emphasized (Unger, 1974). Using this approach, it has been argued that even moderately severe diabetics have inappropriately high serum glucagon concentrations, and that in diabetic ketoacidosis, the glucagon concentration may be very high indeed.

Disorders due to pancreatic glucagon-secreting tumours occur (Bloom, 1975), but are very rare. This is at present the only diagnostic situation in which the estimation of serum glucagon concentration is of clinical value. The syndrome associated with such tumours includes a characteristic rash, mild diabetes, normochromic normocytic anaemia, weight loss, painful glossitis and angular stomatitis. It may be diagnosed by an elevated fasting serum glucagon concentration, and is apparently cured by removal of the pancreatic glucagonoma.

4.6. DIAGNOSIS AND MANAGEMENT OF SOME CONDITIONS AFFECTING GLUCOSE METABOLISM

4.6.1. Diabetes mellitus

The diagnosis of diabetes mellitus is most frequently achieved by means of an oral glucose tolerance test as discussed in section 4.3.1.1. This procedure is not necessary if there is hyperglycaemia after an overnight fast, and it merely provides an arbitrary division of the range of glucose tolerances present in the population.

4.6.1.1. Definitions

In the past, considerable confusion has arisen because of the ill-defined use of various terms relating to diabetes. As a result, the Medical and Scientific Section of the British Diabetic Association has proposed the following definitions and their use is strongly recommended.

Potential diabetic: an individual with normal glucose tolerance who on statistical grounds has an increased risk of developing diabetes. The risk factors concerned are genetic (e.g. identical twin who is diabetic; both parents diabetic) or obstetric (e.g. delivery of an inappropriately heavy baby). The term "pre-diabetic" has been used in this context, but it is best restricted to a retrospective description of the period prior to the development of diabetes. Many individuals with a strong genetic predisposition to diabetes never actually become diabetic.

Latent diabetic: an individual who has at one time been overtly diabetic but who at the time of investigation has a normal glucose tolerance test. The most common examples of this situation are following delivery in a women who has been diabetic during pregnancy, or after weight reduction in a previously mildly diabetic subject.

Asymptomatic diabetic: an individual whose glucose tolerance test falls above the arbitrary range defined as normal, but who has no symptoms or signs of diabetes or its complications. The other term which is often used to describe this situation is "chemical diabetes".

4.6.1.2. Population screening

The apparent prevalence of diabetes is of course governed by the method of testing and the criteria used; it also varies with the population studied. Most surveys have indicated that general populations contain approximately equal numbers of diagnosed and undiagnosed diabetics. Elderly subjects who are screened by testing of oral glucose tolerance may yield as many as 20% "diabetics" by the usual criteria. Very little is known about the significance of mild abnormalities of glucose tolerance in this age group. The question therefore arises as to whether intensive screening for diabetes is valuable. Unfortunately, simple and cheap methods of screening such as those based on self-testing for glucosuria are unreliable. They reveal large numbers of subjects who have glucosuria during a normal glucose tolerance test, and miss a number of people with frankly diabetic glucose tolerance who do not have glucosuria. The former situation would be unimportant if it were true, as has been claimed, that individuals with renal glucosuria later develop diabetes, but the significance of renal glucosuria as a pre-diabetic phenomenon remains a matter of dispute. It is likely that at least part of the disagreement is due to variations in the definition of renal glucosuria. True renal glucosuria, in which there is abnormally large urinary excretion of glucose with a normal fasting blood glucose concentration, is rare, and is almost certainly benign. The situation with glucosuria during a "normal" glucose tolerance test is less clear. It most frequently occurs with the so called "lag-storage" type of test in which blood glucose concentrations are relatively high in the early part of the test but are normal at the end of the test. However, as far as the renal threshold is concerned, it is the arterial glucose concentration which is important, and this is not normally measured. It is therefore highly likely that a number of subjects described as showing "renal glucosuria" on the results of glucose tolerance tests in which venous glucose concentrations are estimated, are incorrectly designated. The capillary blood glucose concentration more nearly approximates to the arterial concentration. Subjects defined as having "lag-storage" curves and who often show glucosuria during this test may go on to develop diabetes (Birmingham Diabetes Survey Working Party, 1970).

In view of the present uncertainty as to the significance and management of mild degrees of diabetes, it seems unnecessary to take a very serious view of glucosuria during a normal glucose tolerance test. Likewise, precise measurements of the renal threshold would not appear to be clinically justifiable except in the context of a prospective research project.

The argument that energetic attempts to discover undiagnosed symptomless diabetes in the general population are unrewarding does not apply to certain situations in which there is predisposition to diabetes, and for which treatment is readily available.

4.6.1.3. Obesity

Obesity imposes an increased requirement for insulin. Although obese subjects with abnormal glucose tolerance commonly have higher plasma insulin concentrations than normal individuals, they are usually found to have lower plasma insulin concentrations than obese subjects with normal glucose tolerance. A measure of weight reduction by dieting is often sufficient to improve glucose tolerance, and it is hard to believe that such treatment is not indicated in this situation. However, it must be recognized that there are severe problems of maintaining weight reduction, and no study has yet clearly demonstrated the long-term benefits of this approach.

4.6.1.4. Oral drug therapy

The publication (Klimpt et al., 1970) of the results of the University Group Diabetes Program Study precipitated a lively discussion of the merits and possible dangers of the drug treatment of symptomatic or asymptomatic diabetes. Further uncertainty concerning oral treatment has been introduced by the advent of the so-called "second generation" sulphonylureas, the dosage of which may be one-hundredth of that of the older compounds. It is not yet clear if the more powerful compounds differ solely in potency, nor is it known if they are qualitatively different in terms of mechanism of action.

In view of the uncertainty surrounding these points, it is suggested that oral treatment should continue to be used with considerable caution. It is possible that if rigorous dietary management could be established and maintained, most patients who are not in need of insulin therapy would have much less requirement for oral hypoglycaemic drugs.

4.6.1.5. Diabetes during pregnancy

The requirement for insulin increases during pregnancy and falls rapidly after delivery. It is possible that this is due to insulin resistance caused by increasing levels of placental lactogen, although other factors cannot be excluded. Some pregnant women show a considerable deterioration of oral glucose tolerance, the change being most marked towards the end of gestation. Diabetes, and the period immediately prior to its onset, are also associated with an increased incidence of abortion, stillbirth, heavy babies and congenital abnormalities. For all of these reasons, the recognition and optimum control of diabetes during pregnancy are extremely important. However, the extent to which dietary or insulin control of diabetes which appears for the first time during pregnancy ("gestational diabetes") improves the outcome of pregnancy is uncertain (British Medical Journal, 1974).

The detection of gestational diabetes is made difficult by the fact that the glomerular filtration rate is increased by 50 to 100% in pregnancy, so that the amount of glucose filtered may exceed the tubular reabsorption capacity. As a result, glucosuria is very common in pregnancy and does not necessarily indicate the presence of diabetes. However, as emphasized above, the detection and optimum management of diabetes during pregnancy is extremely important because of the risks to the foetus. If glucosuria is detected on separate occasions in two random specimens of urine, a full glucose tolerance test should be carried out. Other indications for the testing of glucose tolerance include a family history of diabetes, a previous infant with a birth weight of more than 4 kg, a bad obstetric history, or the presence of hydramnios. On these grounds, the optimum time for testing would appear to be about 28 weeks, since this is late enough for a major effect of pregnancy on glucose tolerance to be manifest, and yet early enough to obtain beneficial effects from careful control. It may be that the ideal procedure would be to subject all pregnant women who have not already shown consistent glucosuria, to an abbreviated glucose tolerance test (i.e. collection of a specimen 2 hours after the glucose load) at 28 weeks, since even the foregoing clinical indications for testing will miss a proportion of gestational diabetics. However, before such a procedure can be established on a sound and economic basis, further prospective studies of the relationship between glucose tolerance, thé outcome of pregnancy and the effects of treatment are needed. The detailed management of the established diabetic who becomes pregnant is beyond the scope of this chapter, and the reader is referred to the monographs which are suggested for further reading.

4.6.1.6. Diabetic ketoacidosis

The treatment of diabetic ketoacidosis remains one of the best illustrations of the need for close integration of laboratory investigation with clinical management (Alberti, 1974). The condition continues to cause potentially preventable loss of life in otherwise fit and active people, so that the rewards for successful treatment are great. It has been estimated that there are 6000 admissions for diabetic coma per year in Great Britain, and the mortality rates range from 5 to 20% between hospitals; these data indicate the possibility of 600 preventable deaths per annum from this condition.

The diagnosis of ketoacidosis, if not immediately obvious from the patient's history, is simply made by the bedside demonstration of hyperglycaemia and ketosis using test strips. A sample of blood should be taken for the laboratory estimation of plasma glucose, urea, electrolytes and blood haematocrit, arterial pH, pO_2 and pCO_2, but treatment for the metabolic disturbance should be initiated immediately, with the aim of correcting the abnormalities in order of priority, and without waiting for the laboratory results. In view of the frequent association of infection with the onset of ketoacidosis, obtaining a throat swab, blood and urine culture and chest radiograph may be advisable. It may be apparent that antibiotics are required at once for treatment or to prevent infection due to the use of venous or urinary catheter.

The most important metabolic disturbance to be corrected is that of dehydration; on average 5 litres of water are needed by the ketoacidotic adult. This may be given as normal saline, since a sodium deficit of 500 mmol, equivalent to 3.5 litres of normal saline, is to be expected. The potassium deficit (400 to 700 mmol), which averages to 10 to 15% of the total body potassium, must also be replaced. Although the initial concentration of plasma potassium may be normal or even high, it will fall rapidly following the administration of insulin, since this causes potassium to be taken up by the tissues. The need for acute replacement of the deficits of phosphate (17 to 34 mmol), calcium (25 to 50 mmol) and magnesium (13 to 25 mmol) is less well established, but should be borne in mind. Administration of alkali is only necessary if the blood pH is less than 7.1, and then only small amounts are necessary.

The requirement for insulin, although urgent, is currently subject to a certain amount of dispute concerning the amount and route of administration. Large amounts of subcutaneous insulin should be avoided, due to the uncertain rate of absorption, the presence of a poor circulation, and the consequent danger of late hypoglycaemia. Very high circulating concentrations of insulin are unnecessary, and it has been shown in vitro that high concentrations of insulin may be ineffective, or may even have actions opposite to those expected. It is also relevant that preparations of insulin contain small amounts of glucagon, and this may alter the efficacy of insulin in vivo. There would seem to be every reason to aim at achieving a plasma insulin concentration in the high physiological range (approximately 100 mU/litre). However, insulin has a short plasma half-life (section 4.4), so that continuous or very frequent administration is required to maintain a plateau concentration. It can be calculated that an intravenous bolus of 100 units of insulin will have disappeared in 36 minutes; therefore, if such treatment were given every 2 hours, there would be no effective therapy for two-thirds of the time.

Where adequate staffing and facilities such as infusion pumps are available, the continuous infusion of insulin at 5 to 8 units/h is ideal. Very occasionally patients are encountered with severe insulin resistance, but these may be detected by a failure to lower the blood glucose concentration within 2 hours of the start of treatment. As an alternative, where there is insufficient staff or facilities for an infusion regime, treatment with 20 units of insulin, given intramuscularly, followed by 5 units/h, has been shown to be very satisfactory.

Hypokalaemia is one of the commonest causes of iatrogenic death in ketoacidosis. Both insulin therapy and the correction of extracellular acidosis cause an increased uptake of potassium by cells. Previous diuretic therapy and potassium loss in the urine may exacerbate the problem of maintaining a normal plasma potassium concentration. Although less difficulty occurs with low-dosage insulin regimes, it is still necessary to administer potassium at a rate of about 13 mmol/h from the start of treatment with insulin, whatever the plasma potassium concentration at that time. The subsequent rate of administration may be modified according to the plasma concentration. A cardiac monitor is advisable, as an indirect indication of changes in extracellular potassium. It is usual to replace about half of the potassium deficit in the first 24 hours, after which oral supplements may be used to complete the replenishment of body potassium over the next few days. If the initial blood pH is below 7.1, a small amount (50 mmol) of intravenous bicarbonate may be administered, but as this will also increase potassium uptake by cells, potassium must be given at the same time.

The general measures which may be taken in the management of diabetic ketoacidosis include aspiration of stomach contents when the level of consciousness is depressed, to prevent the inhalation of vomit; the use of antibiotics; administration of plasma or blood in the treatment of severe hypotension which has not responded to saline; and the accurate measurement of urine production (for which catheterization may be necessary), since the administration of fluid and potassium is hazardous in the absence of an adequate output of urine. These aspects of treatment are dictated by the individual problems confronting the physician. Specific measures include the use of heparin, which may be required to prevent diffuse intravascular coagulation and deep venous thrombosis in the elderly unconscious or the severely hyperosmolar patient.

4.6.2. Other conditions associated with hyperglycaemia

There are many conditions which may lead to hyperglycaemia or abnormal glucose tolerance. These usually present with obvious symptoms and signs of the primary disturbance, but it is beyond the scope of this chapter to describe the diagnosis and management of this wide range of disorders. However, the manner of presentation may focus attention on disturbed glucose metabolism in the first instance, so that a list of possible primary conditions is included here (Table 4.2). The list is by no means exhaustive.

4.6.2.1. Trauma

Severe illnesses, including trauma and overwhelming infections, cause profound metabolic changes. The most important of these, in the context of this chapter, are the increase in the overall rate of metabolism, which may double in the case of major burns, and the unrestrained breakdown of protein for gluconeogenesis. The endocrine basis of the latter change is that of increase in the concentrations of corticosteroids, catecholamines and glucagon, and depression of insulin. The administration of glucose and aminoacids – even in amounts adequate to cope with the protein and calorie requirements of the patient – may not reverse the negative nitrogen balance consequent upon the marked endocrine changes. Thus starvation leading to 40% weight loss is invariably fatal, and the figure associated with a fatal outcome drops to 25 or 30% if the weight loss is associated with serious injury. Patients with extensive burns may require as many as 5000 calories a day to compensate for their increased metabolic requirements. Therefore, in addition to the regimes required for the maintenance of fluid and electrolyte balance, it is necessary to monitor nitrogen balance and provide adequate calories (Allison, 1974).

TABLE 4.2.

SOME CONDITIONS OTHER THAN DIABETES MELLITUS ASSOCIATED WITH FASTING HYPERGLYCAEMIA OR ABNORMAL GLUCOSE TOLERANCE

Endocrine disorders	Acute severe illness	Hepatic disease
acromegaly	infection	cirrhosis
Cushing's syndrome		
thyrotoxicosis	trauma	tumours
phaeochromocytoma	cerebrovascular accident	
glucagonoma	acute coronary insufficiency	
Pancreatic disease	Drug therapy or overdosage	
pancreatitis	salicylates	
haemochromatosis	oral contraceptives	
carcinoma	corticosteroids	
	thiazide diuretics	

In an attempt to overcome the catabolic state associated with the endocrine changes in severe trauma, insulin has been administered in large doses, together with glucose. It has thus been possible to produce dramatic and beneficial changes in nitrogen balance, with consequent improvement in wound healing, resistance to infection and mortality. One such regime employs a solution of 50% glucose containing 40 mmol potassium and 120 units soluble insulin per litre. When severe insulin resistance is encountered, it may be necessary to increase the amount of insulin 4-fold (Allison, 1974).

The precise role and indications for the use of insulin and glucose regimes in various conditions, including acute coronary care and heart failure, are still matters for continuing investigation. Nevertheless there is little doubt that the use of this type of regime may be life-saving.

4.6.3. Hypoglycaemia

Hypoglycaemia is commonly defined as a blood glucose concentration of less than 2.2 mmol/litre (40 mg/dl) in an infant after the postnatal period, or in a child or adult. In the newborn, the lower limit of normal blood glucose is 1.7 mmol/litre (30 mg/dl) in a term infant, and 1.1 mmol/litre (20 mg/dl) in a pre-term infant.

The biochemical definition of hypoglycaemia is precise, but it has little significance unless it is considered in the context of glucose as an obligatory fuel for brain metabolism. The term "neuroglycopaenia" is cumbersome, but it accurately describes the clinician's preoccupying concern when faced with a patient suffering from hypoglycaemia. It is conventional teaching that the adult brain is an obligatory consumer of glucose, and that cerebral uptake of glucose is not influenced by insulin, although there is some evidence to the contrary. Acute cerebral deprivation of glucose produces symptoms which are commonly experienced in their mildest form, and which are relieved by a mid-morning snack. More severe hypoglycaemia can lead to abnormal neurological signs, coma and death. Chronic lack of substrate leads to alterations in the pattern of fuel used by the brain, resulting in a greater consumption of ketone bodies and less dependence upon glucose. Preliminary results suggest that the human foetal brain may metabolize ketones and fatty acids as an important source of fuel under normal circumstances. If this persists to the perinatal period, it may partly explain the low range of normal blood glucose levels in newborn infants and the frequent occurrence of asymptomatic hypoglycaemia. A rapid fall in blood glucose to normoglycaemic levels, such as occurs when a diabetic is given insulin intravenously, may produce symptoms of hypoglycaemia. This is an example of neuroglycopaenia co-existing with normoglycaemia, and serves to illustrate the importance of a clear distinction between the two concepts.

Hypoglycaemia may be considered in various ways of which two will be dealt with here: one traditionally aetiologic, the other pragmatic, according to age. The subdivision of hypoglycaemia by aetiology occurs in every major review of the subject (e.g. Williams, 1968; Marks, 1974) and is worthwhile because it illustrates the pathophysiology. But this approach is not the most helpful to the clinician faced with a hypoglycaemic patient. Because of the changing pattern of differential diagnosis with physical development, a useful practical classification of hypoglycaemia is by age: the newborn infant, the child, and the adult. The hypoglycaemic child or adult, but not the newborn, may then be classified according to whether hypoglycaemia occurs during fasting, or in response to a stimulus. This approach is obviously inappropriate for the newborn, who should not be without food for more than 3 or 4 hours.

4.6.3.1. Classification by aetiology

A clear understanding of the normal homeostasis of glucose (section 4.2) is necessary for the proper appreciation of an aetiological classification of hypoglycaemia. Glucose precursors may not reach the cells in which storage and gluconeogenesis take place, or they may be lost from the body in abnormal amounts. Precursor deficiency may occur in starvation at any age, but particularly in protein-calorie malnutrition and in newborn infants who are fed inappropriately to their needs. Increased losses may occur, despite adequate ingestion, due to malabsorption or because of glucosuria or lactation. Whatever the reason, however, chronic undernutrition results in an inadequate delivery of gluconeogenic substrate from fat and muscle. In these circumstances, important readjustments of fuel homeostasis take place in the adult (Cahill, 1970). When a normal adult fasts, there is a modest fall in blood glucose concentration, but the subject does not become hypoglycaemic. If fasting is imposed on a diseased adult, on a normal child, or on a newborn infant in particular, clinically apparent hypoglycaemia may occur, with potential neurological sequelae.

As emphasised in section 4.2, the liver plays a central role in glucose homeostasis, being the major site for gluconeogenesis and glucose storage. Hepatocellular damage from whatever cause may be associated with hypoglycaemia. Hepatic injury may be generalized, as in infection or heart failure, or localized to the hepatocytes as in ethanol intoxication or in the inborn metabolic errors of fructose intolerance and galactose intolerance. As well as generalized hepatocellular damage, the glycogenoses may cause hypoglycaemia due to a metabolic block in glycogen synthesis or to breakdown in liver or muscle.

Hypoglycaemia is a characteristic finding in certain endocrine diseases, such as growth hormone deficiency and adrenocortical deficiency, in which the regulatory hormones of glucose homeostasis are lacking. By the same token, catecholamine deficiency has been implicated in some examples of paediatric hypoglycaemia, and lack of glucagon is a much discussed – but poorly documented – cause of hypoglycaemia.

If delivery of glucose to the circulation is normal, hypoglycaemia may result if the rate of removal is excessive in clinical terms – excessive means fast enough to cause neuroglycopaenia, with symptoms and abnormal signs. Asymptomatic hypoglycaemia, which commonly occurs in the newborn, and less commonly in the fasting adult, is not so fraught. Abnormally rapid disappearance of glucose from the circulation may occur with or without increased secretion of insulin. The rapid disappearance of an intravenous glucose load in the very ill, and the hypoglycaemia of catabolic states such as exist in prolonged exercise, hyperpyrexia or burns, is not associated with increased secretion of insulin.

Hypoglycaemia in the fasting state is often associated with hyperinsulinaemia, and in these circumstances increased secretion of insulin is usually the cause. Inappropriate release of insulin characteristically occurs in a β-cell tumour or insulinoma of the pancreas. These may be benign or malignant, and if the latter, the metastases may also secrete insulin. Benign insulin adenomata may be single or multiple and vary widely in size; a microscopic tumour which is detectable only by histological examination may be capable of producing profound hypoglycaemia. The spectrum of β-cell neoplasia merges into hyperplasia and includes a number of developmental anomalies, some of which may regress spontaneously, but others may be permanent. Nesidioblastosis is characterized by a pancreas which contains a normal complement of islets, together with β-cells scattered singly or in small groups. The diagnosis is made at operation on a young infant who is suspected of having an insulin-secreting tumour. Islet hyperplasia occurs in Beckwith's syndrome, in which newborn infants are as likely to present surgically with an omphalocoele as in a medical ward. Reversible islet hyperplasia occurs in infants born to diabetic mothers who have hypertrophy and hyperplasia of β-cells, and in infants, suffering from erythroblastosis foetalis, who have large islets due to hyperplasia of all endocrine cell types. The aetiology of hyperinsulinism in the infant of a diabetic mother is thought to be the consequence of prolonged exposure to intermittent hyperglycaemia in utero, but the reason for islet hyperplasia in the erythroblastotic infant is poorly understood.

Other neoplasms, particularly mesenchymal tumours such as fibrosarcomata, may be associated with hypoglycaemia. In these cases, the tumour mass is usually large, and excessive metabolism of glucose by the tumour has been thought to be the explanation of the hypoglycaemia. From some tumours, material has been extracted which has insulin-like activity when tested by bioassay; a few have been shown to contain immunoreactive insulin. Multiple endocrine adenomata or the polyglandular syndrome should be considered, especially in a patient with fasting hypoglycaemia, hyperinsulinaemia and other biochemical disturbances such as hypercalcaemia.

Reactive hypoglycaemia is due to an imbalance between the response of the β-cell mass and the signals of insulin secretion. The signal may be normal in kind, but abnormal in size, as in the rapid glucose absorption of tachyalimentation. This is characteristically a sequel of partial gastrectomy or gastroenterostomy, in which abnormally rapid absorption of glucose from the gut causes oversecretion of insulin and rebound hypoglycaemia. Normal absorption of glucose may also cause reactive hypoglycaemia if the β-cell mass is increased, as in islet hyperplasia or adenoma. Hypoglycaemia may be a presenting sign in undiagnosed diabetes mellitus (section 4.6.1.) and is not uncommon as a late sequel to oral glucose or to a meal when there is a delayed but exaggerated insulin response to the signal.

Abnormal response of the β-cell mass to a normal signal occurs in leucine-sensitive hypoglycaemia. No consistent morphological abnormality of the endocrine pancreas has been described in children with this condition, and speculation that there is a defect in β-cell handling of leucine is complicated by the fact that the patients often outgrow their clinical illness.

Finally, to an aetiologic classification of hypoglycaemia, there has to be added a group of causes due to the absorption of drugs or toxins. A comprehensive account of these is given by Seltzer (1972) and examples will be given here to illustrate the diversity of mechanisms of action. Ethanol intoxication is thought to cause a greater proportion of alanine to be converted into α-glycerophosphate, and thence into triglyceride glycerol, than to glucose in the hepatocyte; the formation of triglyceride accounts for the fatty infiltration and ultimate hepatic cirrhosis of chronic alcoholism. Ethanol hypoglycaemia may occur as an isolated phenomenon, but it is more commonly associated with undernutrition or overdosage of insulin or sulphonylureas in diabetics (Madison, 1968). Salicylate intoxication is the commonest cause of drug-induced hypoglycaemia during childhood in Western society, but the mechanism is poorly understood. A toxin, cycloleucine, which is present in unripe ackee fruit, is responsible for vomiting sickness in young Jamaican children; the associated hypoglycaemia is in part caused by excessive stimulation of insulin secretion. Excess administration of insulin, which is the commonest cause of hypoglycaemia in diabetics, is self-explanatory; so also is overdosage with insulinotropic sulphonylureas which are used in the treatment of maturity onset diabetes.

4.6.3.2. Classification by age

The newborn, unlike the child or adult, is unable to communicate symptoms due to hypoglycaemia and so the clinician must be especially vigilant in considering the diagnosis in this group of patients. The paediatrician screens certain groups of infants who are known to be at risk by performing routine measurements of blood glucose until they are known to be able to maintain a normal concentration. The groups include small-for-dates infants; pre-term infants; the smaller of twins, who may lack gluconeogenic substrate or the ability to synthesize glucose; infants of diabetic mothers; and those suffering from erythroblastosis foetalis who are known to secrete an excess of insulin due to islet hyperplasia. Unremitting hypoglycaemia which lasts for days usually signifies an insulinoma, nesidioblastosis or, rarely, maternal prenatal therapy with a sulphonylurea. Equally rare diagnosis – but ones in which there are clinical clues – include Beckwith's syndrome and inborn metabolic errors such as the glycogenoses and galactose or fructose intolerance. Leucine intolerance may manifest in the newborn and is a characteristic of infants who have been prenatally exposed to sulphonylureas.

Hypoglycaemia in the newborn or in infancy and childhood may occur for reasons which are not self-limiting, such as the inborn metabolic errors, leucine sensitivity and pancreatic neoplasia. Overall, the most frequent cause of hypoglycaemia in childhood is protein-calorie malnutrition, but ketotic hypoglycaemia is the commonest cause in Western societies. The aetiology of ketotic hypoglycaemia is not clearly defined, but both catecholamine deficiency and alanine deficiency have been implicated. Endocrinopathies such as hypopituitarism are rare, but important, causes of hypoglycaemia; hypoglycaemia from drug or toxin ingestion (section 4.6.3.1.) is more common.

There are some causes of hypoglycaemia which are more common in adults than in younger patients, e.g. the hypoglycaemia of overdosage with insulin or sulphonylurea, or due to chronic liver damage. Tachyalimentation and non-pancreatic tumours are characteristically found in adults, as is hypoglycaemia due to the synergistic actions of drugs such as propranolol, bishydroxycoumarin, the tetracyclines and sulphonylureas.

4.6.3.3. Diagnosis

The diagnosis of hypoglycaemia occurs in three stages: the appreciation that certain symptoms and signs may be caused by a low blood glucose concentration; confirmation, by measurement, of the low concentration; and finally the elucidation of the cause.

The clinical picture produced by hypoglycaemia is the product of stimulation of the sympathetic nervous system and depression of central nervous system function.

Sympathetic overactivity causes pallor, sweating, anxiety, tremulousness, pupillary dilatation and tachycardia. Cortical depression causes confusion, personality changes, memory loss and psychotic thinking and behaviour. More profound hypoglycaemia results in loss of consciousness, primitive movements such as sucking, grasping and grimacing, clonic and tonic spasms, decorticate posture and ultimately death. Many patients are able to give a history suggestive of hypoglycaemia, but the diagnosis must be borne in mind in every unconscious patient and in those presenting with psychiatric disturbance.

The signs of hypoglycaemia in the newborn differ in some respects from those in later life and should be noted separately. Autonomic nervous system manifestations are less prominent, and central nervous system signs are different. Infants characteristically show abnormal movements termed "jitteriness", which are clonic movements of the distal parts of the limbs, 3 to 5 cycles/s and lasting for 15 to 30 seconds at a time. In between periods of movement, the infant may be hypotonic and have shallow respirations. These signs may be associated with apathy, refusal to feed and cyanosis. More severe signs are convulsions and apnoiec attacks.

As the pattern of causes of hypoglycaemia changes with age, so must the plan of investigation. Again, newborn infants are distinguished from other age groups more clearly than infants; children and adults are distinguished from one another.

The commonest form of hypoglycaemia in the newborn is asymptomatic, and is associated with a clinical diagnosis such as prematurity, small-for-dates, or the smaller of twins. These patients are often not investigated further but are managed by 6-hourly monitoring of blood glucose concentrations with increasing intake of food by mouth. Glucose measurements are usually made at the bedside by stick test and confirmed in the laboratory when necessary. Should asymptomatic hypoglycaemia persist, or become symptomatic, immediate correction with intravenous glucose is necessary. This therapeutic measure can be put to diagnostic use by giving the initial injection of 10 or 20% glucose, in a dose of 0.5 g/kg body weight, via a peripheral vein over 30 to 60 seconds. Blood specimens (0.5 ml) are collected before, and at accurately timed intervals up to 1 hour after the injection, for the measurement of blood glucose and plasma insulin concentrations. Suitable times are 2, 10, 20, 30, 40 and 60 minutes after the injection is complete. Ideally blood samples are taken from an indwelling umbilical arterial catheter; an umbilical venous catheter is less satisfactory, as pancreatic effluent blood with a high plasma insulin concentration may be sampled if the catheter tip is in the porta hepatis. It is not, however, always possible to collect blood from an indwelling catheter, and if repeated heel stabs are used 0.5 ml samples are taken for the 2-, 30- and 60-minute specimens, the others being smaller (0.1 ml) and used for blood glucose measurement only. Preoccupation with the volume of blood samples is commonplace to the neonatal paediatrician, but it is important to emphasize this point for those more accustomed to dealing with larger patients.

By means of the challenge of the intravenous glucose tolerance test, the plasma insulin response and the glucose disappearance rate can be measured. The normal rate of glucose disappearance in the newborn is less than that in older infants and adults, and the plasma insulin response on the first day is characterized by a small spike and a large wave. Hyperinsulinaemia, both before and in response to the glucose challenge, is characteristic of the infant of the gestational diabetic in erythroblastosis, β-cell neoplasia or hyperplasia, and in some small-for-dates infants. The presence of insulin antibodies in the plasma of infants of insulin-dependent diabetic mothers invalidates measurements of plasma insulin by conventional radioimmunoassay. Normal plasma insulin levels do not, however, exclude the diagnosis of insulinoma, and undue reliance should not be placed upon this facet of a case presentation. A high glucose disappearance rate raises the suspicion of hyperinsulinism, but it is by no means diagnostic of it; a high rate has also been reported in infants with cyanotic congenital heart disease and infection, and in those who are very ill from other causes (Gentz et al., 1969).

The initial intravenous glucose load is continued as an infusion, the strength and rate of which are determined by the infant's caloric and water requirements. Most forms of neonatal hypoglycaemia are self-limiting, and persistence of hypoglycaemia after four days, or the recurrence of hypoglycaemia which has apparently remitted, should raise suspicion of β-cell neoplasia, leucine sensitivity hyperplasia or an inborn metabolic error. These diagnoses are rare in the neonatal period and are considered in more detail below.

The investigation of hypoglycaemia in childhood and in the adult involves a variety of provocative tests (Zuppinger, 1975), each of which is summarized below. Ketotic hypoglycaemia accounted for over one-third of the cases in two large series (Sauls and Ulstrom, 1966; Zuppinger, 1975). Children with ketotic hypoglycaemia are more often male, have a history of having been small-for-dates, and may have suffered neonatal hypoglycaemia. The age of onset is between one and five years. Hypoglycaemic attacks occur with fasting or may be provoked by a low carbohydrate–high fat diet (ketogenic diet), but they are readily corrected by carbohydrate. The long-term prognosis is good, with spontaneous remission occurring in late childhood or at puberty, but the potential danger of each hypoglycaemic attack is serious. As ketonaemia and hypoglycaemia can occur in normal children after a 24-hour fast, the response to a ketogenic diet is more informative than starvation, and more acceptable to the patient.

In all provocative tests it is important that the patient should be correctly prepared. The minimum caloric intake for infants under one year of age is 100 kcal/kg; over one year of age it is 1000 kcal, plus 100 kcal per year of age up to puberty. Half the calories should come from carbohydrate, and the investigator should ensure that such a diet has been followed for at least three days prior to testing. A standard ketogenic diet (1 cal/g) consists of 67% fat, 16% carbohydrate and 17% protein made up as 800 g whole milk, 285 g 20% cream, 17 g casein hydrolysate and 102 g water. This is given in three equal parts at 08.00, 12.00 and 17.00 h at the rate of 1200 kcal/1.73 m^2 with water ad libitum. Activity is not restricted, and all urine which is voided is tested for acetone. Blood is drawn for glucose and free fatty acid determinations at 4-hourly intervals for 24 hours. In most children, acetonuria occurs after 12 hours, and in the child with ketotic hypoglycaemia, a fall in blood glucose and symptoms are noted within the second 12-hour period. At the onset of symptoms, blood should be drawn for glucose and free fatty acid determinations and, if possible, a glucagon tolerance test should be performed. A blunted or absent rise in blood glucose concentration after glucagon is characteristic.

A glucagon tolerance test is performed by giving 30 μg therapeutic glucagon per kg body weight intramuscularly, to a total not exceeding 1 mg. Blood is collected for glucose determinations before and at 15, 30, 45, 60 and, if possible, at 90 and 120 minutes after the injection. A normal response involves maximum rise in blood glucose of not less than 1.4 mmol/litre (25 mg/dl) and usually more than 2.8 mmol/litre (50 mg/dl) which occurs in the 15-, 30- or 45-minute sample, with a return to pre-inejction levels by 60 or 90 minutes. In ketotic hypoglycaemia, an abnormal response occurs because of a deficiency in gluconeogenesis which may be due to impaired release of alanine from muscle or a failure of release of catecholamine. These patients have a normal response to glucagon postprandially, as do those with glycogen storage disease type III or synthetase deficiency. An impaired response to glucagon under all conditions suggests a generalized abnormality of hepatocellular function or type I glycogen storage (von Gierke's) disease. Glucagon stimulates insulin secretion as well as hepatic phosphorylase and, if possible, it is worth measuring the plasma insulin response to glucagon, as hyperinsulinaemia coupled with hypoglycaemia in the latter half of the test may arouse the suspicion of β-cell neoplasia or hyperplasia.

No other single cause of hypoglycaemia is common, but many carry clues in the clinical presentations. Among the endocrinopathies, congenital adrenal hyperplasia is likely to present with symptoms other than hypoglycaemia, as are cretinism and growth hormone deficiency. Corticotrophin deficiency and Addison's disease are more difficult to recognize clinically, but characteristic plasma electrolyte changes will lead to the appropriate investigations and diagnosis. The concept of "idiopathic hypoglycaemia" no longer has a place in paediatric practice. The pathology of this biochemical anomaly is clear when appropriate diagnostic tests are applied, although the physician may not always be able to investigate fully and may be obliged to settle for a diagnosis of "hypoglycaemia – aetiology not proven".

Leucine-sensitive hypoglycaemia is suspected when the history suggests an association between the attacks and protein feeding. This may occur at any time from the neonatal period onwards, milk formulations being potent stimuli to susceptible infants. A leucine tolerance test is performed by giving a solution of 150 mg L-leucine/kg body weight by mouth after an overnight fast. Leucine is more soluble in weak alkali, but may be dissolved immediately before administration in water which has been freed of carbon dioxide by boiling for 30 minutes. The solution may be flavoured with saccharin to make it more palatable; for small infants it may be given by stomach tube. Blood samples are taken before and at 15, 30, 45, 60, 90 and 120 minutes after oral leucine for measurement of glucose and insulin concentrations. If there are facilities for preparing sterile solutions of leucine suitable for intravenous injection, the test may be performed by giving 75 mg/kg intravenously, and then collecting blood samples at the same intervals as in an intravenous glucose tolerance test. Leucine sensitivity is defined as a fall in blood glucose concentration to less than 50% of the fasting value. A weakness of the definition is that sensitivity may co-exist with a low fasting blood glucose concentration, in which case symptoms of hypoglycaemia may be provoked by leucine without the demonstration of the required fall in blood glucose concentration. Clinical hypoglycaemia provoked by leucine can be quickly averted by parenteral glucose or adrenaline; it is advisable to have an intravenous infusion of saline established before the test begins, by means of which glucose may be given. Since many infants and children with leucine-sensitive hypoglycaemia do not come to operation, the incidence of β-cell hyperplasia in this condition cannot be stated. The characteristic presentation in the first six months of life is often coupled with an inappropriate delay in making the diagnosis.

Another important, but uncommon, cause of hypoglycaemia in childhood without clinical stigmata is diabetes mellitus. Such children may be confused with those suffering from leucine sensitivity, as their attacks are also post-prandial but are not related to the ingestion of protein. An oral glucose tolerance test should be performed, the loading dose decreasing with age: up to 18 months, 2.5 g/kg; 18 months to 3 years, 2.0 g/kg; 3 to 12 years, 1.75 g/kg; over 12 years, 1.25 g/kg. The glucose is given as a 25% solution which is chilled and flavoured to reduce nausea. Blood samples for glucose and insulin determinations are collected before and at 0.5, 1, 1.5, 2, 3, 4 and 5 hours afterwards. The results of the test are interpreted as in the adult patient. The findings appropriate to hypoglycaemia are: a flat curve due to malabsorption; reactive hypoglycaemia due to unduly rapid absorption; a diabetic curve coupled with late hypoglycaemia, due to delayed but excessive release of insulin.

Hypoglycaemia in an infant or child with hepatomegaly should lead the investigator to consider certain inborn metabolic errors. Abnormal hepatic storage of glycogen occurs in glycogenoses type I (von Gierke, glucose-6-phosphatase deficiency), type III (Cori, amylo-1,6-glucosidase deficiency) and type VI (Hers, phosphorylase deficiency). In galactose and fructose intolerance, hepatomegaly results from generalized hepatocellular damage. Although enzymatic assays of biopsy material are required for precise diagnosis of the glycogenoses, certain provocative tests are a necessary preamble. The glucose and lactate responses to intramuscular glucagon, intravenous galactose and fructose are the most informative; adrenaline provocation of glycogenolysis is undesirable because of side-effects. Galactose (1 g/kg body weight) or fructose (0.5 g/kg body weight), as a 25% solution, is infused over 2 to 3 minutes and blood samples are withdrawn from an indwelling cannula at 10-minute intervals for 1 hour for the determination of glucose, lactate and galactose or fructose. The fast preceding the test should not last longer than 6 hours.

In type I glycogen storage disease, intramuscular glucagon may cause a fall in blood glucose concentration, no change, or a modest rise to not more than 50% above the fasting value in 30 minutes. This spectrum of response is due partly to the stimulation of insulin by glucagon, and partly to the variation in glucose-6-phosphatase deficiency. There is a rise in plasma lactate concentration which may be coupled with a fall in bicarbonate and pH. Intravenous fructose or galactose disappears rapidly from the circulation, coupled with a rise in plasma lactate concentration but no change in that of glucose. The enzyme deficiency can be demonstrated in gut mucosa, and a duodenal biopsy may be considered less hazardous than a liver biopsy.

Type III glycogenosis is clinically similar to type I but pursues a milder course, with hypoglycaemia and acidosis being less marked. The glycaemic response to glucagon is greater with a significant rise after a 4 to 6 hour fast, but usually no rise after an overnight fast. There is a rise in blood glucose after administration of galactose or fructose. Erythrocytes contain excessive glycogen and the leucocytes also share the deficiency in debranching enzyme.

In type IV glycogenosis, hepatic phosphorylase levels are low but not absent (Hers, 1964). This results in a clinical picture, and responses to glucagon, galactose and fructose, which are similar to those in type III. Phosphorylase in muscle or leucocytes is normal, and the diagnosis rests on enzymatic analysis of a liver biopsy.

Galactosaemia may be suspected in the infant who has prolonged jaundice, hepatomegaly and reducing substances in the urine. A positive Clinitest coupled with a negative response to Clinistix provides a useful bedside clue that a hexose other than glucose is in the urine. If seen late, the infant may have cataracts and splenomegaly as a result of progressive hepatic deterioration. Glucose or fructose tolerance is normal, but oral galactose, given as the sugar itself or as lactose in milk, disappears slowly from the circulation. Hypoglucosaemia has been reported following intravenous galactose but this is not a consistent observation. If the diagnosis is suspected from a reasonably clear-cut clinical presentation, there is no need to impose provocative tests on the patient, for the diagnosis can be made from the raised red cell content of galactose-1-phosphate.

Hereditary fructose intolerance is due to a hepatic deficiency of fructose-1-phosphate aldolase, and hypoglycaemia results in a block in hepatic glucose release; cirrhosis develops later. The first symptoms are noted in infants who vomit on being given sucrose-supplemented feeds or fruit juices, and then show failure to thrive and hypoglycaemia with neurological sequelae. Examination reveals hepatosplenomegaly and sometimes jaundice. Withdrawal of fructose from the diet results in prompt improvement. In the older child and adult there is a self-taught avoidance of fructose-containing foods which produce epigastric pain, nausea, vomiting and even diarrhoea. A carefully drawn clinical history is often the best guide to the diagnosis. Benign fructosuria is excluded by an intravenous fructose tolerance test, which causes a fall in plasma phosphate due to the accumulation of hepatic fructose-1-phosphate, and prolonged hypoglycaemia.

The spectrum of hypoglycaemia in the adult differs from that in earlier life, as has been described earlier. Perhaps the most important diagnostic difference is that the adult is usually able to give an account of his symptoms. The first important discriminant is whether the attacks of hypoglycaemia are thought to be fasting or reactive. If the history is suggestive of fasting hypoglycaemia, then this should be confirmed by measuring blood glucose and insulin concentrations after 24 hours starvation, or longer. An inappropriately high plasma insulin concentration suggests hypersecretion, and the diagnosis of an insulinoma must be considered (Peacock et al., 1974).

Patients with insulin-secreting tumours may have an exaggerated hypoglycaemic and insulin secretory response to intravenous tolbutamide. The test is performed by injecting 1 g tolbutamide dissolved in 20 ml 0.9% saline intravenously over 2 minutes, and collecting venous blood samples at 2, 5, 10, 20, 30, 40 and 60 minutes after the end of injection. Children are given 20 mg/kg body weight with a maximum of 1 g.

Reactive hypoglycaemia is first suspected on the basis of a careful history, and can be confirmed by provocation with the typical meal or oral glucose. The late reactive hypoglycaemia of unrecognized, or maturity onset, diabetes mellitus is also clearly defined by an oral glucose tolerance test, if plasma insulin measurements are made as well.

REFERENCES

Alberti, K.G.M.M. (1974) Diabetic ketoacidosis: aspects of management. In Tenth Symposium on Advanced Medicine (Ed. J.G.G. Ledingham) pp. 68–82, Pitman, London.

Allison, S.P. (1974) Metabolic aspects of intensive care. British Journal of Hospital Medicine, 11, 860–872.

Birmingham Diabetes Survey Working Party (1970) Five-year follow-up report on the Birmingham diabetes survey of 1962. British Medical Journal, 3, 301–305.

Bloom, S.R. (1975) Glucagon. British Journal of Hospital Medicine, 13, 150–158.

British Medical Journal (1974) Leading article. Gestational diabetes. British Medical Journal, 1, 167–168.

Brown, J.C. (1974) "Enterogastrone" and other new gut peptides. Medical Clinics of North America, 58, 1347–1358.

Cahill, Jr., G.F. (1970) Starvation in man. New England Journal of Medicine, 282, 668–675.

Campbell, A.K. and Hales, C.N. (1976) Some aspects of intercellular regulation in the cell. In Medical Science IV (Ed. J.B. Lloyd and F. Beck) pp. 106–151, Academic Press, London.

Dixon, K., Exon, P.D. and Malins, J.M. (1975) Insulin antibodies and the control of diabetes. Quarterly Journal of Medicine, 44, 543–553.

Exton, J.H. (1972) Gluconeogenesis. Metabolism, 21, 945–990.

Felig, P. (1973) The glucose–alanine cycle. Metabolism, 23, 179–207.

Gentz, J., Persson, B. and Zetterstrom, R. (1969) On the Diagnosis of Symptomatic Neonatal Hypoglycemia. Acta Pediatrica Scandinavica, 58, 449–459.

Hers, H.G. (1964) Glycogen Storage Disease. Advances in Metabolic Disorders, 1, 1–44, 335–336.

Holdsworth, C.D. (1969) The gut and oral glucose tolerance. Gut, 10, 422–427.

Klimt, C.R., Knatterud, G.L., Meinert, B.L. and Prout, T.E. (1970) A study of the effect of hypoglycemic agents on vascular complications in patients with adult-onset diabetes. I. Design, methods and baseline results. II. Mortality results. Diabetes, 19, 747–783, 785–830.

Madison, L.L. (1968) Ethanol induced hypoglycaemia. Advances in Metabolic Disorders, 3, 85-109.

Marks, V. (1969) Practical aspects of the investigation of disorders of carbohydrate metabolism. Journal of Clinical Pathology, 22, suppl. 2, 42–47.

Marks, V. (1974) The investigation of hypoglycaemia. British Journal of Hospital Medicine, 11, 731–743.

McIntyre, N., Holdsworth, C.D. and Turner, D.S. (1964) New interpretation of oral glucose tolerance. Lancet, 2, 20–21.

Peacock, M., Gallagher, J.C. and Nordin, B.E.C. (1974) Action of 1α-hydroxy vitamin D_3 on calcium absorption and bone resorption in man. Lancet, 1, 385–386.

Robertson, R.P. and Porte, D. (1973) Adrenergic modulation of basal insulin secretion in man. Diabetes, 22, 1–8.

Sauls, Jr., H.S. and Ulstrom, R.A. (1966) In Brenneman's Practice of Pediatrics, Vol. 1 (Ed. V.C. Kelly) Chap. 40, pp. 1–68, W.S. Prior Co., Hagerstown.

Seltzer, H.S. (1972) Drug-induced hypoglycemia – a review based on 43 cases. Diabetes, 21, 955–966.

Simpson, H.W. (1976) A new perspective – chronobiochemistry. In Essays in Medical Biochemistry, Vol. 2. (Ed. V. Marks and C.N. Hales) The Biochemical Society and the Association of Clinical Biochemists, London.

Snell, C.R. and Smyth, D.G. (1975) Proinsulin: a proposed 3-dimensional structure. Journal of Biological Chemistry, 250, 6291–6295.

Steiner, D.F., Kemmler, W., Clarke, J.L., Oyer, P.E. and Rubenstein, A.H. (1972) The biosynthesis of insulin. In Handbook of Physiology, Section 7, Vol. I, Endocrine Pancreas (Eds. D.F. Steiner and N. Freinkel) pp. 175–198, American Physiological Society, Washington, D.C.

Symposium on Insulin Metabolism (1973) Postgraduate Medical Journal, 49, suppl., 931–963.

Unger, R.H. (1974) Alpha- and beta-cell interrelationship in health and disease. Metabolism, 23, 581–593.

Williams, R.H. (1968) Hypoglycaemia and hypoglycemoses. In Textbook of Endocrinology (Ed. R.H. Williams) pp. 803–846, W.B. Saunders, Philadelphia.

Zuppinger, K.A. (1975) Hypoglycaemia in Childhood, 135 pp., S. Karger, Basel.

FURTHER READING

Malins, J. (1968) Clinical Diabetes Mellitus. Eyre and Spottiswoode, London.

Oakley, W.G., Pyke, D.A. and Taylor, K.W. (1968) Clinical Diabetes and its Biochemical Basis. Blackwell Scientific Publications, Oxford and Edinburgh.

Marble, A., White, P., Bradley, R.F. and Krall, L.P. (Eds.) (1971) Joslins Diabetes Mellitus, 11th edition. Lea and Febiger, Philadelphia.

Keen, H. and Jarrett, J. (Eds.) (1975) Complications of Diabetes. Edward Arnold, London.

Cornblath, M. and Schwartz, R. (1976) Disorders of Carbohydrate Metabolism in Infancy, 2nd edition. W.B. Saunders, Philadelphia and London.

Sutherland, H.W. and Stowers, J.M. (Eds.) (1975) Carbohydrate Metabolism in Pregnancy and the Newborn. pp. 252, Churchill Livingstone, Edinburgh, London and New York.

ADDENDUM

In the 2½ years since this Chapter was completed naturally a large number of new publications have appeared which it is not possible to summarize in a few words. However, probably the most important single advancement has been the recognition that the measurement of glycosylated haemoglobin gives important information about the long-term control of diabetes. This subject has been recently reviewed: Gonen, B. and Rubenstein, A.H. (1978) Haemoglobin A1 and diabetes mellitus. Diabetologia, 15, 1–8.

Chapter 5

Lipids

Barry Lewis

Department of Chemical Pathology and Metabolic Diseases, St Thomas's Hospital, London SE1 7EH, England

CONTENTS

Chemical diagnosis of disease, edited by S.S. Brown, F.L. Mitchell and D.S. Young

5.1. INTRODUCTION

The concentrations of the several lipids of plasma are widely variable, both between and within normal populations. Florid disorders of the lipoprotein system are uncommon; but recent epidemiological evidence is persuasive that even minor degrees of certain hyperlipidaemias are prominent among the risk factors for ischaemic heart disease (Keys, 1966; Stamler et al., 1972; Carlson and Böttiger, 1972; Wilhelmsen et al., 1973; Lewis et al., 1974a). For this reason, chiefly, clinical interest in plasma lipid disorders has burgeoned in the past decade, and numerous specialized lipid clinics are being set up. Pathologists have had to come to terms with this growing subspeciality, in which clinical and laboratory medicine are highly interdependent and in which knowledge is advancing and concepts are changing at a formidable rate. Because of these developments some comments on basic chemistry and physiology are especially necessary.

5.2. THE LIPOPROTEINS OF PLASMA

5.2.1. Characteristics and composition

Lipids are by definition poorly soluble in water. Virtually all of the plasma lipid, totalling about 0.4 to 0.8 g/dl in the fasted state, is held in solution in the form of lipoproteins. These complex proteins, all somewhat variable in composition, comprise specific apoproteins, cholesterol, cholesteryl esters, triglycerides and phospholipids, in differing proportions. Separation methods include flotation in the ultracentrifuge or under gravity, taking advantage of the uniquely low density conferred by their lipid content. Electrophoretic separation is also commonly employed; it is technically less demanding but also less easily quantitated. Table 5.1 lists some of the properties and the approximate compositions of the four major lipoprotein classes, as operationally defined.

Subclasses of these lipoprotein groups can be separated, the compositions and other properties of which represent a series of small stepwise differences in properties; for example, the densest subclass of VLDL resembles the less dense component of LDL. The latter, of density 1.006 to 1.019 g/ml, is richer in triglyceride and contains apolipoprotein C; it has become known as intermediate density lipoprotein, (I.D.L. or LDL_1).

About 60% of the cholesterol in plasma is present in LDL (i.e. β-lipoprotein), and at least 50% of the triglyceride of fasting plasma is present in VLDL (i.e. pre-β-lipoprotein). While changes in the concentration of any lipoprotein could in theory produce hypercholesterolaemia and hypertriglyceridaemia, the compositions of the four classes are such that increased triglyceride levels are most often due to a raised concentration of VLDL, and occasionally to chylomicronaemia, while raised cholesterol levels are commonly the result of a high concentration of LDL. Raised concentrations of HDL (α-lipoprotein) can also produce mild hypercholesterolaemia.

TABLE 5.1.

CHARACTERISTICS AND COMPOSITION OF THE MAJOR LIPOPROTEINS OF PLASMA

Ultracentrifugation	Density range (g/ml)	Electrophoresis	Triglycerides (%)	Cholesteryl esters (%)	Cholesterol (%)	Phospholipids (%)	Protein (%)	Major apoproteins
Chylomicrons	<0.95	Largely immobile	85	4	2	7	1–2	A,B,C
Very low density lipoproteins (VLDL)	0.95–1.006	pre β (α–2)	52	17	7	15	9	B,C,E
Low density lipoproteins (LDL)	1.019–1.063	β	10	37	8	23	22	B
High density lipoproteins (HDL)	1.063–1.21	α (α–1)	4	18	2	25	51	A,E

5.2.2. The apoproteins

The apoproteins, which can be immunochemically defined, in some ways afford a better means of distinguishing groups of lipoproteins than the less specific physical properties which are conventionally used. HDL contains two major polypeptides (AI and AII), small quantities of apoprotein C and traces also of apoprotein B, and a functionally minor component, apoprotein D or apoprotein CIII. Apo AI activates the enzyme lecithin:cholesterol acyltransferase (LCAT, EC 2.3.1.43). LDL_2 contains apolipoprotein B; LDL_1 has apoprotein B and apoprotein C, and also an arginine-rich apoprotein E which may have a special role in the transport of cholesterol. VLDL and chylomicrons contain apoprotein B and apoprotein C, the latter having four components, of which CII is the specific activator of the enzyme lipoprotein lipase (EC 3.1.1.3); nascent chylomicrons have a substantial content of Apo A peptides. The arginine-rich peptide is present in VLDL, IDL and HDL.

5.2.3. Synthesis and catabolism

Chylomicrons carry triglycerides of exogenous (dietary) origin and are synthesized in the small intestinal mucosa. The synthesis of triglyceride in the small bowel chiefly involves the monoglyceride pathway, i.e. absorbed monoglyceride reacts serially with two molecules of fatty acyl-CoA, the esterification being catalyzed by an acyltransferase. Apoprotein B, and also the apoprotein A group, are synthesized in the endoplasmic reticulum of mucosal cells and there combine with the triglyceride and other lipids to form nascent chylomicrons. The carbohydrate moiety is added in the Golgi apparatus. After release from the cell, the chylomicron acquires its full apoprotein C moiety by transfer from HDL. VLDL, which is secreted by the liver, carries endogenous triglyceride; in health this is synthesized from the plasma free fatty acids, which are produced in adipose tissue, but in obesity and other abnormal circumstances other precursors are also utilized. The main synthesis of triglyceride in the liver occurs by esterification of glycerol-3-phosphate with two acyl-CoA molecules to form phosphatidic acid; addition of a further molecule of acyl-CoA yields triglyceride. The subsequent assembly of nascent and "mature" VLDL is analogous to that of the chylomicrons. Some dietary triglyceride is carried in VLDL of intestinal origin.

These lipoproteins undergo compositional changes after their secretion. VLDL triglyceride is largely hydrolyzed by lipoprotein lipase, which is present in the capillary endothelium of muscle, adipose tissue and other organs. Most fatty acid so produced is taken up by these tissues, while VLDL remnants containing cholesterol and phospholipid remain in the circulation, probably forming smaller VLDL particles and intermediate density lipoprotein. VLDL appears to be ultimately converted almost completely into LDL in normal subjects (Sigurdsson et al., 1975). This requires extensive remodelling, involving transfer of apoprotein C and some free cholesterol and lecithin from VLDL and LDL to HDL. Thus in normal subjects LDL is derived, probably entirely, from the catabolism of VLDL. The conversion involves the enzymes lipoprotein lipase and lecithin:cholesterol acyltransferase, and HDL plays an important role. An analogous process appears to exist by which chylomicrons are catabolized to chylomicron remnants, which are then metabolized by the liver.

In man consuming a Western diet (>400 mg cholesterol per day), dietary cholesterol contributes substantially to the cholesterol in plasma; however, it exchanges rapidly with the cholesterol of the liver, red cells and intestine, and more slowly with that of skin, muscle and connective tissue. Endogenous cholesterol is synthesized from acetyl-CoA, the major rate-limiting step being the reduction of β-hydroxy-β-methylglutaryl-CoA to mevalonic acid. Condensation of three C-5 units gives rise to farnesyl pyrophosphate, two molecules of which condense to form squalene, a C-30 hydrocarbon. This cyclizes to produce the four-ring sterol configuration, loses three methyl groups and after further modifications gives rise to cholesterol (C-27). Cholesterol regulates the rate of its own synthesis by repression of hydroxymethylglutaryl-CoA reductase (EC 1.1.1.34/88). Consequently, sterol biosynthesis is enhanced by restricting dietary cholesterol, or by drugs which increase the rate of catabolism of cholesterol to bile salts.

5.2.4. Transport

Thus the plasma lipoproteins are not independent entities of constant composition, but are best regarded as often-labile components of a dynamic system for lipid transport. Triglyceride is carried from the small intestine and the liver to peripheral tissues in chylomicrons and VLDL. Cholesterol is transported centrifugally from the liver and small intestine as VLDL, and from the latter also in chylomicrons; most of the cholesteryl ester which remains within the particle as VLDL is converted into LDL. LDL is then catabolized extravascularly. There is evidence to suggest that this takes place in non-hepatic tissues; cell lines which can catabolize LDL in vitro include fibroblasts, smooth muscle cells, adipocytes and lymphocytes. "Internalization" of LDL by these cells appears to be mediated by cell-surface receptors which can "recognize" Apo B and, probably, the arginine-rich apolipoprotein. Synthesis of receptor protein may be regulated in a manner which stabilizes intracellular content of free cholesterol (Brown and Goldstein, 1976). After internalization, LDL is catabolized in lysosomes, the apoprotein being hydrolyzed.

There is also a distinct mechanism for centripetal transport of free cholesterol from peripheral tissues, where it becomes redundant during the course of cell turnover, to the liver; free cholesterol is transferred to HDL, and becomes esterified by lecithin:cholesterol acyltransferase. It then transfers largely to VLDL, and thence to LDL. Hepatic cholesterol is either catabolized to bile acid, or excreted in the bile, or incorporated into newly synthesized lipoproteins.

5.3. DEFINITIONS OF NORMAL LIPID CONCENTRATIONS

Major problems, both technical and conceptual, hinder the recognition of reference values for serum lipid and lipoprotein concentrations, and the positive identification of risk factors for associated diseases.

5.3.1. Factors which influence reference intervals

5.3.1.1. Geographical differences

Large geographical differences in serum lipid concentrations have been shown. Apparently healthy subjects in various communities show as much as a 2- to 3-fold difference between age- and sex-specific mean concentrations of serum cholesterol and triglyceride. The lower levels are seen in rural populations in the developing world, and also in Japan; these populations have a low incidence of ischaemic cardiovascular diseases and, with few exceptions, consume low average intakes of saturated fats. Higher serum concentrations of both lipids are characteristic of western societies in which ischaemic heart disease is common (Keys, 1966). A major determinant of these differences appears to be dietary, and is probably related chiefly to intake of saturated fats and cholesterol.

In practice, this variability makes it impossible to derive universally applicable reference ranges for serum lipids from population studies. It is necessary for the hospital laboratory to use norms appropriate for the populations which it serves.

5.3.1.2. Effects of age

The concentrations of serum lipids vary in a complex manner with age. They are low in umbilical cord blood, rise steeply in early childhood, then increase very slowly to early adult life. This pattern appears to be quite general, but changes of lipid concentrations in later life are less consistently observed. In western communities, e.g. U.S.A. and Western Europe, cholesterol and triglyceride increase during adult life to a maximum in the sixth or seventh decade, then level off or decrease (Figure 5.1) (Lewis et al., 1974b). The peaks in late middle age may be 40% or more above the values in the decade 20 to 29 years. However, this rise of cholesterol and triglyceride concentrations with adult age is not seen in apparently normal populations living in developing countries. At the present time, it is not clear whether the increase in lipid concentrations in the fourth, fifth and sixth decades should be regarded as physiological, in which case reference ranges should be age-adjusted. The alternative view is to regard it as reflecting a rising prevalance of hyperlipidaemia with age; if so, reference ranges might be better based upon findings in younger adults, aged 20 to 29 or 20 to 39 years.

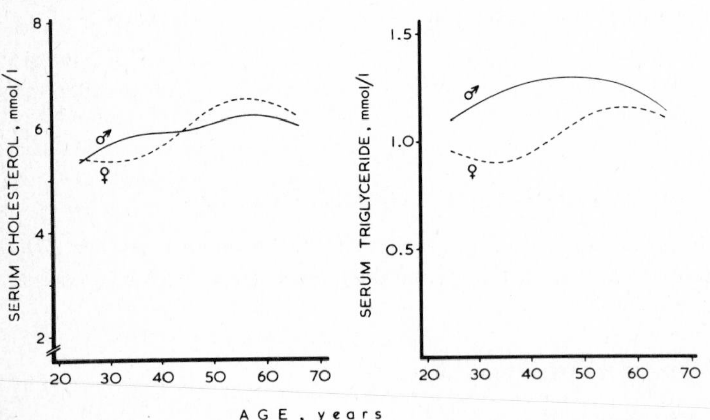

Fig. 5.1. Age trends and sex differences in serum cholesterol and triglyceride concentrations in a London population. (Reproduced, by permission, from Lewis et al., 1974b).

5.3.1.3. Sex differences

Serum lipid concentrations show sex differences which are more pronounced in the case of triglyceride than cholesterol. Serum triglyceride concentrations in men are higher at all ages than in women; in the age group 20 to 39 years, values in males are about 40% higher than those in females, the difference becoming less with advancing age (Carlson and Lindstedt, 1969; Lewis et al., 1974b). Although it is not common practice to use different references ranges for men and women, the sex difference in triglyceride concentrations is probably large enough to justify doing so.

The concentration of serum cholesterol is slightly but significantly higher in young men than in young women. The rise in women during the fourth and fifth decades is much steeper than that in men; as a result, older women have moderately higher cholesterol concentrations than men. The sex difference is seldom allowed for in defining a reference range for serum cholesterol concentration.

5.3.1.4. Other sources of variability

Inter-laboratory variation in lipid analyses is substantial, partly due to differences in the methods employed. Strictly speaking, a reference range is tied to the analytical method used, though there is probably little systematic variation between laboratories using automated methods on lipid extracts. Further sources of variation relate to the conditions under which the blood sample is drawn. These should be standardized as far as possible, to ensure that the analyses are representative of the subjects' usual metabolic state. Blood samples are normally drawn after a 12 to 14 hour fast, and it is advisable for the subject to avoid alcoholic drinks on the evening prior to sampling, as alimentary lipaemia is markedly prolonged by ethanol. Prolonged venous stasis during venesection can introduce a substantial artefactual rise in lipid concentrations (Koerselman et al., 1961). The subject should take his usual diet for 2 to 3 weeks prior to sampling, as lipid levels are sensitive to caloric restriction, to the quantity and type of fat consumed, and to the intake of carbohydrate or alcohol. Similarly, drugs affecting lipid metabolism should be discontinued for at least 3 weeks before lipid measurements are performed. Recent illness can disturb the metabolism of plasma lipids, cholesterol levels often falling steeply, and triglyceride levels either rising or falling. Lipid analyses should be deferred for 2 to 3 weeks after minor illness, and for 3 months or more after major illness, surgery or trauma; this is particularly important in the investigation of patients after myocardial infarction.

The effect of many of these sources of clinical and laboratory variability is of course minimized by analyzing two or more blood specimens obtained on separate occasions. For clinical purposes, two or three samples must be analyzed before committing the patient to lifelong therapy.

Lipid analyses on specimens from patients should be carried out in the ambulant state or on the morning after admission. It should be noted that hospitalization is commonly associated with an unexplained fall in serum lipid concentrations. When the concentrations are initially high, the fall may be due partly to regression towards the mean, but the response also occurs within the reference range.

5.3.1.5. Frequency distribution curves

The frequency distribution curves for serum cholesterol and triglyceride concentrations are not Gaussian; there is a greater or lesser degree of skewing to the right. In most reports, the asymmetry of cholesterol distributions is not pronounced, though some workers have improved the symmetry by logarithmic transformation of the data. Triglyceride distributions are grossly skewed, and the curves are rendered more normal by logarithmic transformation.

It is preferable to employ cut-off points based on percentiles in defining the normal ranges; commonly the 10th and 90th percentiles are used, though the 5th and 95th percentiles may be chosen.

5.3.2. Some reference intervals

The reference intervals for serum lipid concentrations as used by the author are shown in Table 5.2 (Lewis et al., 1974b). They are based on a carefully screened normal population in London, with due regard to the variables mentioned in section 5.3.1.4. The age range was 20 to 39 years. Samples were collected during a 2-year period to avoid bias due to seasonal variation in lipid concentrations, which tend to rise in the winter and fall in the summer. Sera were extracted with isopropanol according to the Technicon N-78 method for serum triglyceride determination (section 5.5.3.), based upon that of Kessler and Lederer (1966). Automated lipid analyses were then performed, using the Technicon N-24a method for cholesterol and the procedure of Cramp and Robertson (1968) for triglyceride. The 10th and 90th percentiles were employed.

Other lipids are seldom measured in clinical practice, and far less information is available concerning reference intervals. There are even fewer data concerning the lipid concentrations in the lipoprotein classes, though some American and British figures have been published (Fredrickson and Levy, 1972; Lewis et al., 1974b).

In umbilical cord blood, the concentration of serum cholesterol ranges from 1.3 to 2.5 mmol/litre (50 to 95 mg/dl), and of triglyceride from 0.11 to 0.74 mmol/litre (10 to 65 mg/dl) (Levy and Rifkind, 1973).

5.3.3. Risk factors

On the basis of certain assumptions, it is possible to define statistical norms for serum lipid concentrations (section 5.3.2). However, the definition of biological norms is far more difficult. The concentrations of serum lipids vary widely between apparently nor-

TABLE 5.2

REFERENCE INTERVALS FOR SERUM CHOLESTEROL AND TRIGLYCERIDE CONCENTRATIONS IN ADULTS (LONDON, ENGLAND)

	mmol/litre	mg/dl
Cholesterol	4.5–6.5	170–250
Triglyceride (men)	0.7–2.1	60–185
Triglyceride (women)	0.6–1.5	55–135.

mal communities. This is not, in the main, due to genetic factors, but reflects differences in diet and possibly other aspects of life style.

Hypercholesterolaemia is unquestionably a risk factor for ischaemic heart disease (Stamler et al., 1972). The status of hypertriglyceridaemia as a risk factor is less well established, but a prospective survey in Stockholm (Carlson and Böttiger, 1972) has provided evidence to indicate that subjects in the top quintile of the population in respect of triglyceride concentrations have a marked increase in risk of ischaemic heart disease. Serum lipid levels appear to confer a graded increase in risk, and no threshold value has been defined below which the disease does not occur. Nevertheless, data from the U.S. Pooling Project (Stamler et al., 1972) suggest that the risk of ischaemic heart disease begins to increase steeply when the concentration of serum cholesterol exceeds 6.5 mmol/litre (250 mg/dl). Clearly the presence of concurrent risk factors, such as cigarette smoking, can confer additional risk at lower levels of serum cholesterol.

If inter-population variation in the incidence of ischaemic heart disease is compared with regional differences in the concentrations of serum cholesterol, it is evident that communities in which the disease is rare have very low mean cholesterol and triglyceride concentrations by western standards. By any criterion based upon observed ranges in "ischaemic heart disease-immune" populations, a high proportion of western populations would be judged to be hyperlipidaemic.

5.4. THE HYPERLIPIDAEMIC STATES (Lewis, 1976)

A large number of metabolic disorders is associated with elevated concentrations of cholesterol or triglyceride, or of both lipids, in plasma. This heterogeneity makes classification necessary; from the clinical viewpoint, a major reason for classifying these disorders is to facilitate an optimal choice of therapy (Tabaqchali et al., 1974). As first emphasized by Fredrickson et al. (1967), and elaborated by Beaumont et al. (1970), classification is made more rational by the concept of hyperlipoproteinaemias than by thinking only in terms of elevated lipid concentrations. The concentrations of lipoproteins vary in plasma, and consequent changes in the concentration of total cholesterol or triglyceride depend on the compostion of the affected lipoproteins (section 5.5.4.). Some lipoprotein disorders are inherited as such, e.g. hyper-β-lipoproteinaemia and α-lipoprotein deficiency; in other conditions, however, it is hyperlipidaemia of one or other type which appears to be inherited, without close correspondence to a particular type of hyperlipoproteinaemia (Goldstein et al., 1973a).

The primary information which affords recognition of a hyperlipoproteinaemic state is usually an abnormality of concentration of serum cholesterol or triglyceride, or both. In this section, therefore, these disorders are grouped as states characterized chiefly by hypercholesterolaemia, those characterized chiefly by hypertriglyceridaemia, and the combined hyperlipidaemias.

The first step is to distinguish primary and secondary hyperlipidaemias; some 15% of patients have hyperlipidaemia secondary to a recognized underlying cause.

5.4.1. Secondary hyperlipidaemias

Secondary hyperlipidaemias more often manifest with hypertriglyceridaemia than hypercholesterolaemia, but in most a variety of abnormalities of serum lipoproteins can develop. Some causes, for example hypothyroidism and nephrotic syndrome, are associated with hyperlipidaemia in the great majority of cases; but only about one-third of uncontrolled diabetics have raised concentrations of serum lipids, and the proportion of alcoholics with hyperlipidaemia is probably even lower. Development of hyperlipidaemia depends upon the interaction between the causal condition and other factors, which appear to include genetic make-up, diet, and associated pathological conditions. The severity and time course of the primary condition are also important. Many patients with hypertriglyceridaemia which is associated with alcohol abuse respond to withdrawal of alcohol by a profound and rapid fall of lipid levels, but these remain somewhat elevated; such patients have a primary hypertriglyceridaemia which is aggravated by alcohol.

Common causes of secondary hyperlipidaemia are uncontrolled diabetes (both insulin-requiring and diet-responsive), chronic renal failure, nephrotic syndrome, alcoholism, hypothyroidism (both primary and secondary), cholestasis and gout. Gout differs from the other conditions listed in that reduction of hyperuricaemia often has no effect on the hypertriglyceridaemia; more often, treatment of the underlying cause corrects the associated hyperlipidaemia. Other causes include partial and total lipodystrophy, glycogenoses types I, III and VI, Werner's syndrome, anorexia nervosa, ideopathic hypercalcaemia and acute intermittent porphyria. Hyper-γ-globulinaemia due to myelomatosis and systemic lupus erythematosus are sometimes associated with pronounced lipaemia. Medication with oestrogens, e.g. high-oestrogen oral contraceptives, usually causes mild hypertriglyceridaemia or an increase of lipid levels within the reference range, but some susceptible individuals, including patients with primary hypertriglyceridaemia, may develop intense lipaemia, with complicating pancreatitis. Primary hepatoma and isolated growth hormone deficiency may be accompanied by hypercholesterolaemia.

In some of these conditions, particularly diabetes, chronic renal disease, gout and hypothyroidism, there is persuasive evidence of a predisposition to ischaemic heart disease. Alcoholism, long regarded as protective, may actually be a risk factor for ischaemic heart disease (Wilhelmsen et al., 1973).

Secondary hyperlipidaemias are often associated with qualitative abnormalities in serum lipoproteins. In obstructive jaundice, hyperlipidaemia is largely due to an abnormal low density lipoprotein which is rich in free cholesterol and phospholipid; this composition is reflected in the pattern of the serum lipid abnormality. This lipoprotein, known as LP-X, has an unusual and low protein content, containing apolipoprotein C and albumin. It occurs in many patients with intrahepatic or extrahepatic cholestasis and in the rare disorder lecithin:cholesterol acyltransferase deficiency. In diabetes, LDL and HDL have a somewhat increased triglyceride content. Qualitatively abnormal VLDL with β mobility on electrophoresis – the hallmark of the type III pattern – may accumulate in plasma in hyperlipidaemia which is secondary to diabetes, hypothyroidism and hyper-γ-globulinaemia.

5.4.2. Primary hypercholesterolaemias and hyper-β-lipoproteinaemias

Primary hypercholesterolaemic states, characterized by a serum cholesterol concentration which consistently exceeds the 90th percentile for the population concerned (triglyceride levels being normal), is most often due to hyper-β-lipoproteinaemia (i.e. type IIa hyperlipoproteinaemia). A few families have been recognized in whom mild hypercholesterolaemia is due to raised concentrations of α-lipoprotein; there appear to be no untoward consequences of this state, and no treatment is required. Its differentiation from hyper-β-lipoproteinaemia is by means of electrophoresis or, preferably, by quantitation of β-lipoprotein.

Although it is not fully established, it is probable that there are at least two forms of hyper-β-lipoproteinaemia. Of these, the commoner is weakly – perhaps polygenically – inherited. Hypercholesterolaemia is usually but not always moderate in degree. Premature arcus and xanthelasmas may occur. The pathogenesis is uncertain. Dietary change – reduction in intake of saturated fat and cholesterol, with increased polyunsaturated fat – often corrects the hyperlipidaemia. Less frequently, hyper-β-lipoproteinaemia is inherited monogenically, as an autosomal dominant trait. In the heterozygote, the serum cholesterol concentration ranges from 7.8. to 14 mmol/litre (300 to 550 mg/dl), and in the very rare homozygous state, from 13 to 31 mmol/litre (500 to 1200 mg/dl). Tendon xanthomas are common, as is premature arcus. Homozygotes have cutaneous xanthomas, usually planar or tubero-planar, and may have episodes of acute arthritis. The hypercholesterolaemia is detectable within the first year of life, and in affected families the concentration of LDL in cord blood plasma is raised.

In both forms of hyper-β-lipoproteinaemia the diagnostic feature is elevation of LDL-cholesterol concentration above a chosen cut-off point, while serum triglyceride or VLDL-triglyceride concentrations are most often normal. This is the likely diagnosis in patients with "pure" hypercholesterolaemia of primary aetiology. The serum is clear in appearance. If electrophoresis is carried out, its main value is to confirm the presence of an increase in β-lipoprotein, often with decreased α- and pre-β-bands; it will reveal the rare alternative of hyper-α-lipoproteinaemia. Where possible, quantitation of LDL-cholesterol concentration may be performed to confirm the diagnosis, but this is not essential.

The pathogenesis of the first ("polygenic") form of hyper-β-lipoproteinaemia is unclear, though it is suspected that it reflects a high degree of responsiveness of cholesterol metabolism to environmental factors, in particular to dietary intake of fat and cholesterol. The monogenic form has been extensively studied. There is no agreement concerning the relative importance of overproduction of LDL or of cholesterol, and of impaired catabolism of LDL or of cholesterol. Absorption is not enhanced, and despite some dispute the consensus is that the excretion of cholesterol and its catabolism to bile acid are not significantly reduced. In the homozygous state, evidence of increased LDL synthesis has been put forward (Simons et al., 1975). In both heterozygotes and homozygotes impaired catabolism of LDL is postulated (Langer et al., 1972). Normal skin fibroblasts and other cell lines grown in tissue culture are believed to have relatively specific mechanisms for uptake of LDL from the medium, which are dependent upon LDL receptors on the cell surface; one concept of monogenic hyper-β-lipoproteinaemia is that these receptors are deficient in number in cells from heterozygotes and are absent in homozygotes (Goldstein and Brown, 1973); in consequence, the catabolism of LDL apoprotein is abnormal. An alternative, but perhaps compatible, view is that a cell membrane defect permits abnormal efflux of cholesterol from the cell (Fogelman et al., 1975). In addition the impaired entry of LDL-cholesterol into the cells releases the biosynthesis of cholesterol from its normal repression. Despite some controversy as to the mechanism involved, it is clear that cells from homozygous patients show grossly deficient LDL uptake (internalization, section 5.2.4) (Stein et al., 1976). Both impaired LDL catabolism and enhanced cholesterol synthesis may, therefore, result from this defect. At sufficiently high plasma LDL levels it is possible that a new steady state is achieved, repression of cholesterol synthesis being restored at the expense of hypercholesterolaemia.

In due course it may be possible to develop an in vitro test for the disorder, based on these findings.

5.4.3. Primary hyperlipidaemias

Primary hyperlipidaemia, characterized chiefly by endogenous hypertriglyceridaemia, is a prevalent group of conditions. It includes an unknown number of metabolic and/or genetic entities. Plasma lipoprotein patterns may be of types IV (most often) or V, i.e., there is pre-β-hyperlipoproteinaemia alone (type IV) or together with chylomicronaemia (type V). It is now accepted that types IV and V not infrequently co-exist in the same family; families with members showing types III and IV have also been described. The inheritance sometimes conforms to the features of a dominant trait but often the disorder appears sporadic or weakly inherited. Polygenic inheritance has been suggested. Onset is most often in adult life.

Associated features include obesity, which is found in the majority of patients. Xanthelasmas may occur. When the hyperlipidaemia is severe, eruptive xanthomas and lipaemia retinalis may be seen, and episodes of severe abdominal pain may develop, sometimes due to acute pancreatitis. (It may be noted that in the presence of lipaemia, there may be interference in the measurement of raised amylase activities leading to false negative results.) Hepatomegaly and sometimes splenomegaly may occur. Hyperuricaemia is common, but it is usually mild. Acute gouty arthritis may be a presenting feature. Glucose intolerance and hyperinsulinism are also common. Fasting hyperglycaemia is unusual, and if it is substantial (e.g. more than 6.6 mmol/litre, 120 mg/dl) it is usual to assign a diagnosis of hypertriglyceridaemia secondary to diabetes rather than that of primary hyperlipidaemia. It is not clear whether glucose intolerance is part of the syndrome of primary endogenous hypertriglyceridaemia or whether these are often co-existing but independent entities; recent evidence tends to favour the latter view.

The diagnosis of primary hyperlipidaemia is suggested by the presence of hypertriglyceridaemia with a normal or moderately increased concentration of serum cholesterol. Exogenous hypertriglyceridaemia, a distinct entity, has similar features but is very much rarer, particularly in adults. The hallmark of most endogenous hypertriglyceridaemias is an elevated concentration of serum VLDL, i.e. VLDL triglyceride (or VLDL cholesterol) concentrations exceed the 90th percentile. The appearance of stored serum (section 5.5.4.1) usually distinguishes between endogenous and exogenous hypertriglyceridaemia.

Serum is lactescent, except in a minority of samples with endogenous hypertriglyceridaemia. In exogenous hypertriglyceridaemia, the excess of triglyceride is present almost entirely in chylomicrons; these particles float under the conditions of the stored serum test, producing a dense creamy layer in the upper part of the sample and leaving the subnatant clear. On present knowledge, this appearance in serum obtained in the fasted state is diagnostic of exogenous hypertriglyceridaemia. In endogenous hypertriglyceridaemia, the specimen remains lactescent throughout, as VLDL does not float under the conditions of the test; sometimes chylomicronaemia accompanies the endogenous hypertriglyceridaemia and gives the appearance of a lactescent sample in which a creamy layer is present at the top of the specimen.

Electrophoresis shows a heavily stained pre-β band in endogenous hypertriglyceridaemia, often with decreased staining in the α- and β-regions. Associated chylomicronaemia results in staining at the origin.

Some workers have attributed endogenous hypertriglyceridaemia to increased production of VLDL, others to a removal defect. Methodological problems abound in this area, and selection of cases may be a factor in a disorder which is probably heterogeneous. Using radio-iodination of VLDL-apoprotein, evidence has been obtained that overproduction of VLDL is common and that there is a positive correlation between production rate and plasma VLDL concentration (Sigurdsson et al., 1976). However, some patients have normal rates of synthesis of VLDL, and here the mechanism must be a removal defect.

Endogenous hypertriglyceridaemia cannot be equated with carbohydrate-induced lipaemia. Some 50% of patients taking a very high carbohydrate diet for 7 days display exaggerated rise in serum triglyceride; but it is not known whether the effect is transient, as it is in normal subjects, or whether persisting hypertriglyceridaemia in some patients is due to sensitivity to carbohydrate consumed at a more normal level. Certainly severe endogenous hypertriglyceridaemia is seldom fully corrected by carbohydrate restriction, though this often ameliorates the lipaemia. Patients with endogenous hypertriglyceridaemia may show a marked increase in lipid levels when they overindulge in alcohol.

5.4.4. Primary hypertriglyceridaemia

Primary exogenous hypertriglyceridaemia is a rare disorder which is induced by dietary fat and corrected by a fat-free diet. There is chylomicronaemia in serum obtained in the fasted state (type I hyperlipoproteinaemia). It is most often of extreme degree, with serum triglyceride levels up to 100 or 180 mmol/litre (8850 to 16,000 mg/dl). The disorder may present with acute abdominal pain or eruptive xanthomas; retinal lipaemia is sometimes observed and hepatosplenomegaly is common. Presentation is most often in infancy or childhood but cases are sometimes recognized de novo in early adult life. The disorder is aggravated by pregnancy and by exogenous oestrogen.

In addition to pronounced hypertriglyceridaemia, the concentration of serum cholesterol is increased, though to a lesser extent. As mentioned in section 5.5.4., stored serum shows marked floating lactescence; the subnatant is clear or, at most, shows traces of lactescence.

The disorder is due to deficiency or absence of a key enzyme in the system for uptake of circulating triglyceride, the lipoprotein lipase of extrahepatic tissues – particularly adipose tissue and muscle. Dietary fat which enters plasma in chylomicrons therefore accumulates in the circulation. VLDL levels are normal or slightly increased in most patients but in some, the levels are distinctly elevated, producing a type V pattern. Although VLDL triglyceride is normally hydrolyzed by extrahepatic lipoprotein lipase, it seems that when this enzyme is deficient, other lipases can take over this role; perhaps hepatic lipase hydrolyzes VLDL sufficiently rapidly to maintain near-normal plasma levels of this lipoprotein.

Diagnosis of the disorder is based upon the demonstration of lipid levels as described, with recognition of fasting chylomicronaemia by the stored serum test. This may be supplemented by lipoprotein electrophoresis or by quantitative ultracentrifugation to determine the chylomicron and VLDL triglyceride concentrations. Lipoprotein lipase is at present assayed in tissues only as a research procedure. It is released into plasma from the capillary endothelium by exogenous heparin (10 to 100 units/kg body weight), and lipolytic activity is assayed in plasma obtained 10 minutes after intravenous injection of heparin (post-heparin lipolytic activity, PHLA, section 5.5.7.).

The final diagnostic feature is a therapeutic response to a diet containing less than 5 g fat per 24 hours. Within 1 to 3 days, chylomicronaemia may be profoundly decreased or disappear, though moderate hypertriglyceridaemia usually persists.

5.4.5. Combined hypertriglyceridaemia and hypercholesterolaemia

This condition refers to a substantial increase in cholesterol as well as triglyceride concentrations. This may be found in apparently healthy subjects and is remarkably common in patients with ischaemic heart disease (Goldstein et al., 1973b; Lewis et al., 1974a). Most often LDL and VLDL levels are increased, constituting type IIb hyperlipoproteinaemia. More rarely, cholesterol-rich VLDL accumulates in plasma, and usually shows atypical β mobility on electrophoresis (section 5.5.4.2.) instead of the pre-β migration of normal VLDL; this abnormality – type III hyperlipoproteinaemia or remnant hyperlipoproteinaemia – is sometimes also known as broad β-disease.

Combined hyperlipidaemia is also sometimes due to an increased concentration of VLDL alone, in which case the increase in triglyceride concentration is relatively greater than that of cholesterol; this is especially so when combined hyperlipidaemia is due to the type V pattern – increased VLDL with chylomicronaemia.

The IIb pattern is itself heterogeneous. Some patients are members of families with monogenic familial hyper-β-lipoproteinaemia; the raised concentration of LDL is due to the underlying familial defect, and the increase in VLDL is sometimes explicable in terms of associated diabetes, alcoholism or obesity. Such patients effectively have two lipoprotein disorders and may require treatment for both. More often, combined hyperlipidaemia may have features in common with familial endogenous hypertriglyceridaemia, with a high frequency of obesity, glucose intolerance and hyperuricaemia; treatment is also similar. There is current disagreement as to whether the genetic basis is polygenic or whether a single dominant gene is responsible. A characteristic feature is that affected members of families show an indeterminate lipoprotein pattern, variably manifesting the type IIb, IV, V or IIa lipoprotein pattern.

Diagnosis of combined hyperlipidaemia is based upon the consistent finding of cholesterol and triglyceride concentrations both exceeding their 90th percentiles, or other chosen cut-off points. The uncommon remnant hyperlipoproteinaemia is suspected clinically when linear planar xanthomas are present in the palmar creases and tuberous xanthomas are seen on the elbows or knees. Serum lipoprotein electrophoresis on agarose, cellulose acetate or paper, which shows a broad band extending from the β- through to the pre-β-region makes the diagnosis probable, but interpretation of this appearance is difficult. Laboratory diagnosis of remnant hyperlipoproteinaemia is preferably based upon preparative ultracentrifugation: the VLDL fraction shows β-mobility on electrophoresis, and has an abnormally high molar ratio of cholesterol/triglyceride (>1.3, i.e. >0.57 in units of mg/dl). Fredrickson et al. (1972) suggest that the diagnosis is readily made on the finding of a molar ratio of VLDL cholesterol to total plasma triglyceride which exceeds 0.7 (i.e. 0.3 in units of mg/dl).

The presence of raised concentrations of LDL and VLDL as a cause of combined hyperlipidaemia is probable when an unequivocal increase in the density of β- and pre-β-bands is seen on electrophoresis. Often, however, qualitative data is inadequate to decide, in the presence of raised VLDL levels, whether LDL levels are normal or also raised. Quantitative lipoprotein measurements by ultracentrifugation or by precipitation methods are necessary. In practice, knowledge of a minor increase in the concentration of LDL, in a patient with a definite increase in VLDL, probably seldom influences management, which is usually that of the endogenous hypertriglyceridaemia group.

The mechanism of this form of combined hyperlipidaemia has been ascribed to overproduction of VLDL and LDL, by studies using radio-iodinated lipoproteins. Evidence from studies of cholesterol and bile acid turnover also suggests that such patients differ from those with "pure" hyper-β-lipoproteinaemia; they have increased turnover of cholesterol, which suggests excessive synthesis of lipoproteins rather than a catabolic defect. Impaired hepatic clearance of remnant particles derived from VLDL and chylomicrons, possibly together with increased VLDL synthesis, may be a major mechanism in remnant (type III) hyperlipoproteinaemia.

As already mentioned, there is a distinct genetic basic for a subgroup of patients with a marked increase in the concentrations of cholesterol and LDL, and some increase in VLDL, often showing tendon xanthomas. Such patients, who belong to families with monogenic hyper-β-lipoproteinaemia, require treatment primarily for this familial disorder, and may need additional therapy for their endogenous hyperglyceridaemia.

5.4.6. Ischaemic heart disease and hyperlipidaemia

Although the pathogenesis of atherosclerotic occlusion of the coronary arteries is incompletely understood, it is now inescapable that certain common forms of hyperlipidaemia increase the risk of developing manifestations of overt ischaemic heart disease, including sudden death. This relationship is greatly potentiated by the co-existence of other risk factors, particularly hypertension, cigarette smoking and glucose intolerance. Hypercholesterolaemia is clearly a major risk factor, although prospective surveys have not taken into account the nature of the lipoprotein abnormalities associated with the hypercholesterolaemia, which are likely to have been types IIa, IIb, IV and, rarely, others. Hypertriglyceridaemia is also a risk factor, but some epidemiologists believe that this association is due to the modest correlation between cholesterol and triglyceride concentrations. The real issue is whether high VLDL levels are a risk factor; this has not been adequately investigated.

These findings must be considered in the light of evidence from a variety of epidemiological, clinical and experimental sources. There is a high risk of early onset of ischaemic heart disease in the affected relatives of patients with hyper-β-lipoproteinaemia (Slack, 1969); and the disease presents at a significantly younger age in patients with increased concentrations of LDL, VLDL, or both lipoproteins, than in those with normal lipoprotein levels (Lewis et al., 1974a). In a study of an asymptomatic "normal" population, Carlson et al. (1975) found a higher frequency of electrocardiographic evidence of cardiac ischaemia in subjects with combined hyperlipidaemia, hypercholesterolaemia or hypertriglyceridaemia than in those with normal lipid levels. The frequency of lipoprotein abnormalities – combined hyperlipidaemia, hypertriglyceridaemia and hypercholesterolaemia – in patients with ischaemic heart disease has been estimated as 30 to 60%; increased concentrations of VLDL, LDL or both lipoproteins occur (Goldstein et al., 1973b; Lewis et al., 1974a).

In several animal species diets which lead to hyperlipidaemia cause gross atherosclerosis. In primates especially such lesions, even if advanced, show slow but substantial regression when diets causing marked reduction in lipid concentrations are fed (Armstrong and Megan, 1972).

The mechanism of these relationships is imperfectly understood. LDL and VLDL, or their metabolic products, can enter the arterial intima (Woolf and Pilkington, 1965; Onitiri et al., 1976). The concentrations of these lipoproteins in the intima are directly correlated with their concentrations in plasma (Smith and Slater, 1972; Onitiri et al., 1976). The deposition of cholesterol in the arterial intima, therefore, appears to occur at a rate determined, inter alia, by factors which alter plasma lipoprotein concentrations.

5.4.7. Lipoprotein deficiency states

Hypolipidaemia may be secondary to undernutrition, as in protein-energy malnutrition (kwashiorkor), and may arise in the malabsorption syndrome, particularly when ileal disease leads to impaired reabsorption of bile salts. It is also seen occasionally in intestinal protein loss of severe degree, e.g. in intestinal lymphangiectasia. End-stage parenchymal liver disease is another cause of subnormal serum lipid concentrations. Hypocholesterolaemia is sometimes present in patients with sideroblastic anaemia, and also in thalassaemia. Severe acute illness, such as myocardial infarction or extensive burns, is commonly associated with hypocholesterolaemia; the concentration of triglyceride responds more variably and sometimes increases, as in Gram-negative septicaemia.

Primary hypolipoproteinaemia occurs in three well-defined genetic disorders, a-β-lipoproteinaemia, hypo-β-lipoproteinaemia and α-lipoprotein deficiency (Fredrickson et al., 1972).

5.4.7.1. A-β-lipoproteinaemia

This is a rare disorder, inherited as an autosomal recessive trait. It may present in infancy with failure to thrive, and steatorrhoea may be overt or, in older patients, inapparent. By the age of 10 years a progressive neurological disorder appears, with ataxia or weakness;

it may be associated with signs of lower and upper motor neurone deficits, proprioceptive and cutaneous sensory loss, and pigmentary retinopathy. Severe disability has usually developed by the third decade of life. Acanthocytosis is present, usually without anaemia. Hypocholesterolaemia and hypotriglyceridaemia are extreme. LDL, VLDL and chylomicrons are not detectable in plasma, the lipid content of which is present in HDL. The concentration of HDL is also somewhat low, and qualitative abnormalities have been described. The diagnosis is based upon the presence of strikingly low serum lipid concentrations (serum cholesterol $<$ 1.8 mmol/litre; 70 mg/dl). Triglyceride is sometimes undetectable by usual methods. Serum electrophoresis (section 5.5.4.2.) shows the absence of all lipoproteins except α-lipoprotein. Immunoelectrophoresis against antiserum to β-lipoprotein is diagnostic. The consensus is that this disorder is due to inability to synthesize apolipoprotein B, a constitutent (sections 5.2.2. and 5.2.3.) of LDL, VLDL and chylomicrons and (in trace amount) of HDL. The neuropathy and retinopathy have not been explained. A plausible hypothesis, not yet supported by substantial evidence, is that the absence of LDL – the transport form of vitamin E – leads to deficiency of this vitamin in the tissues; local accumulation of lipid peroxides might therefore develop and might lead to nervous tissue damage.

Malabsorption of fat is evidently due to the inability of the intestinal mucosa to synthesize chylomicrons and VLDL in the absence of apolipoprotein B. Dietary fat is digested; the products enter the mucosal cell and are esterified to triglyceride. This accumulates in the lipid droplets which are a conspicuous feature of mucosal cells as seen in jejunal biopsy.

5.4.7.2. Hypo-β-lipoproteinaemia

This is a distinct entity, being an autosomal dominant trait in most published pedigrees. It is likely that this abnormality is not as infrequent as other inherited lipoprotein deficiences. The disorder may be clinically silent and may not shorten life, but a few patients have had neuropathy and fat accumulation in mucosal cells. In the family studies by Sigurdsson et al. (1977) the affected members were short in stature, but malabsorption was not a feature. In this family, two affected members were shown to have low rates of synthesis of LDL, and in one case in which it was studied, the synthesis of VLDL was also low. The mechanism of this disorder appears to be an impairment of secretion of VLDL, which leads in turn to decreased production of LDL. Serum cholesterol concentration is below 3.5 mmol/litre (140 mg/dl). The best diagnostic criterion is the finding of a low concentration of LDL cholesterol, e.g. less than the fifth percentile, in the absence of known causes of secondary hypolipidaemia.

5.4.7.3. α-Lipoprotein deficiency

This deficiency – Tangier disease – is an extremely rare disorder, evidently due to an autosomal recessive gene which is partly expressed in the heterozygous state. Tissue accumulation of cholesteryl esters leads to marked enlargement of the tonsils, which are orange in colour; lymph glands, spleen and liver may also be enlarged. Peripheral sensory and motor neuropathies affect many patients. Hypocholesterolaemia is invariable, while the serum triglyceride concentration may be moderately increased or normal. The concentration of HDL is extremely low and the lipoprotein is undetectable on electrophoresis. In the β- and pre-β-region, a broad lipoprotein band is seen. On ultracentrifugation, LDL is found to be present, and it may have an abnormally high triglyceride content. The protein composition is abnormal in the trace quantity of HDL which is present in plasma. Normally apolipoprotein AI and apolipoprotein AII predominate among the several proteins of HDL, apolipoprotein AI being the major one. In Tangier disease, the concentration of apolipoprotein AI is reduced some 600-fold in plasma, and the abnormal HDL in this condition has apolipoprotein AII as its major polypeptide (Lux et al., 1972). However, the composition of apolipoproteins AI and AII have not been shown to be abnormal in patients with Tangier disease. Diagnosis is based on the clinical findings, and on hypocholesterolaemia with normal or raised concentration of triglyceride in whole serum. Serum lipoprotein electrophoresis shows a broad β-band with the absence of α-lipoprotein. On preparative ultracentrifugation, extremely low levels of lipids are present in the HDL density range. When immunoelectrophoresis of whole serum against antiserum to HDL is performed, no precipitation line appears, although the HDL fraction after ultracentrifugation yields a barely detectable line. The disorder appears to be a genetically determined defect in the rate of synthesis of apolipoprotein AI, which affects the compositions of HDL and of VLDL. Low concentrations of HDL may be responsible for impaired centripetal transport of cholesterol from tissues, resulting in its accumulation in reticuloendothelial and other tissues. The activity of lecithin:cholesterol acyltransferase and plasma post-heparin lipolytic activity have been variously reported as normal and low.

Lecithin:cholesterol acyltransferase deficiency is also an extremely rare genetic disorder, not appropriately classified amongst the lipoprotein deficiency states except that the composition of most plasma lipoproteins is grossly abnormal. There is hypercholesterolaemia, due to very high concentrations of free cholesterol in plasma, with extremely low concentrations of cholesteryl esters. Hypertriglyceridaemia is usual. Severe renal failure associated with deposition of lipid in the kidney is a major aspect of the clinical picture.

5.5. METHODS FOR LIPID AND LIPOPROTEIN ANALYSIS

There is no consensus as to the range of investigations which is necessary for the diagnosis and management of patients with plasma lipoprotein disorders. The high prevalence of these disorders and the expense of procedures such as lipoprotein analysis by ultracentrifugation make it necessary to perform the minimum number of investigations commensurate with good clinical practice.

5.5.1. General principles

Probably the majority of hyperlipidaemic patients can be managed satisfactorily on the basis of accurate measurements of serum cholesterol and triglyceride concentrations on two or three blood samples taken in the fasted state, with the precautions outlined in section 5.3.1.4. (Tabaqchali et al., 1974; Fredrickson, 1975; Lewis, 1976). This identifies the major groups of patients with hypercholesterolaemia, hypertriglyceridaemia or combined hyperlipidaemia. This information should be supplemented by qualitative or quantitative data concerning the pattern of lipoproteins in serum; the extent to which it is necessary to pursue these findings is dependent on the clinical requirements. For the investigation and treatment of the common forms of hyperlipidaemia, it usually suffices to note the appearance of stored serum (section 5.5.4.1.), though most laboratories at present can perform qualitative electrophoresis of serum lipoproteins.

For the specialized lipid clinic, these methods are supplemented by several others. Quantitative preparative ultracentrifugation of plasma lipoproteins is available, with lipid analyses and sometimes also electrophoresis, of the fractions. Enzyme measurements, particularly of post-heparin lipolytic activity, are provided. Function tests such as the assessment of the response of serum triglyceride concentration to high carbohydrate diets may be performed.

Cholesterol and triglyceride determinations should be monitored by internal quality control procedures; in addition it is important to assess laboratory performance by participation in an external quality control scheme. The Lipid Standardization Laboratory of the Center for Disease Control (U.S. Department of Health, Education and Welfare, Atlanta, Ga., U.S.A.) operates an extensively used scheme for total serum cholesterol and triglyceride analyses.

5.5.2. Determination of cholesterol

Serum cholesterol is tradiationally determined by colorimetric assay. In addition, fluorometric, enzymatic, gas chromatographic and gravimetric procedures are available; of these, enzymatic methods show promise on account of their relatively great specificity, and may supplant colorimetric procedures, which lack specificity. Cholesterol is largely separable from major non-specific chromogens by solvent extraction, and methods in which this procedure is used before colour development give lower and more accurate results than those in which the colour reagent is added directly to serum. Non-specific chromogens include bilirubin, haemoglobin and certain drugs; sterols other than cholesterol may also react.

Cholesteryl esters have greater chromogenicity than free cholesterol, and since free cholesterol is usually used for calibration, the magnitude of the consequent error varies according to the somewhat inconstant ratio of free to esterified cholesterol. The problem may be overcome by introducing a saponification step into the method, so ensuring that the colour reaction is performed on unesterified cholesterol. With the ferric chloride–sulphuric acid reagent, the difference is minimized in automated procedures by ensuring that the reagent is at 95 to 100 °C as it mixes with the lipid extract (Siegel and Bowdoin, 1971).

Another widely used colour reaction is that of Zak et al. (1954) in which the reagent consists of ferric chloride and sulphuric acid; it provides a stable colour maximum. In this method, the precipitation of cholesterol with digitonin is employed, but alternative procedures employ direct addition of the colour reagent to serum. Mann (1961) has combined the Abell extraction procedure with the ferric chloride colour reagent; its advantages are the hydrolysis of cholesteryl esters, the extraction procedure which enhances the specificity of the method, and the stability of the colour maximum.

Automated procedures have employed the Liebermann–Burchard reagent directly on serum as in the Technicon SMA system, employing a serum calibrator; it is also used in conjunction with manual extraction of serum lipids with isopropanol (Technicon Auto-Analyzer II method). In the Technicon N-24a AutoAnalyzer I method, an isopropanol extract of serum is prepared manually. The ferric chloride–sulphuric acid reagent is added on-stream at an elevated temperature. The results of both of these extraction procedures generally conform well with reference methods of analysis.

Enzymatic and gas chromatographic methods give slightly lower values for serum cholesterol concentration than colorimetric methods, suggesting a measure of non-specificity in the latter. Enzymatic procedures, e.g. that of Richmond (1973), employing cholesterol oxidase are coming into widespread use. They have been coupled to a hydrolysis step using cholesterol esterase (Allain et al., 1975) and have been successfully automated. Cholesterol oxidase is relatively specific, but saturated sterols present in serum may also be oxidized.

A most necessary precaution in any methodology is that of checking the purity of the primary cholesterol standard by melting point and thin-layer chromatography (Williams et al., 1970).

The major reference methods for the assay of cholesterol are those of Sperry and Webb (1950) and Abell et al. (1952). In the former, the lipid extract is saponified and cholesterol is isolated as its insoluble digitonide. The Abell method involves a combined saponification–extraction procedure in which serum is heated with dilute alkali to hydrolyze the cholesteryl esters; unsaponifiable material is extracted with hexane and the cholesterol is measured colourimetrically by the Liebermann–Burchard reaction with acetic anhydride and sulphuric acid. The work-simplified micro-modification (Anderson and Keys, 1956) of the Abell method has been an acceptable routine manual method for the smaller laboratory. However, the convenience, accuracy and precision of the enzymic method have led many laboratories to change to procedures based on the use of cholesterol oxidase.

5.5.3. Determination of triglyceride

Serum triglycerides is measured by colorimetric, fluorometric or enzymatic methods, all of which are designed to be specific for the glycerol moiety. Such methods have been introduced relatively recently, and earlier "difference" methods based upon the supposition: triglyceride = total lipid – (phospholipid + cholesterol + cholesteryl esters) have been superceded. Typically, phospholipid is removed by a preliminary extraction so that glyceride is the major source of glycerol; free glycerol in plasma does, however, contribute slightly (up to 0.3 mmol/litre) to the result. When colorimetric or fluorometric methods are employed, it is also necessary to remove glucose. One commonly used extraction–purification procedure employs isopropyl ether as solvent, with silicic acid as the absorbent for phospholipid and glucose; a widely used alternative employs isopropanol with a mixture of zeolite, Lloyd's reagent, cupric sulphate and calcium hydroxide. Nonane–isopropanol or heptane have been shown to provide adequately selective extraction of triglyceride (Gottfried and Rosenberg, 1973).

After saponification of the triglyceride extract, free glycerol is measured, either chemically or enzymatically. In the usual chemical methods, glycerol is oxidized to formaldehyde, which is measured colorimetrically with chromotropic acid and sulphuric acid, or fluorometrically by the Hantsch condensation with acetylacetone and ammonium acetate. In the enzymatic methods, glycerol reacts with ATP in the presence of glycerate kinase (EC 2.7.1.31) to yield glycerol-3-phosphate. Coupled reactions permit spectrophotometric measurement by reaction rate or end-point methods. A widely used example of enzymatic triglyceride measurement is the manual procedure of Timms et al. (1968). Enzymatic methods are also available in kit form and may be automated (Bell et al., 1970).

Manual colorimetric methods have undergone progressive simplication. The procedure of Carlson (1963) is now an accepted reference method, and that of Laurell (1966) is well suited to routine use in the small laboratory.

Automated fluorometric methods are extensively employed and compare satisfactorily with Carlson's method. In the author's laboratory the Technicon N-78 extraction procedure has been employed; after the adsorption step the extract is analyzed in a two-channel system for cholesterol (Technicon N-24a) and triglyceride (Cramp and Robertson, 1968).

With the availability of direct chemical and enzymatic procedures for measurement of serum triglyceride, indirect methods such as those based upon nephelometry do not appear to offer any advantage.

The preferred standards for triglyceride measurement are triolein (for methods using isopropanol as solvent) or tripalmitin, the purity of which may be assessed by thin-layer chromatography. The use of glycerol or corn oil as standards is obsolete.

5.5.4. Qualitative methods for serum lipoproteins

5.5.4.1. The stored serum test

The appearance of stored serum in the various hyperlipoproteinaemic states was described by Fredrickson et al. (1967) and was used in a formal diagnostic technique by Havel (1969). About 4 ml of serum, obtained in the fasted state, is stored in a clear glass tube, placed vertically, at 4 °C for 18 hours. Vibration must be avoided. When the tube is inspected against a dark background (Figure 5.2) it shows one of four appearances:

(a) it may be clear, indicating normal lipid concentrations or raised levels of β-lipoprotein, α-lipoprotein or LP-X; mild pre-β-hyperlipoproteinaemia does not impart detectable lactescence;

(b) it may show a lactescent layer confined to the upper part of the specimen, with clear subnatant, which indicates chylomicronaemia, i.e. exogenous hypertriglyceridaemia;

(c) there may be lactescence distributed evenly throughout the specimen; this suggests endogenous hypertriglyceridaemia, due to pre-β-hyperlipoproteinaemia or remnant hyperlipoproteinaemia (type III); or

(d) there may be diffuse lactescence with a floating "cream line" which results from endogenous hypertriglyceridaemia associated with chylomicronaemia; this is seen in the type V pattern (increased pre-β-lipoproteins with chylomicronaemia), and also in type III (commonly accompanied by slight chylomicronaemia).

This test is remarkably informative and, together with a knowledge of cholesterol and triglyceride concentrations, it provides sufficient information to allocate appropriate

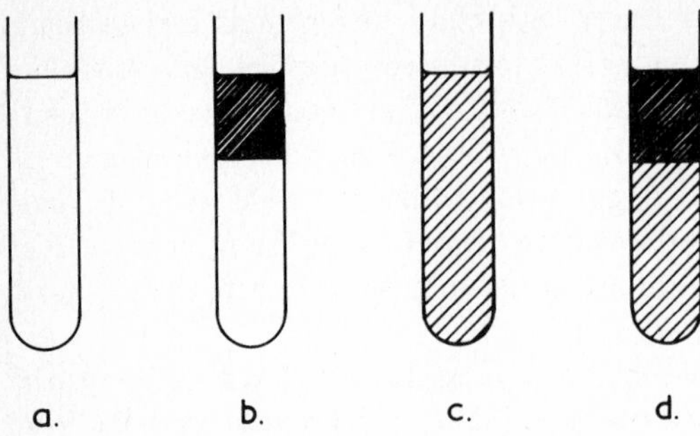

Fig. 5.2. The stored-serum test (see section 5.5.4.).

therapy for the majority of hyperlipidaemic patients (Tabaqchali et al., 1974). A few difficulties may arise in its interpretation. Occasional specimens with quite pronounced endogenous hypertriglyceridaemia (e.g. 5 mmol/litre) may appear clear; the diagnosis of exogenous hypertriglyceridaemia can sometimes be missed when chylomicrons fail to float to the meniscus in intensely lipaemic serum. The latter problem can be averted if a duplicate test using a 1 : 50 dilution of serum is set up; the diluent is sodium chloride of density 1.006 g/ml.

5.5.4.2. Lipoprotein electrophoresis

Although semi-quantitative versions have been published, this is best employed as a qualitative technique, relating the appearance of the strip (Figure 5.3) to cholesterol and triglyceride concentrations. A control strip, employing a pool of normal once-frozen serum and run and stained in the same batch, should be used for comparison. Qualitative and semi-quantitative electrophoretic procedures are most reliable when deviations from normality are pronounced. Free electrophoresis, and the use of filter paper as supporting medium, have largely been replaced by agarose gel (0.5 to 1.2%) or gelatinized cellulose acetate. The convenience of the latter is offset by difficulty in storage, in contrast to agarose gels which may readily be dried and stored. Although adsorption on to the supporting medium is less of a problem with these media than with filter paper, addition of albumin to the buffer system improves resolution on all three media. Satisfactory – but expensive – agarose plates are commercially available; preparation in the laboratory is cheaper and permits incorporation of albumin into the gel buffer. Polyacrylamide gel affords an excellent medium in which separation is determined by particle size as well as by charge. It is somewhat more time consuming unless commercial gels are purchased; moreover, VLDL may form a rather diffuse region in the stacking gel.

Lipoprotein bands may be detected after electrophoresis and fixation by staining with lipophilic dyes, e.g. Fat Red 7B or Sudan Black, or by Schiff staining with cellulose acetate. Pre-staining has also been employed, particularly on polyacrylamide gel. A promising method (Seidel et al., 1973) uses precipitation of lipoproteins by dextran sulphate and Ca^{2+}.

Chylomicrons largely remain at the application line on electrophoresis, their size

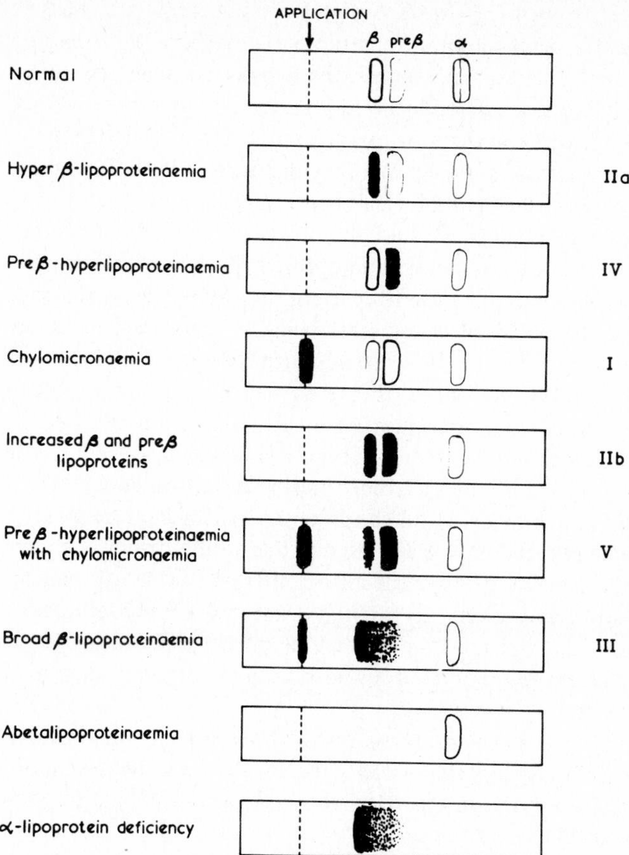

Fig. 5.3. Patterns of plasma lipoprotein abnormalities as seen on electrophoresis on agarose gel (see section 5.5.4.2.).

limiting migration. Smaller chylomicrons possibly migrate to the pre-β (α_2) position. Exogenous hypertriglyceridaemia (type I hyperlipoproteinaemia) is therefore characterized by a dense band at the application line, often with decreased staining in the α- and β-regions. In non-fasting samples, chylomicron and pre-β bands increase in quantity. LDL migrates as a sharply defined band in the β position, its main component, LDL_2, migrating slightly slower than the minor, triglyceride-richer component, LDL_1. A clear-cut increase in the intensity of this band, together with hypercholesterolaemia and a normal triglyceride concentration, indicates the presence of hyper-β-lipoproteinaemia. The α- and pre-β bands are often faint.

VLDL runs as one or more bands in the pre-β (α_2) position. On agarose or cellulose acetate, it is completely resolved from β-lipoprotein. In the presence of hypertriglyceridaemia with a normal or relatively minor increase in cholesterol concentration, a heavy pre-β band constitutes the type IV pattern of endogenous hypertriglyceridaemia.

When there is a marked increase in pre-β-lipoprotein levels, the staining may trail back to the origin, obscuring the β-band and rendering differentiation from the type III pattern difficult. In patients with severe hypertriglyceridaemia, the increase in pre-β-lipoprotein is sometimes accompanied by staining at the application line, i.e. by chylomicronaemia, comprising the type V pattern. A well-stained, slow pre-β band which is associated with normal serum triglyceride concentration is usually due to a high titre of the polymorphic variant lipoprotein Lp(a), of no established pathological significance.

When there is a substantial increase in both cholesterol and triglyceride concentrations – combined hyperlipidaemia – the commonest lipoprotein pattern on electrophoresis is an increase in β- and pre-β-lipoprotein – the IIb pattern. In a hypertriglyceridaemic sample it may be difficult to decide by electrophoresis whether associated moderate hypercholesterolaemia is due to the IIb or IV pattern; quantitation of LDL is then required. More rarely combined hyperlipidaemia is due to remnant hyperlipoproteinaemia; the characteristic appearance on electrophoresis of serum is the broad β-band, extending as a single band through the β- to pre-β-region. However, this appearance is not always unequivocal and confirmation by ultracentrifugal analysis is required.

In summary, electrophoresis may provide useful confirmatory evidence of the lipoprotein abnormality in hyperlipidaemia. Hypercholesterolaemia due to the common abnormality hyper-β-lipoproteinaemia may be distinguished from the rare, evidently benign, hyper-α-lipoproteinaemia. Distinction between hypertriglyceridaemia of endogenous or exogenous origin may be confirmed, and the type III may be provisionally diagnosed if appearances are unequivocal. Electrophoretic analysis is, or course, highly informative in identifying the lipoprotein deficiency states.

Satisfactory procedures using agarose gel are those of Noble (1968) and of Houtsmuller (1970). Among the many cellulose acetate methods that of Chin and Blanckenhorn (1968) is widely employed, and the procedure of De Baets and Lezy (1971) gives good results on gelatinized cellulose acetate.

5.5.5. Lipoprotein quantitation

The classical quantitative procedure is preparative ultracentrifugation, although recent advances in instrumentation may make analytical ultracentrifugation more accessible for clinical use. The uniquely low densities of the lipoproteins make it possible to isolate them serially under a high gravitational field by a stepwise increase in the density of the medium. VLDL is isolated by flotation, as the fraction of density less than 1.006 g/ml. An LDL class may then be floated in the density range 1.006 to 1.063 g/ml; alternatively, lipoproteins of intermediate density (1.006 to 1.019 g/ml) are first collected and LDL_2 is subsequently floated in the density range 1.019 to 1.063 g/ml. The subnatant then contains HDL. Fractions are most reproducibly isolated by a tube-slicing technique. A fixed-angle rotor is normally used, but for isolation of the chylomicron fraction a swing-out rotor is preferable. Fractions are made up to standard volume and analyzed for cholesterol and triglyceride content, or submitted to electrophoresis. If the ferric chloride colour reagent is used in the measurement of cholesterol, bromide (which is employed in adjusting the background density) must first be removed from the lipid extract by adsorption onto anion exchange resin. Recoveries during preparative ultracentrifugation should be in the range 90 to 105%.

A detailed account of preparative ultracentrifugation of serum lipoproteins is that of Carlson (1973). The method is of clinical use in confirming the diagnosis of remnant hyperlipoproteinaemia, as discussed in section 5.4.5. Quantitation of LDL concentration is sometimes necessary to distinguish the type IIb and IV patterns. Possibly a major value of lipoprotein quantitation is in monitoring the changes in the individual lipoproteins during therapy. When severe endogenous hypertriglyceridaemia is treated with clofibrate or nicotinic acid, the concentration of LDL sometimes rises substantially, as that of VLDL falls; lipoprotein quantitation is desirable to monitor for this potentially untoward effect. Sometimes the concentration of VLDL rises during the treatment of increased LDL concentration with cholestyramine.

Precipitation of lipoproteins may be used in quantitative separations, either alone or in conjunction with ultracentrifugation. In one procedure, as employed by Fredrickson et al. (1967) and described by Carlson (1973), VLDL is isolated by a single run in the preparative ultracentrifuge. LDL is then precipitated from the subnatant using heparin and Mn^{2+}. Results are closely comparable with those obtained by two-stage ultracentrifugation. A technique for precipitating VLDL has been used by Wilson and Spiger (1973) in a quantitative procedure in which LDL and HDL are separated by dextran sulphate and Ca^{2+}. Ononogbu and Lewis (1976) have used precipitation techniques to provide direct analyses of VLDL and HDL cholesterol and triglyceride, LDL being estimated by difference. This procedure provides results which compare closely with preparative ultracentrifugation, and is of promising simplicity for routine use. In the current modification heparin–Mn^{2+} is used in place of dextran sulphate–Ca^{2+}.

5.5.6. Laboratory investigation of secondary hyperlipidaemia

Detection of this important subgroup of hyperlipidaemias is largely clinical. It is usual to obtain a biochemical profile on hyperlipidaemic patients to define associated abnormalities and to test for common underlying causes. Data include fasting blood glucose, and serum urea, uric acid, creatinine, albumin, globulin and bilirubin concentrations. Serum alkaline phosphatase, gamma-glutamyl transferase and lactate dehydrogenase activities are assayed. As an index of hypothyroidism, serum thyroid-stimulating hormone levels may be measured; in the present author's experience, hypothyroidism causing hyperlipidaemia is usually clinically evident.

Obstructive jaundice lipoprotein, LP-X, was discussed in section 5.4.1. It is by no means invariably present in cholestasis and opinions differ as to the diagnostic value of its detection. It is most easily demonstrated by electrophoresis on agar in which SO_4^{2-} is present; on such a medium the migration of LP-X is cathodal, a unique and diagnostic characteristic. Detection may be effected by use of formal immunoelectrophoresis against a specific antiserum to LP-X, or can be performed without the antiserum by precipitation using dextran sulphate (Seidel et al., 1973).

5.5.7. Plasma post-heparin lipolytic activity (PHLA)

Deficiency of the extrahepatic component of this group of enzymes is the hallmark of primary exogenous hypertriglyceridaemia as presently defined. A variety of methods for

PHLA assay exists, and none has been universally accepted as the standard procedure. Until recently total PHLA was assayed in plasma obtained 10 minutes after intravenous injection of heparin (usually 10 units of heparin per kg body weight), e.g. in the methods of Schotz and Garfinkel (1972) and Fredrickson et al. (1963).

Other authors, e.g. Boberg (1969), have recommended doses of up to 100 units/kg. To facilitate the assay it has been common practice to prepare an artificial emulsion of radioactive triglyceride in the laboratory. However, variation in the properties of such substrates is considerable, particularly when inhibitors such as protamine sulphate are employed (Riley and Robinson, 1974). A suitable substrate is the parenteral fat emulsion Intralipid 10% (Vitrum Labs.), activated by pre-incubation with serum. Lipolysis is measured by the release of glycerol in the Boberg method, which requires a glycerol-free substrate. More often the release of fatty acid is measured, e.g. by the colorimetric assay of Novak (1965), which is readily performed and depends on the formation of a cobalt soap with fatty acids.

When total PHLA is unequivocally low, lipoprotein lipase deficiency is probable. However, the assay of PHLA may be unreliable as heparin releases substantial quantities of an hepatic triglyceride lipase. If this enzyme forms a large component of total PHLA, deficiency of extrahepatic lipoprotein lipase may be masked when total lipolytic activity is assayed. Krauss et al. (1974) have attempted to assay extrahepatic and hepatic PHLA by differential inhibition, the former being inhibited by protamine sulphate. This general approach is likely to prove more informative than assay of total PHLA, but an optimal substrate has not been agreed upon, and Riley and Robinson (1974) prefer Intralipid to the sonicated radioactive triglyceride emulsion used by Krauss et al.

REFERENCES

Abell, L.L., Levy, B.B., Brodie, B.B. and Kendall, F.E. (1952) A simplified method for the estimation of total cholesterol in serum and demonstration of its specificity. Journal of Biological Chemistry, 195, 357–366.

Allain, C.C., Poon, L.S., Chan, C.S.G., Richmond, W. and Fu, P.C. (1974) Enzymatic determination of total serum cholesterol. Clinical Chemistry, 20, 470–475.

Anderson, J.T. and Keys, A. (1956) Cholesterol in serum and lipoprotein fractions: its measurement and stability. Clinical Chemistry, 2, 145–159.

Armstrong, M.L. and Megan. M.B. (1972) Lipid depletion in atheromatous coronary arteries in rhesus monkeys after regression diets. Circulation Research, 30, 675–680.

Beaumont, J.L., Carlson, L.A., Cooper, G.R., Fejfar, Z., Fredrickson, D.S. and Strasser, T. (1970) Classification of the hyperlipidaemias and hyperlipoproteinaemias. Bulletin of the World Health Organization, 43, 891.

Bell, J.L., Atkinson, M. and Baron, D.N. (1970) An AutoAnalyzer method for estimating serum glyceride glycerol using a glycerokinase procedure. Journal of Clinical Pathology, 23, 509–513.

Boberg, J. (1969) Quantitative determination of heparin-released lipoprotein lipase activity in human plasma. Lipids, 5, 452–456.

Brown, M.S. and Goldstein, J.G. (1976) Receptor-mediated control of cholesterol metabolism. Science, 191, 150–154.

Carlson, K. (1973) Lipoprotein fractionation. Journal of Clinical Pathology, 26, suppl. 5, 32–37.

Carlson, L.A. (1963) Determination of serum triglycerides. Journal of Atherosclerosis Research, 3, 334–336.

Carlson, L.A. and Böttiger, L.E. (1972) Ischaemic heart disease in relation to fasting values of plasma triglycerides and cholesterol. Stockholm Prospective Study. Lancet, 1, 865–868.

Carlson, L.A., Ekelund, L.G. and Olsson, A.G. (1975) Frequency of ischaemic exercise ECG changes in symptom-free men with various forms of primary hyperlipaemia. Lancet, 2, 1–3.

Carlson, L.A. and Lindstedt, S. (1969) The Stockholm Prospective Study. 1. Initial values for plasma lipids. Acta Medica Scandinavia, 195, suppl. 493, 1–135.

Chin, H.P. and Blanckenhorn, D.H. (1968) Separation and quantitative analysis of serum lipoproteins by means of electrophoresis on cellulose acetate. Clinica Chimica Acta, 20, 305–314.

Cramp, D.C. and Robertson, G. (1968) The fluorimetric assay of triglyceride by a semi-automated method. Analytical Biochemistry, 25, 246–251.

De Baets, J. and Lezy, W. (1971) Improved method for lipoprotein electrophoresis on Cellogel. Clinica Chimica Acta, 32, 142–144.

Fogelman, A.M., Edmond, J., Seager, J. and Popjak, G. (1975). Abnormal induction of 3-hydroxy-3-methylglutaryl coenzyme A reductase in leucocytes from subjects with heterozygous familial hypercholesterolemia. Journal of Biological Chemistry, 250, 2045.

Frederickson, D.S., Gotto, A.M. and Levy, R.I. (1972) Familial lipoprotein deficiency. In The Metabolic Basis of Inherited Disease, 3rd edition. (Eds. J.B. Stanbury, J.B. Wyngaarden and D.S. Frederickson) Chapter 26, McGraw-Hill, New York.

Fredrickson, D.S. (1975) It's time to be practical. Circulation, 51, 209–211.

Fredrickson, D.S. and Levy, R.I. (1972) Familial hyperlipoproteinaemia. In The Metabolic Basis of Inherited Disease, 3rd edition (Eds. J.B. Stanbury, J.B. Wyngaarden and D.S. Fredrickson). pp. 545–614, McGraw-Hill, New York.

Fredrickson, D.S., Levy, R.I. and Lees, R.S. (1967) Fat transport in lipoproteins: an integrated approach to mechanisms and disorders. New England Journal of Medicine, 276, 32–44, 94–103, 148–156, 215–226, 273–281.

Fredrickson, D.S., Ono, K. and Davis, L.L. (1963) Lipolytic activity of post-heparin plasma in hyperglyceridaemia. Journal of Lipid Research, 4, 24–27.

Goldstein, J.L. and Brown, M.S. (1973) Familial hypercholesterolaemia: identification of a defect in the regulation of 3-hydroxy-3-methylglutaryl coenzyme A reductase activity associated with overproduction of cholesterol. Proceedings of the National Academy of Sciences, 70, 2804–2808.

Goldstein, J.L., Schrott, H.G., Hazzard, W.R., Bierman, E.L. and Motulsky, A.G. (1973a) Hyperlipidaemia in coronary heart disease. II. Journal of Clinical Investigation, 52, 1544–1568.

Goldstein, J.L., Hazzard, W.R., Schrott, H.G., Bierman, E.L. and Motulsky, A.G. (1973b) Hyperlipidaemia in coronary heart disease. I. Journal of Clinical Investigation, 52, 1533–1543.

Gottfried, S.P. and Rosenberg, B. (1973) Improved manual spectrophotometric procedure for determination of serum triglycerides. Clinical Chemistry, 19, 1077–1078.

Havel, R.J. (1969) Pathogenesis, differentiation and management of hypertriglyceridaemia. Advances in Internal Medicine, 15, 117–154.

Houtsmuller, A.J. (1970) Agarose-Gel-Electrophoresis of Lipoproteins: A Clinical Screening Test, Van Gorcum and Co., Assen.

Kessler, G. and Lederer, H. (1966) Fluorometric measurement of triglycerides. In Technicon Symposium on Automation in Analytical Chemistry. (Ed. L.T. Skeggs) Mediad, New York.

Keys, A. (Ed.) (1966) Epidemiological Studies Related to Coronary Heart Disease: Characteristics of Men Aged 40–59 in 7 countries. Acta Medica Scandinavica, 181, suppl. 460, 1–392.

Koerselman, H.B., Lewis, B. and Pilkington, T.R.E. (1961) The effect of venous occlusion on the level of serum cholesterol. Journal of Atherosclerosis Research, 1, 85–87.

Krauss, R.M., Levy, R.I. and Fredrickson, D.S. (1974) Selective measurement of two lipase activities in post heparin plasma from normal subjects and patients with hyperlipoproteinaemia. Journal of Clinical Investigation, 54, 1107–1124.

Langer, T., Strober, W. and Levy, R.I. (1972) The metabolism of low density lipoprotein in familial type II hyperlipoproteinaemia. Journal of Clinical Investigation, 51, 1528–1537.

Laurell, S. (1966) A method for routine determination of plasma triglycerides. Scandinavian Journal of Clinical and Laboratory Investigation, 18, 668–672.

Levy, R.I. and Rifkind, B.M. (1973) Diagnosis and management of hyperlipoproteinaemia in infants and children. American Journal of Cardiology, 31, 547–556.

Lewis, B. (1973) Classification of lipoproteins and lipoprotein disorders. Journal of Clinical Pathology, 26, suppl. 5, 26–31.

Lewis, B. (1976) The Hyperlipidaemias: Clinical and Laboratory Practice. Blackwell, Oxford.

Lewis, B., Chait, A., Oakley, C.M., Wootton, I.D.P., Krikler, D.M., Onitiri, A., Sigurdsson, G. and February, A. (1974a). Serum lipoprotein abnormalities in patients with ischaemic heart disease: comparison with a control population. British Medical Journal, 3, 489–493.

Lewis, B., Chait, A., Wootton, I.D.P., Oakley, C.M., Krikler, D.M., Sigurdsson, G., February, A., Maurer, B. and Birkhead, J. (1974b) Frequency of risk factors for ischaemic heart disease in a healthy British population with particular reference to serum lipoprotein levels. Lancet, 1, 141–146.

Lux, S.E., Levy, R.I., Gotto, A.M. and Fredrickson, D.S. (1972) Studies on the protein defect in Tangier disease. Journal of Clinical Investigation, 51, 2505–2519.

Mann, G.V. (1961) A method for measurement of cholesterol in blood serum. Clinical Chemistry, 7, 275–284.

Noble, R.P. (1968) Electrophoretic separation of plasma lipoproteins in agarose gel. Journal of Lipid Research, 6, 693–700.

Novak, M. (1965) Colorimetric ultramicro-method for the determination of free fatty acids. Journal of Lipid Research, 6, 431–433.

Omitiri, A.C., Lewis, B., Bentall, H., Jamieson, C., Wisheart, J. and Faris, I. (1976) Lipoprotein concentrations in serum and in biopsy samples of arterial intima: a quantitative comparison. Atherosclerosis, 23, 513–519.

Ononogbu, I.C. and Lewis, B. (1976) Lipoprotein fractionation by a precipitation method. A simple quantitative procedure. Clinica Chimica Acta, 71, 397–402.

Richmond, W. (1973) Preparation and properties of a cholesterol oxidase from Nocardia sp. and its application to the enzymatic assay of total cholesterol in serum. Clinical Chemistry, 19, 1350–1356.

Riley, S.E. and Robinson, D.S. (1974) Studies on the assay of clearing factor lipase (lipoprotein lipase). Biochimica et Biophysica Acta, 369, 371–386.

Schotz, M.C. and Garfinkel, A.S. (1972) A simple lipase assay using trichloracetic acid. Journal of Lipid Research, 13, 824–826.

Seidel, D., Wieland, H. and Ruppert, C. (1973) Improved techniques for assessment of plasma lipoprotein patterns. I. Precipitation in gels after electrophoresis with polyanionic compounds. Clinical Chemistry, 19, 737–739.

Siegel, A.L. and Bowdoin, B.C. (1971) Modification of an automated procedure for serum cholesterol which permits the quantitative estimation of cholesterol esters. Clinical Chemistry, 17, 229–230.

Sigurdsson, G., Nicoll, A. and Lewis, B. (1975) Conversion of very low density lipoprotein to low lipoprotein: a metabolic study of apolipoprotein B kinetics in human subjects. Journal of Clinical Investigation, 56, 1481–1490.

Sigurdsson, G., Nicoll, A. and Lewis, B. (1976) Metabolism of very low density lipoproteins in hyperlipidaemia: studies of apolipoprotein B kinetics in man. European Journal of Clinical Investigation, 6, 167–177.

Sigurdsson, G., Nicoll, A. and Lewis, B. (1977) Turnover of apolipoprotein in two subjects with familial hypobetalipoproteinaemia. Metabolism, 26, 25–31.

Simons, L.A., Reichl, D., Myant, N.B. and Mancini, M. (1975) The metabolism of the apoprotein of plasma low density lipoprotein in familial hyperbetalipoproteinaemia in the homozygous form. Atherosclerosis, 21, 283–298.

Slack, J. (1969) Risk of ischaemic heart disease in familial hyperlipoproteinaemic states. Lancet, 2, 1380–1384.

Smith, E.B. and Slater, R.S. (1972) Relationship between low density lipoprotein in aortic intima and serum lipid levels. Lancet, 1, 463–469.

Sperry, W.M. and Webb, M. (1950) A revision of the Schoenheimer–Sperry method for cholesterol determination. Journal of Biological Chemistry, 187, 97–106.

Stamler, J., Berkson, D.M. and Lindberg, H.A. (1972) Risk factors: their role in the etiology and pathogenesis of the atherosclerotic disease. In Pathogenesis of Atherosclerosis. (Eds. R.W. Wissler and J.C. Geer) pp. 41–119, Williams and Wilkins, Baltimore.

Stein, O., Weinstein, D.B., Stein, Y. and Steinberg, D. (1975) Binding, internalization and degradation of low density lipoproteins by normal human fibroblasts and by fibroblasts from a case of homozygous familial hypercholesterolemia. Proceedings of the National Academy of Sciences, U.S.A., 73, 14.

Tabaqchali, S., Chait, A., Harrison, R. and Lewis, B. (1974) Experience with a simplified scheme of treatment of hyperlipidaemia. British Medical Journal, 3, 377–380.

Timms, A.R., Kelly, L.A., Spirito, J.A. and Engstrom, R.G. (1968) Modification of Hofland's colorimetric semi-automated serum triglyceride determination, assessed by an enzymatic glycerol determination. Journal of Lipid Research, 9, 675–680.

Wilhelmsen, L., Wedel, H. and Tibblin, G. (1973) Multivariate analysis of risk factors for coronary heart disease. Circulation, 48, 950–958.

Williams, J.H., Kuchmak, M. and Witter, R.F. (1970) Evaluation of the purity of cholesterol primary standards. Clinical Chemistry, 16, 423–426.

Wilson, D.E. and Spiger, M.J. (1973) Actual precipitation method for quantitative plasma lipoprotein measurement without ultracentrifugation. Journal of Laboratory and Clinical Medicine, 82, 473–482.

Woolf, N. and Pilkington, T.R.E. (1965) The immunohistochemical demonstration of lipoproteins in vessel walls. Journal of Pathology and Bacteriology, 90, 459–463.

Zak, B., Dickenman, R.C., White, E.G., Burnett, H. and Cherney, P.J. (1954) Rapid estimation of free and total cholesterol. American Journal of Clinical Pathology, 24, 1307–1315.

FURTHER READING

Brown, S.S. (1973) Notes on the quality of performance of serum cholesterol assays. Annals of Clinical Biochemistry, 10, 146–154.

Fredrickson, D.S., Gotto, A.M. and Levy, R.I. (1972) Familial lipoprotein deficiency. In The Metabolic Basis of Inherited Disease, 3rd edition. (Eds. J.B. Stanbury, J.B. Wyngaarden and D.S. Fredrickson) pp. 493–530, McGraw-Hill, New York.

Gjone, E. and Norum, K.R. (1974) Recent research on lecithin:cholesterol acyltransferase. Scandinavian Journal of Clinical and Laboratory Research, 33, suppl. 137.

Havel, R.J. (1972) Mechanism of hyperlipoproteinaemia. Advances in Experimental Medicine and Biology, 26, 57.

Lewis, B. (1976) The Hyperlipidaemias: Clinical and Laboratory Practice. Blackwell, Oxford.

McGowan, G.K. and Walters, G. (Eds.) (1973) Disorders of Lipid Metabolism. Journal of Clinical Pathology, 21, suppl. 5.

Smellie, R.M.S. (Ed.) (1971) Plasma lipoproteins, Biochemical Society Symposium No. 33. Academic Press, London.

Tonks, D.B. (1967) The estimation of cholesterol in serum: a classification and critical review of methods. Clinical Biochemistry, 1, 12–29.

Witter, R.F. and Whitner, V.S. (1971) Determination of serum triglycerides. In Blood Lipids and Lipoproteins. (Ed. G.J. Nelson) pp. 75–112, Wiley-Interscience, New York.

ADDENDUM

Since submission of this manuscript, significant advances have been made in several aspects of lipoprotein metabolism, including the following.

(1) The characteristics of the cell-surface lipoprotein receptor on extrahepatic cells have been clearly established (Anderson et al., 1976; Goldstein and Brown, 1977). The primary defect in familial hypercholesterolaemia is deficiency of functional impairment of these receptors; but a full understanding of the in vivo consequences of defective receptor function is still lacking.

(2) The metabolic defects in genetic hyperlipidaemias have been clarified by kinetic studies of VLDL- and LDL-apolipoprotein B (Lewis et al., 1978). Familial combined hyperlipidaemia is characterized by over-production of VLDL- and LDL-apoB. In familial hypercholesterolaemia, reduced fractional catabolism of LDL-apoB is present; and there is over-production of LDL, not from VLDL, but possibly by direct hepatic secretion. Remnant hyperlipoproteinaemia (type III) is associated with a low fractional catabolic rate of IDL (Chait et al., 1977); apolipoprotein composition is abnormal in this disorder, with a subnormal ratio of $apoE_3$ to $apoE_2$ (Uterman et al., 1975).

(3) The inverse relationship between HDL-cholesterol concentration and risk of ischaemic heart disease has evoked very great interest (Gotto et al., 1978). A role for HDL in centripetal transport of cholesterol is suggested by the negative correlation between HDL levels and tissue cholesterol pool size (Miller et al., 1979) and by the evidence that HDL cholesterol may be a major precursor of biliary cholesterol and bile acids (Halloran et al., 1978). HDL has several subclasses. HDL_{2a}, HDL_{2b} and HDL_3 differ in composition and, it appears, in regulation (Anderson et al., 1978). HDL-I, a small apoE-containing subclass, has the ability to compete with LDL for binding to cell surface lipoprotein receptors (Gotto et al., 1978). From these experimental findings, an understanding of the seemingly protective role of HDL may develop.

(4) The rate of transfer of LDL from plasma into human arterial intima has been shown to correlate strongly with plasma LDL levels (Niehaus et al., 1977). This is in agreement with the concept that cholesterol deposition in the artery, and atherogenesis, are accelerated by hypercholesterolaemia due to elevated LDL concentration.

Anderson, R.G.W., Goldstein, J.L. and Brown, M.S. (1976) Localization of LDL receptors on plasma membranes of normal human fibroblasts and their absence in cells from a familial hypercholesterolemia homozygote. Proceedings of the National Academy of Sciences, USA, 73, 2434–2438.

Anderson, D.W., Nichols, A.V., Pan, S.S. and Lindgren, F.T. (1978) High density lipoprotein distribution – resolution and determination of three major components in a normal population sample. Atherosclerosis, 29, 161–179.

Chait, A., Brunzell, J.D., Albers, J.J. and Hazzard, W.R. (1977) Type III hyperlipidemia ("remnant removal disease"). Lancet, i, 1176–1178.

Goldstein, J.L. and Brown, M.S. (1977) The low density lipoprotein pathway and its relation to atherosclerosis. Annual Reviews of Biochemistry, 46, 897–930.

Halloran, L.G., Schwarts, C.C., Vlahcevic, Z.R., Nisman, R.M. and Swell, L. (1978) Evidence for high-density lipoprotein free cholesterol as the primary precursor for bile-acid synthesis in man. Surgery, 84, 1–6.

Gotto, A.M., Jr., Miller, N.E. and Oliver, M.F. (1978) High Density Lipoproteins and Atherosclerosis. Elsevier/North-Holland Biomedical Press, Amsterdam.

Lewis, B., Nicoll, A., Janus, E., Wootton, R. and Turner, P. (1978) In Proceedings of International Conference on Atherosclerosis (Eds. L.A. Carlson, R. Paoletti, C.R. Sirton and G. Weber) pp. 275–277, Raven Press, New York.

Miller, N.E., Nestel, P.J. and Clifton-Bligh, P. (1976) Relationships between plasma lipoprotein cholesterol concentrations and the pool size and metabolism of cholesterol in man. Atherosclerosis, 23, 535–547.

Niehaus, C.E., Nicholl, A., Wootton, R., Williams, B., Lewis, J., Coltart, D.J. and Lewis, B. (1977) Influence of lipid concentrations and age on transfer of plasma lipoprotein into human arterial intima. Lancet, ii, 469–471.

Utermann, G., Jaeschke, M. and Menzel, J. (1975) Familial hyperlipoproteinemia type III: deficiency of a specific apolipoprotein (apoE-III) in the very low density lipoproteins. FEBS Letters, 56, 352–355.

Chapter 6

Proteins

Theodore Peters, Jr.

The Mary Imogene Bassett Hospital, Cooperstown, New York, NY 13326 U.S.A.

CONTENTS

Chemical diagnosis of disease, edited by
S.S. Brown, F.L. Mitchell and D.S. Young

6.1. THE NATURE OF PROTEINS

Proteins are the essence of life. They include the enzymes which conduct metabolism, the structural framework of cell membranes and of the protective coverings skin and hair, the moving elements of muscles and cilia, and the guardian substances which recognize "foreign" molecules and take action against them. Most proteins are locked up in cells and are inaccessible to sampling, but others occur in the blood, either for a specific purpose or merely through leakage, and their measurement can give useful information to the clinician. This Chapter concerns mainly those proteins which are purposefully secreted into the blood; the circulating enzymes are dealt with in Chapter 7.

6.1.1. Amino acids

Proteins are chain-like polymers of L-α-amino acids, linked in a specific, predetermined sequence. In a protein chain, amino acid residues have the structure:

$$-\mathrm{NH}-\overset{\displaystyle \mathrm{R}}{\underset{\displaystyle \mathrm{H}}{\mathrm{C}}}-\mathrm{CO}-$$

where the unattached dashes indicate *peptide bonds* to adjacent amino acid residues. Thus a chain of amino acid residues would appear as:

$$-\mathrm{NH}-\overset{\displaystyle R_1}{\underset{\displaystyle \mathrm{H}}{\mathrm{C}}}-\mathrm{CO}-\mathrm{NH}-\overset{\displaystyle \mathrm{H}}{\underset{\displaystyle R_2}{\mathrm{C}}}-\mathrm{CO}-\mathrm{NH}-\overset{\displaystyle R_3}{\underset{\displaystyle \mathrm{H}}{\mathrm{C}}}-\mathrm{CO}-\mathrm{NH}-\overset{\displaystyle \mathrm{H}}{\underset{\displaystyle R_4}{\mathrm{C}}}-\mathrm{CO}-\mathrm{NH}-\overset{\displaystyle R_5}{\underset{\displaystyle \mathrm{H}}{\mathrm{C}}}-\mathrm{CO}-$$

A short chain is called a *peptide,* a longer one (50 residues or more) a *protein.* The length of peptide chains in proteins varies from about 100 residues in ribonuclease (EC 3.1.4.22) or cytochrome c to about 1000 in collagen.

The "R" groups appended to the peptide chain backbone may be any of 20 different species shown in Table 6.1. Some of these groups are polar in nature – serine, threonine, asparagine, glutamine, cysteine, histidine, and those with charged groups, aspartic and glutamic acids, lysine, and arginine. Others – valine, leucine, isoleucine, proline, phenylalanine, and methionine – are non-polar or hydrophobic. Asparagine and glutamine are

TABLE 6.1.

THE AMINO ACIDS

Name	Structure of R group	pK of R group	Average plasma concentration (various reports) (μmol/litre)	Daily requirement if essential (grams)
Glycine	H–	–	210	–
Alanine	CH_3–	–	350	–
Serine	$HOCH_2$–	–	150	–
Cysteine	$HSCH_2$–	10.3	0	–
Cystine	$S–CH_2$– | $S–CH_2$–	–	80	–
Aspartic acid	$^-OOCCH_2$–	3.8	5	–
Glutamic acid	$^-OOCCH_2CH_2$–	4.3	30	–
Asparagine	NH_2COCH_2–	–	50	–
Glutamine	$NH_2COCH_2CH_2$–	–	500	–
Proline	$CH_2CH_2CH_2$–	–	225	–
Threonine	CH_3CHOH–	–	150	0.5
Methionine	$CH_3SCH_2CH_2$–	–	20	1.1
Valine	$CH_3CH(CH_3)$–	–	200	0.8
Isoleucine	$CH_3CH_2CH(CH_3)$–	–	55	0.7
Leucine	$CH_3CH(CH_3)CH_2$–	–	110	1.1
Tyrosine	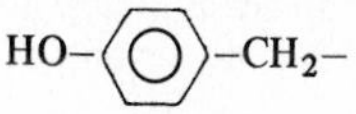 HO–C_6H_4–CH_2–	10.1	55	1.1 (Tyrosine + Phenylalanine)
Phenylalanine	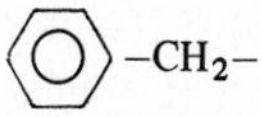 C_6H_5–CH_2–	–	53	
Tryptophan	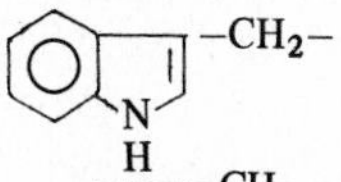 indolyl–CH_2– (N–H)	–	40	0.25
Histidine	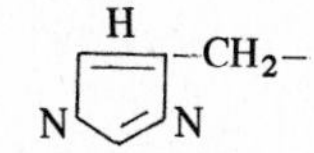 imidazolyl–CH_2– (N, N)	6.0	90	–
Lysine	$^+H_3NCH_2CH_2CH_2$–	10.5	170	0.8
Arginine	$^+H_2N{=}C(NH_2)NHCH_2CH_2CH_2$–	12.3	90	–
Ornithine	$^+H_3NCH_2CH_2CH_2$–	10.8	75	–

the uncharged amide forms of aspartic and glutamic acids. The three aliphatic species: valine, leucine, and isoleucine, are called the *branched-chain amino acids* because of their homologous structure and similarities in their metabolism. The residues most plentiful in many proteins are aspartic and glutamic acids, leucine, and lysine. In the structural protein, collagen, however, glycine and proline are the most abundant. An amino acid found in the free state but not in proteins is ornithine, the five-carbon analogue of lysine (Table 6.1). Ornithine is a participant in urea synthesis.

When a protein is fully hydrolyzed, by acid, alkali, or a protease, peptide bonds are cleaved to give free amino acids:

$$NH_2{-}\underset{H}{\overset{R}{C}}{-}COOH \quad \text{or} \quad {+}NH_3{-}\underset{H}{\overset{R}{C}}{-}COO^-$$

The ionized forms of these acids predominate at neutral pH. Being ionic compounds, amino acids are generally soluble in body fluids. The exception is cystine, the disulphide of cysteine, which is soluble only to the extent of 0.2 g/litre; it precipitates renal stones when present in excess, as in the congenital condition *cystinuria* (Chapter 18).

6.1.2. The structure of proteins

The peptide chains of a protein are linear – they may cross-link internally (as in albumin, Figure 6.1) or to other chains, but they never branch. If there is no hindrance by interactions between R groups, the hydrogen atom of an –NH– may be shared with the O atom of a nearby –CO– to form a *hydrogen bond.* Although hydrogen bonds are very weak, a large number of them can stabilize the formation either of a coil called the α-helix (as in lysozyme, Figure 6.2), or of a parallel alignment called a β-pleated sheet. The order of the amino acid residues in the peptide chain is termed the *primary structure,* whereas the α-helix or β-sheet is termed *secondary structure.* Most globular proteins have 40 to 80% of their structure in the helical form, and less than 30% in the β form.

Even a helical coil would be an unwieldy structure for a long protein chain, and in most globular proteins the coiled regions fold back on themselves in a specific manner to form a more compact molecule. This folding gives the protein *tertiary structure,* which is also illustrated by the model of lysozyme in Figure 6.2. The lysozyme chain has five helical segments and is folded into the form of a compact globule by four cross-linking disulphide (S-S) bonds. The tertiary structure is stabilized by hydrogen bonds, by electrostatic attractions between positive and negatively charged R groups, and by van der Waal's forces between hydrophobic residues.

The result of the folding is to place the hydrophilic (polar) groups on the outer surface of the folded molecule, and to create in the interior of the molecule a hydrophobic environment. The almost limitless permutations of the order of the 20 diverse amino acid residues (Table 6.1) permit the formation of specific sites with biological activities, such as binding of substrate by an enzyme or of antigen by an antibody. In the case of an enzyme, the binding results in conformational changes which allow the substrate(s) to react in a manner otherwise unlikely to occur. This is the basis of the catalytic activity of enzymes. For the reader interested in further pursuit of the intricacies of protein structure the short monograph of Dickerson and Geis (1969) is recommended.

Thus far *simple proteins,* those containing only amino acid residues, have been considered. Many proteins, particularly extracellular ones, have chains of carbohydrate residues attached, and are termed *glycoproteins* or *proteoglycans.* Others have prosthetic groups such as haem, flavin coenzymes, or iron, and are called *haemoproteins, flavoproteins,* and *metalloproteins,* respectively. *Nucleoproteins* or *lipoproteins* contain nucleic acid or lipid constituents. These are all examples of *complex proteins.*

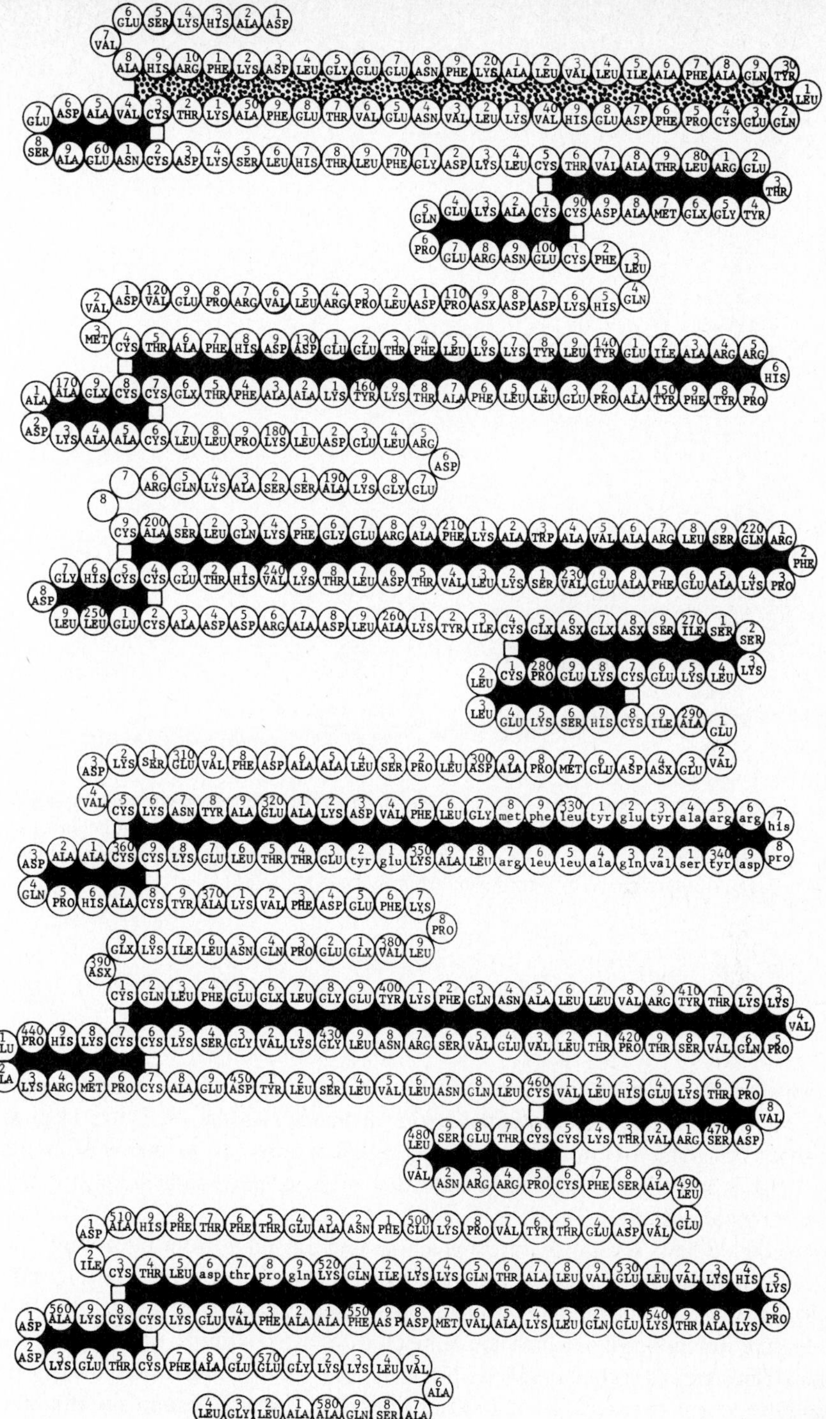

Figure. 6.1. Sequence of amino acid residues in human serum albumin. The residues are shown as circles and are identified by the first three letters of their names, except ASN = asparagine, GLN = glutamine, ILE = isoleucine nad TRP = tryptophan. The shaded areas indicate the loops formed by disulphide bonds between Cys–Cys residues. (Reproduced, by permission, from Behrens et al., 1975). The sequence determined independently by Meloun et al. (1975) differs very little, except that residues 278–281 are Cys–Glu–Lys–Pro instead of Lys–Glu–Pro–Cys.

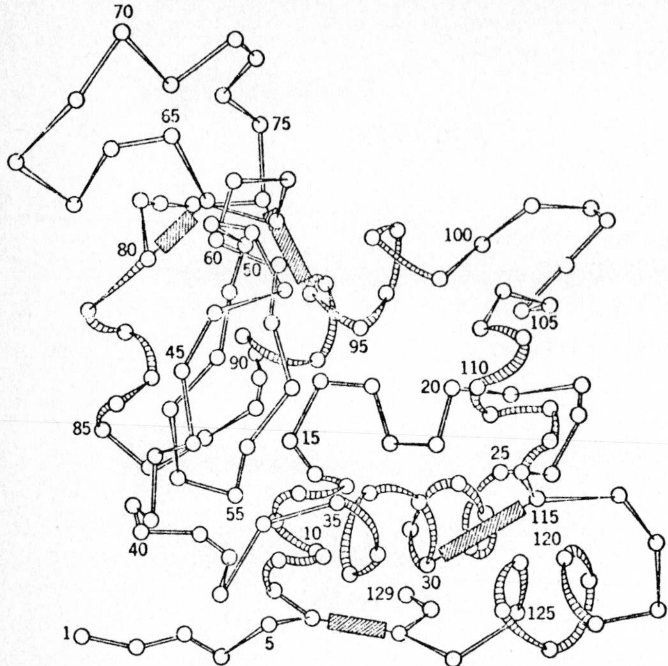

Figure 6.2. Three-dimensional structure of the peptide chain of egg white lysozyme. Each circle indicates an amino acid residue, numbered from the amino to the carboxyl ends. Five short helical regions are shown by cross hatching. Cross-linking by disulphide bonds is indicated by the four shaded rectangles. (By W.L. Bragg – Reproduced, by permission, from Blake et al., 1965)

6.1.3. The proteins of blood plasma

The proteins of plasma help to retain fluid within the vascular bed, transport poorly soluble nutrients, and inactivate potential toxins or invasive agents. In 1 litre of plasma there is about 75 grams of protein; of this, 42 grams is albumin, 11 grams is immunoglobulin G (IgG), and the remainder is a collection of 50 or more individual proteins in lower concentrations (Table 6.2).

Plasma proteins have several features which distinguish them from intracellular proteins. Characteristically they contain disulphide bonds (Figure 6.2) and rarely have free thiol (–SH) groups. The disulphide bonds provide stability against denaturation, an important feature for molecules which are subjected to the continual turbulence of the circulation. Thiol groups, often found on intracellular enzymes, might be subject to oxidation at the oxygen tensions found outside the cells. The thiol group on albumin is unique; it is apparently protected from oxidation by its sheltered position in the albumin molecule, and may have a specific transport role.

A second feature of plasma proteins is that nearly all of them are proteoglycans (Spiro,

TABLE 6.2.

PROPERTIES OF PLASMA PROTEINS

Name	Abbreviation	Mol. mass $\times 10^{-3}$	% carbohydrate	Concentration in normal plasma: average (g/litre) [a]	Concentration in normal plasma: range (g/litre) [a]	% intravascular	$t_{1/2}$ (days)	Functions
1. Prealbumin	PA	55	0	0.25	0.1–0.4			Binds retinol binding protein (1 : 1, 0.38 g/g); binds thyroxine
2. Albumin	SA	66	0	42	35–50	40	19	Osmotic, nutritional; binds fatty acids, bilirubin, tryptophan, hormones, etc.
3. α_1-Lipoprotein	αLP	200	1.5 [b]	3.6	2.9–7.7		4.5	Lipid transport
4. Orosomucoid	Oro	44	41	0.9	0.6–1.4		5	Inactivate progesterone?; tissue repair
5. α_1-Antitrypsin	AT	53	12.4	2.9	1.8–4		3–5	Inhibits proteases; binds trypsin (2 : 1, 0.91 g/g)
6. α_2-Macroglobulin	α_2M	725	8.4	2.4	1.5–3.5	90	7	Binds
7. Haptoglobin (1–1)	Hp	85 [c]	22.7	1.7	1.2–2.6	50	2	Binds haemoglobin (1 : 1, 0.80 g/g)
8. Caeruloplasmin	Cp	151	7.0	0.32	0.16–0.6	40	4.5	Oxidize neurogenic amines?; aid iron binding to Tn?
9. Haemopexin	Hpx	57	21	0.8	0.5–1.0		7	Binds haem (1 : 1, 11 mg/g)
10. Transferrin	Tn	76.5	5.3	2.3	1.8–2.7	40	8.5	Transports iron (2 : 1, 1.5 mg/g); bacteriostasis
11. β-Lipoprotein	βLP	3200	1.8 [d]	3.2	2.6–3.8	45	3.2	Lipid transport
12. Complement C'3	C3	185	2.7	1.1	0.8–1.4		2.5	Inactivate infectious agents
13. Fibrinogen	Φ	341	2.5	2.9	2–4.5	80	2.5	Clot formation
14. Immunoglobulin A	IgA	175–500	7.5 [e]	2.0	1–4	40–45	6	In secretions; agglutinins; esp. diphtheria, tetanus, typhoid, parathyroid B
15. Immunoglobulin M	IgM	900	12 [f]	1.2	0.6–2.6	75	5	Primary response; agglutinins; cell lysis; Rh factor
16. Immunoglobulin G	IgG	150	2.9 [g]	11	8–16	40	24	Secondary responses; neutralizes toxins; binds bacteria, viruses
17. Total serum protein	TSP	–	3.7	72	62–82			

[a] 10 g/litre = 1 g/dl = 1 g/100 ml
[b] 41% lipid
[c] Mol. mass of Hp 2–1 and 2–2 is 220,000; if Hp is 2–1, normal level is about 41% higher
[d] 79% lipid
[e] 1 g/litre of IgA = 5.95 I.U./ml
[f] 1 g/litre of IgM = 115 I.U./ml
[g] 1 g/litre of IgG = 11.5 I.U./ml

1973). The proportion of carbohydrate, by weight, varies from 0% in albumin and 2.5% in fibrinogen to 41% in orosomucoid. The 2.7 grams of protein-bound carbohydrate in 1 litre of plasma includes 1.2 grams of hexoses, 0.8 grams of aminosugars, 0.6 grams of sialic acid, and 0.09 grams of fucose. Proteoglycans containing less than 4% (w/w) hexosamine are termed *glycoproteins*; those with more than 4% are *mucoproteins.* Typically the carbohydrate units are chains of molecular mass 2000 to 3000 (11 to 16 residues of hexose), attached at the amide group of asparagine residues or the hydroxyl groups of serine residues of peptide chains. The number of carbohydrate chains varies from two per molecule of transferrin or IgG, to 31 per molecule of α_2-macroglobulin. Carbohydrate chains of many plasma proteins have the structure:

(sialic acid–galactose–*N*-acetylglucosamine)$_4$–mannose$_n$–*N*-acetylglucosamine–asparagine

Fucose occurs in some of the chains.

Mucopolysaccharides are chains of sugar units of 10,000 to 30,000 molecular mass, containing sulphate and uronic acid groups which give them acidic properties. They are components of the intercellular ground substance and are not normally detectable in plasma, but appear there in certain pathological conditions in conjunction with the C-reactive protein (section 6.3.2.5).

The proteoglycans of plasma were once thought to have a common function, related to the sharp rise in protein-bound carbohydrate in plasma following inflammation or trauma – the *acute phase reaction* (section 6.3.2.5). This rise has now been shown to be due largely to increases in specific proteins (e.g. orosomucoid and haptoglobin) which are high in carbohydrate, and so it seems more appropriate to consider the proteoglycans as individual proteins rather than as a group. The function of the carbohydrate chains is still unknown. Their attachment may be obligatory for secretion from cells; they may serve to increase the solubility of the proteins to which they are attached; or they may be important in interaction with specific recognition sites on target cell membranes.

6.1.4. Assay of total protein

The amount of protein in a mixture such as serum or plasma may be determined by several approaches. Since protein constitutes most of the solid content of plasma, measurement of total nitrogen or of refractive index gives a reasonable estimate of the amount of protein present. Fair specificity for the peptide chain is found in the biuret reaction or in the optical absorbance peak near 185 nm. Other techniques are based on chemical reactions of particular R groups of the amino acids, most commonly the aromatic groups of tyrosine, tryptophan, and phenylalanine, or the amino groups of lysine residues.

Total nitrogen measurement, usually conducted by the Kjeldahl digestion method, is a tedious procedure which is now reserved largely for standardization efforts. Nitrogen is not restricted to the peptide chain – some of the carbohydrate components and prosthetic groups such as haem contain nitrogen – and the nitrogen content varies even among peptide chains, depending upon their proportions of arginine, histidine, lysine, and tryptophan. An average nitrogen content for serum proteins is 16% (w/w).

Refractometry is a simple measurement which is widely used with serum. It requires only a drop of liquid in a refractometer such as is used for urine specific gravity determination. Pre-calibration by the manufacturer against solutions of known protein content is required. Since refractometry measures total solids, in practice the instrument is calibrated to allow for the non-protein solids usually found in normal serum, about 17 g/litre; errors can obviously result if refractometry is employed with specimens having an abnormally high concentration of non-protein solids, such as glucose in diabetes mellitus or urea in severe uraemia. Highly lipaemic specimens will also give erroneous results by refractometry, since the refractive index increment for lipoproteins is less than that for most plasma proteins (1.71×10^{-4} compared to 1.88×10^{-4}).

Another common protein assay in the clinical laboratory uses the biuret reaction (see Henry et al., 1974). Named for its early use with biuret, $NH_2CONHCONH_2$, a pyrolysis product of urea, the reaction is the formation of a stable purple colour between copper ions (Cu^{2+}) and the nitrogen atoms of peptide bonds in an alkaline solution. The biuret reaction has been readily adapted to automation, and gives values which are almost constant from protein to protein. Human albumin and immunoglobulin G, for instance, have biuret colour intensities within ±2% when compared on a peptide basis. The biuret reaction is relatively insensitive – the absorbance at 540 nm of a 1 g/litre solution of albumin in a biuret reagent is 0.30 ± 1% (Doumas, 1975) – but insensitivity is not a serious problem when measuring serum protein concentration. Specimens which are haemolyzed, icteric, or lipaemic will give falsely high values unless suitable blanks are included. The method must be standardized against a solution of known protein content, since it has not yet been possible to standardize the colour yield for the variety of biuret reagents and spectrophotometers which are in use. A suitable standard solution can be prepared in the laboratory by dissolving crystalline bovine plasma albumin and measuring its absorbance at 280 nm, using the factor $A_{280}^{1\,g/litre} = 0.661$. Several commercial preparations contain human or bovine albumin standardized by nitrogen assay, assuming 16.0% (w/w) nitrogen. The U.S. National Bureau of Standards offers a Standard Reference Material (SRM 927) suitable for calibrating total protein assays – 70 g/litre solution of pure bovine albumin standardized gravimetrically. This preparation should improve the agreement of protein assays among laboratories by providing a reference against which secondary protein standard solutions can be assessed.

Measurement of optical absorbance near 185 nm, is highly sensitive and specific for the peptide chain. The absorbance at 205 nm, for instance, is about 100 times as intense as that of the biuret reaction, but most spectrophotometers give only marginal performance in this region of the ultraviolet, and the potential of this non-destructive approach has not yet been realized.

Measurement of proteins by chemical reactions of the amino acid R groups suffers from variation in the proportions of the R groups in individual proteins. Thus the Lowry assay, a reaction with phosphomolybdic acid and copper (Cu^{2+}) largely measures phenolic compounds, and the colour yield varies with the tyrosine content. Its chemistry is more complex and the composition of its reagents is more critical than the biuret reaction, but it is appreciably more sensitive.

The three aromatic residues absorb ultraviolet light near 280 nm, giving a non-destructive measurement which has been useful in assaying the proteins in flowing streams such as effluents from column chromatographs. There are large differences between the factors for different proteins ($A^{1\,g/litre}_{280\,nm}$ for human albumin and immunoglobulin G are 0.53 and 1.34, respectively), so that the results are highly dependent on the composition of the protein mixture. The amino groups of lysine may be reacted with suitable chromogens – ninhydrin, trinitrobenzenesulphonate, certain wool dyes – or more recently, with the fluorogen Fluorescamine (Hoffman La Roche). Coupling with dyes is useful in visualizing protein bands after fractionation on solid supports, such as electrophoretic separations.

The total protein concentration of normal serum, assayed as peptide material by the biuret method, is 72 (62 to 82) g/litre. For plasma, containing about 3 g/litre of fibrinogen, the concentration is correspondingly higher. This increase is not observed if salts such as oxalates are used as anticoagulants, since water is drawn from red cells and dilutes the plasma so that its protein concentration is about the same, or even less, than that of serum.

The total serum protein concentration is low at birth, about 46 to 70 g/litre, and lower still, 36 to 60 g/litre, in premature infants. By about 3 years of age, the concentration observed in the adult is reached. With increasing age past maturity, the protein level drops slowly, to about 66 g/litre in persons over 80 years. There is little difference between the concentrations in men and in women, and no recorded change post-prandially or with different seasons of the year. Diurnal variation is 5 g/litre or less. The concentration is affected by activities which cause fluid to enter or leave the circulation; there is an increase of 4 to 8 g/litre within an hour of assuming an upright posture, and a similar increase after vigorous exercise. In pregnancy, the total protein normally falls by about 8 g/litre during the last trimester. Variations with disease are considered in section 6.2.5.

6.1.5. Characterization of individual plasma proteins

Characterization of the proteins in plasma or serum for many years utilized crude fractionation procedures. *Albumin* remained soluble in salt-free solution whereas *globulin* did not. The scheme of Howe, which was introduced in 1921, used 11%, 15%, 18% and 22% (w/v) sodium sulphate to precipitate progressively fibrinogen and three mixtures of globulins, leaving albumin largely in solution. Ammonium sulphate solutions of 25%, 33%, and 50% saturation were employed in the same manner. Such techniques have largely been supplanted by either (a) fractionation into groups of proteins of like charge or size or (b) direct determination of specific proteins by immunochemical or ligand-binding techniques.

6.1.5.1. Separations based on charge

The different charges among proteins allow proteins to be separated by the technique of *electrophoresis* – the migration of charged molecules in an electric field. Applied to proteins in solution by Tiselius in 1937, electrophoresis is now conducted mainly on solid supports such as cellulose acetate films or agarose gels. The cellulose acetate films (Kohn, 1957) have largely supplanted paper, because of shorter drying times and a lesser tendency for albumin to be absorbed by the support and leave a trail which affects the interpretation. In studying plasma or serum, the pH of the system is usually maintained between 8.5 and 9, so that all of the proteins present will have a net negative charge and hence will migrate in the same direction, although at rates depending on their charge-to-mass ratios. The time of the run can be as short as 20 minutes. After the separation, the proteins are visualized by fixation to the support using organic solvents, heat, or precipitants such as trichloroacetic acid, then staining with various dyes. The red dye, Ponceau S, a product of the wool industry, is widely used. The stained bands may be scanned photoelectrically to give quantitative results.

Examples of the electrophoretic separation of plasma are shown in Figure 6.3. Tiselius' original system, at pH circa 7, demonstrated albumin, fibrinogen, and three globulin fractions, which he termed α, β, and γ (alpha, beta, and gamma). With the introduction of barbital buffers at pH 8.5 to 9, the α-globulin was resolved into two bands, termed α_1 and α_2. Values for electrophoretic fractions in healthy individuals are listed in Table 6.3. Observation of electrophoretic patterns is useful to detect deficiencies of albumin and immunoglobulins (sections 6.3.1 and 6.3.3), the presence of paraproteins (section 6.3.3.4), the occurrence of acute phase and chronic reactions (sections 6.3.2 and 6.3.3), and the degree of protein loss via kidney or gut. A summary of the relevant considerations is found in section 6.4.

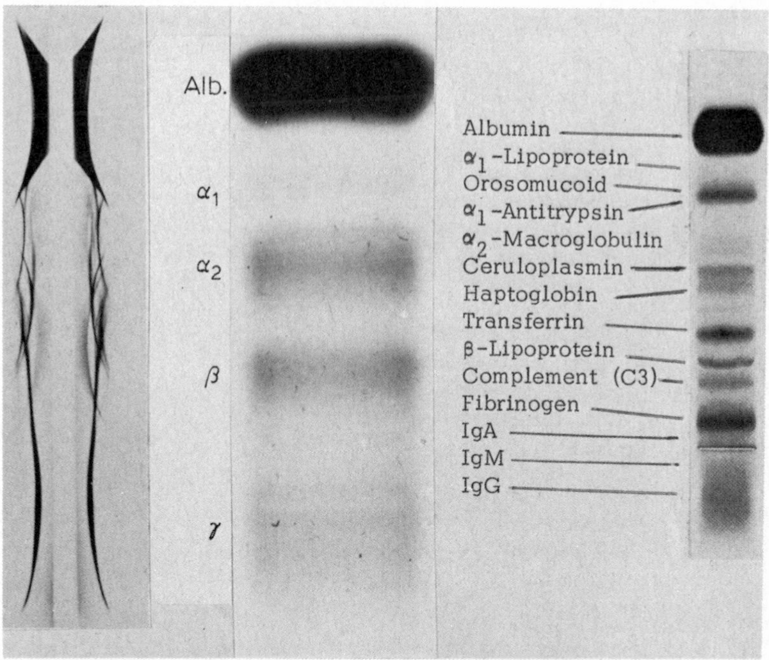

Fig. 6.3. Comparison of electrophoretic separations of serum or plasma proteins. Centre: cellulose acetate electrophoresis of serum, stained for proteins. Right: agarose gel electrophoresis of plasma, stained for proteins (reproduced, by permission, from Laurell, 1972); note the greater resolving power of agarose gel compared to cellulose acetate. Left: immunoelectrophoresis, showing bands of precipitate corresponding to individual serum proteins (courtesy of Millipore Biomedica).

TABLE 6.3.

NORMAL DISTRIBUTION OF SERUM PROTEINS UPON ELECTROPHORESIS ON CELLULOSE ACETATE

Notes: Values are a composite of selected reports. Values obtained with paper electrophoresis differ mainly in showing a lower percentage of albumin because of trailing. The figures for the bands do not necessarily correlate with the calculated totals of their constituent proteins shown in Table 6.2 because staining indicates mainly the peptide portion of the proteins, and certain proteins such as orosomucoid and haemopexin stain very weakly.

Band	Albumin	$alpha_1$	$alpha_2$	beta	gamma	Total
% of total	59	4.1	10.2	12.2	15	100
range	45–69	2–5.4	7.5–12.9	6.8–16.3	9.5–17.7	
g/liter	42	3	7.5	9	11	72
range	33–51	1.5–4	5.5–9.5	5–12	7–13	

Electrophoresis on supporting media offers the option of staining non-peptide constituents, such as glycoproteins with Schiff's reagent or lipoproteins with Oil Red O. Staining for glycoproteins has received only limited use, but lipoproteins (Chapter 5) are widely measured by this technique.

Proteins with many charges are hydrophilic and tend to be highly soluble, whereas those with few charges are hydrophobic and tend to be insoluble. At the *isoelectric point,* where positive and negative charges balance so the net charge is zero, the solubility is at a minimum, a phenomenon which is useful in isolating proteins from mixtures. Solubility may be decreased by lowering the polar nature of the solvent through the removal of salt or the addition of alcohol. Thus a hydrophilic protein such as albumin remains soluble at pH 6 in distilled water, but the more hydrophobic immunoglobulins, particularly the macroglobulins, do not. This property is the basis of the simple Sia test for macroglobulins, which are precipitated when a drop of serum is added to a little water. The general principles of manipulation of alcohol and salt concentrations, pH, and temperature were evolved by Cohn and his colleagues (1950) at the Harvard Physical Chemical Laboratory to meet the need for plasma substitutes during World War II and they are still the basis for most large-scale methods of fractionating plasma proteins.

Protein chemists have learned to treat proteins gently during isolation. Secondary and tertiary structure can be disrupted by conditions which alter the weak hydrogen bonds. Disruption leaves the protein in a random configuration without biologically active sites, and the protein is said to be *denatured*; in most cases denaturation is irreversible. The possibility of denaturation mandates the use of temperatures near the freezing point when proteins are placed in non-polar solvents such as those containing alcohol; the avoidance of extremes of pH; and precautions against foaming, since even spreading of protein molecules into the thin film of a bubble causes irreversible conformational changes, just as does the whipping of egg white.

Differences of charges among proteins are also the basis of separation by *ion exchange chromatography.* Negatively charged proteins bind with varying affinities to positively charged solid supports, for instance, and can be eluted in order of increasing protein charge by gradual changes in salt concentration or pH. The most commonly used medium with plasma is diethylaminoethylcellulose. Ion exchange chromatography is a powerful tool, widely used in research, and which is entering the clinical field as a simple method of separating enzymes that are similar but have different charges, such as the isoenzymic forms of lactate dehydrogenase (EC 1.1.1.27) or creatine kinase (EC 2.7.3.2).

6.1.5.2. Separations based on molecular size

Proteins may also be separated on the basis of their molecular size. Two simple physical techniques have been widely used. By ultracentrifugation, a technique developed by Svedberg and Pedersen about 1940, normal serum separates into bands designated 4S, which is mainly albumin and smaller α- and β-globulins, 7S, which is largely immunoglobulin G, and 19S, which is largely immunoglobulin M or macroglobulin. S is the unit of sedimentation rate, or Svedberg number, Ultracentrifugation is not a routine measurement with plasma, but is useful in the separation of lipoproteins which, being of lower density, rise rather than sediment in solutions of the density of plasma. Lipoproteins are rated by the S_f, or Svedberg flotation number, rather than a sedimentation constant, and are considered in Chapter 5.

The newer technique of *gel filtration,* also termed molecular exclusion chromatography, utilizes beads of a gel, usually polymerized dextran (Sephadex, Pharmacia Fine Chemicals, Inc.), formed with uniform pores such that small molecules may diffuse into the gel beads but larger molecules are excluded. During passage through a bed of these beads, the smaller molecules are retarded while the larger ones, which are restricted to the

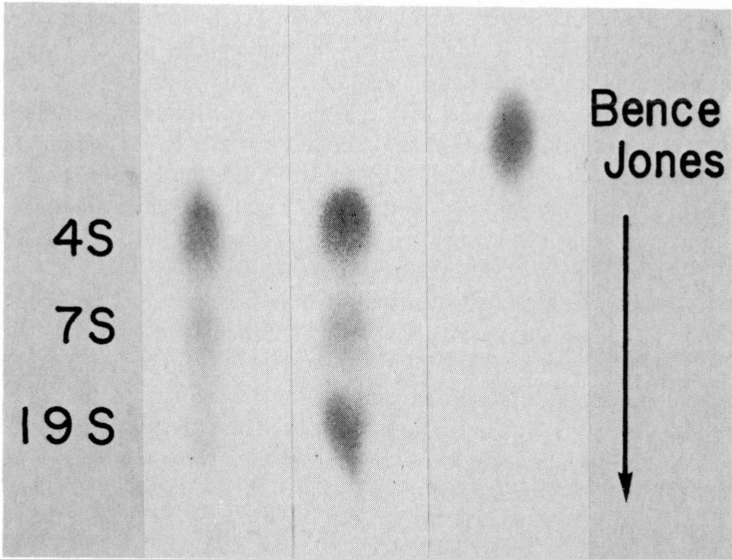

Figure 6.4. Separation of proteins on the basis of molecular size using a thin layer of dextran gel (Sephadex G-200). The larger molecules have migrated farther toward the bottom of the sheet. Left: normal serum; middle: serum showing elevated IgM (19S); right: urine showing Bence Jones protein.

space outside the beads, emerge first. The porosity of the gels can be regulated in manufacture to permit separation in molecular size ranges between 500 and 2,000,000. Serum distributes into three components corresponding to the 4S, 7S and 19S ultracentrifugal fractions. Gel filtration has been more widely employed than ultracentrifugation, and is applicable either on a preparative scale in columns or analytically on thin-layer sheets. The sheets can be stained to show the proteins as spots, and are useful to detect macroglobulins (section 6.3.3.3) or Bence Jones proteins (section 6.3.3.4), as demonstrated in Figure 6.4.

Gels are also used to increase the resolving power of electrophoresis by modifying the migration of larger molecules. Starch, polyacrylamide, or agarose are commonly employed, agarose electrophoresis in particular having been adapted to the analysis of serum and plasma (Figure 6.3). By this technique, the α_1-, α_2-, β- and γ-globulin zones are further resolved, in some cases into bands representing single proteins.

6.1.5.3. Assays based on biological properties

Individual proteins may be measured by their biological properties such as ligand binding, catalysis (Chapter 7), or combination with specific antibody. These tests have the advantage of not requiring prior separation of the protein in question – they may be applied directly to serum – and are gradually replacing electrophoretic fractionation as the usefulness of specific protein measurements in diagnosis becomes appreciated.

A pitfall is that the biological property may not be fully active. Inhibitors may be present, or the active sites of some of the protein molecules may have been damaged through denaturation. On the other hand, frequently it is the biological activity of the protein which is of primary interest to the clinician. The requirement for fully active materials as standards for these assays is a difficult one, and poses one of the main concerns in assays of biological properties. Recommendations concerning the applications of assays for specific proteins are given in sections 6.3 and 6.4.

In testing ligand-binding ability, an excess of the ligand is usually added. A colour change which is characteristic of the ligand–protein complex, as seen in the binding of bromcresol green by albumin, may be measured directly. Otherwise the unbound ligand may be removed and the ligand–protein complex measured. Examples are the determination of transferrin by loading with iron, of haptoglobin by loading with haemoglobin, or of thyroxine-binding globulin by loading with radioactive thyroxine.

The introduction of immunochemical techniques into the clinical laboratory in the last decade has provided simple and sensitive assays for specific individual proteins. Only the availability of suitable antisera appears to limit the usefulness of this approach. For quantitative results, there are three techniques in clinical use. In two of these, the bands of precipitate (*precipitins*) between protein (antigen) and specific antibody are observed in gels. The most widely used technique, and the simplest, is *radial immunodiffusion*, in which the concentration of antigen is related to the distance it diffuses into agar gels containing antibody by measuring the diameter of the circle of precipitate formed (Fahey and McKelvey, 1965; Mancini et al., 1965). The drawback is that diffusion takes one to three days for good results. Application of an electric field speeds the movement of antigen so that results can be obtained within an hour. The resulting parabolic arcs of precipitate have prompted the name *rocket electrophoresis* for this technique (Laurell, 1966).

Both radial immunodiffusion and rocket electrophoresis require a supply of prepared gel plates for each protein to be measured. These are now available from a number of commercial sources.

The third approach uses a nephelometer to measure the Tyndall scattering of light when the colloidal antigen–antibody complex first forms in solution. It can be performed manually (Deaton et al., 1976) or in mechanized equipment, where it is called *automated immunoprecipitation* (Ritchie et al., 1973; Buffone et al., 1974). This technique is capable of high throughput and rapid output of results but requires a separate channel of automation with a blank, or a separate run, for each antigen determined, and its standardization calls for careful attention and some degree of skill.

In standardizing immunochemical assays, Hobbs (1971) recommended the use of a pool of normal adult serum, which had been assayed against freshly prepared pure preparations of individual proteins. The pooled serum should be frozen in small batches so that a container need be thawed only once. Precision of immunochemical techniques is only about ±10%, but can be improved to ±3% with replicate analyses.

For identification of a protein, *immunoelectrophoresis* is useful. In this technique (Figure 6.3) fractions separated by electrophoresis in agar gel are allowed to diffuse laterally toward antibodies applied in a trough in the gel, producing precipitin arcs for each antigen–antibody system present. Immunoelectrophoresis is of particular aid in identifying immunoglobulins.

The limit of detection of proteins has been extended downward significantly by measuring the competition of an antigen for binding sites on an antibody by using a radioactive form of the same antigen, in the technique called *radioimmunoassay* (Henry et al., 1974). This is applicable even to non-precipitating antigen–antibody systems, for instance digoxin or many other drugs, as well as to protein antigens, but it has the disadvantage of requiring radioactive tracer techniques and expensive reagents. It gives results in the picogram (10^{-12} g) range for antigens of interest.

6.2. METABOLISM OF PROTEINS

The metabolism of plasma proteins is intertwined closely with that of tissue protein. Both tissue and plasma proteins arise from, and break down to, the same amino acid pool, and chronic changes in one group are in time reflected in the other. Hence this section will consider overall protein metabolism, including that of both plasma and tissue proteins (Munro and Allison, 1970).

6.2.1. Distribution

In the 6 litres of blood in a 70-kg person there are 3.5 litres of plasma, which, at a concentration of 75 grams of protein per litre (including fibrinogen), contains just over 250 grams of protein. According to Starling's hypothesis, the proteins are the chief substances in plasma which are too large to pass through the capillary walls, and thus they exert an osmotic effect, in this case a colloid osmotic effect. This effect draws filtered water back into the capillaries at their venous ends, where hydrostatic pressure between capillary and tissue is low (Chapter 2, section 2.4.6). The magnitude of the colloid osmotic pressure, measured in a collodion sack, is about 35 cm of water (25 mm Hg).

The capillary is not a collodion sack, however, and the situation is less simple than that just indicated. The capillary wall is permeable to plasma proteins to varying degrees, roughly inversely to their molecular sizes, so that some proteins enter the interstitial fluid and counteract the colloid osmotic pressure as measured in the collodion bag. This extravasated protein does not re-enter the capillary, but finds its way back to the circulation through the lymph channels, a slow and easily interrupted route. The result is that a considerable amount of "plasma" protein is outside the plasma at any one time. This amount is about 350 grams, or 1.5 times as much as the intravascular protein. The total exchangeable plasma protein pool is 250 g + 350 g = 600 g. This contrasts with about 1.5 kg of tissue protein in the same 70-kg individual. The proportion which is extravascular is about 60% for albumin and IgG, and only 20% for large molecules such as fibrinogen and α_2-macroglobulin (Table 6.2). Equilibration of tracer proteins between the intra- and extravascular compartments requires 2 to 3 days, but most of the transfer takes place during the first day. Hence in acute changes – haemorrhage, consumption of circulating antibody by an antigen, administration of a protein-bound drug or toxin – only the intravascular protein pool need be considered, whereas for longer-acting changes, including metabolic degradation, the extravascular pool must be considered as well.

6.2.2. Biosynthesis

The molecules of plasma proteins do not circulate for the life of the host but are continually being destroyed and replaced even though their number at any one time remains constant. The rate of replacement varies for different proteins as shown by the half-lives ranging from 2 to 24 days which are listed in Table 6.2. Tissue proteins are also continually replaced, at high rates for enzymes of metabolically active tissues and very low rates for structural proteins such as collagen. The total daily turnover of plasma protein is about 25 grams; that of total tissue protein is about 150 grams. Thus the plasma proteins, which are only 4% of the total protein of the body, account for about 15% of the protein turnover.

Most plasma proteins are produced by the parenchymal cells of the liver. A major exception is the immunoglobulins, which are found in plasma cells and B lymphocytes. Some lipoprotein is made by the intestinal mucosa, and some transferrin is formed in the intestine and the bone marrow. But the liver is by far the major producer both of quantity and of numbers of protein species.

Plasma proteins are assembled by the same mechanisms that synthesize intracellular proteins. Energy in the form of ATP and GTP is required. The synthesis of a polypeptide chain typically requires 1 to 2 minutes. If a newly formed protein is destined for export (or circulation) it proceeds through the membranous channels of the cytoplasm to reach the circulation; during their passage the glycoproteins receive carbohydrate chains, and lipoproteins acquire their lipid moieties. Secretion takes 20 to 40 minutes and is continuous – there is no storage of plasma proteins in cells.

6.2.3. Degradation

More is known about the source of plasma proteins than about their fate. Labelled molecules added to plasma disappear in a random or first-order manner, that is, the age of molecules does not influence their selection for destruction. The plasma proteins are broken down to free amino acids which mix with the active plasma amino acid pool, and are almost immediately available for re-incorporation or oxidation at any point in the body. The first-order type of disappearance can be explained by a random imbibition of tiny portions of plasma by cells, with the proteins therein being digested by lysosomal enzymes. What this mechanism does not explain, however, is the fact that different proteins of plasma have different turnover rates (Table 6.2). At some point a mechanism of specificity or recognition of individual proteins must be invoked. This recognition may be of forms of a protein which have been slightly altered by proteases, chemical changes, or loss of ligands.

The sites of plasma protein breakdown are widespread. Plasma proteins, particularly albumin, leak into the lumen of the gastrointestinal tract where they are digested, but this probably represents less than 10% of the total catabolism in normal persons. Neither the liver nor the kidney accounts for more than this proportion in the healthy individual, and it appears that plasma proteins are taken up by most tissues of the body, probably according to the metabolic rates of the tissues. The 25 grams of plasma protein which is broken down daily contributes about one-seventh of the amino acids used to replace protein in tissues. In this sense, the plasma proteins have a nutritional role, and one which is probably more significant in post-absorptive periods when the free amino acid concentration is somewhat decreased.

6.2.4. Amino acid metabolism

The immediate source of proteins is the intracellular pool of free amino acids. These are in rapid equilibrium with the free amino acids of plasma; the interchange is so fast that the average time an amino acid molecule spends in the circulation is about 1 minute. Regulation of the composition of the plasma amino acid pool is primarily the function of the liver. Situated as it is at the head of the portal circulation, this organ has the first selection of the amino acids which are absorbed following a meal. It takes up 50 to 90% of the portal amino acids in a single passage.

An amino acid molecule in the plasma normally has an equal chance of becoming part of a protein or of being catabolized. When protein intake is high, the proportion catabolized is larger. In this situation, the liver forms additional enzymes to degrade amino acids which are present in excess or to convert them into non-essential amino acids which are in short supply. When the need for these enzymes declines they, too, are degraded and their amino acids enter the pool. There is no mechanism to store protein for future need other than by maintaining a full measure of plasma proteins and active tissue proteins.

Dietary protein is required for growth and to replace amino acids which are unavoidably catabolized in the course of protein turnover. Man cannot produce the essential amino acids (Table 6.1) and these (or their deaminated congenors) must be supplied in the diet. The normal daily requirement for protein in the adult has been established at

0.5 g/kg; more is needed for growing children, pregnant women, and especially infants. The normal intake of protein in Western countries is 0.7 to 1.5 g/kg (50 to 100 g/day), varying with religious custom and economic status; in Eastern nations it is generally less.

The amino acids which are most important in nitrogen transfers within the body are glutamine and alanine. These are also the two species which have the highest concentrations in venous blood, about 0.5 mmol/litre (Table 6.1). The inter-relationships between the portal and peripheral circulations are protrayed in Scheme 6.1. Glutamine formed in liver from glutamic acid and ammonia releases its ammonia in the kidney. Nitrogen from amino acids which are catabolized in peripheral tissues enters the venous circulation in the form of alanine. In the liver, the nitrogen of alanine is formed into urea and the remaining pyruvate is rebuilt into glucose. The amount of alanine recycled in this manner, the "alanine cycle", has been estimated as equivalent to 50% of the amount of pyruvate or lactate which moves from muscle to liver in the Cori cycle (Felig and Wahren, 1974; Felig, 1975).

Insulin is important in amino acid metabolism as well as in carbohydrate metabolism. It is apparently required for effective protein synthesis by the liver; it should be noted that the insulin released from the pancreas proceeds directly to the liver, which consumes about 90% of this hormone as it passes. The well-known effect of carbohydrate administration in lowering plasma amino acid concentrations can be attributed to the insulin release it evokes. Insulin promotes the entrance of amino acids and glucose into muscle cells and retards the breakdown of proteins into amino acids by lysosomes (Mortimore et al., 1973). Corticosteroids also affect protein metabolism, by accelerating protein breakdown and providing amino acids for gluconeogenesis. Increases in the amount of one amino acid, leucine, can cause release of insulin which serves to counterbalance the action of corticosteroids.

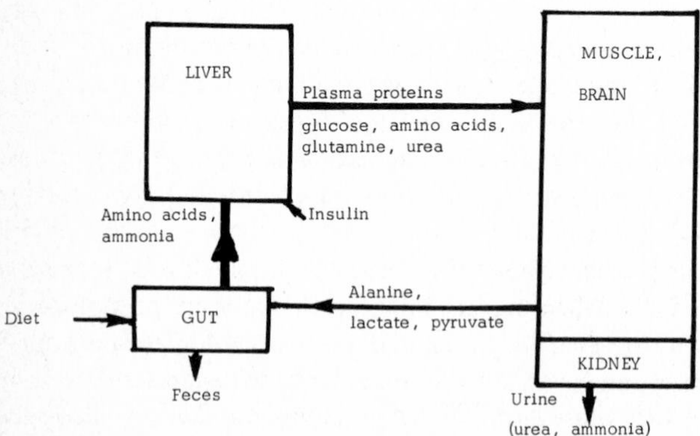

Scheme 6.1. Inter-relationships of nitrogen metabolism in the portal and peripheral circulations. Nitrogen from the breakdown of plasma protein and muscle protein leaves muscle largely as alanine. In the liver, alanine loses its nitrogen to form urea, and the remaining pyruvate is reformed into glucose as part of the Cori cycle. Other nitrogen in the form of ammonia from intestinal bacterial action also goes to urea in the liver, or is transported as glutamine to the kidney. Insulin, released into the portal circulation, aids amino acid uptake in muscle and slows protein breakdown.

6.2.5. Metabolism in pathological states

Protein deficiencies are grouped by nutritionists under the term "protein–calorie malnutrition" (Olson, 1975). The extremes are *kwashiorkor,* a condition observed in infants after weaning in regions of Africa and the West Indies where the diet consists only of high-carbohydrate fruits and vegetables and protein is almost completely lacking, and *marasmus,* a generalized starvation in which there is a deficit of calories plus protein (Waterlow and Alleyne, 1971).

Nitrogen depletion results when the protein intake is inadequate to meet minimum needs to replace amino acids lost in metabolism. If sufficient energy is available through intake of fats or carbohydrates, amino acids are "spared" for essential needs, and the body can adapt to an appreciably decreased intake of protein. One saving is in the enzymes which are needed for the catabolism of amino acids themselves; the burning of fats and carbohydrates utilizes simpler pathways. Vegetarians, it may be noted, suffer no ill effects from their reduced protein intake provided that the proteins they consume furnish the essential amino acids. This is easily accomplished by inclusion of some "complete" proteins from animal sources such as eggs, dairy products, or seafood. In kwashiorkor, however, the lack of protein can lead to a loss of 50% of body weight and 30% of muscle protein mass. There is little loss of stable proteins such as collagen, as evidenced by normal urinary hydroxyproline excretion. Loss of 20 to 40% of body protein generally portends the death of an afflicted infant.

In starvation or marasmus, there is a deficit even of foodstuffs for energy, so that the body is left to consume its own substance. A total fast, of course, will bring on demise more rapidly than will protein restriction. The body undergoes a series of adaptations starting with consumption of carbohydrate (glycogen) stores for about a day, then a few days of catabolism mainly of protein, and then a prolonged and variable period when primarily fat stores are consumed. A second spurt of protein catabolism may occur in the immediately pre-mortem phase.

In contrast to protein deficiency, a high-protein intake can be readily accommodated – man can adapt to the carnivorous state. Most of the absorbed amino acids are burned within 2 or 3 hours after a meal, producing a feeling of warmth from "specific dynamic action", which is traceable to the metabolic effort of converting the excess amino acids into urea, fat, and carbohydrate, primarily in the liver. The chief danger in a high-protein diet is that it is usually rich in lipids, with an associated risk of atherosclerosis.

Disturbances of protein metabolism also occur with diseases of organs which regulate amino acid concentration or remove nitrogenous waste products, chiefly the gastrointestinal organs, liver, and kidney. The pathology of these organs is discussed more fully in Chapters 16, 10, and 9, respectively. Metabolic diseases also may affect protein metabolism. In diabetes, for instance, the lack of insulin prevents utilization of glucose for energy, so that the tissues are in effect fasting; uptake of amino acids into muscle is decreased and the catabolism of muscle proteins accelerates.

When malnutrition is the result of problems of the digestive tract, patients may be maintained in fairly satisfactory protein nutrition through intravenous feeding of free amino acid mixtures (Heird and Winters, 1975). Adequate calories must be supplied from glucose or lipid emulsions in order to spare the amino acids from being consumed for energy. Most of the guidelines for such therapy, sometimes inappropriately called "hyperalimentation" ("total parenteral nutrition" is a better term), have evolved on a empirical basis. The need is greatest for the essential amino acids, as there will always be some protein catabolism to provide starting material to form the non-essential amino acids.

6.2.5.1. Total protein of plasma

The concentration of total plasma protein falls in severe protein depletion, but this is not a sensitive indicator since the amounts of some individual proteins increase, and dehydration may raise the concentration thus masking a fall in the actual quantity of intravascular protein. The quantity of plasma proteins decreases faster than does that of total body protein – after consuming a minimal intake of 10 grams of protein per day for 3 to 6 weeks, the circulating albumin and γ-globulin of adult males falls by 13 to 18%, while the total body protein falls by only 10%. The extravascular plasma protein mass declines as proteins are drawn into the circulation in depleted states, whether these are nutritional or wasting in origin. In effect, the extravascular protein pool furnishes a minor reserve for deficiency states. This does not occur if the capillary permeability is increased, or if lymphatic return channels are blocked. Then an increase of extravascular protein is more likely.

Depressed concentrations of total plasma protein occur also with haemorrhage, chronic diseases, or malnutrition of malabsorption from any cause. The fall is not as great in starvation as in nitrogen depletion alone. Concentrations below 40 g/litre are often accompanied by oedema.

Elevated concentrations of total protein are found only in the presence of dehydration, in hyperimmune conditions, including kala azar and lymphogranuloma venereum, or in paraproteinaemia (section 6.3.3.4) when abnormal proteins are present in high concentrations.

6.2.5.2. Urea

Normal serum urea concentrations in healthy adults are 3 to 7 mmol/litre (80 to 200 mg N/litre), but a distinction should be made between those of men (3.5 to 8 mmol/litre) and of women (2 to 6.5 mmol/litre). The concentration is generally higher at birth (3 to 10 mmol/litre), but promptly declines to that of the adult as the neonatal liver responds. It decreases by about 25% in the first two trimesters of pregnancy. With advancing age, the "normal" urea concentration increases gradually. A slight (circa 10%) elevation can be detected after meals containing protein; larger elevations occur with increased protein catabolism, whether the result of a high-protein diet, of internal haemorrhage, shock, fever, infection, or other stress; and with impaired glomerular filtration, which can be the result of kidney disease, post-renal obstruction, or poor circulation to the kidney. Abnormally low blood urea concentrations occur in about 1% of patients. Most commonly, these are the result of forced oral or intravenous fluids, of protein malnutrition or wasting disease, or of overwhelming parenchymal liver failure without attendant renal damage. Unexplained is the occurrence of a low urea concentration with neuroses, psychoses, and anxiety states (Casey et al., 1973); an associated elevation of serum albumin and depression of creatinine suggests that the situation is not one of simple overhydration.

The serum urea concentration is a useful index of the rate of protein breakdown, since urea is derived from ammonia which arises primarily from amino acid catabolism. The urinary excretion of urea offers a more sensitive measure. Urea excretion drops from about 21 grams (10 grams of N) per day, to as low as 0.6 grams after several weeks on a protein-free diet; the other nitrogenous components of urine such as creatinine (section 6.2.5.3) change much less, so that the proportion of urea N to total N falls from 90% to less than 20%.

6.2.5.3. Creatinine

Creatinine, $NHC(NH)N(CH_3)CH_2CO$, is the internal anhydride of creatine. The normal serum concentration is 45 to 90 μmol/litre (5 to 10 mg/litre) for females and 55 to 105 μmol/litre (6 to 12 mg/litre) for males. The concentration is slightly higher at birth, in infancy and in the elderly. Urinary creatinine excretion offers a measure of muscle mass, since creatinine is primarily formed in muscle from creatine phosphate. Males excrete 1 to 2 g/day, females 0.8 to 1.8 g/day. The creatinine coefficient, $mg \cdot kg^{-1} \cdot day^{-1}$, is 20 to 26 for males, 14 to 24 for females, and 5 to 15 in infancy.

The serum creatinine concentration is a better index of renal glomerular function than is the serum urea concentration, since it is less influenced by urinary flow rate and by protein catabolism. A molar ratio of urea to creatinine above 40 (mass ratio of urea N to creatinine above 10) suggests increased protein catabolism or decreased urinary flow (glomerular filtration rate); a lower ratio occurs with diarrhoea, vomiting, low protein intake, or haemodialysis. Like the serum creatinine, urinary creatinine excretion falls much less in protein depletion than that of urinary urea.

Conventional methodology for creatinine determination is relatively more difficult and less specific than that of urea. Protein removal by precipitation or dialysis is required for accurate results, and specificity for creatinine must be enhanced by suitable pre-treatment or choice of reaction conditions. Advances in high pressure liquid chromatography are likely to overcome some of these difficulties.

6.2.5.4. Amino acids

Normal plasma concentrations of individual free amino acids are listed in Table 6.1. The total amino acid concentration is now little used. There is a diurnal cycle, variable between individuals, in which essential amino acids are decreased 10 to 50% in the afternoon hours. With advancing age, the concentrations of essential amino acids decline somewhat. A slight increase in the amino acids of the peripheral circulation occurs 2 to 4 hours after a protein-containing meal.

The changes in pathological conditions are still under study, but certain patterns are apparent (Felig, 1975). In severe protein depletion, the total amino acid concentration, like that of the total protein, shows little change. There is a fall in the essential amino acids, especially those of the branched-chain groups, and an increase in glycine and (in venous blood) alanine. These changes probably reflect the net movement of nitrogen from muscle proteins to the liver and other essential organs. In fasting, there is a rise in the concentration of branched-chain amino acids during the first week as proteins are utilized for energy; concentrations of leucine, isoleucine, and valine behave distinctively because the liver, lacking the necessary transaminases, cannot catabolize this group of amino acids. The concentrations of most other amino acids decrease, excepting glycine which climbs steadily. It has been postulated that glycine is in excess because many of the synthetic processes in which it is involved are markedly suppressed.

Decreases are seen in most individual amino acids, particularly of glutamine, in infections and following administration of insulin; alanine, however, is an exception. In liver disease, with associated circulatory shunting, the concentrations of the branched-chain amino acids are decreased, while tryptophan, methionine, tyrosine, phenylalanine, and histidine are increased, particularly if hepatic coma impends. In uraemia, alanine and glycine increase but the essential amino acids decline. Upon haemodialysis, amino acids as well as urea pass from the plasma through the extra-corporeal semipermeable membrane. A single dialysis has been estimated to remove 7 grams of amino acids; tryptophan, being largely bound to albumin, is an exception. The urinary excretion of hydroxyproline is useful as a measure of osteolysis attendant to bone growth or of disorders of collagen in general.

The only useful assay procedure for free amino acids is ion exchange chromatography, although gas chromatography offers potential for the future.

6.2.5.5. Ammonia

The blood ammonia concentration is normally 10 to 50 μmol/litre. Arterial values are about 20% less than venous, and are a better indication of liver function. At birth and in the newborn the ammonia concentration is about twice the adult value.

Hyperammonaemia is generally associated with liver disease, and is an ominous sign of declining hepatic functional capacity. Ammonia also builds up with portocaval shunting, either surgically performed or as an outcome of development of collateral circulation in cirrhosis; then ammonia produced by intestinal bacteria no longer passes directly to the liver for conversion into urea. Hyperammonaemia without obvious liver disease, particularly when an individual is on a high-protein diet, has in rare but interesting cases been traced to the congenital absence of one of the four enzymes of the urea cycle; this has been reviewed by Levin (1971) and Hsia (1974).

Ammonia may be assayed enzymatically, or chemically after isolation from blood by diffusion or ion exchange procedures (Henry et al., 1974). The enzymatic method is not yet in general use. Testing is complicated by the lability of amide groups on proteins, which contribute ammonia if the specimen is allowed to remain at room temperatures for more than a few minutes. The diffusion method gives somewhat higher values than the other procedures.

6.3. SOME SPECIFIC PLASMA PROTEINS

There are over 50 individual proteins which are truly plasma proteins, i.e., which have a presumed function in plasma in contradistinction to tissue proteins that have leaked into the circulation. This Chapter will of necessity largely restrict its coverage to the 16 individual proteins listed in Table 6.2, but observations on a few others will be made.

The individual plasma proteins are grouped below on a broad assignment of their primary functions as (a) those which assist the organism in its normal metabolism and (b) those which act to protect the organism from harmful substances or help it to respond to trauma. The normal metabolic role includes transport of nutrients, transport of hormones, and maintaining the flow of the circulation within the vessels. Harmful substances which are inactivated either by sequestration or by lysis include normal catabolic products like haemoglobin and bilirubin, errant intracellular components such as proteases, and invaders such as foreign proteins, viruses, and micro-organisms. With trauma comes the need for haemostasis and subsequent tissue repair. The protective proteins are subdivided into those which respond promptly to acute inflammation or trauma – the acute phase reactants – and those which characteristically increase in chronic conditions. Some proteins have multiple functions; albumin both transports fatty acids and sequesters bilirubin. For others – caeruloplasmin and orosomucoid – any function is but a conjecture at present, so their assignment to groups is a matter of convenience. For further information see Laurell (1972), Schultze and Heremans (1966), and Putnam (1975, 1976).

6.3.1. Proteins of normal metabolism and nutrition

Most nutrients and hormones reach tissue cells in free solution in the blood, but some require assistance from carrier molecules owing to insolubility or instability, e.g. lipids, steroid hormones, thyroxine, vitamin A, pyridoxal, iron, copper, and the amino acids tryptophan and cystine. In addition, plasma proteins contribute to the amino acid supply of tissues (section 6.2.3).

All plasma proteins contribute to the colloid osmotic pressure of plasma (section 6.2.1), but albumin is responsible for 75 to 80% of the total effect. This is due to the relatively low molecular mass and the Donnan effect of the high negative charge of albumin as well as to its abundance. In rare cases of analbuminaemia or extreme hypoalbuminaemia, the osmotic and other functions of albumin can apparently be assumed by the augmented mixture of globulins.

6.3.1.1. Serum albumin

Specific functions of albumin include the binding of bilirubin and haem (beyond that bound by haemopexin, section 6.3.2.2), the transport of these compounds to the liver for disposition, the transport of steroid hormones and thyroxine when these overflow their normal carrier proteins, and the transport of various nutrients. Among these nutrients are fatty acids (less than 0.1% of the "free" fatty acids are actually free in plasma), ionic copper, and tryptophan. There is evidence that cystine and pyridoxal are also transported on albumin, in this case linked via covalent bonds rather than through associative forces. In severe neonatal jaundice the binding capacity of albumin may be inadequate, so that large amounts of free bilirubin circulate, necessitating exchange transfusion, administration of extra albumin, and/or photo-oxidation of the bilirubin. Qualitative changes in binding properties have been reported in renal failure, perhaps due to competing metabolites (DeTorrente et al., 1974), and the effects of such changes plus a decreased concentration may be highly significant in determining effective dosages of those drugs which are largely bound to albumin. The binding of bilirubin or anionic drugs (aspirin, penicillin) can be observed as a broadening – or even splitting – of the albumin band on electrophoresis. Reviews on albumin are found in Watson (1965), Peters (1970, 1975, 1977), and Rothschild et al. (1973).

The normal concentration of albumin is 42 ± 3.5 g/litre, with a range of 35 to 50. Upon electrophoretic separation, albumin comprises 60 ± 4% of the total serum protein. Albumin concentrations in men are about 2 g/litre higher than in women. Between the ages of 20 and 70 years the average concentration gradually falls about 3 g/litre, faster in men than women, so that at age 70 the sex differential has disappeared. The daily variation in an individual is about equal to the analytical variation of 2.5% C.V. (Winkel et al., 1976). In the foetus, albumin concentrations rise from about 18 to 36 g/litre between 26 and 40 weeks of gestation. The concentration at birth is usually slightly higher in the baby than in the mother. Adult values are reached by about 3 months of age. In the later months of pregnancy, or while a women is taking oral contraceptives, albumin concentrations fall 8 to 10 g/litre.

Albumin is formed in the liver at the rate of about 14 g/day. Its formation is highly dependent upon the supply of amino acids brought by the portal vein, more so than is the production of the other plasma proteins excepting transferrin and prealbumin. During a 10-day period of protein depletion in the rat, albumin production falls by 60%, but accelerates within a half hour after re-feeding amino acids. The concentration of albumin is not a sensitive indicator, however, since the rate of albumin catabolism also falls when amino acids are lacking, and albumin is drawn from the extravascular space, so that the amount in the plasma is protected and does not indicate the full extent of the nutritional deficit. No change in plasma albumin concentration is detected with meals, and a 1-day fast lowers the concentration by only about 1 g/litre.

In times of illness, albumin tends to move toward the extravascular compartment, in contrast to its movement from this compartment with malnutrition alone. Increased permeability of the capillary wall to molecules of the size of albumin, and impaired venous return, are probable causes; the resulting lowered concentration of albumin is the most common change in the plasma protein pattern in pathological states. Concentrations less than 31 g/litre usually signify serious organic disease. The most common conditions associated with hypoalbuminaemia are malignant disease, particularly those affecting the colon, bronchi, or pancreas, and liver disease including alcoholism. Diseases of the lungs, kidney, cardiovascular system, and gastrointestinal system, also rheumatoid arthritis, diabetes, protein-calorie malnutrition, and acute infections, are next in frequency. The lowest values, 10 to 20 g/litre, occur in the nephrotic syndrome and protein-losing enteropathy. In these conditions, the major loss occurs in the urine or intestine; in the latter case, the amino acids are actually not lost but are caught in a rapid enterohepatic cycle as the albumin is digested in the gut and re-synthesized in the liver (section 6.2.2). The liver can respond with increased synthesis of albumin to about double the normal rate, but there is still a continuous drain on the albumin supply. Albumin concentrations persistently below 22 g/litre have been reported by Muehrcke (1956) to be associated with thin, paired white lines on the fingernails. Concentrations below 20 g/litre generally are accompanied by oedema.

Hyperalbuminaemia is rarely encountered. It is usually the result of dehydration, although an overshoot of the regulatory mechanism after a hypoalbuminaemic state has been proposed.

Tests for albumin utilize either (a) removal of globulins and quantitation of the remaining protein, usually by the biuret reaction; (b) indirect assay by subtraction of the content of globulins from the total protein; (c) electrophoretic separation followed by quantitation; (d) colour changes of indicator dyes when bound to albumin; (e) immunochemistry (Henry et al., 1974). Dye-binding methods are in widespread use, since they involve a minimum of manipulation and are readily adaptable to mechanization. Bromcresol green is superior in specificity to dyes formerly used, such as methyl orange and 2-(4′-hydroxyazobenzene)-benzoic acid ("HABA"), but even bromcresol green has been shown to bind to some α_2- and β-globulins (probably lipoproteins) as well as to albumin, and to give falsely high values for albumin compared with those obtained by electrophoresis (Webster, 1974). This is particularly troublesome when the albumin is in low and the globulins in high concentration, a frequent situation in renal disease and enteropathies. There is evidence that albumin reacts promptly with bromcresol green, whereas the interfering globulins react much more slowly, so that making readings as early as 10 seconds after mixing dye and serum may provide reliable results (Corcoran and Durnan, 1977). Only with such a reservation can the widely used bromcresol green procedure of Doumas and Biggs (1972) be recommended.

6.3.1.2. Transferrin

Transferrin, also formerly called siderophilin or simply iron-binding protein, is a single-chain protein of about the size of albumin which can bind two atoms of iron (Fe^{3+}) per molecule. The normal serum concentration of transferrin is 2.3 g/litre; with a molecular mass of 76,000 this corresponds to a capacity to bind 3.4 mg of iron/litre, or 1.46 mg of Fe^{3+} per gram transferrin. Actual measurements on serum yield values about 1.3 mg Fe^{3+}/g. Normally the transferrin is about 33% saturated with iron. There are no significant differences between the concentrations in men and in women, nor in women during phases of the menstrual cycle. The diurnal change which is observed in the serum iron concentration is not reflected in transferrin (Winkel et al., 1976); only the relative saturation of transferrin with iron changes. At birth, the transferrin concentration is about 55% of the adult value, but in infancy and childhood the values are about 20% higher than in the adult. The values decline slightly after about 60 years of age. During pregnancy or use of oral contraceptives, transferrin concentrations rise about 50%.

The sole apparent function of transferrin is the transport of iron between the intestine and the sites of synthesis and degradation of haemoglobin and other iron-containing proteins. Unsaturated transferrin has a bacteriostatic action which is attributed to sequestration of iron required by micro-organisms. Transferrin is formed largely in the liver, but there is also evidence for transferrin synthesis in bone marrow, spleen, and lymph nodes, perhaps by lymphocytes. The half-life of transferrin is shorter than that of albumin, but it is not degraded merely upon delivery of its iron. Its extravascular distribution and its susceptibility to loss through the kidney are similar to those of albumin. Decreases of transferrin concentrations parallel those of albumin in many pathological conditions – protein or caloric malnutrition, malignancy or other wasting disease, the nephrotic syndrome, hepatic cirrhosis, and acute illness such as trauma and myocardial infarction. Transferrin decreases even more than does albumin with acute or chronic infections, and appears to be more sensitive to amino acid supply. Concentrations of transferrin correlate most closely with the probability of survival of children with kwashiorkor (McFarlane et al., 1970) and of persons with leukaemia and haemolytic anaemias, perhaps due to its bacteriostatic effect. Transferrin concentrations change inversely with the irong stores of the body, rising in iron deficiency and falling in haemolytic and aplastic anaemias, haemochromatosis, or transfusion-induced haemosiderosis. Transferrin as it relates to iron metabolism is discussed in Chapter 16, section 16.2.

Transferrin is determined either immunochemically or by the amount of iron retained by serum after saturation with inorganic iron and removal of the excess iron by ion exchange adsorption. The two approaches have agreed well in several studies; follow-up of cases in which the iron saturation procedure gave higher values led to the discovery that the iron-storage protein, ferritin (Chapter 16, section 16.2.3) also circulates in plasma, normally in traces but in increased amounts when iron stores are high.

6.3.1.3. Lipoproteins

Lipoproteins may be measured immunochemically or by their lipid content, usually by use of lipid stains after electrophoretic separation. Their role in lipid transport is more properly considered in Chapter 5, section 5.2.4. The peptide portions of the α-(high density) and β-(low density) lipoproteins, which correspond to 55% and 21% of the mass respectively, are antigenically distinct and can be detected by immunodiffusion or immunonephelometric techniques. Difficulties are encountered, however, with samples showing chylomicronaemia.

Lipoproteins are formed both in the liver and in the intestinal mucosa. Their measurement has chiefly been of interest in the evaluation of lipid disorders (Chapter 5). When the protein components are observed in other pathological conditions, the α-lipoprotein has been found to decrease with liver disease, malnutrition, and acute conditions, similar to the behavior of albumin and transferrin, whereas the β-lipoprotein tends to rise in acute conditions. Both lipoproteins are found in high concentration in the nephrotic syndrome, since they are among the largest proteins in the plasma and remain behind when other proteins are lost through enlarged glomerular pores. For inter-relations of the lipoproteins see Frederickson (1973).

6.3.1.4. Caeruloplasmin

The copper-protein caeruloplasmin has no clearly defined function but boasts several unique features. It contains 0.34% copper (Cu^{2+}), totalling over 90% of the total serum copper, it is blue in colour (hence its name), and it is an oxidative enzyme (Poulik and Weiss, 1975; Frieden and Hsieh, 1976). The copper content corresponds to eight atoms of Cu^{2+} per caeruloplasmin molecule.

In the normal adult male, the plasma contains 0.32 (0.16 to 0.6) g/litre of caeruloplasmin. Values in newborns are only about one-third as high; they rise to the adult value by the end of the first year, and are generally higher than the adult value until about puberty. The concentration in females is about 20% higher than in males. Caeruloplasmin is one of the plasma proteins most sensitive to oestrogens; it rises 3-fold during pregnancy or intake of contraceptive pills.

Inorganic copper is incorporated into newly-formed caeruloplasmin in the liver. The survival of the protein in the plasma parallels that of its copper, with a half-life of about 4.5 days. Whether caeruloplasmin has a function in the blood is uncertain; it has ascorbate oxidase (EC 1.10.3.3), amine oxidase (histaminase, EC 1.4.3.6), and ferroxidase

(EC 1.16.3.1) activities. It has been suggested that it inactivates neurogenic amines, that it assists in the conversion of Fe^{2+} into Fe^{3+} during its uptake by transferrin, and that it transports copper to be used in formation of copper-containing enzymes of peripheral tissues. It does not seem likely that caeruloplasmin is a re-usable carrier of copper in the sense that transferrin is a carrier of iron for haemoglobin synthesis – the copper is more tightly bound and its removal probably entails the destruction of the caeruloplasmin.

Caeruloplasmin concentration is characteristically elevated in acute inflammation (see section 6.3.2) and elevations have been reported in chronic inflammation and acute myelogenous or lymphatic leukaemia. It is low in protein-losing situations such as the nephrotic syndrome and enteropathies, in the presence of hepatitis or severe liver damage, and in multiple sclerosis. A specific deficit of caeruloplasmin occurs in Wilson's disease, a familial condition characterized by damage to the liver and central nervous system. The defect appears not to be in the production of the peptide portion of caeruloplasmin, since apocaeruloplasmin can still be detected in liver cells, but may involve copper transport or copper incorporation within the liver. Treatment is aimed not at increasing the caeruloplasmin but in removing excess copper through the urine by administering copper-chelating compounds such as penicillamine. For further consideration of the clinical significance of copper measurements see Chapter 19, section 19.3.

Serum may be assayed for caeruloplasmin by measuring the tightly bound copper, i.e., that portion not removed from proteins by acidity alone. More specific and sensitive is the enzymatic oxidation of aromatic diamines such as *p*-phenylenediamine: immunochemical detection is equally specific and sensitive. The choice between the enzymatic and immunochemical procedures is one of convenience. If the scope of the laboratory routine already includes immunochemical assays, the addition of another specific protein assay is a simple matter.

6.3.1.5. Other proteins

The protein *prealbumin* was named for its location preceding albumin upon cellulose acetate electrophoresis. It is determined by the staining of this electrophoretic band or, more specifically, by immunoassays. It is present in serum at only 0.25 (0.1 to 0.4) g/litre in normal persons over about 10 years of age. The concentration is markedly decreased in the newborn and somewhat decreased in pregnancy, but rises during intake of oral contraceptives.

The complete amino acid sequence of prealbumin (molecular mass 55,000) is now known. It is believed to bind the smaller-sized (21,000 dalton) retinol-binding protein, preventing its loss and that of retinol through the kidneys. It also binds thyroxine (Chapter 13, section 13.1.2) in an overflow manner similar to albumin, but with greater affinity (Nilsson et al., 1975).

Measurement of prealbumin has little clinical use at present. Its concentration falls in many conditions which affect the serum albumin also – malnutrition, malignancy, burns, and liver diseases of many kinds. It has been suggested to be a more sensitive indicator of liver disease, protein malnutrition, and acute inflammation (section 6.3.2) than is albumin or transferrin (Ingenbleek et al., 1975).

There are numerous other proteins circulating in plasma which play a role in normal metabolism. These are present in small quantities and function in specific aspects of metabolic control, so that they are more appropriately treated in other chapters, rather than as proteins. Some of these proteins are hormones – insulin (Chapter 4, section 4.4.1) and small gastrointestinal hormones (Chapter 11, section 11.5) are examples. Others are transport vehicles. These include thyroxine-binding globulin (Chapter 13, section 13.1.2), an α_2-globulin of molecular mass 36,500, present at 0.01 to 0.02 g/litre; transcortin or cortisol-binding globulin, of α_1 mobility, molecular mass 55,700, and present at 0.07 g/litre (Chapter 14, section 14.4); and transcobalamins I and II, α_1- and β-globulins of molecular mass 121,000 and 35 to 38,000, respectively, carriers of vitamin B_{12}, of which transcobalamin II is the more important.

6.3.2. Protective proteins: the acute phase

Under sudden stress such as major surgery, trauma, infarction, or acute infection, characteristic changes occur in the plasma proteins. In the electrophoretic pattern, albumin decreases slightly and α_1- and α_2-globulins increase, beginning within 1 to 2 days and continuing for 2 to 3 weeks. Analysis of individual proteins permits identification of the components which are responsible for the increases. These have been termed "acute phase reactants" (Kelley, 1952), to distinguish them from the proteins of the immune system which accumulate more slowly in the blood.

Appearance of these acute phase reactants is apparently an integral part of the stress reaction, by which the body responds to meet potential demands for available glucose, oxygen and amino acids, and to stimulate the leucocytic defence system (Cuthbertson and Tilstone, 1969). Stress brings a period of obligatory protein catabolism, with the inescapable wastage of some amino acids, an increase in urea concentrations, and a brief period of negative nitrogen balance. Efforts to stem this tide by pre-loading the individual with protein have been unsuccessful.

The effects of these changes, and a concomitant increase in leakage of plasma proteins to the extravascular spaces, are registered to some extent in the concentrations of all of the plasma proteins, although the total protein concentration varies only slightly, if at all. Proteins whose synthesis is not stimulated tend to decrease with the increase in catabolic rate and the loss to interstitial spaces. One group of proteins rises promptly, within a matter of hours – C-reactive protein, haptoglobin and fibrinogen (Figure 6.5). Another rises at intermediate rates – orosomucoid and antitrypsin – while complement (C′3) and caeruloplasmin rise at slower rates. The acute phase proteins have in common that they are glycoproteins; they are synthesized in the liver and they are induced by injury. Their functions are diverse, and complications of the disease process modify the plasma concentrations of some more than of others, so that there is justification for measuring several of these indicators in the evaluation of an acute disease.

6.3.2.1. Fibrinogen

Fibrinogen, the final component of the clotting cascade which protects the circulation against loss of blood, is the only member of this chain which occurs in plasma in sufficient quantity to make a significant contribution to the total proteins. Clotting is discussed in Chapter 16, and fibrinogen has been reviewed by Doolittle (1973). In the electrophoretic pattern of plasma, fibrinogen appears as a sharp peak between the β- and

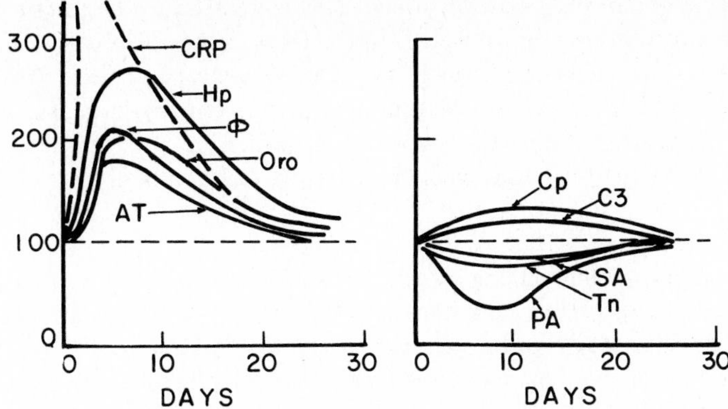

Figure 6.5. Changes in plasma protein concentrations during a typical acute phase reaction, compiled from data for uncomplicated surgery or myocardial infarction from Aronsen et al. (1972), Johansson et al. (1972), and Werner and Cohnen (1969). The abbreviations (from Table 6.2) are: CRP, C-reactive protein; Hp, haptoglobin; ϕ, fibrinogen; Oro, orosomucoid; AT, α_1-antitrypsin; Cp, ceruloplasmin; C3, C′3 of complement; SA, albumin; Tn, transferrin; PA, prealbumin. The ordinate indicates % of normal concentration.

γ-globulins (Figure 6.3). Because its presence obscures the interpretation of the pattern, electrophoresis is usually conducted with serum. Fibrinogen can readily be assayed by one of the immunochemical procedures; if none of these is in use, fibrinogen may be determined chemically by causing a clot to form with thrombin, washing it, and measuring the total protein of the fibrin clot by the biuret method. The fibrinopeptides lost upon the conversion to fibrin amount to only about 3% of the mass of the fibrinogen.

The normal concentration of fibrinogen is 2.9 g/litre: even at birth it is near this figure. Fibrinogen rises about 80% in pregnancy. As shown in Figure 6.5, it is one of the first plasma proteins to respond in the acute phase reaction, and tends to remain above the normal concentration throughout the course of the illness, so that fibrinogen measurements are useful in following the progress of the disease.

The erythrocyte sedimentation rate (ESR) correlates directly with the concentration of fibrinogen and inversely with that of albumin. Hence this test provides a simple means of estimating the occurrence and persistence of inflammation or a response to stress. Sedimentation is an empirical test, however, and the ESR also rises in conditions such as congestive heart failure, malignancy, sickle cell anaemia, and paraproteinaemia (section 6.3.3.4). Not only fibrinogen but also caeruloplasmin, haptoglobin, and immunoglobulin G accelerate the ESR, particularly in liver disease. The normal upper limits of ESR as per formed by the Westgren procedure are 15 mm/h for men and 25 mm/h for women. Above age 50 years, the ESR increases by about 5 mm/h.

In addition to the acute phase reaction, fibrinogen increases in the nephrotic syndrome, where there is a selective loss of smaller-size proteins through the kidney. Low concentrations of fibrinogen are uncommon: they occur as a consequence of severe hepatic disease, when fibrinogen biosynthesis is compromised or, more specifically, in the presence of pronounced fibrinolysis or disseminated intravascular coagulation, when fibrinogen is consumed much faster than it is produced. Indeed, the failure to observe an increase in plasma fibrinogen during illness should be suggestive that one of these processes is at work. Premature separation of the placenta (abruptio placentae) during pregnancy is associated with a reduced plasma fibrinogen concentration in more than one-third of cases. The loss of fibrinogen may lead rapidly to a massive loss of blood.

6.3.2.2. Haptoglobin and haemopexin

Haptoglobin, the specific haemoglobin-binding protein, normally occurs at a concentration of 1.7 g/litre (1.2 to 2.6) in plasma, and constitutes about one-fourth of the α_2-globulin peak. This amount of haptoglobin in the blood system could bind about 3 g of haemoglobin, a little less than half of the amount which is degraded daily. The haptoglobin is 30% lower in women than men, being increased by administration of androgens. Only about 15% of newborn infants have detectable haptoglobin, but by 2 weeks it makes an appearance, and the adult concentration is attained by 4 months. Unlike caeruloplasmin and fibrinogen, there is no elevation during pregnancy; the plasma concentration tends to decrease during oral contraceptive therapy.

Haptoglobin contains two α and two β chains. Polymorphism occurs in the α chains, producing haptoglobin types 1–1, 2–1, and 2–2, with various subtypes discernible upon closer study. The homozygous form, 1–1, occurs in 38% of Caucasians and 55% of Negroes, and gives a single sharp band on starch gel electrophoresis, the usual technique for identification of the haptoglobin allotypes. On cellulose acetate or agarose electrophoresis (Figure 6.3), Hp 1–1 appears as a sharp band in the α_2-globulin zone. The 2–1 and 2–2 allotypes show multiple bands in starch gel, and are distributed broadly through the α_2-globulin zone on the simpler supporting media. They tend to associate in a dimer form. Type 2–2 occurs in 53% of Japanese, and geographically appears to centre in India. All of the polymorphic forms bind haemoglobin in a 1 : 1 ratio (2 : 1 for the dimers). The binding is primarily to the α chain of haemoglobin; haemoglobins such as Haemoglobin$_{\mathrm{BART}}$, which contain only β chains, are transported poorly by haptoglobin.

Haptoglobin serves to bind haemoglobin which reaches the plasma and transports it to reticuloendothelial sites of destruction. When haemoglobin is bound to haptoglobin, the complex is rapidly cleared from the blood, with a half-life of only 8 minutes. The haptoglobin is destroyed along with its cargo. About 10% of the normal turnover of haemoglobin occurs in this manner. This accounts for about half of the haptoglobin turnover; the other half proceeds through the usual catabolic processes, with a half-life of 4 days.

Conditions which accelerate red cell breakdown act to lower haptoglobin concentrations. These are sudden haemolytic events, such as paroxysmal nocturnal haemoglobinuria, resolving haematoma, congenital or acquired haemolytic anaemias, or pernicious anaemia. After lysis of only 25 ml of blood, the haptoglobin concentration falls within 6 to 10 hours and remains low for 2 or 3 days. Haptoglobin concentrations are normal in aplastic anaemia, iron-deficiency anaemia, and leukaemias. Decreased values are also found in infectious mononucleosis and severe liver injury.

In acute phase reactions which are uncomplicated by haemolysis, haptoglobin concentrations rise promptly (Figure 6.5), and then decline with an estimated half-life of 5 to 6 days. Haptoglobin is a good indicator of many kinds of inflammation, for instance glomerulonephritis; peak values are usually nearly 3 times normal, but can reach 10 times normal. If there is concurrent haemolysis, the expected rise is not seen, so that the detection of unsuspected haemolysis is one of the most useful features of haptoglobin assay.

Haptoglobin is best assayed by saturating serum with haemoglobin and determining the bound haemoglobin by means of a peroxidation reaction; the free haemoglobin is first separated, usually by electrophoresis. Immunochemical assays are complicated by the polymorphism of haptoglobin. For further information on haptoglobin, the reader is referred to the monograph by Putnam (1975).

A companion protein, the β_1-globulin haemopexin (Table 6.2), binds free haem which is encountered in plasma. Haemopexin forms a 1 : 1 complex with haem, from which the haem is released to the liver for degradation, with a half-life of 7 to 8 hours. At the normal concentration of 0.8 g/litre, the total haemopexin suffices to bind 25 mg of haem, the equivalent of 0.7 grams of haemoglobin or about 10% of the daily turnover.

Unlike haptoglobin, haemopexin is not an acute phase reactant; even with major fractures or severe infections there is no rise in its concentration in plasma. Haemopexin concentrations decline in haemolytic conditions, and haemopexin has been proposed as a better index of the presence of haemolysis during inflammation or injury than is haptoglobin. Thus, a normal haptoglobin concentration following trauma might be the result of increased haptoglobin synthesis due to an acute phase reaction and of increased haptoglobin loss as the haemoglobin complex; the haemopexin concentration would decline because of the haemolysis.

Haemopexin also declines in malnutrition and with protein loss. It increases in diabetes and with some malignancies, particularly melanomas. For further details the reader is referred to the review by Müller-Eberhard and Liem (1974).

6.3.2.3. α_1-Antitrypsin and α_2-macroglobulin

Plasma contains inhibitors which are active against the "serine" proteases such as trypsin, chymotrypsin, plasmin, thrombin, and elastase, as well as against cathepsins and collagenase. They function to protect tissue membrane surfaces from destruction by enzymes of bacterial, leucocytic, or intestinal origin. Of these, α_1-antitrypsin and the α_2-macroglobulin have been most widely measured.

α_1-Antitrypsin, or simply antitrypsin, occurs normally at a concentration of 2.9 g/litre (range 1.8 to 4). It is only about 10% lower at birth, and is about 15% higher in women than in men. The action of oestrogens elevates the concentration about 2-fold in pregnancy and during intake of oral contraceptive pills.

Antitrypsin is a polymorphic protein of an autosomal recessive nature. As many as 23 alleles of Pi (protein inhibitor) types have now been detected by starch gel electrophoresis. The alleles are designated by letters such as F, I, M, S, V, X, Z. The homozygous MM phenotype is the most common. About 5% of individuals show the MZ or MS heterozygous forms; in them the concentration of antitrypsin in plasma is only about 60% of normal. Rarer still, are those homozygous for SS or ZZ genes, who have 10% or less of the normal antitrypsin concentration (Sveger, 1976). These persons also have glycoprotein inclusion bodies in their hepatic parenchymal cells which have been shown to contain a form of antitrypsin which is deficient in the acidic carbohydrate component, sialic acid (Eriksson and Larsson, 1975). The cause of the low plasma concentrations may thus be a block in a sialation step necessary for secretion. Even the phenotypes may be the result of defective sialation, since sialic acid affects the net charge on the protein and hence its electrophoretic migration.

As an acute phase reactant, serum antitrypsin rises to about twice its normal value during most inflammatory states. Its rise is not as abrupt as are those of fibrinogen and haptoglobin (Figure 6.5). It is particularly sensitive to liver disease. Congenital deficiency, at least the homozygous state, causes an emphysema, affecting women more than men and usually evident by 40 years of age, which is attributed to damage of the alveolar membranes by uninhibited proteases. It is more pronounced in the lower lobes of the lungs. In the infant, the homozygous deficiency state (ZZ) may produce hepatitis, presumably owing to damage to the liver by congestion of the cytoplasm with unsecreted antitrypsin. Hepatic cirrhosis in the juvenile and the adult may ensue, and a case has been reported of associated intestinal mucosal atrophy. Antitrypsin concentrations are low in neonates with respiratory distress syndrome. The findings of studies are conflicting as to whether the milder heterozygous deficiency (MZ) is associated with chronic obstructive lung disease: as many as 25% of patients with idiopathic emphysema have depressed antitrypsin concentrations, however, so that the measurement of antitrypsin is of considerable interest for aetiological reasons. Phenotyping by starch gel electrophoresis is required for a reliable diagnosis. Unfortunately, no specific therapy is available.

In addition to the immunochemical procedures, antitrypsin may be determined chemically by measuring the amount of added trypsin which it binds and inactivates. Various substrates may be used to measure the remaining trypsin activity; the synthetic peptide, benzoylarginine-*p*-nitroanilide, is one of the most convenient (Erlanger et al., 1961). One mol of antitrypsin inactivates 2 mol of trypsin so that 1 gram of antitrypsin is equivalent to 0.91 gram of trypsin; antitrypsin is sometimes reported in its trypsin equivalents, e.g. mg trypsin inhibited per ml serum. Hopefully, these units will give way to direct reporting of the quantity of the inhibitor. It is active against most of the proteases found in plasma. Antitrypsin contributes about 90% of the protein of the α_1-globulin electrophoretic peak, so a reduction in its concentration can often be detected on screening. For a general review see Talamo (1975).

The α_2-macroglobulin (Tunstall et al., 1975) makes up about one-third of the α_2-globulin band. It binds trypsin as well as many other proteases, but inactivates only the proteolytic activity of trypsin and does not inhibit the esterase activity. Hence it can be assayed by measuring the esterase activity which remains when trypsin and then an excess of soybean trypsin inhibitor are added. α_2-Macroglobulin is the only plasma inhibitor active against pepsin and cathepsin D. The normal concentration of α_2-macroglobulin is 2.4 (1.5 to 3.5) g/litre in men and about 30% higher in women. In the newborn, the concentration is 1.5 times that of the adult male, decreasing only in the teens, and increasing again above 70 years of age. Increased concentrations occur in pregnancy and in women on oral contraceptive drugs.

Although it is not a typical acute phase protein, α_2-macroglobulin rises following severe burns, but returns to normal within 7 days. It is elevated in systemic lupus erythematosus with associated renal disease, in enteropathy, diabetes, and cirrhosis, but no consistent change has been noted in rheumatoid arthritis, malignancy, or leucocytic dyscrasias. The greatest increases occur with the nephrotic syndrome.

Four other protease inhibitors are generally recognized as being present in serum. α_1-Antichymotrypsin, molecular mass 69,000, normal concentration range 0.3 to 0.6 g/litre, is active only against chymotrypsin. Antithrombin III, molecular mass 65,000, concentration range 0.2 to 0.7 g/litre, is the only inhibitor which has been clearly shown to inactivate thrombin, and it is also effective against several other clotting factors as well as trypsin. Inter-α-trypsin inhibitor, molecular mass 90,000 and concentration range 0.17 to 0.7 g/litre, is active both against trypsin and the chymotrypsin-like cathepsin G. C′1 inactivator, molecular mass 104,000, concentration range 0.15 to 0.35 g/litre, is an α_2-globulin which inactivates plasmin (fibrinolysin), Hageman factor, and C1s, the first element of the complement cascade (section 6.3.2.5).

6.3.2.4. Orosomucoid

Earlier called seromucoid or α_1-acid glycoprotein, orosomucoid is one of the most reliable indicators of acute inflammation. Seromucoid was originally defined as the glycoprotein fraction which is soluble in 1.8 mol/litre perchloric acid and is precipitated by 5% (w/v) phosphotungstic acid. With a carbohydrate content of 41%, orosomucoid is largely responsible for the changes in the seromucoid fraction in various pathological conditions. On electrophoresis it stains weakly, and so it is usually determined immunochemically.

Normal concentrations in men and women are about 0.9 g/litre (0.6 to 1.4), but at birth, only about one-third of this value. In pregnancy, or with intake of contraceptive drugs the concentration falls about 15%. Both day-to-day and inter-individual variations are high – 11% and 43% C.V., respectively (Statland et al., 1976).

Orosomucoid consistently rises in acute or chronic inflammatory disease, as well as in cirrhosis and many malignant conditions. The response is slower than that of haptoglobin, reaching a peak of nearly twice the initial concentration at about 5 days, but persisting throughout the illness; in Crohn's ileitis, the value reaches 8 times normal. Abnormally low concentrations occur in generalized hypoproteinaemic conditions such as hepatic disease, cachexia and malnutrition, and the nephrotic syndrome. Orosomucoid binds progesterone and perhaps functions as a transport agent for this hormone. It has also been proposed that it serves to carry needed carbohydrate constituents to the sites of tissue repair following injury. Its turnover is rapid, with a half-life of 2 days. The reader is referred to Schmid (1975) for further details.

6.3.2.5. Complement and C-reactive protein

The complement system (Müller-Eberhard, 1971; Ruddy et al., 1972) is a complex group of 11 proteins in plasma which act to complete, or complement, the action of antibodies in defending against cellular infectious agents. Antibodies are considered in the following section. The proteins of the complement system, named C1q, C1r, C1s, and C2–C9, are shown in Figure 6.6 in relation to their electrophoretic mobilities, molecular masses, and concentrations. In its action, $C1\overline{qrs}$ combines as the *recognition unit,* binding to an antibody which has formed a complex with an antigen (Sim et al., 1977). This attracts the *activation unit,* consisting of C4, C2, and C3 in sequence, which are activated and then bind at a nearby site. Proteins C5–C9 comprise the *attack unit*; a complex $C\overline{567}$ is activated by $C\overline{423}$ and attaches at another nearby site, attracting C8 which, accelerated by C9, punctures a hole in the membrane causing lysis of the microorganism. An *alternate*

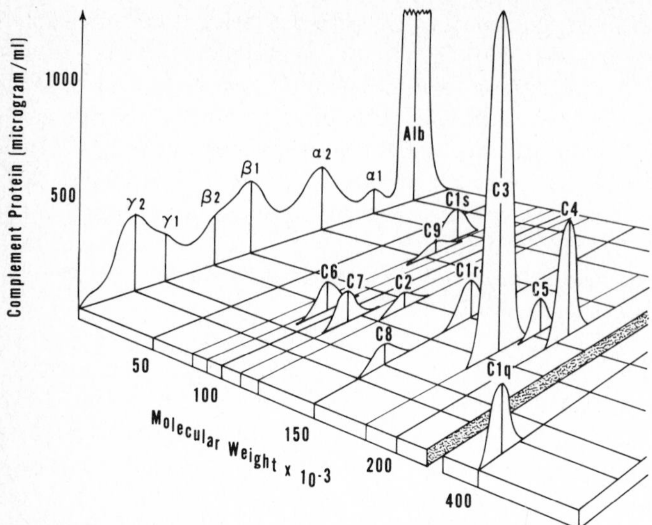

Figure 6.6. Schematic representation of the molecular masses, electrophoretic mobilities, and serum concentrations of the human complement proteins. The scale is 20 times that of the peaks in the electrophoretic pattern of serum shown in the background. (Reproduced, by permission, from Müller-Eberhard, 1971)

pathway of activation of $\overline{C56789}$ involves a serum glycoprotein, properdin, and is triggered by membrane surface constituents such as lipopolysaccharides rather than by specific immunoglobulin complexes. Deleterious side reactions can occur. The recognition and activation units may bind to antigen–antibody complexes deposited in the renal glomerulus, in joints, membranes, or in vessel walls; there they attract leucocytes which cause tissue damage seen in association with glomerulonephritis, rheumatoid arthritis, polyarteritis, or systemic lupus erythematosis. Small anaphylotoxic peptides also appear during activation, particularly from C2, C3, and C5, which evoke release of histamine from mast cells, contraction of smooth muscles, increased capillary permeability, and platelet aggregation. Obviously the complement system can have far-reaching effects in addition to defending against invading organisms.

Only the two proteins of the complement system which are present in highest concentration, C3 and C4, are commonly assayed; C3 is considered further as it has received more attention. In some studies the term "complement" is used to mean only this one constituent. Formerly called β_{1C} globulin, or C′3, the term C3 is now accepted. Assay is by immunochemical detection using antibodies prepared against pure C3; more sensitive procedures and tests for other complement proteins utilize the haemolysis of red cells as an end result.

Fresh serum contains about 1.1 g/litre of C3 and about a third as much C4. If the serum is allowed to stand, the C3 is converted into a smaller protein form, C3c; the smaller size allows C3c to diffuse faster through agar and gives higher values in radial immunodiffusion methods. In women, the C3 concentration is about 80% of that in men;

in the infant at birth, serum concentrations are 50% to 75% of those in the adult.

C3 is produced by the liver, as are most of the other proteins of complement, but C1 is produced by the columnar epithelium of the gut, and C2 and C4 are in part made by macrophages. The half-life of circulating C3 is about 2.5 days.

C3 increases with inflammation as do acute phase proteins; its rise is slow and not as marked, seldom exceeding 120% of the initial value (Figure 6.5). Serum concentrations are high in biliary obstruction, polyarteritis, amyloidosis, rheumatic fever, and gout. Depressed values occur in malnutrition which is complicated by infection, in severe hepatic cirrhosis, and in conditions where the C3 is consumed, such as disseminated intravascular clotting, coagulation, serum sickness, Sjögren's syndrome, acute glomerulonephritis, paroxysmal nocturnal haemoglobinuria, and systemic lupus erythematosis. C3 concentration rises before that of transferrin, prealbumin, or albumin upon refeeding children suffering from protein-calorie malnutrition. Characteristically, the C3 concentration is lowered in diseases involving autoimmunity, presumably because of the loss of C3 through binding as part of the activation unit to antibody which is deposited on membranes.

A prompt acute phase reactant is the C-reactive protein (CRP) (Mortensen et al., 1975). It is barely detectable in normal serum (about 0.5 mg/litre), but rises very rapidly following injury (Figure 6.5). Named for the classical method of its assay – the appearance of a precipitate when the C-polysaccharide of pneumococcus is added – it is now more commonly determined by reaction with antisera. The immune reaction can be detected by latex particle agglutination, by microprecipitation in a tube or in agar, or by radioimmunoassay. CRP is synthesized in the liver during the day following trauma. Two electrophoretic forms appear on immunoelectrophoresis: CRP alone in the γ-band, and a CRP complex with an acidic mucopolysaccharide, termed m-CRP, in the β region.

The function, if any, of CRP is not clear. It can bind haem, and bears some chemical and antigenic relation to liver catalase. It binds to T lymphocytes and activates complement. A role in the formation of haem proteins or as an opsonin in augmenting immunity has been proposed. CRP is certainly a sensitive, if non-specific, indicator of the early phase of an inflammatory process. It remains increased in the presence of solid tumours, but not in conditions which impair the immune response such as leukaemia or Hodgkin's disease.

6.3.2.6. Other proteins

Many other proteins deserve mention, but it is impractical to list more than a few of the individual proteins which have been detected in plasma. The functions of some of these have been obvious, of others suspected, and of others unknown.

The blood clotting system is considered in Chapter 16. Aside from fibrinogen (factor I) (section 6.3.2.1) three of the most-studied are pro-enzymes. Prothrombin (factor II), is a protein of molecular mass 60,000, concentration 0.05 to 0.1 g/litre, which migrates as an α_1-globulin. Fibrin stabilizing factor (FSF, factor XIII), a transamidase which strengthens newly polymerized fibrin by formation of cross linkages, is a β-globulin of molecular mass 320,000, concentration 0.01 to 0.04 g/litre. Plasminogen, or profibrinolysin, is the inactive form of the fibrin-lysing enzyme, plasmin. It has a molecular mass of 87,000, α_2 mobility and concentration 0.02 g/litre.

Two active enzymes, in addition to caeruloplasmin, are found in more than trace amounts in plasma. Lysozyme, a basic protein of molecular mass 15,000, migrates even more slowly on electrophoresis than the γ-globulins. It is probably of leucocytic origin, and aids the body's defences by lysis of bacteria. The cholinesterase of serum (formerly called pseudocholinesterase to distinguish it from a similar enzyme in red cells) is a much larger protein (348,000) which catalyzes the hydrolysis of acetylcholine and other choline esters, but has no clearly defined biological function.

Two α_2-glycoproteins which are also of uncertain function are α_2-heat-stable glycoprotein, molecular mass 49,000, and Zn-α_2-glycoprotein, molecular mass 41,000. Their concentrations are 0.6 and 0.05 g/litre, respectively. The former may act as an opsonin to attract leucocytes (Van Oss et al., 1974). Gc-globulin, or group-specific component, is an α_2-globulin of molecular mass 50,800, and also without a known function, but which has proved useful in genetic typing owing to its electrophoretic polymorphism. Its concentration is 0.25 to 0.55 g/litre. α_1-Foetoprotein, molecular mass 68,000, is found in significant amounts in the foetus or in the presence of hepatomas (Chapter 25). It bears some sequence homology to albumin.

6.3.3. Immunoprotective proteins: chronic states

As inflammation becomes prolonged or chronic, responses are seen in the immunoglobulins of plasma. The term *immunoglobulins* includes all proteins with specific antibody activities, and is preferred over earlier terms such as γ-globulin, which was applied because antibodies were found mainly in the γ-globulin band on electrophoresis: actually their mobilities may extend well into the β-globulin region.

The structure of immunoglobulins is shown diagrammatically in Figure 6.7. The basic monomeric structure (IgG) contains two heavy (H) chains and two light (L) chains, with molecular masses of 22,000 and 53,000 to 75,000 respectively, coupled into a Y configuration by disulphide bonds at the "hinge" region. Sites for binding to a specific antigen are situated at the tip of each arm of the Y, rather like the claws of a lobster; when antigens are bound the arms open from a Y to a T configuration. The specificity of these sites at the tips of the arms is related to the sequence of amino acids in the amino-terminal portions of the H and L chains. The upper half of the arms, containing the upper half of the L chain and the upper quarter of the H chain, is highly variable in amino acid sequence (the V or variable region), whereas the rest of the chains is more constant (the C or constant region). By some mechanism, as yet unclear, the antibody-forming cells are able to insert amino acid sequences tailored to the particular antigen into these V regions.

The stem of the Y and, in some immunoglobulins, the bottom portion of the arms of the Y, contain carbohydrate chains attached to asparagine residues. The lower half of the stem of the Y contains sites which can bind or "fix" complement (section 6.3.2.5) after the immunoglobulin couples to an antigen.

There are two classes of L chains, termed kappa (κ) and lambda (λ); only one class occurs in a given molecule. Of the H chains there are five or six classes, γ, α, μ, δ, ϵ, and possibly ϕ; these define the immunoglobulins which contain them as G, A, M, D, E, or F. The monomeric structure of IgG (Figure 6.7) is "7S" (160,000 molecular mass) in the ultracentrifuge. IgA tends to dimerize or trimerize to structures sedimenting at 9 to 11S.

IgM, sedimenting at 19S, is a pentameric molecule in which the parts are joined by small links called J, or joining, pieces (Figure 6.7). The classes of immunoglobulins may be designated either as IgG, IgD, IgM, etc., or more specifically as $\gamma_2\kappa_2$, $\delta_2\lambda_2$, $(\mu_2\lambda_2)_5$, etc., to indicate the peptide chain classes which are included. Electrophoretically, IgG moves as a true "γ-globulin", IgM slightly faster, and IgA between β- and γ-globulins (Figure 6.3). IgG is further divided into four subclasses (Figure 6.7 and Table 6.4), termed IgG_1, IgG_2, etc., on the basis of differences in their chains. Likewise there are two subclasses of IgA and IgM. The immunoglobulin classes differ considerably with respect to their functions and responses to stimuli.

Immunoglobulins are determined by immunochemical means, but care is required in the selection of the antisera for this purpose. The best are reported to be made against a mixture of isolated Fc fragments, which comprise the stem of the Y and include only the constant region of the H chains, thus avoiding the complexities of the variable regions. Caution must also be observed in applying the radial immunodiffusion technique in the presence of forms having unexpected alterations in molecular mass, such as secretory IgA (section 6.3.3.2) or IgMs which are larger or smaller than 19S. These species will diffuse at different rates than the typical IgA or IgM used for calibration and can give false results.

To type specific immunoglobulins, antisera directed against only single classes of L or H chains are employed. These should not be prepared against a single or idiotypic protein, but against a pool of normal immunoglobulin chains of the desired class, carefully absorbed to remove unwanted antibodies. Antisera against L chains, in particular, should be capable of reacting both with the free L chain and with the L chain bound in protein. Methodology for immunoglobulin detection is reviewed by Grant and Butt (1970), Hobbs (1971), and Ritzmann and Daniels (1975); pathology is covered by Hobbs (1971),

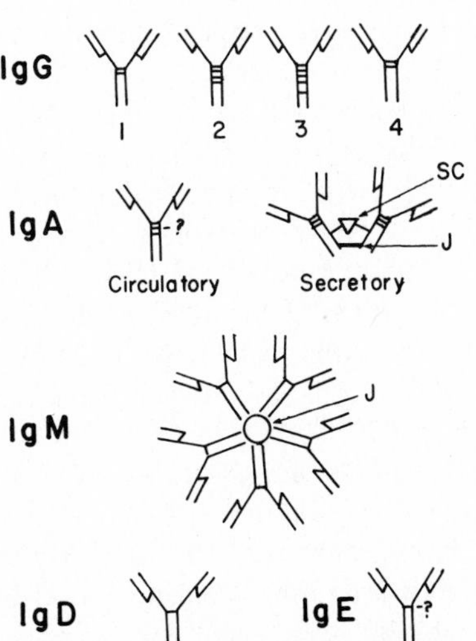

Figure 6.7. Diagrams of the peptide chains of immunoglobulins. Cross-bars indicate the inter-chain disulphide bonds; SC = secretory component of IgA; J = J (joining) piece. Adapted from Hong (1972).

TABLE 6.4.

SUBCLASSES OF IMMUNOGLOBULIN G (IgG)

Subclass	Concentration in normal serum		No. of S–S bonds in H chain	Relative electro-phoretic mobility	$t_{\frac{1}{2}}$ (days)	Binding of complement
	average (g/litre) [a]	range				
IgG_1	7.3	6.7–10.5	2	slow	22	++++
IgG_2	2.8	2.5–4.2	4	fast	22	+
IgG_3	0.6	0.5–1.0	5	slow	7	++
IgG_4	0.4	0.3–0.7	2	fast	22	0

[a] 1 g/litre of IgG = 11.5 I.U./ml.

LoGrippo et al., (1971), and Leonardy and Peacock (1972); structure and function by Hong (1972) and Putnam (1977); and normative values by Maddison and Reimer (1976). Immunoglobulin concentrations are given in terms of mass (g/litre, mg/litre) or in International Units (I.U./ml). The latter are referred to standard preparations of the five major immunoglobulin classes which are distributed by the World Health Organization. The correspondence between mass and I.U. is noted in Tables 6.2 and 6.4 and in the text for each immunoglobulin class.

6.3.3.1. *Immunoglobulin G (IgG)*

Normally the most abundant immunoglobulin, IgG, or γG, occurs at a concentration of 11 (8 to 16) g/litre (= 127 I.U./ml) in normal adults. The concentration is relatively stable in an individual, varying by only ±20%when measured at weekly intervals over a long period. The concentrations of the four identified IgG subclasses decrease in numerical order (Table 6.4). There is minimal synthesis of IgG in the foetus, starting at 5 months of gestation; most of the IgG is derived from the mother through placental transfer. In fact, IgG is the only plasma protein which has this ability to cross the placenta. It is interesting that the concentration in the newborn infant, 10 g/litre, is even higher than that of the mother, which has declined to 7 g/litre at the puerperium. As this store of protective protein is catabolized, the IgG concentration falls to a minimum value of about 3 g/litre at about 3 months (Figure 6.8), and then rises slowly as the infant's antibody-forming cells become active. The adult concentration is reached for the second time at 4 to 7 years of age. In babies born before 22 weeks of gestation, the IgG concentration is much reduced, since the placental transfer has not yet occurred.

IgG functions chiefly by coupling with circulating soluble antigens to speed their removal from the circulation. It enters the extravascular space (Table 6.2) to almost the same extent as albumin. Hence IgG is said to be the main protector of the body fluids, whereas IgA protects body surfaces, and IgM protects primarily against organisms which invade the bloodstream. Complement "fixes" or binds strongly to IgG subclasses 1 and 3, weakly to 2, and apparently not at all to 4 (Table 6.4). IgG is much less effective than IgM in binding to surfaces in vitro.

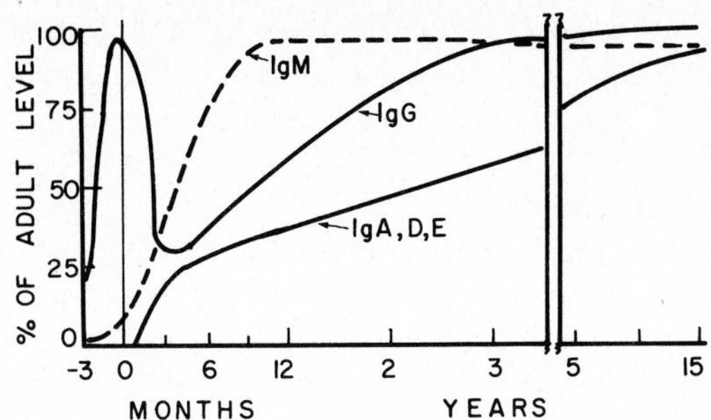

Figure 6.8. Changes in serum immunoglobulin concentrations with age; IgA, IgD, and IgE do not reach adult values until adolescence. (Plotted from data of Hobbs, 1971)

IgG is one of the most stable plasma proteins, having a half-life of 24 days at a normal concentration (Table 6.2). The catabolism is slow because tissue receptors protect IgG molecules from random destruction. At an increased concentration, a saturation point appears, however, at about 25 g/litre, above which the proportion of IgG broken down per day increases. The turnover of subclass IgG_3 is faster than that of the other subclasses (Table 6.4).

The serum concentration of IgG characteristically rises in chronic disease. IgG antibodies are formed by plasma cells derived from B lymphocytes; in the early stages of an immune response IgM is formed, but with interaction of T lymphocytes synthesis switches to IgG. These are the slowest of the antibodies to respond, appearing after about 10 days and remaining for a matter of weeks. The early response may show evidence of several bands within the γ-globulin zone (Figure 6.9, pattern 3); these are believed to be "oligoclonal" antibodies, arising from only a few strains of lymphocytes. They occur more frequently in infection which is restricted to a compartment such as the cerebrospinal fluid or aqueous humour. As the illness progresses, the γ-globulin pattern becomes broader and the "polyclonal" pattern develops (Figure 6.9, pattern 4). Together with IgA and IgM, elevations of IgG occur in most infections, and the concentrations of these proteins are characteristically found to be higher in the blood of persons from under-developed countries, who have been exposed to more infections in childhood. In Martinique, for example, values are higher in Indians than in whites, and in Bantus than in Indians. The difference is environmental, not genetic. All three classes also rise in subacute bacterial endocarditis, persistent hepatitis, and secondary biliary cirrhosis, but not in simple biliary obstruction. The increases in IgA and IgM cause "β-γ bridging" in the electrophoretic pattern. IgG and IgA rise in alcoholic cirrhosis, haemochromatosis, rheumatic fever, Wilson's disease, and Sjögren's syndrome. A variable IgM response is seen with IgG in systemic lupus erythematosus, chronic aggressive hepatitis, sarcoid, and scleroderma. Serum IgG concentration is high, but that of IgM is low in uraemia and with reticuloendothelial neoplasms.

Decreased concentrations of IgG occur in generalized hypoproteinaemic conditions such as depressed nutrition from any cause; in toxic conditions, such as overwhelming infections and multiple myeloma; and in protein-losing situations including enteropathies and the nephrotic syndrome. Being the smallest-size immunoglobulin class, IgG is readily lost through the injured glomerulus, and its normally slow production shows no compensatory increase as that of albumin often does; thus very low concentrations of IgG are seen in the nephrotic syndrome (Figure 6.9, pattern 9).

Congenital lack of IgG occurs in 1% of newborns. Persons with this formerly fatal condition can be brought to reasonably normal adulthood through the judicious use of antibiotics and parenteral immunoglobulin preparations. Acquired hypogammaglobulinaemia can develop at any stage of life due to marrow disorders or toxic causes, and it is encoun-

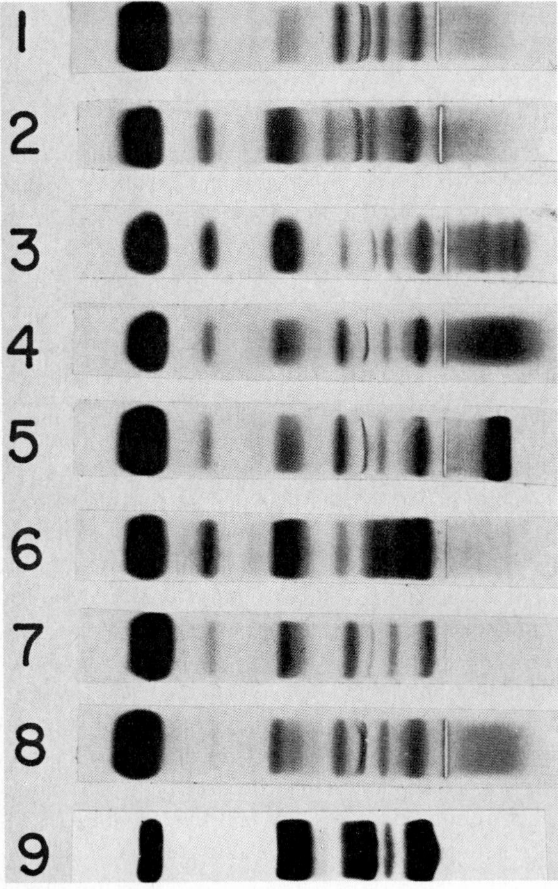

Figure 6.9. Agarose gel electrophoretic patterns of plasma in selected disease conditions – (1) normal; (2) acute phase; (3) oligoclonal hyper-γ-globulinaemia; (4) polyclonal hyper-γ-globulinaemia; (5) paraprotein of the IgG type; (6) paraprotein of the IgA type covering the fibrinogen zone, in an acute inflammatory response; (7) extreme hypo-γ-globulinaemia; (8) α-antitrypsin deficiency of ZZ type; (9) nephrotic syndrome. (Reproduced, by permission, from Laurell, 1972)

tered in 2 to 4% of hospital patients. Again the parenteral administration of immunoglobulins is helpful.

6.3.3.2. Immunoglobulin A (IgA)

IgA, or γA, also formerly called β_2A and γ_1A, occurs in serum at an average concentration of 2.0 g/litre (Table 6.2). This is the monomeric form or *circulatory IgA*, which is synthesized in spleen, marrow, and lymph nodes. It is absent in the newborn, as it does not cross the placenta and synthesis is minimal before birth. By 3 months there has been appreciable synthesis (Figure 6.8), but the concentration reaches that of the adult only at adolescence, or even as late as 40 years of age. If the mother has been afflicted with rubella, syphilis, or some pneumococcal infections, circulatory IgA may be found in the newborn.

IgA is more characteristically an antibody of secretions than of the bloodstream. *Secretory IgA* occurs as a dimer or trimer containing the J chain (Figure 6.7). It is synthesized by plasma cells within the lamina propria of mucous membranes, and in passing through the cells of the mucosa acquires an additional protective "secretory piece" (Figure 6.7) which protects the IgA from destruction by proteases of the gut. This protected form of IgA is the major antibody of colostrum, tears, saliva, and enteric secretions (Tomasi et al., 1965; Tomasi, 1972). The adult concentration of IgA in secretions is reached within the first few months of life, in contrast to the delayed appearance of circulatory IgA.

The serum concentration of IgA rises together with that of IgG in chronic infections. Elevations of IgA without parallel increases of IgG are seen in diseases of body surfaces such as respiratory diseases (asthma, emphysema, and tuberculosis), skin diseases, and enteric diseases including Crohn's ileitis and ulcerative colitis. IgA is also elevated in early hepatic cirrhosis, nephritis, rheumatoid arthritis, and some cases of sarcoid and lupus erythematosus. Because of their large size and rapid replacement rates IgA and IgM tend to remain in serum in the nephrotic syndrome and in protein-losing enteropathies when smaller proteins and those more slowly replaced become depleted. IgA and IgM also rise in malnutrition when the concentrations of most proteins fall, probably stimulated by concomitant exposure to various infections.

Deficiencies of IgA occur with lymphoid neoplasia and myelomatosis, as well as in rheumatoid arthritis and in association with chronic sinusitis, bronchitis, and otitis media. If IgA is deficient in serum, secretions should be examined, and this is most easily done with saliva. If IgA is deficient in secretions, tests for the presence of intestinal parasites should be performed. For further discussion the reader is referred to section 12.1.4.

6.3.3.3. Immunoglobulin M (IgM)

The pentameric IgM (Figure 6.7), or γM, formerly γ_1M or β_2M, is largely restricted to the blood plasma owing to its size (Table 6.2). In adults, IgM concentration averages 1.2 g/litre, and is about 20% higher in women than in men. Its synthesis begins in the foetus at about 5 weeks of age, but only about 0.15 g/litre is found at birth, after which the concentration rises rapidly (Figure 6.8), starting by about 10 days and reaching the adult value by about one year. Like IgG, the "normal" values are somewhat higher in economically poor countries. Concentrations which are greater than 0.2 g/litre at birth are suggestive, but not conclusive, evidence of intrauterine infection.

Manufactured by B lymphocytes, IgM, by virtue of its large size and numerous (ten) antibody-binding sites, is particularly effective in binding to foreign surfaces and causing agglutination or fixation of complement, with resultant cell lysis. In these respects, IgM is about 7000 times as effective as IgG. It is the first antibody to appear following an acute infection, and constitutes the initial line of defence of the bloodstream against alien organisms. Like IgA, the concentration of IgM is low compared to that of IgG, but the turnover rate is 4 to 5 times as high (Table 6.2), so that the production of IgA and IgM together about equals that of IgG.

Increases of IgM occur in most infections, particularly in the early phases. Rheumatoid factors are commonly IgMs, and IgM values are increased in 65% of patients with rheumatoid arthritis. Elevations of IgM are also found in malaria, mononucleosis, rubella, syphilis, histoplasmosis, infectious hepatitis, and primary biliary cirrhosis. IgM is not elevated in alcoholic cirrhosis as are IgG and IgA. IgM levels are low in uraemia and with lymphoid neoplasia.

6.3.3.4. Paraproteins

Paraprotein is the term used to refer to a monoclonal form of immunoglobulin (i.e. one produced by a single lymphocyte or plasma cell, or clone). The term "M protein" should be discarded, since it is easily confused with IgM or γM, and not all paraproteins are IgMs. The presence of a paraprotein signifies a dyscrasia in immunoglobulin synthesis by a B lymphocyte or plasma cell strain which is not under control. It is usually characterized by an imbalance of H and L chain production which can lead to L chain, L chain dimers, or fragments of L chains appearing in blood and, because of their small size (22,000 daltons or less), are excreted rapidly in urine as Bence Jones protein (Solomon, 1976).

The incidence of paraproteinaemia is about 1% of the adult population, rising to 3% in those over 65 years of age and 6% over 80 years. Paraproteins are nearly always first detected as a narrow band on electrophoresis (Figure 6.9 pattern 5; Figure 6.10). Most,

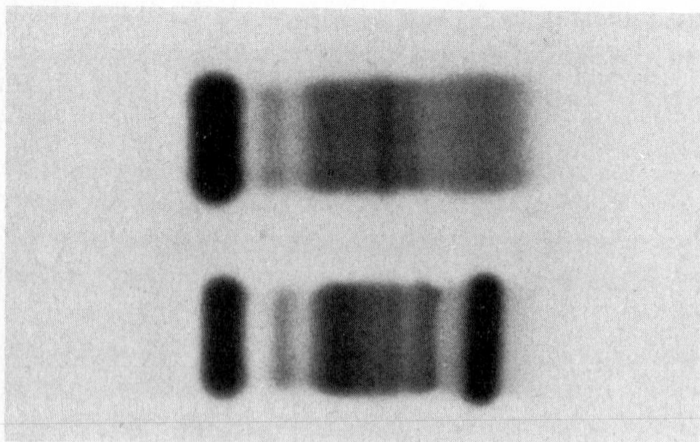

Figure 6.10. A monoclonal paraprotein seen on cellulose acetate electrophoresis. Upper: normal serum; lower: serum showing paraprotein in mid-γ region, and near absence of normal γ-globulins. The direction of migration was from right to left. (Courtesy of Millipore Biomedica)

but not all, are in the γ region; surveys show about 80% migrate with γ mobility, 6% intermediate (β to γ), 13% β, and 1% α. About 20% of all paraproteins are IgMs; of these IgM paraproteins, 50% occur with Waldenström's macroglobulinaemia, 25% with lymphomas, 2% with multiple myeloma, and 10% are apparently benign. The occurrence of paraproteins has been reviewed by Hobbs (1971) and by Ameis et al. (1976).

Of all cases of paraproteinaemia, about 65% occur with multiple myeloma, 7% with plasmacytomas of soft tissues rather than bone, 10% with macroglobulinaemia, 7% with various sarcomas, leukaemias, and Hodgkin's disease, and 12% are "benign" or idiopathic. Such idiopathic *secondary* paraproteinaemia is seen especially with cirrhosis, diabetes, connective tissue disorders, or chronic infections. It should not be assumed that a paraprotein is benign without at least 10 years of annual follow-up, because many cases develop myeloma or other immunocytomata at a late stage. If the concentrations of the normal immunoglobulins are low, there is a higher probability that a paraprotein is of malignant origin.

In most cases of multiple myeloma, the paraprotein is IgG (55% of cases), but in 22% it is an IgA, 1% an IgM, 1% an IgD, and rarely an H chain or a fragment of it (Franklin's disease). The occurrence of the IgG subclasses as paraproteins is not significantly different from the prevalence of these subclasses in plasma (Table 6.4). About 20% of patients with multiple myeloma will show no paraprotein in their blood, but will still have Bence Jones protein or a monomeric immunoglobulin in their urine. About 70% of all myeloma patients and 60% of patients with paraproteinaemia have Bence Jones proteinuria.

In the detection of paraproteins, a narrow band which is seen upon electrophoresis may be confused with fibrinogen owing to incomplete coagulation (Figure 6.9, pattern 6), with haemoglobin (in the β region), or with α-lipoprotein. If myeloma or paraproteinaemia is suspected, electrophoresis of urine, after concentration, should always be carried out, as well as a test for Bence Jones protein. Hobbs (1971) has found that the usual heat coagulation test will miss one-third of Bence Jones proteins in urine, and that immunochemical testing is unsure owing to the many small L-chain fragments which may appear. The most sensitive test (99% positive) is the simple procedure of Bradshaw (see Hobbs, 1971), in which clear urine is layered over concentrated HCl; 0.01 g/litre of globulin can be detected. Even in the absence of a paraprotein in the serum, it is recommended that the urine of any patient showing proteinuria should be studied by electrophoresis, since Bence Jones protein or leakage of a paraprotein through the kidney can be the first evidence of multiple myeloma or other immunocytomata. Bence Jones protein is an ominous sign; it almost invariably portends malignancy.

Quantitation of a paraprotein in serum may be achieved by immunochemical means, unless the paraprotein fails to react in the normal fashion with the antisera used. Because of this problem, it is more reliable to follow paraprotein concentrations by quantitation of cellulose acetate electrophoresis patterns. Often the paraprotein band appears in an isolated region since the malignant cells suppress the synthesis of normal immunoglobulins. If the paraprotein band or "spike" is on top of a normal, broad γ region, estimates may be made of the amounts due to the paraprotein and to the normal γ-globulin. Both figures are useful, the first to estimate the response of the plasmacytoma to therapy and the latter to indicate the probable degree of immunoresistance remaining. A concentration of 30 g/litre of paraprotein corresponds to about 30% replacement of bone marrow by plasma cells. The sizes of paraproteins and urinary proteins may be estimated by thin-layer gel chromatography (Figure 6.4). They may be classified by immunoelectrophoresis or by quantitative immunochemical tests with a battery of antisera against IgG, IgA, IgM, H and L chain types, etc.

There are several corollary features of paraproteinaemia. The viscosity of blood may be increased, causing difficulty with its circulation through capillaries – a phenomenon particularly noticeable in the extremities. Like fibrinogen, the large IgM molecule contributes to viscosity out of proportion to its concentration, so that hyperviscosity is often observed with an increased IgM concentration, above 30 g/litre. In addition, about 4% of IgG paraproteins and some IgA paraproteins tend to aggregate and thus increase the serum viscosity. About 6% of IgM paraproteins are cryoglobulins, which can interfere with the circulation in extremities upon exposure to cold. Cryoglobulins precipitate, reversibly, when serum is refrigerated, but for their detection in this way the blood must be allowed to clot while warm, and must be kept warm until serum is separated; if plasma is tested, oxalate should be used as anticoagulant, since some cryoglobulins are precipitated by heparin.

Amyloid disease, which is characterized by deposits thought by Virchow to be starch-like because they stained with iodine, is frequent (20%) in myeloma and other conditions showing paraproteinaemia, although it also occurs with leprosy, rheumatoid arthritis, tuberculosis, chronic infection, and (in about half of all cases) idiopathically. Rather than being of carbohydrate nature, the amyloid deposits mainly contain either fibrils formed of L chains or the variable portion of L chains (Glenner et al., 1973) or a non-immunoglobulin protein of molecular mass about 8000 (Levin et al., 1972). Both forms have been isolated and their amino acid sequences determined. The mechanism is believed to be an increased activation of lysosomal enzymes, causing breakdown of proteins which polymerize and form fibrils in tissue. The earlier differentiation of primary and secondary amyloidosis does not now appear as clear-cut; monoclonal proteins almost invariably appear in the serum or urine in both forms (Kyle and Bayrd, 1975).

6.3.3.5. Other immunoglobulins

Immunoglobulins D and E (Figure 6.7) are monomeric proteins which are present in trace amounts in serum (30 mg/litre and 0.1 mg/litre, respectively). One mg/litre of IgD corresponds to about 0.75 I.U./ml; 1 mg/litre of IgE corresponds to about 500 I.U./ml. No antibody function has yet been assigned to IgD, but IgE comprises the reagins of allergic responses. IgE is the responsible agent in skin sensitivity reactions, causing the release of histamine, of serotonin, and of bradykinins (Ishizaka, 1977). IgE molecules are transient, their half-life in plasma being only 2 to 3 days. Serum IgE is increased in atopic diseases – asthma (60%), hay fever (30%), eczema, and parasitic infections. Radioimmunoassays can now detect IgE antibodies against specific allergens such as ragweed or mouse hair. Desensitization to such an allergen can be effected by repeated injections so as to produce IgG antibodies to the same allergen, which outnumber the scarcer and weaker-affinity IgE molecules in competition for the available sites on antigens (Johansson et al., 1972).

Another protein fragment of considerable interest is β_2-microglobulin, which is not usually detectable in serum (0.8 to 2.4 mg/l) but is found in significant amounts in urine following cadmium poisoning and in other renal diseases. This has been shown to be a single chain of about 100 amino acids with one disulphide bond forming a 60-residue internal loop. Its sequence is homologous to the constant domains of immunoglobulin heavy chains, particularly the H chain of IgG_1. It is bound to the surface of heterologous lymphocytes and polymorphonuclear leucocytes (mouse, rat, guinea-pig) but not to human white cells. β_1-Microglobulin has also been shown to be the smaller of two peptide chains comprising the human lymphocyte antigen (HLA), a finding which suggests that tissue antigens and immunoglobulins arose from a common precursor gene during evolution (Anderson et al. 1975).

6.4. SUMMARIZED INDICATIONS FOR SCREENING OR FOR SPECIFIC TESTS

In this section the use of protein assays in diagnosis and follow-up of therapy is outlined, summarizing some of the information of the preceding sections. Good practice requires that such assays, or any laboratory data, be only supportive and suggestive, and that a diagnosis should be arrived at by consideration of the complete clinical picture. Where a specific test is suggested, a more complete description of the significance of its results will usually be found in the pertinent preceding subsection.

The selection of tests will, of course, depend upon the scope of the available laboratories. Tests for urea, creatinine, ESR, total protein, and albumin are hopefully so commonplace that this information will generally be on hand. Electrophoretic separation by either the cellulose acetate or agarose gel technique is highly recommended, even if only qualitative in nature. Testing for individual plasma proteins is in its infancy. A recommended order of priority for their introduction would be: fibrinogen, immunoglobulins IgG, IgA, and IgM, transferrin (or total iron-binding capacity), complement (C3), orosomucoid, haptoglobin, and antitrypsin. Laurell (1973) uses caeruloplasmin routinely, but mainly to assess the effect of oestrogens (caused by pregnancy or "the pill") on the concentrations of the other proteins.

A qualitative electrophoretic pattern will permit detection of the following: presence of a *paraprotein*, seen as a sharp extra band (Figure 6.9, patterns 5 and 6; Figure 6.10) for which purpose no other method is as reliable; *hypo- or a-γ-globulinaemia* (Figure 6.9, pattern 7); *protein loss* via the kidney (Figure 6.9, pattern 9) or via the intestine, in which case there is a similar pattern of depressed albumin and γ-globulin, but with less elevation of α_2-M; occurrence of an *acute phase reaction* with elevation of α- and β-globulins (Figure 6.9, pattern 2); or the status of a *chronic inflammatory response* (Figure 6.9, pattern 4) with a relative rise in γ-globulin and β-γ bridging (the bridging between β- and γ-globulins is a rough estimate of the elevation of IgA). Oligoclonal patterns (e.g. Figure 6.9, pattern 3) suggest an early infection or one sequestered in an isolated compartment such as the cerebrospinal fluid. A diminished α_1-globulin band is suggestive, but by no means conclusive, evidence for antitrypsin deficiency. Obviously analyses for specific proteins will give more precise evaluations, but serum protein electrophoresis will still retain value in the conditions above and as a screening test in most of those listed below. Electrophoresis of urine (after concentration by ultrafiltration) is likewise recommended to assess the degree of glomerular damage and to detect Bence Jones protein or paraproteins in the urine.

6.4.1. Protein assays in diagnosis

Suggestions as to the most suitable tests are grouped in this section on a basis of initial complaints or findings.

Diarrhoea, indigestion, weight loss, "failure to thrive", oedema, anaemia. Serum albumin and total protein concentrations, together with urea and creatinine, will help to evaluate the degree of protein deficit. Transferrin, prealbumin, and C3 are reportedly even better indices of malnutrition. The protein loss with enteropathies appears as lowered albumin, transferrin, and IgG concentrations. Immunoglobulin assays will help to assess the role of chronic inflammation in the disease process. In diarrhoea, specific testing for IgA, in secretions if possible, may suggest a basis for the abnormality or promote a further search for parasitic organisms. In anaemia, haptoglobin should be determined as a test for haemolysis; elevated urea concentrations suggest internal haemorrhage.

Ascites, jaundice, hepatomegaly. A "liver profile" would normally include bilirubin, certain enzymes, and albumin. Tests for immunoglobulins can aid in determining the severity of chronic hepatitis and in the differentiation of jaundice. Thus, IgM tends to be elevated in primary biliary cirrhosis whereas IgG and IgA rise in alcoholic cirrhosis, and all three rise in secondarv biliary or mixed cirrhosis and in persistent hepatitis. In simple biliary obstruction, the immunoglobulins remain at normal concentrations.

Lymphadenopathy, splenomegaly, recurrent infections, prolonged ESR elevation, neonatal infection, fever of unknown origin, allergy, or atopy. In this group of conditions, immunoglobulin assays are indicated, as well as serum electrophoresis, to detect paraproteinaemia, with urinary electrophoresis if possible. Characteristic findings are considered in section 6.3.3. In differentiating a febrile condition as chronic or acute, orosomucoid and other acute phase reactants are helpful (Figure 6.5), including haptoglobin to test for haemolysis. Increased C3 suggests an acute phase reaction; decreased C3 suggests an autoimmune condition such as lupus erythematosus or glomerulonephritis.

Emphysema, chronic lung disease. Antitrypsin and immunoglobulins are recommended. For positive diagnosis of antitrypsin deficiency, phenotyping by gel electrophoresis is required.

Oliguria, proteinuria. The albumin concentration and electrophoresis will indicate the degree of protein loss. Depression of C3 will aid in the diagnosis of glomerulonephritis, but may also be caused by urinary loss in nephrosis.

Obscure pain, including bone pain, back pain, neck pain. Electrophoresis for possible paraproteinaemia is recommended (see section 6.3.3.4).

6.4.2. Protein assays in follow-up and during therapy

Trauma, infarction, inflammation, fever, burns. The course of the acute phase reaction can be followed by electrophoresis or, more closely, by individual protein assays (Figure 6.5). Orosomucoid and haptoglobin, in conjunction with the ESR and C-reactive protein, are most useful. Immunoglobulin measurements are suggested if the situation appears more chronic. The fibrinogen concentration and other clotting parameters will aid in detecting disseminated intravascular coagulation or extensive fibrinolysis.

Nutritional problems in malabsorption or systemic disease, including carcinomatosis. Protein nutrition can be followed by electrophoresis and by quantitation of C3, pre-albumin, albumin, transferrin, and serum and urine urea. If available, the amino acid pattern of plasma (section 6.2.4) will aid in differentiating starvation from liver failure.

Hepatic failure, hepatic function. Immunoglobulins are useful, together with the other liver function tests indicated in section 6.4.1. Depressed urea serum concentrations are an ominous sign in failure; ammonia and amino acid concentrations may predict the degree of by-pass of the liver and the severity of liver failure.

Amyloid, sarcoid, rheumatic arthritis, lupus erythematosus, myelomatosis, lymphoid diseases, haemolytic processes. Electrophoresis for paraproteinaemia and paraproteinuria plus immunoglobulin and C3 assays are indicated at 3 to 12 month intervals. In detecting haemolysis or suspected transfusion reaction, a haptoglobin measurement is useful. Hobbs (1975) recommends haemoglobin, albumin and urea measurements as well in monitoring myelomatosis.

Nephrotic syndrome, uraemia. The degree and nature of protein loss can be estimated by electrophoresis of serum and urine, as well as by specific tests for albumin, transferrin, and IgG.

REFERENCES

Ameis, A., Ko, H.S. and Pruzanski, W. (1976) M components – a review of 1242 cases. Canadian Medical Association Journal, 114, 889–895.

Anderson, C.L., Kubo, R.T. and Grey, H.M. (1975) Studies on the cytophilic properties of human β_2-microglobulin. Journal of Immunology, 114, 997–1000.

Aronsen, K.-F., Ekelund, G., Kindmark, C.-O. and Laurell, C.-B. (1972) Sequential changes of plasma proteins after surgical trauma. Scandinavian Journal of Clinical and Laboratory Investigation, 29, suppl. 124, 127–136.

Behrens, P.Q., Spiekerman, A.M. and Brown, J.R. (1975) Structure of human serum albumin. Federation Proceedings; Federation of American Societies for Experimental Biology, 34, 591, (abstr.).

Blake, C.C.F., Koenig, D.F., Mair, G.A., North, A.C.T., Phillips, D.C. and Sarma, V.R. (1965) Structure of hen egg-white lysozyme. Nature, 206, 757–761.

Buffone, G.J., Savory, J. and Cross, R.E. (1974) Use of a laser-equipped centrifugal analyzer for kinetic measurement of serum IgG. Clinical Chemistry, 20, 1320–1323.

Casey, A.E., Gilbert, F.E., Copeland, H., Downey, E.L. and Casey, J.G. (1973) Albumin, $alpha_{1,2}$, beta, and gamma globulins in cancer and other diseases. Southern Medical Journal, 66, 179–185.

Cohn, E.J., Gurd, F.R.N., Surgenor, D.M., et al. (1950) A system for the separation of the components of human blood. Journal of American Chemical Society, 72, 465–474.

Corcoran, R.M. and Durnan, S.M. (1977) Albumin determination by a modified bromcresol green method. Clinical Chemistry, 23, 765–766.

Cuthbertson, D. and Tilstone, W.J. (1969) Metabolism during the post-injury period. Advances in Clinical Chemistry, 12, 1–55.

Deaton, C.D., Maxwell, K.W., Smith, R.S. and Creveling, R.L. (1976) Use of laser nephelometry in the measurement of serum proteins. Clinical Chemistry, 22, 1465–1471.

DeTorrente, A., Glazer, G.B. and Gulyassy, P. (1974) Reduced in vitro binding of tryptophan. Kidney International, 6, 222–229.

Dickerson, R.E. and Geis, I. (1969) In The Structure and Action of Proteins. Harper and Row, New York.

Doolittle, R.F. (1973) Structural aspects of the fibrinogen to fibrin conversion. In Advances in Protein Chemistry, Vol. 27 (Eds. C.B. Anfinsen and J.T. Edsall) pp. 1–109, Academic Press, New York.

Doumas, B.T. (1975) Standards for total serum protein assays – a collaborative study. Clinical Chemistry, 21, 1159–1166.

Doumas, B.T. and Biggs, H.G. (1972) Determination of serum albumin. Standard Methods in Clinical Chemistry, 7, 175–188.

Eriksson, S. and Larsson, C. (1975) Purification and partial characterization of PAS-positive inclusion bodies from the liver in $alpha_1$-antitrypsin deficiency. New England Journal of Medicine, 292, 176–180.

Erlanger, B.F., Kokowsky, N. and Cohen, W. (1961) The preparation and properties of two new chromogenic substrates of trypsin. Archives of Biochemistry and Biophysics, 95, 271–278.

Fahey, J.L. and McKelvey, E.M. (1965) Quantitative determination of serum immunoglobulins in antibody-agar plates. Journal of Immunology, 94, 84–90.

Felig, P. (1975) Amino acid metabolism in man. Annual Reviews of Biochemistry, 44, 933–953.

Felig, P. and Wahren, J. (1974) Protein turnover and amino acid metabolism in the regulation of gluconeogenesis. Federation Proceedings; Federation of American Societies for Experimental Biology, 33, 1092–1097.

Fredrickson, D.S. (1973) Plasma lipoproteins and apolipoproteins. The Harvey Lectures, Series 68, 185–237.

Frieden, E. and Hsieh, H.S. (1976) Ceruloplasmin: the copper transport protein with essential oxidase activity. Advances in Enzymology, 44, 187–236.

Glenner, G.G., Terry, W.D. and Isersky, C. (1973) Amyloidosis: its nature and pathogenesis. Seminars in Hematology, 10, 65–86.

Grant, G.H. and Butt, W.R. (1970) Immunochemical methods in clinical chemistry. Advances in Clinical Chemistry, 13, 383–466.

Harris, R.I. and Kohn, J. (1974) The pre-albumin fraction: a useful parameter in the interpretation of routine protein electrophoresis. Journal of Clinical Pathology, 27, 986–989.

Heird, W.C. and Winters, R.W. (1975) Total parenteral nutrition in pediatrics. Pediatrics, 56, 17–23.

Henry, R.J., Cannon, D.C. and Winkelman, J.W. (1974) Clinical Chemistry: Principles and Techniques, 2nd edn., Harper and Row, Hagerstown, Maryland.

Hobbs, J.R. (1971) Immunoglobulins in clinical chemistry. Advances in Clinical Chemistry, 14, 219–317.

Hobbs, J.R. (1975) Monitoring myelomatosis. Archives of Internal Medicine, 135, 125–130.

Hong, R. (1972) The Immunoglobulins. In Clinical Immunobiology, Vol. 1, (Eds. F.H. Bach and R.A. Good) pp. 29–46, Academic Press, New York.

Hsia, Y.E. (1974) Inherited hyperammonemic syndromes. Gastroenterology, 67, 347–374.

Ingenbleek, Y., van den Schrieck, H.-G., De Nayer, P. and de Visscher, M. (1975) Albumin, transferrin and the thyroxine-binding pre-albumin/retinol-binding protein (TBPA–RBP) complex in assessment of malnutrition. Clinica Chimica Acta, 63, 61–67.

Ishizaka, K. (1977) Structure and biologic activity of immunoglobulin E. Hospital Practice, 12, 57–67.

Johansson, B.G., Kindmark, C.-O., Trell, E.Y. and Wollheim, F.A. (1972) Sequential changes of plasma proteins after myocardial infarction. Scandinavian Journal of Clinical and Laboratory Investigation, 29, suppl. 124, 117–126.

Johansson, S.G.O., Bennich, H.H. and Berg, T. (1972) The clinical significance of IgE. In Progress in Clinical Immunology, Vol. 1. (Ed. R.S. Schwartz) pp. 157–181, Grune and Stratton, New York.

Kelley, V.C. (1952) Acute phase reactants. I. Serum nonglucosamine polysaccharides in patients with rheumatic fever and related conditions. Journal of Pediatrics, 40, 405–412.

Kohn, J. (1957) A cellulose acetate supporting medium for zone electrophoresis. Clinica Chimica Acta, 2, 297–303.

Kyle, R.A. and Bayrd, E.A. (1975) Amyloidosis: a review of 236 cases. Medicine, 54, 271–299.

Laurell, C.-B. (1966) Quantitative estimation of protein by electrophoresis in agarose gel containing antibodies. Analytical Biochemistry, 15, 45–52.

Laurell, C.-B. (1972) Composition and variation of the gel electrophoretic fractions of plasma, cerebrospinal fluid and urine. Scandinavian Journal of Clinical and Laboratory Investigation, 29, suppl. 124, 71–82.

Laurell, C.-B. (1973) Electrophoresis, specific protein assays, or both in measurement of plasma proteins? Clinical Chemistry, 19, 99–102.

Leonardy, J.G. and Peacock, L.B. (1972) An evaluation of quantitative serum immunoglobulin determinations in clinical practice. Annals of Allergy, 30, 378–390.

Levin, B. (1971) Hereditary metabolic disorders of the urea cycle. Advances in Clinical Chemistry, 14, 66–143.

Levin, M., Franklin, E.C., Frangione, B. and Pras, M. (1972) The amino acid sequence of a major non-immunoglobulin component of some amyloid fibrils. Journal of Clinical Investigation, 51, 2773–2776.

LoGrippo, G.A., Anselm, K. and Hayashi, H. (1971) Serum immunoglobulins and five serum proteins in extrahepatic obstructive jaundice and alcoholic cirrhosis. Immunoglobulins and proteins in liver diseases. American Journal of Gastroenterology, 56, 357–363.

Maddison, S.E. and Reimer, C.B. (1976) Normative values of serum immunoglobins by single radial immunodiffusion. A review. Clinical Chemistry, 22, 594–601.

Mancini, G., Carbonara, A.O. and Heremans, J.F. (1965) Immunochemical quantitation of antigens by single radial immunodiffusion. Immunochemistry, 2, 235–254.

McFarlane, H., Reddy, S., Adcock, K.H., Adeshina, H., Cooke, A.R. and Akene, J. (1970) Immunity, transferrin, and survival in kwashiorkor. British Medical Journal, 4, 268–270.

Melou, B., Moravek, L. and Kostka, V. (1975) Complete amino acid sequence of human serum albumin. FEBS Letters: Federation of European Biochemical Societies, 58, 134–137.

Mortensen, R.F., Osmand, A.P. and Gewurz, H. (1975) Effects of C-reactive protein on the lymphoid system. I. Binding to thymus-dependent lymphocytes and alteration of their functions. Journal of Experimental Medicine, 141, 821–839.

Mortimore, G.E., Neely, A.N., Cox, J.R. and Guinivan, R.A. (1973) Proteolysis in homogenates of perfused rat liver: responses to insulin, glucagon and amino acids. Biochemical and Biophysical Research Communications, 54, 89–95.

Muehrcke, R.C. (1956) The finger-nails in chronic hypoalbuminaemia; a new physical sign. British Medical Journal, 1, 1327–1328.

Muller-Eberhard, H.J. (1971) The molecular basis of the biological activities of complement. The Harvey Lectures, Series 66, 75–104.

Muller-Eberhard, U. and Liem, H.H. (1974) Hemopexin, the heme-binding serum β-glycoprotein. In Structure and Function of Plasma Proteins, Vol. 1 (Ed. J.B. Allison) pp. 35–53, Plenum Press, London.

Munro, H.N. and Allison, J.B. (Eds.) (1970) Mammalian Protein Metabolism, 4th edn., pp. 299–387. Academic Press, New York.

Nilsson, S.F., Rask, L. and Peterson, P.A. (1975) Studies on thyroid hormone-binding proteins. II. Binding of thyroid hormones, retinol-binding protein, and fluorescent probes to prealbumin and effects of thyroxine on prealbumin subunit self association. Journal of Biological Chemistry, 250, 8554–8563.

Olson, R.E. (1975) Protein-Calorie Malnutrition. Academic Press, New York.

Peters, T., Jr. (1970) Serum albumin. Advances in Clinical Chemistry, 13, 37–111.

Peters, T., Jr. (1975) Serum albumin, In The Plasma Proteins, Vol. 1, 2nd edn. (Ed. F.W. Putnam) pp. 133–181, Academic Press, New York.

Peters, T., Jr. (1977) Serum albumin: recent progress in the understanding of its structure and biosynthesis. Clinical Chemistry, 23, 5–12.

Poulik, M.D. and Weiss, W. (1975) Ceruloplasmin. In The Plasma Proteins, Vol. II, 2nd edn. (Ed. F.W. Putnam) Chapter 2, Academic Press, New York.

Putnam, F.W. (Ed.) (1975) The Plasma Proteins, Vols. I and II, 2nd edn. Academic Press, New York.

Putnam, F.W. (Ed.) (1977) The Plasma Proteins, Vol. III, 2nd edn. Academic Press, New York.

Ritchie, R.F., Alper, C.A., Graves, M.A., Pearson, N. and Larson, C. (1973) Automated quantitation of proteins in serum and other biologic fluids. American Journal of Clinical Pathology, 59, 151–159.

Ritzmann, S.E. and Daniels, J.C. (1975) Serum Protein Abnormalities. Little, Brown and Co. Boston.

Rothschild, M.A., Oratz, M. and Schreiber, S.S. (1973) Albumin metabolism. Gastroenterology, 64, 324–337.

Ruddy, S., Gigli, I. and Austen, K.F. (1972) The complement system of man. New England Journal of Medicine, 287, 489–495; 545–549; 592–596; 642–646.

Schmid, K. (1975) α_1-Acid glycoprotein. In The Plasma Proteins, Vol. 1, 2nd edn. (Ed. F.W. Putnam) Chapter 4, Academic Press, New York.

Schultze, H.E. and Heremans, J.F. (Eds.) (1966) Molecular biology of human proteins, with special reference to plasma proteins. In Molecular Biology of Human Proteins, Vol. 1. Elsevier, Amsterdam.

Schur, P.H. (1972) Human gamma-G subclasses. Progress in Clinical Immunology, 1, 71–104.

Sim, R.B., Porter, R.R., Reid, K.B.M. and Gigli, I. (1977) The structure and enzymic activities of the C1r and C1s subcomponents of C1, the first component of human serum complement. Biochemical Journal, 163, 219–227.

Solomon, A. (1976) Bence-Jones proteins and L chains of immunoglobulins. New England Journal of Medicine, 294, 17–23; 91–98.

Spiro, R.G. (1973) Glycoproteins. Advances in Protein Chemistry, 27, 349–467.

Statland, B.E., Winkel, P. and Killingsworth, L.M. (1976) Factors contributing to intra-individual variation of serum constituents: 6. Physiological day-to-day variation in concentrations of 10 specific proteins in sera of healthy subjects. Clinical Chemistry, 22, 1635–1638.

Sveger, T. (1976) Liver disease in alpha$_1$-antitrypsin deficiency detected by screening of 200,000 infants. New England Journal of Medicine, 294, 1316–1321.

Talamo, R.C. (1975) Basic and clinical aspects of the alpha$_1$-antitrypsin. Pediatrics, 56, 91–99.

Tomasi, T.B., Jr. (1972) Secretory immunoglobulins. New England Journal of Medicine, 287, 500–506.

Tomasi, T.B., Tan, E.M., Solomon, A. and Prendergast, R.A. (1965) Characterstics of an immune system common to certain external secretions. Journal of Experimental Medicine, 121, 101–124.

Tunstall, A.M., Merriman, J.M.L., Milne, I. and James, K. (1975) Normal and pathological serum levels of α_2-macroglobulins in men and mice. Journal of Clinical Pathology, 28, 133–139.

Van Oss, C.J., Gillman, C.F., Bronson, P.M. and Border, J.R. (1974) Opsonic properties of human serum α_2-HS-glycoprotein. Immunological Communications, 3, 329–335.

Waterlow, J.C. and Alleyne, G.A.O. (1971) Protein malnutrition in children: advances in knowledge in the last ten years. Advances in Protein Chemistry, 25, 117–241.

Watson, D. (1965) Albumin and "total globulin" fractions of blood. Advances in Clinical Chemistry, 8, 237–303.

Webster, D. (1974) A study of the interaction of bromocresol green with isolated serum globulin fractions. Clinica Chimica Acta, 53, 109–115.

Werner, M. and Cohnen, G. (1969) Changes in serum proteins in the immediate postoperative period. Clinical Science, 36, 173–184.

Winkel, P., Statland, B.E. and Nielsen, M.K. (1976) Biologic and analytic components of variation of concentration values of selected serum proteins. Within-day variation in a group of healthy young men. Scandinavian Journal of Clinical and Laboratory Investigation, 36, 531–537.

FURTHER READING

Dickerson, R.E. and Geis, I. (1969) The Structure and Action of Proteins. Harper and Row, New York.

Fredrickson, D.S. (1973) Plasma lipoproteins and apolipoproteins. The Harvey Lectures, Series 68, 185–237.

Hershko, C. (1975) The fate of circulating haemoglobin. British Journal of Haematology, 29, 199–204.

Hobbs, J.R. (1971) Immunoglobulins in clinical chemistry. Advances in Clinical Chemistry, 14, 219–317.

Kawai, T. (1973) Clinical Aspects of the Plasma Proteins. 1st. edn., Igaku Shoin Ltd., Tokyo, J.B. Lippincott Co., Philadelphia and Toronto.
Putnam, F.W. (Ed.) (1975) The Plasma Proteins, Vols. I and II, 2nd edn. Academic Press, New York. (1977) Vol. III.
Ritzmann, S.E. and Daniels, J.C. (1975) Serum Protein Abnormalities, Little, Brown and Co., Boston.
Schultze, H.E. and Heremans, J.F. (Eds.) (1966) Molecular biology of human proteins, with special reference to plasma proteins. In Molecular Biology of Human Proteins, Vol. 1. Elsevier, Amsterdam.
Sharp, H.L. (1976) The current status of α-1-Antitrypsin, a protease inhibitor in gastrointestinal disease. Gastroenterology, 70, 611–621.
Spiro, R.G. (1973) Glycoproteins. Advances in Protein Chemistry, 27, 349–467.
Talamo, R.C. (1975) Basic and clinical aspects of the alpha$_1$-antitrypsin. Pediatrics, 56, 91–99.

ADDENDUM

Since this chapter was written, newer information pertinent to several sections has been encountered.

6.2.4. Amino acid metabolism

Glutamine is now recognized as an important energy source for the gut (Windmueller and Spaeth, 1978). Much of the consumed glutamine is converted by the gut to alanine, which then goes to the liver. Scheme 6.1 should be altered in this respect.

6.2.5.5. Ammonia

The enzymatic assay of blood ammonia with glutamic dehydrogenase has proven highly satisfactory and has been adapted to automatic instruments (e.g. Bruce et al., 1978).

6.3.1.1. Serum albumin

A dye-binding assay for albumin using bromocresol purple has been proposed which appears to avoid some of the problems of specificity inherent in the bromocresol green method (Pinnell and Northam, 1978). More experience with the new procedure will be awaited.

6.3.1.2. Transferrin

Measurement of serum ferritin concentrations in order to assess iron stores is increasing in popularity (Munro and Linder, 1978). This test appears to be more specific although not more sensitive than iron transferrin saturation as a measure of iron deficiency of iron stores.

6.3.1.5. Other proteins of normal metabolism and nutrition

A vitamin D-binding protein has been isolated from rat serum (Bouillon et al., 1978). It is an α_2-globulin of molecular weight 52,000, present at about 13 μmol/litre, which binds all three forms of the vitamin – vitamin D_3, 25-hydroxyvitamin D_3, and 1,25-dihydroxyvitamin D_3.

Bouillon, R., van Baelen, H., Rombants, W. and de Moor, P. (1978) The Isolation and characterization of the vitamin D-binding protein from rat serum. Journal of Biological Chemistry, 253, 4426–4431.

Bruce, A.W., Leiendecker, C.M. and Freier, E.F. (1978) Two-point determination of plasma ammonia with the centrifugal analyzer. Clinical Chemistry, 24, 782–787.

Munro, H.N. and Linder, M.C. (1978) Ferritin: structure, biosynthesis, and role in iron metabolism. Physiological Reviews, 58, 317–396.

Pinnell, A.E. and Northam, B.E. (1978) New automated dye-binding method for serum albumin determination with bromcresol purple. Clinical Chemistry, 24, 80–86.

Windmueller, H.G. and Spaeth, A.E. (1978) Identification of ketone bodies and glutamine as the major respiratory fuels in vivo for postabsorptive rat small intestine. Journal of Biological Chemistry, 253, 69–76.

Chapter 7

Enzymes

Mogens Hørder and J. Henry Wilkinson

Department of Clinical Chemistry, Odense University Hospital, DK-5000 Odense, Denmark and Department of Chemical Pathology, Charing Cross Hospital, Fulham Palace Road, London W6 8RF, England

CONTENTS

Chemical diagnosis of disease, edited by
S.S. Brown, F.L. Mitchell and D.S. Young

INTRODUCTION

Although the digestive enzymes have been studied as aids to diagnosis since the beginning of the present century, and the plasma phosphatases became established as useful tests in the clinical laboratory about 1934, it was the discovery of the transient elevation of aspartate transaminase (then known as glutamate oxaloacetate transaminase) in serum after myocardial infarction by LaDue, Wróblewski and Karmen in 1954 that led to the present upsurge of interest in clinical enzymology. This observation demonstrated that tissue damage leads to the liberation into the plasma of intracellular enzymes. Enzyme tests are now regularly used to assist the diagnosis of a variety of cardiac, hepatic, muscular, neoplastic, haematological and hereditary diseases. Currently, 10 to 15% of all tests performed in clinical chemistry laboratories are enzyme determinations.

7.1. MATERIALS

The various materials in which enzyme activities can be measured are listed in Table 7.1.

7.1.1. Enzymes in blood

7.1.1.1. Serum or plasma

The vast majority of enzyme tests are performed on specimens of serum or plasma – mainly serum, because of the problems posed by the presence of anticoagulants in plasma. Many of the commonly used anticoagulants are enzyme inhibitors: thus, ethylenediamine-tetraacetic acid (EDTA) almost completely inhibits the plasma alkaline phosphatase by removing Mg^{2+} ions which are essential activators of this enzyme; oxalate inhibits lactate dehydrogenase. When plasma is used heparin is the preferred anticoagulant; although it does have a slight inhibitory action on some enzymes, this does not usually exceed 10%.

On the other hand, if the separation of serum is delayed more than an hour or two after blood collection, there is a risk of leakage of enzymes from the blood cells even in the absence of overt haemolysis. The lactate dehydrogenase of serum is usually greater than that of the corresponding heparinized plasma, the discrepancy being attributed by Cohen and Larson (1966) to release of the enzyme from platelets. Nevertheless, enzyme tests are usually performed on serum, but it is important to separate it from the cells as soon as possible and to reject haemolyzed specimens since the erythrocytes may contain more than 100 times the enzyme activity of the serum.

The serum (or plasma) enzymes of established clinical values are listed in Table 7.2;

TABLE 7.1

CLINICAL MATERIALS FOR ENZYME ASSAY

Blood	Serum or plasma Erythrocytes Leucocytes Platelets
Other body fluids	Urine Cerebrospinal fluid Semen Amniotic fluid Sputum Pleural fluid Ascitic fluid Synovial fluid
Tissues	Skeletal muscle Liver Kidney Brain Skin Intestinal mucosa
Tissue cultures	Skin fibroblasts Amniotic cells

several others have been investigated but have found only limited applications in diagnosis. In some cases, enzymes whose assay is potentially valuable (e.g. ornithine carbamoyltransferase and sorbital dehydrogenase, which are highly specific for hepatocellular damage), are not commonly assayed because increases in their concentrations are much less sensitive markers than when other established enzymes are measured, e.g. alanine transaminase. Technical difficulties have prevented the widespread investigation of potentially useful enzymes such as argininosuccinase, an enzyme of the urea cycle which is believed to be highly specific for the detection of liver damage.

The occurrence of many enzymes in multiple forms has added greatly to the diagnostic value of enzyme tests, especially in the serum or plasma. The term *isoenzyme* has been applied to each of the multiple forms of enzymes, but the International Union of Biochemistry has recommended that the word should be used only for those forms of enzymes which are genetically determined. In clinical laboratories, however, the term has been applied to enzymes catalyzing the same reaction, but occurring in different physicochemical forms, irrespective of the mechanism involved in forming the catalytic structure.

TABLE 7.2.

SERUM (OR PLASMA) ENZYMES OF ESTABLISHED CLINICAL VALUE

Enzyme	EC No. *	Principal clinical applications
Lactate dehydrogenase	1.1.1.27	Myocardial infarction Megaloblastic and haemolytic anaemias Malignant disease
Isocitrate dehydrogenase	1.1.1.42	Liver diseases
Glutamate dehydrogenase	1.4.1.3	Liver diseases
γ-Glutamyltransferase	2.3.2.1	Hepatobiliary diseases
Aspartate transaminase	2.6.1.1	Myocardial infarction Liver diseases Muscle diseases
Alanine transaminase	2.6.1.2	Liver diseases
Creatine kinase	2.7.3.2	Myocardial infarction Muscle diseases
Cholinesterase	3.1.1.8	Suxamethonium sensitivity Liver diseases Organophosphorus insecticide poisoning
Alkaline phosphatase	3.1.3.1	Bone diseases Hepatobiliary diseases
Acid phosphatase	3.1.3.2	Carcinoma of the prostate Bone diseases
Amylase	3.2.1.1	Epidemic parotitis (mumps) Pancreatitis
Leucine aminopeptidase	3.4.11.1	Hepatobiliary diseases
Aldolase	4.1.2.13	Myocardial infarction Muscle diseases Liver diseases

* Enzyme Classification [Enzyme Nomenclature: Recommendations (1972) of the International Union of Pure and Applied Chemistry and the International Union of Biochemistry. Elsevier, Amsterdam, 1973.]

Five different isoenzymes of lactate dehydrogenase occur in most human tissues, but the proportions vary considerably from one tissue to another. This enzyme is a tetramer composed of four subunits which are of two types, usually designated as H (heart) or M (muscle). The subunits combine to form the set of isoenzymes: H_4, H_3M, H_2M_2, HM_3 and M_4. The H subunit contains a higher proportion of acidic aminoacids than the M subunit and on electrophoresis the H_4 isoenzyme migrates fastest towards the anode. This has led to the numbering of the isoenzymes, LD-1, LD-2, etc. (or LD_1, LD_2, etc.) in order of decreasing mobility towards the anode.

The creatine kinase molecule consists of only two subunits, but these also may be of two types: B (brain) or M (muscle). In addition to the BB and MM forms, there is also a hybrid MB isoenzyme which is found as a minor, although diagnostically important, component of the heart muscle enzyme.

The multiple forms of lactate dehydrogenase, creatine kinase and a number of other enzymes owe their occurrence to their subunit structures, the syntheses of which are controlled by separate genes; consequently they may be described as isoenzymes as defined by the International Union of Biochemistry. The mitochondrial and cytosolic forms of aspartate transaminase also qualify for description as isoenzymes since they have been shown to have quite different aminoacid compositions (section 7.3.1), but the various forms of alkaline phosphatase are more difficult to classify. The placental and intestinal mucosal enzymes differ from each other, and from other tissue phosphatases, in their physicochemical and kinetic properties; they may well be distinct entities, but the liver and bone enzymes show only slight differences from each other. The different electrophoretic mobilities of the various alkaline phosphatases appear to be due largely to differences in their sialic acid contents, since treatment with neuraminidase before electrophoresis reduces the mobility of all except the intestinal mucosal enzyme (Fishman and Ghosh, 1967).

The occurrence of serum cholinesterase in multiple forms is under genetic control, as several different phenotypes have been described (Harris et al., 1962), but up to seven interconvertible forms have been separated by starch-gel electrophoresis of a diluted human serum. On concentration, however, all these bands were converted into a single component, a phenomenon attributed to reversible polymerization (LaMotta et al., 1968).

Electrophoretic separation and other methods of investigation of the isoenzymes of lactate dehydrogenase, creatine kinase and alkaline phosphatase in serum have added greatly to the diagnostic value of these enzymes. The observed patterns reflect the isoenzyme composition of their tissues of origin (Table 7.3).

For further discussion of the multiple forms of enzymes the reader is referred to the monographs by Latner and Skillen (1968) and Wilkinson (1970a).

7.1.1.2. Erythrocytes

The erythrocytes are rich sources of enzymes, especially those concerned with glycolysis and the pentose phosphate shunt. Red cell enzymes have been extensively investigated in hereditary haematological diseases, some of which are associated with defects in the synthesis of particular enzymes, notably glucose-6-phosphate dehydrogenase and pyruvate kinase (Beutler, 1976). Many red cell enzymes exhibit genetic polymorphism and there

TABLE 7.3

DISTRIBUTION OF COMMONLY MEASURED ISOENZYMES IN HUMAN TISSUES

Enzyme	Isoenzyme	Tissue
Lactate dehydrogenase	LD-1 (most anionic)	Heart, erythrocytes, brain, kidney
	LD-3	Leucocytes, adrenal, thyroid
	LD-5 (most cationic)	Skeletal muscle (white fibres), liver
Creatine kinase	BB (most anionic)	Brain, lung, thyroid
	MB	Heart (minor component)
	MM (most cationic)	Skeletal muscle, heart
Alkaline phosphatase	Liver (most anionic)	Liver
	Bone (mobility close behind liver isoenzyme)	Bone
	Placenta (heat-stable, L-phenylalanine-sensitive)	Placenta
	Intestinal (most cationic, L-phenylalanine-sensitive)	Intestinal mucosa

are numerous examples of the association between the electrophoretic or kinetic abnormalities of a particular enzyme and congenital non-spherocytic haemolytic anaemia or sensitivity to drugs. The occurrence of variant phenotypes in the healthy population, however, sometimes poses problems of interpretation.

Since the erythrocyte is devoid of a nucleus and hence cannot synthesize proteins, its enzyme complement cannot be replaced during its life. Consequently, during the ageing process, enzyme activity tends to fall. This is particularly well marked in the case of hexokinase and aspartate transaminase, the activities of which are significantly higher in young cells than in aged cells. Thus erythrocytic enzyme activities tend to be increased above the normal range in patients with a reticulocytosis.

Although red cells are readily available for study, their use in diagnostic enzymology is limited for the reasons summarized above.

Leucocytes are also readily available, although the numbers present in a 10 to 15 ml specimen of blood limit the range of enzyme determinations which can be carried out in an individual patient. Nevertheless, they have proved useful in confirming the presence of glycogen storage disease and identifying the type. In this instance, enzyme studies on leucocytes often avoid the necessity for tissue biopsy (Ryman, 1976). Neutrophil alkaline phosphatase activity has proved useful in the diagnosis of Down's syndrome (mongolism), which is characterized by increased activity, which is usually demonstrated cytochemically. This technique has also found application in various forms of leukaemia and other haematological diseases.

Hitherto few reports have appeared on the assay of enzymes in platelets, and at the present time the clinical value of such measurements is doubtful.

7.1.2. Enzymes in other body fluids

7.1.2.1. Urine

Urine is of course the most accessible body fluid, but as a medium for enzyme study it has many drawbacks. In the absence of renal disease, only those enzymes with a molecular mass of less than 55,000 (e.g. amylase, uropepsin) appear in the urine in significant quantities. No more than traces of lactate dehydrogenase or aspartate transaminase can be detected in normal urine, although in renal disease markedly increased amounts may be observed (Wilkinson, 1968).

Owing to its acid pH and the presence of high concentrations of urea and certain other enzyme inhibitors, urine is a hostile environment for enzymes. Moreover, the involuntary incubation of urine at body temperature in the bladder for several hours tends to enhance the effects of inhibitors. Urinary enzyme measurements are therefore of only limited value as aids to diagnosis, but in certain instances they may be useful. In the differential diagnosis of the acute abdomen, an increased serum amylase activity is indicative of acute pancreatitis, but the elevation is transient, and a raised urinary activity may give useful information after the serum activity has returned to normal. Other examples are the raised urinary lactate dehydrogenase and alkaline phosphatase activities which occur in benign and malignant diseases of the urinary tract.

The presence in urine of urea and oxalate, which preferentially inhibit LD-5 and LD-1 respectively, casts doubt upon the reliability of measurements of lactate dehydrogenase isoenzymes in urine. Nevertheless, Ringoir (1967) has reported favourably on the value of urinary LD-5 as an index of impending rejection in patients receiving kidney transplants; Wellwood et al. (1973) measured the urinary N-acetylglucosaminidase activity for this purpose.

Dubach (1966) has suggested that the urinary lactate dehydrogenase originates largely in urinary deposits, cells, casts, etc., but Rosalki and Wilkinson (1960) reported high activities in cell- and cast-free urines of patients with renal disease, and considered the urinary enzyme to originate in the damaged kidney. Another possibility is that the damaged glomerulus might permit serum enzymes to pass into the urine. It is likely that in some patients all three mechanisms might operate simultaneously, but examples can be quoted where one or other may be excluded.

7.1.2.2. Other body fluids

Although there are several reports in the literature, enzyme studies on other body fluids have not yet proved to be of diagnostic value except in rare instances.

No more than traces of enzyme activity can be detected in normal cerebrospinal fluid; in cerebrovascular disease, increased enzyme activity is rarely encountered unless the protein concentration is markedly elevated. The blood–brain barrier appears to be impermeable to plasma enzymes.

The semen is of interest from the enzymological viewpoint mainly because it contains a sixth lactate dehydrogenase isoenzyme (LD-X) which is not found elsewhere. This isoenzyme appears to be associated with spermatogenesis, since it accounts for about 70% of the total lactate dehydrogenase activity of the spermatozoa, and is not found in the prepubertal testis. The semen is also rich in acid phosphatase, derived very largely from the prostate. Although measurement of the activities of these enzymes has found application in forensic medicine, seminal fluid enzymes have not established a role in clinical diagnosis.

While amniotic fluid enzymes have not proved to be of direct interest in diagnosis, the enzymes of amniotic cells have assisted the pre-natal diagnosis of certain hereditary diseases, especially the lethal Type II (Pompe) glycogen storage disease (Ryman, 1976).

7.1.3. Enzymes in tissues

Enzymes tests on biopsy specimens are usually performed to confirm the diagnosis of a congenital enzyme anomaly, but wherever possible such tests are carried out on blood cells in order to avoid subjecting the patient to unnecessary trauma. Liver and muscle biopsy specimens, for example, are required to confirm the absence of liver glucose-6-phosphatase and muscle phosphorylase in Types I (von Gierke) and V (McArdle) glycogen storage diseases, respectively (Ryman, 1976). Biopsy specimens of the intestinal mucosa are essential to establish disaccharidase deficiencies, because these enzymes are confined to the brush border and are not normally released into the succus entericus (Gowenlock, 1976).

Diagnosis of the enzyme defect in certain mucopolysaccharidoses, lipidoses and other herditary diseases can sometimes be made in cultured skin fibroblasts, thus obviating the need for biopsy of the liver or other internal organ (Raine and Westwood, 1976).

7.2. METHODOLOGY

7.2.1. Enzyme assay

Since enzymes are catalytically-active proteins, their concentrations may, in principle, be determined by any of the methods commonly employed for non-catalytically-active proteins, e.g. measurement of specific absorbance, refractive index, etc. In practice it is generally difficult to employ such methods owing to the presence of relatively large concentrations of other proteins, enzymic or non-enzymic, in the available samples, usually serum or plasma. Some enzymes, however, such as caeruloplasmin, have characteristic absorption spectra which can be utilized for measuring their concentrations in the presence of other proteins.

Alternatively, immunological techniques may be employed when specific antisera are available. Immunodiffusion in agar-gel on Ouchterlony plates is commonly employed for protein determination, and such a procedure may be used for enzyme assays. However, in most body fluids the enzyme concentration may be extremely low, and immunodiffusion is consequently rather insensitive. Radioimmunoassay techniques in which a radioactively labelled antigen competes with the unlabelled antigen for binding sites on an antibody have the required sensitivity, but hitherto have not been extensively employed for the assay of enzymes in clinical material. The main problem is the poor correlation observed between measurements of catalytic activity and radioimmunoassay procedures, owing to the fact that inactivated enzyme protein may still be immunologically reactive.

The catalytic sites of enzymes can in some cases be titrated with suitable reagents. Thus reactive thiol groups at the active centre may be titrated with such reagents as iodoacetate or a heavy metal. These procedures have been extensively used for the study of the structures of active sites, but pure enzymes are required and there is the possibility that the reagent may couple with groups on the enzyme molecule at positions outside the active site. Titration of active sites is not suitable for clinical purposes because it is rarely practicable to isolate and purify the enzyme concerned.

In general the methods discussed above are too time consuming for use in the clinical laboratory, apart from their other limitations, and measurement of the catalytic activities of enzymes is universally employed for diagnostic purposes. The reaction rate is measured by determining the amount of product formed, or substrate consumed, over a timed period, but the conditions under which the reaction is carried out are critical. Measurement of reaction rates has the important advantage of being independent of the presence of other proteins and consequently it can be applied to serum, plasma or tissue extracts, although care must be taken to ensure the absence of competing reactions.

7.2.2. Measurement of enzyme activities

The unit of catalytic activity which is recommended by the International Union of Biochemistry is the *katal* i.e. that amount of enzyme activity which converts one mol of substrate or forms one mol of product per second. At the present time this unit has not been generally accepted, as it is inconveniently large for clinical purposes, but it is widely used in Scandinavia. Thus Dybkaer (1975, 1977) has described its application, pointing out that concentrations of enzyme activity (catalytic ability) should be expressed in katals (or submultiples) per litre (kat/litre).

Elsewhere, the earlier International Unit (U) is widely used. This unit is defined as that amount of catalytic activity which converts one micromol of substrate per minute, i.e. 6×10^7 U = 1 katal. The reference volume is usually the litre, so that enzyme activities are expressed as U/litre.

The introduction of the International Unit and the katal has disappointed those who hoped that the replacement of many earlier units, e.g. the King–Armstrong and Bodansky units for alkaline phosphatase, and the Karmen unit for aspartate transaminase, would lead to greater comparability between the results reported by different laboratories. Discrepancies are due to differences in methodology and to variations in the conditions employed. It is generally accepted that in the clinical laboratory enzyme determinations should be performed under optimal conditions, so that the highest possible activity is measured.

Methods can broadly be divided into two classes: those involving measurement of product or substrate concentrations before and after a fixed incubation period (two-point assays), and those in which the concentration of a reactant is monitored continually or intermittently over a period of time (continuous monitoring methods).

7.2.2.1. Two-point assays

Two-point assays are exemplified by the King–Armstrong method for alkaline phosphatase as re-defined by Moss et al. (1971). In this procedure the enzyme preparation (usually serum) is incubated at 37 °C in a carbonate–bicarbonate buffer at pH 10.0 with the substrate, phenyl phosphate, and the amount of phenol liberated after 15 minutes is determined colorimetrically with the Folin–Ciocalteu or amino-antipyrine reagents. The problem which is exemplified by this technique is that while it is known how much phenol is liberated over the reaction period, there is no means of ascertaining whether the rate is constant throughout, i.e. whether the reaction obeys zero-order kinetics, so that the reaction rate is independent of the substrate concentration and hence depends solely on the enzyme concentration. While enzyme activities can be derived from first-order and mixed-order kinetics (Statland and Louderback, 1972), the mathematics and the equipment required are necessarily more complicated, and for clinical purposes the aim is to use reactions involving zero-order kinetics. In a two-point assay such as that outlined above, there is no means of checking that product formation is indeed rectilinear with time. This limitation applies equally to semi-automated (e.g. AutoAnalyzer) procedures depending upon one or two measurements. However, there is a wealth of evidence establishing that the alkaline phosphatase reaction follows a rectilinear course, within certain limits, with serum specimens from a variety of patients, but this requirement is not met by many other two-point assay procedures.

7.2.2.2. Continuous monitoring techniques

The introduction of the recording spectrophotometer has enabled the course of an enzyme reaction to be followed and its initial reaction rate to be measured. Allowances can be made,for deviations from rectilinearity, due to an initial lag phase or to substrate or coenzyme exhaustion, which are not possible when a two-point assay system is employed. Continuous monitoring techniques are readily applied to the measurement of the activities of enzyme dependent on the reduction of NAD^+ or $NADP^+$ or the oxidation of the corresponding reduced co-enzymes, since the reduced forms have specific absorbance peaks at about 340 nm. Fluorometric techniques may also be used for following the course of such reactions since NADH and NADPH are fluorescent under certain conditions (Lowry and Passonneau, 1972).

Many clinically important non-NAD(P)-dependent enzymes may be determined spectrophotometrically (or fluorometrically) by coupling their reactions with one which is catalyzed by an NAD^+- or NADP-dependent dehydrogenase. Typical examples are aspartate and alanine transaminases and creatine kinase:

Aspartate transaminase (Karmen, 1955)

(1) Aspartate + 2-oxoglutarate ⇌ glutamate + oxaloacetate

$$\text{(2) Oxaloacetate} + \text{NADH} + \text{H}^+ \underset{\text{dehydrogenase}}{\overset{\text{malate}}{\rightleftharpoons}} \text{malate} + \text{NAD}^+$$

Alanine transaminase (Wróblewski and LaDue, 1956)

(1) Alanine + 2-oxoglutarate ⇌ glutamate + pyruvate

$$\text{(2) Pyruvate} + \text{NADH} + \text{H}^+ \underset{\text{dehydrogenase}}{\overset{\text{lactate}}{\rightleftharpoons}} \text{lactate} + \text{NAD}^+$$

Creatine kinase (Oliver, 1955; Rosalki, 1967)

(1) Creatine phosphate + ADP ⇌ ATP + creatine

$$\text{(2) ATP} + \text{glucose} \xrightarrow{\text{hexokinase}} \text{glucose 6-phosphate} + \text{ADP}$$

$$\text{(3) Glucose-6-phosphate} + \text{NADP}^+ \underset{\text{dehydrogenase}}{\overset{\text{glucose-6-phosphate}}{\rightleftharpoons}} \text{6-phosphogluconate} + \text{NADlH} + \text{H}^+$$

When using a technique involving an auxiliary or indicator enzyme, it is essential that sufficient activity be present in the reaction mixture to ensure that reactions (2) and (3) do not become rate-limiting.

7.2.2.3. Reaction conditions

Enzyme activity is of course dependent upon enzyme concentration, but direct proportionality cannot be assumed unless the conditions under which the reaction is performed are rigidly controlled. Among the variables to be considered are the substrate and coenzyme concentrations; the nature of the buffer, its strength and pH; the temperature; the presence of activators in adequate concentration; freedom from inhibitors; and the presence of auxiliary and indicator enzymes in adequate concentration. Discussion will be restricted to brief considerations of the roles of the substrate concentration and the reaction temperature.

The typical Michaelis curve illustrates that enzyme activity increases asymptotically with increasing substrate concentration, and consequently the theoretical maximum velocity (V_{max}) can never be reached in practice. Degeller and Sandifort (1973) have recommended that for clinical purposes the aim should be to use a substrate concentration of $20 \times K_m$, which should give reaction velocities of 95% of the V_{max}. In practice this is difficult to achieve owing to the limited solubility, or the high cost, of some substrates. Furthermore, some enzymes are inhibited by excess substrate; thus lactate dehydrogenase is inhibited by excess pyruvate and determinations must therefore be performed with the optimum concentration, even though the observed reaction rate is appreciably lower than the V_{max}.

Enzyme determinations should be performed at a fixed temperature, preferably with a tolerance not greater than ±0.1 °C, but in recent years much controversy has arisen over the choice of temperature. The International Union of Biochemistry initially recommended 25 °C, but later changed this to 30 °C because of the difficulty experienced in cooling reaction vessels to 25 °C in hot countries. However, 30 °C was not widely accepted in clinical laboratories where in general 37 °C was preferred. The situation has been complicated by the introduction of certain mechanized instruments for the spectrophotometric determination of enzymes, which are factory-set to operate at 35 °C or 37 °C. The Expert Panel on Enzymes of the International Federation of Clinical Chemistry has reconsidered the question, and it is understood that 30 °C is favoured owing to the risk of denaturation of certain enzyme proteins during pre-incubation at 37 °C. It is expected that in due course all laboratories will be recommended to carry out enzyme determinations at 30 °C. Meanwhile the Scandinavian Clinical Chemistry Societies have recommended 37 °C, and the German Society, 25 °C.

7.2.2.4. Calibration of enzyme determinations

The most widely used method of calibration of enzyme activity measurements involves use of the molar absorptivity of the reduced forms of NAD^+ or $NADP^+$ since many of the enzymes commonly determined are either dependent upon one or other of these co-enzymes, or their reactions can be coupled with an indicator enzyme which is NAD^+- or $NADP^+$-dependent. The molar absorptivity of these reduced co-enzymes at 340 nm is generally taken to be 6220 litre · mol^{-1} · cm^{-1}, but a slightly higher figure may be more accurate (6317 litre · mol^{-1} · cm^{-1}, McComb et al., 1976; 6292 litre · mol^{-1} · cm^{-1}, Ziegenhorn et al., 1976).

The molar absorptivity of *p*-nitrophenol may be used to calibrate determinations of alkaline *p*-nitrophenylphosphatase activity (Wilkinson et al., 1969), but the King–Armstrong method (section 7.2.2.1), depends upon the colorimetric determination of a phenol standard.

Another approach to calibration involves the use of commercial "enzyme standards". These are preparations, the enzyme activity of which has been determined by accepted methods. On the basis of these measurements, a value for the activity is assigned and the material is supplied for use as a "secondary standard". While such "standards" may give satisfactory results (Ellis, 1976), their use is open to the objections that errors in the primary and secondary calibrations are summated, and that it is difficult to guard against random deterioration during distribution, e.g. by exposure to heat or sunshine.

It is generally agreed that temperature conversion factors should not be used. Transaminase activities determined at 37 °C average approximately twice those measured at 25 °C, but different specimens vary appreciably in their temperature coefficients (Rosalki et al., 1975).

7.2.3. Current analytical reliability

The precision which is found in replicate analyses of enzyme activities in an individual laboratory rarely approaches that achieved for the analysis of electrolytes or of relatively simple organic compounds such as urea or glucose. This is due to the difficulties inherent in the determination of reaction rates which are affected by minor variations in the conditions mentioned above. At the upper limit of the reference interval, the transaminases can be determined with a standard deviation of ±1.5 U/litre, i.e. a coefficient of variation of about ±7%, under the most favourable conditions. The standard deviation increases only slightly with marginally raised activities, and the coefficient of variation consequently falls to about ±5%, i.e. there is a 95% probability that the true value of a result reported as 100 U/litre will lie between 90 and 110 U/litre. This represents the present "state of the art", but with improved instrumentation and better procedures it is to be hoped that during the next decade this degree of uncertainly will be reduced.

The "between-laboratory" precision of enzyme tests, however, is much worse, even when the same technique is employed. For example, the *Ringversuche* of the German Society for Clinical Chemistry regularly reports coefficients of variation for transaminase determinations ranging from 15 to 20% despite the fact that the majority of German laboratories use a standardized procedure. Similar variances have been reported in other countries for a particular procedure, but the scatter of results when different techniques are employed is often much greater. Certain of the less precise techniques, such as those depending on the colorimetric measurement of a dinitrophenylhydrazone, should no longer be used. Increasing attention is being paid to the causes of these discrepancies, and a number of reference methods have been proposed. International co-operation in devising and checking such procedures will undoubtedly improve the situation, but at present it is difficult to compare the results obtained in one laboratory with those observed in another. In this book, we have favoured the presentation of enzyme data with reference to a "normal" limit, in preference to indicating actual values that are subject to this method dependency.

7.2.4. Identification and measurement of isoenzymes

In most clinical laboratories, isoenzymes are separated by electrophoresis on a suitable medium, e.g. cellulose acetate. This at best is only semi-quantitative owing to the impracticability of using optimum reaction conditions for detecting individual isoenzymes, and to the "nothing dehydrogenase" phenomenon which is due, it seems, to the reaction of traces of alcohol in the reagents with alcohol dehydrogenase (Beutler, 1967; Shaw and Koen, 1967). In general, the isoenzyme present in largest amount tends to be under-estimated, particularly when tetrazolium-staining techniques are employed. Scanning of electropherograms thus gives a set of figures of rather dubious value, and too much reliance should not be placed upon the results so obtained. A marked increase in the concentration of a particular isoenzyme can usually be detected by visual inspection, e.g. an increase in LD-1 and LD-2 is suggestive of myocardial infarction, and a rise in LD-5 is indicative of hepatocellular damage.

The qualitative electrophoretic study of the alkaline phosphatase of serum frequently provides information on the tissue of origin of a raised serum activity, and the presence of the MB isoenzyme of creatine kinase is a valuable means of confirming myocardial infarction. A semi-quantitative scanning technique based upon the fluorescence of NADPH has been devised by Konttinen and Somer (1972) for demonstrating the presence of this isoenzyme in serum, but a method dependent upon the inhibition of the M sub-unit by a specific antibody (Jockers-Wretou and Pfleiderer, 1975) appears even more promising for clinical purposes.

Several non-electrophoretic techniques have been devised for the estimation of the relative proportions of lactate dehydrogenase isoenzymes in serum, but they all suffer from the disadvantage of being unable to differentiate concurrent increases in LD-1 and LD-5 from an increase in LD-3. These are based upon the use of substrate analogues, of heat inactivation or of urea inactivation (Wilkinson, 1970a). Similar techniques have been used to aid the differentiation of liver and bone alkaline phosphatases (Moss et al., 1972).

7.3. BIOCHEMISTRY AND PHYSIOLOGY OF ENZYMES

7.3.1. Subcellular localization of enzymes

The internal organization of a cell is such as to permit a complex series of inter-related enzymically catalyzed chemical reactions to proceed in an orderly fashion. If all enzymes were to be distributed solely in the cell sap (cytosol), interference with the reactions of one by another would be inevitable, and competition for common substrates would occur in a chaotic manner. Glucose-6-phosphate, for example, is a key intermediate in the glycolytic pathway where it serves as a substrate for glucose phosphate isomerase and glucose-6-phosphate dehydrogenase, but it is also attacked by glucose-6-phosphatase and alkaline phosphatase. The phosphatases would interfere with glycolysis if they were present in the cell sap, but glucose-6-phosphatase is almost exclusively confined to the microsomes of the liver, while alkaline phosphatase is membrane-bound, though occurring in a variety of tissues.

It follows that the distribution of enzymes throughout the various subcellular organelles (Figure 7.1) is a vital factor in the maintenance of metabolic processes. Those enzymes which are primarily concerned with respiratory processes occur in the mitochondria, while those believed to be involved in transport mechanisms are usually bound to the relevant membranes. Table 7.4 lists the subcellular organelles with which some of the enzymes of diagnostic interest are associated.

Some enzymes occur in different forms in different organelles. The mitochondrial form of malate dehydrogenase, for example, differs in several of its properties from that found in the cytosol. The latter form appears to be more suited to the reduction of oxaloacetate to malate which can freely enter the mitochondrion, where the enzyme is more effective in catalyzing the reverse reaction. The net result is the transfer of hydrogen from cytoplasmic NADH to mitochondrial NAD^+ (Kaplan, 1963).

Mitochondrial aspartate transaminase has been shown to differ in its aminoacid composition, and thus to be a quite different protein, from the cytosolic enzyme (Martinez-Carrion and Tiemeier, 1967).

The nature of the subcellular binding of an enzyme is sometimes of diagnostic value. The release of mitochondrial enzymes, e.g. glutamate dehydrogenase, or the mitochondrial form of aspartate transaminase, into the plasma is considered to be a useful indicator of cellular necrosis (see section 7.3.3.1), while an increase of certain microsomal enzymes, particularly γ-glutamyltransferase, may be due to enzyme induction by alcohol or certain drugs (Rosalki and Rau, 1972).

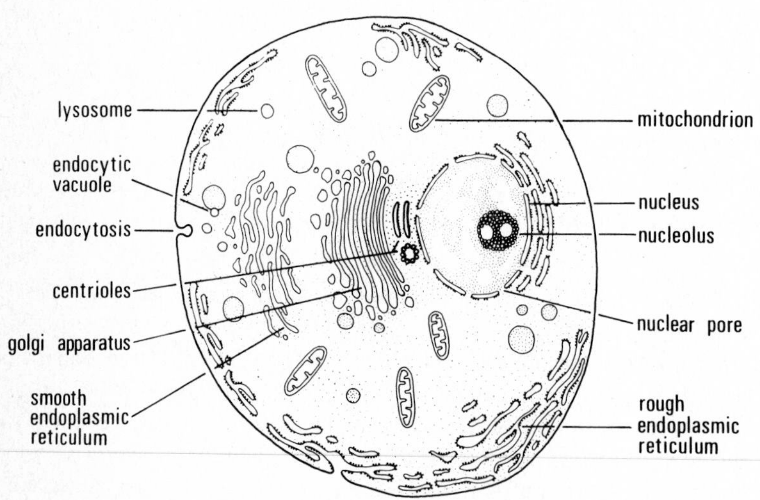

Figure 7.1. Diagram of a typical cell showing the main subcellular organelles. (Kindly provided by Dr. A.C. Allison)

TABLE 7.4

SUBCELLULAR LOCALIZATION OF THE PRINCIPAL INTRACELLULAR ENZYMES OF CLINICAL IMPORTANCE

Enzyme	Subcellular fraction				
	Cytosol	Mitochondria	Micro-somes	Nucleus	Membrane
Sorbitol dehydrogenase	+				
Lactate dehydrogenase	+				
Malate dehydrogenase	+	+	+		
Isocitrate dehydrogenase (NAD^+)		+			
Isocitrate dehydrogenase (NADP)	+				
Glucose-6-phosphate dehydrogenase	+				
Glutamate dehydrogenase		+			
Ornithine carbamoyltransferase	+				
γ-Glutamyltransferase			+		
Aspartate transaminase *	+	+			
Alanine transaminase	+				
Creatine kinase	+				
Phosphoglucomutase	+				
Alkaline phosphatase			+		+
Acid phosphatase		+			
5′-Nucleotidase		+	+	+	
Glucose-6-phosphatase			+		
Leucine aminopeptidase	+				
Arginase		+	+	+	
Aldolase	+			+	

* Different forms of aspartate transaminase occur in the cytosol and mitochondria

7.3.2. Synthesis of enzymes and its regulation

Like other proteins, enzymes are synthesized in the ribosomes of the endoplasmic reticulum on specific RNA templates, themsleves translated from coded DNA sequences in individual genes in the nucleus. Individual aminoacids are transported by specific transfer RNA to the template, where they are assembled in the sequence laid down by the genetic code. A detailed discussion of the processes involved in protein synthesis would be out of place in this Chapter, but reference must be made to genetic defects which result in failure to synthesize a particular enzyme and hence to inherited disease, e.g. galactosaemia due to deficiency of hexose-1-phosphate uridylyltransferase, or phenylketonuria due to deficiency of phenylalanine-4-oxygenase (phenylalanine hydroxylase). In such conditions, the gene responsible for coding the enzyme protein is absent or defective.

Some enzymes are synthesized at multiple gene loci. An example is lactate dehydrogenase, the H and M subunits of which are synthesized independently and subsequently undergo homopolymerization or heteropolymerization to form the series of tetrameric isoenzymes, H_4, H_3M, H_2M_2, HM_3 and M_4. There is evidence that hypoxic conditions lead to a relative increase in the synthesis of the M subunit (Goodfriend et al., 1966; Hellung-Larsen and Anderson, 1968). Since the H and M subunits have different aminoacid sequences (though they have similar molecular weights), the five isoenzymes differ in their physicochemical and catalytic properties, though they are all capable of reversibly oxidizing lactate in the presence of the appropriate form of the co-enzyme (NAD^+).

Other enzymes owe their occurrence in multiple forms to the presence of alleles at a single gene locus.

Regulation of enzyme synthesis in response to an excess or a deficiency of substrate occurs, but the process is relatively slow. In untreated diabetes mellitus, enzymes concerned with gluconeogenesis are synthesized in increased amounts, but treatment with insulin gradually reverses this process. Reference has already been made to the increased biosynthesis of γ-glutamyltransferase in response to the administration of alcohol, but the synthesis of other enzymes is also induced by drugs, e.g. UDP glucuronyltransferase which converts bilirubin into its soluble ester glucuronides.

7.3.3. The origin and fate of plasma enzymes

The elevated activities of enzymes found in the plasma in disease states are due to leakage from damaged tissues, but until recently the mechanisms involved have not been studied very extensively. The early literature of clinical enzymology contains many references which attributed raised serum enzyme activities to cell necrosis. Although necrosis undoubtedly leads to the discharge of the cell contents, including enzymes, into the circulation, there are several clinical situations in which the elevations of serum enzyme activities are disproportionately high in relation to the extent of cell necrosis. Raised serum enzyme activities are also associated with a variety of inflammatory disorders, and it must be concluded that factors other than cell death are involved in the release of intracellular enzymes through the cell membrane.

In acute disorders, such as myocardial infarction and acute hepatitis, serum enzyme activities rise to a peak and then gradually return to normal levels. Clearly the body has mechanisms for removing enzymes from the circulation but, with a few exceptions, excretion in the urine or bile is negligible. Most enzymes are proteins with relatively high molecular mass and the majority of those of clinical interest cannot by filtered by the glomerulus and, apart from amylase and pepsinogen (with molecular masses of 48,000 and 42,500, respectively), no more than trace amounts can be detected in normal urine. The elevated serum alkaline phosphatase associated with obstructive jaundice was for many years explained by the theory that it normally originates in the bones and is excreted in the bile (Gutman, 1959), but this hypothesis has since proved untenable (Posen, 1970).

Whatever the mechanisms involved, the circulating concentration of a given enzyme is the resultant of two opposing processes: release from a damaged tissue and removal from the plasma. The activity which is normally found in the plasma of healthy individuals is regarded as being derived from "wear-and-tear" cell breakdown.

7.3.3.1. Release of intracellular enzymes

Cell necrosis is followed by disintegration of the cell membranes, so permitting intracellular enzymes to be released into the extracellular fluid. Since both cell membranes and mitochondrial membranes are disrupted, cytosolic and mitochondrial enzymes are likely to be present in the plasma in necrotic conditions. Thus in myocardial infarction both the cytosolic and mitochondrial forms of aspartate transaminase can be detected in the plasma (Boyde, 1968; Murros et al., 1973). Both of these isoenzymes occur in the plasma of patients with severe hepatitis or acute exacerbations of cirrhosis (Schmidt et al., 1967), conditions in which the liver mitochondrial enzyme, glutamate dehydrogenase, can also be detected in the plasma (Schmidt and Schmidt, 1962). Cell necrosis is a feature of all three disorders. Since mitochondrial enzymes can rarely be detected in the plasma in inflammatory states, measurement of cytosolic and mitochondrial enzyme activities may indicate whether the tissue damage is mainly inflammatory or predominantly necrotic.

The increased membrane permeability which is associated with inflammatory disorders has been investigated experimentally. Enzyme release from tissues slices has been described, but mechanical damage could lead to enzyme leakage in such preparations. Zierler (1958), however, showed that the efflux of aldolase from intact rat muscles was markedly increased by such factors as anoxia, deprivation of glucose, the presence of metabolic inhibitors and electrolyte imbalance. The release of lactate dehydrogenase from human leucocytes during incubation was demonstrated by Englhardt et al., (1969) to be associated with a reduction in the intracellular ATP concentration, and Wilkinson and Robinson (1974a, b) showed that incorporation of ATP into the medium markedly reduced the loss of intracellular enzymes from rat lymphocytes and human leucocytes. It seems, therefore, that the integrity of the membrane is dependent upon the ATP (i.e. energy) content of the cell, and it has been suggested that a common factor in tissue damage due to virus infections, chemical or mechanical trauma, hypoxia, etc., is failure to synthesize ATP in adequate amounts (Wilkinson and Robinson, 1974b). A similar suggestion was made by Sweetin and Thomson (1973) to explain their observation that in human erythrocytes significant loss of enzymes did not occur until the glucose content of the medium was exhausted.

Other high-energy phosphates, such as UTP and phosphoenolpyruvate, also exert protective effects which are due, it seems, to the availability of enzymes capable of converting them into ATP (Wilkinson and Robinson, 1974b). While the energy content of the cell appears to be an important factor in maintaining the integrity of the membrane and so preventing loss of intracellular enzymes, there is evidence that adenosine nucleotides may have a direct action on the membrane. ADP and AMP protect human lymphocytes and erythrocytes against enzyme leakage, whereas in rat lymphocytes ADP has little effect while AMP increases enzyme loss (Wilkinson et al., 1975; Hallak and Wilkinson, 1976).

7.3.3.2. Disappearance of enzymes from the circulation

The disappearance of enzymes from the circulating plasma has been studied clinically and experimentally in a variety of ways, but until recently most of the information gained has been of a rather negative nature. Thus Strandjord et al. (1959) found that the rates of disappearance of lactate and isocitrate dehydrogenases from the plasma of dogs which had been injected with the pure enzymes were unaffected by removal of the liver, kidneys or spleen – a finding which appears to exclude an excretory mechanism. Similar conclusions were reached by Rosalki and Wilkinson (1959) who found that, in the absence of renal disease, enzymes occur in the urine in trace amounts only, except those with low molecular mass.

There is abundant clinical evidence that the rates at which enzymes disappear from the plasma differ considerably from one enzyme to another. Thus, despite peak elevation to about 10 times the upper limit of normal after myocardial infarction, the plasma creatine kinase returns to the normal range by about the third day, while the more modest elevations of aspartate transaminase and lactate dehydrogenase (mainly LD-1) persist for about 5 and 10 days, respectively. It is difficult to deduce reliable figures for the biological half-lives of enzymes in the plasma from clinical tests, because it can rarely be established when discharge of enzymes from the damaged tissue ceased. However, a number of acute cases have been recorded in which very high plasma enzyme activities have followed an exponential course during their return to normal. For example, serial determination on the serum of a patient with idiopathic myoglobinuria gave the following biological half-lives: creatine kinase, 1.4 days; aspartate transaminase, 2.0 days; alanine transaminase, 6.3 days (Wilkinson, 1970b).

As already indicated, many investigators have injected purified enzymes into experimental animals and have followed the rates at which the corresponding activities in the plasma disappear. Amelung (1960), for example, determined the biological half-lives of muscle lactate dehydrogenase, and other enzymes, from the biphasic disappearance curves observed after injection of enzymes into the rabbit. The first rapid phase is attributed to distribution throughout the extracellular fluid, while the second slower phase represents catabolism of the enzyme. Aspartate and alanine transaminases were found to disappear from the plasma of the dog according to a triphasic catenary system (Fleisher and Wakim, 1963; Wakim and Fleisher, 1963a; b), and similar results have been reported for lactate dehydrogenase in the sheep (Boyd, 1967). Wakim and Fleisher (1963b) suggested that the reticuloendothelial system might be involved in the removal of enzymes from the circulation.

Breakdown in the circulation was first suggested by Schmidt and Schmidt (1960) who observed a gradual loss of substrate affinity, evidenced by a progressive increase in the Michaelis constant (K_m) of malate dehydrogenase in successive serum samples taken from a patient with myocardial infarction. On the other hand, however, Wakim and Fleisher (1963a) were unable to detect any change in the K_m value for aspartate transaminase injected into a dog, and it seems that the change in the K_m value for malate dehydrogenase noted above might have been due to alterations in the proportions of circulating isoenzymes.

Studies of the rates of disappearance of injected enzymes cannot give any indication of their catalytic fate, in the absence of measurements of the concentrations of enzyme proteins in the plasma as well as their catalytic activities. The disappearance rates for several radioactively labelled enzymes have now been reported, but a number of problems are inherent in this approach. In addition to the difficulty encountered in labelling the enzyme without seriously impairing its catalytic activity (Bär et al., 1972), the question arises as to whether the body handles the labelled protein in the same manner as the endogenous enzyme.

In most cases enzymes have been labelled with ^{131}I or ^{125}I, but the oxidizing conditions required for iodination cause marked inactivation, and recoveries of catalytic activity average about 15%. However 80 to 85% recoveries were obtained when solid-state lactoperoxidase on Sepharose beads was used in the radio-iodination of lactate dehydrogenase-1 with ^{125}I (Wilkinson and Qureshi, 1976). Similar yields of active enzyme were also obtained by Bär et al. (1972) when lactate dehydrogenase-5 was labelled with [^{14}C]acetic anhydride.

Both Schapira et al. (1962), who studied the catabolism of injected ^{131}I-labelled aldolase in the rabbit, and Massarat (1965) who injected ^{131}I-labelled aspartate and alanine transaminases into the pig, reported that radioactivity and catalytic activity disappeared at similar rates, from which they concluded that the enzyme protein is not inactivated in the plasma. However, Posen (1970) suggests that similar disappearance rates for catalytic activity and radioactivity do not necessarily exclude the possibility of intravascular inactivation if the interval between inactivation and removal of the products is very short.

Recently, however, strong evidence in support of the intravascular inactivation theory has been obtained from studies in which ^{125}I-labelled lactate dehydrogenase-5 was injected into the rabbit (Qureshi and Wilkinson, 1976). The catalytic activity was found to disappear from the plasma at a faster rate than the radioactivity (Table 7.5). Though it disappears at a much slower rate than isoenzyme 5, ^{125}I-labelled lactate dehydrogenase-1 also appears to be catabolized in the circulation in the rabbit (Table 7.5) (Wilkinson and Qureshi, 1976).

In experiments with both isoenzymes, appreciable radioactivity was subsequently detected in the intestinal contents, and Qureshi and Wilkinson (1976) suggested that after inactivation in the circulating plasma, the radioactive, but catalytically inactive, products discharged into the intestine in a similar manner to the plasma albumin (Wetterfors et al., 1960). This recalls the earlier demonstration by Fleisher and Wakim (1968) that the small intestine contributes to the clearance of injected alanine transaminase from the plasma of the dog.

TABLE 7.5

DISAPPEARANCE RATES FOR THE CATALYTIC ACTIVITY AND RADIOACTIVITY AFTER THE INTRAVENOUS INJECTION OF ^{125}I-LABELLED LACTATE DEHYDROGENASE ISOENZYMES-1 AND -5: RADIOACTIVITY MEASURES AMOUNT OF ENZYME PROTEIN: CATALYTIC ACTIVITY MEASURES ENZYME ACTIVITY IN THE RABBIT

Based upon Wilkinson and Qureshi (1976) and Qureshi and Wilkinson (1976)

Enzyme	Phase and time span	Mean biological half-life (hours)
LD-1	Distribution	0.95 (radioactivity)
	1 to 4 hours	0.73 (catalytic activity)
	Enzyme catabolism	31 (radioactivity)
	4 to 34 hours	18 (catalytic activity)
LD-5	Distribution	1.2 (radioactivity)
	1 to 4 hours	0.70 (catalytic activity)
	Enzyme catabolism	12 (radioactivity)
	4 to 12 hours	3.6 (catalytic activity)

Further evidence in support of this theory is provided by the demonstration that rabbit lactate dehydrogenase-5 is inactivated during incubation in vitro at 37 °C in rabbit whole blood at rates comparable with those observed in vivo. It seems that the leucocytes are responsible, since white cell suspensions in rabbit plasma inactivate the enzyme at similar rates to those found with whole blood (Qureshi and Wilkinson, 1977), though the effect of the platelets cannot be excluded.

It seems, therefore, that lactate dehydrogenase isoenzymes-1 and -5 are inactivated in the circulating plasma, and that the products are discharged into the intestine where they are digested like dietary proteins into their constituent aminoacids which are reabsorbed and enter the aminoacid pool. It remains to be seen whether this hypothesis applies to the catabolism of other enzymes, and also to other species including man.

7.4. APPLICATION OF ENZYME MEASUREMENTS IN CLINICAL MEDICINE

7.4.1. General considerations

The application of enzyme measurements in the management and diagnosis of human diseases is usually referred to as "clinical" or "diagnostic" enzymology. Although studies of enzyme structure, enzyme reaction mechanisms and the metabolic regulation by enzymes have all provided important background knowledge for the development of clinical enzymology, this is generally not reflected in the way the results of enzyme measurements are interpreted in the clinical context. This, of course, applies not only to enzyme measurements but to biochemical measurements in general. Biochemical measurement is only one of several "tools" used by the clinician in the management of disease. He uses a combination of these tools to detect disease ("screening"), to establish a diagnosis ("confirmation") and a prognosis, and to direct treatment. He requires to have information on the cost, clinical sensitivity and specificity, and the predictive value of a test before he can optimize its value. Formalization of the diagnostic process has made progress in recent years through the development of computer-assisted "pattern recognition" (Lusted, 1968). This and other logic procedures have provided a means of assessing the clinical value of new methods, and have been successfully applied to enzyme measurements.

If the clinician wishes to classify disease processes in terms of biological phenomena, in order to understand the mechanism of action of a drug, or to protect the human organism from disease-causing agents ("preventive medicine"), then a deeper understanding of processes at the cellular level is necessary. This includes a knowledge of the theory of the action of enzymes, and of the mechanisms for their release, distribution and catabolism, as already discussed in section 7.3.

The demonstration of congenital enzyme defects as the cause of disease in more than 100 inborn errors of metabolism is the best illustration of a rational usage of enzymology in medicine. Other examples are the use of encapsulated or matrix-bound enzymes in the treatment of diseases due to defective naturally occurring enzymes. Knowledge of an enzyme system as the link between hormone action and metabolic response, has been utilized in the diagnosis and treatment of diseases of bone and liver.

Both the empirical ("pattern recognition") and the rational usage of enzyme measurements in medicine are illustrated in the following section although emphasis has been placed on the empirical approach due to its prominent role in current medical practice.

7.4.2. Heart and lung diseases

Heart and lung tissues contain many enzymes necessary for their normal function, and enzyme assays in relation to diseases of these organs are used mainly as biochemical markers of tissue destruction. Enzyme measurements have not yet been successfully utilized for demonstrating the state of, or changes in, the metabolism of the intact organs.

7.4.2.1. Acute myocardial infarction

Changes of enzyme activities in the blood have become established diagnostic criteria for confirmation of suspected myocardial infarction. Three enzymes are currently used – lactate dehydrogenase, aspartate transaminase and creatine kinase – but none of these are specific markers for heart tissue. By direct evidence from experiments on dogs, it appears that myocardial creatine kinase depletion accompanies, and is proportional to, ischaemic necrosis (Sobel, 1975). It has also been well documented that the pattern of change in creatine kinase activity in the blood correlates with the myocardial depletion of the enzyme and thus reflects the extent of myocardial necrosis. The findings obtained so far for creatine kinase can also be expected to be true for aspartate transaminase and lactate dehydrogenase, although this has not been proved by experiment. Creatine kinase measurement has the advantage over measurement of the other two enzymes in that its distribution in the heart is confined mainly to myocardial tissue proper, rather than to the connective tissue and blood elements of the heart. This relative specificity may become more prominent if current attempts to develop quantitative methods for the measurement of the MB isoenzyme of creatine kinase in the blood succeed. The MB isoenzyme constitutes approximately 15% of the total creatine kinase activity in heart tissue, and in man it is confined almost exclusively to the heart.

For establishing the diagnosis of acute myocardial infarction, serial changes in the activities of two or more of the enzymes are required. The time dependence and magnitude of changes in enzyme activities are indicated in Table 7.6. These data and those following apply in cases of infarction without re-infarction and without later complications possibly involving the lungs, the liver, and the pump function of the heart as regards to peripheral perfusion.

Creatine kinase is the first enzyme for which increased activity in the blood can be shown, usually within 3 to 6 hours of infarction. The peak value is reached at about 20 to 30 hours, being about 5 to 20 times the upper limit of normal. The creatine kinase activity returns to normal, on average, by the fourth day. The changes in the MB-isoenzyme of creatine kinase follow very closely the changes in total creatine kinase, provided that no complications occur. The combined measurements of the MB isoenzyme and total creatine kinase could provide the basis for distinguishing between re-infarction and the involvement of extracardial tissues as the source of a late and prolonged increase in creatine kinase activity (Klein et al., 1973).

TABLE 7.6

SERIAL CHANGES IN THREE ENZYMES IN BLOOD FOLLOWING AN UNCOMPLICATED EPISODE OF ACUTE MYOCARDIAL INFARCTION

Hours after onset of chest pain	Enzyme activities, expressed as multiples of the upper limit of normal		
	Creatine kinase	Aspartate aminotransferase	Lactate dehydrogenase
7	1.2	0.7	0.9
11	2.0	1.0	1.0
17	3.9	2.0	1.1
20	4.9	2.5	1.3
24	6.9	3.3	1.6
30	8.5	4.4	1.9
35	7.9	4.6	2.5
39	7.0	4.5	2.7
45	5.6	3.9	3.0
49	4.4	3.3	3.1
55	3.5	3.1	2.7
60	2.7	2.6	2.6
77	1.2	1.6	2.0
101	0.7	1.5	1.5
115	0.3	0.8	1.1

Aspartate aminotransferase activity begins to increase 6 to 8 hours after infarction, reaching a peak value of 3 to 10 times the upper limit of normal after 25 to 40 hours; it returns to normal after 4 to 5 days. Prolonged increase is often found, due to blood stasis in the lungs and the liver.

Elevation of lactate dehydrogenase activity starts 10 to 20 hours after infarction. The peak value, which tends to be at a plateau, is reached after 4 to 6 days. The maximum value does not usually exceed 5 times the upper limit of normal. Return to normal values occurs after 8 to 12 days. Measurement of LD-1 by electrophoresis improves the specificity with regard to heart tissue, as the source of enzyme. Slight elevations of lactate dehydrogenase may then be properly classified as being of cardiac or non-cardiac origin. Activity of the LD-1 isoenzyme usually returns to normal after 6 to 8 days, indicating that the late rise in total lactate dehydrogenase even in uncomplicated myocardial infarction may be of non-cardiac origin.

After two decades of the routine use of enzyme measurements in the confirmation of suspected myocardial infarction, they are now utilized in the early detection, in the quantification, in the projection of the evolution, and in the prognosis of infarction (Sobel, 1975). In the first 24 hours following onset of chest pain the determination of the MB-isoenzyme of creatine kinase seems to have the highest predictive value (Blomberg et al., 1975) of different enzyme tests. The combined use of creatine kinase and lactate dehydrogenase isoenzyme measurements would appear to provide the greatest discrimination between myocardial infarction and non-myocardial infarction, independent of the time of the first blood sampling (Galen et al., 1975). The cumulative activity of MB-creatine kinase released by the heart can be estimated from serial measurements of the enzyme activity in blood after compensating for the continuous disappearance of the enzyme (Sobel, 1975). This index can give a reliable estimate of infarct size, and may therefore be used as a prognostic guide and for the evaluation of therapeutic interventions which are designed to reduce infarct size.

The interpretation of enzyme measurements is complicated when myocardial infarction is concurrent with, or followed by, a number of events or conditions. These will be indicated by deviations from the typical serial changes of the three enzymes which are indicated in Table 7.6; for this reason two or more of the enzymes should be followed. Cardioversion seldom gives rise to changes in the enzyme pattern. Cardiac catheterization and angiography will result in minor changes only, provided dissection of heart tissue is avoided. In the first week following myocardial infarction there is no elevation, or only a slight one, of alanine transaminase. A moderate increase in the second and third week is often found without clinical signs of liver involvements. More pronounced elevation of alanine transaminase and aspartate transaminase indicates liver damage, and is usually found if congestive heart failure arises after the infarct.

7.4.2.2. Cardiac disorders other than myocardial infarction

In pericarditis, levels of enzyme activities in serum are usually within normal limits. Pericarditis and myocarditis accompanied by increases in lactate dehydrogenase and creatine kinase activities may be found, indicating slight myocardial necrosis. In cardiac arrhythmias with acute congestive heart failure and in chronic congestive heart failure, the LD-5 fraction of lactate dehydrogenase, and aspartate transaminase as well as alanine transaminase are usually increased due to liver damage, whereas creatine kinase remains normal.

Intravascular, mechanical haemolysis liberates lactate dehydrogenase from the erythrocytes. An assessment of the function of heart ball-valve prostheses can therefore be made by measurement of lactate dehydrogenase immediately following the operation. Long-term function may also be monitored in this way.

7.4.2.3. Lung diseases

Enzyme measurements play a minor role in the diagnosis and treatment of lung diseases. In pulmonary infarction and in pneumonia, reported changes in aspartate transaminase and lactate dehydrogenase activities probably indicate a haemolysis of red cells in lung tissues, and secondary liver involvement, rather than damage to lung tissue.

Increased activity and abnormal fractions of alkaline phosphatases have been found in primary tumours of the lung due to de novo enzyme–protein synthesis in the neoplastic tissue.

7.4.3. Liver diseases (see also Chapter 10, section 10.2.4).

Diseases of the liver may be classified according to the clinical features, to the results of histological examination of liver biopsies, to radiological findings, and to a description of the functional state of the liver in biochemical and physiological terms. None of these approaches alone allows a detailed and unequivocal classification, and combinations of the diagnostic procedures are therefore common. An assessment of the value of enzyme measurements in liver diseases may be biased because the classification of the disease involves the measurement of enzymes.

Prerequisites for the understanding of changes in the enzyme content of blood which accompany diseases of the liver are knowledge of the locations and concentrations of enzymes in the liver, of their release mechanisms, and of their distribution and catabolism. Information of this kind is very limited, and therefore any rational interpretation of changes in enzyme activities accompanying liver diseases must be incomplete. Fortunately, however, the pragmatic approach does yield useful results.

The alternative approach of pattern recognition, by which a defined disease entity is characterized by changes in one or more enzymes, is of limited value because of the fact that very few enzymes are confined only to liver tissues. Differential diagnosis may therefore be difficult.

The following discourse should be considered as almost entirely empirical, and has not been wholly confirmed by experiment.

7.4.3.1. Toxic and inflammatory diseases of the liver

Toxic side reactions of drugs on liver tissue are increasingly important. Liver cell necrosis is indicated by increases in lactate dehydrogenase, alanine transaminase, aspartate transaminase and glutamate dehydrogenase, with the greatest increase in the first of these enzymes and the least increase in glutamate dehydrogenase. The ratio of aspartate transaminase to alanine transaminase is usually less than one. If the toxic drug reaction involves other organs, e.g. the muscles, this pattern of changes in enzyme activities in the blood is altered. Measurement of ornithine carbamoyltransferase may be of value in such cases, due to its occurrence in liver tissue only. In toxic drug effects which are mainly cholestatic, increases in alkaline phosphatase, 5′-nucleotidase and γ-glutamyltransferase are dominant, although elevated activities of transaminases are often found also. An assessment of the severity of the toxic effect is not possible from the degree of increase in enzyme activity, but the course of liver involvement is reflected in the fluctuations of enzyme activities.

In acute (viral) hepatitis, elevations of the transaminases occur before the patient shows clinical jaundice. Maximum activities of these enzymes in blood are usually reached shortly after the onset of jaundice. If the increase persists beyond 6 weeks, active hepatitis or the onset of chronic hepatitis is indicated. The magnitude of the rises in transaminase activities in acute inflammatory hepatitis is rarely seen in any other clinical situation. Activities of 30 times the upper limit of normal are the rule, and the assay of these enzymes in icteric hepatitis is particularly useful.

Several other enzymes have been used as markers for liver cell necrosis: lactate dehydrogenase (especially the slowest moving fraction by electrophoresis, LD-5), alcohol dehydrogenase, guanase, sorbitol dehydrogenase, isocitric dehydrogenase, aldolase, and arginase. Measurement of none of these activities, however, seems to provide a better diagnostic reliability than the transaminase assays. Another argument in favour of the transaminases is the high degree of analytical reliability by which these enzymes can be measured at present. Ornithine carbamoyltransferase may prove of some value because of its organ specificity.

7.4.3.2. Cholestasis

The excretion of bile can be obstructed by intra- and extrahepatic causes, but it is not possible, by using enzyme measurements, to localize the site of obstruction. In both types of obstruction, increases in non-specific alkaline phosphatases, 5′-nucleotidase, leucine aminopeptidase and γ-glutamyltransferase can be expected. None of these enzymes is increased in jaundice caused by hepatocellular necrosis. The transaminases usually have increased activities in cholestasis except perhaps during the early stages, and in clinically mild cases. To discriminate between cholestatic and parenchymal damage, the ratio between alanine transaminase (as marker for the parenchymatous liver tissue) and alkaline phosphatase or γ-glutamyltransferase (as marker for cholestasis) seems to be of some diagnostic value. γ-Glutamyltransferase alone has been used as a sensitive indicator of alcoholic liver tissue damage. Leucine aminopeptidase and 5′-nucleotidase are of little value in differential diagnosis and confirmation of liver diseases.

7.4.3.3. Chronic and regenerative liver disease

The most important disease that shows regeneration of liver tissue is cirrhosis. Enzyme measurements are generally of little value in establishing the diagnosis, but may be of prognostic value in following the progression of disease and the effects of therapy. Alkaline phosphatase and γ-glutamyltransferase both serve as markers for regeneration.

7.4.3.4. Malignancy

The presence of metastases in the liver can often be detected before any other sign of liver involvement by measurement of alkaline phosphatase in serum. Even slight elevations should be evaluated by isoenzyme determination in order to rule out the liver as the source of elevated alkaline phosphatase if metastases are suspected.

In summary, enzyme measurements in diseases of the liver should be evaluated only in conjunction with clinical and other investigations of the patient. Their main role is in differential diagnosis and in following the progress of the disease. Although many enzymes which originate in liver tissue can be measured in the blood, clinicians should obtain experience with the measurement of a few: alanine and aspartate transaminases, γ-glutamyl-transferase and alkaline phosphatase. They should know which changes are physiological and which are pathological in nature and in collaboration with the clinical biochemist, they should define sampling and storage conditions and take part in the development of sub-classes of reference intervals. By such combined efforts, the empirical use of enzyme measurements will be valuable to the clinician, pending the development of a more rational basis for their use.

7.4.4. Pancreatic diseases

Enzyme assays which are used in the management of pancreatic diseases are those of trypsin and chymotrypsin in duodenal juice, following exogenous stimulation by secretin or pancreozymin; and amylase, lipase, and proteolytic enzymes in blood and urine. The measurement of trypsin and chymotrypsin in faeces may be used in screening for defective secretion of the proteolytic enzymes, but this approach is less sensitive than the use of the above tests, including gastric stimulation.

7.4.4.1. Cystic fibrosis of the pancreas

Determination of trypsin in faeces has been used as a screening test for this disease, but is now replaced by measurements of electrolytes in sweat and of α_1-antitrypsin in serum.

7.4.4.2. Acute pancreatitis

Determinations of amylase in blood and in urine are still of decisive importance in the diagnosis of acute pancreatitis. These assays do have a rather low clinical specificity and sensitivity, but no other diagnostic procedure has been developed that can replace them for the differential diagnosis of acute abdominal pain and acute pancreatitis. Increased activity of amylase in the blood may also be seen in perforated ulcer, biliary tract diseases and in intestinal obstructions. Except for acute pancreatitis, it is rare, however, to find values higher than 10 times the upper limit of normal. The time course of the changes usually enables detection of increased values of amylase activity in blood, and excretion in urine, 3 to 5 hours after the onset of abdominal pain. Maximum values are reached within 20 to 30 hours. Amylase is normally excreted in the urine, but complexes of amylase with immunoglobulins in serum may occur (macroamylasaemia), and in such cases the excretion of amylase in urine is low or zero, and the concentration in serum is very high. The salivary glands also produce amylase, as demonstrated in mumps where amylase activity in blood is usually increased.

Lipase in blood is also of diagnostic value in pancreatitis, especially in combination with the determination of amylase. However, the analytical reliability of lipase measurements alone is lower than that for amylase, which tends to make amylase the preferred test in acute pancreatitis.

7.4.4.3. Chronic pancreatitis

The main feature of chronic pancreatitis is defective digestion. This is well illustrated by low or zero concentrations of trypsin and chymotrypsin in jejunal juice after stimulation.

7.4.4.4. Tumours of the pancreas

Enzyme determinations are of little value in the detection of malignancy of the pancreas. Elevated activities of amylase, lipase and γ-glutamyltransferase in the blood may be obtained, but very often they are normal, even in the late stages of the disease.

7.4.5. Diseases of the gastrointestinal tract

Enzyme measurements generally play no role in the diagnosis and treatment of gastrointestinal tract diseases. An exception is the classification of malabsorption due to disaccharidase deficiencies. Although the diagnosis can be made by lactose-, sucrose-, or maltose-tolerance tests, the measurement of relevant enzymes (Table 7.7) in jejunal biopsies has enabled a detailed classification of the type of deficiency. The enzyme activity in question will be low, but the wide variation which is found in biopsies from normal jejunal tissue should be taken into consideration.

Temporary impairment of disaccharidases is common, particularly of lactase in infants and young children; it may occur also in non-tropical and tropical sprue. A relative deficiency in lactase is normally found in persons from Asia and Africa, whereas persons of

TABLE 7.7.

DISACCHARIDASES IN JEJUNAL TISSUE

Enzyme	Substrate	Component of diet
Lactase	Lactose	Milk
Iso-maltase	Iso-maltose	Starch (bread, potatoes)
	Maltose	Glycogen (meat, liver)
Sucrase	Sucrose	Sugar, fruits
Maltase	Maltose	Starch and glycogen

European origin keep an intact lactase activity in adult life. This difference correlates with the presence of milk in the diet of most European adults, whereas adults from some other areas do not usually drink milk.

7.4.6. Bone diseases

The measurement of serum alkaline phosphatase, one of the first assays of a circulating enzyme to find diagnostic applications, is still one of the most useful tests in the investigation of bone disease. It has long been known to be concerned in the ossification of cartilage, though its exact role in the mineralization of bone remains uncertain (Moss, 1976). Its association with the calcification of bone is illustrated by the correlation between the rate of bone growth and the serum alkaline phosphatase during childhood and adolescence (Clark and Beck, 1950). In children, the serum enzyme activity is about twice that found in healthy adults. A considerable increase in alkaline phosphatase occurs at the site of a fracture. This is associated with the repair process, but the local increase is rarely reflected in the serum enzyme activity.

The alkaline phosphatase activity of bone can be shown by histochemical studies to be largely confined to the osteoblasts. Consequently in diseases of bone, raised serum enzyme activities are indicative of processes involving the formation of bone, whereas osteolytic lesions, characterized by the breakdown of bone, are associated with normal serum phosphatase activity unless there is concurrent bone repair.

It must be borne in mind, however, that elevated serum alkaline phosphatase activity also occurs in hepatobiliary diseases. While the liver enzyme can be distinguished by electrophoresis from that originating in bone, their electrophoretic mobilities are similar, and the faster liver enzyme often overlaps with the slower, more diffuse, bone enzyme. Many laboratories, therefore, prefer to rely on other enzyme tests, notably 5′-nucleotidase and γ-glutamyltransferase, the serum levels of which are not elevated in bone disease in the absence of hepatobiliary complications.

7.4.6.1. Paget's disease (Osteitis deformans)

Marked elevation of serum alkaline phosphatase activity is usually found in Paget's disease, sometimes reaching about 15 times the upper limit of normal when the disease is extensive; in small localized lesions the enzyme activity may not greatly exceed the normal range. About 3 to 5% of patients with Paget's disease develop osteogenic sarcoma, which leads to a rapid increase in the serum alkaline phosphatase activity. In either case, the affected bone is rich in osteoblasts which accounts for the rise in the serum enzyme activity.

Successful treatment of Paget's disease with calcitonin (Woodhouse et al., 1971) or diphosphonates (Smith et al., 1973) leads to a fall in the serum alkaline phosphatase activity.

7.4.6.2. Rickets and osteomalacia

The increase in uncalcified osteoid matrix which occurs in rickets in children and osteomalacia in adults leads to increased osteoblastic activity and hence to elevation of the serum alkaline phosphatase. Rickets and osteomalacia may result from deficient dietary vitamin D; from various malabsorption syndromes, especially those associated with steatorrhoea; and from hereditary and acquired renal disease. In renal disease, a defect in the hydroxylase system which converts 25-hydroxycholecalciferol into 1,25-dihydroxycholecalciferol, the most active form of vitamin D, appears to be the cause of the failure to absorb sufficient calcium from the gut.

In early rickets, the serum alkaline phosphatase activity may not greatly exceed the values normally found in children of comparable age, but in severe cases the serum enzyme levels may reach 8 or 10 times the upper limit of the adult normal. In adult osteomalacia, however, the elevation is usually less pronounced.

7.4.6.3. Hyperparathyroidism

The marked elevation in serum alkaline phosphatase activity in primary or secondary hyperparathyroidism, once frequently reported in the literature, is rarely encountered today, presumably because most cases are now diagnosed before bone changes have occurred. Since elevation of the alkaline phosphatase activity is derived from the osteoblasts, the enzyme level remains normal in the absence of bone lesions. Thus the enzyme measurement is no longer reliable as a test for hyperparathyroidism, and demonstration of the characteristic hypercalcaemia is a more appropriate biochemical procedure.

7.4.6.4. Malignant disease of bone

Since osteosarcomata originate in the osteoblasts, the tumours may be osteogenic, in which case markedly elevated serum alkaline phosphatase activity may be observed, particularly when the primary tumour has metastasized. Some forms of osteosarcomata, however, are mainly osteolytic, and in such cases the serum alkaline phosphatase shows normal activity or only slight elevation.

The response of the serum alkaline phosphatase to infiltration by metastases from tumours of other tissues depends upon whether the secondaries are predominantly osteoblastic or osteolytic. In the former, the serum enzyme activity is elevated, such as for example in bone metastases secondary to carcinoma of the prostate, but the bone metastases associated with carcinoma of the breast and the bone lesions of multiple myeloma are mainly osteolytic in character, so that the serum alkaline phosphatase is generally within the normal range. In certain tumours, however, ectopic production of a parathyroid hormone-like substance occurs, in which case the serum alkaline phosphatase activity may be raised in parallel with an elevated serum calcium concentration, which is similar to the findings in primary or secondary hyperparathyroidism.

Since elevation of serum alkaline phosphatase activity may occur as the result of secondary infiltration of either the liver or bone, or both, it is sometimes necessary to perform other tests to enable a decision to be made. If the 5′-nucleotidase or γ-glutamyl-transferase is normal, metastatic activity is confined to bone, but if either of these enzymes shows raised activity, liver metastases are likely to be present, though the presence of bone metastases cannot be excluded. In such cases, determination of the urinary excretion of hydroxyproline may be helpful, since raised excretion often accompanies bone involvement. Separation of serum alkaline phosphatase isoenzymes by electrophoresis may show the presence of both liver and bone components when both tissues are involved.

The serum acid phosphatase is sometimes raised in the presence of certain bone diseases, including Paget's disease and secondary deposits due to carcinoma of the breast. Acid phosphatase appears to originate in the osteoblasts, and reduction of osteolytic activity by removal of a tumour usually leads to a fall in the serum acid phosphatase activity. Unlike the prostatic enzyme, bone acid phosphatase is not sensitive to inhibition by L(+)tartrate (Moss, 1976). The serum acid phosphatase has long been used to aid the diagnosis of a metastasizing carcinoma of the prostate, but in this case the enzyme is inhibited by L(+)tartrate.

7.4.7. Diseases of skeletal muscle

Skeletal muscle is a rich source of enzymes and, since it accounts for about 40% of the adult body mass, considerable amounts of enzyme protein may be released into the circulating blood in widespread disease of muscle. Among the muscle enzymes, creatine kinase is the most abundant, and determination of serum creatine kinase activity is therefore the most sensitive biochemical index of muscle fibre damage. Muscle also contains appreciable amounts of aldolase, aspartate and alanine transaminases and lactate dehydrogenase (particularly LD-5), the serum activities of which are often elevated in muscle disease.

Most primary myopathies are associated with marked elevations of serum enzyme activities, whereas in muscle disease which is secondary to an innervation disorder, the serum activities remain within the normal range or are only slightly elevated. Thus, serum enzyme determination may aid the differentiation of a primary myopathy from neurogenic muscular atrophy, and is especially useful in the diagnosis of muscular dystrophy (Rosalki, 1976).

7.4.7.1. Muscular dystrophy

Marked elevation of the serum creatine kinase, up to 50 to 100 times the upper limit of the normal range, is found soon after the onset of the severe sex-linked (Duchenne) form of muscular dystrophy, but the serum aldolase, aspartate transaminase and lactate dehydrogenase activities are also elevated, though to a lesser extent. As the disease progresses, muscle fibres are replaced by connective tissue and fat, and the elevation of the serum enzyme levels becomes less marked; in the terminal phase they may not greatly exceed the upper limit of the normal range. Although muscle creatine kinase is predominantly of the MM type, the MB isoenzyme can be demonstrated in the sera of about 90% of patients with Duchenne type dystrophy (Somer et al., 1973). This suggests a reversion to the foetal type (Schapira et al., 1968).

Like the severe form, the benign form of Duchenne dystrophy also affects males, but the disease is generally of later onset. The lifespan is longer and the serum enzyme abnormalities are less marked, though the serum creatine kinase activity may reach 10 times the upper limit of normal. The severe and benign forms, however, cannot be differentiated by means of serum tests (Shaw, 1971).

One of the main applications of serum enzyme tests in muscular dystrophy is to aid detection of the carrier state. Since this disease is characterized by a high mutation rate, it cannot be assumed that the mother of an affected son is a carrier. Creatine kinase measurement is of most value in this connection since about 75% of definite carriers show raised activities in their sera (Rosalki, 1976). The incidence approaches 100% in young carriers, but care is required to eliminate the effect of previous vigorous exercise which is known to cause elevation of the serum enzyme in healthy non-carriers. Raised activities occur in about half of the carriers of the benign form of the disease.

Other forms of muscular dystrophy are characterized by raised serum creatine kinase activities, but the values observed are not so high as in the Duchenne type. In the limb-girdle form of the disease, the serum levels are about 10 to 20 times normal and the incidence of raised values is about 70%. This form of muscular dystrophy appears to be transmitted by autosomal recessive inheritance, but serum enzyme measurements usually fail to detect the heterozygous carrier state, except possibly in children (Thomson, 1971). In the autosomal dominant form, facioscapulohumeral dystrophy, the serum creatine kinase is only slightly or moderately elevated. The degree of elevation and the incidence of raised activities in the serum of other enzymes originating in muscle are much less than those of creatine kinase in these forms of muscular dystrophy.

Slight or moderate elevation of the serum creatine kinase has also been reported in several of the rarer genetically determined myopathies, e.g. hyperkalaemic periodic paralysis, ocular dystrophy and congenital dystrophy (Rosalki, 1976).

7.4.7.2. Polymyositis

About 70% of patients with polymyositis have increased serum creatine kinase and aldolase activities, the highest values being observed in children, where they may resemble those found in Duchenne dystrophy. In polymyositis, however, steroid treatment usually brings about a reduction in the serum enzyme activities while having little or no effect on those in muscular dystrophy.

7.4.7.3. Muscle trauma

The effect of exercise on the serum creatine kinase activity has already been briefly mentioned. Marked elevation may follow prolonged vigorous exercise, especially in untrained subjects (Griffiths, 1966), but the rise is much less pronounced when the severity of the exercise is adjusted to the exercise capacity of the individual (Shapiro et al., 1973: Rosalki, 1976).

Raised activities of creatine kinase and other muscle enzymes may be transiently observed after surgical trauma (Marmar et al., 1969; Penneys and Wilkinson, 1970) and after intramuscular injections (Hess et al., 1964). Repeated injections, however, may cause moderate elevation which may persist up to a week afterwards (Nevins et al., 1973). Crush injuries involving extensive muscle trauma also result in raised serum enzyme activities.

There have been several reports of the release of muscle enzymes into the plasma following the administration of drugs, particularly those given over long periods, e.g. chloroquine (Rewcastle and Humphrey, 1965). Markedly raised serum creatine kinase activities have been reported after overdosage of hypnotic drugs resulting in coma (Maclean et al., 1968; Henderson et al., 1970), and after prolonged excessive alcohol consumption (Nygren, 1966). A value 500 times the upper limit of normal was found in a patient with idiopathic myoglobinuria precipitated by acute ethanol poisoning (Griffith, quoted by Wilkinson, 1970b).

Malignant hyperpyrexia, a rare but frequently fatal disorder which follows anaesthesia, particularly with halothane, is also a drug-induced condition in which marked elevation of the serum creatine kinase (up to 300 times the upper limit of normal) is observed (Denborough et al., 1970). Sensitivity to anaesthetics is transmitted as an autosomal dominant character, and the skeletal muscle creatine kinase isoenzyme patterns of patients and their sensitive relatives may be abnormal. Zsigmond et al. (1972) have reported the BB component to be the main component of the muscle and serum enzyme, but Rosalki (1976) has found members of affected families to have elevated serum enzyme activities, with normal isoenzyme patterns.

7.4.7.4. Myxoedema

Skeletal muscle appears to be the source of the raised serum creatine kinase activities found in hypothyroidism (Graig and Ross, 1963; Griffiths, 1963), and an inverse relationship has been reported between the serum enzyme activity and the serum protein-bound iodine concentration in thyroid disease (Graig and Smith, 1965; Doran and Wilkinson, 1971). It seems that thyroid hormone controls the membrane permeability in muscle, but Doran and Wilkinson (1975) obtained evidence that muscle is not the only tissue affected by increased permeability in myxoedema. Owing to the large muscle mass and its high creatine kinase activity, this is the most sensitive enzyme test in hypothyroidism.

7.4.7.5. Neurogenic muscle disease

In contrast to the high values frequently encountered in myopathies, serum enzyme activities generally remain within normal limits or are only slightly elevated in muscle diseases which are due to an underlying nerve defect. Normal serum creatine kinase activities are almost invariably found in infantile spinal muscular atrophy (Werdnig–Hoffman disease), multiple sclerosis, poliomyelitis and myasthenia gravis, but a proportion of patients with Friedreich's ataxia and motor neurone disease exhibit slightly increased levels, usually in the early stages of the disease (Rosalki, 1976).

7.4.8. Diseases of the kidney and urinary tract

7.4.8.1. Serum enzyme activities

Measurements of serum enzyme activities are generally of little diagnostic value in diseases of the kidney and urinary tract. It has long been known that the serum amylase may be elevated in renal failure due to impaired renal clearance of the enzyme. The serum lactate dehydrogenase shows the greatest incidence of raised activities in acute and chronic glomerulonephritis, acute renal failure, systemic lupus erythematosus and other diseases involving the kidney, but the serum aspartate transaminase activity is usually normal (West and Zimmerman, 1958). Among other enzyme tests which have been proposed for the investigation of renal disease are the serum tripeptidase (Richet et al., 1957) and the serum transaminidase (Horner et al., 1965). Since the latter is not usually detectable in normal serum, the reported high activities in acute glomerulonephritis and acute renal failure merit further study.

Transient elevations of the serum lactate dehydrogenase, aspartate transaminase and alkaline phosphatase activities have been reported after renal infarction, a condition in which, unlike myocardial infarction, the serum creatine kinase remains within the normal range (Gault and Steiner, 1965).

7.4.8.2. Urinary enzyme activities

Certain enzymes, such as amylase and uropepsinogen, have molecular masses which are small enough to permit their filtration by the glomerulus, but most enzymes of clinical interest have molecular masses exceeding 70,000 and hence are not filterable by the healthy kidney. Normal urine, therefore, contains no more than traces of lactate dehydrogenase and aspartate transaminase. In renal disease, especially acute glomerulonephritis and acute tubular necrosis, significant amounts of these enzymes were found in the urine by Rosalki and Wilkinson (1959), who considered the urinary enzymes to originate in the damaged kidney. It has also been suggested that filtration through the damaged glomerulus may be a factor responsible for the appearance of enzymes in the urine (Crockson, 1961; Coltorti et al., 1962), and a third possibility is release of enzymes from leucocytes, erythrocytes or other components of the urinary deposit (Gelderman et al., 1965; Dubach, 1966).

Determination of the urinary lactate dehydrogenase or alkaline phosphatase has been proposed as a screening test for malignant disease of the urinary tract (Wacker and Dorfman, 1962; Amador et al., 1963; Macalalag and Prout, 1964). Similar raised values in non-malignant diseases, however, limit the value of such tests for this purpose, and Dubach (1965) has concluded that they are of little diagnostic significance, except that normal values may exclude the presence of a carcinoma, but 6 out of 22 patients with carcinomas of the urinary tract were found by Emerson and Morgan (1966) to have normal urinary enzyme excretion. Mirabile et al., (1966) consider that urinary enzyme determinations lack specificity in the evaluation of kidney masses and bladder tumours.

Urinary enzyme determination has found limited application in the early detection of impending rejection of a renal transplant. Lactate dehydrogenase was one of the first enzymes to be studied in this context, and a rise in the urinary output, especially of LD-5, generally precedes a change in the creatinine clearance (Prout et al., 1964; Ringoir, 1968). Increased excretion of alkaline phosphatase (Dossetor et al., 1964), lysozyme (Noble et al., 1965) and alanine aminopeptidase (Dutz et al., 1968) have also been reported during impending rejection, but the most promising enzyme test in this connection appears to be measurement of the urinary N-acetyl-β-D-glucosaminidase (Wellwood et al., 1973).

7.4.9. Haematological diseases

Hereditary enzyme anomalies in the erythrocyte form an important group of haematological disorders in which enzyme determinations have found applications. Haemolytic anaemia is commonly associated with such inherited enzyme defects, although many of the affected individuals remain symptom-free. The role of enzymes is uncertain in the aetiology of such forms of haemolytic anaemia as hereditary spherocytosis, in which the cell membrane is defective, or the haemoglobinopathies, in which abnormal haemoglobins are synthesized. However, haemolytic episodes following the ingestion of certain drugs, and certain forms of congenital non-spherocytic haemolytic anaemia, have been shown to be due to deficiencies of glucose-6-phosphate dehydrogenase or other erythrocytic enzymes (Beutler, 1976).

7.4.9.1. Glucose-6-phosphate dehydrogenase deficiency

Glucose-6-phosphate dehydrogenase deficiency is the commonest of the known red cell enzyme defects. It is a sex-linked disorder affecting about 11% of male American Negroes, but it also occurs in Mediterranean peoples and populations in other parts of the world. About 150 variants of the enzyme differing in their catalytic and physicochemical properties have been recorded (Beutler, 1976). The best known variant is the A+ form, whcih occurs in about 20% of American Negroes, and differs from the usual Caucasian form (B+) in exhibiting faster electrophoretic mobility towards the anode.

Many variants exhibit normal activity and are not manifested by any clinical effects, but the deficient variants display a spectrum ranging from clinical normality to severe or even fatal haemolysis, usually in response to stress induced by infections or the administration of drugs, or the ingestion of fava beans. Among the drugs to which affected individuals may be sensitive are many antimalarials, sulphonamides, other antibacterial agents and various oxidizing agents. Other variants, however, lead to shortening of the lifespan of the red cell in the absence of such stresses, and to the syndrome of congenital non-spherocytic haemolytic anaemia.

Enzyme activity may be determined in washed erythrocytes, but a number of simple screening tests for glucose-6-phosphate dehydrogenase deficiency have been developed (Beutler, 1976). These usually prove adequate in males, but are less satisfactory in female heterozygotes (Beutler, 1969) and immediately after haemolytic episodes in males when the older, deficient cells are preferentially destroyed.

7.4.9.2. Other red cell enzyme defects

Although glucose-6-phosphate dehydrogenase deficiency is the commonest known cause of congenital non-spherocytic haemolytic disease, it must be emphasized that in the vast majority of cases the underlying defect is unknown (Beutler, 1976). In certain cases, however, the disorder is due to deficiency of pyruvate kinase, glucose phosphate isomerase, hexokinase or other erythrocytic enzymes. Of these defects, pyruvate kinase deficiency ranks second to that of glucose-6-phosphate dehydrogenase as a known cause (Tanaka and Paglia, 1971), but differs from the latter in having an autosomal recessive rather than a sex-linked mode of inheritance. Characterization of the abnormal pyruvate kinase is extremely complex owing to the inheritance of two different mutant genes for the enzyme and also to its allosteric activation by fructose-1,6-diphosphate (Niessner and Beutler, 1973).

When measuring pyruvate kinase activity in erythrocytes, it is important to exclude leucocytes since they are rich sources of this enzyme. Moreover, the white cell enzyme appears to be under separate genetic control from that of the red cells. Some of the problems involved in confirming the diagnosis of erythrocytic pyruvate kinase deficiency and the use of screening techniques are discussed by Beutler (1976).

7.4.9.3. Plasma enzymes in anaemia

Although measurements of plasma (or serum) enzyme activities are of only limited value in the differential diagnosis of anaemia, their determination has certain applications, especially in megaloblastic anaemias due to either vitamin B_{12} or folic acid deficiency, when the serum lactate dehydrogenase activity may be markedly elevated. The degree of elevation appears to be related to the severity of the anaemia, and a rapid return towards normal values generally follows the initiation of specific therapy (Emerson and Wilkinsson, 1966). The increase is mainly in the anionic isoenzymes, reflecting the difference between the isoenzyme patterns of normal and megaloblastic bone marrows.

By contrast, the serum lactate dehydrogenase activity is only slightly or moderately elevated in haemolytic anaemias, and remains within the normal range in iron-deficiency anaemia even when the blood haemoglobin concentration is less than 40 g/litre.

7.4.9.4. Alkaline phosphatase in leucocytes

Histochemical assessment of the alkaline phosphatase activity in leucocytes has found a number of applications in haematological diseases. Low values occur in chronic myeloid (granulocytic) leukaemia, acute myeloblastic leukaemia (Grossbard and Marks, 1970), and paroxysmal nocturnal haemoglobinuria (Lewis and Dacie, 1965), while raised activities are found in acute lymphocytic leukaemia (Grossbard and Marks, 1970), Down's syndrome (mongolism) (Phillips et al., 1967), and Hodgkin's disease (Bennett et al., 1968).

7.4.10. Genetic disorders

More than 140 diseases which are inherited by a recessive or sex-linked mechanism are known in which the primary defect is due to deficiency or abnormality of a particular enzyme (McKusick, 1975). It is not possible in this context to give more than a brief survey, and for more information the reader is referred to Chapter 18. As shown by the examples listed in Table 7.8, practically any metabolic system may be primarily involved.

Some of these metabolic disorders, e.g. benign pentosuria, are symptomless and are compatible with a normal lifespan, but the majority have serious, even fatal, consequences if untreated. Severe mental retardation is characteristic of both phenylketonuria and galactosaemia, and the latter also leads to cirrhosis and cataracts; however, reduction of the dietary intake of phenylalanine or galactose respectively during early infancy prevents these consequences and enables the patient to develop normally. Early investigation is therefore vital and enzyme measurements play an important part in confirmation of the diagnosis.

TABLE 7.8

SOME EXAMPLES OF CONGENITAL DISEASES WHICH ARE DUE TO ENZYME DEFECTS

For further details see Raine and Westwood (1976) and Ryman (1976).

Metabolic system	Disorder	Enzyme defect	EC No.
Aminoacids	Alkaptonuria	Homogentisate oxidase	1.13.11.5
	Phenylketonuria	Phenylalanine oxidase	1.14.16.1
	Aspartylglycosaminuria	Aspartylglucosaminidase	3.5.1.26
Carbohydrates	Fructosuria	Fructokinase	2.7.1.3
	Galactosaemia	Hexose 1-phosphate uridylyltransferase	2.7.7.12
	Glycogen storage diseases, e.g. Type I (Von Gierke)	Glucose 6-phosphatase	3.1.3.9
	Mucopolysaccharidoses, e.g. Type 3B (Sanfilippo B)	N-Acetylglucosaminidase	3.2.1.50
Lipids	Norum's disease	Lecithin: cholesterol acyltransferase	2.3.1.43
	Wolman's disease	Lipase	3.1.1.3
	Niemann–Pick disease	Sphingomyelinase	3.1.4.3
	Gaucher's disease	β-D-Glucosidase	3.2.1.21
Urea cycle	Hyperargininaemia	Arginase	3.5.3.1
	Argininosuccinic aciduria	Argininosuccinate lyase	4.3.2.1
Miscellaneous	Lesch–Nyhan syndrome	Hypoxanthine-guanine phosphoribosyltransferase	2.4.2.8
	Suxamethonium sensitivity	Cholinesterase	3.1.1.8

Although excess phenylalanine can be demonstrated in the plasma and (with its metabolite phenylpyruvate) in the urine of patients with phenylketonuria, liver biopsy specimens are required for the detection of phenylalanine oxidase deficiency (Friedman et al., 1973). In galactosaemia, however, deficiency of hexose-1-phosphate uridylyltransferase can be detected in the erythrocytes, which of course are much more accessible.

The glycogen storage diseases illustrate the necessity to select appropriate tissues for demonstration of the enzyme defect. While the glucose-6-phosphatase deficiency of Type I (Von Gierke's disease) is demonstrable only in liver biopsy specimens, and that of phosphorylase of Type V (McArdle's disease) only in muscle biopsy specimens, the lack of lysosomal α-glucosidase in Type II (Pompe's disease) and of branching enzyme in Type IV (Andersen's disease) can be detected in leucocytes, cultured fibroblasts and other tissues (Ryman, 1976).

7.4.11. Pregnancy

Although an increase in the serum alkaline phosphatase during the second half of pregnancy was first observed about 40 years ago, the value of enzyme tests in monitoring the course of pregnancy remains inconclusive. Since the placenta is peculiarly rich in heat-stable alkaline phosphatase, cystyl aminopeptidase (oxytocinase) and diamine oxidase (histaminase), the activities of these enzymes in the serum have been extensively explored as indicators of placental function and foetal development.

After the discovery that placental alkaline phosphatase differs from the phosphatases of other tissues in being unusually stable to heat (56 or 60°C), it soon became apparent that the placenta was the source of the excess serum activity in pregnant women (McMaster et al., 1964; Neale et al., 1965). During normal pregnancy, heat-stable alkaline phosphatase gradually increases to reach a maximum shortly before term, but disappears shortly after delivery. Abnormally high values have been reported in pre-eclampsia, while abnormally low values occur in pregnancies which are at risk due to diabetes mellitus or hypertension. The normal range or reference interval, however, is very wide and single values are difficult to interpret. Successive measurements showing a fall may indicate poor placental development while high values are suggestive of placental damage, but the test appears to be insufficiently sensitive to serve routinely as an index of placental dysfunction (Watney et al., 1970; Curzen, 1971).

Similar problems are encountered in interpreting the serum cystyl aminopeptidase which also increases as pregnancy progresses. Here again the reference interval shows a wide scatter. Serial determinations appear to be of value in detecting intrauterine death of the foetus or imminent abortion; failure to rise indicates that the foetus is at risk. Chapman et al. (1971) concluded that this enzyme test is a valuable guide in patient management, but further experience is needed to assess its ultimate status in obstetrics.

Owing to the difficulties of determining the serum diamine oxidase by conventional biochemical techniques, the assessment of this enzyme test in monitoring pregnancy had to await the development of a convenient radioactive procedure (Okuyama and Kobayashi, 1961). This enzyme differs from heat-stable alkaline phosphatase and cystyl aminopeptidase in showing a marked increase during the first half of pregnancy and then remaining more or less constant until term. Again the normal range is very wide, but failure of the serum diamine oxidase to rise during early pregnancy, or a rapid fall, indicates a poor prognosis. Weingold and Southren (1968) found serum diamine oxidase determinations to be helpful in monitoring pregnancies which were at risk due to diabetes, habitual abortion or poor obstetric histories, but Resnik and Levine (1969) were unable to confirm its value in this connection.

It must be concluded that, at the present time, enzyme tests have only limited applications in detecting abnormalities of pregnancy.

7.4.12. Malignant diseases

The role of enzyme tests in the diagnosis of malignant diseases and in following the response to therapy is discussed in Chapter 25.

7.5. BIOLOGICAL VARIABILITY OF ENZYMES

General considerations of the sources and degrees of variability in the concentrations of serum constituents have already been discussed (Chapter 2). Until recently, poor analytical reliability of enzyme measurements has delayed the study of the true biological variability. This situation is now rapidly changing.

Certain factors associated with specimen collection can affect the final measurement. In general, the fasting state need not be specified. Physical activity prior to sampling will result in an increase in serum creatine kinase activity, and to a lesser degree in that of lactate dehydrogenase and of aspartate aminotransferase. Prolonged venous stasis should be avoided because enzymes – in common with other macromolecules – will concentrate in the blood following transcapillary diffusion of water.

Provided that the above requirements are fulfilled, the true intra- and inter-individual variability can be studied. This has been done for a few enzymes, e.g. alkaline phosphatase and aspartate aminotransferase. For both of these enzymes, it has been found that the long-term (months) intra-individual variability is small (coefficient of variation about 5%) and not higher than for non-enzyme constituents in plasma. It is to be expected that most enzymes in the blood will show the same low degree of intra-individual variability.

The degree of inter-individual variability determines the distribution of values defining the reference interval. Most reference intervals for enzymes are very broad and reflect the variation with age, sex, weight, etc. No actual values will be cited here because of the strong dependence on methodology, and the reader should refer to the local laboratory for this kind of information. However, irrespective of the actual values the following generalizations may be made. For creatine kinase, the values are higher among men than women, reflecting the greater muscle mass, but the age of the patient is usually of little importance, except in infancy and in the early detection of carriers of Duchenne-type muscular dystrophy. For the transaminases the same is true, but alanine aminotransferase activity seems to be greater in obesity, while lactate dehydrogenase shows no important variation with age, sex and weight. Alkaline phosphatase activity is much higher in childhood and in adolescence than in adult life.

Except for the foregoing variations, most reference intervals will include, and thus make unimportant, any variation of enzyme activities with age, sex, weight, and to some extent, race. The clinician should, however, consult the literature and the local laboratory for further information, especially if there is a special interest in particular diseases or sub-classes of reference populations. Further discussion of the effects of demographic factors on serum enzyme activity is given by Goldberg and Winfield (1974).

REFERENCES

Amador, E., Zimmerman, T.S. and Wacker, W.E.C. (1963) Urinary alkaline phosphatase activity. I. Elevated urinary LDH and alkaline phosphatase activities for the diagnosis of renal adenocarcinomas. Journal of the American Medical Association, 185, 769–775.

Amelung, D. (1960) Untersuchungen zur Grösse der Eliminations-Geschwindigkeit von Fermenten aus dem Kaninchen-Serum. Hoppe-Seylers Zeitschrift für Physiologische Chemie, 218, 219–228.

Bär, U., Fiedel, R., Heine, H., Mayer, D., Ohlendorf, S., Schmidt, F.W. and Trautschold, I. (1972/3) Studies on enzyme elimination. III. Distribution, transport and elimination of cell enzymes in the extracellular space. Enzyme, 14, 133–156.

Bennett, J.M., Nathanson, L. and Rutenburg, A.M. (1968) Significance of leukocyte alkaline phosphatase in Hodgkin's disease. Archives of Internal Medicine, 121, 338–341.

Beutler, E. (1967) "Galactose dehydrogenase", "nothing dehydrogenase" and alcohol dehydrogenase. Science, 156, 1516–1517.

Beutler, E. (1969) G-6-PD activity of individual erythrocytes and X-chromosomal inactivation. In Biochemical Methods in Red Cell Genetics (Ed. J.J. Yunis) pp. 95–113, Academic Press, New York.

Beutler, E. (1976) Enzyme tests in haematological diseases. In The Principles and Practice of Diagnostic Enzymology (Ed. J.H. Wilkinson) pp. 423–455, Edward Arnold, London.

Blomberg, D.J., Kimber, N.D. and Burke, M.D. (1975) Creatine kinase isoenzymes. Predictive value in the early diagnosis of acute myocardial infarction. American Journal of Medicine, 59, 464–469.

Boyd, J.W. (1967) The rates of disappearance of L-lactate dehydrogenase isoenzymes from plasma. Biochimica et Biophysica Acta, 132, 221–231.

Boyde, T.R.C. (1968) Serum levels of the mitochondrial isoenzyme of aspartate aminotransferase in myocardial infarction and muscular dystrophy. Enzymologia Biologica et Clinica, 9, 385–392.

Chapman, L., Silk, E., Skupny, A., Tooth, E.A. and Barnes, A. (1971) Spectrofluorimetric assay of serum cystine aminopeptidase in normal and diabetic pregnancy compared with total oestrogen excretion. Journal of Obstetrics and Gynaecology of the British Commonwealth, 78, 435–443.

Clark, L.C. Jr. and Beck, E. (1950) Plasma "alkaline" phosphatase activity. I. Normative data for growing children. Journal of Pediatrics, 36, 335–341.

Cohen, L. and Larson, L. (1966) Activation of serum lactic dehydrogenase. New England Journal of Medicine, 275, 465–470.

Coltorti, M., Ascione, A., Giusti, G. and Di Simone, A. (1962) Eliminazione urinaria di alcuni enzimi in soggetti a rene integro ed in nefropatici: correlazione con l'entita della proteinuria. Riforma Medica, 47, 1313–1318.

Crockson, R.A. (1961) Lactic dehydrogenase in renal disease. Lancet, i, 140–142.

Curzen, P. (1971) Enzyme assays in the management of pregnancy. In Enzyme Assays in Medicine (Eds. G.K. McGowan and G. Walters). Journal of Clinical Pathology, 24, Suppl. 4, 90–95.

Deggeller, K. and Sandifort, C.R.J. (1973) Comments on the "Recommendations of the German Society for Clinical Chemistry, Standardization of Methods for the Estimation of Enzyme Activity in Biological Fluids". Clinical Chimica Acta, 43, 13–22.

Denborough, M.A., Ebeling, P., King, J.O. and Zapf, P. (1970) Myopathy and malignant hyperpyrexia. Lancet, i. 1138–1140.

Doran, G.R. and Wilkinson, J.H. (1971) Serum creatine kinase and adenylate kinase in thyroid disease. Clinica Chimica Acta, 35, 115–119.

Doran, G.R. and Wilkinson, J.H. (1975) The origin of the elevated activities of creatine kinase and other enzymes in the sera of patients with myxoedema. Clinica Chimica Acta 62, 203–211.

Dossetor, J.B., Gault, M.H., Oliver, J.A., Inglis, F.G., MacKinnon, K.J. and MacLean, L.D. (1964) Cadever renal homotranplants. Canadian Medical Association Journal, 91, 733–742.

Dubach, U.C. (1965) Diagnostischer Wert von Enzymbestimmungen im Urin bei Tumoren des Urogenitalsystems. Oncologia, 19, 254–258.

Dubach, U.C. (1966) On the origin of lactic dehydrogenase isoenzymes in urine. Helvetica Medica Acta, 33, 139–150.

Dutz, W., Schneider, G., Gawellek, F., Dietrich, G. and Erdmann, T. (1968) Zur Rejektionsdiagnostik bei Nierentransplantationen. Deutsche Gesundheitswesen, 23, 783–785.

Dybkaer, R. (1975) Problems of quantities and units in enzymology. Enzyme, 20, 46–64.

Dybkaer, R. (1977) Quantities and units in enzymology. Enzyme, 22, 91–123.

Ellis, G. (1976) Quality control of serum alkaline phosphatase assays: project report and discussion of some factors affecting the assay. Annals of Clinical Biochemistry, 13, 327–335.

Emerson, P.M. and Morgan, M.N. (1966) Lactate dehydrogenase in urinary tract disease. British Journal of Urology, 38, 551–555.

Emerson, P.M. and Wilkinson, J.H. (1966) Lactate dehydrogenase in the diagnosis and assessment of response to treatment in megaloblastic anaemia. British Journal of Haematology, 13, 678–688.

Englhardt, A., Schmidt-Sodingen, G. and Lange, H. (1969) Metabolitgehalt und Enzympermeabilität isolierter menschlicher Blutzellen bei Substratmangel und Zusatz von Stoffwechselgiften. Enzymologia Biologica et Clinica, 10, 258–280.

Fishman, W.H. and Ghosh, N.K. (1967) Isoenzymes of human alkaline phosphatase. Advances in Clinical Chemistry, 10, 255–370.

Fleisher, G.A. and Wakim, K.G. (1963) The fate of enzymes in body fluids – an experimental study. I. Disappearance rates of glutamic-pyruvic transaminase under various conditions. Journal of Laboratory and Clinical Medicine, 61, 76–85.

Fleisher, G.A. and Wakim, K.G. (1968) The role of the small intestine in the disposal of enzymes. Enzymologia Biologica et Clinica, 9, 81–96.

Friedman, P.A., Fisher, D.B., Kang, E.S. and Kaufman, S. (1973) Detection of hepatic phenylalanine-4-hydroxylase in classical phenylketonuria. Proceedings of the National Academy of Sciences of the U.S.A., 70, 552–556.

Galen, R.S., Reiffel, J.A. and Gambino, S.R. (1975) Diagnosis of acute myocardial infarction. Relative efficiency of serum enzyme and isoenzyme measurements. Journal of the American Medical Association, 232, 145–147.

Gault, M.H. and Steiner, G. (1965) Serum and urinary enzyme activity after renal infarction. Canadian Medical Association Journal, 93, 1101–1105.

Gelderman, A.H., Gelboin, H.V. and Peacock, A.C. (1965) Lactic dehydrogenase isoenzymes in urines from patients with malignancies of the urinary bladder. Journal of Laboratory and Clinical Medicine, 65, 132–142.

Goldberg, D.M. and Winfield, D.A. (1974) Relationship of serum enzyme activities to demographic variables in a helathy population. Clinica Chimica Acta, 54, 357–368.

Goodfriend, T.L., Sokol, D.M. and Kaplan, N.O. (1966) Control of synthesis of lactate acid dehydrogenases. Journal of Molecular Biology, 15, 18–31.

Gowenlock, A.H. (1976) Diseases of the alimentary tract. In The Principles and Practice of Diagnostic Enzymology (Ed. J.H. Wilkinson) p. 361, Edward Arnold, London.

Graig, F.A. and Ross. G. (1963) Serum creatine phosphokinase in thyroid disease. Metabolism, 12, 57–59.

Graig, F.A. and Smith, J.C. (1965) Serum creatine phosphokinase activity in altered thyroid states. Journal of Clinical Endocrinology, 25, 723–731.

Griffiths, P.D. (1963) Creatine phosphokinase levels in hypothyroidism. Lancet, i, 894.

Griffiths, P.D. (1966) Serum levels of A.T.P., creatine phosphotransferase (creatine kinase). The normal range and effect of muscular activity. Clinica Chimica Acta, 13, 413–420.

Grossbard, L. and Marks, P.A. (1970) Enzymes in hematologic disease. In Diagnostic Enzymology (Ed. E.L. Coodley) p. 73, Lea and Febiger, Philadelphia.

Gutman, A.B. (1959) Serum alkaline phosphatase activity in diseases of the skeletal and hepatobiliary systems. American Journal of Medicine, 27, 875–901.

Hallak, G.J. and Wilkinson, J.H. (1976) Action of metabolic inhibitors on the release of intracellular enzymes from human and rat lymphocytes and human erythrocytes. Clinica Chimica Acta, 66, 251–261.

Harris, H., Hopkinson, D.A. and Robson, E.B. (1962) Two-dimensional electrophoresis of pseudocholinesterase components in normal human serum. Nature (London), 196, 1296–1298.

Hellung-Larsen, P. and Anderson, V. (1968) Lactate dehydrogenase isoenzymes of human lymphocytes cultured with phyto-haemagglutinin at different oxygen tensions. Experimental Cell Research, 50, 286–292.

Henderson, L.W., Metz, M. and Wilkinson, J.H. (1970) Serum enzyme elevation in glutethimide intoxication. British Medical Journal, 3, 751.

Hess, J.W., MacDonald, R.P., Frederick, R.J., Jones, R.N., Neely, J. and Gross, D. (1964) Serum creatinine phosphokinase (CPK) activity in disorders of heart and skeletal muscle. Annals of Internal Medicine, 61, 1015–1028.

Horner, W.H., Chambliss, J.F. and Mahanand, D. (1965) Serum transaminidase in renal disease. Proceedings of the Society for Experimental Biology and Medicine, 118, 65–69.

Jockers-Wretou, E. and Pfleiderer, G. (1975) Quantitation of creatine kinase isoenzymes in human tissues and sera by an immunological method. Clinica Chimica Acta, 58, 223–232.

Kaplan, N.O. (1963) Multiple forms of enzymes. Bacteriological Reviews, 27, 155–169.

Karmen, A. (1955) A note on the spectrophotometric assay of glutamic-oxalactic transaminase in human blood serum. Journal of Clinical Investigation, 34, 131–133.

Klein, M.S., Shell, W.E. and Sobel, B.S. (1973) Serum creatine phosphokinase (CPK) isoenzymes following intramuscular inejctions, surgery, and myocardial infarction: experimental and clinical studies. Cardiovascular Research, 7, 412–418.

Konttinen, A. and Somer, H. (1972) Determination of serum-creatine-kinase isoenzymes in myocardial infarction. American Journal of Cardiology, 29, 817–820.

LaDue, J.S., Wróblewski, F. and Karmen, A. (1954) Serum glutamic oxalacetic transaminase activity in human acute transmural myocardial infarction. Science, 120, 497–499.

LaMotta, R.V., McComb, R.B., Noll, C.R., Jr., Wetstone, H.J. and Reinfrank, R.F. (1968) Multiple forms of serum cholinesterase. Archives of Biochemistry and Biophysics, 124, 299–305.

Latner, A.L. and Skillen, A.W. (1968) Isoenzymes in Biology and Medicine. Academic Press, London.

Lewis, S.M. and Dacie, J.V. (1965) Neutrophil alkaline phosphatase in paroxysmal nocturnal haematuria. British Journal of Haematology, 11, 549–556.

Lowry, O.H. and Passonneau, J.V. (1972) A Flexible System of Enzymatic Analysis. Academic Press, New York.

Lusted, L.B. (1968) Introduction to Medical Decision Making. C.C. Thomas, Springfield, Illinois.

Macalalag, E.V., Jr. and Prout, G.R., Jr. (1964) Confirmation of the source of elevated urinary lactic dehydrogenase in patients with renal tumor. Journal of Urology, 92, 416–423.

MacLean, D., Griffiths, P.D. and Elmslie-Smith, D. (1968) Serum enzymes in relation to electrocardiographic changes in accidental hypothermia. Lancet, ii, 1266–1270.

Marmar, J.L., Karafin, L. and Kendell, A.R. (1969) The activity of serum enzymes following prostatic operation. Journal of Urology, 102, 84–87.

Martinez-Carrion, M. and Tiemeier, D. (1967) Mitochondrial glutamate-aspartate transaminase. I. Structural comparison with the supernatant enzyme. Biochemistry, 6, 1715–1722.

Massarat, S. (1965) Enzyme kinetics, half-life, and immunological properties of iodine-131-labelled transaminases in pig blood. Nature (London), 206, 508–509.

McComb, R.B., Bond, L.W., Burnett, R.W., Keech, R.C. and Bowers, G.N., Jr. (1976) Determination of the molar absorptivity of NADH. Clinical Chemistry, 22, 141–150.

McKusick, V.A. (1975) Mendelian Inheritance in Man: Catalogs of Autosomal Dominant, Autosomal Recessive and X-linked Phenotypes, 4th edn. John Hopkins, Baltimore.

McMaster, Y., Tennant, R., Clubb, J.S., Neale, F.C. and Posen, S. (1964) The mechanism of the elevation of serum alkaline phosphatase in pregnancy. Journal of Obstetrics and Gynaecology of the British Commonwealth, 71, 735–739.

Mirabile, C.S., Bowers, G.N., Jr. and Berlin, B.B. (1966) Urinary lactic dehydrogenase: a report based on 250 hospitalized patients. Journal of Urology, 95, 79–82.

Moss, D.W. (1976) Enzyme tests in disease of bone. In The Principles and Practice of Diagnostic Enzymology (Ed. J.H. Wilkinson) pp. 399–422. Edward Arnold, London.

Moss, D.W., Baron, D.N., Walker, P.G. and Wilkinson, J.H. (1971) Standardisation of clinical enzyme assays. Journal of Clinical Pathology, 24, 740–743.

Moss, D.W., Shakespeare, M.J. and Thomas, D.N. (1972) Observations on the heat stability of alkaline phosphatase isoenzymes in serum. Clinica Chimica Acta, 40, 35–41.

Murros, J., Konttinen, A. and Somer, H. (1973) An electrophoretic method for the quantitation of aspartate aminotransferase isoenzymes. Clinica Chimica Acta, 41, 263–268.

Neale, F.C., Clubb, J.S., Hotchkis, D. and Posen, S. (1965) The heat stability of human placental alkaline phosphatase. Journal of Clinical Pathology, 18, 359–363.

Nevins, M.A., Saran, M., Bright, M. and Lyon, L.J. (1973) Pitfalls in interpreting serum creatine phosphokinase activity. Journal of the American Medical Association, 224, 1382–1387.

Niessner, H. and Beutler, E. (1973) Fluorometric analysis of glycolytic intermediates in human red blood cells. Biochemical Medicine, 8, 123–134.

Noble, R.E., Najarian, J.S. and Brainerd, H.D. (1965) Urine and serum lysozyme measurement in renal homotransplantation. Proceedings of the Society for Experimental Biology and Medicine, 120, 737–740.

Nygren, A. (1966) Serum creatine phosphokinase activity in chronic alcoholism, in connection with acute intoxication. Acta Medica Scandinavica, 179, 623–630.

Okuyama, T. and Kobayashi, Y. (1961) Determination of diamine oxidase activity by liquid scintillation counting. Archives of Biochemistry, 95, 242–250.

Oliver, I.T. (1955) A spectrophotometric method for the determination of creatine phosphokinase and myokinase. Biochemical Journal, 61, 116–122.

Penneys, R. and Wilkinson, J.H. (1970) Elevation of serum creatine kinase following amputation of the leg. Surgery, 67, 302–305.

Phillips, J., Herring, R.M., Goodman, H.O. and King, J.S., Jr. (1967) Leucocyte alkaline phosphatase and erythrocyte glucose 6-phosphate dehydrogenase in Down's syndrome. Journal of Medical Genetics, 4, 268–273.

Posen, S. (1970) Turnover of circulating enzymes. Clinical Chemistry, 16, 71–84.

Prout, G.R., Jr., Macalalag, E.V. and Huma, D.M. (1964) Serum and urinary lactic dehydrogenase in patients with renal homotransplants. Surgery, 56, 283–295.

Qureshi, A.R. and Wilkinson, J.H. (1976) The fate of circulating lactate dehydrogenase-5 in the rabbit. Clinical Science and Molecular Medicine, 50, 1–14.

Qureshi, A.R. and Wilkinson, J.H. (1977) Inactivation in vitro of lactate dehydrogenase-5 in blood. Annals of Clinical Biochemistry, 14, 48–52.

Raine, D.N. and Westwood, A. (1976) Congenital enzyme anomalies. In The Principles and Practice of Diagnostic Enzymology (Ed. J.H. Wilkinson) pp. 518–567, Edward Arnold, London.

Resnik, R. and Levine, R.J. (1969) Plasma diamine oxidase activity in pregnancy: a reappraisal. American Journal of Obstetrics and Gynecology, 104, 1061–1066.

Rewcastle, N.B. and Humphrey, J.G. (1965) Vacuolar myopathy. Archives of Neurology, 12, 570–582.

Richet, G., Villiers, H. and Ardaillou, R. (1957) Activité tripeptidasique du plasma au cours de l'insufficiance rénale. Revue Francaise d'Études Cliniques et Biologiques, 2, 808–819.

Ringoir, S. (1967) LDH Isoenzymen bij Nieraandoeningen Experimentele en Klinische Studie. Arscia, Brussles.

Ringoir, S. (1968) Correlations between kidney, serum and urinary enzyme activity. In Enzymes in Urine and Kidney (Ed. U.C. Dubach) p. 177, Verlag Hans Huber, Berne.

Rosalki, S.B. (1967) An improved procedure for creatine phosphokinase determination. Journal of Laboratory and Clinical Medicine, 69, 696–705.

Rosalki, S.B. (1976) Enzymes in diseases of skeletal muscle. In The Principles and Practice of Diagnostic Enzymology (Ed. J.H. Wilkinson) pp. 263–302. Edward Arnold, London.

Rosalki, S.B., Brown, S.S., Fleck, A., McCormack, J.J., Padmore, G.R.A., Smith, A.F. and Wilkinson, J.H. (1975) Investigation of the validity of temperature correction factors for serum aspartate and alanine transaminases. Annals of Clinical Biochemistry, 12, 78–82.

Rosalki, S.B. and Rau, D. (1972) Serum γ-glutamyl transpeptidase activity in alcoholism. Clinica Chimica Acta, 39, 41–47.

Rosalki, S.B. and Wilkinson, J.H. (1959) Urinary lactic dehydrogenase in renal disease. Lancet, ii. 327–328.

Rosalki, S.B. and Wilkinson, J.H. (1960) Reduction of α-ketobutyrate by human serum. Nature (London), 188, 1110–1111.

Ryman, B.E. (1976) The glycogen storage diseases. In The Principles and Practice of Diagnostic Enzymology (Ed. J.H. Wilkinson) pp. 503–517, Edward Arnold, London.

Schapira, F., Dreyfus, J.C., Allard, D. and Grégori-Lauer, C. (1968) Les isozymes de la créatine kinase et de l'aldolase du muscle foetal et pathologique. Clinica Chimica Acta, 20, 439–447.

Schapira, F., Dreyfus, J.C. and Schapira, G. (1962) La durée de séjour dans le plasma de l'aldolase chez le lapin: étude à l'aide d'une aldolase marquée à l'iode radioactif. Revue Francaise d'Études Cliniques et Biologiques, 7, 829–832.

Schmidt, E. and Schmidt, F.W. (1960) Über Änderungen der Substrat-Affinität von Malat-Dehydrogenase. Klinische Wochenschrift, 38, 810–811.

Schmidt, E. and Schmidt, F.W. (1962) Methode und Werte der Bestimmung der Glutaminsäure-Dehydrogenase-Aktivität im Serum. Ein Beitrag zur Bedeutung der Untersuchung von Enzym-Relationen im Serum. Klinische Wochenschrift, 40, 962–969.

Schmidt, E., Schmidt, F.W. and Otto, P. (1967) Isoenzymes of malic dehydrogenase, glutamic oxaloacetic transaminase and lactic dehydrogenase in serum in diseases of the liver. Clinica Chimica Acta, 15, 283–289.

Shapiro, Y., Magazanik, A., Sohan, E. and Reich, C.B. (1973) Serum enzyme changes in untrained subjects following a prolonged march. Canadian Journal of Physiology and Pharmacology, 51, 271–276.

Shaw, C.R. and Koen, A.L. (1967) "Galactose dehydrogenase", "nothing dehydrogenase" and alcohol dehydrogenase. Science, 156, 1517–1518.

Shaw, R.F. (1971) Serum enzymes and prognosis in muscular dystrophy. Lancet, i, 856–857.

Smith, R., Russell, R.G.G., Bishop, M.C., Woods, C.G. and Bishop, M. (1973) Paget's disease of bone. Experience with a diphosphonate (disodium etidronate) in treatment. Quarterly Journal of Medicine, 42, 235–256.

Sobel, B.E. (1975) Applications and limitations of estimation of infarct size from serial changes in plasma creatine phosphokinase activity. Acta Medica Scandinavica, Suppl. 587, 151–167.

Somer, H., Donner, M., Murros, J. and Konttinen, A. (1973) A serum isozyme study in muscular dystrophy. Archives of Neurology, 29, 343–345.

Statland, B.E. and Louderback, A.L. (1972) Nonlinear regression analysis approach for determining "true" lactate dehydrogenase activity in serum with the centrifugal analyser ("Rotochem"). Clinical Chemistry, 18, 845–849.

Strandjord, P.E., Thomas, K.E. and White, L.P. (1959) Studies on isocitric and lactic dehydrogenases in experimental myocardial infarction. Journal of Clinical Investigation, 38, 2111–2118.

Sweetin, J.C. and Thomson, W.H.S. (1973) Enzyme efflux and clearance. Clinica Chimica Acta, 48, 403–411.

Tanaka, K.R. and Paglia, D.E. (1971) Pyruvate kinase deficiency. Seminars in Haematology, 8, 367–396.

Thomson, W.H.S. (1971) Serum enzyme studies in inherited disease of skeletal muscle. Clinica Chimica Acta, 35, 183–191.

Wacker, W.E.C. and Dorfman, L.E. (1962) Urinary lactate dehydrogenase activity. I. Screening method for detection of cancer of kidneys and bladder. Journal of the American Medical Association, 181, 972–978.

Wakim, K.G. and Fleisher, G.A. (1963a) The fate of enzymes in body fluids – an experimental study. II. Disappearance rates of glutamic-oxalacetic transaminase I under various conditions. Journal of Laboratory and Clinical Medicine, 61, 86–97.

Wakim, K.G. and Fleisher, G.A. (1963b) The fate of enzymes in body fluids – an experimental study. IV. Relationship of the reticuloendothelial system to activities and disappearance rates of various enzymes. Journal of Laboratory and Clinical Medicine, 61, 107–119.

Watney, P.J.M., Hallum, J., Ladell, D. and Scott, P. (1970) The relative usefulness of methods of assessing placental function, Journal of Obstetrics and Gynaecology of the British Commonwealth, 77, 301–311.

Weingold, A.B. and Southren, A.L. (1968) Diamine oxidase as an index of the fetoplacental unit. Clinical applications. Obstetrics and Gynecology, 32, 593.

Wellwood, J.M., Ellis, B.G., Hall, J.H., Robinson, D.R. and Thompson, A.E. (1973) Early warning of rejection. British Medical Journal, 2, 261–265.

West, M. and Zimmerman, H.J. (1958) Serum enzymes in disease. IV. Lactic dehydrogenase and glutamic oxalacetic transaminase levels in renal disease. Journal of Laboratory and Clinical Medicine, 52, 185–192.

Wetterfors, J., Gullberg, R., Liljedahl, S.O., Plantin, L.O., Birke, G. and Olhagen, B. (1960) Role of the stomach and small intestine in albumin breakdown. Acta Medica Scandinavica, 168, 347–363.

Wilkinson, J.H. (1968) Diagnostic significance of enzyme determinations in urine. In Enzymes in Urine and Kidney (Ed. U.C. Dubach) p. 207, Verlag Hans Huber, Berne.

Wilkinson, J.H. (1970a) Isoenzymes, 2nd edn. Chapman and Hall, London.

Wilkinson, J.H. (1970b) Clinical significance of enzyme activity measurements. Clinical Chemistry, 16, 882.

Wilkinson, J.H., Boutwell, J.H. and Winsten, S. (1969) Evaluation of a new system for the kinetic measurement of serum alkaline phosphatase. Clinical Chemistry, 15, 487–495.

Wilkinson, J.H. and Qureshi, A.R. (1976) Catabolism of plasma enzymes, as studied with ^{125}I-labelled lactate dehydrogenase-1 in the rabbit. Clinical Chemistry, 22, 1269–1276.

Wilkinson, J.H. and Robinson, J.M. (1974a) Effect of adenosine triphosphate on the release of intracellular enzymes from damaged cells. Nature (London), 249, 662–663.

Wilkinson, J.H. and Robinson, J.M. (1974b) Effect of energy-rich compounds on the release of intracellular enzymes from human leukocytes and rat lymphocytes. Clinical Chemistry, 20, 1331–1336.

Wilkinson, J.H., Robinson, J.M. and Johnson, K.P. (1975) Factors affecting the release of haemoglobin and enzymes from human erythrocytes. Annals of Clinical Biochemistry, 12, 58–65.

Woodhouse, N.J.Y., Reiner, M., Bordier, Ph., Kalu, D.N., Fisher, M., Foster, G.V., Joplin, G.F. and MacIntyre, I. (1971) Human calcitonin in the treatment of Paget's bone disease. Lancet, i, 1139.

Wróblewski, F. and LaDue, J.S. (1956) Serum glutamic-pyruvic transaminase in cardiac and hepatic disease. Proceedings of the Society for Experimental Biology and Medicine, 91, 569–571.

Ziegenhorn, J., Senn, M. and Bücher, T. (1976) Molar absorptivities of β-NADH and β-NADPH. Clinical Chemistry, 22, 151–160.

Zierler, K.L. (1958) Increased muscle cell permeability to aldolase produced by depolarisation and by metabolic inhibitors. American Journal of Physiology, 193, 534–538.

Zsigmond, E.K., Starkweather, W.H., Duboff, G.S. and Flynn, K.A. (1972) Abnormal creatine-phosphokinase isoenzyme pattern in families with malignant hyperpyrexia. Anesthesia and Analgesia, 51, 827–840.

FURTHER READING

Bodansky, O. (1972) Acid phosphatase. Advances in Clinical Chemistry, 15, 44.

Coodley, E.L. (1970) Diagnostic Enzymology, xiv + 323 pp. Lea and Febiger, Philadelphia.

Moss, D.W. and Butterworth, P.J. (1974) Enzymology and Medicine. vii + 175 pp. Pitman Medical, London.

Rosalki, S.B. (1975) Gamma-glutamyl transpeptidase. Advances in Clinical Chemistry, 17, 53.

Wilkinson, J.H. (1970) Isoenzymes, 2nd edn. Chapman and Hall, London. Paperback edition, 1974.

Wilkinson, J.H. (1976) The Principles and Practice of Diagnostic Enzymology, xvi + 592 pp. Edward Arnold, London.

ADDENDUM

In 1978 agreement was reached among several professional organizations on nomenclature, kind of quantity and units of enzyme measurements.

Catalytic activity and the katal

The *catalytic activity* of an enzyme is the property measured by the increase in the rate of reaction. The *katal* (symbol: kat) is that catalytic activity that will raise the rate of reaction by one mol per second in a specified assay system. The old enzyme unit (U) may be related to the katal by the following: 1 U catalyzes a rate of 1 μmol/min = 1.60 μmol/sec ≈ 16.67 nmol/sec. Therefore 1 U corresponds to 16.67 nkat.

Catalytic activity concentration

This is the unit katal per litre (symbol: kat/litre, kat · litre^{-1}). The name may be shortened to "catalytic concentration". 1 U/litre = 16.67 nkat/litre.

Clinica Chimica Acta (1979) Approved Recommendation of the International Federation of Clinical Chemistry on General Considerations Concerning the Determination of the Catalytic Concentration of an Enzyme in the Blood Serum or Plasma of Man. In press.

Chapter 8

Calcium and magnesium

Kay W. Colston, Imogen M.A. Evans, Peter B. Greenberg *, Richard G. Larkins * and Iain MacIntyre

*Endocrine Unit, Royal Postgraduate Medical School, Hammersmith Hospital, Ducane Road, London W12 OHS, England and * The Royal Melbourne Hospital, Melbourne, Australia.*

CONTENTS

Chemical diagnosis of disease, edited by
S.S. Brown, F.L. Mitchell and D.S. Young

INTRODUCTION

The last 15 years have seen great advances in our overall understanding of calcium and magnesium homeostasis, with particular emphasis on the hormonal regulation of these ions by parathyroid hormone, calcitonin and 1,25-dihydroxycholecalciferol. Ionized calcium can now be measured directly in biological fluids (Ross, 1967), and it has become apparent that, as well as potent effects on neuromuscular tissue and on blood coagulation, calcium ions participate directly in many physiological phenomena, including hormone secretion (Douglas, 1968) and action (Rasmussen, 1970). It is likely that measurements of serum ionized calcium will allow more precise evaluation of disorders of calcium metabolism (Ladenson and Bowers, 1973).

Magnesium ions also have been shown to participate intimately in many cellular reactions and they are of prime importance as enzyme activators.

The diagnosis of disorders of calcium and magnesium metabolism rests on clinical examination with biochemical, radiological and possibly histological investigations. Because of the nature of this book, emphasis will be placed on the biochemical features associated with the relevant diseases, with passing reference only to the other characteristics. To help understand the significance of current biochemical tests, a brief summary of recent advances in physiology will be given.

8.1. BIOCHEMICAL PHYSIOLOGY OF CALCIUM

8.1.1. Intestinal absorption

Calcium intake in the diet varies widely. On average, about 1 gram is ingested per day. Of this, only about 200 mg is absorbed, although increased proportional absorption occurs under conditions of increased demand, such as in growth or pregnancy (Dowdle et al., 1960), or after a preceding period of dietary calcium deficiency (Rottenstein, 1938; Nicolaysen, 1943).

Calcium and phosphorus absorption is dependent on the presence of adequate amounts of vitamin D. Excessive phosphate in the diet interferes with calcium absorption in the rat (Bethke et al., 1932), but this seems less important in man (Malm, 1953). Phytate, which is found in cereals, can depress calcium absorption, but this is probably of importance only when calcium intake is marginal. A small obligatory faecal excretion of endogenous calcium and phosphate occurs (Nicolaysen, 1937).

8.1.2. Renal excretion

The urinary excretion of calcium varies in different parts of the world, between sexes, and from day to day. Up to 6 mmol/24 hours in females and up to 8 mmiol/24 hours in males is normal, and much of the calcium is complexed with phosphate, citrate and oxalate. The slope relating urinary calcium excretion to dietary intake is fairly flat in normal individuals, but steeper in patients with "idiopathic hypercalciuria" and hyper-absorption (Nordin et al., 1972). There is a direct relationship between excretion of calcium and that of sodium (Walser, 1961b), and a high intake of magnesium increases urinary calcium excretion (Heaton and Parsons, 1961). Systemic acidosis tends to increase, and systemic alkalosis to decrease, urinary calcium excretion (Nordin et al., 1972). Hypercalcaemia of any cause will lead to increased urinary calcium excretion; however, when hypercalcaemia is due to hyperparathyroidism, the urinary calcium excretion is less than occurs with comparable hypercalcaemia of non-parathyroid origin (Nordin and Peacock, 1969). Vitamin D and its metabolites probably have a minor direct effect in enhancing calcium reabsorption from the tubular fluid (Puschett et al., 1972). Thiazides decrease urinary calcium excretion (Lamberg and Kuhlbäck, 1959), whereas frusemide enhances it (Hanze and Seyberth, 1967).

8.1.3. Calcium in bone

The skeleton contains 99% of the total calcium (1 kg) in the body; about 5 grams of this exists in a form which is readily exchangeable (Bauer et al., 1957), presumably at the surface of the bone crystal. Exchange of the remainder is slower, and probably requires bone remodelling involving osteoblastic, osteoclastic and osteocytic activity (Albright, 1947). The relative rates of bone formation and resorption are determined by age, plasma calcium and phosphate concentrations, pH, parathyroid hormone, calcitonin and 1,25-dihydroxycholecalciferol concentrations.

8.1.4. Calcium in soft tissues

About 4 grams of calcium is contained in soft tissues. It is not known in what form it exists, although the ionized fraction performs specialized functions in muscle, nerve, neuromuscular junction and secretory tissues.

8.1.5. Calcium in blood plasma

Calcium exists in the plasma partly as free calcium ions, partly bound to protein, and partly complexed to phosphate, citrate and other anions (Table 8.1). The proportion of

TABLE 8.1.

DISTRIBUTION OF CALCIUM IN NORMAL HUMAN PLASMA

Reproduced and modified, by permission, from Walser (1961a).

	mmol/litre	% total
Free calcium ions	1.18	47.5
Protein bound	1.14	46.0
Calcium phosphate	0.04	1.6
Calcium citrate	0.04	1.7
Unidentified	0.08	3.2
Total	2.48	100

calcium which is protein bound depends on the plasma protein concentration and the pH of the blood. The concentration of calcium is subject to complex metabolic control, involving parathyroid hormone, calcitonin and 1,25-dihydroxycholecalciferol which act on intestine, kidney and bone.

8.1.6. Measurement of serum calcium

The classic method for estimation of total serum calcium involved precipitation of calcium as the oxalate (Kramer and Tisdall, 1921). Flame photometric methods have suffered from interferences, both chemical and spectral, although these can be overcome (MacIntyre, 1957). Atomic absorption spectrometry provides a reliable and precise method, providing sufficient care is taken, and a reference method based on this technique has been described (Cali et al., 1973). However, because of the relative expense of atomic absorption spectrometers, compleximetric methods (e.g. chelation with ethylenediamine tetraacetic acid) are widely used in automated laboratories (Pickup and Brown, 1973). Interlaboratory variation, partly dependent on techniques, should be taken into account when serum calcium values from different centres are compared (Pickup et al., 1975).

Significant changes in serum calcium occur with changes in concentration of the serum proteins (particularly albumin), and various methods of correcting for these changes have been suggested (McLean and Hastings, 1935; Dent, 1962; Parfitt, 1974). However, there appears to be much individual variation in the effect of alterations in protein concentration on total serum calcium concentration in different patients, and it may be necessary to calculate individual regression coefficients by studying the effect of venous occlusion on serum albumin and calcium estimations (Pain et al., 1975). The median regression coefficient for serum calcium concentration on serum albumin concentration is 0.025 mmol/g.

Blood should be collected for serum calcium without a tourniquet, and after a standard period (e.g. 30 minutes) of supine posture, to avoid the effects of extravasation of fluid into the extracellular space (Husdan et al., 1973). Intake of food has a variable effect on serum calcium (Fourman and Royer, 1968), and it is therefore preferable to take the sample fasting. Because of differences in plasma protein concentration, uncorrected total calcium concentrations tend to be slightly lower in women than in men (Goldsmith, 1972).

By standardizing the technique by which blood is taken, the normal range becomes more narrow, and the usefulness of serum calcium concentration as a diagnostic aid is correspondingly enhanced. Greater diagnostic precision is likely to result from the use of ionized rather than total, calcium concentrations, when this determination becomes generally available.

8.2. PARATHYROID HORMONE

Certain aspects of the chemistry and physiology of parathyroid hormone are particularly relevant to appreciating current laboratory tests of parathyroid function.

8.2.1. Chemistry, synthesis and secretion

Purified bovine, porcine and human parathyroid hormones each consist of a single chain of 84 aminoacids. The complete aminoacid sequence of human parathyroid hormone is not yet known; two independent sequence determinations have produced conflicting results at three of the residues in the first 34 aminoacids (Keutmann, 1974). Biological activity appears to be associated with the first 34 aminoacids, and requires the 2–27 sequence counting from the amino-terminal.

Several isohormones of parathyroid hormone, with similar immunological, but different physiochemical properties, are synthesized by human parathyroids. Normal glands (Chu et al., 1973) and adenomata (Habener et al., 1972) incorporate isotopically labelled aminoacids initially into pro-parathyroid hormone, which is slightly larger than parathyroid hormone; subsequently, conversion of pro-parathyroid hormone into parathyroid hormone occurs. The relative contents of newly synthesized pro-parathyroid hormone and parathyroid hormone apparently vary in different adenomas. Hyperplastic parathyroid glands also synthesize a number of these larger isohormones (Wong and Lindall, 1973). Bovine pro-parathyroid hormone contains six basic aminoacids attached to the amino-terminal end of parathyroid hormone (Cohn et al., 1974).

The main peptide secreted is parathyroid hormone but a number of the larger isohormones are secreted as well. Bigger peptides are found in the venous effluent of some parathyroid adenomas (Habener et al., 1971) and a basic peptide with the properties of pro-parathyroid hormone is sometimes released into the medium, along with parathyroid hormone, when human parathyroid adenomas are grown in cell culture (Martin et al., 1973). In contrast, peptides smaller than parathyroid hormone do not appear to be released.

The secretion of parathyroid hormone is dependent upon the concentration of ionized calcium, and possibly also upon the rate at which this changes (Potts and Deftos, 1969); magnesium concentration may also be relevant. Secretion appears to be independent of the serum concentrations of phosphate and of calcitonin, although it may be promoted by the associated hypocalcaemia. Vitamin D and its active metabolites may also regulate secretion.

In vitro studies with human parathyroid tissue have suggested that the secretion of parathyroid hormone by adenomas – unlike hyperplastic glands – may be less responsive to changes in calcium concentration (Sherwood et al., 1971).

8.2.2. Metabolism

Although tissues from several organs are capable of degrading parathyroid hormone, only the kidney has been shown to play a significant role in vivo (Martin et al., 1969).

In contrast to the findings in parathyroid venous effluent, peripheral plasma contains smaller isohormones in addition to parathyroid hormone (Habener et al., 1971), but the site at which these smaller fragments are produced is unknown.

8.2.3. Actions

Parathyroid hormone binds specifically to receptors on the membranes of target cells (Sutcliffe et al., 1973). Early effects include the activation of adenyl cyclase, the production of cyclic AMP, and the uptake of calcium by the cell (Robinson, 1974).

The major actions are due to the changes produced in renal, skeletal and gastrointestinal tissues, but other tissues including liver may be responsive (Robinson, 1974).

8.2.3.1. Renal effects

Phosphaturia is due to inhibition of proximal tubular reabsorption of phosphate; increased urinary excretion of cyclic AMP precedes the phosphaturia. Distal tubular reabsorption of calcium is enhanced, and this effect contributes to its long-term hypercalcaemic action. The net effects on urinary calcium excretion, however, are also dependent on the increased filtered load of calcium which follows hypercalcaemia produced by parathyroid hormone. Inhibition of urinary excretion of hydrogen and magnesium ions, and increased excretion of sodium ions, are also produced.

8.2.3.2. Skeletal effects

The acute increase of serum calcium which is produced by parathyroid hormone is mainly due to its action on bone. Enhanced bone resorption is mediated by osteoclasts and probably by osteocytes as well; hydroxyproline is released, in addition to the mineral components of bone, indicating that bone matrix is also resorbed. A second mechanism for calcium release from bone may involve changes in the cellular transport of calcium which are independent of bone resorption; dissociation of calcium and phosphate release from bone may therefore occur.

Prolonged exposure to parathyroid hormone may actually stimulate osteoblast numbers, and net bone formation can increase (Rasmussen and Bordier, 1974).

8.2.3.3. Gastrointestinal effects

Parathyroid hormone appears to increase the absorption of calcium by the gastrointestinal tract. It is still not certain whether this effect is directly due to the active fragment of parathyroid hormone, or whether it is mediated by other mechanisms.

8.2.4. Laboratory assessment of parathyroid status

Parathyroid function is assessed by determining the circulating concentration of parathyroid hormone and the apparent biological effects of endogenous or exogenous parathyroid hormone.

8.2.4.1. Assay of parathyroid hormone

The least sensitive, but most specific, assays for parathyroid hormone measure the degree of hypercalcaemia or phosphaturia produced in laboratory animals. More sensitive, but less specific, assays measure the release of ^{47}Ca from pre-labelled mouse calvaria, the stimulation of adenyl cyclase, or the inhibition of binding of highly purified, radioactively labelled parathyroid hormone to receptors in cell membrane fractions. Unfortunately, none of these biological assays has sufficient sensitivity for clinical use; the plasma concentrations of parathyroid hormone are approximately 100th of the limit of sensitivity of the best of these assays.

Radioimmunoassays (Buckle, 1974a) are sufficiently sensitive to detect the presence of immunologically reactive parathyroid hormone in normal plasma. As indicated in section 8.2.1, a number of parathyroid hormone-like isohormones may be present in plasma, representing molecules secreted by the glands, and fragments formed by degradation after secretion. The net concentration of immunologically reactive parathyroid hormone in plasma is a function of the concentration and the immunological reactivity of each of the various parathyroid hormone isohormones present.

The apparent concentration will therefore depend upon: the secretion rate of parathyroid hormone, and its precursors and fragments, into the particular plasma pool sampled; the metabolic clearance of each of these species from that plasma pool; and the particular properties of the immunoassay system.

The types of molecules which are detected by a radioimmunoassay depend on the nature of the highly purified peptide used for labelling, the type of hormone preparation used as a reference standard, the antiserum, and the conditions under which the peptide is reacted with antibody.

Certain implications are apparent from a consideration of these factors. There may be poor correlation between the concentration of immunologically reactive parathyroid hormone and the apparent biological activity of the hormone. Only about 40% of the parathyroid hormone molecule is needed for biological activity. Immunoassays may not detect this region of the molecule at all; they may *only* detect this fragment, or as is most usual, they may partially react with this portion. Furthermore, if the biologically active peptide sequence is rapidly cleared from plasma, the concentration may be so small as to be undetectable. It may not always be correct to assume that the plasma level is indeed an index of the secretion rate, for differences in the clearances of various peptides may occur in disease.

(a) *Parathyroid hormone radioimmunoassay in normal subjects.* With most radioimmunoassays, parathyroid hormone in the peripheral plasma of normal adults is measurable, although some subjects have concentrations which are below the detection limit of the assays. The absolute concentrations of parathyroid hormone are usually not known, for the reference standard is rarely human parathyroid hormone; either bovine parathyroid hormone or a standard prepared from human parathyroid adenomas or hyperparathyroid plasma are most commonly used.

Assays which are relatively specific for a particular portion of the parathyroid hormone molecule have been developed by four techniques:

(i) by preparation of antibodies against one particular portion of the molecule (aminoacids 1–34) and incubation of the antibody with the same labelled peptide as tracer (Fischer et al., 1974);

(ii) by blocking a portion of antibody prepared against the entire parathyroid hormone molecule with synthetic fragments of (bovine) parathyroid hormone (Segre et al., 1974);

(iii) by selecting antibodies and labelled hormone systems which are found by experiment to react only with certain portions of the parathyroid molecule (Arnaud et al., 1974);

(iv) by using an assay system that measures carboxy-terminal reactivity in molecules isolated from plasma by a method which selects fragments with amino-terminal reactivity (O'Riordan et al., 1972).

Studies with such assays indicate that the peripheral venous plasma of normal adults contains molecules which react with both the amino- and carboxy-terminal regions of parathyroid hormone; there is relatively less amino- than carboxy-terminal peptide. Detailed characterization of the molecular species in peripheral plasma by a combination of gel filtration and radioimmunological techniques has not as yet been possible, due to the small concentrations of hormone present.

Parathyroid hormone is also measurable in infancy, and the concentrations increase in the early postnatal period (Tsang et al., 1973). A circadian rhythm is apparent (Arnaud et al., 1971; Jubiz et al., 1972) and concentrations increase during pregnancy (Cushard et al., 1971). The values which are found in thyroid venous effluent of patients without disorders of calcium metabolism exceed the values in peripheral blood by 2 to 20 times (Shimkin and Powell, 1973).

During calcium infusion, peripheral parathyroid hormone levels are suppressed, but the rate and extent of this suppression depend upon the relative clearances of the peptides measured by the particular assay used, as well as by the secretion rate of parathyroid hormone. In normal subjects, there is an inverse correlation between the concentration of parathyroid hormone and that of serum calcium (Arnaud et al., 1971).

(b) *Radioimmunoassay in diseases with increased concentrations of circulating parathyroid hormone* (Buckle, 1974b; Parfitt, 1974). In primary hyperparathyroidism, the peripheral venous levels of parathyroid hormone tend to be higher than normal. There is, however, considerable variation in the capacity of various radioimmunoassay systems to identify hyperparathyroidism in this way. In clinical practice, the most useful assay (Reiss and Canterbury, 1973) provides excellent discrimination, but with most other immunoassay systems a number of patients with primary hyperparathyroidism appear to have peripheral concentrations which are well into the normal range, and are sometimes so low as to be undetectable (Buckle, 1974b). It is of particular interest that assays which measure the biologically active portion of the molecule actually result in poorer differentiation than those which measure the carboxy-terminal fragment (Fischer et al., 1974; Arnaud et al., 1974); this apparent paradox is probably accounted for by a much faster clearance of the amino-terminal peptides.

Better discrimination between hyperparathyroid subjects and normals is possible if the serum calcium concentration is also taken into account (Arnaud et al., 1971). In hyperparathyroid subjects with normal peripheral immunoreactive parathyroid hormone concentrations, serum calcium is usually elevated, and circulating parathyroid hormone is therefore inappropriately increased. Furthermore, parathyroid hormone levels correlate with adenoma size (Purnell et al., 1971) and with the concentration of osteoclasts on bone surfaces (Arnaud et al., 1974).

In hyperparathyroidism as well, the peripheral plasma contains greater quantities of peptides which react with carboxy-terminal assays than amino-terminal assays, and most of this material elutes later than intact parathyroid hormone from gel filtration columns, suggesting that hormone fragments are involved (Arnaud et al., 1974; Segre et al., 1974). Such fragments may be biologically active (Canterbury et al., 1973). It is also possible that species which are larger than parathyroid hormone may be present in hyperparathyroidism (Fischer et al., 1974). Pro-parathyroid hormone has not been identified as yet, and the separation of hyperparathyroid subjects from normals on the basis of peripheral pro-parathyroid hormone levels, analogous to proinsulin in insulinoma, is not yet possible.

In theory, stimulation of the release of parathyroid hormone by hypocalcaemia would be expected to result in higher parathyroid hormone concentrations in hyperparathyroidism than in normals. Also, measurement of parathyroid hormone during calcium infusion would be expected to be useful, by indicating the degree of acute suppression of parathyroid activity. In practice, suppression tests have given variable results, probably reflecting the differences in the types of fragments detected by different assays; clinically they have not been found to help in the diagnosis of hyperparathyroidism or in differentiating adenoma from hyperplasia (Buckle, 1974b).

The measurement of parathyroid hormone in samples collected from the major neck veins and their branches may be useful in the localization of parathyroid tissue (Buckle, 1974b). The precision of localization depends on the ability to sample selected veins; screening under fluoroscopic control with injection of appropriate dyes, by allowing selective catheterisation of thyroid veins, enhances the diagnostic potential. A significant gradient (at least 3-fold) between parathyroid and peripheral values suggests the presence of parathyroid tissue proximally; the larger the vein sampled, and the further from the parathyroids, the smaller is the likelihood of showing a significant gradient, as parathyroid hormone will be diluted with blood from non-parathyroid tissues. Failure to show a significant gradient may be due to difficulty in sampling from appropriate veins and does not exclude the presence of a parathyroid adenoma.

These procedures are most useful in the localization of parathyroid tissue following previous neck exploration for hyperparathyroidism. Unfortunately, the distortion of the venous anatomy in the neck which follows previous surgery may make catheterization relatively more difficult. The results of neck vein sampling do not contribute to the diagnosis of hyperparathyroidism, for high parathyroid hormone concentrations can be found in the thyroid veins of euparathyroid subjects. Some groups have advocated selective venous catheterisation with parathyroid hormone measurements, as a routine investigation in the pre-operative evaluation of patients with primary hyperparathyroidism (Eisenberg et al., 1974). In view of the finite risk of complications, the time and expense of the procedure, and the good results of experienced surgeons in finding abnormal parathyroid tissue during operation, the present authors do not routinely undertake selective venous studies.

It has been suggested that amino-terminal assays may produce wider gradients between parathyroid and peripheral values (Arnaud et al., 1974). In theory, measurement of a peptide with a rapid clearance secreted only by parathyroid tissue would be ideal, but further studies are required to substantiate a specific role for amino-terminal assays for this purpose.

In renal failure, the fact that renal tissue makes a substantial contribution to the clearance of parathyroid hormone complicates the interpretation of plasma immunoreactive parathyroid hormone levels. As previously discussed, peripheral concentrations are a net measure of the rate of secretion of parathyroid hormone *and* its clearance from peripheral plasma. Therefore it cannot be assumed that the higher concentrations which are found in renal failure are only due to increased parathyroid secretory activity.

In addition, there are important consequences of radioimmunoassay techniques which are particularly relevant in renal failure. In radioimmunoassay, the inhibition of binding of labelled hormone to antibody by hormone standards is compared to that of plasmas with unknown concentrations. Valid measurements are only possible if the pattern of inhibition produced by increasing concentrations of "unknowns" and of standards are similar ("parallel"). The plasmas of some patients with renal failure react differently from standard hormone, so that precise quantitation is not possible. This problem may not be recognized if only one volume or dilution of plasma is used in the assays, and meaningless results may be obtained, especially if different volumes or dilutions are compared.

In general, plasma parathyroid hormone concentration is commonly elevated in patients with renal failure, even if there is no other evidence for hyperparathyroidism. The values are often much greater than those found in primary hyperparathyroidism. Analysis of the particular fragments indicates that, as in primary hyperparathyroidism, the main increase is in carboxy-terminal, rather than amino-terminal reactive peptide (Arnaud et al., 1974). Before the significance of multiple immunologically reactive forms with different clearances was appreciated, it was not possible to account for the differing responses of peripheral parathyroid hormone to calcium infusion found by various groups (Buckle, 1974b). Apparent suppression of parathyroid hormone during calcium infusion will be demonstrable if parathyroid hormone secretion is reduced *and* if the clearance of the major peptide determined by the particular assay is rapid enough for a significant fall in plasma concentration to occur during the period of study (Arnaud et al., 1974).

Non-parathyroid tumours, usually carcinomas, in hypercalcaemic patients may be associated with increased concentrations of circulating parathyroid hormone (Buckle, 1974b). Measurements of veno-arterial gradients in vivo, and parathyroid hormone production in vitro, suggest that some non-parathyroid cancers can synthesize and release parathyroid hormone. Normocalcaemic patients with bronchial carcinoma may also have increased concentrations (Berson and Yalow, 1966).

The parathyroid hormone present in such patients may have different immunological properties from that in hyperparathyroidism due to parathyroid disease; comparison of the properties using several different antisera may reveal differences in immunoreactivity (Buckle, 1974b). It is not known whether these differences are due to alterations in the aminoacid sequence of the ectopic parathyroid hormone molecule, or to differences in the types and quantities of parathyroid isohormones present. The differential diagnosis of ectopic from parathyroid hyperparathyroidism cannot always be made confidently by immunoassay. Normal or increased concentrations of circulating parathyroid hormone may occur in both, and the immunological differences referred to above may not always be present. Using a number of antisera, however, it has become evident that the concentration of circulating parathyroid hormone is generally lower for a given concentration of serum calcium in the ectopic parathyroid hormone syndromes (Roof et al., 1971; Benson et al., 1974).

In vitamin D deficiency, increased concentrations of circulating parathyroid hormone are commonly found; the values, however, are not always raised, even in hypocalcaemic subjects (Buckle, 1974b). High concentrations slowly return to normal during treatment with vitamin D (Lumb and Stanbury, 1974).

Other diseases which are associated with increased concentrations of circulating parathyroid hormone include pseudohypoparathyroidism (Tashjian et al., 1966), idiopathic hypercalciuria (Coe et al., 1973), Zollinger–Ellison syndrome (Jaffe et al., 1973), fluorosis (Teotia and Teotia, 1973), spinal cord trauma (Arnstein et al., 1973), pseudogout (Phelps and Hawker, 1973), idiopathic osteoporosis (Riggs et al., 1973) and familial medullary thyroid carcinoma (Melvin et al., 1971).

(c) *Radioimmunoassay in diseases with lower than normal concentrations of circulating parathyroid hormone.* Most parathyroid hormone immunoassays are not sufficiently sensitive to detect parathyroid hormone in all normal subjects. The hormone is usually undetectable in hypoparathyroidism but some patients may have normal concentrations (Nusynowitz and Klein, 1973). Values are low in patients with sarcoidosis even in the presence of renal failure (Cushard et al., 1972). Non-parathyroid hypercalcaemia, in the absence of renal failure, is often associated with a low concentration of parathyroid hormone, especially when the concentration of serum calcium is also taken into account (Buckle, 1974b).

8.2.4.2. Indirect tests of parathyroid function

The effects of endogenous parathyroid hormone in relation to assays of serum calcium, phosphate, chloride, bicarbonate and alkaline phosphatase, and urinary excretion of calcium, phosphate and cyclic AMP, are considered in the differential diagnosis of hypercalcaemia in section 8.5.1.4, and in relation to assays of urinary phosphate and cyclic AMP in hypocalcaemia in section 8.5.2.4.

8.2.4.3. Diagnosis of hyperparathyroidism

Hyperparathyroidism may present as recurrent renal calculi, bone disease, chronic renal failure, or as symptomatic or asymptomatic hypercalcaemia in the investigation of other diseases or in the screening of healthy individuals. The selection of appropriate tests for differential diagnosis depends on the type of presentation. The diagnosis of hyperparathyroidism which presents as symptomatic or asymptomatic hypercalcaemia is discussed in section 8.5.1.

(a) *Diagnosis of hyperparathyroidism presenting as recurrent renal calculi.* Chemical analysis of the calculus permits diagnosis of the less common types of nephrolithiasis: uric acid, cystine or xanthine stones (Nordin, 1973). Urinary tract infection, often associated with urine stasis due to anatomical changes within the urinary tract, or to urinary obstruction, may lead to magnesium ammonium phosphate stones containing varying amounts of calcium. However, the majority of renal stones contain only calcium oxalate and/or calcium phosphate, and in patients forming recurrent renal stones of this variety, primary hyperparathyroidism must be distinguished from idiopathic hypercalciuria and from the situation in individuals who have no demonstrable biochemical disorder of calcium metabolism.

If serum calcium concentration is clearly elevated, the presumptive diagnosis is hyperparathyroidism, but it is important to exclude sarcoidosis and vitamin D intoxication by a hydrocortisone suppression test (section 8.5.1.4) and possibly by parathyroid hormone immunoassay if renal function is normal. The administration of thiazide diuretics to reduce urinary calcium excretion can produce mild hypercalcaemia, even in the absence of hyperparathyroidism (Parfitt, 1969) and specimens for serum calcium determination should be taken in the untreated state.

Diagnosis is much more difficult if the concentration of serum calcium is normal. In general, a very high urinary calcium excretion suggests idiopathic hypercalciuria or sarcoidosis, but calcium intake (Peacock et al., 1967) and renal function must also be taken into consideration. Patients who are subsequently shown to have hyperparathyroidism will almost always have hypercalcaemia at some stage of their illness, but as hypercalcaemia may only be intermittent, repeated determinations of serum calcium should be made. Rarely, the total serum calcium concentration is normal and only the ionized fraction is elevated (Muldowney et al., 1973). If concomitant vitamin D deficiency is a possibility, repletion with vitamin D may unmask latent hypercalcaemia (Woodhouse et al., 1971). The assay of parathyroid hormone is seldom helpful, for the concentration may not be higher than normal in hyperparathyroidism and can be elevated in idiopathic hypercalciuria.

Measurements of urinary phosphate clearance in relation to creatinine clearance may be of some value in making the diagnosis of hyperparathyroidism in this situation (Nordin and Smith, 1965). The determination of phosphate excretion index (Nordin and Fraser, 1960) is technically simple, involving the simultaneous measurement of serum and urine phosphate and creatinine concentrations; the test must be performed fasting and although a standard time or urine collection (e.g. between 07.00 and 09.00 hours) improves reproducibility, at least three measurements on consecutive days should be made. Any degree of renal insufficiency increases the excretion of phosphate relative to creatinine and invalidates the test. Care to avoid haemolysis, which will increase the apparent serum phosphate concentration, is essential. In normocalcaemic patients with recurrent renal calculi, the finding of an increased phosphate excretion index makes hyperparathyroidism likely; failure of the phosphate excretion index to be suppressed into the normal range during 4 days administration of calcium and aluminium hydroxide, especially if such treatment produces hypercalcaemia (Adams et al., 1970), is further evidence for hyperparathyroidism. Urinary cyclic AMP (Schmidt-Gaye and Roher, 1973) and possibly urinary hydroxyproline determinations may facilitate the diagnosis of parathyroid disease without sustained hypercalcaemia.

(b) *Diagnosis of hyperparathyroidism presenting as bone disease.* Radiological changes of osteitis fibrosa are always due to hyperparathyroidism. Osteitis fibrosa is unusual in primary hyperparathyroidism and may depend upon concomitant vitamin D deficiency (Keynes and Caird, 1970; Woodhouse et al., 1971); vitamin D repletion may heal the bone disease and unmask latent hypercalcaemia. In secondary hyperparathyroidism associated with vitamin D depletion, osteitis fibrosa occurs with normo- or hypocalcaemia, and hypo- or normo- and more rarely hyperphosphataemia (Lumb and Stanbury, 1974). In the secondary hyperparathyroidism of renal failure, osteitis fibrosa is found, together with biochemical evidence of frank uraemia, and hyperphosphataemia with normo- or hypocalcaemia. Treatment of renal osteodystrophy with aluminium hydroxide may, however, reduce the serum phosphate and increase the serum calcium concentration into the normal range. Tertiary hyperparathyroidism is best defined as hyperparathyroidism due to renal failure or vitamin D depletion in which the serum calcium concentration is elevated; it may be accompanied by radiological evidence of osteitis fibrosa. Increases in serum alkaline phosphatase activity and/or the concentration of plasma hydroxyproline are found in patients with osteitis fibrosa; urinary hydroxyproline excretion is increased if renal function is not severely impaired. Only one case of hyperparathyroidism associated with non-parathyroid tumour has shown osteitis fibrosa (Scholz et al., 1973).

Very rarely, hyperparathyroid bone disease can present with radiological appearances similar to those of osteoporosis. The diagnosis of hyperparathyroidism can be made by similar procedures to those described for recurrent renal calculi. Again the diagnosis is substantiated by the finding of hypercalcaemia, which may be intermittent, or masked by vitamin D deficiency. Multiple myeloma and thyrotoxicosis should also be excluded. As parathyroid hormone concentrations can be increased in idiopathic osteoporosis, this investigation may not prove helpful.

(c) *Diagnosis of hyperparathyroidism presenting with uraemia.* As well as rendering interpretation of the concentrations of immunoreactive parathyroid hormone difficult, the presence of uraemia complicates the interpretation of serum calcium, phosphate and bicarbonate concentrations and urinary excretion of calcium, phosphate and cyclic AMP. The distinction between tertiary hyperparathyroidism due to renal failure, and primary hyperparathyroidism complicated by moderate to severe uraemia, is virtually impossible without determining serum calcium concentration and renal function. In the absence of osteitis fibrosa, vitamin D intoxication, milk alkali syndrome and sarcoidosis should be excluded by corticosteroid administration.

8.2.5. Laboratory assessment of treatment in parathyroid disease

8.2.5.1. Parathyroidectomy

Hypocalcaemia, and less commonly hypomagnesaemia, may occur within hours of parathyroidectomy; severe hypocalcaemia and hypomagnesaemia are common when hyperparathyroidism is associated with radiological evidence of osteitis fibrosa. Renal function may also deteriorate temporarily after parathyroidectomy. Serum calcium concentration should be monitored during long-term follow-up after parathyroidectomy, in order to detect recurrence or hypoparathyroidism.

8.2.5.2. Hypoparathyroidism

Serum calcium and phosphate concentrations should be measured at intervals of not more than 3 months during treatment of hypoparathyroidism. The minimum dose of calcium and/or vitamin D which is required to maintain a normal serum calcium concentration in hypoparathyroidism varies from patient to patient. Changes in the bioavailability of commercial vitamin D preparations cannot always be anticipated (Parfitt and Frame, 1972), and alterations in the dosage of other drugs (section 8.4.1) may modify the metabolism of vitamin D. More frequent determinations should be made during immobilisation and at times of physiological stress, including pregnancy.

Urinary excretion of calcium should also be monitored, especially in infants and children, in order to avoid the possible consequences of hypercalciuria.

8.2.5.3. Hyperparathyroidism

Repeated measurements of serum calcium concentration and, if there is bone disease, alkaline phosphatase activity, are useful in following the course of hyperparathyroidism and in assessing the results of medical treatment. Serum phosphate and indices of renal function should also be monitored frequently during treatment of secondary hyperparathyroidism in renal failure.

8.3. CALCITONIN

Human calcitonin has been extracted from tissues obtained from patients with medullary carcinoma of the thyroid gland in sufficient quantities to allow purification and structural analysis. The molecule consists of a chain of 32 aminoacids with a disulphide bond between cystine residues near the amino-terminal (Neher et al., 1968). Human thyroid calcitonin has similar immunological and biological properties to that from medullary carcinoma (Clark et al., 1969), but precise identity has not yet been established. Non-human calcitonins (porcine, bovine, ovine and salmon), extracted and purified from the animal thyroid glands or the ultimobranchial body of the salmon, contain a similar number of aminoacids, but the sequence is different.

In the human, most calcitonin is present within the thyroid gland. Hypocalcaemic activity is also present in extracts of parathyroid glands and thymus (Galante et al., 1968) and cells in these organs may take up fluorescein-labelled antibody to calcitonin. Immunologically reactive calcitonin is also present in extracts of some non-thyroid carcinomas (Hillyard et al., 1975), and these tumours can also synthesize and release calcitonin.

Thyroidectomized subjects who are maintained on thyroxine have slight impairment of calcium tolerance and tend to have higher serum calcium concentrations after calcium loading, but this biochemical finding does not appear to be associated with any disease state.

Most of the effects of calcitonin are due to its action on the skeleton, and to a smaller extent on kidney and possibly the gastrointestinal tract. Structural changes in osteoclasts are apparent within minutes of calcitonin administration (Holtrop et al., 1974) and the hypocalcaemia so produced is due to acute inhibition of bone resorption (MacIntyre and Parsons, 1966). The administration of calcitonin is also associated with hypophosphataemia, but the mechanism of this effect is obscure. As with other polypeptide hormones, binding by cytoplasmic receptors followed by adenyl cyclase activation and transcellular calcium fluxes mediate its effects. The metabolic clearance of human calcitonin is considerably lower in patients with severe renal failure, suggesting that the kidneys play a significant role in degradation (Ardaillou et al., 1970).

8.3.1. Biological assay of calcitonin

Calcitonin activity is defined by the hypocalcaemic effect which is produced in laboratory animals. No fragments have yet been shown to be hypocalcaemic, and oxidation of the cystine bridge removes biological activity. In patients with medullary carcinoma and very high circulating concentrations of calcitonin (~10 ng/ml), measurement of calcitonin by bioassay is feasible, but the bioassay does not have sufficient sensitivity for routine clinical use. Biological activity can also be measured by the inhibition of binding of highly purified, radioactively labelled calcitonin to receptors in cell membrane fractions (Aurbach and Heath, 1974), or by determining the inhibition of bone resorption in tissue culture (Raisz et al., 1972); however, the sensitivity of these assays is comparable to the hypocalcaemia bioassay and problems of specificity may arise.

8.3.2. Radioimmunoassay of calcitonin

Radioimmunoassays for human calcitonin measure the inhibition of binding of radioactively labelled synthetic human calcitonin to antibodies prepared against either synthetic human calcitonin or extracts of medullary thyroid carcinoma tissue; the inhibitory effect of plasma is compared to that of synthetic human calcitonin standards.

8.3.2.1. Physiological concentrations of calcitonin
The normal range of circulating immunoreactive calcitonin depends on the properties of the particular radioimmunoassay system. With most assays, the plasma calcitonin in healthy adults is found to be less than 0.10 ng/ml, which is the minimum detectable concentration. With some assays, normal plasmas may contain up to 1.0 ng/ml and this value largely reflects differences in the particular immunologically reactive calcitonin-like molecules which are detected by different assay systems. Another source of variation is the type of plasma used as blank for standard curves and for dilutions of unknown plasmas. Calcitonin-free plasma can be prepared by adsorption of calcitonin on to micro-fine silica, glass beads, or charcoal, but this procedure removes other material as well. With some assays, plasma from totally thyroidectomised patients is used as blank, but it is still uncertain whether this is truly calcitonin-free.

The infusion of calcium may increase immunoreactive calcitonin concentrations in normal adults, but this finding is variable and differing results probably reflect the particular properties of the immunoassay systems used.

Calcitonin concentrations in umbilical cord blood have been reported to be higher than those in the circulating blood of normal adults (Samaan et al., 1973). Immunoreactive calcitonin concentrations are slightly higher in late pregnancy than in non-pregnant adults of the same age, and return towards normal post-partum (Samaan et al., 1974).

8.3.2.2. Levels of calcitonin in disease
Patients who have chronic hypocalcaemia tend to have higher than normal quantities of calcitonin within the thyroid gland (Deftos et al., 1974) and hypercalcitoninaemia may also occur. Patients with chronic hypercalcaemia usually have undetectable concentrations, but hyperparathyroid patients may have high values. Increased concentrations are also found in the Zollinger–Ellison syndrome (Sizemore et al., 1973), and in some patients with chronic renal failure (Heynen and Franchimont, 1974); intermittently high high concentrations have been reported in one patient with pycnodysostosis (Baker et al., 1973).

Hypercalcitoninaemia is common in patients with non-thyroid tumours, even in the absence of hypercalcaemia (Coombes et al., 1974). Ectopic production of calcitonin by carcinoma of the lung has been reported (Silva et al., 1974; Ellison et al., 1975). The finding of a plasma concentration exceeding 10 ng/ml in a patient with metastatic disease and unknown primary tumour, suggests medullary carcinoma of the thyroid gland. It is possible that ectopic calcitonin will prove immunologically distinguishable from thyroid calcitonin.

Medullary carcinoma of the thyroid gland (Hazard et al., 1959) is consistently associated with hypercalcitoninaemia. The tumour produces large quantities of calcitonin which, like calcitonin in the parafollicular cells of the normal thyroid, is stored within granules (Bussolati et al., 1969). Medullary carcinoma is a relatively uncommon form of thyroid carcinoma which is characterized histologically by being anaplastic and containing amyloid in its stroma. Fasting plasma concentrations are usually raised, but a normal value does not exclude the diagnosis of medullary thyroid carcinoma. In equivocal cases, assays should be carried out in association with provocative testing by the standard calcium infusion, short calcium infusion (Parthemore et al., 1974) or after glucagon (Melvin et al., 1971) and pentagastrin (Hennessy et al., 1974) infusion, or oral whisky (Dymling et al., 1976). The assay of samples during provocative testing may also provide a guide to the mass of calcitonin which is present within the tumour cells.

Calcitonin assay may be indicated for several reasons in patients with suspected or proven medullary carcinoma.

(a) *To assist in establishing a diagnosis.* The finding of hypercalcitoninaemia is not pathognomic of medullary carcinoma of the thyroid. Even in the patients with a strong family history of medullary carcinoma, hypercalcitoninaemia may reflect excess production of calcitonin from *hyperplastic* C cells (Tashjian et al., 1974). In patients presenting with thyroid nodules or goitre, the finding of hypercalcitoninaemia is suggestive of medullary carcinoma, but confirmation requires histological diagnosis; the small fraction of patients presenting with thyroid enlargement which is due to medullary carcinoma, and the need for histological confirmation of diagnosis anyway, means that calcitonin assay is not generally helpful in these patients. By contrast, in patients presenting with other manifestations of syndromes associated with medullary carcinoma, e.g. multiple mucosal neuromata and Marfanoid habitus, the finding of hypercalcitoninaemia is particularly helpful in diagnosis. In familial medullary carcinoma of the thyroid, often associated with phaeochromocytoma and usually with a normal habitus, hypercalcitoninaemia defines those members at most risk of developing illness from either disease (Melvin et al., 1971; Greenberg and MacIntyre, 1974).

(b) *To follow the course of the disease and the effect of treatment.* Serial calcitonin estimations, particularly after provocative stimulation, provide an index of the change in the activity and magnitude of the calcitonin-producing cell population. The assay of single samples may be inadequate, for up to 10-fold fluctuation in concentration may occur in fasting specimens collected over several days from patients who are not receiving specific treatment (Deftos, 1974; Dymling et al., 1976). Comparisons of calcitonin concentrations before and after surgical treatment assist in confirming the adequacy of treatment; persistent hypercalcitoninaemia suggests residual tumour, and may antedate morphological evidence of recurrence (Goltzman et al., 1974).

(c) *In localization of metastases.* Higher calcitonin concentrations are found in the veins draining medullary carcinomas than in the systemic circulation (Deftos, 1974; Goltzmann et al., 1974). Selective venous catheterization may permit localization of metastatic tissue.

8.4. VITAMIN D

Vitamin D activity is generated partly by the synthesis of vitamin D_3 (cholecalciferol) in the skin under the influence of ultraviolet irradiation, and partly from ingested foodstuffs such as vitamin D_2 (ergocalciferol) or vitamin D_3. The structural formulae of vitamins D_3 and D_2 and of their precursors are shown in Figures 8.1 and 8.2. Endogenously synthesized cholecalciferol is the predominant source of vitamin D_3 under usual circumstances (Haddad and Hahn, 1973; Stamp and Round, 1974).

8.4.1. Vitamin D metabolism

The major circulating form of vitamin D_3 is 25-hydroxycholecalciferol (Blunt et al., 1968) which is formed from cholecalciferol in the liver. 25-Hydroxycholecalciferol is relatively inactive, and for full biological activity it must be converted into 1,25-dihydroxycholecalciferol by a further hydroxylase enzyme which is found only in the kidney (Fraser and Kodicek, 1970). Preliminary evidence indicates that this highly active metabolite acts in a manner analogous to steroid hormones by interacting with cytosolic and nuclear receptors to initiate transcriptional changes leading to the synthesis of new protein. Other metabolites of cholecalciferol, such as 24,25-dihydroxycholecalciferol, and 1,24,25-trihydroxycholecalciferol have also been identified, but their physiological significance has not yet been clarified.

Ingested vitamin D is absorbed in the small intestine, in both jejunum and ileum, and bile appears to play an important role. After absorption via the lymphatics into the blood stream, vitamin D and its metabolites are carried in association with a specific transport protein which has greatest affinity for the 25-hydroxy derivatives, but also binds the parent compound. Binding proteins for vitamin D metabolites have also been characterized from kidney and many other sites.

The disappearance of vitamin D from the circulation follows a biphasic pattern. The early phase, with a half-life of 20 to 30 hours represents uptake and storage by the tissues, whereas the slow phase, with a half-life of several weeks, reflects the eventual biotransformation and excretion of the vitamin and its metabolites (Mawer et al., 1969).

The liver participates in early uptake of vitamin D, but skeletal muscle and adipose tissue are more important storage sites, which presumably act as sources during periods of deprivation. The eventual excretion of vitamin D occurs largely in the faeces, after inacti-

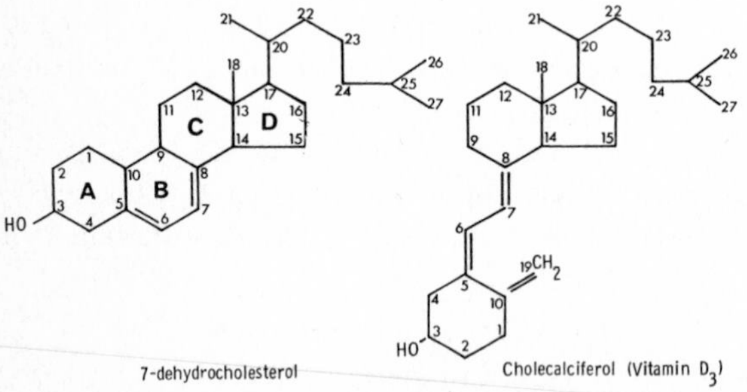

Figure 8.1. Chemical structures of 7-dehydrocholesterol and cholecalciferol (vitamin D_3); 7-dehydrocholesterol is converted into cholecalciferol by exposure to ultraviolet irradiation. Full activation of cholecalciferol is achieved by introduction of hydroxy-groups in the 1 and 25 positions.

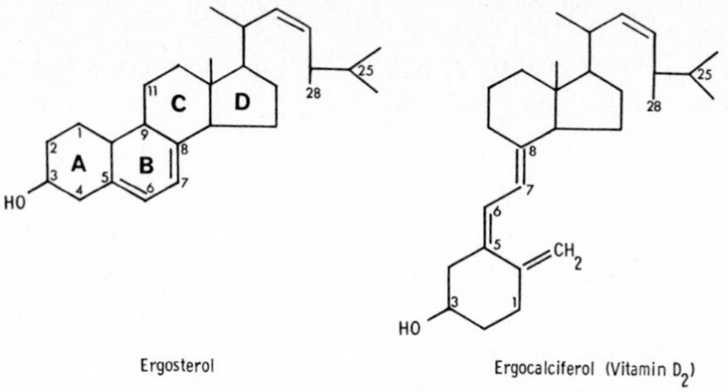

Ergosterol

Ergocalciferol (Vitamin D_2)

Figure 8.2. Chemical structure of ergosterol and ergocalciferol (vitamin D_2); ergosterol is converted into ergocalciferol by exposure to ultraviolet irradiation.

vation in the liver and excretion in the bile (Kodicek, 1963). Some urinary excretion of metabolically altered, water soluble metabolites, including a glucuronide conjugate (Avioli et al., 1967), also occurs. The final stages of hepatic biotransformation are enhanced by drugs such as phenobarbitone and diphenylhydantoin which induce liver microsomal enzymes (Hahn et al., 1972b). This probably accounts for the low plasma concentrations of 25-hydroxycholecalciferol which are found in patients chronically receiving anticonvulsant therapy (Hahn et al., 1972a).

8.4.2. Actions of vitamin D metabolites

1,25-Dihydroxycholecalciferol enhances the absorption of calcium and phosphate from the intestine, the mobilization of calcium from bone, and probably the reabsorption of calcium and phosphate from the urine. Vitamin D_2 and vitamin D_3, together with their 25-hydroxy-derivatives, probably have a similar effect, but at much higher concentrations. A direct action on muscle is also likely. There has been controversy about whether vitamin D and its metabolites have a direct action on bone formation in vivo, and this has not been totally resolved. Certainly the net effect of administration of vitamin D and its metabolites in states of vitamin D deficiency is to enhance the deposition of calcium in bone.

8.4.3. Measurement of vitamin D metabolites

A competitive protein binding assay for 25-hydroxy-chole/ergo-calciferol has been developed. Unlabelled 25-hydroxy-chole/ergo-calciferol competes with a small fixed amount of radioactively labelled compound for binding to the specific protein (section 8.4.1) found in kidney cytosol (Haddad and Chyu, 1971) or serum (Belsey et al., 1971). Rat binding proteins do not differentiate between 25-hydroxycholecalciferol and 25-hydroxyergocalciferol, whereas chick binding proteins bind the former much more avidly than the latter (Greenberg et al., 1974; Belsey et al., 1974), so allowing differential assays for the two compounds.

Depending on ethnic factors, 25-hydroxycholecalciferol concentrations in serum have

TABLE 8.2.

25-HYDROXY-CHOLE/ERGO-CALCIFEROL CONCENTRATIONS IN DIFFERENT CONDITIONS ASSOCIATED WITH DISTURBANCES OF CALCIUM METABOLISM

Low	Normal	High
Dietary osteomalacia	Sarcoidosis	Vitamin D intoxication
Biliary and portal cirrhosis	Some cases of renal osteodystrophy	Excessive exposure to sunlight
Anticonvulsant osteomalacia	Vitamin D-resistant rickets	
Some cases of renal osteodystrophy		
Osteitis fibrosa cystica		
Osteomalacia in Asian immigrants to Great Britain		

been found to be of the order of 5 to 30 ng/ml, with low values found in nutritional osteomalacia, cirrhosis, or chronic anticonvulsant ingestion; variable concentrations occur in chronic renal failure, and high values after excessive exposure to sun (Table 8.2).

To be of real value in understanding the biochemical basis of metabolic bone disease, it is necessary to measure the most active metabolite, 1,25-dihydroxycholecalciferol, the circulating level of which is of the order of 0.1 ng/ml (Brumbaugh et al., 1974). This assay depends on a competitive interaction with a cytosolic and then a nuclear receptor isolated from intestinal cells. Preliminary results suggest that the concentration of 1,25-dihydroxycholecalciferol is indeed low in patients with chronic renal failure. These competitive binding assays for metabolites are very much more sensitive than bioassay techniques such as the "line-test" (McCollum et al., 1922), which depends on the deposition of a line of calcification in cartilage from rachitic rats on a standard diet, or on tests depending on the ability of active vitamin D metabolites to enhance intestinal calcium absorption in vivo or in vitro.

8.5. DISORDERS OF CALCIUM HOMEOSTASIS

8.5.1. Hypercalcaemia

Hypercalcaemia may manifest itself in many different ways. It may present with classical symptoms, including weakness, tiredness, lassitude, thirst, polyuria, nausea, vomiting, constipation and vague psychological disorders. Alternatively, the first suggestion of this biochemical disturbance may come from a history of recurrent renal calculi. Occasionally the patient presents in a hypercalcaemic crisis, with dehydration and depressed conscious state (sometimes coma) or with delayed complications of hypercalcaemia such as chronic renal failure and peptic ulceration. However, it is increasingly common to detect hypercalcaemia incidentally as the result of biochemical screening procedures in people without symptoms, or who have been hospitalized for conditions not primarily involving calcium homeostasis.

The major causes of hypercalcaemia are listed in Table 8.3. The most common are those associated with neoplastic disorders, with or without metastases to bone, and primary hyperparathyroidism. Prostaglandins or sterols may contribute to hypercalcaemia by causing bone resorption, which in some cases is associated with malignancy, while ectopic production of parathyroid hormone-like peptides may occur in other cases (section 8.2.4.1).

When sought, mild degrees of hypercalcaemia are quite commonly found in thyrotoxicosis, probably in association with increased bone resorption. In sarcoidosis, hypercalcaemia is mainly a result of increased intestinal absorption of calcium due to increased sensitivity to vitamin D, although increased bone resorption probably also contributes. Hypercalciuria is an even more common manifestation of these two disorders. The hypercalcaemia of the "milk-alkali syndrome" is due partly to increased calcium load from the intestine, and partly to impaired urinary excretion of calcium which accompanies the systemic alkalosis from ingestion of soluble alkali. There is also the possibility that the hypercalcaemia in this condition is due to some other cause (e.g. parathyroid adenoma) and that a peptic ulcer has occurred secondary to the hypercalcaemia. Paget's disease rarely produces hypercalcaemia except when it is extensive and associated with immobilization. Thiazide diuretics can cause mild hypercalcaemia by enhancing tubular reabsorption of calcium. Hypercalcaemia is being recognized with increasing frequency as a self-limiting phenomenon of unknown mechanism which occurs during the diuretic phase of acute renal failure. Hypercalcaemia in acromegaly may be due to co-existent parathyroid adenoma, or to the elevated growth hormone itself.

The steps taken in the elucidation of a case of hypercalcaemia can be summarized as follows.

TABLE 8.3.

CAUSES OF HYPERCALCAEMIA

I.	Primary and tertiary hyperparathyroidism
II.	Malignant disease with bone involvement, in particular – metastatic carcinoma of breast, lung, kidney, multiple myeloma, lymphomas and leukaemia
III.	Malignant disease without bone involvement, in particular – squamous cell carcinoma of lung, carcinoma of kidney
IV.	Sarcoidosis
V.	Vitamin D intoxication
VI.	Milk-alkali syndrome
VII.	Paget's disease with immobilization
VIII.	Thyrotoxicosis
IX.	Acromegaly
X.	Thiazide diuretics
XI.	Diuretic phase of acute tubular necrosis
XII.	"Idiopathic" hypercalcaemia of infancy

8.5.1.1. History

Particular attention should be paid to the duration of symptoms (a malignant cause would be unlikely with a prolonged history); the nature of the symptoms (renal calculi together with hypercalcaemia suggest hyperparathyroidism); and a history of excessive antacid, calcium or vitamin D intake. Symptoms of malignant disease, renal disease, Paget's disease, thyrotoxicosis, sarcoidosis or Addison's disease should be sought. Symptoms suggesting a co-existent insulinoma or pituitary tumour may be found in primary hyperparathyroidism, and occasionally there is a family history.

8.5.1.2. Examination

Clinical examination may reveal evidence of the underlying cause in cases secondary to malignancy, Paget's disease, thyrotoxicosis, Addison's disease or acromegaly. In hyperparathyroidism (particularly secondary or tertiary), corneal calcification may occur. In the now rare cases where hyperparathyroidism is accompanied by overt osteitis fibrosa, bones may be tender or deformed. Hypertension and proteinuria may be present, and occasionally myopathy may occur. It is rare for a parathyroid adenoma to be palpable.

8.5.1.3. Radiology

Radiological findings may give evidence of metastatic tumours, or a primary carcinoma of the lung, kidney or other organ. The radiological signs of osteitis fibrosa cystica may be present, and the finding of subperiosteal erosions of the phalanges and of the terminal digital tufts is particularly useful in establishing a diagnosis of hyperparathyroidism. Paget's disease may be revealed.

8.5.1.4. Biochemical tests

(a) *Serum calcium.* Blood must be collected as described in section 8.1.6, and the estimated serum calcium concentration should be corrected, if necessary, to allow for abnormal protein concentration. In marginal cases, repeated estimations or a determination of ionized calcium may be required, but adequate care with sampling and standardization considerably reduces the number of hyperparathyroid patients who are found to have normal serum calcium concentrations (Watson, 1974).

(b) *Serum phosphate.* Parathyroid hormone decreases the tubular reabsorption of phosphate, leading to a low serum phosphate concentration in hyperparathyroidism, providing that renal function is normal. However, the discriminative value of a low serum phosphate concentration is not high, as hypercalcaemia of any cause will increase the loss of renal phosphate (Schussler et al., 1972). Serum phosphate may be normal or raised if there is co-existent renal impairment, and it may also be high in metastatic carcinoma of the breast.

(c) *Urinary calcium.* In patients with normal renal function, hypercalcaemia is accompanied by increased urinary excretion of calcium. Because of the effect of parathyroid hormone in enhancing the tubular reabsorption of calcium, the increase in urinary excretion of calcium is less in hypercalcaemia due to hyperparathyroidism than for a comparable degree of hypercalcaemia due to other causes. However, because of the difficulty in defining appropriate degrees of hypercalciuria in the presence of variable degrees of hypercalcaemia, this distinction has little value in differential diagnosis. In sarcoidosis and thyrotoxicosis, hypercalciuria is often present even if the serum calcium concentration is normal.

(d) *Urinary phosphate.* Because of the effects of hypercalcaemia of any cause on the tubular reabsorption of phosphate, tests based on the urinary excretion of phosphate have not found widespread use in the investigation of hypercalcaemia.

(e) *Serum alkaline phosphatase.* The concentration is often increased in hypercalcaemia accompanying malignant disease with bone involvement, in Paget's disease of bone, and in hyperparathyroidism accompanied by bone involvement. It may be increased in thyrotoxicosis, but is usually normal in hyperparathyroidism without bone involvement, in milk-alkali syndrome, and in sarcoidosis and vitamin D intoxication. Alkaline phosphatase can be assumed to have originated from bone – and not liver – if there is no concurrent elevation of 5′-nucleotidase; alternatively, specialized methods can be used to distinguish the bone isoenzyme from that arising from liver. The interpretation of the alkaline phosphatase activity must be related to the appropriate reference interval for sex, and particularly for age, as serum alkaline phosphatase is considerably higher during growth.

(f) *Serum bicarbonate.* Hyperparathyroidism tends to be accompanied by a hyperchloraemic renal tubular acidosis (Wills and McGowan, 1964). Thus in this condition, but not in most other conditions causing hypercalcaemia, serum bicarbonate is lower than normal, and serum chloride tends to be high. Multivariate analysis of serum chloride, bicarbonate, urea, alkaline phosphatase and phosphate values in hypercalcaemia has been described, and a high level of diagnostic accuracy claimed (Fraser et al., 1971).

(g) *Urinary cyclic AMP excretion.* In the majority of patients with hyperparathyroidism, urinary excretion of cyclic AMP is raised (provided that renal function is normal), whereas in hypercalcaemia of other causes, the excretion tends to be low (Dohan et al., 1972).

(h) *Parathyroid hormone.* The scope and limitations of the assay of parathyroid hormone are discussed in section 8.2.4.

(i) *Hydrocortisone suppression test* (Dent and Watson, 1968). The administration of hydrocortisone (40 mg) every 8 hours for 10 days produces a marked fall in serum calcium concentration in immobilized patients or those with sarcoidosis, vitamin D intoxication, milk-alkali syndrome, Addison's disease or thyrotoxicosis. Patients with metastatic tumours or non-metastatic malignant disease show a variable response. Patients with primary or tertiary hyperparathyroidism rarely show a significant response. As fluid retention may produce some dilutional fall in serum calcium, correction for protein concentration should be made.

(j) *25-Hydroxycholecalciferol.* In cases of vitamin D intoxication, the assay of 25-hydroxycholecalciferol may reveal high blood concentrations. In other causes of hypercalcaemia (Table 8.3), 25-hydroxycholecalciferol concentrations are normal or low.

(k) *Other tests.* In general, studies of calcium absorption, calcium balance, calcium infusion with measurement of phosphate excretion, hydroxyproline concentration, parathyroid scanning and quantitative bone histology, have not found general usefulness in the differential diagnosis of hypercalcaemia. When indicated, serum thyroxine, or plasma or urinary cortisol estimations, may provide the diagnosis.

In spite of the number of tests available, in some cases neck exploration must be undertaken without a firm diagnosis of hyperparathyroidism being made pre-operatively. The aim of investigation should be to reduce these cases to a minimum.

8.5.2. Hypocalcaemia

It is important to allow for the effect of changes in plasma protein concentration and pH before assessing the importance of hypocalcaemia. Total calcium is lowered in cases of hypoalbuminaemia, and in chronic acidosis (e.g. in chronic renal failure), because of a decrease in protein-bound calcium; ionized calcium is often normal in these situations. The main causes of hypocalcaemia are listed in Table 8.4. The patients may present with acute symptoms, or after the gradual onset of symptoms such as paraesthesiae, epilepsy, mental changes, dry scaly skin and brittle nails, cataract, or growth retardation with or without tetany.

The elucidation of the cause of a case of hypocalcaemia may be summarized as follows.

8.5.2.1. History

Particular note should be taken of the severity and duration of symptoms, family history (often present in pseudohypoparathyroidism), diet or episodes of diarrhoea (which may suggest malabsorption). A history of previous neck surgery would strongly suggest the possibility of hypoparathyroidism.

8.5.2.2. Examination

This would be directed particularly towards looking for a scar in the neck, characteristic skeletal abnormalities of pseudohypoparathyroidism (round face, short neck, thick set, short, stocky build, short metacarpals or metatarsals), manifestations of malabsorption, subcutaneous calcification (common in pseudohypoparathyroidism), cataracts, and epithelial changes (found in both hypoparathyroidism and pseudohypoparathyroidism). Hyperirritability of the facial nerve (Chvostek's sign) and carpal spasm on occluding arterial blood flow in the upper limb (Trousseau's sign) should be sought.

TABLE 8.4.

CAUSES OF HYPOCALCAEMIA

I.	Idiopathic and surgical hypoparathyroidism
II.	Pseudohypoparathyroidism
III.	Vitamin D deficiency, in particular – nutritional malabsorption
IV.	Chronic renal failure
V.	Magnesium deficiency
VI.	Prolonged anticonvulsant therapy
VII.	Acute pancreatitis
VIII.	Massive blood transfusion

8.5.2.3. Radiology

Radiological features of osteomalacia may be apparent. Short metacarpals or metatarsals can be confirmed. Occasionally increased density of bone in the skeleton or calvarium can be detected in hypoparathyroidism. Basal ganglia calcification is found in about one-half of cases of pseudohypoparathyroidism, and in about one-third of cases of idiopathic hypoparathyroidism.

8.5.2.4. Biochemistry

(a) *Serum calcium.* By definition, the total serum calcium concentration is low in all these conditions, although osteomalacia (commonly) and chronic renal failure can occur with normal serum calcium concentrations, presumably due to compensatory parathyroid hypersecretion. The skeletal abnormalities of pseudohypoparathyroidism can occur without hypocalcaemia; in this situation, the condition is sometimes termed "pseudopseudohypoparathyroidism". Ionized calcium is also low in hypoparathyroidism, pseudohypoparathyroidism, vitamin D deficiency, and magnesium deficiency. However, it may be normal or only slightly reduced in chronic renal failure, if significant acidosis has contributed to the low total calcium concentration by interference with protein binding.

(b) *Serum phosphate.* This assay is useful in distinguishing malabsorption and vitamin D deficiency from hypoparathyroidism, pseudohypoparathyroidism and hypocalcaemia of renal failure. In the first group, the serum phosphate concentration is usually low, whereas in the second group it is high. However, severe osteomalacia may occasionally be accompanied by high serum phosphate concentration, perhaps due to impaired parathyroid hormone secretion.

(c) *Urinary calcium excretion.* This is low in all conditions associated with hypocalcaemia. However, when related to serum calcium, the decrease of calcium excretion in hypoparathyroidism is less marked than in other causes of hypocalcaemia. This test has little practical value in differential diagnosis.

(d) *Urinary phosphate excretion.* Phosphate-losing renal tubular disorders, such as familial hypophosphataemic rickets and the Fanconi syndrome may be associated with radiological evidence of osteomalacia, but the serum calcium concentration is usually normal. In disorders which are associated with hypocalcaemia, the urinary phosphate excretion is variable, e.g. in vitamin D deficiency the low serum phosphate concentration tends to be associated with a low urinary phosphate excretion, but compensatory parathyroid overactivity may raise urinary phosphate excretion and thus the test is of little discriminative value.

(e) *Serum alkaline phosphatase.* As discussed later (section 8.6.1), the serum alkaline phosphatase activity is raised when vitamin D deficiency is associated with osteomalacia (or rickets) and in chronic renal failure with bone disease. It is normal in hypoparathyroidism, pseudohypoparathyroidism, and magnesium deficiency.

(f) *Serum magnesium.* An association between hypocalcaemia and hypomagnesaemia has been recognized for many years (Randall et al., 1959), but the mechanism for this effect has been debated. Unresponsiveness to parathyroid hormone has been claimed (Estep et al., 1969), although more recent work has suggested that inhibition of parathyroid hormone secretion in hypomagnesaemia may be more important (Anast et al., 1972; Suh et al., 1973). In any case, correction of the hypomagnesaemia leads to restoration of the normal serum calcium concentration. Thus serum magnesium should be measured in every patient with hypocalcaemia of indeterminate cause.

(g) *Urinary excretion of cyclic AMP and phosphate in response to parathyroid hormone.* In normal subjects and in patients with hypoparathyroidism, the infusion of parathyroid extract (200 units) causes a prompt increase in urinary excretion of phosphate and of cyclic AMP. The cyclic AMP response can be measured in plasma as well as in urine, and the effect of parathyroid extract should be compared with the response to a control, inactive preparation. Patients with pseudohypoparathyroidism do not, in general, respond to parathyroid hormone by increasing urinary excretion of cyclic AMP (Chase et al., 1968). A second type of pseudohypoparathyroidism has been described in which a normal cyclic AMP response to parathyroid extract occurs, but with a decreased phosphaturic response.

(h) *Parathyroid hormone.* In vitamin D deficiency, pseudohypoparathyroidism or chronic renal failure, parathyroid hormone concentrations are raised. In chronic renal failure, the immunoreactive parathyroid hormone often does not behave in an identical manner to, extracted parathyroid hormone standards, as much of the immunoreactivity is contributed by fragments of variable size (section 8.2.4.1). In hypoparathyroidism and hypomagnesaemia, immunoreactive parathyroid hormone is barely detectable.

(i) *25-Hydroxycholecalciferol.* The concentration of this metabolite (section 8.4.1) is low in vitamin D deficiency. Variable values, often lower than normal, have been reported in chronic renal failure (Bayard et al., 1973), but the main defect of vitamin D metabolism in this condition lies in the subsequent conversion of 25-hydroxycholecalciferol into 1,25-dihydroxycholecalciferol (section 8.4.3). Normal concentrations are found in hypoparathyroidism.

8.6. METABOLIC BONE DISEASES

Biochemical investigations aid in the diagnosis and differential diagnosis of many metabolic bone diseases and assist in following the course of the disease and the effects of treatment.

8.6.1. Osteomalacia and rickets

These disorders (Table 8.5) are best defined by morphological criteria. Diagnostic histological changes include an increase in both the volume and extent of osteoid, or unmineralized bone, *and* a reduction in the amount of osteoid surface bearing a calcification front (Rasmussen and Bordier, 1974). With advanced disease, increase in osteoid produces the characteristic radiological features: widening of the gap between metaphysis and epiphysis and cupping of the metaphysis in rickets, and pseudofractures in osteomalacia (Fourman and Royer, 1968). In both adults and children the bones also become more radiolucent; there may be histological and radiological evidence of secondary hyperparathyroidism.

TABLE 8.5.

CLASSIFICATION OF OSTEOMALACIA AND RICKETS

I.	Vitamin D deficiency –
	inadequate diet
	inadequate sunlight
	malabsorption syndromes [a]
	drugs
II.	Uraemic osteodystrophy [a] ("renal rickets" – rickets or osteomalacia associated with uraemia)
III.	Renal tubular diseases [a] –
	renal tubular acidosis
	multiple renal tubular defects (Fanconi syndrome)
IV.	"Familial" hypophosphataemic rickets or osteomalacia [a] (primary hypophosphataemic rickets)
V.	Vitamin D-dependent rickets [a]
VI.	Fibrogenesis imperfecta ossium [a]
VII.	Iatrogenic phosphate depletion [a]
VIII.	Tumour-related osteomalacia [a] –
	neurofibromatosis
	angioma
IX.	Hypophosphatasia [a]

[a] Vitamin D-"resistant"

8.6.1.1. Diagnosis

In assessing the results of the following biochemical tests in hospitalised patients, it is important to allow for the changes attributable to alterations in the vitamin D content of diet. Hospital diets are usually adequate in vitamin D, and in patients with nutritional osteomalacia, the characteristic biochemical changes may be partially or completely corrected by the time specimens are collected.

(a) *Serum calcium.* This may be subnormal in advanced cases, but initially the tendency to hypocalcaemia is corrected by increased parathyroid activity, so that a normal serum calcium concentration is not uncommon. Occasionally hypercalcaemia occurs due to the development of tertiary hyperparathyroidism.

(b) *Serum phosphate.* Except in uraemic patients, the serum phosphate concentration is usually in the low-normal or sub-normal range but some patients with vitamin D deficiency show hyperphosphataemia. Serum phosphate concentrations are higher in childhood, and comparisons must be made with appropriate normal ranges.

(c) *Serum alkaline phosphatase.* This is generally elevated, because increased osteoblastic activity produces an increase in the bone isoenzyme. Some patients do not have increased serum activities so that a normal result does not exclude osteomalacia or rickets. As with serum phosphate, the normal ranges are higher in childhood and adolescence.

(d) *Urinary calcium excretion.* Because parathyroid hormone is secreted in response to hypocalcaemia, the urinary excretion of calcium is usually low, even if the serum calcium concentration returns to normal.

Except in renal tubular acidosis and familial hypophosphataemia, the finding of normal urinary calcium excretion for a particular patient's dietary calcium intake is rare; in practice, a 24-hour excretion of calcium which exceeds 1.2 mmol makes osteomalacia unlikely. Hypocalciuria loses its significance if renal function is impaired.

(e) *Urinary phosphate excretion.* With secondary hyperparathyroidism, the urinary excretion of phosphate may be high relative to the serum phosphate concentration, but measurement does not aid diagnosis (section 8.5.2.4).

(f) *Urinary hydroxyproline excretion.* This is usually increased if renal function is normal, but the determination is of diagnostic value only if there is no increase in serum alkaline phosphatase activity or if concomitant liver disease leads to an increase in serum activity of liver alkaline phosphatase.

8.6.1.2. Differential diagnosis

The following chemical tests may assist the differential diagnosis, but the clinical and radiological features are generally more helpful.

(a) *Plasma 25-hydroxycalciferol.* In vitamin D deficiency due to poor nutrition, inadequate sunlight or malabsorption, plasma 25-hydroxycalciferol (section 8.4.1) is reduced. Patients with renal failure may also have sub-normal concentrations (Bayard et al., 1973), but the values are normal in familial hypophosphataemic osteomalacia (Haddad et al., 1973).

(b) *Renal disease.* In renal rickets or osteomalacia, renal function, as assessed by serum urea and serum creatinine concentrations, is always impaired (section 8.6.3).

When renal tubular acidosis is suspected (Nordin, 1973) because of a family history or associated disease causing hyper-γ-globulinaemia, or a history of renal stones or nephrocalcinosis, chemical tests may be diagnostic: random urine samples with pH less than 5.4 exclude renal tubular acidosis, and the finding of metabolic acidosis with urine pH greater than 5.5 is diagnostic. A short acid-loading test is sometimes indicated in doubtful cases (Wrong and Davies, 1959). Hypokalaemia, sometimes severe enough to produce muscular weakness or paralysis, may also occur in renal tubular acidosis; if renal function is normal, hyperchloraemia with a low serum bicarbonate concentration suggests renal tubular acidosis.

In patients with osteomalacia or rickets due to renal tubule disease, renal tubular acidosis may not be the only abnormality. In the Fanconi syndrome, which may be familial and is usually due to cystine storage disease in children, biochemical testing reveals renal glycosuria and – if creatine clearance is normal – increased phosphate clearance as well as renal tubular acidosis. A similar pattern of tubular malfunction may occur with heavy metal intoxication and cirrhosis. Aminoaciduria is a common concomitant of multiple renal tubule defects; in contrast to the aminoaciduria of vitamin D deficiency, it may persist in spite of vitamin D repletion.

(c) *Familial hypophoshataemia (simple hypophosphataemic rickets).* Diagnosis is often suspected from the family history and clinical features (Fourman and Royer, 1968; Nordin, 1973). A definite biochemical diagnosis from other types of rickets or osteomalacia cannot be made, but hypocalcaemia is unusual, hypophosphataemia is invariable and the urinary excretion of calcium may be normal. In spite of the hypophosphataemia, there is relative hyperphosphaturia, but this finding is of no diagnostic assistance. The varied results of extensive biochemical investigations do not at present provide a clear picture of the pathogenesis, and the syndrome can probably be produced by a number of different disorders involving intestinal and renal phosphate, and possibly calcium transport. To date, there is no evidence to suggest that abnormal vitamin D metabolism occurs in these conditions. Hypophosphataemia without bone disease is common in the female relatives of affected patients.

(d) *Hypophosphatasia* (Fraser, 1957). The radiological changes resemble those of osteomalacia or rickets; dental lesions accompany the skeletal changes. Chemical tests help in making the diagnosis of this rare disease. The serum alkaline phosphatase activity is in the low-normal or frankly sub-normal range and the neutrophil alkaline phosphatase activity is also low. Urinary excretion of phosphoethanolamine is increased, but this finding is not specific for hypophosphatasia; urinary pyrophosphate and calcium excretion may also be increased and some infants show hypercalcaemia.

8.6.1.3. Response to treatment

The response of osteomalacia and rickets to treatment with vitamin D is assessed clinically, biochemically, histologically and radiologically. In nutritional vitamin D deficiency, treatment may be associated with further reductions in serum calcium concentration and urinary excretion of calcium in the first 2 weeks, during which time the serum phosphate concentration usually becomes normal. The serum calcium concentration usually increases to normal during the first 3 weeks. Serum alkaline phosphatase activity may transiently increase, with values reaching a peak at about the second month (Morgan et al., 1965), before falling slowly towards normal, which may not be reached for 6 to 12 months.

A number of types of rickets and osteomalacia may be "resistant" to small daily oral doses of vitamin D, as indicated in Table 8.5. The finding of vitamin D resistance has diagnostic and therapeutic implications.

The vitamin D deficiency of malabsorption syndromes is corrected by small doses of parenteral vitamin D, but also tends to improve without vitamin D supplements once the cause of malabsorption (e.g. coeliac disease) is treated. Vitamin D-dependent rickets is resistant to small doses of vitamin D, but complete remission occurs with large doses of the vitamin or with very small doses of 1,25-dihydroxycholecalciferol (Fraser et al., 1973). In contrast, patients with familial hypophosphataemia show no response to small doses, and only partial response to large doses, of vitamin D or its active metabolites. To some extent, vitamin D resistance in renal tubular acidosis improves with alkali treatment, but supplementary vitamin D is often required to heal the bone disease.

8.6.2. Paget's disease of bone

This is a common skeletal disorder with characteristic clinical, radiological and histological features and with biochemical evidence of increased bone turnover.

8.6.2.1. Diagnosis

Serum alkaline phosphatase activity is increased because of enhanced osteoblast activity (Rasmussen and Bordier, 1974). The values may be so high in active Paget's disease with extensive skeletal involvement as to exceed the working analytical range. Normal serum alkaline phosphatase does not, however, exclude active Paget's disease. In active disease, the level is normal if only a small fraction of the skeleton is involved; extensive disease may be clinically as well as biochemically inactive.

Urinary total hydroxyproline excretion is increased because of increased osteoclast activity (Rasmussen and Bordier, 1974). Hydroxylation of proline occurs during the synthesis of collagen, and when collagen is catabolized, some hydroxyproline is released into the circulation, resulting in increased plasma concentration and enhanced urinary excretion. Proteins other than collagen contain relatively smaller proportions of hydroxyproline. Although hydroxyproline may be released from extra-skeletal collagen as well, large increases are due to bone destruction (Prockop and Kivirikko, 1967). If care is taken to restrict hydroxyproline in the diet by avoiding gelatin-containing foods, increased hydroxyprolinuria is a more sensitive index of high bone turnover than serum alkaline phosphatase activity; urinary hydroxyproline may be elevated without increase of serum alkaline phosphatase. In general, the increase in serum alkaline phosphatase activity is proportional to the increase in urinary hydroxyproline excretion, but in very active disease, the serum alkaline phosphatase activity tends to be relatively higher. Plasma hydroxyproline concentrations are also increased in active Paget's disease (Smith et al., 1973).

Hypercalcaemia may occur in active Paget's disease but it is often intermittent and is not usually sustained. Immobilization, particularly after fractures, is prone to produce hypercalcaemia and hypercalciuria. Serum phosphate concentration is normal, and the urinary excretion of calcium is usually appropriate for the dietary intake. In patients with very high levels of alkaline phosphatase and hydroxyproline excretion, serum acid phosphatase activity may also be increased.

8.6.2.2. Differential diagnosis

Biochemical evidence of high bone turnover is not specific for Paget's disease. Increased serum alkaline phosphatase activity and urinary excretion of hydroxyproline may occur in a number of skeletal diseases, but very marked increases are confined to patients with the clinical and radiological features of Paget's disease.

8.6.2.3. Response to treatment

Serial measurements of serum alkaline phosphatase activity and/or urinary hydroxyproline excretion are useful in following the course of the disease and the effects of treatment. However, considerable fluctuations in both values are usual (Nagant de Deuxchaisnes and Krane, 1964) so that serial estimations should be performed before treatment to permit assessment of spontaneous changes in the progress of the disease.

During treatment with calcitonin, a lowering of the urinary excretion of hydroxyproline is apparent from the first day (Singer et al., 1972). Reduction in serum alkaline phosphatase activity takes at least 2 to 3 weeks; this is probably due to the relatively slow clearance of alkaline phosphatase from the circulation (Posen, 1970). Prolonged treatment with calcitonins or sodium etidronate usually produces parallel reductions in both of these levels, but the two may be dissociated on treatment with porcine calcitonin (de Rose et al., 1974).

Acute reductions in serum calcium and phosphate concentrations 2 to 6 hours after a dose of calcitonin indicate that the patient is manifesting a response to that dose. Failure to show an effect does not necessarily imply that the patient will fail to show a clinical response, as a hypocalcaemic and hypophosphataemic effect is unusual unless serum alkaline phosphatase activity is at least moderately increased. Loss of a hypocalcaemic response in a patient who was previously responsive may be due to remission of the disease, with reduction of turnover to normal or near-normal levels, or to the development of neutralizing antibodies (Haddad and Caldwell, 1972).

8.6.3. Chronic renal osteodystrophy

As kidney function deteriorates, serum phosphate concentration tends to increase because of reduced glomerular filtration. This increase is associated with a reduction in serum calcium, and parathyroid secretion is stimulated. In mild renal failure, the renal response to parathyroid hormone, by reducing tubular resorption of phosphate, serves to reverse the tendency for hyperphosphataemia and to increase serum calcium concentrations to normal. Increased serum alkaline phosphatase activity and plasma hydroxyproline concentration reflect the action of parathyroid hormone on bone, but these may not be raised in mild cases; plasma concentration of immunoreactive parathyroid hormone (section 8.2.4) is elevated.

With further deterioration of renal function, frank hyperphosphataemia and hypocalcaemia result. The development of vitamin D resistance, due in part to defective 1-hydroxylation of calciferol, may also contribute to the hypocalcaemia. The concentration of ionized calcium may be less than that expected from the corrected serum calcium concentration as an increase in the proportion of complexed calcium may occur. Progressive elevations of serum alkaline phosphatase activity and plasma hydroxyproline concentration reflect the increase in turnover of bone.

The therapeutic effect of oral aluminium hydroxide may be monitored by determining the reduction in serum phosphate and increase in serum calcium concentrations. The effect of vitamin D may be reflected by changes in serum alkaline phosphatase activity and calcium concentration; serial determinations of renal function should also be made in order to detect deterioration. Renal haemodialysis with fluids high in calcium concentration may improve the biochemical as well as the clinical and radiological features of secondary hyperparathyroidism. Late in the course of uraemic osteodystrophy, persistent hypercalcaemia may result, due to progressive increase in parathyroid gland mass and inappropriate suppression by ionized calcium (section 8.2.1). Hypercalcaemia may follow renal transplantation and may persist until the hyperplastic parathyroid glands have involuted; soon after renal transplantation, hypophosphataemia may also be associated with hypercalcaemia.

8.6.4. Osteoporosis

In histological terms, osteoporosis is characterized by a reduction in the actual volume of bone tissue within the volume occupied by a particular bone; in generalized osteoporosis, trabecular bone is affected more than cortical bone (Nordin, 1973). The radiological diagnosis of spinal osteoporosis depends on the presence of vertebral crush fractures as well as relative radiolucency and a tendency for selective preservation of the vertical rather than the horizontal trabeculae.

8.6.4.1. Diagnosis

Chemical tests are of little help in making a positive diagnosis of osteoporosis. Serum calcium and phosphate concentrations are normal; serum alkaline phosphatase activity and urinary excretion of hydroxyproline are normal, except in the first 10 weeks following fracture, when transient increases are usual. In some patients with osteoporosis, marginal increases of urinary hydroxyproline excretion, reflecting slightly increased bone turnover, may be found; particular attention must be paid to minimizing the dietary intake of gelatin-containing foods when assessing slight elevations of hydroxyproline excretion.

8.6.4.2. Differential diagnosis

A syndrome identical to spinal osteoporosis may occur in protracted and mild thyrotoxicosis. Cushing's syndrome, with relatively few other clinical features, may also present as a spinal osteoporosis. Appropriate chemical tests may be required to exclude these diseases, as well as multiple myeloma or hyperparathyroidism.

8.6.4.3. Response to treatment

The course of osteoporosis is followed by clinical and radiological assessment. Chemical assays (e.g. of serum calcium concentration) are indicated when large doses of vitamin D are administered.

8.6.5. Other metabolic bone diseases

8.6.5.1. Osteopetrosis

In osteopetrosis, which may occur at all ages, there is a generalized increase in bone density. The bones are brittle and tend to fracture easily; extramedullary haemopoiesis resulting in splenomegaly and anaemia is common. Biochemically, no defect is usually demonstrable, but serum acid phosphatase activity may be raised.

8.6.5.2. Osteogenesis imperfecta

Thin and fragile bones are associated with conduction deafness and blue sclerae. Serum alkaline phosphatase activity may be raised after fractures, and urinary excretion of hydroxyproline can sometimes be higher than normal, even if there has been no recent fracture.

8.6.5.3. Fibrous dysplasia of bone

The presence of hypercalcaemia suggests osteitis fibrosa cystica, rather than fibrous dysplasia, as a cause of cysts which expand bone. Increased bone turnover, reflected in high serum alkaline phosphatase activity, is not uncommon, even without recent fracture (Pritchard, 1951).

8.7. BIOCHEMICAL PHYSIOLOGY OF MAGNESIUM

8.7.1. Body content and tissue distribution

Magnesium is the fourth most abundant cation in the body, exceeded only by calcium, sodium and potassium. The total body content of magnesium in the normal adult is approximately 1000 mmol. About 1% of the total is in the extracellular fluid, 35% is localized within cells, and the remainder is concentrated in bone.

8.7.2. Intestinal absorption

A normal adult daily diet contains about 12.5 mmol magnesium, much of which is obtained from green vegetables which have large amounts of the ion as a constituent of the chlorophyll molecule. Approximately one-third of the ingested magnesium is absorbed while the remainder is excreted in the stool. Absorption occurs along the entire small intestine but is most active proximally, in the area where calcium absorption is maximal; it appears that the two ions are handled by transport mechanisms which have some factors in common. Colonic absorption is usually negligible, but increased plasma concentrations may be observed in individuals who receive magnesium-containing enemas. Factors such as protein intake, parathyroid hormone, exogenous growth hormone, large doses of vitamin D and antibiotics (e.g. neomycin) have been shown to influence gut absorption, but no single factor has been shown to play a dominant role in magnesium absorption similar to that of vitamin D in calcium absorption. The absorption of magnesium is impaired by substances which form sparingly soluble compounds of the ion, e.g. phytate, fatty acids and excess of phosphate.

8.7.3. Renal excretion

The approximate range of urinary excretion of magnesium in the normal adult is from 3 to 10 mmol/24 hours. In the event of diminished intake or deficiency of magnesium, renal conservation is highly efficient so that the urine concentration can fall to less than 0.5 mmol/litre. The filtered portion of plasma magnesium represents that fraction (60 to 70%) which is not protein-bound; this is mainly ionized and complexed magnesium. Reabsorption occurs chiefly in the proximal tubule so that the amount excreted represents only 1 to 5% of the filtered load. Adrenocorticosteroids and aldosterone facilitate tubular excretion and there is evidence that magnesium may be actively secreted in the distal tubule. Reabsorption may be reduced by the administration of magnesium, certain carbohydrates (glucose, galactose, fructose), ethanol, acid load, various hormones (including glucagon and growth hormone), and by osmotic diuresis, natriuresis, increased calcium excretion, and diuretics. Reabsorption is enhanced by diminished dietary intake of magnesium, by extra-renal losses, and by parathryoid hormone.

8.7.4. Magnesium in bone

In bone, magnesium is mainly combined with calcium and phosphate and small amounts of other ions (e.g. sodium, potassium, chloride and fluoride) in complex salts. A variable amount of bone magnesium, located on the osseous crystal surfaces as either magnesium ion or as an hydroxide complex, represents a labile fraction which can be readily mobilised.

8.7.5. Magnesium in soft tissues

About 350 to 500 mmol magnesium is found in soft tissues and it is the second most abundant intracellular cation after potassium. Those tissues with the highest concentrations are liver (10 mmol/kg), straited muscle (10 mmol/kg), brain (8.5 mmol/kg) and kidney (6.5 mmol/kg). The ionized fraction is of crucial importance in the activation of many enzymes, and at several steps in the pathway of protein synthesis.

8.7.6. Magnesium in blood

Only a very small proportion (1%) of total body magnesium is located extracellularly, but despite this the physiological plasma concentration is maintained between 0.75 and 0.9 mmol/litre (1.5 and 1.8 mEq/litre) (Alcock et al., 1960; MacIntyre, 1967). Approximately one-third of this is protein bound at physiological pH so that, like calcium, the concentration of protein influences the distribution in plasma. The erythrocyte level averages one-third to one-quarter of that found in most other cells and is maintained within close limits at around 2.7 ± 0.27 mmol/litre.

8.8. MEASUREMENT OF SERUM MAGNESIUM

In the past, the lack of suitably precise analytical methods gave normal serum magnesium values ranging from 0.7 to 1.25 mmol/litre. Application of the techniques of flame spectrophotometry, first flame emission spectroscopy and subsequently atomic absorption, made possible the accurate determination of the low concentrations of magnesium in blood, urine and tissues (Alcock and MacIntyre, 1966). Of the two methods, atomic absorption is now most widely used. In addition, the application of these simple and precise methods has led to a better appreciation of aberrations in magnesium metabolism in a wide variety of clinical settings. Using these techniques it has become apparent that the normal range is much narrower than was formerly thought, the reference interval for serum, for example, being from 0.75 to 0.9 mmol/litre (Alcock et al., 1960).

8.9. DISORDERS OF MAGNESIUM HOMEOSTASIS

8.9.1. Hypermagnesaemia

Symptomatic hypermagnesaemia occurs most frequently in patients with renal failure. In the other conditions (Table 8.6), clinical manifestations of hypermagnesaemia are usually absent.

At serum concentrations of 2.5 to 5 mmol/litre a retarding effect on the cardiac con-

TABLE 8.6.

CAUSES OF HYPERMAGNESAEMIA

I.	Renal insufficiency (chronic and acute renal failure)
II.	Uncontrolled diabetes mellitus
III.	Adrenocortical insufficiency
IV.	Adrenalectomy
V.	Hypothyroidism
VI.	Excessive ingestion; magnesium poisoning; increased colonic absorption (magnesium-containing enemas)

duction system is manifest and hypermagnesaemia potentiates the cardiac effect of hyperkalaemia. Deep tendon reflexes are lost at about 5 mmol/litre and respiratory paralysis occurs near 7.5 mmol/litre at which level, general anaesthesia may also be observed. At levels in excess of 12.5 mmol/litre, cardiac arrest occurs in diastole (Wacker and Parisi, 1968). Hypermagnesaemia is treated with intravenous calcium, but artificial respiration, dialysis and a cardiac pacemaker may be indicated.

8.9.2. Hypomagnesaemia

The diagnosis of hypomagnesaemia (Table 8.7) is often overlooked, because deficiency of this ion may not be considered in a given clinical setting. It must be remembered that only a small fraction of body magnesium is located intravascularly, hence the serum magnesium concentration does not always reflect the status of total body magnesium.

TABLE 8.7.

CAUSES OF HYPOMAGNESAEMIA

I.	Disorders associated with inadequate intake and/or impaired absorption of magnesium – malabsorption syndromes kwashiorkor and protein calorie malnutrition alcoholism
II.	Disorders associated with increased magnesium requirement and inadequate replacement – prolonged or severe loss of body fluids excessive lactation
III.	Disorders associated with impaired renal conservation of magnesium – hypercalcaemia of any cause, e.g. hyperparathyroidism hyperaldosteronism diabetic acidosis hyperthyroidism diuretic therapy inappropriate secretion of antidiuretic hormone unclassifiable

8.9.2.1. Clinical manifestations
Magnesium deficiency, as might be expected, leads to widespread neuromuscular dysfunction. The patients are hyperexcitable and may manifest a variety of behavioural disturbances. Tetany, tremors, ataxia, vertigo, muscular weakness and non-specific electroencephalographic and electrocardiographic changes may be present either separately or in various combinations. However, the most important manifestation of magnesium deficiency is seizure activity, both generalized and focal in nature. Indeed, the tendency to unheralded and potentially fatal convulsions can be considered the cardinal feature of this condition.

8.9.2.2. Biochemistry
The initial test is measurement of serum magnesium; symptomatic magnesium deficiency is seen with serum concentrations of less than 0.5 mmol/litre although some patients fail to show any overt clinical manifestations even with such low values. If the serum magnesium is normal but the diagnosis remains likely on clinical grounds, then 24-hour urinary excretion, erythrocyte content, or tissue concentration in muscle or bone might be measured. Magnesium depletion is said to be present when with adequate hydration, normal physiological pH, electrolyte balance and renal function, the 24-hour urine volume contains less than 1 mmol magnesium. Definite deficiency is indicated by the excretion of less than 0.5 mmol/24 hours. Deficiency can also be assessed on the basis of urinary excretion of a test dose of magnesium. An individual with adequate magnesium stores will excrete within 16 hours more than 80% of a parenterally administered dose of 20 mmol, and most of this amount is eliminated within the first 4 hours. Excretion of less than 70% within 16 hours after such a dose generally indicates magnesium deficiency. Normal renal function is a prerequisite of this test.

8.9.2.3. Disorders associated with inadequate intake and/or impaired absorption of magnesium

(a) *Malabsorption syndromes.* The diseases comprising this syndrome represent the most common cause of hypomagnesaemia. It has been estimated that about 40% of cases are associated with low serum magnesium concentration (Booth et al., 1963), and the cause of hypomagnesaemia is an abnormally high faecal loss of magnesium. In coeliac disease, the loss of magnesium can rise to 4 times the normal dietary intake; this loss can be reversed by the institution of a gluten-free diet (Goldman et al., 1962).

Steatorrhoea itself causes loss of magnesium through the excretion of large amounts of magnesium soaps. A low-fat diet can restore a positive magnesium balance without the administration of magnesium supplements. The therapeutic use of oral calcium supplements can also contribute to excessive faecal loss of magnesium, possibly because calcium competes with magnesium for a common intestinal transport system (Alcock and MacIntyre, 1962).

In acute pancreatitis, the serum magnesium concentration is commonly decreased although tetany is an infrequent accompaniment.

(b) *Kwashiorkor and protein calorie malnutrition.* Magnesium deficiency is now known to be an important factor in these syndromes. In less severe cases, the serum and erythrocyte magnesium concentrations are usually normal but muscle magnesium content and urinary magnesium excretion are decreased (Montgomery, 1960). In severely affected children, serum magnesium concentration may be low and signs of neuromuscular irritability evident.

(c) *Alcoholism.* Hypomagnesaemia commonly occurs in patients with alcoholism, either with or without delirium tremens or cirrhosis (Heaton et al., 1962). There seems to be a relationship between the decrease in serum magnesium concentration and the appearance of withdrawal symptoms in chronic alcoholics. Usually the lowest values are encountered in the more severe cases, but severe withdrawal symptoms may occur without a fall in the serum magnesium concentration. The most likely explanation for the magnesium deficiency is inadequate dietary intake accompanied by increased urinary excretion, the reason for which has not been firmly established.

8.9.2.4. Disorders associated with increased magnesium requirements and inadequate replacement

Hypomagnesaemia due to excessive loss of body fluids is most often seen in the post-operative patient. Thus, the fluid aspirated by nasogastric tube contains about 0.5 mmol/litre of magnesium; hence prolonged nasogastric suction, if accompanied by parenteral replacement with magnesium-free fluids, may lead to significant hypomagnesaemia. An unusual cause of magnesium loss in body fluids is excessive lactation; in one such case a serum magnesium concentration of 0.2 mmol/litre was recorded (Greenwald et al., 1963).

8.9.2.5. Disorders associated with impaired renal conservation of magnesium

Several conditions are associated with magnesium deficiency due to impaired renal conservation. The most important is hyperparathyroidism, and abnormalities of magnesium metabolism in this disorder are often overlooked.

In hyperparathyroidism, increased urinary excretion of magnesium may occur and sometimes the serum magnesium concentration is low. Such hypermagnesiuria is especially prominent in patients with marked hypercalcaemia in whom there is an increased tubular calcium load and excessive reabsorption of calcium. This renal effect induced by the hypercalcaemia outweighs any effects of parathyroid hormone in increasing the tubular reabsorption of magnesium. A post-operative fall in serum magnesium concentration is usually seen after removal of a parathyroid tumour; this is particularly marked in patients with severe bone disease and pre-operative hypomagnesaemia, and is presumably due to the rapid deposition of magnesium in bone (Heaton and Pyrah, 1963).

Hypomagnesaemia is also seen in patients with hypoparathyroidism and is usually associated with hyperphosphataemia. Urinary excretion of magnesium is not increased, and it is possible that a shift of magnesium from the extracellular fluid to other sites is responsible for the decreased serum concentration.

REFERENCES

Adams, P., Chalmers, T.M., Hill, L.F. and Truscott, B.McN. (1970) Idiopathic hypercalciuria and hyperparathyroidism. British Medical Journal, 4, 582–585.

Albright, F. (1947) The effect of hormones on osteogenesis in man. Recent Progress in Hormone Research, 1, 293–353.

Alcock, N., MacIntyre, I. and Radde, I. (1960) The determination of magnesium in biological fluids and tissues by flame spectrophotometry. Journal of Clinical Pathology, 13, 506–510.

Alcock, N. and MacIntyre, I. (1962) Interrelation of calcium and magnesium absorption. Clinical Science, 22, 185–193.

Alcock, N.W. and MacIntyre, I. (1966) Methods for estimating magnesium in biological materials. Methods of Biochemical Analysis, 14, 1–52.

Anast, C.S., Mohs, J.M., Kaplan, S.L. and Burns, T.W. (1972) Evidence of parathyroid failure in magnesium deficiency. Science, 177, 606–608.

Ardaillou, R., Sizonenko, P., Meyrier, A., Vallee, G. and Beaugad, C. (1970) Metabolic clearance rate of radioiodinated human calcitonin in man. Journal of Clinical Investigation, 49, 2345–2352.

Arnaud, C.D., Goldsmith, R.S., Bordier, P.J., Sizemore, G.W., Larsen, J.A. and Gilkinson, J. (1974) Influence of immunoheterogeneity of circulating parathyroid hormone on results of radioimmunoassays of serum in man. American Journal of Medicine, 56, 785–793.

Arnaud, C.D., Tsao, H.S. and Littledike, T. (1971) Radioimmunoassay of human parathyroid hormone in serum. Journal of Clinical Investigation, 50, 21–34.

Arnstein, A.R., Blumenthal, F.S. and McCann, D.S. (1973) Increased immunoreactive parathyroid hormone levels after spinal cord trauma. Clinical Research, 21, 615.

Aurbach, G.D. and Heath, D.A. (1974) Parathyroid hormone and calcitonin regulation of renal function. Kidney International, 6, 331–345.

Avioli, L.V., Lee, S.W., McDonald, J.E., Lund, J. and DeLuca, H.F. (1967) Metabolism of vitamin D_3-^3H in human subjects: distribution in blood, bile, faeces and urine. Journal of Clinical Investigation, 46, 983–992.

Baker, R.K., Wallach, S. and Tashjian, A.H. (1973) Plasma calcitonin in pycnodysostosis: intermittently high blood levels and exaggerated responses to calcium and glucagon infusion. Journal of Clinical Endocrinology and Metabolism, 37, 46–55.

Bauer, G.C.H., Carlsson, A. and Lindquist, B. (1957) Bone salt metabolism in humans studied by means of radiocalcium. Acta Medica Scandinavica, 158, 143–150.

Bayard, F., Bec, P.H., Ton-that, H. and Louvet, J.P. (1973) Plasma 25-hydroxycholecalciferol in chronic renal failure. European Journal of Clinical Investigation, 3, 447–450.

Belsey, R., DeLuca, H.F. and Potts, J.T. (1971) Competitive binding assay for vitamin D and 25-OH vitamin D. Journal of Clinical Endocrinology and Metabolism, 33, 554–557.

Belsey, R.E., DeLuca, H.F. and Potts, J.T. (1974) Selective binding properties of vitamin D transport proteins in chick plasma in vitro. Nature (London), 247, 208–209.

Benson, R.C., Riggs, B.L., Pickard, B.M. and Arnaud, C.D. (1974) Radioimmunoassay of parathyroid hormone in hypercalcaemia patients with malignant disease. American Journal of Medicine, 56, 821–826.

Berson, S.A. and Yalow, R.S. (1966) Parathyroid hormone in plasma in adenomatous hyperparathyroidism, uraemia and bronchogenic carcinoma. Science, 154, 907–909.

Blunt, J.W., DeLuca, H.F. and Schnoes, H.K. (1968), 25-Hydroxycholecalciferol. A biologically active metabolite of vitamin D_3. Biochemistry, 7, 3317–3322.

Booth, C.C., Babouris, N., Hanna, S. and MacIntyre, I. (1963) Incidence of hypomagnesaemia in intestinal malabsorption. British Medical Journal, 2, 141–144.

Brumbaugh, P.F., Haussler, D.H., Bresser, R. and Haussler, M.R. (1974) Radioreceptor assay for 1α,25-dihydroxyvitamin D_3. Science, 183, 1089–1091.

Buckle, R. (1974a) Measurement of parathyroid hormone. Clinics in Endocrinology and Metabolism, 3, 345–387.

Buckle, R. (1974b) Ectopic PTH syndrome, pseudohyperparathyroidism, hypercalcaemia of malignancy. Clinics in Endocrinology and Metabolism, 3, 237–251.

Bussolati, G., Foster, G.V., Clark, M.B. and Pearse, A.G.E. (1969) Immunofluorescent localisation of calcitonin in medullary (C cell) thyroid carcinoma, using antibody to the pure porcine hormone. Virchow's Archives Abt. B. Zellpath, 2, 234–238.

Cali, J.P., Bowers, G.N. and Young, D.S. (1973) A referee method for the determination of total calcium in serum. Clinical Chemistry, 19, 1208–1213.

Canterbury, J.M., Levey, G.S. and Reiss, E. (1973) Activation of renal cortical adenylate cyclase by circulating immunoreactive parathyroid hormone fragments. Journal of Clinical Investigation, 52, 524–527.

Chase, L.R., Melson, G.L. and Aurbach, G.D. (1968) Metabolic abnormality in pseudohypoparathyroidism, defective renal excretion of cyclic 3′,5′-AMP in response to parathyroid hormone. Journal of Clinical Investigation, 47, 18a.

Chu, L.L.H., MacGregor, R.R., Liu, P.I., Hamilton, J.W. and Cohn, D.V. (1973) Biosynthesis of proparathyroid hormone and parathyroid hormone by human parathyroid glands. Journal of Clinical Investigation, 52, 3089–3094.

Clark, M.B., Byfield, P.G.H., Boyd, G.W. and Foster, G.V. (1969) A radioimmunoassay for human calcitonin M. Lancet, ii. 74–77.

Coe, F.L., Canterbury, J.M., Firpo, J.J. and Reiss, E. (1973) Evidence for secondary hyperparathyroidism in idiopathic hypercalciuria. Journal of Clinical Investigation, 52, 134–142.

Cohn, D.V., MacGregor, R.R., Chu, L.L.H., Huang, D.W.Y., Anast, C.S. and Hamilton, J.W. (1974) Biosynthesis of proparathyroid hormone and parathyroid hormone. American Journal of Medicine, 56, 767–773.

Coombes, R.C., Hillyard, C., Greenberg, P.B. and MacIntyre, I. (1974) Plasma immunoreactive calcitonin in patients with non thyroid tumours. Lancet, i, 1080–1083.

Cushard, W.G., Creditor, M.A., Canterbury, J.M. and Reiss, E. (1971) Physiological hyperparathyroidism in pregnancy. Journal of Clinical Endocrinology and Metabolism, 34, 767–771.

Cushard, W.G., Simon, A.B., Canterbury, J.M. and Reiss, E. (1972) Parathyroid function in sarcoidosis. New England Journal of Medicine, 286, 395–398.

Deftos, L. (1974) Radioimmunoassay for calcitonin in medullary thyroid carcinoma. Journal of the American Medical Association, 227, 403–406.

Deftos, L., Powell, D., Parthemore, J.G. and Potts, J.T. (1974) Secretion of calcitonin in hypocalcaemic states in man. Journal of Clinical Investigation, 52, 3109–3114.

Dent, C.E. and Watson, L. (1968) The hydrocortisone test in primary and tertiary hyperparathyroidism. Lancet, ii, 662–664.

Dent, C.E. (1962) Some problems of hyperparathyroidism. British Medical Journal, 2, 1419–1425.

deRose, J., Singer, F.R., Auramides, A., Flores, A., Dziadiw, R., Baker, R.K. and Wallach, S. (1974) Response of Paget's disease to porcine and salmon calcitonins. Effects of long term treatment. American Journal of Medicine, 56, 858–866.

Dohan, P.H., Yamashita, K., Larsen, P.R., Davis, B., Deftos, L. and Field, J.B. (1972) Evaluation of urinary cyclic 3′5′-adenosine monophosphate excretion in the differential diagnosis of hypercalcaemia. Journal of Clinical Endocrinology and Metabolism, 35, 775–784.

Dymling, J.F., Ljungberg, D., Hillyard, C., Greenberg, P.B., Evans, I.M.A. and MacIntyre, I. (1976) Whisky: a new provocative test for calcitonin secretion. Acta Endocrinologica, 82, 500–509.

Eisenberg, H., Pallotta, J. and Sherwood, L.M. (1974) Selective arteriography, venography and venous hormone assay in diagnosis and evaluation of parathyroid lesions. American Journal of Medicine, 56, 810–819.

Ellison, M., Woodhouse, D., Hillyard, C., Dowsett, M., Coombes, R.C., Gilby, E.D., Greenberg, P.B. and Neville, A.M. (1975) Immunoreactive calcitonin production by human lung carcinoma cells in culture. British Journal of Cancer, 32, 373–379.

Estep, H., Shaw, W.A., Watlington, C., Hobe, R., Holland, W. and Tucker, S.G. (1969) Hypocalcaemia due to hypomagnesmia and reversible parathyroid hormone unresponsiveness. Journal of Clinical Endocrinology and Metabolism, 29, 842–848.

Fischer, J.A., Binswanger, U. and Dietrich, F.M. (1974) Human parathyroid hormone. Journal of Clinical Investigation, 54, 1382–1394.

Fourman, P. and Royer, P. (1968) Calcium Metabolism and the Bone. Blackwell Scientific Publications, Oxford, 2nd edn.

Fraser, D.R. and Kodicek, E. (1970) Unique biosynthesis by kidney of a biologically active vitamin D metabolite. Nature (London), 228, 764–766.

Fraser, D., Kooh, S.W. Kind, H.P., Holick, M.F., Tanaka, Y. and DeLuca, H.F. (1973) Pathogenesis of hereditary vitamin D-dependent rickets. New England Journal of Medicine, 289, 817–822.

Fraser, P., Healy, M., Rose, N. and Watson, L. (1971) Discriminant functions in the differential diagnosis of hypercalcaemia. Lancet, i, 1314–1319.

Galante, L., Gudmundsson, T.V., Matthews, E.W., Williams, E.D., Tse, A., Woodhouse, N.J.Y. and MacIntyre, I. (1968) Thymic and parathyroid origin of calcitonin in man. Lancet, ii, 537–538.

Goldman, A.S., Van Fossan, D.D. and Baird, E.E. (1962) Magnesium deficiency in celiac disease. Paediatrics, 29, 948–952.

Goldsmith, R.S. (1972) Laboratory aids in the diagnosis of metabolic bone disease. Orthopaedic Clinics of North America, 3, 545–560.

Goltzman, D., Potts, J.T., Ridgway, E.C. and Malouf, F. (1974) Calcitonin as a tumour marker. New England Journal of Medicine, 290, 1035–1039.

Greenberg, P.B., Hillyard, C.J., Galante, L., Colston, K.W., Evans, I.M.A. and MacIntyre, I. (1974) Affinity of calciferol analogues for 25-hydroxycholecalciferol receptor. Clinical Science and Molecular Medicine, 46, 143–147.

Greenberg, P. and MacIntyre, I. (1974) Serum calcitonin and thyroid carcinoma. British Medical Journal, 3, 256.

Greenwald, J., Dubin, A. and Cardon, L. (1963) Hypomagnesemic tetany due to excessive lactation. America Journal of Medicine, 35, 854–860.

Habener, J.F., Kemper, B., Potts, J.T. and Rich, A. (1972) Proparathyroid hormones: biosynthesis by human parathyroid adenomas. Science, 178, 630–633.

Habener, J.F., Powell, D., Murray, T.M., Mayer, G.P. and Potts, J.T. (1971) Parathyroid hormone: secretion and metabolism in vivo. Proceedings of the National Academy of Sciences, 68, 2986–2991.

Haddad, J.G. and Caldwell, J.G. (1972) Calcitonin resistance: clinical and immunologic studies in subjects with Paget's disease of bone treated with porcine and salmon calcitonins. Journal of Clinical Investigation, 51, 3133–3141.

Haddad, J.G., Chyu, K.J., Hahn, T.J. and Stamp, T.C.B. (1973) Serum concentrations of 25-hydroxy vitamin D in sex-linked hypophosphataemic vitamin D-resistant rickets. Journal of Laboratory and Clinical Medicine, 81, 22–27.

Haddad, J.G. and Chyu, K.J. (1971) Competitive protein-binding radioassay for 25-hydroxycholecalciferol. Journal of Clinical Endocrinology and Metabolism, 33, 992–995.

Haddad, J.G. and Hahn, T.J. (1973) Natural and synthetic sources of circulating 25-hydroxyvitamin D in man. Nature (London), 244, 515–516.

Hahn, T.J., Hendin, B.A., Scharp, C.R. and Haddad, J.G. (1972a) Effect of chronic anticonvulsant therapy on serum 25-hydroxycholecalciferol levels in adults. New England Journal of Medicine, 287, 900–904.

Hahn, T.J., Birge, S.J., Scharp, C.R. and Avioli, L.V. (1972b) Phenobarbital-induced alterations in vitamin D metabolism. Journal of Clinical Investigation, 51, 741–748.

Hanze, S. and Seyberth, H. (1967) Untersuchungen zur Wirkung der diuretica Furosemid, Etacrynsaüre, and Triamteren auf die renale Magnesium und Calcium-ausscheidung. Klinische Wochenschrift, 45, 313–314.

Hazard, J.B., Hawk, W.A. and Crile, G. (1959) Medullary (solid) carcinoma of the thyroid – a clinicopathologic entity. Journal of Clinical Endocrinology and Metabolism, 19, 152–161.

Heaton, F.W. and Parsons, F.M. (1961) The metabolic effect of high magnesium intake. Clinical Science, 21, 273–284.

Heaton, F.W., Pyrah, L.N., Beresford, C.C., Bryson, R.W. and Martin, D.F. (1962) Hypomagnesaemia in chronic alcoholism. Lancet, ii, 802–805.

Heaton, F.W. and Pyrah, L.N. (1963) Magnesium metabolism in patients with parathyroid disorders. Clinical Science, 25, 475–485.

Hennessy, J.F., Wells, S.A., Ontjes, D.A. and Cooper, C.W. (1974) A comparison of pentagastrin injection and calcium infusion as provocative agents for the detection of medullary cell carcinoma of the thyroid. Journal of Clinical Endocrinology and Metabolism, 39, 487–495.

Heynen, G. and Franchimont, P. (1975) Human calcitonin and serum phosphate. Lancet, i, 527.

Hillyard, C.J., Coombes, R.C., Greenberg, P.B., Galante, L.S. and MacIntyre, I. (1976) Calcitonin in breast and lung cancer. Clinical Endocrinology, 5, 1–8.

Holtrop, M.E., Raisz, L.G. and Simmons, H.A. (1974) The effects of parathyroid hormone, colchicine and calcitonin on the ultrastructure and the activity of osteoclasts in organ culture. Journal of Cell Biology, 60, 346–355.

Husdan, H., Rapoport, A. and Locke, S. (1973) Influence of posture on the serum concentration of calcium. Metabolism, 22, 787–797.

Jaffe, B., Peskin, G.W. and Kaplan, E.L. (1973) Serum levels of parathyroid hormone in the Zollinger Ellison syndrome. Surgery, 74, 621–625.

Jubiz, W., Canterbury, J.M., Reiss, E. and Tyler, F.H. (1972) Circadian rhythm in serum parathyroid hormone concentrations in human subjects. Journal of Clinical Investigation, 51, 2040–2046.

Keutmann, H.T. (1974) The chemistry of parathyroid hormone. Clinics in Endocrinology and Metabolism, 3, 173–197.

Keynes, W.M. and Caird, F.I. (1970) Hypocalcaemic primary hyperparathyroidism. British Medical Journal, 1, 208–211.

Kodicek, E, (1963) Turnover and distribution of vitamin D and its mode of action. In The Transfer of Calcium and Strontium across Biological Membranes (Ed. R.H. Wassermann) pp. 185–196, Academic Press, New York.

Kramer, B. and Tisdall, F.F. (1921) A simple technique for the determination of calcium and magnesium in small amounts of serum. Journal of Biological Chemistry, 47, 475–481.

Ladenson, J.H. and Bowers, G.N., Jr. (1973) Free calcium in serum II. Rigor of homeostatic control, correlations with total serum calcium, and review of data on patients with disturbed calcium metabolism. Clinical Chemistry, 19, 575–582.

Lamberg, B.A. and Kuhlback, B. (1959) Effect of chlorothiazide and hydrochlorothiazide on the excretion of calcium in urine. Scandinavian Journal of Clinical and Laboratory Investigation, 11, 351–357.

Lumb, G.A. and Stanbury, S.W. (1974) Parathyroid function in human vitamin D deficiency and vitamin D deficiency in primary hyperparathyroidism. American Journal of Medicine, 56, 833–839.

MacIntyre, I. (1957) The flame-spectrophotometric determination of calcium in biological fluids and an isotopic analysis of the errors in the Kramer–Tisdall procedure. Biochemical Journal, 67, 164–172.

MacIntyre, I. and Parsons, J.A. (1966) Blood–bone calcium equilibrium in the perfused cat tibia and the effect of thyroid calcitonin. Journal of Physiology, 183, 31–33.

MacIntyre, I. (1967) Magnesium metabolism. In Advances in Internal Medicine (Eds. W. Dock and I. Snapper) Year Book Medical Publishers Inc.

Martin, T.J., Greenberg, P.B. and Michelangeli, V. (1973) Synthesis of human parathyroid hormone by cultured cells: evidence for release of prohormone by some adenomata. Clinical Science, 44, 1–8.

Martin, T.J., Melick, R.A. and DeLuise, M. (1969) The effect of nephrectomy on the metabolism of labelled parathyroid hormone. Clinical Science, 37, 137–142.

Mawer, E.B., Lumb, G.A. and Stanbury, S. (1969) Long biological half-life of vitamin D_3 and its polar metabolites in human serum. Nature (London), 222, 482–483.

McCollum, E.V., Simmonds, N., Shipley, P.G. and Park, E.A. (1922) Studies on experimental rickets. XVI. A delicate biological test for calcium-depositing substances. Journal of Biological Chemistry, 51, 41–49.

McLean, F.C. and Hastings, A.B. (1935) Clinical estimation and significance of calcium ion concentrations in the blood. American Journal of Medical Science, 189, 601–613.

Melvin, K.E.W., Tashjian, A.H. and Miller, H.H. (1971) Studies in familial (medullary) thyroid carcinoma. Recent Progress in Hormone Research, 28, 399–470.

Montgomery, R.D. (1960) Magnesium metabolism in infantile protein malnutrition. Lancet, ii, 74–75.

Morgan, D.B., Paterson, C.R., Woods, C.G., Pulvertaft, C.N. and Fourman, P. (1965) Osteomalacia after gastrectomy: a response to very small doses of vitamin D. Lancet, ii, 1089–1091.

Muldowney, F.P., Freaney, R., Spillane, E.A. and O'Donohoe, P. (1973) Ionised calcium levels in 'normocalcaemic' hyperparathyroidism. Irish Journal of Medical Science, 142, 223–229.

Neher, R., Riniker, B., Maier, R., Byfield, P.G.H., Gudmundsson, T.V., and MacIntyre, I. (1968) Human calcitonin. Nature (London), 220, 984–986.

Nicolaysen, R. (1937) Studies upon the mode of action of vitamin D. II. The influence of vitamin D on the faecal output of endogenous calcium and phosphorus in the rat. Biochemical Journal, 31, 107–121.

Nordin, B.E.C. (1973) Metabolic Bone and Stone Disease. Churchill-Livingstone, London.

Nordin, B.E.C. and Fraser, R. (1960) Assessment of urinary phosphate excretion. Lancet, i, 947–950.

Nordin, B.E.C. and Smith, D.A. (1965) Diagnostic Procedures in Disorders of Calcium Metabolism. Churchill-Livingstone, London.

Nordin, B.E.C. and Peacock, M. (1969) The role of the kidney in the regulation of plasma calcium. Lancet, ii, 1280–1283.

Nagant de Deuxchaisnes, C. and Krane, S.M. (1964) Paget's disease of bone: clinical and metabolic observations. Medicine, 43, 233–266.

Nusynowitz, M.L. and Klein, M.H. (1973) Pseudoidiopathic hypoparathyroidism. American Journal of Medicine, 55, 677–686.

O'Riordan, J.L.H., Woodhead, J.S., Addison, G.M., Keutmann, H.T. and Potts, J.T. (1972) Localisation of antigenic sites in parathyroid hormone. In Endocrinology 1971, Proceedings of the Third International Symposium (Ed. S. Taylor) pp. 386–392, Heinemann, London.

Pain, R.W., Rowland, K.M., Phillips, P.J. and Duncan, B.McL. (1975) Current 'corrected' calcium concept challenged. British Medical Journal, 4, 617–619.

Parfitt, A.M. (1969) Chlorothiazide-induced hypercalcaemia in juvenile osteoporosis and hyperparathyroidism. New England Journal of Medicine, 218, 55–59.

Parfitt, A.M. (1974) Investigation of disorders of the parathyroid glands. Clinics in Endocrinology and Metabolism, 3, 451–474.

Parfitt, A.M. and Frame, B. (1972) Treatment of rickets and osteomalacia. Seminars in Drug Treatment, 2, 83–115.

Parthemore, J.G., Bronzert, D., Roberts, G. and Deftos, L.J. (1974) A calcium infusion in the diagnosis of medullary thyroid carcinoma. Journal of Clinical Endocrinology and Metabolism, 39, 108–111.

Peacock, M., Nordin, B.E.C. and Hodgkinson, A. (1967) Importance of dietary calcium in the definition of hypercalciuria. British Medical Journal, 3, 469–471.

Phelps, P. and Hawker, C.D. (1973) Serum parathyroid hormone levels in patients with calcium pyrophosphate crystal deposition disease (chondrocalcinosis, pseudogout). Arthritis and Rheumatism, 16, 590–595.

Pickup, J.F. and Brown, S.S. (1973) Scope of automation in the analysis of body fluids. In Automated Analysis of Drugs (Eds. C.T. Rhodes and R.E. Hone) pp. 106–158, Butterworth, London.

Pickup, J.F., Jackson, M.J., Price, E.M., Healy, M.J.R. and Brown, S.S. (1975) Use of the reference method for determination of serum calcium in a quality-assurance survey. Clinical Chemistry, 21, 1416–1421.

Posen, S. (1970) Turnover of circulating enzymes. Clinical Chemistry, 16, 71–84.

Potts, J.T. and Deftos, L.J. (1969) Parathyroid hormones, thyrocalcitonin, vitamin D, bone and bone mineral metabolism. In Duncan's Diseases of Metabolism (Eds. P.K. Bondy and L.E. Rosenberg) Saunders, Philadelphia.

Pritchard, J.E. (1951) Fibrous dysplasia of the bones. American Journal of Medical Sciences, 222, 313–332.

Prockop, D.J. and Kivirikko, K.I. (1967) Relationship of hydroxyproline excretion in urine to collagen metabolism. Annals of Internal Medicine, 66, 1243–1266.

Purnell, D.C., Smith, L.H., Scholz, D.A., Elveback, L.R. and Arnaud, C.D. (1971) Primary hyperparathyroidism, a prospective clinical study. American Journal of Medicine, 50, 670–675.

Puschett, J.B., Moranz, J. and Kurnick, W.S. (1972) Evidence for a direct action of cholecalciferol on the renal transport of phosphate, sodium and calcium. Journal of Clinical Investigation, 51, 373–385.

Raisz, L.G., Au, W.Y.W., Simmons, H. and Mandelstam, P. (1972) Calcitonin in human serum. Archives of Internal Medicine, 129, 889–893.

Randall, R.E., Rossmeisl, E.C. and Bleifer, R.H. (1959) Magnesium depletion in man. Annals of Internal Medicine, 50, 257–287.

Rasmussen, H. and Bordier, Ph. (1974) The Physiological and Cellular Basis of Metabolic Bone Disease. Williams and Wilkins, Baltimore.

Rasmussen, H. (1970) Cell communication, calcium ion and cyclic adenosine monophosphate. Science, 170, 404–412.

Reiss, E. and Canterbury, J.M. (1973) Blood levels of parathyroid hormone in disorders of calcium metabolism. Annual Review of Medicine, 23, 217–232.

Riggs, B.L., Arnaud, C.D., Jowsey, J., Goldsmith, R.S. and Kelly, P.J. (1973) Parathyroid function in primary osteoporosis. Journal of Clinical Investigation, 5, 181–189.

Robinson, C.J. (1974) The physiology of parathyroid hormone. Clinics in Endocrinology and Metabolism, 3, 389–417.

Roof, B.S., Carpenter, B., Fink, D.J. and Gordon, G.S. (1971) Some thoughts on the nature of ectopic parathyroid hormone. American Journal of Medicine, 50, 686–691.

Ross, J.W. (1967) Calcium-selective electrode with liquid ion exchanger. Science, 156, 1378–1379.

Samaan, N.A., Hill, C.S., Beceiro, J.R. and Schultz, P.N. (1973) Immunoreactive calcitonin in medullary carcinoma of the thyroid and in maternal and cord serum. Journal of Laboratory and Clinical Medicine, 81, 671–681.

Samaan, N.A., Wigoda, C. and Castillo, E.G. (1974) Human serum calcitonin and parathyroid hormone levels in the maternal, umbilical cord blood and postpartum. In Endocrinology 1973, Proceedings of the Fourth International Symposium (Ed. S. Taylor) Heinemann, London.

Schmidt-Gaye, H. and Roher, H.D. (1973) Urinary excretion of cyclic adenosine monophosphate in the detection and diagnosis of primary hyperparathyroidism. Surgery, Gynaecology and Obstetrics, 137, 439–444.

Scholz, D.A., Riggs, B.L., Purnell, D.C., Goldsmith, R.S. and Arnaud, C.D. (1973) Ectopic hyperparathyroidism with renal calculi and subperiosteal bone resorption. Mayo Clinic Proceedings, 48, 124–126.

Schussler, G.C., Verso, M.A. and Nemoto, T. (1972) Phosphaturia in hypercalcaemic breast cancer patients. Journal of Clinical Endocrinology and Metabolism, 35, 497–504.

Segre, G.V., Niall, H.D., Habener, J.F. and Potts, J.T. (1974) Metabolism of parathyroid hormone. American Journal of Medicine, 56, 774–784.

Sherwood, L.M., Lundberg, W.G., Targovnik, J.H., Rodman, J.S. and Seyfer, A. (1971) Synthesis and secretion of parathyroid hormone in vitro. American Journal of Medicine, 50, 658–669.

Shimkin, P.M. and Powell, D. (1973) Parathyroid hormone levels in thyroid vein blood of patients without abnormalities of calcium metabolism. Annals of Internal Medicine, 78, 714–716.

Silva, O.L., Becker, K.L., Primack, A., Doppman, J. and Snider, R.H. (1974) Ectopic secretion of calcitonin by oat-cell carcinoma. New England Journal of Medicine, 1122–1124.

Singer, F.R., Keutmann, H.T., Neer, R.M., Potts, J.T. and Krane, S.M. (1972) Pharmacological effects of salmon calcitonin in man. In Calcium, Parathyroid Hormone and the Calcitonins (Eds. R.V. Talmage and P.L. Munson) Excerpta Medica International Congress Series, Excerpta Medica, Amsterdam.

Sizemore, G.W., Go, V.L.W., Kaplan, E.L., Sanzenbacher, L.J., Holtermuller, K.H. and Arnaud, C.D. (1973) Relation of calcitonin and gastrin in the Zollinger–Ellison syndrome and medullary carcinoma of the thyroid. New England Journal of Medicine, 288, 641–644.

Smith, R., Russell, R.G.G., Bishop, M.C., Woods, C.G. and Bishop, M. (1973) Paget's disease of bone: experience with a diphosphonate (disodium etidronate) in treatment. Quarterly Journal of Medicine, 47, 235–256.

Stamp, T.C.B. and Round, J.M. (1974) Seasonal changes in human plasma levels of 25-hydroxyvitamin D. Nature (London), 247, 563–565.

Suh, S.M., Tashjian, A.H., Matsuo, N., Parkinson, D.K. and Fraser, D. (1973) Pathogenesis of hypocalcaemia in primary hypomagnesemia: normal end-organ responsiveness to parathyroid hormone, impaired parathyroid gland function. Journal of Clinical Investigation, 52, 153–160.

Sutcliffe, H.S., Martin, T.J., Eisman, J.A. and Pilczyk, R. (1973) Binding of parathyroid hormone to bovine kidney-cortex membranes. Biochemical Journal, 134, 913–921.

Tashjian, A.H., Frantz, A.G. and Lee, J.B. (1966) Pseudohypoparathyroidism: assays of parathyroid hormone and calcitonin. Proceedings of the National Academy of Science, 56, 1138–1142.

Tashjian, A.H., Wolfe, H.J. and Voelkel, E.F. (1974) Human calcitonin. American Journal of Medicine, 56, 840–849.

Teotia, S.P.S. and Teotia, M. (1973) Secondary hyperparathyroidism in patients with endemic skeletal fluorosis. British Medical Journal, I, 637–640.

Tsang, R.C., Wen Chen, I., Friedman, M.A. and Chen, I. (1973) Neonatal parathyroid function: role of gestational age and postnatal age. Journal of Paediatrics, 83, 728–738.

Wacker, W.E. and Parisi, A.F. (1968) Magnesium metabolism. New England Journal of Medicine, 278, 712–715.

Walser, M. (1961a) Ion association. VI. Association between calcium, magnesium, inorganic phosphate, citrate and protein in normal human plasma. Journal of Clinical Investigation, 40, 723–730.

Walser, M. (1961b) Calcium clearance as a function of sodium clearance in the dog. American Journal of Physiology, 200, 1099–1104.

Watson, L. (1974) Primary hyperparathyroidism. Clinics in Endocrinology and Metabolism, 3, 215–235.

Wills, M.R. and McGowan, G.K. (1964) Plasma chloride levels in hyperparathyroidism and other hypercalcaemic states. British Medical Journal, I, 1153–1156.

Woodhouse, N.J.Y., Doyle, F.H. and Joplin, G.F. (1971) Vitamin D deficiency and primary hyperparathyroidism. Lancet, ii, 283–286.

Wong, E.T. and Lindall, A.W. (1973) Preliminary evidence for a microsomal precursor to human parathyroid hormone. Proceedings of the National Academy of Sciences, 70, 2291–2294.

Wrong, O. and Davies, H.E.F. (1959) The excretion of acid in renal disease. Quarterly Journal of Medicine, 28, 259–313.

FURTHER READING

Fourman, P. and Royer, P. (1968) Calcium Metabolism and the Bone. Blackwell, Oxford.

MacIntyre, I. (Ed.) (1972) Calcium Metabolism and Bone Disease, Clinics in Endocrinology and Metabolism, Vol. 1, No. 1. Saunders, London.

Nordin, B.E.C. (1973) Metabolic Bone and Stone Disease. Churchill-Livingstone, London.

Rasmussen, H. and Bordier, P. (1973) Bone Cells, Mineral Homeostasis and Skeletal Remodelling. Williams and Wilkins, Baltimore.

Wacker, W.E.C. and Parisi, A.F. (1968) Magnesium metabolism. New England Journal of Medicine, 278, 658–663, 712–717, 772–776.

ADDENDUM

Calcitonin

It is now known that there is a large sex-difference in plasma calcitonin levels (Hillyard et al., 1978). This difference was previously unappreciated because of technical difficulties and for two further reasons. These are that the contraceptive pill produces a rise from the depressed levels found in young women to those present in healthy men. The other reason for failure to appreciate these differences has been that the diurnal rhythm present in plasma calcitonin levels (Hillyard et al., 1977) was often not taken into adequate account. The practical consequences of these new findings are that the time of sampling must be rigidly controlled when plasma calcitonin is measured and that the sex of the subject must also be taken into account. However, the theoretical implications of these findings are far from clear. It seems natural to suspect that the sex hormones, oestrogen and testosterone, may be involved and that the greater liability of women to bone loss may be connected with a depleted calcitonin reserve. Thus, while the rapid loss of bone shortly after the menopause is undoubtedly connected with oestrogen deficiency, it may also be related to calcitonin metabolism. However, further work is necessary to assess these interesting possibilities (MacIntyre et al., 1977; MacIntyre, 1978).

Vitamin D

Regulation of the metabolism of 25-OH-D_3 to 1,25$(OH)_2D_3$ by the kidney has recently become clearer. It now appears that both growth hormone (Spanos et al., 1978) and prolactin (MacIntyre et al., 1978) are of major importance in enhancing production of this highly active metabolite of vitamin D; how this is achieved remains unknown.

It now seems that plasma calcitonin and plasma 1,25$(OH)_2D_3$ levels are elevated together in the times of major physiological calcium stress: growth, pregnancy and lactation. It is possible that a major function of calcitonin is to protect the integrity of the skeleton as well as to help in regulating plasma calcium levels. Calcitonin will inhibit the bone-resorbing action of 1,25$(OH)_2D_3$ without affecting the action of that metabolite in increasing calcium absorption from the gut. Calcitonin plays an essential part in the action of 1,25$(OH)_2D_3$ in increasing calcium absorption without increasing bone destruction.

Hillyard, C.J., Cooke, T.J.C., Coombes, R.C., Evans, I.M.A. and MacIntyre, I. (1977) Normal plasma calcitonin: circadian variation and response to stimuli. Clinical Endocrinology, 6, 291–298.

Hillyard, C.J., Stevenson, J.C. and MacIntyre, I. (1978) Relative deficiency of plasma-calcitonin in normal women. Lancet, 1, 961–962.

MacIntyre, I. (1978) Review article. The action and control of the calcium-regulating hormones. Journal of Endocrinological Investigation, 1, 277–284.

MacIntyre, I., Evans, I.M.A. and Larkins, R.G. (1977) Review article. Vitamin D. Clinical Endocrinology, 6, 65–79.

MacIntyre, I., Colston, K.W., Robinson, C.J. and Spanos, E. (1978) Vitamin D: introduction and recent studies on regulation. In Molecular Endocrinology, Proceedings of Endocrinology '77 (Eds. I. MacIntyre and M. Szelke) pp. 73–85, Elsevier/North-Holland Biomedical Press, Amsterdam.

Spanos, E., Barrett, D., MacIntyre, I., Pike, J.W., Safilian, E.F. and Haussler, M.R. (1978) Effect of growth hormone on vitamin D metabolism. Nature, 273, 246–247.

Chapter 9

Renal function

Douglas A.K. Black and J. Stewart Cameron

Royal College of Physicians, Regent's Park, London NW1 4LE and Clinical Science Laboratories, Guy's Tower, Guy's Hospital, London Bridge SE1 9RT, England

CONTENTS

9.1. NORMAL FUNCTION

Much has been learnt of kidney function since Homer Smith in the 1940s stated "the only thing we know for sure about the kidney is that it makes urine". He was one of the pioneers in moving from this situation, but the implied emphasis on excretion, important as it is, has to be balanced by Cannon's concept of the homeostatic (or regulatory) function of the kidney; put more crudely, what the kidney leaves in the body is as important as what it puts in the pot. In very general terms, the excretion of waste products is achieved by the physical process of glomerular filtration, with energy supplied by the heart; whereas regulation is accomplished by variations in tubular reabsorption of particular constituents, including water. Energy required for the reabsorption of solute accounts for by far the greater part of the kidney's own consumption of oxygen: the reabsorption of water is largely passive, in pursuit of solute; but the ability to form a concentrated urine depends also on the counter-current arrangement of blood vessels and hairpin tubular loops in the renal medulla. In addition to its major normative function in relation to body fluid, the kidney has endocrine and metabolic functions of some importance. For detailed coverage of the physiological anatomy and function of the kidney see Robinson (1972a), and Brenner and Rector (1976).

9.1.1. Excretory function

Although the two kidneys together account for less than 0.5% of body weight, they receive more than 20% of the cardiac output. In total, over one litre of blood per minute is distributed to two million glomerular tufts, whose combined filtering area is of the order of 1 m^2. The glomerular filter retains cells and almost all of the protein of plasma, but allows the passage of water and solutes, to an extent limited by the fall in hydrostatic pressure and the increase in colloid oncotic pressure as the capillary is traversed. The product of glomerular filtration, containing only traces of protein, amounts to 120 ml/min, so that in the course of a day nearly 60 times the entire volume of plasma in the body has been filtered in the kidneys (Robinson, 1972a). The normal efficiency of renal excretion is based on this very large volume of "raw material", and therefore the excretory process is very vulnerable to a decrease in cardiac output, to a fall in blood pressure, or to any local factor which impedes renal circulation. By comparison with changes in perfusion pressure, alterations in capillary permeability are not recognized as important hindrances to effective filtration, short of the situation where glomeruli are totally destroyed; but they are responsible for the abnormal leakage of protein which can occur in disease.

For a waste product to be excreted it is essential that it should, at least in part, be exempted from that process of tubular reabsorption which reduces the 120 ml/min of glomerular filtrate to the much smaller volume of urine finally excreted, usually 1 to 2 ml/min, but exceptionally from 0.5 to 20 ml/min. To take urea, the quantitatively major substance excreted, as an example, about one-third of that filtered is reabsorbed when large volumes of urine are excreted, and about two-thirds with a low rate of urine excretion (e.g. <800 ml/24 h). Given the diffusibility of urea, it is not surprising that back-diffusion should occur; the problem is rather why much larger amounts of urea are not reabsorbed along with water and other solutes. The answer is not completely known, but part of the explanation may lie in the counter-current arrangement in the renal medulla, which allows a concentration of urea in the deep medullary tissue comparable to that in urine (Black, 1965).

The dual mechanism involving massive filtration and restricted reabsorption appears to be the predominant selective mode of excretion of natural waste products – in the main urea, but also phosphate and sulphate derived from protein catabolism. Some foreign substances, such as inulin, escape reabsorption, and their clearance can thus be used as a measure of glomerular filtration. A component of active tubular secretion enters into the excretion of other substances, such as creatinine and uric acid. A number of important drugs are excreted in part by the mechanism of "non-ionic diffusion" (Milne et al., 1958). The unionized form of some drugs is lipid-soluble and can diffuse through the tubular wall; but the water-soluble ions formed within the tubules, at a pH different from that within cells, cannot freely diffuse, so there can be massive pH-dependent excretion, given the appropriate urinary acidity. A few substances, such as *p*-aminohippurate, are quantitatively cleared from blood at low plasma concentrations, and can thus be used as measures of renal blood-flow.

9.1.2. Regulatory function

The large volume of glomerular filtrate contains both substances to be excreted and substances whose loss from the body must be controlled. Clearly, fine regulation is needed to achieve the right balance between excretion and conservation. This essential principle was first clearly enunciated by Cushny, in his theory of an "ideal reabsorbate", whose composition would be that of a "perfected Locke's Fluid". His generalization was of value at the time when it was made, in establishing the filtration–reabsorption pattern of renal function; but it neglected the influence of renal function on intracellular composition. It has been displaced by study of the separate mechanisms which regulate urinary output of the major substances concerned and stabilize the internal environment of the body with regard to sodium, potassium, water and hydrogen ions. The large mass of minerals in the skeleton is determined, in the main, by controlled absorption, and by endocrine action on skeletal mineralization and reabsorption; but parathormone has an effect in increasing phosphate excretion. In the space available, and taking account of the main emphasis of this book, only an outline can be given of the regulatory mechanisms for major constituents, giving for each, key references which can be consulted for detail.

9.1.2.1. Water (Diamond, 1965; Berliner and Bennett, 1967; Dicker, 1970).
About four-fifths of the filtered water is reabsorbed passively, concurrently with the active reabsorption of solute during transit of the proximal convoluted tubule, in that segment of the nephron. Any regulation of water output in this phase is indirect, being dependent on the factors influencing solute reabsorption, and in line with Gamble's concept of the "companionship" of solute and water in body fluid. Direct regulation of water output is exerted on the remaining one-fifth of tubule fluid which enters the distal tubule. This fluid is essentially iso-osmolar as it leaves the proximal tubule, but in the loop of Henle in the medulla it passes through a zone of hyperosmolality; later, however, because of active sodium reabsorption in the ascending limb of Henle's loop, the fluid entering the distal tubule is hypo-osmolar. In the absence of antidiuretic hormone, this low osmolality persists into the final urine, and is even enhanced by active absorption of solute in the distal segment. On the other hand, when antidiuretic hormone is active, the hyperosmolality of medullary tissue is further increased, together with the permeability to water of the collecting ducts, enabling the final urine to reflect the increased hyperosmolality of the medulla. The operation of this basic mechanism is enhanced in states of dehydration by alterations in renal haemodynamics, which lessen the wash-out of solute from the renal medulla. Yet another determinant of urinary osmolality is the amount of solute which is being excreted.

9.1.2.2. Sodium (de Wardener, 1972)
In contrast to the passive nature of water reabsorption in the proximal tubule, this is a site of active sodium reabsorption, which can take place against an electrochemical gradient, and is linearly related to the oxygen consumption of the kidney. The amount of sodium involved is substantial – of the filtered load of some 15 mmol/min, about 80% is reabsorbed in this way. The bulk of electrolyte reabsorption takes place in the proximal tubule, and is "driven" by active sodium reabsorption, generating a potential difference

of 2 to 4 mV, the lumen being negative to the renal tissue (Burg and Orloff, 1970). Burg and Green (1973) have produced evidence that in the thick ascending limb of Henle's loop the active process is one of the chloride reabsorption, the potential difference in this segment being positive in the lumen, of the order of 20 to 25 mV. In the distal tubule, the 3 mmol/min of sodium which enters is further reduced to amounts of the order of 0.1 mmol/min. In this segment, sodium ions are reabsorbed in exchange for potassium and, to a less extent, hydrogen ions; the activity of this process is enhanced by aldosterone, and diminished by thiazide diuretics and spironolactone. Surprisingly perhaps, the filtered load of sodium does not appear to be a major determinant of ultimate sodium excretion by the normal kidney. Changes in glomerular filtration are compensated for by cognate changes in tubular reabsorption; this situation of "glomerulotubular balance" may be departed from in the diseased kidney, leading to sodium retention or to sodium loss. Although it is difficult to exclude haemodynamic factors, there is increasing evidence in favour of a "natriuretic hormone" which inhibits proximal sodium reabsorption when the volume of extracellular fluid is expanded.

9.1.2.3. Potassium (Wesson, 1969)

Potassium is present in glomerular filtrate in a concentration of approximately 5 mmol/litre. There is, however, considerable reabsorption of potassium in the proximal tubule and loop of Henle, so that only 5% or less of filtered potassium enters the distal tubular system. The potassium which appears in the final urine represents, in the main, potassium which has been added to the fluid in the distal tubules and collecting ducts. This view is consistent with clearance studies and observations on the excretion of isotopically labelled potassium, and is supported more directly by the findings on tubular micropuncture (Giebisch and Windhager, 1964). Much of the potassium added in the distal tubule is exchanged for sodium, and this process is stimulated by aldosterone. The remainder of distally added potassium may represent a passive leak from tubular cells whose potassium concentration is of the order of 100 mmol/litre, but a more active secretory process has not been excluded.

Potassium loading leads to an increase in potassium excretion, while potassium depletion leads to progressive decline in the output of potassium in the urine. This regulation of potassium excretion in response to changes in potassium balance occurs more slowly and is less complete than in the case of sodium. Whereas the kidneys operate directly on extracellular fluid, which contains most of the sodium in the body, their contact with the cellular stores of potassium is indirect, and the mechanisms whereby potassium regulation is achieved are still uncertain. Among the factors known to influence potassium excretion are the level of aldosterone activity; the potassium content of plasma and of cells, including those of the renal tubules; the pH of extracellular and intracellular fluid; and the amount of sodium reaching the distal tubule, and thus available for exchange with potassium.

9.1.2.4. Hydrogen ion (Robinson, 1972b; Rector, 1976)

Leaving aside the much larger amount of "volatile" hydrogen ion which is disposed of by the lungs as carbon dioxide (Chapter 3, section 3.2.3), in a normal man the kidneys are called upon to retrieve some 5000 mmol/24 h of filtered bicarbonate, and to dispose of some 70 mmol/24 h of "non-volatile" * hydrogen ion generated by the catabolism of sulphur-containing proteins, phospholipids and phosphoproteins; in addition, the diet may occasionally contain strong mineral acid such as hydrochloric acid. Hydrogen ions are secreted into the tubular fluid throughout the nephron in sufficient amount to neutralize the filtered bicarbonate, and to eliminate the much smaller amounts of "non-volatile" hydrogen ion requiring excretion, so as to titrate the body fluids to their constant low concentration of hydrogen ion (35 mmol/litre).

The filtered bicarbonate is used up by combination with the secreted hydrogen ion, forming carbon dioxide, which diffuses back into the tubular cell where it reforms bicarbonate to replenish the body's store of this buffer. When all the bicarbonate is neutralized, then the hydrogen ion concentration of the tubular fluid further down the nephron increases, with a corresponding fall in pH; the fall in pH is limited by the secreted hydrogen ion titrating other urinary buffers, principally phosphate; and by the ability of the tubule to generate a gradient of hydrogen ion from tubular lumen to blood, which is about 600:1 at maximum. About half of the hydrogen ion in the urine is present in this buffered form, and can be measured as titratable acid, i.e. adding alkali to urine on the bench until the pH returns to that of the blood (Chapter 3, section 3.3.4.2).

In the case of the strong acids (sulphuric, hydrochloric and the third hydrogen of phosphoric) which may require excretion, negligible quantities of hydrogen ion can be excreted at the minimum pH (4.8) attainable by the tubule. This would result in sulphate, some phosphate and some chloride being excreted in association with other cations, such as sodium, potassium and calcium, which would need to be replenished. It also requires the excretion of hydrogen ion in a form other than buffered hydrogen ion. This task is accomplished by the formation of ammonia in the nephron. This diffuses across into the tubular lumen where, if the pH is low, it will combine with free hydrogen ions to form ammonium ion (NH_4^+), and is "trapped". This allows further hydrogen ion to be secreted without further change in pH; or in the case of a maximally acid urine, permitting its excretion in the only form possible. About half of the excretion of hydrogen ion is normally accomplished in this fashion, and increases in states of acidosis.

9.1.3. Endocrine function (Peart, 1972; Penington, 1972)

Although renin was discovered in 1898, attention was almost totally concentrated on the excretory aspects of renal function until Goldblatt's studies on hypertension induced by renal ischaemia re-awakened interest in what Selye has called "the endocrine kidney". The second major humoral agent of renal origin, erythropoietin, was not discovered until 1950.

Substances with renin-like activity have been extracted from other organs, but the main source of renin is the juxtaglomerular cells of the afferent arteriole to the glomerulus. Its production and release are stimulated by a fall in pressure in the afferent arteriole, or by a fall in the sodium concentration of tubular fluid at the level of the macula densa in the distal tubule, which closely adjoins the juxtaglomerular body. On release into the circulation, renin is effective in generating active angiotensin from its precursor

* So called because, unlike carbonic acid (H_2CO_3) which has a volatile anhydride (CO_2), sulphuric, phosphoric and hydrochloric acids do not have respirable anhydrides.

(angiotensinogen) in plasma. The angiotensin so produced has a direct pressor action on arterioles, and stimulates the secretion of aldosterone by the adrenal glands, with important consequent effects on the sodium-potassium exchange in distal tubules, as noted in section 9.1.2.2.

As with renin, the kidney is the main, but not the only source of erythropoietin, the exact site of production of which, within the kidney, has not been firmly established. Its production is stimulated by reduction in the oxygen content of blood, and the kidney appears to be more sensitive to this than are other organs. As its name suggests, its action is to stimulate production of red cells in the bone marrow.

The renal medulla has been shown to synthesize a number of vasodepressor lipids related to or identical with known prostaglandins; McGiff et al. (1971) discussed the possible role of these substances in the haemodynamics of the medulla and in modulating the action of antidiuretic hormone. Another important metabolic activity of the kidney is the second step in the conversion of cholecalciferol (vitamin D_3) into its biologically active form (Kodicek et al., 1970). Cholecalciferol is hydroxylated in the liver first to 25-hydroxycholecalciferol, and then in the kidney to 1,25-dihydroxycholecalciferol. Failure of the second step, in renal failure or in anephric man, is responsible for certain of the defects in renal osteodystrophy, which can be reversed by treatment with the active agent (De Luca, 1974).

9.1.4. Metabolic aspects (Wesson, 1969)

As might be expected from the high blood flow, conditioned by the needs of excretion, the renal cortex is an active site of aerobic metabolism. The renal medulla, on the other hand, with its sluggish blood supply, derives most of its energy requirement anaerobically. It has already been mentioned that most of the oxygen consumed in the kidney is related to the active proximal reabsorption of solute, but the kidney is also an important metabolic organ (Metcoff, 1975) and slices have been much used in metabolic studies. Provided that oxygen is freely available, the cortex of the kidney uses free fatty acid as its main source of energy, but glucose is also utilized to some extent as an energy source. Glucose, however, is the main source of energy utilized by the medulla: in the outer medulla, glycolysis is both anaerobic and aerobic, but in the inner medulla and papilla it is almost exclusively anaerobic. Glucose is produced in the cortex (gluconeogenesis) and used in the medulla. Ammoniagenesis also occurs in the outer medulla and cortex in parallel with gluconeogenesis. Acidosis increases the activity of pyruvate carboxylase, phosphoenolpyruvate (PEP) carboxykinase and phosphofructokinase, all of which favour gluconeogenesis rather than glycolysis. Acidosis also influences the balance between NAD^+ and NADH in favour of NAD^+, which in turn favours the deamination of glutamate to α-ketoglutarate (Pitts, 1964) with the generation of ammonia. α-Ketoglutarate is an important substrate in the kidney for gluconeogenesis. Under anaerobic conditions, it may undergo a coupled decarboxylation with oxaloacetate to yield phosphoenolypyruvate and carbon dioxide. This carbon dioxide dissolves to form carbonic acid, and hence hydrogen ion, for secretion into the renal tubule. Thus, although oxidative decarboxylation is available, oxygen is not an obligatory requirement in the generation of hydrogen ion in the tubule.

9.2. ASPECTS OF RENAL PATHOLOGY (Heptinstall, 1974)

The kidney is subject to general pathological processes – tumours, infections, vascular changes, intoxications – as are other organs of the body. As a major organ of excretion, with a very high blood supply relative to its mass, it is specially vulnerable both to toxic effects and to deprivation of its blood supply. It is also one of the organs most liable to be affected in the collagen disorders, and by general vascular disorders such as atheroma and diabetic arterial disease. This section, however, deals with the special ways in which the kidney reacts to immunological insult and to infection.

9.2.1. Glomerulonephritis – a group of immunological disorders

The group of conditions known collectively as glomerulonephritis, accounts for a major proportion of patients with renal disease who require chemical investigation. All have in common structural and functional alterations in the glomeruli. Some of these lead only to transient alterations in renal function, but others produce progressive changes ending in chronic renal failure, often together with hypertension. Glomerulonephritis not only presents in any of the major syndromes of renal disease, as described below, but also exhibits a bewildering variety of histopathological appearances at both biopsy and autopsy, and a confusing multiplicity of underlying pathogenesis. Much effort has been put into this field, however, and some unifying ideas have now emerged.

Attention was first drawn to the probable importance of abnormal immune responses in relation to glomerulonephritis by the recognition that acute nephritis following streptococcal infection was not a direct infection of the kidney, but a sequel to the primary infection related in time to the development of antistreptococcal immunity; later, by the quite similar involvement of the kidney in diseases such as disseminated lupus erythematosus, whose basis in abnormal immune reactions is now clearly established. Recognition of autoimmunity in the context of Hashimoto's disease and acquired haemolytic anaemia, led to interest in the possibility that the immune mechanisms of the body might be responsive to renal antigens. This mechanism is applicable in the uncommon disorder of lung purpura with nephritis – sometimes known as Goodpasture's syndrome – in which there is a destructive immune response to antigens derived from capillary basement membranes. Antigens derived from renal tubule cells are the basis of one form of experimental nephritis, and may also be relevant to some forms of human disease. Present evidence strongly suggests, however, that the great majority of patients with glomerulonephritis are suffering, in immunological terms, from one or other form of "soluble-complex disease" (type III reaction – Gell and Coombs, 1968).

Underlying many varieties of glomerulonephritis appears to be a relative immunodeficiency, (Germuth and Rodriguez, 1973; Peters, 1974) leading to partial failure of elimination of circulating antigens, both endogenous and exogenous. These antigens lead to the formation of small, potentially injurious, circulating soluble complexes, containing both antigen and antibody, which localize in the kidney in preference to other parts of the capillary circulation, because of its large blood flow, and the peculiarly high permeability of the glomerular capillaries. The immunodeficiency in most patients has not yet been characterized, but may be related either to complement, to quantity or quality (i.e. avidity or affinity) of antibody, or to T-lymphocyte function. There is good evidence that T-cell deficiency leads to glomerulonephritis both in man and animals, that complement deficiencies in man are associated with glomerulonephritis and that, in animals, nephritis-prone strains make antibody in smaller quantities, or of poorer affinity, than those animals who do not develop nephritis in response to antigen load. The complexes formed in moderate intermittent antigen excess appear to be responsible for most forms of glomerulonephritis. The role of the kidney is that of an "innocent bystander" becoming involved in a general immune reaction to antigens which is unrelated to the kidney itself.

The antigens so far incriminated in human glomerulonephritis (Table 9.1) include streptococcal and staphylococcal antigens, viral and plasmodial antigens, tumour antigens, altered DNA, Australia antigens, and thyroglobulin (Wilson and Dixon, 1972). In about 95% of those cases of human glomerulonephritis which have been examined by immunofluorescent techniques, evidence of soluble-complex disease has been found; but in many cases, the antigen responsible for initiating the process is unidentified, and there seems little doubt that further antigenic precipitants of glomerulonephritis will be discovered, including drugs and poisons. The variability in nature – and probably also in dosage – of antigen no doubt represents one factor in producing the diversity of histological appearances found in glomerulonephritis.

TABLE 9.1.

SOME ANTIGENS BELIEVED TO BE IMPORTANT IN THE GENESIS OF GLOMERULONEPHRITIS

Exogenous	bacterial	streptococci
		staphylococci
		pneumococci
		m. leprae
	rickettsial	coxiella
	viral	EB virus
		hepatitis B
		ECHO 9
		measles
	treponemal	syphilis
	parasitic	*P. malariae*
		P. falciparum
		S. haematobium
		S. mansoni
		filariasis
	drugs	mercury
		mercurials
		gold
		penicillamine
		tridione
Endogenous		DNA
		thyroglobulin
		carcinoembryonic and other tumour antigens
		renal tubular antigen
		IgG

The localization of potentially inflammatory complexes in the glomerular capillaries is not always followed by even a transient nephritis. The removal of this material by the phagocytic mesangial (axial) cells of the glomerulus is crucial and little understood. In addition, complexes formed with various antigens by antibodies of various classes and subclasses differ in their ability to evoke inflammatory responses. To take an example where the source of antigens is known, the spectrum of acute post-streptococcal nephritis ranges from a mild illness with minimal cellular proliferation in the glomerular mesangium, to acute anuria with massive destruction of glomeruli and extension of the inflammatory process beyond the glomerular tuft, in the shape of epithelial crescents. The onset phase of the majority of cases of human glomerulonephritis can reasonably be ascribed to soluble-complex disease; many of these patients get well after an acute illness, but a proportion of them, and in one series even the majority (Baldwin, 1977), show residual and even progressive renal damage. The factors which determine progression of renal damage may well be quite different from immunological mechanisms which initiate it; they are obscure, but may include vascular damage, and scarring of the interstitium of the kidney.

The acute inflammatory responses include the complement system. Immune complexes can activate complement, with the release of soluble factors and the generation of cell-fixed components which together attract leucocytes, induce immune adherence at the site of complement activation, and bring about the release of cell components from mast cells, leucocytes and possibly platelets, with increase in capillary permeability and release of proteolytic enzymes. Immune complexes can also cause platelet aggregation and release of platelet factors directly, without the intervention of complement, again leading to release of factors which increase permeability, and secondarily to activation of the coagulation cascade. In any injury where the collagen component of the capillary basement membrane is exposed, again platelets are aggregated to form a plug, and in addition the collagen will activate the coagulation cascade, with formation of fibrin. Secondarily, the kinin system and fibrinolysis are activated with release of kinins from kinogen fibrinopeptides – themselves inflammation-inducing – and fibrin degradation products from fibrinogen. These in turn are capable of affecting complement and platelet function, and were it not for a system of inhibitors limiting the active lives of all these components the inflammation would be explosive.

There is good evidence that all the above mechanisms operate both in clinical nephritis in man (Wilson and Dixon, 1974) and in experimental nephritis in animals, although the evidence is much more secure in the case of acute reversible disease than in chronic disease. Complement levels fall, complement turnover increases, and products of complement activation may be found in the plasma. Complement and polymorph depletion protects animals to a considerable extent in some forms of induced nephritis. Platelet turnover is accelerated and renal uptake of platelets enhanced in human glomerulonephritis. Fibrinolysis is indicated by the finding of fibrin degradation products in excess in the urine of patients with active nephritis. Morphologically, complement components and fibrinogen may be found in the glomeruli, although inflammatory cells, and especially platelets, are difficult to find.

The second immune mechanism involved in human glomerulonephritis, i.e. antibody specifically directed against glomerular components, may be important as a secondary mechanism determining chronicity. The antibody may be directed either against damaged glomerular components, or against foreign material fixed as complexes in the glomeruli (Van Es et al., 1977).

The clinical features of the various stages of glomerulonephritis are outlined later, in discussing the syndromes which they produce. The histological features are so varied as to have aroused the sorting instincts of distinguished nephrologists from Volhard through Dorothy Russell to Ellis and Longcope. The technique of renal biopsy has brought a new dimension to renal pathology, both by making tissue available in the early stages of renal disease, and by providing fresh material for study by immunofluorescence and electron microscopy. One of the present authors (Cameron, 1979) has reviewed the natural history of glomerulonephritis, taking into account the new evidence obtained in this way, and has proposed what is no doubt an interim classification of the histological patterns seen in what must be regarded as a group of diseases rather than a single entity.

The immunological processes described above lead to a variety of alterations in the glomerular architecture. Although valuable in predicting response to treatment and likely outcome, they are not specific: the same aetiological agent may lead to a variety of glomerular appearances, presumably as the result of variations in antigen load and host response, and each glomerular appearance may be found in a variety of circumstances. It follows that in considering glomerulonephritis, it is necessary to specify not only the clinical presentation, but also the glomerular reaction, and – if possible – the aetiology. Although this is possible in a growing number of patients, the aetiology remains unknown in the majority.

The various histological appearances of the glomeruli result both from alterations in the various glomerular components, and from additional features not normally present, such as material believed to represent immune deposits. A detailed description of these various histological appearances and their clinical correlations can be found elsewhere (Heptinstall, 1974) but the following classification is one widely adopted –

(a) *Minimal charges.* No evidence of immune involvement, and only minor or no glomerular alteration.

(b) *Focal (segmental) glomerulosclerosis*. The prominent lesion is a segmental sclerosis of some glomeruli, but with diffuse mesangial and minor alterations.

(c) *Membranous nephropathy*. Capillary wall lesions showing deposits on the outer aspect of the basement membrane diffusely throughout all glomeruli; no or minor glomerular proliferation.

(d) *Proliferative glomerulonephritis.* Characterized by proliferation of at least one cellular element of the glomerular tuft, sometimes more; occasionally with exudation of polymorphs; either endo-capillary, extra-capillary or both; if prominent capillary wall thickening by deposits, termed mesangiocapillary; occasionally focal and segmental, often in association with systemic arteritis.

To any of these descriptions may be added the effects of hypertension.

In terms of renal function, the crucial event in glomerulonephritis is the fall-off in glomerular function; measurement of this aspect is essential for the diagnosis and treatment of the condition.

It is worthwhile drawing attention to the variety of histological appearances which have been found to underly a somewhat smaller number of clinical syndromes; but the pathological chemistry of renal disease is more closely correlated with the clinical syndromes than with histological appearances, so it will be considered under the clinical syndromes. In due course, it is likely that further connections between histology and identifiable chemical phenomena will be discovered, similar to the link between mesangiocapillary proliferative glomerulonephritis and hypocomplementaemia, and that between minimal change nephropathy and highly "selective" proteinuria.

9.2.2. Infection and the kidney – the enigma of chronic pyelonephritis

The preceding section has indicated the significance in glomerulonephritis of the role played by bacterial or viral infection in initiating soluble-complex disease. There are several other ways in which the kidney may be damaged by infective processes – the formation of pyaemic abscesses, the development of interstitial nephritis, and the extension of inflammation from the renal pelvis, which constitutes pyelonephritis. The first two of these conditions occur in association with generalized infection with a variety of organisms, but the clinical picture is dominated by the primary infection. The use of antibiotics has considerably lowered the incidence of these conditions, and indeed, when a biopsy shows the cellular infiltration supposedly characteristic of interstitial nephritis, the condition is much more likely to be a manifestation of analgesic nephropathy or of pyelonephritis, in which interstitial involvement is common. Heptinstall (1967) has given a lucid critical review of the difficulties which occur in the histological diagnosis of pyelonephritis.

In terms of practical importance, as well as of theoretical interest, the paramount renal manifestation of infection is acute pyelonephritis. Although infection can reach the kidney by the blood stream, or even by lymphatic spread, the clinical condition of pyelonephritis is overwhelmingly associated with ascending infection of the urinary tract. This occurs most frequently in infants wearing diapers, in sexually active and pregnant women, and in older men with prostatic urinary stasis. It can however, occur at any age and in either sex. The syndrome of urinary infection is briefly described later (section 9.3.6).

The salient pathological feature of chronic pyelonephritis is its localized character, in contrast to the diffuse involvement which is seen in all the common forms of glomerulonephritis. Chronic pyelonephritis may be limited to one kidney, and indeed to one segment of the kidney, a finding which greatly lessens the value of renal biopsy in its diagnosis, but enhances the importance of pyelography. This can reveal differences in cortical thickness between different parts of the kidney, as well as demonstrating localized atrophy of the pyramids of the renal medulla. Radiology may also reveal evidence of urinary obstruction or ureteric reflux, which are important predisposing factors to the establishment of infection in the kidney. In acute pyelonephritis, polymorphs are found both in the interstitial tissue and in the tubular lumina of the affected segment of the kidney.

Coarse scarring of kidneys visible to the naked eye, together with diffuse scarring microscopically visible throughout the whole kidney, have been recognized since the nineteenth century. Unlike the contracted kidney which is produced by chronic glomerulonephritis, the scarring is patchy, and under the microscope it can be seen to affect predominantly the interstitium and tubules; the glomeruli show only ischaemic, or intrarenal hydronephrotic changes suggesting obstruction further down the nephron. The interstitium is greatly increased in area, often with dense patchy infiltrate of chronic inflammatory cells, mostly plasma cells and lymphocytes. The tubules show thickened basement membranes, flat tubular epithelium, and are sometimes greatly dilated and filled with coagulated protein. Finally the histological features associated with chronic, or occasionally malignant, hypertension may be seen.

On occasion, these appearances are found in a patient with a structural lesion of the lower urinary tract, vesicoureteric reflux of urine on micturition, and a history of recurrent urinary tract infections with documented bacteriuria. These patients are considered below. However, in the majority of adults with small, coarsely scarred kidneys there is no reflux and the urine is sterile although it may contain an excess of leucocytes. Because of the undoubted association with infection in a disordered urinary tract, and the occasional finding of bacteriuria, this type of kidney disease has usually been termed "*chronic pyelonephritis*" in the United Kingdom and the United States, although the *interstitial* element has always received emphasis on the continent of Europe. More correctly the terminology should be "small scarred kidneys of unknown aetiology". Three possibilities arise –

(a) Although there are no longer any bacteria present and multiplying in either urine or kidney, the changes represent the result of a now burnt-out infection. This possibility has received recent support in the suggestion that the persistence of *bacterial antigen* alone in the renal parenchyma may lead to inflammation, probably by an immune mechanism (Aoki et al., 1969).

(b) The primary cause of the scarring in all cases was originally reflux of urine (see below) which was never severe and has now ceased. It is known that in children the natural history of vesicoureteric reflux is to become less or disappear, but its course in adult life has not been charted. This would leave a small, scarred but non-refluxing kidney (Bailey, 1975).

(c) Certain agents can cause coarse diffuse renal interstitial scarring. Uric acid, phenacetin contained in analgesic drugs and lead are known to be capable of this, and some antibiotics such as the penicillins and cephalosporins can produce a more acute interstitial nephritis. There may be other substances in the environment, of which we are ignorant, which could cause similar scarring.

In constrast, it appears that recurrent bacteriuria is a very common finding, especially in women, and that without a primary structural disorder of the urinary tract it does not lead to renal scarring, at least in adults. It is contestable whether even in the growing kidney, bacteriuria without reflux can produce renal scarring. Any suggestion that repeated acute urinary tract infections lead eventually to coarse renal scarring now appears untenable. If the term "chronic pyelonephritis" continues in use it should be with the understanding that it refers to a coarsely scarred kidney, without reflux of urine, for which no explanation is available.

9.2.3. Analgesic nephropathy

It was noticed about 20 years ago that the consumption of excessive amounts of analgesic drugs was associated with both an interstitial nephritis leading to renal failure, and a necrosis of the papillae of the kidney with separation and sloughing of the affected tissue (papillary necrosis). Particular attention was directed at mixed analgesics containing phenacetin, and it appears that the cumulative or total consumption of more than 1.5 kg of phenacetin is necessary to induce the changes. The weight of epidemiological evidence favours phenacetin – or its metabolites – as the main agent responsible in man, although the concurrent ingestion of aspirin and perhaps caffeine may enhance this toxicity. Paracetamol (acetominophen), which is also one metabolite of phenacetin, is not above suspicion, but other metabolites such as *N*-acetophenetedin are more probably responsible. Aspirin alone can produce similar changes in rodents, but the rodent kidney differs anatomically and in terms of concentrating power from the human kidney. Few patients have been described with analgesic nephropathy apparently induced by aspirin alone, despite the large amount of aspirin consumed throughout the world. Aspirin does, however, have an acute effect on the human kidney, producing a fall in glomerular filtration rate and a sloughing of tubular cells and other debris into the urine.

The state of hydration appears important in the induction of analgesic nephropathy in both man and animals. Dehydration enhances the toxic effects, and the highest incidence of analgesic nephropathy has been reported from countries like Australia, (especially in Queensland) and South Africa, where analgesics are widely publicised and the climate is hot.

The quantity of analgesic which must be consumed to cause the effect is far beyond normal usage. Two groups of patients are vulnerable: those with minor but important chronic pain, such as sufferers from osteoarthritis; and those who take the analgesics in a manner consistent with a drug dependence, usually to calm or stimulate, to induce sleep, or for other less obvious reasons, all unrelated to the actual pharmacology of the drugs in question. This second group forms the great majority of patients.

In terms of *renal function*, tubular function tends to be more profoundly affected than glomerular function for the greater part of the illness, with inability to acidify or concentrate the urine and with salt losses at a high level independent of intake. Later, falls in glomerular filtration rate are seen, but severe destruction of the medulla is demonstrable by radiology with almost normal filtration rates.

9.3. THE SYNDROMES OF RENAL DISEASE

The term "syndrome" was originally used to denote a grouping of symptoms or signs characteristic of a single disease process. As it became appreciated that such patterns could be produced by more than one pathological process, the meaning of the term was extended to include such situations. For example, chronic renal failure represents the end-stage of a considerable number of renal diseases; but clinically there is virtue, both for recognition and for practical management, in concentrating attention on the outward manifestation in the first instance, leaving the more academic question of the underlying cause for later decision. This section summarizes the clinical features and the associated pathological chemistry of the major renal syndromes. There are also a number of important syndromes which may be caused either by renal disease, or by diseases of other systems of the body. Table 9.2 lists the syndromes of primary renal disease, including their salient features; Table 9.3 lists syndromes of which renal disease is an important, but by no means the only, cause. In patients presenting with syndromes listed in Table 9.3, the

TABLE 9.2.

SYNDROMES OF DOMINANTLY RENAL ORIGIN

Syndrome	Salient features
Acute nephritic syndrome	Haematuria and oliguria, moderate oedema
Nephrotic syndrome	Massive proteinuria, hypoproteinaemia, oedema
Asymptomatic proteinuria	Detected on routine testing
Acute renal failure	Oliguria, azotaemia, following "shock"
Chronic renal failure	Polyuria, azotaemia, clinical "uraemia"
Urinary infection	Dysuria, bacilluria, pyuria
Calculous nephropathy	Colic, haematuria
Obstructive nephropathy	Urological symptoms and findings
Renal tubular syndromes	Aminoaciduria, tubular acidosis, glycosuria, phosphaturia

TABLE 9.3.

SYNDROMES WITH BOTH RENAL AND "NON-RENAL" CAUSES

Syndrome	Examples of "non-renal" causes
Hypertension	"Essential" hypertension, endocrine hypertension
Osteodystrophy	Hyperparathyroidism, rickets, steatorrhoea
Sodium depletion	Gastrointestinal losses, Addison's disease
Potassium depletion	Gastrointestinal losses, diuretic abuse
Acidosis	Metabolic and respiratory causes
Polyuria	Diabetes insipidus, compulsive water drinking
Anaemia	Blood disorders
Oedema	Cardiac and hepatic failure

clinical requirement in relation to renal disease is in the main to exclude it; this can be done on the basis of a normal urine and urine-sediment, normal plasma urea and serum creatinine concentrations, and the absence of any history or signs suggestive of renal disease.

9.3.1. Acute nephritic syndrome

In addition to acute glomerulonephritis, this can be simulated by polyarteritis nodosa, Henoch–Schönlein purpura, systemic lupus, Wegener's granuloma, lung purpura with nephritis, recurrent haematuria and accelerated hypertension. The patient complains of puffiness of the face, and of dark cloudy urine or of overt haematuria. The urine is notably scanty in amount, grossly albuminous, and with a sediment containing red cells, leucocytes, and granular and blood casts. Examination of the patient confirms the presence of some oedema, and of a modest rise in blood pressure. There may be some discomfort in the loins, but there is little malaise during the course of the illness, provided that the intake of salt and water is decreased; if this is not done, the situation may be complicated by the paroxysmal dyspnoeas of left ventricular failure, or the convulsions of cerebral oedema. Exceptionally, the oliguria may amount to virtual anuria, so that the syndrome becomes effectively one of acute renal failure.

Clinically, there is only a moderate rise in the plasma urea concentration, or in creatinine, particularly if protein intake is restricted soon after onset of the disease. There is depression of the clearance of inulin and *p*-aminohippurate. Patients with anuria, and those with generalized vascular disease have considerable azotaemia, and are clinically uraemic. Most patients with primary glomerulonephritis make a good recovery, passing through a phase of spontaneous diuresis. A minority do not clear up in this way; the persistence of albuminuria or of microscopic haematuria or cylindruria indicates continued activity which may lead ultimately to renal failure.

9.3.2. Nephrotic syndrome (Robson, 1972)

Approximately 75% of patients with the nephrotic syndrome are suffering from one or other form of primary glomerulonephritis. Causes of the syndrome in the remaining patients include systemic lupus, renal amyloidosis, diabetic nephropathy, myelomatosis, infections and tumours, and the toxic effects of poisons and drugs. The primary event leading to the syndrome is massive proteinuria, which causes depletion of the plasma protein, and ultimately generalized oedema. Hyperlipidaemia is a frequent, but not a necessary, concomitant of the syndrome, and is associated with atheroma. Some patients have a normal blood pressure and renal excretory function, while in others the picture is complicated by varying degrees of renal insufficiency, with or without significant hypertension. It is usually possible to control the oedema by salt restriction and diuretics. There is a variable response to corticosteroids and to immunosuppressive agents.

The plasma albumin concentration is commonly below 30 g/litre, and may be as low as 5 g/litre. Of the globulin fractions, α_1- and γ-globulin are reduced, while the α_2- and β-fractions, and also fibrinogen, are normal or increased. The reason for the hypoproteinaemia is the massive loss of protein in the urine, not less than 5.0 g/24 h, and sometimes in excess of 30 g/24 h. The pattern of protein loss is different in different patients. In some, it is limited to albumin and other proteins of low molecular mass, this pattern of "high selectivity" being associated with minimal histological changes in the renal glomeruli. In other patients, proteins of larger molecular mass are also lost, and such "low selectivity" is associated with florid glomerular changes, either proliferative or membranous. This and other evidence suggest that the mechanism of protein loss lies in an increase in glomerular permeability, and not necessarily in any change in tubular secretion or reabsorption of protein. The level of excretory renal function in the syndrome is very variable, depending on the nature of the renal lesion; in minimal-change nephrotic syndrome, glomerular filtration rate may be unusually high, possibly because of the low osmotic pressure which is exerted by the diminished plasma proteins.

The depletion of the plasma protein pool may cause hypovolaemia as well as hypoproteinaemia, and this may be relevant to the increased secretion of aldosterone which is one factor in the salt retention characteristic of the nephrotic syndrome. Cholesterol and phospholipid fractions of plasma lipids are commonly much increased, whereas triglycerides are normal or less markedly raised; there is an increase in pre-β- and β-lipoproteins, and sometimes a fall in α-lipoproteins (Chopra et al., 1971). Aminoaciduria, glycosuria, potassium-wasting and renal tubular acidosis have been described in individual patients with the nephrotic syndrome.

9.3.3. **Symptomless proteinuria** (Hardwicke, 1970)

The clinical significance of proteinuria in the absence of symptoms lies mainly in two directions – it may, when relatively small in amount, indicate the presence of unsuspected renal disease; or it may represent, when massive in amount, the presymptomatic phase of the nephrotic syndrome. An indication of the latter possibility might be found in depression of the plasma albumin concentration, which would imply that substantial protein loss had been present for some time.

Normal urine contains about 100 mg/24 h of protein, which is partly Tamm–Horsfall protein, of high molecular weight, derived from the renal tubular cells; it also represents in part a failure completely to reabsorb the traces of albumin (10 to 20 mg/litre) found in normal glomerular filtrate. Failure of reabsorption of this filtered protein is the basis of the "tubular proteinuria" found in the Fanconi proximal tubular syndrome, in tubular necrosis, and in cadmium poisoning. Bence Jones proteinuria represents an overflow of abnormal protein with low molecular weight. In renal vein thrombosis and orthostatic proteinuria, the protein is present because of raised capillary pressure in the glomeruli. In the majority of cases of pathological proteinuria, however, the basis is an increase in glomerular permeability, as in the nephrotic syndrome, and likewise due to a wide variety of glomerular lesions, generally separable only on the basis of renal biopsy. Considerable uncertainty still remains about the significance of the proteinuria, which may or may not be orthostatic, and which is not uncommonly found in apparently healthy young people. On the one hand, a variety of glomerular changes has been observed when renal biopsy has been performed; on the other, a 10 year follow-up of such patients seldom shows evidence of renal functional impairment, even when the proteinuria is persistent (R.R. Robinson, 1972).

9.3.4. **Acute renal failure** (Kerr, 1979)

It has already been noted that acute renal failure is occasionally produced by fulminant destruction of glomeruli in a small minority of patients with the acute nephritic syndrome. Much more commonly, it arises from damage to the kidneys due to impaired renal circulation, or to the action of nephrotoxins, and the primary events leading to such damage are legion. Ischaemic renal damage can occur in any form of severe shock, whether its cause be medical (e.g. haematemesis, hepatic necrosis, Gram-negative septicaemia), surgical (trauma, haemorrhage, incompatible transfusion), or obstetric (eclampsia, antepartum haemorrhage, septic abortion). The causes of toxic damage to the kidney are likewise numerous; Kerr (1979) lists the types of drug and poisons which have been known to cause damage to various parts of the nephron. The degree of ischaemia and the amount of a drug or poison reaching the kidney are both examples of graded phenomena; it is not surprising that the same applies to the consequent renal damage. At one end of the scale is a transient diminution of glomerular filtration, with no apparent structural damage to renal tissue, the scanty urine which is formed being of normal or even high osmolality. Moderate doses of nephrotoxins can cause necrosis of tubular epithelial cells, which may be shed and lead to transient tubular blockage, but no more radical interference with renal architecture. Larger doses of nephrotoxins, and prolonged ischaemia, lead to more radical tubular damage, with rupture, a process described by Jean Oliver as "tubulorrhexis". Here, the urine is commonly hypo-osmolar to plasma, and amounts to less than 500 ml/24 h. The most severe degrees of damage are represented by partial or complete cortical necrosis. The clinical picture is correspondingly varied, ranging from transient oliguria and elevation of the plasma urea concentration to complete and irreversible anuria. Some patients, in circumstances where renal ischaemia is likely, show an elevated plasma urea concentration, with notable oliguria, but this is exceptional. It is of the utmost practical importance to rule out mechanical obstruction to the outflow of urine, before regarding urinary suppression as evidence of acute renal failure of ischaemic or toxic origin.

Acute renal failure is characterized biochemically by retention in the blood of waste products, mainly those derived from protein. The plasma urea and serum creatinine concentrations have both been used as indices; the two factors which mainly determine the rate at which the concentration of *urea* rises are the degree of renal damage and – perhaps more importantly – the rate of protein catabolism, which is commonly much increased by virtue of the severity of the clinical situations which are likely to give rise to acute renal failure. In a patient with no extra-renal cause of protein breakdown, and whose protein catabolism is minimized by a diet which is adequate in carbohydrate and containing only 20 grams of high quality protein per day, the rate of rise in plasma urea concentration can be as little as 20 mg/dl per day. In severely ill patients, however, this rate may be increased 5-fold. The serum *creatinine* concentration is less affected by tissue catabolism, and disparity in the increases of creatinine and of urea concentrations is an indicant of tissue damage outside the kidneys. Retention of hydrogen ions occurs, and is important both in itself as a cause of clinical acidosis with Kussmahl breathing; and as one of the determinants of the plasma potassium concentration. Since there are some 4000 mmol of *potassium* in the body the mere retention of the daily potassium intake of around 100 mmol would take many days to raise the plasma concentration to 8 mmol/litre or more, at which cardiac toxicity becomes threatening. Some potassium is no doubt released from damaged tissue, but the main factor in the rapid rise in concentration of plasma potassium which occurs in acute renal failure, is the shift of potassium from cells to extracellular fluid which occurs in acidosis. *Water* and *sodium* are likewise retained in acute renal failure. When they are retained concomitantly, oedema develops, the dangerous clinical manifestation being oedema of the lungs, which was a common cause of death before the need to restrict sodium intake was appreciated. Water restriction is as necessary as sodium restriction, and is also more difficult to achieve, since the restriction is not uncommonly evaded by thirsty patients or over-solicitous attendants. The best index of adequate or inadequate water restriction is the plasma sodium concentration, which should not be allowed to fall unduly. Dilution of body fluid carries the hazard of convulsions. Many of the regular constituents of blood, including glucose, show some elevation in acute renal failure; but calcium and protein concentrations tend to be low, unless special factors are operating, e.g. hyperparathyroid over-activity may prevent the fall in serum calcium concentration.

Acute renal failure is an anxious condition for all concerned, especially, perhaps, when it is partly iatrogenic; some of this load of anxiety has been lessened by the general adoption of peritoneal and other forms of dialysis, which also allows a somewhat more relaxed regime of food and fluid than was required in the days when a patient had to sit out a week or more of anuria.

9.3.5. Chronic renal failure (Bricker et al., 1972)

There are at least 40 recognized causes of chronic renal failure; the most common are glomerulonephritis, pyelonephritis, vascular nephropathy in severe hypertension, and obstructive nephropathy. Vascular and obstructive nephropathy have practical importance over and above their frequency, since they can be arrested or improved in their early stages. The same applies to analgesic nephropathy, which ranks as a common cause of chronic renal failure in a number of countries. Although a raised plasma urea concentration is one of the hallmarks of chronic renal failure, it is also found in other conditions, notably extra-renal uraemia and acute renal failure. The terms uraemia, chronic renal failure and terminal (or end-stage) renal failure do indeed lead to confusion, but it is important to distinguish them. *Uraemia* is a chemical term, referring to an increase in the plasma urea concentration, but it has come into use, sometimes modified to "clinical uraemia", as a blanket term for the complex of symptoms observed both in acute and chronic renal failure, as a consequence of nitrogen retention; in either acute or chronic renal failure, the complex of symptoms can be relieved by dialysis. *Chronic renal failure* should mean the whole course of progressive renal impairment, from its asymptomatic phase to its latest stages, which alone should be termed *terminal renal failure,* in which life can only be maintained by restoration of renal function through dialysis or transplantation.

The symptomatology of chronic renal failure is complicated by a lack of correspondence between the degree of uraemia or azotaemia and the clinical state; by the special features of the many disorders which cause it; by its varying effects on mineral balance; and by the effects of hypertension, which commonly but not constantly accompanies renal failure. We are still far from understanding some of the features of clinical uraemia, e.g. uraemic pericarditis, but for practical purposes it is perhaps best to concentrate on those symptoms whose pathogenesis is reasonably understood, as this points the way to appropriate measures of alleviation. The widespread use of dialysis has clarified the issue of what features of uraemia can be attributed to excretory failure; these features include lethargy followed by coma, thirst and gastrointestinal irritation, muscle twitching, skin pigmentation and the urea frost. These "toxic" aspects of uraemia are probably not due to the retention of urea itself, but of other nitrogenous wastes such as methylguanidine; the search for a single uraemic toxin has not been successful and may be illusory. The progressive loss of the regulatory functions of the kidney is responsible for another group of symptoms. Sodium depletion produces clinical dehydration; sodium excess, with oedema, is uncommon except as a manifestation of hypertensive cardiac failure. Potassium excess is not common, except in patients maintained on a low-protein diet for long periods; potassium depletion is likewise uncommon, except in patients with primary tubular syndromes. Water depletion is common, but only as a concomitant of sodium depletion; water retention also occurs, in response to water loads, and can cause convulsions. Some lowering of the plasma sodium concentration is common in uraemic patients, probably indicating latent water depletion. Acidosis is general in the later stages, leading to over-breathing, and possibly contributing to coma in some patients. These disturbances of body fluid are generally features of quite advanced renal failure, but before they arise spontaneously, there is a stage of intolerance to any deviation from the normal intake of water and minerals. The osteodystrophy of chronic renal failure is complex in its pathogenesis, since patients can show varying combinations of osteoporosis, osteomalacia (related to diminished production of the active metabolite of vitamin D), and osteitis fibrosa (related to parathyroid overreaction), which may also be responsible for bicarbonate-wasting (Muldowney et al., 1971). The serum calcium concentration is low, and tetany may occur in spite of the acidaemia. The anaemia is largely attributable to deficiency of erythropoietin, but gastrointestinal blood loss and a more general haemorrhagic diathesis, contribute to it in some patients. When hypertension is present, it contributes notably both to the speed of progression of the renal damage, and to the symptomatology, including heart failure, hypertensive retinopathy, and cerebrovascular accidents.

The pathological chemistry of chronic renal failure is as varied as the symptomatology. Those of its features which can be fairly well related to symptoms have already been mentioned. The clearances of urea and of creatinine decline progressively over a number of years, but the decline in excretory function can be sharply accelerated by hypertensive renal damage, by sodium depletion and possibly by intercurrent infection. There are, however, several mechanisms which prevent any substantial rise in the blood concentrations of renally excreted substances until renal impairment is far advanced; for example, patients who have lost an entire kidney have plasma urea and creatinine concentrations which are well within the reference ranges. One mechanism limiting the rises in these values is increased function of those nephrons which survive, and which are in a state of osmotic diuresis, in that a normal amount of osmotically active excreted substances is distributed to many fewer nephrons; thus the osmotic load delivered to each surviving tubule is greater. Another factor is increased elimination of substances by extra-renal channels, notably the gut; for example, in renal failure the rise in the plasma urate concentration is diminished by excretion of urate into the bowel, in which bacterial degradation of urate prevents re-cycling. Adaptive hormonal mechanisms also diminish the rise in plasma concentrations – phosphate excretion is stimulated by the increased parathyroid activity in renal failure, and stimulation of sodium losing factors may be responsible, in addition to osmotic diuresis, for preventing sodium retention in spite of loss of nephrons which diminishes the load of sodium available for excretion. The relationship between plasma urea concentration and urea clearance is appreciably modified by changes in urea production – a low-protein diet is effective in lowering the plasma urea concentration at any given clearance value, whereas an infective episode can raise it markedly by increased tissue breakdown. Urate is retained to a limited extent in chronic renal failure, and it may be deposited in renal tissue, but clinical gout is only a rare complication of chronic renal failure; indeed, where the two conditions are found together, the gouty diathesis is usually the cause and not the consequence of renal failure. The electrolyte pattern in plasma is the resultant of the balance between a variable intake of water and salts, spontaneous or imposed as part of a regime, and a variable pattern of urinary output. In most cases, the dominant feature of the urine produced is *isosthenuria,* so that at the expense of polyuria and nocturia the patient can maintain himself in approximate electrolyte balance. However, the normal plasticity of renal homeostatic performance has gone, and he is defenceless against high intakes of water and electrolytes, and also against the abnormal losses in the vomiting and diarrhoea which are common in the terminal stages of chronic renal failure. While this is the general picture, there are important variants of water and electrolyte excretion which indicate aberrations in tubular function over and above those imposed by the osmotic diuresis which results from the need to eliminate a normal solute load through a greatly reduced population of nephrons. These unusual states have been summarized in the terms: water-losing, sodium-losing, and potassium-losing kidney. The acidosis associated with chronic renal failure is generally related to diminished excretion of buffer and to reduced formation of ammonia in the diminished renal mass. Some patients, however, show prominent bicarbonate-wasting, and this has been associated with excessive parathormone activity; other patients, with predominantly tubular disease, fail to produce a urine of appropriately low pH.

Phosphate retention, hypocalcaemia, raised serum alkaline phosphatase activity and raised parathormone concentration, are indicants of disordered metabolism of skeletal minerals. Renal excretion of therapeutic agents, including antibiotics and salts of magnesium and aluminium, is impaired in chronic renal failure, both from diminished filtration, and by altered urinary pH where the mechanism of excretion is by non-ionic diffusion.

As renal failure approaches its terminal stages, with filtration rates of 10 ml/min or less, the protein intake diminishes, either from anorexia or by therapeutic restriction. General metabolic changes appear at this stage, with protein depletion and, at times, diminished tolerance of carbohydrate, with hyperglycaemia. When the filtration rate falls below 2 ml/min, life can only be maintained by dialysis or transplantation. Each of these has its particular hazards, and those associated with biochemistry predominate in patients on chronic dialysis, largely because the prolongation of life with diminished renal function allows complications to develop after the patient has been rescued from uraemic coma. Short-term hazards of dialysis include the significant protein losses which occur in peritoneal dialysis, and the disequilibrium syndrome of cerebral oedema, when urea is removed so rapidly as to outpace transfer of urea from the brain to the circulation. Longer-term hazards, reviewed by Gordon et al. (1972), include metastatic calcification, osteodystrophy, hypokalaemia, and fluid overloading or depletion.

9.3.6. Urinary infection

Though it has high incidence and clinical importance, urinary infection will be dealt with here only insofar as it is one of the common causes of chronic renal failure. The typical clinical picture of an acute urinary infection is easy to recognize, with the frequent and painful passage of small amounts of turbid urine, fever and malaise, and some pain over the bladder or in the loins. There are, however, problems in the recognition of urinary infection when these symptoms are absent, as is common in chronic urinary infection. The diagnosis in the acute stages rests on clinical and microbiological evidence, but in the chronic stage, in addition to such evidence, radiological investigation is needed to establish whether the infective process is involving the kidneys, and producing scarring. In evaluating the impact of the disease on renal function, chemical tests become paramount, but the chemical picture is essentially that of chronic renal failure. Since pyelonephritis tends to involve the medulla at an early stage, there is a greater inability to concentrate the urine than there is with patients with glomerulonephritis at the same stage of glomerular failure. Sodium-, potassium-, and bicarbonate-losing states are more common in pyelonephritis than in glomerulonephritis, with bicarbonate wastage leading to hyperchloraemic acidosis. These evidences of greater tubular involvement than in comparable stages of glomerulonephritis are perhaps of theoretical rather than practical diagnostic interest, as is the tendency of proteinuria to be less in pyelonephritis than in glomerulonephritis.

9.3.7. Calculous nephropathy (Nordin and Hodgkinson, 1973)

About 80% of all renal stones contain calcium, combined with oxalate or with phosphate, usually in the form of apatite; other commonly occurring stones are composed of cystine, of uric acid or of magnesium ammonium phosphate. Small calculi are liable to be passed as "gravel", but may also become impacted, leading to renal colic with haematuria, especially with the harder irregular stones such as those composed of calcium oxalate. Larger calculi, mainly of magnesium ammonium phosphate, may remain in the renal pelvis and grow to form stag-horn calculi. These are associated with persistent infection and lead, in time, to loss of renal function on the affected side. Cystine and calcium-containing stones are radio-opaque, whereas those containing uric acid and magnesium ammonium phosphate are initially radiolucent, though calcium salts may later be added, so making them radio-opaque.

Cystine stones are most commonly found in patients with the familial metabolic anomaly of cystinuria, in which cystine is the least soluble member of a group of aminoacids which are excreted in grossly abnormal amount, the others being lysine, arginine, and ornithine. The solubility of cystine decreases with increase in urine acidity. Normally, less than 70 mg of cystine is excreted daily; in cystinuria, the amount excreted ranges from 100 to 1000 mg/day, stone formation being likely only in those excreting the larger amounts. Uric acid stones are similarly associated with increased formation and excretion of uric acid, whether in primary gout or in states of increased nucleic acid breakdown; e.g. the Lesch–Nyhan syndrome (Chapter 21) or leukaemia treated with cytotoxic agents. The occurrence of calculi in gout is not, however, simply related to excessive output, since only about 25% of gouty patients, unless treated by uricosuric agents, excrete uric acid in amounts above the normal range of 400 to 500 mg/day. One additional factor, as with cystine calculi, is the formation of concentrated urine, especially at night. But in the case of uric acid calculi, since the solubility of uric acid is much less in acid urine, a more important factor is the tendency in some patients to produce urine of greater than normal acidity; this anomaly has been ascribed to diminished ammonia formation, such that the proportion of hydrogen ions which is excreted as titratable acid increases. Magnesium ammonium phosphate stones are characteristically associated with infection by urea-splitting organisms, which increase both the alkalinity and the ammonium concentration of urine.

The most clearly established factor in the causation of calcium-containing stones is *hypercalciuria,* which need not necessarily be associated with hypercalcaemia. While most normal men show a daily calcium excretion of 300 mg or less (250 mg or less in women), variations in dietary intake and intestinal absorption make somewhat higher figures not uncommon. There are, of course, a number of conditions which unequivocally lead to increased excretion of calcium, derived from either increased absorption (the "milk-alkali" syndrome, vitamin D intoxication, sarcoidosis), or from increased bone resorption (hyperparathyroidism, myelomatosis, metastatic tumours, osteoporosis – including that from prolonged immobilization). Many of these disorders are associated with calculus formation, and also with deposition of calcium in the substance of the kidney (nephrocalcinosis). More difficulty arises in relation to apparently healthy people who repeatedly form calcium stones, sometimes over many years; one explanation put forward by Nordin is that these patients absorb more calcium than is normal, a state which has been described as "absorption hypercalciuria". Other factors, aside from the rare familial disease of oxaluria, which may be associated with calcium stone formation, include persistent urinary infection, urinary stasis, low urine volume (e.g. in the tropics), and high urinary pH.

9.3.8. Obstructive nephropathy (Bricker, 1967)

Obstruction of the urinary tract may manifest itself in various ways, some obvious such as suppression of urine, ureteric colic, renal enlargement and pain; others less immediately obvious, such as acute or chronic renal failure, persistent infection, and even polyuria, which may alternate with periods of partial suppression when the obstruction is partial and intermittent. Investigation and treatment of the causes of urinary obstruction are in the hands of the urological surgeon, but its effects on the kidney are of importance to the physician and clinical chemist.

Sudden and complete obstruction of the lower urinary tract, or bilaterally of the ureters, produces the syndrome of acute renal failure already described. Chronic obstruction leads to dilatation of the pelvis of one or both kidneys, with an increased liability to infection, and progressive loss of renal function. Initially, tubular function is affected more prominently than glomerular function, and is manifest in defective concentrating ability – which accounts for the polyuria sometimes encountered in partial obstruction – and in defective acidification, based on inability to achieve the normal maximal hydrogen ion gradient between plasma and tubular fluid. If the obstruction continues unrelieved, atrophy of renal tissue progresses around the hydronephrotic sac, and excretory function is progressively lost, the rate of loss being increased by any infection of the remaining renal tissue.

Effects similar to those of urinary obstruction can be produced by *vesicoureteric reflux* (which may also be induced by obstruction to outflow from the bladder). Vesicoureteric reflux is most easily demonstrated by voiding cystography after radio-opaque dye has been introduced into the bladder by catheterization. *Transient* reflux occurs during acute infections in children, and also in animals in whom sterile inflammation of the bladder has been induced. It is of little significance. *Persistent* reflux, on the other hand, may be bilateral or unilateral, and if associated with intrarenal reflux of urine into the kidney substance, is followed by scarring of the growing kidney, whether or not associated infection is present, in both children and experimental animals (pigs). Reflux may be present alone, or associated with one of the obstructive conditions mentioned above, or with neurological disorders affecting the bladder, whether leading to a "spastic" or an atonic bladder. Secondary infection is common, but by no means invariable, and may be the event which brings the disordered urinary tract to notice. Diagnosis is particularly important in young children, since the growing kidney is especially susceptible to the combination of infection and reflux, or reflux alone. The natural history of reflux unaccompanied by obstruction in children is one of improvement, and in these circumstances it is usually best to wait, doing serial measurements of renal size (by radiology or, better, scanning) and renal function before considering reimplantation of the ureter into the bladder. If obstruction or a neurogenic bladder is present, however, the treatment will first be aimed at the obstruction, and, in a minority of patients, urinary diversion will have to be performed into a "bladder" constructed of ileum and draining externally.

9.3.9. **Tubular syndromes** (Stanbury et al., 1972; Brodehl and Bickel, 1973)

Numerous examples of altered tubular function have been noted in the accounts of syndromes so far described. This present note concerns a group of disorders in which the tubular dysfunction appears to be primary, although in some of the syndromes there is later progression to glomerular damage. In *proximal tubular syndromes,* there is excretion of excessive amounts of aminoacids, phosphates, or glucose. Renal aminoaciduria has to be distinguished from "overflow aminoaciduria", in which the abnormality lies in excessive production of aminoacids (Frimpter, 1973); the blood concentrations of aminoacids are normal or reduced in renal aminoaciduria, but increased in overflow aminoaciduria. There are at least five separate gene-controlled systems for the reabsorption of aminoacids (Table 9.4), and the number of familial aminoacidurias is considerable (see Chapter 18, section 18.11) (Smart, 1973). They include cystinuria, the de Toni–Debré–Fanconi syndrome, Hartnup disease, glycinuria and glycine-iminoaciduria. Aside from these familial syndromes, aminoaciduria occurs in renal damage from heavy metals,

TABLE 9.4.

GENETICALLY DETERMINED SYSTEMS FOR AMINOACID REABSORPTION IN THE RENAL TUBULE

System	Aminoacids involved	Syndrome of renal aminoaciduria
dibasic	cystine, arginine, ornithine, lysine	cystinuria
dicarboxylic	aspartic and glutamic	none [1]
αI	proline, hydroxyproline, glycine	iminoglycinuria
αII	remaining α-aminoacids (13)	Hartnup disease
β-amino	alanine, aminoiso-butyric acid, taurine	none [1]

[1] No specific defect of the systems has yet been described; in the generalized defect of the Fanconi syndrome (multiple proximal tubular defects) these, along with all the other aminoacids, may be found in the urine.

and in some patients with the nephrotic syndrome. Renal glycosuria can occur as an isolated familial anomaly of good prognosis, or in association with other proximal tubular defects. Abnormal phosphaturia occurs in multiple defects, but also as an isolated familial anomaly which manifests itself as one form of vitamin D-resistant rickets.

Renal tubular acidosis is an uncommon condition, with infantile, adult and occasionally familial forms, and sometimes associated with other tubular defects. It is often complicated by abnormally high excretion of phosphate and of potassium, and by hypercalciuria with stone formation and nephrocalcinosis. Morris (1969) has suggested two forms, different in mechanism – "bicarbonate-wasting renal tubular acidosis" in which defective proximal tubule function leads to flooding of the distal tubule with bicarbonate; and "classical renal tubular acidosis", in which the main defect is inability to establish the normal hydrogen ion gradient across the tubule wall, so that the urine pH is high (5.7 or more), even in the presence of acidosis. Wrong and Davies (1959) clearly distinguish this from the renal acidosis associated with general renal failure, in which ammonia production is reduced. They also identified the syndrome of "incomplete tubular acidosis", in which ammonia production suffices to compensate for the inability to lower the urinary pH to a normal extent, as demonstrable on acid-loading. Generalized renal failure is liable to follow renal tubular acidosis in many cases.

9.3.10. Cystic disease of the kidneys (Gardiner, 1976)

A number of conditions result in cysts which are visible to the naked eye or on careful radiological examination. The origin and nature of these is almost always unknown, but several different conditions can be distinguished. Of these, the *adult form of polycystic kidney* is by far the most important. This is an inherited disorder, probably an autosomal dominant with variable, incomplete penetrance. Occasionally the liver is also cystic. The whole substance of the kidneys is replaced by innumerable cysts of various sizes. The condition usually presents in early adult life with gradual enlargement of the kidneys; hypertension is common. In terms of renal function, tubular impairment is often early and disproportionate, with failure of concentration and acidification, and often a salt-losing polyuria which occasionally may affect potassium as well. The evolution of the disease is slow, but renal failure eventually ensues. *Infantile polycystic kidneys,* in contrast, are rare; they are present at birth or shortly afterwards, and are always associated not only with hepatic cysts but also hepatic fibrosis. The condition is inherited and recessive, with the morphology of the cysts differing from the adult form. Survival is unusual. The third form of cystic disease leading to renal failure is also relatively rare: *nephronophthisis* (uraemic medullary cystic disease). This presents in childhood with polyuria and polydipsia, is familial in the majority of patients, and leads to renal failure in childhood or adolescence. *Medullary sponge kidney,* however, is benign. The cysts are confined to the medulla and frequently communicate with the calyces. Stones form in situ with or without infection. There is often hypercalciuria, for unknown reasons, and prominent failure of acidification amounting to tubular acidosis.

Finally, many *dysplastic kidneys* are cystic in part, along with the elements of primitive tissue such as cartilage that may be present. They are often associated with other anomalies of the renal tract as well as vesicoureteric reflux.

There now follows a group of disorders, listed in Table 9.3, which has renal disease as one possible cause, but which can also be produced in a variety of other ways. Some of these, e.g. electrolyte depletion and oedema, are covered elsewhere (Chapters 3 and 14), so only brief notes are given here on their relationship to renal disease. Hypertension, however, will be treated more fully.

9.3.11. Hypertension (Peart, 1972)

The question is avoided as to whether hypertension is a "disease" or a disadvantageous variant of normality. Criteria of what constitutes hypertension are distinctly arbitrary. The much-used figure of a diastolic pressure of 100 mm Hg is less tenable as evidence increases that life expectancy may be improved by hypotensive treatment of patients whose blood pressure is lower than this value. The increase of "normal" blood pressure with ageing is a further incentive, were any needed, to caution in defining hypertension too rigidly. Looked at more practically, a large number of people in the older age groups are regarded as hypertensive, and a considerable proportion of these show such ill effects as cardiac failure, renal damage, retinopathy and cerebrovascular accidents. In the great majority, no specific cause for their hypertension can be found, and they are labelled as suffering from "essential hypertension". A much smaller, but clinically very important, group is found to have one of the recognized conditions which lead to hypertension. These include vascular disorders (coarctation of the aorta, polyarteritis nodosa), endocrine disorders (Cushing's syndrome, Conn's syndrome, pheochromocytoma) and a variety of renal disorders. Although chemical evidence plays little part in the investigation of the vascular disorders, it is critical in establishing the presence of the foregoing endocrine disorders, through estimation of corticosteroids, aldosterone and catecholamines in blood and urine.

There is a dual relationship between hypertension and the kidneys. On the one hand, severe hypertension leads to vascular damage to the kidneys, and this attains its most florid expression in the rapidly progressive renal failure of accelerated (or malignant) hypertension. On the other hand, interference with the blood supply to the renal glomeruli stimulates the release of renin and leads to hypertension. The Goldblatt experiment, with the appearance of vascular changes in the kidney contralateral to that which had been clipped, was the first clear demonstration of the vicious spiral set up by the summation of these two mechanisms, with the clear practical consequence that therapeutic intervention directed at either of them must be early, if it is to be successful.

Renal hypertension can be due to stenosis of major renal arteries, which is sometimes amenable to surgery. More commonly it is due to multiple vascular lesions within the kidney itself, in the course of a variety of nephropathies, including the common glomerulonephritis and pyelonephritis; the less common diabetic nephropathy and the collagenoses; and the rare scleroderma and irradiation nephritis. In the course of routine study, chemical evidence of a renal cause for the hypertension may be found in the shape of any degree of proteinuria, combined in the case of diabetic nephropathy with glycosuria; of any of the indices of nitrogen retention in the body; or of hypoproteinaemia, which is then found to be due to massive proteinuria. When there is any suspicion that the hypertension may be due to unilateral – and so potentially remediable – renal disease, some help can be obtained from separate assessment of the renal function on the two sides. When one kidney is ischaemic, it produces a smaller volume of urine, with lower sodium concentration, than that produced from its fellow. This can be demonstrated by obtaining urine from each side by catheterization of both ureters. The procedure is exacting but it is important, using creatinine clearance or some comparable index, to assess the functions of both kidneys, and perhaps particularly of the "non-ischaemic" kidney which is at hazard from the hypertension. Its function must be shown to be normal, or at least adequate, if the ischaemic kidney is to be removed, or plastic reconstruction carried out on a stenosed renal artery.

It is, however, possible to identify a hypo-perfused kidney and to evaluate its contribution to overall renal function by using radiological and radioisotope techniques. Since the ischaemic kidney produces much more concentrated urine with respect to most solutes except sodium, the nephrogram seen on IVP is slower to develop, much denser, and persists longer than in the normal kidney. Radioisotope imaging permits computer analysis of the entry into each kidney separately of the radiolabelled chelate used, and hence calculation of differential renal function.

Renin and angiotensin measurements have perhaps contributed less to the detection of renal hypertension than might be expected. In peripheral blood, the concentrations may be normal, and if raised, to no greater extent than in severe hypertension not of renal origin. Detection of a higher concentration of renin in one renal vein is certainly good evidence that the corresponding kidney is ischaemic; but this does not fully prove that it is causing the hypertension, as it might merely reflect a combination of reduced blood flow and normal renin secretion, i.e. a rise in concentration, but not in total amount.

The renin–angiotensin mechanism is not the sole factor in the relationship between primary renal disease and hypertension. Vasodilator substances, possibly kinins, can be extracted from the kidney, and particularly from the medulla. It has often been shown experimentally that total nephrectomy is followed by a rise in blood pressure, and the concept of "renoprival hypertension", possibly related to loss of renal vasodilators, has gained some currency. This concept has certainly not been disproved, but studies in patients with minimal renal function, maintained on dialysis, suggest that the major factor in determining the level of blood pressure is the state of salt balance. These patients have no effective feed-back control of sodium balance by the renin–angiotensin–aldosterone mechanism, and may further be unable to excrete sodium in significant amounts because of grossly diminished glomerular filtration. In these circumstances, a small positive balance of sodium is associated with significant hypertension, which can be corrected by subsequent salt-depletion. A difficult decision can arise when a small functionless pair of kidneys is pouring out pressor material, so that the blood pressure can be controlled only by a degree of salt restriction which implies materially reduced plasma volume. Bilateral nephrectomy in such circumstances may actually improve the quality of life.

9.3.12. Osteodystrophy

This has many causes, of which the commonest, apart from primary bone lesions, is probably gluten-sensitive enteropathy. However, nutritional rickets is still prevalent in

Asian immigrant populations in the North of Britain, for example, because of nutritional habits and the relatively small exposure to sunlight. The cause of osteodystrophy most likely to be confused with renal disease is primary hyperparathyroidism, given that secondary hyperparathyroidism is general in advanced renal disease, and that parathyroid hyperplasia, originally secondary to renal disease, may assume the form of autonomous adenomata, sometimes described as tertiary hyperparathyroidism. The distinction cannot be made solely on the basis of the extent of renal function, since in primary hyperparathyroidism the kidneys are subject to nephrolithiasis, nephrocalcinosis and pyelonephritis; nor can the distinction be made by assay of parathormone or of alkaline phosphatase, since these are increased in both conditions. If primary hyperparathyroidism has not yet led to impaired renal function, the distinction is relatively easy, based on a low plasma phosphate concentration, a high phosphate excretion, and a plasma calcium concentration above the upper limit of the reference range. In primary renal disease, on the other hand, there is typically a raised plasma phosphate concentration, low phosphate excretion, and a low or normal plasma calcium concentration. However, when the renal disease is complicated by osteitis fibrosa, the plasma calcium concentration can rise above normal, and the phosphate concentration is less unequivocally raised. The chemical findings may then come to be similar in primary hyperparathyroidism complicated by renal failure, on the one hand, and on the other in primary renal disease complicated by osteitis fibrosa. When there is such doubt, parathyroidectomy should probably be carried out, with the chance of arrest of renal damage if the parathyroid condition is primary, and with relief of bony symptoms, and easier management of any osteomalacic component, if the renal disease is primary.

9.3.13. Sodium and potassium depletion

The various non-renal causes of these depletions are considered in Chapter 14. Here attention need only be drawn to the important point that normal kidneys will retain both these cations, when they are depleted and their plasma concentrations are low. If, under such circumstances, the urine is found to contain substantial amounts of the cations, abnormal urinary loss is a likely cause of the depletion. This cannot necessarily of course be equated to a primary renal cause without further evidence of renal disease. In the case of sodium, there may be a lack of aldosterone, as in Addison's disease; or a state of sustained osmotic diuresis, as in diabetic pre-coma; or the use of natriuretics may not be disclosed by the followers of weight-reducing regimes. Intrinsic failure of the kidneys to conserve sodium is usually part of general renal disease, and is usually mild in degree, related to the osmotic diuresis which is imposed by a reduced number of functioning nephrons; but it may be severe enough to deserve the term "salt losing nephritis". A few cases have now been described, under the term Bartter's syndrome, in which the primary lesion may be impairment of the active reabsorption of sodium in the proximal tubule; however, the consequent sodium depletion leads to secondary aldosteronism of such degree that the dominant clinical feature is potassium depletion, with hypokalaemia.

In the case of potassium, abnormal urinary losses can likewise occur in the absence of primary renal disease. Excess of aldosterone, the most potent kaliuretic hormone, may be due to primary aldosteronism; but much more commonly to secondary aldosteronism related to depleted plasma volume in states of hypoalbuminaemia, sodium depletion and the abuse of diuretics, which are themselves also kaliuretic. Glucocorticoids have a less pronounced kaliuretic action. Kaliuretic drugs include carbenoxolone, glycyrrhitinic acid, and of course diuretics. Osmotic diuresis entails losses of potassium. Potassium-wasting of primary renal origin occurs in the renal tubular syndromes, in a small proportion of patients with chronic renal failure, and during the recovery phase of acute tubular necrosis. Potassium depletion is itself a cause of renal tubular damage in the form of a vacuolar nephropathy.

9.3.14. Acidosis

The characteristic feature of renal acidosis, as distinct from metabolic and respiratory acidosis, lies in the failure of the kidneys to respond adequately to the systemic acidosis. In circumstances where the urine would be expected to be of high ammonium content, and free of bicarbonate, it may instead be found to have a relatively high pH, a low content of ammonium, and to contain bicarbonate. As already noted, the failure of response is different in generalized renal failure and in the tubular syndromes. When there is marked systemic acidosis, defects in the renal response can be demonstrated simply by obtaining a timed specimen of urine for analysis of pH, titratable acidity and ammonia concentration. However, it may be necessary, particularly in the syndrome of incomplete tubular acidosis, to place the acidifying mechanisms of the kidney under stress, before the nature of the defect can be clearly delineated.

9.3.15. Polyuria

Polyuria due to osmotic diuresis is characterized by the osmolality of the urine being greater than 300 mOsm/litre. However, as the urine volume rises, the excess of osmolality over that of plasma becomes less, until at really high urine volumes it is little if any higher than that of plasma. This situation of isosthenuria (section 9.3.5) is found in most patients with advanced renal failure, and the mechanism of its production may well be similar. A minority of patients with generalized renal disease, especially pyelonephritis, pass large volumes of urine of an osmolality lower than that of plasma. A possible mechanism here is interference with the architecture of the counter-current system of the medulla, which would reach its extreme in patients with necrosis of the papilla. Alternatively, there could be impairment of active sodium reabsorption in the thick part of the ascending limb of Henle's loop. Failure to concentrate the urine adequately is also found in hypercalcaemia, Fanconi's syndrome, potassium depletion, and sickle-cell anaemia. Further, there is a specific syndrome of nephrogenic diabetes insipidus, determined by a recessive sex-linked gene transmitted by female carriers, and finding expression in males. In the absence of clear general evidence of renal disease or other indications of their nature (e.g. the detection of disorders causing hypercalcaemia), these states of renal diabetes insipidus have to be distinguished from true diabetes insipidus and from the syndrome of compulsive water drinking. This is most conveniently done by giving 5 units of vasopressin tannate intramuscularly, which abates the diuresis to some extent both in true diabetes insipidus and in compulsive water drinking, but has little or no affect in nephrogenic diabetes insipidus. Concurrently, search should be made for other evidence of renal disease, and particularly of tubular anomalies (aminoaciduria, glycosuria), or for evidence of hypercalcaemia or hypokalaemia. When positive evidence of this kind can be obtained, it clearly has greater force than the negative evidence of unresponsiveness to Pitressin. If there is no evidence of a renal cause for sustained hypotonic diuresis, a test involving prolonged water deprivation is usually necessary to distinguish between true diabetes insipidus and compulsive water drinking.

9.3.16. Anaemia and oedema

Renal disease is only one of the many causes of anaemia and oedema but their importance lies in their being possible modes of initial presentation and also in the distress which they may cause to the patient at end-stage of renal disease.

The investigation of *anaemia* is primarily haematological, but when the cause of anaemia is obscure, evidence of renal disease is worth seeking. At present, the assay of erythropoietin is biological, using rodents which are made polycythaemic by anoxia or transfusion so that their endogenous production of erythropoietin is minimized. Purification of erythropoietin has not so far been adequate to provide the basis for a radioimmunoassay or other non-biological method. Losses of blood in repeated haemodialyses have been reduced by using dialysers of smaller capacity, by rinsing blood back into the circulation at the end of the procedure, and by lessening the frequency of blood tests. Dialysis patients do, however, have some inevitable blood loss, and need oral iron; but transfusion is to be avoided, in view of the risk of hepatitis and of introducing leucocyte antigens which would prejudice later transplantation. At the other end of the scale, some patients with renal tumours or with hydronephrosis have presented with polycythaemia.

Oedema associated with renal disease arises in several ways, which have already been indicated and need only to be summarized here. In acute nephritis and acute renal failure, salt and water retention is the main cause. In the nephrotic syndrome, salt and water retention is much greater, but is secondary to the hypoproteinaemia and hypovolaemia which lead to secondary aldosteronism. In chronic renal failure, the copious flow of urine tends in itself towards dehydration rather than to oedema; but with the concurrent hypertension, oedema does in fact occur on a basis of cardiac failure. The distinction between different forms of oedema associated with renal disease is largely clinical; but biochemical evidence is important also, in establishing the presence of massive proteinuria and of hypoproteinaemia in the nephrotic syndrome, and of nitrogen retention in chronic renal failure.

9.3.17. Renal function in non-renal disease

Renal function is strongly influenced by extra-renal events, so that changes in renal function may be seen in many states of extra-renal disease. These changes principally relate to alterations in hormone concentrations which affect the kidney, for example aldosterone and other corticosteroids, and antidiuretic hormone; or to alterations in the renal circulation which may involve diversion of blood flow from cortex to medulla in states of low cardiac output and during catecholamine drive, or global renal ischaemia. Thus any cause of a falling cardiac output, of a contraction in effective circulating volume, or of alteration in the state of constriction of the peripheral vascular bed, will influence renal blood flow and hence renal function, usually in the direction of a diminution of glomerular filtration. The renal circulation is also sensitive to circulating vasoactive substances in disease states, for example endotoxins from Gram-negative bacteria and in liver disease.

A few conditions are associated with an increase in glomerular filtration rate. It is worth noting that in acromegaly there is an increase in renal blood flow and glomerular filtration rate, along with the increase in kidney size which is observed radiographically and at post-mortem. An increase in growth hormone has also been evoked to explain the increase in glomerular filtration rate which is seen in the early stages of juvenile-onset diabetes (Ditzel and Junker, 1972).

9.3.18. Drugs and renal function

Renal function, being so dependent upon blood flow, is influenced by many drugs which affect the circulation, and by situations with secondary effects on the circulation. However, some drugs act specifically upon the kidney, the most important being diuretics. Their mode of action is summarized by Lant and Wilson (1972).

9.4. TESTS USED IN THE INVESTIGATION OF RENAL DISEASE

The amount of a substance excreted through the kidneys is the product of the urine volume (V), and the urinary concentration of that substance (U). The quantity UV is of importance in the context of metabolic balance, but by itself it does not define renal performance in respect of that substance. For that purpose, it is also necessary to know the plasma concentration (P). As a convenient way of expressing the renal handling of a substance, the concept of *clearance* was introduced. Clearance (C) is given by the expression UV/P, representing a notional volume of plasma which would be completely "cleared" of the given substance in a defined time period. This is usually expressed as ml/min, but sometimes as litres/24 hours. The power of the clearance concept lies in its applicability to any substance excreted in the urine. The handling of a given substance can be established in health and in disease; comparison may be made with different substances and in some cases, the clearance of a particular substance corresponds to an important parameter of renal function, such as glomerular filtration rate or renal plasma flow.

9.4.1. Excretory (glomerular) function

The glomerular filtration rate (usually abbreviated as GFR) is the most important function of the kidney from a clinical viewpoint, and considerable attention has been given towards measuring it as accurately as possible.

The clearance (C = UV/P) of a substance which is not metabolized either by renal or extra-renal tissues, is freely filterable at the glomerulus, and is neither reabsorbed nor secreted by the renal tubules, would equal the rate of filtration at the glomerulus. Unfortunately, no substance yet described exactly satisfies these conditions, and the major problem in the clinical measurement of the GFR is the interpretation of data using endogenous substances such as creatinine, which fall short of this ideal; or infusing or injecting foreign substances (such as inulin or [^{51}Cr]edetate) which approach it much more exactly. Until recently, this involved infusions over several hours and catheterization for accurate urine collections, but recently interest has been attracted once again to the practical advantages of single injection methods without urine collection, despite their theoretical problems.

9.4.1.1. The inulin clearance as a measure of GFR

The clearance of inulin (or inulin-like polyfructosans) using continuous intravenous infusion, together with bladder catheterization to ensure accurate urine collections, has for long been the reference method for the measurement of the GFR (Shannon and Smith, 1935; Smith, 1951). Although rigorously and very extensively validated in *normal* man (and many other species) it is often forgotten that it is still uncertain whether the inulin clearance corresponds exactly to the GFR in *diseased* kidneys. It must be assumed that inulin can penetrate the diseased glomeruli equally with water as in health; and that the diseased tubule, like the normal tubule, does not handle inulin. In infants, it is known that the relatively impermeable neonatal glomerular filter excludes to some extent polymers with molecules which are only a little larger than inulin (Arturson et al., 1971). Another factor often forgotten is that to ensure accurate urine collections, a water or osmotic diuresis is usually induced; in some species, including man (Smith, 1951), this leads to a rise in the GFR. Finally, the subject with an indwelling catheter and intravenous infusion in place is necessarily at rest, and most investigators attempt to standardize the conditions while they measure an average GFR over several hours. These conditions probably give a false impression of the constancy of the GFR from minute to minute, and under conditions of exercise or excitement.

Inulin, prepared from dahlia tubers, is a polymer of fructose with a molecular weight of about 5000. Commercial preparations inevitably contain some free fructose, which may be increased by the heating necessary to obtain a solution of 100 g/litre. Since the method of inulin estimation depends upon the measurement of free fructose following acid hydrolysis, the plasma and urine "blanks" are of particular importance. Now, automated methods for the measurement of inulin are available (Dawborn, 1965; Rose, 1969; Wilson et al., 1969), with coefficients of variation as low as 1% (Rose and Durbin, 1967). Davies and Shock (1950), using a manual method for inulin estimation, suggested that half of their coefficient of variation of 8% in replicate determinations of inulin clearance was due to the errors in measuring the inulin concentrations. Nowadays, the coefficient of variation in inulin clearances is probably about 5% using automated methods. This would suggest that two clearances differing by 14% have a 95% chance of representing a real difference in GFR.

In attempts to eliminate the need for accurate urine collections, and hence catheterization, both single injection (Robson et al., 1949) and infusion equilibrium (Rose, 1969; Cole et al., 1972) methods have been explored. The single injection technique is discussed below (section 9.4.1.5). That described by Rose (1969) involves an accurately determined infusion of inulin lasting several hours. After equilibrium has been reached, and thorough mixing of inulin throughout the extracellular fluid has taken place, then

$$C_{in} = \frac{I_{in} \cdot V}{P_{in}}$$

where C_{in} = clearance of inulin
V = rate of infusion
I_{in} = inulin concentration in infusion liquid
P_{in} = inulin concentration in plasma

All that is required, therefore, is a knowledge of the rate of infusion and the inulin concentration in the infusion liquid, and a single determination of inulin concentration in a specimen of blood plasma. The disadvantage is that a very accurate – and therefore expensive – infusion pump must be used, and the infusion must be maintained for 4 hours or more. Moreover, in oedematous subjects or those with renal failure, the time required to reach equilibrium may be different from normal, and is not known unless repeated samples are taken.

Reference ranges (95% confidence limits) for the GFR given by Smith et al. (1943) and Smith (1951) are 88 to 174 ml/min for males, and 87 to 147 ml/min for females, corrected to 1.73 m^2 surface area. However, the effect of age is important (Table 9.5), since up to the age of 2 years the GFR rises steadily (even when corrected for surface area); moreover, from the age of 40 years, the GFR steadily falls. These data are not surprising in view of the anatomical changes described by Darmady et al. (1973). Watkin and Shock (1955) related C_{in} to age as follows: $C_{in} = 157 - 1.16 \times$ age in years.

TABLE 9.5.

GLOMERULAR FILTRATION RATES MEASURED AS INULIN CLEARANCE AT VARIOUS AGES

Data for children are as collected by Barratt and Chantler (1975). Data for adults derived from the collected data of Wesson (1969).

Age	GFR (C_{inulin}, ml/min per 1.73 m^2 of surface area)			
	Mean		Range ± 2 S.D.	
newborn	38		26– 60	
3 months	58		30– 86	
6 months	77		41–103	
1 year	103		49–157	
2–12 years	127		89–165	
12–30 years	131 (male)	117 (female)	88–174 (male)	87–147 (female)
20–29	132	119	90–174	84–156
30–39	128	116	88–168	82–150
40–49	120	114	78–162	82–146
50–59	110	104	68–152	66–142
60–69	97	94	57–137	58–130
70–79	82	83	42–122	45–121
80–89	67	–	39–105	–

9.4.1.2. Creatinine clearance

Ever since the suggestion of Popper and Mandel (1937) that the clearance of endogenous creatinine approximates to the GFR, this test has been popular in clinical medicine in one form or another. However its performance and interpretation present formidable difficulties which centre round three problems:

(a) the accurate measurement of creatinine, particularly in plasma;

(b) the handling of creatinine by the renal tubule;

(c) the difficulty of obtaining complete urine collections.

These important problems will be examined in turn.

(a) *The measurement of plasma creatinine* – Plasma creatinine concentrations vary little throughout the day (Sirota et al., 1950) but are slightly raised in the afternoon; they have the principal advantage of being almost independent of protein intake (Addis et al., 1951).

Creatinine is usually measured by the Jaffé reaction with alkaline picrate (Bonsnes and Taussky, 1945; Husdan and Rapaport, 1968). Unfortunately other chromogens which react to give an identical colour are present in plasma but not in urine; overestimation takes place, so that the calculated creatinine clearance is therefore underestimated. This is particularly important at normal concentrations, and above all in paediatrics.

Cook (1975) reviewed the factors which influence the assay of creatinine by different methods, and concluded that chemical alternatives to the Jaffé reaction are not more convenient or specific than the reaction itself; enzyme methods are in principle available, but the present high cost and limited availability of specific enzymes prevent their widespread use. The Jaffé reaction, therefore, is still the most practicable method for the estimation of plasma creatinine.

With manual Jaffé methods, the attempted removal of interfering chromogens by adsorption methods has the disadvantage of being time consuming and of requiring relatively large plasma volumes.

Reaction rate methods give promise of greater accuracy provided that the reaction conditions and measurement period are carefully selected. If dilution is used as a means of reducing the influence of interfering substances, there is a marked fall in the sensitivity of the methods, and this restricts the range of suitable measuring equipment.

AutoAnalyzer methods are more precise than manual methods, and this may be due to the more uniform quality of reagents as well as to the reproducibility of the timing sequence for performing the Jaffé reaction. However, the failure to eliminate interfering substances means that the standard AutoAnalyzer methods are inaccurate. Whilst obtaining values which are less than those for "total" chromogens, measurements with this technique are usually 0 to 0.2 mg/dl higher than "true" creatinine.

(b) *Renal handling of creatinine* – Varying degrees of secretion are shown in the renal handling of creatinine by different species, and the kidneys of many do not appear to transport it in either direction. In the adult rat or dog there is even a difference between the sexes, but this is not true of humans (Harvey et al., 1966). In man, infused creatinine is secreted by the renal tubule (Shannon, 1935) but it is by no means established that secretion also occurs at endogenous concentrations in health although many studies have been carried out both in health and in renal disease. Usually, the creatinine clearance equals or exceeds the GFR as measured by inulin clearance by a factor of 1.1 to 1.2, at clearances above 80 to 90 ml/min (Doolan et al., 1962; Goldman et al., 1967; Healy, 1968; Kim et al., 1969). In children, creatinine clearances showed a ratio of 0.98:1 in relation to inulin clearance at GFRs above 100 ml/min, and 1.1:1 at figures less than this (Arrant et al., 1971). The ratio, however, is regularly increased as the GFR falls, to as much as 2.0 (Miller et al., 1952; Mandel et al., 1953; Doolan et al., 1962; Schirmeister et al., 1964; Dodge et al., 1967; Healy, 1968; Lavender et al., 1969), although not all authors have found this to be the case (Bennett and Porter, 1971) for reasons which are unclear. A further area of controversy is the effect of proteinuria on the creatinine clearance. Brod and Sirota (1948) showed that in the presence of profuse proteinuria, the creatinine clearance could be double the inulin clearance, but equality could be achieved if carinamide (a blocking agent for the proximal tubule) was given. Although Berlyne et al. (1965) confirmed this, several other authors have found no relation between proteinuria and creatinine clearance (Tobias et al., 1962; Breckenridge and Metcalfe-Gibson, 1965; Rapaport and Husdan, 1968; Hilton et al., 1969; Cameron et al., 1970). Rosenbaum (1970) noted no difference with proteinuria, but the presence of a full nephrotic syndrome, including oedema, was associated with higher creatinine/inulin clearance ratios. It must be remembered that an acute water diuresis may increase the clearance temporarily, probably by "washing-out" all or part of the medullary pool of creatinine (Porter et al., 1966).

(c) *Accurate urine collections* – Because creatinine clearances are usually measured in ambulant in-patients or outpatients, the problem of achieving complete collections of urine is crucial. The exact period is immaterial providing the criteria for a good collection are adhered to. The difficulties are well known: patients "lose" specimens of urine and may forget or be afraid to report this. The start and finish of the collection may not be noted precisely, and the bladder not emptied at the beginning and end of the study.

Some check on completeness of collection can be made by measuring the total creatinine output in the specimen (Wibell and Bjørsell-Östling, 1973); overnight urines may be used in children. However, some patients, such as those with urinary tract anomalies and vesicoureteric reflux of urine, or those with prostatic obstruction, cannot provide accurate collections however careful they may be. The value of testing the completeness of urine collections by creatinine excretion depends upon the assumption that the excretion of creatinine is relatively constant in an individual from day to day, and is related simply to body weight. The data of Kampmann et al. (1974) show clearly that the change in body composition with age is an important factor: a fit muscular 25-year-old person weighing 60 kg may excrete more than twice as much creatinine as an obese 60-year-old with the same body weight. Creatinine excretion is not as constant from day to day as has been assumed since the original work of Folin (Scott and Hurley, 1968; Edwards et al., 1969). The coefficient of variation in creatinine excretion in a single individual is never less than 6%, and may exceed 20%. In some studies of nitrogen excretion, including Folin's original work, the variance in the excretion of urea is *less* than that of creatinine. It is usual to correct creatinine clearances by surface area, but Masarei (1975) has shown that in adults, correction by body weight reduces variance by a similar amount.

Consecutive 24-hour collections may increase the accuracy (Wibell and Bjørsell-Östling, 1973) and give some indication as to how good a patient may be at collecting specimens. Chantler and Barratt (1972) found that in well motivated adults, the coefficient of variation in replicate estimations in a single individual was 11%. This implies that two estimates of creatinine clearance must differ by 31% if there is to be a 95% chance that a real change in GFR has taken place.

Despite its many problems and disadvantages, the creatinine clearance is the most widely used test for estimating the GFR in clinical practice. Table 9.6 gives reference intervals from the literature for children and adults. It is necessary to consider these values in relation to the class of analytical method since each will give different results.

TABLE 9.6.

CREATININE CLEARANCES MEASURED AT DIFFERENT AGES IN NORMAL INDIVIDUALS

Author(s)	Age of subjects	Creatinine clearance ml/min per 1.73 m² surface area				Period	Method of estimation[1]
	yr	mean	male range ± 2 S.D.	mean	female range ± 2 S.D.		
Barratt and Chantler (1975)	3–13		113		94–142		true
Roscoe (1958)	adults	108	83–142	75	47– 96	?	true
van Pilsum and Seljeskog (1958)	adults	135	107–163	127	91–153	1–24 h	true
Edwards and Whyte (1959)	adults	108	76–140	204	86–132	4 h	true
Doolan et al. (1962)	adults 20–59	123	84–162	114	84–146	24 h	true
Sirota et al. (1950)	adults	106	76–146	–	–	24 h	total
Hopper (1951)	adults	105	72–141	95	74–130	12 h	total
Camara et al. (1951)	adults	95	81–108	95	79–110	12 h	total
Roscoe (1958)	adults	80	64–101	55	40–64	?	total
Doolan et al. (1962)	adults	103	71–135	97	77–117	24 h	total
Tobias et al. (1962)	adults	105	77–133	95	59–131	24 h	total
Wibell et al. (1973)	17–36	117	49–185	114	74–154	2 × 24 h	AutoAn.
	37–56	111	59–163	104	74–134	2 × 24 h	AutoAn.
	57–76	94	58–130	94	38–150	2 × 24 h	AutoAn.
Kampmann et al. (1974)	patients [1]						
	20–29	110	64–156	95	57–133	24 h	AutoAn.
	30–39	97	19–175	103	53–153	24 h	AutoAn.
	40–49	88	44–132	81	29–133	24 h	AutoAn.
	50–59	81	39–123	74	26–122	24 h	AutoAn.
	60–69	72	28–116	63	33– 93	24 h	AutoAn.
	70–79	64	34– 94	54	30– 78	24 h	AutoAn.
	80–89	47	17– 77	46	18– 74	24 h	AutoAn.
	90–99	34	16– 52	39	23– 55	24 h	AutoAn.

[1] "without known renal disease"

[1] true = plasma creatinine absorbed and eluted from Fuller's earth or resin; total = total Jaffé-positive chromogens measured without adsorption; AutoAn. = dialysable Jaffé-positive chromogens measured in AutoAnalyzer.

The profound effect of age upon creatinine clearance – greater than that on the GFR because of the fall in creatinine excretion with age (see below) – is often forgotten.

9.4.1.3. Plasma creatinine concentration as an indicator of GFR

Because it is difficult to make accurately timed urine collections, the possibility of predicting the GFR from measurements of the plasma creatinine concentration alone has been explored. Creatinine excretion is only relatively constant for each individual, as indicated, and it varies with muscle mass. Hence if, as before (section 9.4.1.1) –

$$C_{cr} = \frac{U_{cr} \cdot V}{P_{cr}} \text{ and } U_{cr}\, V = k, \text{ then}$$

$$C_{cr} \propto \frac{1}{P_{cr}}$$

The measurement of "true" plasma creatinine concentration has a coefficient of variation for replicates on specimens from the same patient of 6% (Winberg, 1959; Doolan et al., 1962). Thus, a change of 17% in successive samples has a 95% chance of representing a real change in GFR. However, the precision of this measurement will vary from method to method and between laboratories. For example, Wibell and Bjørsell-Östling (1973) mention a coefficient of variation as low as 2%. In view of the importance of this measurement, it is essential to assess what degree of accuracy is available locally.

In children, complete urine collections are particularly difficult to obtain, and muscle mass can be predicted with some accuracy from height and weight (Graystone, 1968). Relevant data from several sources are summarized in Table 9.7. In adults, the position is somewhat different; urine collections are easier to obtain, but several problems are evident, as already discussed. Firstly, the variation in excretion of creatinine; secondly, as the GFR falls, it is exceeded by the creatinine clearance by an increasing amount, possibly because relatively more creatinine is secreted at higher plasma creatinine concentrations. Although both the creatinine clearance (Wibell and Bjørsell-Östling, 1973) and the GFR (Wesson, 1969) fall steadily with increasing age during adult life, the plasma creatinine concentration does not show a corresponding rise (Josephson, 1963; Dubach et al., 1967; Siersback-Nielson et al., 1971; Kampmann et al., 1974). This presumably results from the fact that, as age increases, muscle mass represents less and less of body mass. Table 9.8 demonstrates that, as age increases, creatinine excretion decreases and plasma creatinine concentration remains substantially constant while creatinine clearance falls. Finally, the rise in plasma concentration with decreasing GFR has been recognized to fall short of that predicted from a constant creatinine production, even allowing for the somewhat enhanced creatinine secretion at high plasma creatinine concentrations (Doolan et al., 1962; Enger and Blegen, 1964). It is possible in fact that creatinine production decreases in uraemia (Goldman and Moss, 1959). However, careful studies using [^{14}C-methyl]creatinine (Jones and Burnett, 1974) in man have shown that creatinine, like urea and uric acid (section 9.4.1.6) is excreted in increasing amounts into the gut in uraemia, where it is broken down by gut bacteria, which are selectively favoured. The creatinine "deficit" of extra-renal excretion varied from 16 to 66% in the five patients studied by

TABLE 9.7.

PLASMA CREATININE CONCENTRATION AT VARIOUS AGES DURING CHILDHOOD

Data collected by Barratt and Chantler (1975) and Chantler (personal communication). Adult data from Doolan et al. (1962) and Edwards and Whyte (1959)

Age	Surface area (m^2)	Height (cm)	"True" plasma creatinine (μmol/litre)		AutoAnalyzer plasma creatinine (μmol/litre)	
			Mean	Range ± 2 S.D.	Mean	Range ± 2 S.D.
Cord blood	–	–	66.3	45.1– 87.5	78.7	57.5– 99.9
0–2 weeks	0.21	50	44.2	30.1– 58.4	56.6	42.4– 70.7
2 weeks–26 weeks	0.28–0.36	60	34.5	20.3– 48.6	46.8	32.7– 61.0
26 weeks–1 year	0.36–0.50	70	28.3	15.9– 40.7	40.7	28.3– 53.0
2 years	0.50–0.60	87	28.3	17.7– 38.9	40.7	30.1– 51.3
4 years	0.60–0.75	101	32.7	22.1– 43.3	45.1	34.5– 55.7
6 years	0.75–0.87	114	30.0	23.9– 52.2	50.4	36.2– 64.5
8 years	0.87–1.00	126	42.4	27.4– 57.5	54.8	39.8– 69.8
10 years	1.00–1.17	137	46.0	30.1– 61.9	58.3	42.4– 74.2
12 years	1.17–1.56	147	52.2	36.2– 69.0	64.5	48.6– 81.3
Adult Male	1.76	174	85.7	63.6–107.8	98.1	76.0–120.2
Adult Female	1.56	163	68.1	46.8– 89.3	80.4	59.2–101.7

TABLE 9.8.

PLASMA CREATININE AND CREATININE EXCRETION IN ADULTS AT DIFFERENT AGES

	Age in years	No.	Serum creatinine mg/dl ± S.D.	Urinary creatinine mg/kg/24 h ± S.D.	C_{creat} ml/1.73 m^2 surface area
Males	20–29	12	0.99 ± 0.16	23.8 ± 2.3	110
	30–39	16	1.14 ± 0.22	21.9 ± 1.5	97
	40–49	32	1.10 ± 0.20	19.7 ± 3.2	88
	50–59	37	1.16 ± 0.17	19.3 ± 2.9	81
	60–69	23	1.15 ± 0.14	16.9 ± 2.9	72
	70–79	18	1.03 ± 0.22	14.2 ± 3.0	64
	80–89	12	1.06 ± 0.25	11.7 ± 4.0	47
	90–99	5	1.20 ± 0.16	9.4 ± 3.2	34
	AutoAnalyzer creatinine estimations, data of Siersback-Nielsen et al. (1971); Kampmann et al. (1974).				
Females	20–29	32	0.89 ± 0.17	19.7 ± 3.9	95
	30–39	14	0.91 ± 0.17	20.4 ± 3.9	103
	40–49	48	1.00 ± 0.24	17.6 ± 3.9	81
	50–59	34	0.99 ± 0.26	14.9 ± 3.6	74
	60–69	23	0.97 ± 0.17	12.9 ± 2.6	63
	70–79	27	1.02 ± 0.23	11.8 ± 2.2	54
	80–89	32	1.05 ± 0.22	10.7 ± 2.5	46
	90–99	9	0.91 ± 0.12	8.4 ± 1.4	39

Jones and Burnett (1974). Simple diagrams relating plasma creatinine to expected GFR, and calculated on the basis of constant creatinine production with age, and equivalence of creatinine and inulin clearance in uraemia, can be found in many reviews of renal function testing. These are of little value, and give a false sense of precision, especially at higher creatinine concentrations.

In summary, the repeated measurement of the plasma creatinine concentration is a useful and simple test of renal function for clinical practice, especially when the GFR is reduced. However, it must be remembered that the GFR may halve without a detectable change in plasma creatinine concentration, and that in both the young and the very old apparently "normal" plasma concentrations may conceal gross renal dysfunction. Siersback-Nielsen et al. (1971) and Kampmann et al. (1974) have published a nomogram (Figure 9.1) which, allowing for age (from 25 to 95 years), enables the creatinine clearance to be estimated from the plasma creatinine up to a concentration of 5 mg/dl: Rowe et al. (1976b) suggest a nomogram which incorporates the change in creatinine clearance with age, presenting the result as a percentile for age. Alternatively, the formula suggested

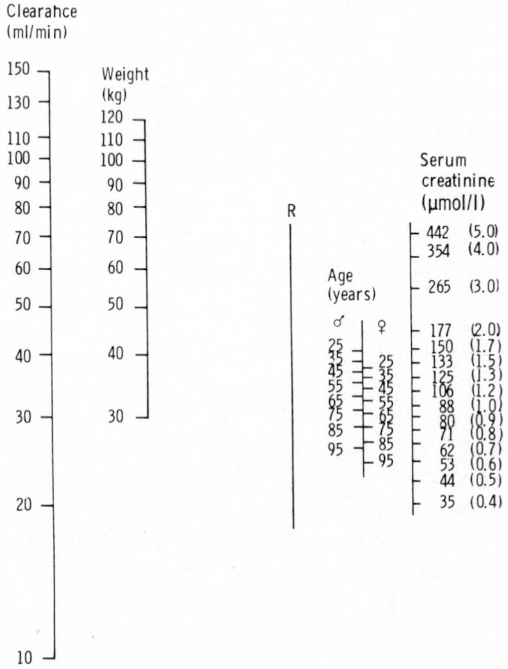

Figure 9.1. Nomogram relating serum creatinine and creatinine clearance, allowing for patient age and body weight. Since allowance is included for body weight, the nomogram is applicable to both adult men and women. With a ruler, connect the patient's age and the patient's weight; note the point at which this line intersects the line R, and keep the ruler on it. Move the right-hand part of the ruler to the point on the scale of serum creatinine measurements corresponding to the observed value. Read off the patient's creatinine clearance from the point where the ruler cuts the scale on the left. (Reproduced, with permission, from Kampmann et al., 1974)

by Cockroft and Gault (1976) may be used –

$$C_{cr} = \frac{(140 - \text{age}\,\{\text{yr}\}) \times \text{wt (kg)}}{72 \times P_{cr}\,(\text{mg/dl})}$$

where P_{cr} is the plasma creatinine concentration as measured by AutoAnalyzer

Edwards and Whyte (1959) correlated the glomerular filtration rate, measured as inulin clearance (in ml/min), with the plasma creatinine concentration and obtained the following regressions –

$$\text{for males: GFR} = \frac{94}{P_{cr}(\text{mg/dl})} - 1.8 \text{ (``true'' creatinine)}$$

$$\text{for females: GFR} = \frac{70}{P_{cr}(\text{mg/dl})} + 2.2 \text{ (``true'' creatinine)}$$

In children, Barratt and Chantler (1975) show that plasma creatinine concentration is directly related to height (which is more reliable than weight in disease) as follows –

$$P_{cr}(\mu\text{mol/litre}) = \text{ht(cm)} \times 0.331 \text{ (``true'' creatinine)}$$

$$P_{cr}(\mu\text{mol/litre}) = \text{ht(cm)} \times 0.331 + 12.4 \text{ (AutoAnalyzer creatinine)}$$

Thus the GFR (in ml/min per 1.73 m^2 of surface area) may be predicted –

$$\text{GFR} = 52.5 \times \frac{\text{ht(cm)}}{P_{cr}(\mu\text{mol/litre})} \text{ (``AutoAnalyzer'' creatinine)}$$

9.4.1.4. Plasma urea concentration as an indicator of GFR

Urea, next to water, is the most diffusible metabolite; hence, unlike creatinine, the concentration in intracellular water is the same as in plasma water. Furthermore, it is well known that, as part of the nitrogen retention of uraemia, the concentration of urea in the blood rises, and it is therefore an indicator of GFR, as is the urea clearance. The actual value of the plasma urea concentration is of interest in its own right, since above 150 or 200 mg/dl symptoms (mainly gastrointestinal) appear, and knowledge of the concentration is of importance to dietary management. The reasons for this are worth summarizing briefly (Kassirer, 1971a; Relman and Levinsky, 1971).

(a) Urea clearance and the plasma urea concentration are very dependent upon the urine flow rate, since urea is reabsorbed in the tubules to a variable extent which depends on flow rate, being greater in states of low urine flow rate, and less in diuresis. Moreover, at the onset of diuresis the medullary pool of urea which is trapped at concentrations above that of the plasma, by the counter-current system, is "washed" out so that the urea clearance temporarily rises. The concentration of urea in plasma thus increases more in states of dehydration and poor urine output than that of creatinine, and the urine passed under these circumstances may have a high urea concentration.

(b) The plasma urea concentration is markedly raised by increase in exogenous protein intake, or in endogenous protein catabolism from starvation, infection, fever or corticosteroid administration.

(c) In nitrogen retention from renal failure, a variable and increasing amount of urea is excreted via the gut (Walser and Bodenlos, 1959).

(d) The urea concentration in the blood does not rise detectably until the GFR is reduced to perhaps 30% of normal.

The plasma urea concentration, therefore, gives more information on the nitrogen intake and fluid balance of the patient than the exact value of GFR. This information – especially when compared to similar data for creatinine (Dossetor, 1966) – may be very useful, for example: in babies fed an excess of nitrogen with insufficient water from cow's milk (Davies and Saunders, 1973); in states of acute, reversible "renal failure" from dehydration, saline depletion or blood loss; and in assessing the effects of diet in patients with renal disease. In this context it is worth noting that the metabolism of each gram of protein leads to the excretion of 0.3 grams of urea.

9.4.1.5. Single injection methods of determining GFR

Although much of the work in this area is at present done by isotope techniques in departments of nuclear medicine, the same principles have been applied, for example, to inulin. Some knowledge of "single shot" clearance is an advantage, since comparisons may be made or asked for between single injection methods and conventional clearances.

Following the intravenous injection of a bolus of a non-metabolized substance such as inulin, it should be possible to derive the GFR from some function of the disappearance curve of the substance in the plasma. This was investigated by Homer Smith (see Smith, 1951) and others (Robson et al., 1949), but the theoretical difficulties led to this approach being abandoned. The introduction of easily assayed radioactive tracer molecules for injection reawakened interest, and after a false start using vitamin B_{12} labelled with ^{57}Co (which proved quite unsatisfactory), the method now seems to have an assured future using compounds such as [^{51}Cr]edetate, [^{125}I]iothalamate and [^{99m}Tc]DPTA.

None of these compounds is ideal; there is considerable tubular secretion of [^{125}I]-sodium diatrizoate (Donaldson, 1968) which led to its virtual abandonment in favour of [^{125}I]iothalamate (Sigman et al., 1966). However, the binding of the iodine is not completely firm in this compound and also it may be secreted in bile. [^{51}Cr]Edetate is reabsorbed in the renal tubule to a certain extent (Favré and Wing, 1968; Chantler, 1971). Again, the stability of the chelates in vivo, although clearly good, is still in question, and their protein binding has not been studied in the detail required.

Despite these objections, there is no doubt that the use of these compounds provides reproducible results which are clinically helpful. The compound most used has been [^{51}Cr]edetate (Stacey and Thorburn, 1966; Favré and Wing, 1968; Heath et al., 1968; Chantler et al., 1969; Chantler, 1971; Chantler and Barratt, 1972; Ditzel et al., 1972; Hagstam et al., 1974), although iothalamate has also been popular (Sigman et al., 1966; Cohen et al., 1969; Harries et al., 1972). Single injection inulin clearances have also been re-examined (Harries et al., 1972).

The material is injected intravenously and it is important to know the exact amount given (which is usually estimated by weighing the syringe before and after injection). Also that all of it has entered the vein; this may be assured by setting up an infusion for a few minutes and injecting into the fluid stream, but this complicates the technique for out-patient use and increases the cost considerably. Following injection, the plasma is sampled from the opposite arm and the concentration plotted against time. Accurate timing of the samples is most important. After 90 to 120 minutes in non-oedematous individuals, the fall-off can be described by a single exponential, and samples may be taken after this time to perform the measurement of the GFR. The number of samples required can be quite small, equally accurate results having been obtained with from two to twelve (Chantler et al., 1969; Chantler, 1971; Ditzel et al., 1972). To obtain the best results, it may be necessary to vary the sampling times in patients with severe renal functional impairment (Maisey et al., 1969). Radioactivity is plotted against time on semi-logarithmic paper, and the slope of the fall-off in counts is extrapolated back to zero time to give a notional volume of distribution at time zero (V_0). The GFR is then derived from –

$$GFR = V_0 \cdot \frac{\log_e 2}{t(1/2)}$$

where: V_0 = notional volume at zero time by extrapolation and t(1/2) = half-time for the fall-off in radioactivity.

This simple monoexponential analysis has inherent disadvantages, although in practice the "clearance" which is obtained is highly reproducible. The calculated result must be multiplied by 0.87 to correct for (a) 22% overestimate of V_0 which arises from over-simplifying in the monoexponential approach; (b) 5% discrepancy from inulin and [^{51}Cr]edetate clearances due to tubular reabsorption of the chelate; and (c) 7% higher concentration of chelate in venous blood compared to arterial (venous blood is used in clinical practice rather than the theoretically necessary arterial blood).

To avoid these corrections, other authors have employed a double exponential analysis, taking samples during the initial equilibrium period (Chantler, 1971; Ditzel et al., 1972; Silkalns et al., 1973) or basing calculations on the area under the whole curve (Harries et al., 1972; Hagstam et al., 1974). Both of these methods have theoretical advantages, but have practical disadvantages in that they require more samples – usually five or six – to obtain a satisfactory analysis.

The simple estimate of GFR using a monoexponential analysis gives confidence limits of ±11% for a 95% possibility that a change in [^{51}Cr]edetate clearance represents a real difference in GFR (Chantler and Barratt, 1972); it is thus more reproducible than even the infusion inulin clearance, and much superior to the creatinine clearance (section 9.4.1.2). Fisher and Veall (1975) have described the use of a single blood sample to determine the GFR, but this is not valid in oedematous patients.

9.4.1.6. Retention of other nitrogen-containing compounds in uraemia

Urea and creatinine are relatively non-toxic compounds, and the body tolerates 30- to 40-fold increases in concentration in uraemia, sometimes with surprising maintenance of health. The patient may have anaemia, itching, nausea, weight loss and bone disease, etc., but it is now apparent that no single compound is responsible for the many complex disorders that arise. Attention has, however, been directed to other nitrogen-containing compounds to see if they possess notable toxicity, even if their molar contribution to the nitrogen retention of uraemia may be slight. At present none of these compounds need be measured for clinical purposes, but it is possible that the assay of such compounds as methylguanidine and guanidinosuccinate (Cohen et al., 1968; Giovannetti et al., 1973) will prove sufficiently important to merit transfer from the research to the service laboratory in the next few years.

Uric acid is however the one other nitrogen-containing compound which deserves attention at present. The renal aspects of its metabolism have been reviewed by Hatfield and Simmonds (1974) and Cameron and Simmonds (1976). More general aspects of uric acid metabolism are dealt with elsewhere (Chapter 21). The excretion of urate is com-

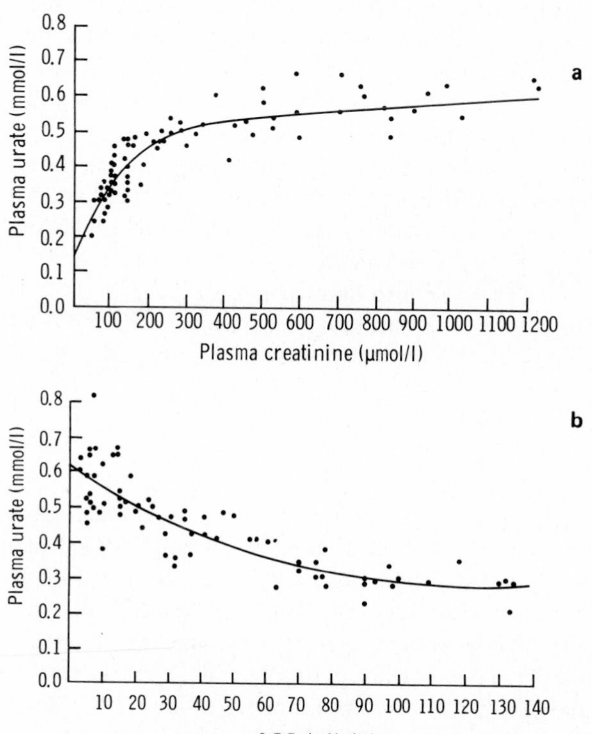

Figure 9.2. a: relationship between plasma creatinine and urate in non-gouty patients with renal failure. As renal function declines, plasma urate rises in step with plasma creatinine until creatinine levels of 3 mg/dl are reached. Thereafter decreasing renal function results in only a small increase in plasma urate. Above plasma urate levels of 0.5 mmol/litre (8 mg/dl) increased normal tubular secretion and extra-renal elimination of uric acid limit the rise in plasma levels. The computer-drawn curve has a correlation of 0.80. (Redrawn, with permission, from Hatfield and Simmonds, 1975) b: relationship between GFR and plasma urate in non-gouty patients with renal disease. With declining renal function, plasma urate levels remain essentially unchanged until the GRF is below 60 ml/min. Even when the GFR is less than 10 ml/min plasma urate levels seldom rise above 0.65 mmol/litre (11 mg/dl). The computer-drawn curve has a correlation coefficient of 0.82. (Redrawn, with permission, from Hatfield and Simmonds, 1975)

plex, since in blood it is protein bound to some extent, it is filtered at the glomerulus, and it is subject to bidirectional transport in the renal tubules. There are important species differences in its renal handling, and only in man and the higher apes (and in the Dalmatian coach hound) does the absence of uricase lead to the end-product of purine metabolism being uric acid, rather than the much more soluble allantoin. The striking feature of urate retention in uraemia is its very limited extent (Figure 9.2). The uric acid concentration increases only 2-, or at most 3-fold in uraemia, in contrast to the large increases in creatinine and urea concentrations already mentioned. The synthesis of urate does not appear to decrease in uraemia but its retention is limited by two processes: its renal tubular secretion increases considerably (Danovitch et al., 1972), and extra-renal elimination of urate becomes the predominant route of excretion. Normally, only about 8% of the filtered urate is excreted in the urine, there being considerable net tubular reabsorption; this diminishes in uraemia in response to unknown stimuli, together with a considerable increase in secretion, so that up to 85% of the filtered urate may be excreted in patients with very low GFRs. Sørensen (1960) showed that the gastrointestinal tract normally excretes one-third of the urate, and that this proportion increases in uraemia.

The data in Figure 9.2 suggest an answer to the vexed question which is often posed: does this patient have simple urate retention from loss of renal tissue, or does he have primary gout with renal failure from gouty nephropathy? At all levels of renal function, patients previously diagnosed as having gout show higher concentrations of uric acid, unless they have received drugs such as allopurinol to limit their uric acid production. It is not yet known whether the raised urate concentrations in uraemia accelerate renal damage from other glomerular or intestinal diseases but it does seem possible (Verger et al., 1967).

9.4.2. Tests of tubular function

Since the tasks achieved by the tubules are so varied, measurement of a single function, as with glomerular filtration, is not attempted. For convenience, tests can be divided into those of "mainly proximal" or "mainly distal" tubular function, but this is an oversimplification: tests of concentrating function depend upon the ability of the whole nephron and the vasa recta to establish the medullary concentration of solute upon which urinary concentration depends, as well as upon the rate of delivery of solute to the distal nephron from the proximal nephron, i.e. upon proximal reabsorption or rejection of solute. Similarly, tests of acidification depend not only upon an ability to establish a hydrogen ion gradient between the tubular lumen and the blood in the distal tubule and collecting duct, but also upon the reabsorption of filtered bicarbonate in the proximal tubule.

9.4.2.1. Tests of mainly proximal tubular function

Because of the diversity of proximal tubular function, there is no single test which gives an overall assessment. Since the proximal tubules reabsorb (in addition to a large volume of water and electrolytes) the bulk of the filtered urate, phosphate, and aminoacids, and almost all the glucose, severe generalized proximal tubular dysfunction or a specific inherited or acquired transport defect leads to excessive excretion of some or all of these compounds, together with relatively low concentrations in the plasma. That is, the clearances, both in absolute terms and in relation to the amount of filtered water (the GFR), rise above normal values.

9.4.2.1.1. The tubular reabsorption of *glucose* can be measured by infusing successively greater amounts of glucose, while measuring the plasma concentrations and urinary excretion of glucose, and the GFR; the tubular maximum reabsorptive capacity (T_m glucose) for glucose will be reached and exceeded, and glucose appears in the urine. This measurement of the T_m for glucose can be made with some accuracy and the shape of the titration curve of plasma concentration multiplied by GFR (i.e. filtered glucose) against excreted glucose may be of importance, especially in the inherited glycosurias mentioned below. It is not a technique that can be applied to routine testing of renal function in clinical situations but, nevertheless, a crude index can be obtained by simply testing for glycosuria, which is present in most situations of multiple proximal tubular dysfunction, and determining the *blood* glucose concentration (the "threshold") at which glycosuria occurs. Anyone showing glycosuria with a blood concentration below 130 mg/dl must have some defect in the proximal tubular reabsorption of glucose. Most commonly this is a part of a generalized defect of proximal tubular function, but there is also a group of inherited specific defects of glucose reabsorption in which isolated glycosuria occurs (Kranes, 1972). This is a relatively common anomaly and may result in confusion with diabetes mellitus. Patients with advanced uraemia may also show glycosuria at relatively normal blood glucose concentrations, if tubular function in some nephrons is depressed to a greater extent than glomerular filtration rate.

9.4.2.1.2. Besides the $T_m$glucose, the virtually complete extraction of *p*-aminohippurate or diodrast has lead to the use of the corresponding T_m measurement as a measure of proximal tubular secretory capacity. In these studies, the plasma concentration of the substance is raised well above the usual values employed in studies of plasma flow, and the tubules are titrated until the *maximum secretory capacity for p*-aminohippurate (T_mPAH) or diodrast (T_mD) is reached. The technique, involving infusions and accurate urine collections, is not suitable for routine clinical use; nor can loss of functioning tubular mass be distinguished from loss of proximal tubular secretory capacity from specific defects. T_mPAH and T_mD fall with age (Davies and Shock, 1950; Watkin and Shock, 1955), the fall-off occurring in parallel with the fall in renal plasma flow.

9.4.2.1.3. In practice, the assessment and diagnosis of defects of proximal tubular function centres on measurement of the urinary excretion of the endogenous metabolites which are normally filtered and reabsorbed in the proximal tubule. Glucose has already been discussed (section 9.4.2.1.1). The full assessment of *aminoaciduria* is complex (Brodehl and Bickel, 1973; Frimpter, 1973; see also Chapter 18, section 18.11.1). All aminoacids except tryptophan are freely filtered at the glomerulus, and about 98% are reabsorbed in the proximal tubule by a complex set of transport systems of varying affinity and specifity. Many aminoacids are handled by more than one system and some, such as cystine and glycine, are apparently reabsorbed by several distinct systems. In young infants, there is normally an aminoaciduria but by 9 months of age the adult level of function is reached. Aminoaciduria may arise when the kidney is quite normal, as a result of overproduction of a normal or abnormal aminoacid – "overflow" aminoaciduria – (Frimpter, 1973). The aminoacidurias resulting from tubular defects may be described as "generalized" (when all aminoacids are present in excess in the urine) or "specific" (when only one, or a defined group of aminoacids is present in excess, the excretion of the remainder being normal (Table 9.4)). The reference method of distinguishing the many aminoacidurias is to measure the clearance of each individual aminoacid using an ion-exchange column chromatography method to estimate their concentrations in blood and urine (Moore and Stein, 1954). In practice, since the plasma concentrations of aminoacids are relatively constant and the defects often gross, use may be made of the urine concentration or rate of excretion of the aminoacids. For screening purposes, two-dimensional paper chromatography (Dent, 1947), thin-layer chromatography (Fahmy et al., 1961) or high-voltage electrophoresis (Mabry and Todd, 1963) on paper or thin-layer cellulose, can all be used. The aminoacid spots can be detected or quantitated by the ninhydrin reaction, or by more specific reactions, of which the only one of clinical importance is the nitroprusside–cyanide test for cystine.

The generalized form of proximal tubular defect is usually called the Fanconi (or Debré–de Toni–Fanconi) syndrome and it is worth digressing at this point to clarify the somewhat confusing terminology in this area. The name Fanconi syndrome is applied to the clinical effect of the proximal tubular defects (glycosuria, aminoaciduria, phosphaturia, tubular proteinuria, hypouricaemia and sometimes acidosis) which usually occur together and have a wide variety of causes (Table 9.9), some of which are unknown. Usually renal function, as judged by GFR, is initially normal, but in the conditions indicated

TABLE 9.9.

CAUSES OF MULTIPLE PROXIMAL RENAL TUBULAR DEFECTS (THE FANCONI SYNDROME)

Type	Condition	Toxic substance (where known)	Inheritance [1]	Renal failure later?
primary	–	?	usually D, some R	some
due to inborn errors of metabolism	cystinosis	cystine	R	yes
	galactosaemia	galactose-1-phosphate	R	no
	Wilson's disease	copper	R	no
	Lowe's syndrome	?	SLR	?
	tyrosinosis	?	R	no
	glycogen storage disease	glycogen	R	no
acquired in course of other diseases	nephrotic syndrome	? protein	–	some
	myeloma	light chain	–	some
acquired from exogenous toxic substances	heavy metals	Pb, Cd, Au, Hg U, Bi	–	some
	antibiotics	streptomycin kanamycin bacitracin polymyxins neomycin degraded tetracycline amphotericin B	–	no
	salicylates			no

[1] R = recessive; D = dominant; SLR = sex-linked recessive.

in the Table, renal failure may occur later. Unfortunately, Fanconi's name is also applied to one of the *causes* of multiple proximal tubular defects – cystinosis, or cystine storage disease – which is sometimes referred to as the Fanconi–Lignac disease. The plasma cystine concentration is usually normal in this condition, but the intracellular concentration is very high. However, since generalized aminoaciduria is often present, the urine contains an excess of cystine along with all the other aminoacids, and will give a positive "spot" test for cystine. This is also true in patients with the specific tubular transport defect causing cystinuria, which may easily be distinguished by aminoacid chromatography.

9.4.2.1.4. The renal excretion of *phosphate* (Lancet, 1970) is increased both as a part of the generalized proximal tubular defect just discussed, or as a result of a specific proximal tubular defect in phosphate transport. In either case, the urinary phosphate loss is of clinical importance, since it may lead to rickets or osteomalacia, especially if there is coincident bicarbonate wasting as part of the generalized defect, and therefore a systemic acidosis (section 9.3.5). The relationship between excreted phosphate and plasma phosphate is complex, since tubular reabsorption varies with a number of influences, including the plasma phosphate concentration itself. However, hypophosphataemia with hyperphosphaturia suggests proximal tubular dysfunction unless hyperparathyroidism be present. Nordin and Fraser (1960) introduced the use of the phosphate excretion index (PEI) to describe the complex relationship between plasma phosphate and phosphate excretion. Because the tubular reabsorption of phosphate varies with the plasma phosphate concentration, it is not sufficient to relate the clearance of phosphate to the GFR (or creatinine clearance) by a simple ratio. The PEI is calculated as follows –

$$\mathrm{PEI} = \frac{C_p}{C_{cr}} - \frac{P_p - 1}{20}$$

where C_p = phosphate clearance, in ml/min
C_{cr} = creatinine clearance, in ml/min
P_p = plasma phosphate concentration in mg/dl.

The normal range in adults is from –0.08 to +0.08. In children (Thalassinos et al., 1970) the value of the PEI is somewhat lower than in adults, usually falling between –0.20 and zero. One advantage of the PEI is that the ratio C_p/C_{cr} eliminates the effects of any inaccuracy in urine collection, since the volume of urine upon which the two clearances are based appears in both the numerator and the denominator. An increased PEI, suggesting increased phosphate loss in the urine, occurs in hyperparathyroidism, sex-linked hypophosphataemic rickets (see Chapter 13) and in the Fanconi syndrome from whatever cause. Calculation of the T_m for phosphate would be more specific, but as in all T_m measurements inulin clearances are involved, together with prolonged infusions of phosphate. Bijvoet (1969) has suggested a method of predicting T_m phosphate from the plasma creatinine and phosphate concentrations and entailing the collection of urine over an unspecified period, and Walton and Bijvoet (1975) gave a nomogram for calculating the renal threshold phosphate concentration from the phosphate clearance and plasma phosphate concentration.

9.4.2.1.5. *Hypouricaemia,* because of reduced renal tubular absorption of urate, may be seen as an isolated, rare, specific transport defect, but it is also frequently present in patients with multiple proximal tubular defects (Hatfield and Simmonds, 1975).

9.4.2.1.6. *Tubular proteinuria*. Some aspects that have been useful in screening for proximal tubular defects are worth consideration here. Proteins of small molecular mass (up to 15000) are normally filtered at a rate comparable to water, and are reabsorbed and catabolized in the renal tubule (Harrison et al., 1968). Thus the excretion of lysozyme (mass 15,000 daltons) has been suggested as a test of proximal tubular function (Barratt and Crawford, 1970). More recently, attention has centred on β_2-microglobulin (mass 11,500 daltons) which can very easily be measured using radial diffusion immunoassay. It appears in the urine in detectable amounts in all tubular proteinurias (Berggard and Bearn, 1968) and its plasma concentration has been shown to be a better indicator of GFR, than that of plasma creatinine, the correlation with inulin clearance being excellent (Wibell et al., 1973).

9.4.2.2. Tests of mainly distal tubular function

9.4.2.2.1. *Concentrating ability* – The ability of the kidney to achieve a urine concentration of a solute in excess of that in plasma is one of the simplest tests of renal function, and if properly performed it affords an accurate guide to overall renal function. In the majority of patients with renal disease, the concentrating ability correlates closely with GFR and the degree of histological change, even in apparently pure glomerular disease (Schainuck et al., 1970). It is also in detecting specific defects in concentrating ability.

The relevant measurement is the *osmolality* of the urine (Dormandy, 1967; Wolf and Pillay, 1970). This, measured by the freezing point depression method, gives an accurate indication of the total number of particles in solution in the urine. Ideally, to test tubular concentrating ability, the absorption of solute-free water under conditions of maximum antidiuresis should be measured. This is usually referred to as $T^c_mH_2O$, since the reabsorption of water is denoted by T^cH_2O. This may be calculated by subtracting the urine volume (V) from the total osmolar clearance which, like any other clearance, may be calculated from –

$$C_{osm} = \frac{U_{osm} \cdot V}{P_{osm}} \quad \text{so that } T^cH_2O = C_{osm} - V$$

In situations of water loading, when the osmolality of the plasma is greater than that of the urine and the volume of urine is high, there is net *excretion* of free water rather than net reabsorption.

The measurement of $T^c_mH_2O$ requires timed urine samples and simultaneous plasma osmolality measurements, and is thus not suitable for clinical use; however, the plasma/urine osmolality ratio has clinical value – especially in situations of oliguria (section 9.4.5.3). It should be noted that the ability to reabsorb this "solute-free" water depends upon the delivery of solute to the distal nephron, and this is also true of the simpler concentration tests which are done clinically. Normally the $T^c_mH_2O$ is about 5 ml/min per 1.73 m^2 of surface area (Boyarsky and Smith, 1957) but may exceed this 2-fold in situations of high solute intake and excretion.

In practice, the osmolality of the urine alone gives much information, since the plasma osmolality remains constant in the majority of clinical situations (but see section 9.4.5.3). The simplest test is to measure the osmolality of a fresh, early morning specimen of urine. This will often exceed 800 mOsm/litre and thus exclude a significant concentrating defect. If it is wished to test concentrating ability more formally, dehydration is the simplest method. After lunch, no further fluid is given, a dry supper is taken and the early morning specimen of urine examined next day. Miles et al. (1954) showed that 18 to 26 hours of fluid deprivation were necessary to achieve the maximum concentrations possible. A check on the efficiency of the dehydration should be made by repeated weighing of the patient on the same scales; a weight loss of 3 to 5% indicates that the concentrating mechanism has been stressed sufficiently, and that water has not been taken surreptitiously. If the patient is known to be very polyuric with very dilute urine, the test may be terminated when regular weighings suggest a 5% weight loss, to avoid unnecessary and possibly dangerous dehydration.

The osmolality of the early morning specimen of urine should be 800 to 1300 mOsm/litre, provided that the patient is taking a normal diet (de Wardener, 1967). Isaacson (1960) used 18 hours' water deprivation and obtained a mean urine osmolality of 1057 mOsm/litre (with 95% confidence limits of 807 to 1407 mOsm/litre) in adults. The maximum specific gravity (see below) attainable after dehydration falls with age (Lewis and Alving, 1938). At 65 years of age, a value of 1026 is still attainable, but by 95 years of age 1023 is the upper limit.

In a population study, Waters et al. (1967) found the following relationship of osmolar concentration to age in early morning urine specimens –

for males: mOsm/litre = $-4.41 \times$ age(yr) + 914

for females: mOsm/litre = $-4.94 \times$ age(yr) + 834

The 60 to 70 year cohort could concentrate only to 650 mOsm/litre overnight, compared with a mean of 950 mOsm/litre at 20 years of age. Rowe et al. (1976a) studied the influence of age on maximum urinary osmolarity after a 12-hour thirst in normal individuals. Those aged 20 to 39, 40 to 49, and 60 to 79 years of age, respectively, achieved maximum osmolarities of 1109 ± 22, 1051 ± 19, and 882 ± 49 mOsm/litre. Edelmann (1967) found that normal children could concentrate their urine as well as adults; a mean urine osmolality of 1089 mOsm/litre was attained (95% confidence limits of 869 to 1309 mOsm/litre). The influence of diet upon concentrating ability is especially important in infancy. The urea provided most of the excreted solute upon which urinary "concentration" depended in the studies of Edelmann et al. (1966), the concentration of non-urea solutes remaining constant on different diets. The apparent failure of some infants to concentrate their urine can be explained by their being in an overall anabolic state, excreting very little urea when fed diets containing only a moderate amount of protein such as breast milk. In contrast, infants fed cow's milk are protein- and solute-loaded. The effects of continued high fluid intake must not be forgotten; prolonged water diuresis leads to a "washing out" of the medullary pool of solute responsible for the medullary hypertonicity, which is necessary if hypertonic urines are to be elaborated (Black, 1967). Thus, compulsive water drinkers may show a concentrating defect which may mimic true diabetes insipidus even in the presence of endogenous or exogenous antidiuretic hormone (Black, 1967; de Wardener, 1967).

An alternative (and complementary) approach is to stress the concentrating capacity with an intramuscular injection of pitressin tannate (ADH) in oil (de Wardener, 1967), combined with simple overnight deprivation of fluid. It may also be necessary to test a patient who shows failure to concentrate his urine after dehydration with an injection of pitressin, to determine whether the defect relates to failure of response to endogenous ADH ("nephrogenic" or renal diabetes insipidus); or to a failure of secretion of endogenous ADH (pituitary diabetes insipidus). The osmolalities achieved during this form of test are slightly lower than those seen after prolonged dehydration (de Wardener, 1967) although 750 to 1150 mOsm/litre can be attained. Winberg (1959a) found a mean osmolality of 1069 mOsm/litre (with 95% confidence limits of 813 to 1327 mOsm/litre) in children given pitressin. The insolubility of the pitressin presents a problem which may be overcome by warming and thoroughly mixing. In children, the risk of the test is not excessive dehydration, as in the water deprivation test, but of water intoxication if the child continues to drink while under the effects of the long-acting ADH. As a result, Black (1965) has advocated the use of aqueous vasopressin in a dose adjusted for body weight in children. Desmopressin would now be used.

Concentrating ability, when carefully tested, closely parallels the drop in GFR in conditions affecting all parts of the nephron, becoming abnormal long before there is any detectable rise in the blood urea or plasma creatinine concentration. In addition, idsproportionate and precocious loss of concentrating power may be seen in conditions affecting the tubules more than the glomeruli, e.g. pyelonephritis with or without reflux of urine up the ureters, polycystic disease, sickle cell and the recovery phase of acute tubular necrosis. In patients with apparently normal kidneys but with loss of concentrating power, the examination of this function by exogenous and endogenous ADH should be the central examination.

Despite the continued advocacy of urinary specific gravity measurements for monitoring the concentrating ability of the kidney (Relman and Levinsky, 1971; Kassirer, 1971b) it does not appear to the present authors that this assessment is adequate. Unlike the osmolality, the specific gravity of the urine is dependent upon the molecular size and species as well as the number of particles in solution, and will correspondingly vary according to the nature of the solute. Galambos et al. (1964) showed that a urine with specific gravity of 1010 has a mean osmolality of 320 mOsm/litre, but the 95% confidence limits for this predicted osmolality are 126 to 510 mOsm/litre. Similarly, Isaacson (1960) took the lower limit of normality in a series of dehydrated adults to be 900 mOsm/litre. This represented a mean specific gravity of 1023, but to be 95% sure that the individual had in fact attained an osmolality of only 900 mOsm/litre, the specific gravity reached had to be above 1029. Miles et al. (1954) and Wolf and Pillay (1969) have also discussed the effects of different solutes and the presence of proteinuria on the relationship of specific gravity to osmolality.

The practical problems of measuring the specific gravity under clinical conditions are often disregarded. Unclean glassware (especially contamination with detergents), uncalibrated urinometers with unfixed scales, the variation of specific gravity with the temperature of the urine (urinometers are usually calibrated at 15 °C, and fresh urine is at 37 °C) and the influence of excreted contrast media or volume expanders must all be taken into account, otherwise a useless (or even worse a misleading) figure will be obtained. Small, relatively cheap osmometers are available, some portable for ward use; and for paediatric use, refractometry has advantages (Wolf and Pillary, 1969) because it can require only a drop of urine. The concentrating and diluting capacity of the kidney is best monitored by measuring urinary osmolality.

Methods have been described for the radioimmunoassay of *vasopressin* (ADH) in plasma (Beardwell, 1971) and in urine (Fressinaud et al., 1974). These methods have potential in the investigation of polyuria and of the syndrome of inappropriate secretion of ADH, but are not yet generally available.

Diluting capacity is quite difficult to assess under clinical conditions. Normal individuals are capable of passing urine of only 40 to 80 mOsm/litre under a water load of 1 to 2 litres taken slowly (Schoen, 1957), provided that they are taking a diet of normal solute content. ADH is not required for urine dilution, so that in states of ADH resistance or absence, dilution is possible without concentrating ability being present. This is also true of potassium depletion, hypercalcaemia and sickle cell disease, all states in which reversible defects of concentrating capacity are present (Black, 1967). Conversely, concentrating ability may be preserved with loss of diluting capacity in adrenal insufficiency, liver disease and cardiac failure (Relman and Levinsky, 1971). In practice the nausea produced by drinking the large quantities of fluid necessary to test diluting capacity often results in ADH secretion and antidiuresis. Diluting ability is therefore rarely assessed.

9.4.2.2.2. *Tests of hydrogen ion excretion* – The ability of the kidney to excrete hydrogen ion is reflected in the pH of the urine, the excretion of ammonium, titratable acid buffered by phosphate and other urinary buffers and, in some situations, the excretion of bicarbonate (absent from normal urine). In general, failure of the kidney to excrete hydrogen ion results from either a failure of secretion of hydrogen ion or ammonium on the one hand, or a failure to reabsorb filtered bicarbonate on the other. To examine these aspects of renal function fully would require examination of excreted hydrogen ion, ammonium, titratable acid and bicarbonate at one time at various values of blood and urine pH, i.e. at rest, and under stress with an acid load, after hydrogen ion equilibrium had been attained. In practice much can be learned by simply measuring plasma bicarbonate concentration and urine pH under stress.

Conditions associated with an inability to excrete hydrogen ion lead to a resting acidosis. Normally this is compensated, and the plasma pH is normal at around 7.37, but there is, however, a decrease in buffering capacity of the blood, with a corresponding fall in bicarbonate concentration and pCO_2. The first step in examining a patient's ability to excrete hydrogen ion is careful measurment of the plasma bicarbonate. This is best done by the Astrup technique using capillary (or better arterial) blood, since manual Van Slyke or AutoAnalyzer estimations on venous blood can give misleading values. If the concentration is below 20 mmol/litre at rest, however, then in all but infants the method of measurement becomes unimportant. The combined finding of a low resting bicarbonate and a urine pH of 5.5 or more indicates with certainty a defect of urinary acidification. Conversely, an early morning urine pH of less than 5.3 excludes almost all patients with failure of hydrogen ion secretion. Urine pH should be measured on fresh specimens since, for a number of reasons, the pH changes after storage.

Further examination involves stressing the system with an acid load. The test described by Wrong and Davies (1959) which involves a single dose of ammonium chloride, has proved popular and useful. This detects an inability to produce a gradient of hydrogen ion between the blood and distal tubular fluid. Normally, hydrogen ion can be concentrated 600-fold (pH 4.7) in the distal tubular fluid when compared with the plasma (pH 7.4). In the Wrong and Davies test, 0.1 g/kg of ammonium chloride is administered to the patient. For an adult, this is approximately 7 grams (84 mmol) of ammonium, while for children, 75 mmol/m^2 has been suggested, with a doubling of the dose if the urine fails to be acidified. Ammonium chloride is nauseating, and should be given 0.5 or 1.0 grams at a time *during* a meal – above all not on an empty stomach; usually the dose can be retained if given in this manner over a half hour period; gelatin capsules or a mixture should be used. Usually the dose is taken during breakfast, and urine specimens are collected at 2, 4 and 6 hours after administration. Normal individuals should pass at least one specimen with a pH of 5.3 or less (representing a tubule/blood hydrogen ion gradient of 125/1 or better). At 4 hours, a capillary or venous blood sample is taken for bicarbonate estimation to ensure that an acidosis has been achieved. If the patient vomits all or part of the ammonium cloride, the test must be repeated.

Newborns and infants in the first year of life present special features. The newborn kidney is much less capable of secreting either ammonium or titratable acid than kidneys in infants, older children or adults (McCance and Hatemi, 1961), and the pH of the urine in premature babies and during the first week of life is normally 6.0 to 7.0 (Edelmann, 1967). By the end of the first week of life, however, the pattern is much nearer normal, and the infant is correspondingly better able to withstand the stress of acidosis. Throughout the whole first year of life the concentration at which plasma bicarbonate appears in the urine (the bicarbonate "threshold") is 17 to 19 mmol/litre, compared with 20 to 26 mmol/litre in older children and adults. This presumably represents a relative immaturity of the proximal tubule for bicarbonate reabsorption and means that infants from one week to about one year of age, although able to reduce the pH of their urine to 5.0 or less, have lower plasma bicarbonate concentrations than expected from studies of older subjects (Edelmann et al., 1967b).

These simple measurements of plasma bicarbonate concentration and urine pH at rest and under the stress of an acid load allow detection of patients with specific defects of hydrogen ion secretion in the distal tubule – so called "distal", "gradient" or "classical" renal tubular acidosis. More recently, it has been realized that patients may have renal tubular acidosis because of a relative inability to reabsorb bicarbonate, either as an isolated defect, or as part of multiple proximal tubular dysfunction (Fanconi syndrome, section 9.4.2.1.3): so-called "proximal" or "threshold" tubular acidosis (Soriano et al., 1967; Rodriguez-Soriano and Edelmann, 1969; Morris, 1969). The presence of this defect was not realized initially because these patients can, under stress of an acid load, generate urine with a low pH; the difference lies in the degree of acidosis (depletion of plasma bicarbonate) which is required to achieve this. Because there is bicarbonate wasting through the proximal tubule, the "threshold" for bicarbonate is lower than normal (Figure 9.3), varying from 16 to 20 mmol/litre instead of the usual 20 to 26 mmol/litre. The ful examination of such patients requires titration of the kidney with a bicarbonate infusion to determine the bicarbonate threshold (Soriano et al., 1967; Morris, 1969) but

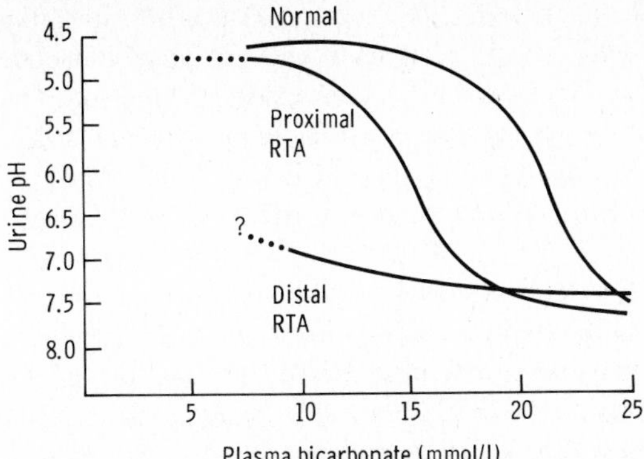

Figure 9.3. The relationship between urinary pH and plasma bicarbonate (Astrup) in normal individuals; and in patients with distal (gradient) and proximal (threshold) renal tubular acidosis. In normal individuals, bicarbonate only spills into the urine when the plasma bicarbonate exceeds 22 mmol/litre, so that the urine only becomes alkaline under normal circumstances if this "threshold" is exceeded. Correspondingly, a fall in the plasma bicarbonate below 18 mmol/litre results in a maximally acid urine being excreted. In patients with a proximal "leak" of bicarbonate, the threshold for the appearance of bicarbonate in the urine may be only 15 to 16 mmol/litre, and correspondingly the urine becomes alkaline at a plasma bicarbonate as low as 16 to 18 mmol/litre. If the plasma bicarbonate is lowered by an acid load, however, when it falls below the low threshold of 15 mmol/litre, then the urine becomes maximally acid to the same extent as in a normal individual. In the case of the patient with distal renal tubular acidosis, the renal bicarbonate threshold is normal, but the distal tubule is incapable of producing the hydrogen ion gradient required to acidify the urine. The urine therefore remains alkaline however low the plasma bicarbonate falls; although for ethical reasons extreme acidosis has not been investigated in these patients. (Modified from the data of Soriano et al., 1967)

the combination of an alkaline urine, a low resting bicarbonate, the ability to lower the urine pH under stress, and finally the very large quantity of oral bicarbonate required to correct the acidosis should make the diagnosis certain. In some patients there will be signs of losses of other metabolites normally conserved by the renal tubule, or a known cause of proximal tubular defects such as cystinosis.

In patients with chronic renal failure, the ability to excrete ammonium is the principal defect (Wrong, 1965) and it is usual for the ability to acidify the urine to be preserved. Indeed, patients in renal failure usually pass urines of acid pH because of the deficiency in urine buffer, principally phosphate. A failure of ammonium excretion also occurs with age (Barzel et al., 1964) and in patients with gout, who normally pass urine of very low pH throughout the 24 hours without the usual diurnal variation (Pak Poy, 1965).

9.4.3. The renin–angiotensin system

9.4.3.1. Measurements related to the system (Beevers et al., 1975)
The relevance of estimations of renin, angiotensin and aldosterone cannot be made clear without some expansion of the brief note on the system which was given earlier in section 9.1.3. Renin is predominantly formed and stored in the kidney, and is released both

into the renal vein and renal lymph. When released into the circulation it acts on renin substrate (angiotensinogen, a large molecular weight protein) to give a relatively inactive decapeptide, angiotensin I, which is then transformed by converting enzyme into the active octapeptide, angiotensin II. In addition to its effect in raising blood pressure, angiotensin II has a major effect in stimulating aldosterone secretion. It also stimulates thirst, ADH secretion, and catecholamine secretion, and it has a direct effect on renal function in addition to that mediated by aldosterone.

The system as a whole is a major factor in the control of sodium balance, being activated by sodium restriction, and inhibited by sodium loading. Conversely, the system is inhibited by potassium loading, which may provide a long delayed explanation of the observation by Bunge (1873) of reciprocity between sodium and potassium balance. The system is also stimulated by water deprivation, by exercise, and even by the assumption of the upright posture after a period of recumbency. It is influenced by drugs, most obviously by natriuretic agents. but also by diazoxide and other hypotensive drugs, by licorice preparations, and by oral contraceptives. Control of such factors is essential if assays of components of the system are to be useful. The necessary practical measures necessary to achieve this are detailed by Beevers et al. (1975).

The assay of *renin* depends on the generation under controlled conditions in vitro, of angiotensin, which is then determined by radioimmunoassay. Since plasma contains varying amounts of renin substrate, and also of angiotensinases, the assay system has to be "purified" in various ways, which include the extraction of renin followed by reaction with prepared substrate, and comparison with a calibration curve using serial dilutions of a standard renin preparation (external calibration); removal of angiotensinases, followed by addition of known amounts of standard renin to all but one aliquot (internal calibration); the addition of excess substrate, to swamp variation in endogenous substrate; and assay independently of endogenous substrate. In spite of these methodological complexities, good agreement was obtained between different centres in the assays of coded unknown plasmas (Bangham et al., 1975). A typical reference range for plasma renin of 4 to 18 units was found by Brown et al. (1964).

Radioimmunoassay methods for *angiotensin* I and II have been described in detail by Morton et al. (1975). In addition to being an integral part of the assay of renin, angiotensin estimation per se is of value. The estimation of angiotensin II, in particular, yields information on the prevailing functional activity of the renin–angiotensin system. An essential step in the assay is the prompt inhibition both of renin activity and of the action of converting enzyme. Typical ranges in peripheral venous plasma are 11 to 88 pg/ml for angiotensin I, and 5 to 50 pg/ml for angiotensin II (Beevers et al., 1975).

The measurement of *aldosterone* and its degradation products is covered in Chapter 14.

9.4.3.2. Clinical value

The clinical use of estimations of renin and angiotensin is discussed in detail by Beevers et al. (1975). In relation to *hypertension*, there have been claims that elevated plasma renin levels are associated with a greater prevalence of complications, and with greater responsiveness to β-adrenergic blocking agents, but these claims are not generally substantiated. At present, apart from research investigations, it seems justified to confine these assays, for which facilities are limited, to patients in whom there is solid evidence to suggest a renal or endocrine cause for the hypertension. A further limitation is that when primary hypertension has entered the malignant phase, high levels of renin and angiotensin are present, due to secondary renal damage.

On the other hand, increased activity of the renin–angiotensin system is a valuable finding in the confirmation of hypertension due to renal ischaemia, or to the rare but curable renin-secreting tumour (Brown et al., 1973). Measurement of the renin concentration in renal venous blood is of particular value in predicting which patients with renal arterial stenosis (or unilaterally scarred kidneys) will benefit from nephrectomy (Stockigt et al., 1972). Better discrimination is obtained by comparing the renin concentration in blood from the renal vein of the affected kidney and the contralateral supposedly normal kidney, and in peripheral venous blood (Arakawa et al., 1973). Despite the blood flow from the affected ischaemic kidney being less than that from the normal kidney, which should increase the renin concentration, good discrimination can be achieved. With careful venous catheterization it is even possible to decide which segment of the kidney is concerned in cases where the stenosis may be intra-renal and possibly multiple (Schambelan et al., 1974). When hypertension is associated with hypokalaemia, aldosterone secretion should be estimated; if this is found to be raised, suppression of the renin–angiotensin system should be sought, as evidence of primary aldosteronism. In this situation, accurate renin assay is a component of the data which, when subjected to quadric analysis, can differentiate between a localized aldosteronoma and diffuse hyperplasia of aldosterone-secreting tissue (Ferriss et al., 1970) (see also Chapter 14.5. and 14.6.6). In *renal failure,* very high activity of the renin–angiotensin system may indicate those patients in whom nephrectomy may be required for the control of hypertension. Renin or angiotensin assay is necessary for diagnosis of the uncommon syndrome of hypoaldosteronism due to renin deficiency, which manifests itself as sodium depletion with hyperkalaemia, similarly to Addison's disease, but may be distinguished by the presence in Addison's disease of raised renin and angiotensin, and of the effects of glucocorticoid deficiency. The combination of hypertension and hypokalaemia is an indication for the assay of *aldosterone secretion* rate, which may then have to be supplemented by assay of the renin–angiotensin system as previously outlined. Other indications for aldosterone assay are hypoadrenalism, and the investigation of hypokalaemia not accounted for by diuretic therapy. Aldosterone assays are not required in oedematous states where there is a clear cause of secondary aldosteronism such as cardiac or hepatic failure, or the nephrotic syndrome.

9.4.4. Renal blood flow

In physiological studies, it is possible to estimate both the total blood flow through the kidneys, and its relative distribution to superficial and to deep zones of the kidney. The knowledge so gained has proved to be useful in interpreting some of the phenomena of renal disease, and also in understanding what happens when sound kidneys are prejudiced in their blood supply by various forms of shock, or by transplant rejection. The direct application of these techniques to human disease is, however, severely limited. The main technique employed for assessment of regional blood flow has been the injection of microspheres of different diameters, usually carrying a radioactive label, with subsequent analysis of the distribution of the spheres in various parts of the kidney either histologically, or by assay of radioactivity. This involves removal of the organ and is obviously not a method for clinical practice. Analysis of "wash out" of an inert gas such as xenon or krypton has, however, been used clinically to assess regional distribution of blood flow in several organs. The solubility of the gas varies from tissue to tissue, and the accummulation is a function of this factor and of the amount of blood flowing through the tissue. The gases are breathed in, or injected in aqueous solution as a bolus, and an external counter records radioactivity continuously over the kidney. A multicomponent decay curve is generated, which can be broken down into several components as detailed in section 9.4.4.2. However, in disease the compartmental analysis has not been shown to be valid.

9.4.4.1. Total blood flow

Even the accurate measurement of plasma flow by clearance methods is not easy to achieve in clinical practice, and the results of such measurements may be difficult to interpret. The renal blood flow may be calculated from the renal plasma flow and the haematocrit, but a problem immediately arises since the haematocrit varies in different parts of the circulation. In practice, the peripheral venous haematocrit is often employed. The determination of renal plasma flow is based upon substances which are not only filtered, but secreted by the renal tubules with such avidity that at low plasma concentrations the blood leaving the kidney in the renal vein is virtually free of the marker. If these conditions are fulfilled, then the clearance of the substance will approach or equal the rate of flow of plasma through the kidney. In fact, only about 92% of the flow perfuses the tubules or glomeruli of the kidney in health, so that clearances measure the "effective renal plasma flow" (ERPF), which is defined as that plasma flow coming into contact with secreting tubules. The extent to which this clearance can fall short of true plasma flow may be determined by passing a catheter into the renal vein, and estimating the proportion of the marker extracted, i.e. (A – V)/A, where A and V are the arterial and renal venous concentrations of the marker, respectively. Most clinical studies which are based on clearance measurements of renal plasma flow involve the assumption that the extraction of the compound is constant and virtually complete, and that the peripheral haematocrit can be used to calculate the renal blood flow. However, the extraction may be less than normal to an unknown extent in disease, and the accuracy of renal plasma flow measurements in disease is therefore uncertain unless renal vein catheterization has been employed. This clearly limits its clinical use.

The substances used include diodone, *p*-aminohippurate and [^{125}I]iodohippurate. The basic method was described by Smith et al. (1945) and resembles that of measuring the clearance of inulin, with a priming dose of *p*-aminohippurate followed by a sustaining infusion, so that the two are often measured together in investigative studies. Normal values for children and adults have been reported by Wesson (1969) and in neonates the apparent ERPF is low (70 ml/min per 1.73 m^2 of surface area). However, the extraction of *p*-aminohippurate is as low as 60% in infants (Calcagno and Rubin, 1963) compared to the figure of about 90% in adults, so that its clearance underestimates the plasma flow in the newborn. If the figures are corrected for this low extraction, the ERPF in infants approaches that of older children or adults. The reasons for this low extraction of *p*-aminohippurate in infants are speculative (Edelmann, 1973) but in puppies, and probably also in human babies, renal blood flow is predominantly to the juxtamedullary glomeruli, whose efferent arterioles pass directly from the glomeruli to the vasa recta of the medulla without perfusing the renal tubules of the inner cortex. At the age of 20 years in man, the ERPF is at its peak of 650 ± 100 (S.D.) ml/min, giving a calculated renal blood flow of 1050 ± 150 (S.D.), but in those aged 80 to 89 years, the blood flow is only 475 ± 141 (S.D.) ml/min (Davies and Shock, 1950). The regression of ERPF on age is 820 – 6.75 × age (in years) (Watkin and Shock, 1955), indicating that the ERPF falls about 70 ml/min for each decade from its peak at 20 to 29 years of age.

There is a wide variation in renal blood flow findings which probably reflects the difficulties of maintaining basal conditions during a procedure which involves infusion and repeated sampling of blood and urine. Renal blood flow is depressed by emotional stress and pain; it is subject to diurnal variation, ERPF being lowest in sleep; it is reduced by moderate exercise and markedly reduced by severe exercise; it is increased by a high protein diet, and during pregnancy; depression occurs in states of shock, irrespective of the cause – haemorrhagic, traumatic, obstetric, cardiogenic or oligaemic, and apparent renal plasma flow is reduced in both acute and chronic glomerulonephritis, except in those patients with the nephrotic syndrome whose glomeruli show only minimal changes.

Attempts have been made to relate the GFR/ERPF ratio (the filtration fraction) to specific renal diseases, especially in hypertensive patients, but with little success, probably because of the imprecision of the measurements and physiological variation.

Measurement of the ERPF has been attempted using a single injection of *p*-aminohippurate or [^{125}I]*o*-iodohippurate and some success has been achieved using a double exponential analysis of the fall-off in plasma concentration (Farmer et al., 1967; Cohen et al., 1971; Silkalns et al., 1973). The agreement with the classical techniques may well have been fortuitous, since *o*-iodohippurate is also excreted by the liver to some extent, arteriovenous concentrations may differ up to 30%, and at no time after the injection can the removal be described by a single exponential; finally the stability of the ^{125}I label in vivo is in doubt.

A radioactive compound can be used for studies involving infusion and extraction of the compound by the kidney with a renal venous catheter in place. Using the extraction of ^{85}Kr, Brun et al. (1955) made the important observation that anuric kidneys are still being perfused at some 20% of normal blood flow.

9.4.4.2. Distribution of blood flow

The curve of disappearance of ^{85}Kr from the kidney may be analyzed into four components, apparently corresponding to blood flow through the outer cortex, the inner cortex and outer medulla, the inner medulla, and peri-renal and hilar fat (Barger and Herd, 1971). Estimates based upon this type of analysis show striking differences in the perfusion rates per minute of the various regions of the kidney as follows –

outer cortex	400 to 500 ml/100 g
inner cortex and outer medulla	120 to 150 ml/100 g
inner medulla	12 to 20 ml/100 g
renal fat	<5 ml/100 g

In a number of circumstances, such as with circulatory overload and some diuretics (e.g. frusemide), cortical blood flow increases; whereas in congestive heart failure and in haemorrhagic shock or nephrotoxic acute renal failure, blood flow through the medulla apparently increases, although the component of the wash-out curve attributed to the outer cortex may disappear altogether. These findings have been studied extensively in dogs, and verified by injection of silastic to confirm the conclusions. However, their applicability to man is still open to some doubt, especially in disease, since man has an outer cortex with a higher proportion of short-loop nephrons, i.e. those with loops of Henle not reaching the medulla, than other species.

9.4.4.3. The phenolsulphonephthalein test

Phenolsulphonephthalein is handled by the kidney similarly to *p*-aminohippurate and a simple test based on its excretion has been in use for some 50 years. However, now that the GFR may be measured with some accuracy in clinical situations by single injection techniques or creatinine clearance, its continuing popularity in North America is a tribute to tradition rather than to precision of clinical diagnosis.

The phenolsulphonephthalein test (Smith, 1951; Relman and Levinsky, 1971) was first introduced as a test of proximal tubular function. Although it is excreted into the urine almost entirely by tubular secretion – because it is 80% protein-bound and inaccessible to filtration – the capacity of tubular secretion only becomes the limiting factor in its excretion at plasma concentrations of 1 mg/dl or above. The peak concentration following the injection of the usual dose of 6 mg is about 0.2 mg/dl, and the limiting factor at these low concentrations in the blood is the rate of delivery to the kidney, i.e. the renal blood flow. The phenolsulphonephthalein excretion test is thus a crude measure of the ERPF, since it is 60% extracted in one transit through the kidney (Smith et al., 1938). The attraction of the test, which probably accounts for its continuing popularity, is the final measurement by spectrophotometry (or even by a visual comparator) after simple alkalinization of the urine; phenolsulphonephthalein is also remarkably non-toxic.

In the test as usually performed (Chapman and Halstead, 1933), the dose of exactly 6 mg is injected intravenously; it is important to see that all the dye is given, since this amount is the standard with which the excretion is compared. The subject then passes urine at 15 minutes, 30 minutes, 1 and 2 hours after the injection; to attain this rate of sampling the subject must be water-loaded before the test. There is no need to empty the bladder when the injection is given, and to do so may render the 15-minute sample unobtainable. The volumes of urine are measured, aliquots are made alkaline, and the absorbance is measured so as to estimate the concentration of phenolsulphonephthalein. The amount excreted as a percentage of that injected is calculated, and normal values (Chapman and Halstead, 1933) are as follows –

Time after injection (minutes)	Excretion	
	Mean	Range
15	35	28–51
30	17	13–24
60	12	9–17
120	6	3–10
Total in 24 hours	70	63–84

The most sensitive index of early renal functional impairment is the 15-minute sample, since even in uraemia the kidney can excrete most of the injected phenolsulphonephthalein within 2 hours. As can be seen from the tabulated data, there is considerable extra-renal excretion, principally into the gut; the test is rendered invalid by concomitant liver disease. Modifications of the test using the rate of fall-off in the first 30 minutes or so, using plasma sampling, have been described (Gault et al., 1966) but these seem to have all the disadvantages of single injection measurement of GFR or ERPF without approximating to any specific renal function. Blood and bile in the urine will also interfere with the estimation. The test cannot be used in children, since rapidly timed urine samples are required, nor is it suitable for patients with urinary tract obstruction or vesicoureteric reflux.

Although, as expected, there is good correlation between the results of the test and clearances of *p*-aminohippurate (Gault et al., 1966), [^{131}I]*o*-iodohippurate (Nanra et al., 1969) and creatinine (Healy, 1968), the role of the phenolsulphonephthalein test seems to be a diminishing one in face of other tests of renal function which are more closely related to glomerular filtration rate.

9.4.5. Miscellaneous tests

9.4.5.1. The general principles of urine testing have been considered in Chapter 2 (section 2.4.1), and are also discussed, with illustrations of casts, by Morrison (1979). A fresh and uncontaminated specimen is essential for bacteriological examination, and for microscopy, and it is highly desirable for simple urine analysis, especially in relation to pH; the practice of batch testing ward urines at some convenient time after the last specimen has been obtained is inadequate. Urine testing is a necessary part of physical examination, and may reveal the presence of renal disease in the absence of any symptoms. If proteinuria is discovered by qualitative testing, the plasma protein should be estimated in a 24-hour specimen, and in young adults, especially, the possibility of intermittent proteinuria should be explored by taking several specimens, some after periods of recumbency. Serial estimations of the 24-hour output of protein are useful as a guide to progress and treatment in the nephrotic syndrome. In patients with persistent proteinuria, even in the absence of symptoms, a test of excretory renal function, such as creatinine clearance measurement, should be done as a guide to prognosis. Positive chemical tests for blood require confirmation by microscopy, in the case of haematuria, or by spectroscopy, in the case of haemoglobinuria or myoglobinuria.

9.4.5.2. The significance of electrolyte determinations in plasma and urine is considered in other chapters, but attention may be drawn here to the value of the 24-hour output of sodium and potassium as a guide to the dietary requirement of these ions, particularly in the terminal stages of renal failure, where a course between dehydration and hypertension may depend on control of the salt intake. These estimations are also necessary to detect the occasional patient with massive urinary losses of sodium and potassium, which call for appropriate supplementation with sodium or potassium salts. They are also useful in determining electrolyte balances in patients with renal functional impairment before or after surgery or other metabolic stress.

9.4.5.3. The 24-hour output of urea is also a useful guide to the dietary management of patients with chronic renal failure. As already noted (section 9.4.1.4), the catabolism of 1 gram of protein leads to the formation of 0.3 grams of urea. Consequently, the urinary excretion of urea, in the rather unvarying situation of chronic renal failure, gives a guide to the amount of endogenous and exogenous protein being catabolized. If the equivalent, in grams of protein, of less than three times the urinary urea output is fed, then normally a fall in blood urea concentration may be anticipated. Conversely, since nitrogen balance cannot be maintained on less than 18 to 21 grams of first class animal protein, the excretion of less than 6 or 7 grams of urea per 24 hours is not compatible with continued existence. If this low level of excretion is not increased, dialysis will be required, irrespective of the plasma concentration of the various nitrogenous metabolites.

The urinary concentrations of electrolytes and urea, and the osmolality of the urine, are also of value in states of oliguria. It is of great importance to be able to distinguish, as early as possible, a patient in established acute tubular necrosis – who will be oliguric for weeks rather than days – from an oliguric patient whose oliguria depends upon renal hypo-perfusion. Both patients may show rapidly rising blood urea concentrations but the latter type of patient will respond to manoeuvres such as infusion of a large volume of colloid or electrolyte solution, which may be dangerous or even fatal in established acute renal failure, where no diuresis in response to any manoeuvre can be expected.

The urinary composition in such patients, together with clinical information such as peripheral perfusion, central venous pressure and other indices of cardiovascular status, enable the clinician to predict with some accuracy which patients will have a prompt diuresis. The urine composition of the two states may be contrasted as follows –

	Renal hypo-perfusion	Established acute renal failure
Na^+	<20 mmol/litre [1]	30– 60 mmol/litre
K^+	40–60 mmol/litre	40– 60 mmol/litre
Urea	>1000 mg/dl	300–500 mg/dl
Ratio of urine-to-plasma osmolalities	>1.3	<1.1

[1] If diuretics have been given, the Na^+ concentration may rise to 100 mmol/litre or more.

In short, the hypo-perfused kidney produces urine which is distinctly more concentrated than plasma, in spite of containing a very low concentration of sodium (Eliahou and Bata, 1965; Luke et al., 1965, 1970). In uraemic states, the plasma osmolality may be much higher than the usual 285 mOsm/litre; values over 400 mOsm/litre may be recorded on occasion if the blood urea concentration is very high, or if there is coincident hyperglycaemia – which may be the case if peritoneal dialysis is carried out using solutions of high glucose content.

In elderly patients, because of generally impaired powers of urinary concentration, it may not be possible to differentiate these two states, on the basis of urine-to-plasma concentration ratios; but even in the elderly, renal hypoperfusion, as opposed to acute renal failure, is still characterized by a low concentration of sodium in the urine (Papper,

1973). In infants, the urine-to-plasma ratio for urea may be a better guide to the reversibility of oliguria than the urine-to-plasma ratio of osmolalities (Gordillo-Paniagua and Velasquez-Jones, 1976).

From these figures, a prediction can be made as to which patients will respond to large doses of powerful diuretics and to volume replacement. The patient with urine which is iso-osmolar to plasma and a moderate or high urinary sodium concentration, will respond rarely, if at all, to these manoeuvres. The combination of low sodium concentration and high urinary osmolality has also been used in comparing the urine from the two kidneys in patients suspected of having unilateral renal hypoperfusion as a cause of hypertension. Since the technique involves bilateral ureteric catheterization, and since other methods are now available for exploring this situation, the technique of divided renal function studies is now little used.

9.4.5.4. The activity, as opposed to the mere presence, of renal disease can only be rather crudely assessed by changes in proteinuria or in microscopic haematuria. Wellwood et al. (1973, 1974) have reported on the usefulness of β-*N*-acetylglucosaminidase (EC 3.2.1.30) determined fluorometrically, as an index of disease activity and of allograft rejection. Patients with glomerulonephritis had raised urinary excretion of this enzyme, in comparison with normal subjects, but those with deteriorating renal function showed higher values than those whose renal function was stable, even if somewhat impaired. Patients with chronic pyelonephritis had raised excretion only when their renal function was deteriorating. Elevated values were found in patients with hypertensive renal damage, in patients with no renal disease during episodes of hypotension and in transplant rejection. A problem with β-*N*-acetylglucosaminidase estimations (which holds for all estimations relating to urinary excretion of tubular enzymes), is that many events, such as acute infection and the administration of antibiotic or analgesic drugs also increase the excretion of the enzyme.

9.4.5.5. The excretion of fibrin degradation products in the urine is supposed to correlate with disease activity. The principal work in this field has been done on patients with glomerulonephritis (Clarkson et al., 1971; Davison et al., 1973; Naish et al., 1974) and correlations have been claimed with histological type, disease activity, and the amount of fibrin seen in immunofluorescent study of the kidney. It has also been claimed that fibrin degradation products in the urine result from fibrinolysis of intra-glomerular fibrin, rather than from filtration of circulating degradation products or fibrinolysis of filtered fibrin in the urine. However, some of these promising claims have come under criticism (Ekert et al., 1972; Hall et al., 1975) since fibrin degradation products in the urine seem to depend upon the quantity and quality of proteinuria, being greatest in patients with heavy proteinuria and with least selectivity of protein clearances. Since these features are characteristics of patients with severe and progressive disease, it may be that the correlations of fibrin degradation products with disease activity are fortuitous; certainly the analytical methods leave much to be desired.

9.5. SUMMARY STATEMENT ON THE PLACE OF BIOCHEMICAL TESTS IN RENAL DISEASE

9.5.1. General principles of diagnosis

The categorization of disease states is of value in communication between doctors, with patients, and as a guide to management. Existing categories are always imperfect, as they are constrained by limitations of knowledge and of the methods of investigation. There is also the difficulty that a disease is not a substantial entity, but an interaction between a pathological process and a person. The purpose of this brief concluding section is to indicate the place of biochemical investigations in the general scheme of management of renal disease. Simply to put a name to a disease is a very incomplete description of an actual clinical situation – the nature of the pathological process needs to be known, together with the extent to which it alters renal function, and any structural changes which it may have produced in the kidney, and secondarily in other organs.

9.5.2. The pathological process

Information on this aspect comes mainly from the natural history of the complaint, from radiological and microbiological investigations, and to an increasing extent, from visual and electron microscopy, fluorescent antibody staining, and microchemical examination of renal biopsy specimens. There are, however, disorders with no known aetiology or structural concomitants, in which the lesion is essentially a biochemical one, such as a genetically determined enzyme defect. In the field of renal disease, this can be exemplified by various tubular syndromes where the characterization of the lesion rests on biochemical evidence.

9.5.3. Functional assessment

Although the advanced stages of renal failure may be suspected on clinical grounds, biochemical confirmation of their presence is essential, both for diagnosis and for deciding on the appropriate type of palliation to be used, whether dietary, by dialysis, by transplantation, or by a combined program involving all three techniques. Less advanced degrees of renal failure can only be detected by biochemical tests. For this overall assessment of renal function, estimations of the plasma urea and serum creatinine concentrations suffice to demonstrate advanced renal failure; but creatinine clearance, preferably over 24 hours, is needed to demonstrate lesser infringements of renal function. The same measure is needed to chart the progress of renal disease, and to assist in the detection of transplant rejection. Serial measures of the serum creatinine concentration are useful in monitoring the effect of dialysis, and are to be preferred to the plasma urea concentration, as being less influenced by changes in the protein content of the diet, or in tissue catabolism. In view of the prevelance of bone disease in patients on maintenance dialysis, plasma calcium and phosphate concentrations, and alkaline phosphatase activity should also be regularly determined. In addition to their central role in the quantitation of renal insufficiency, biochemical tests are crucial in the detection of unsuspected renal disease; in the investigation of tubular syndromes and of polyuria; in the investigation of endocrine and other forms of hypertension; and in the characterization of renal osteodystrophy. These applications have been detailed in the preceding sections.

While renal units vary in their selection of tests, there is merit in having a standard scheme, for the routine testing of renal function. One such scheme for comprehensive one-day testing is set out by Györy et al. (1974).

REFERENCES

Addis, T., Barrett, E., Poo, L.J., Ureen, H.J. and Lippman, R.W. (1951) The relation between protein consumption and diurnal variations of the endogenous creatinine clearance in normal individuals. Journal of Clinical Investigation, 30, 206–209.

Aoki, S., Imamura, S., Aoki, M. and McCabe, W.R. (1969) Abacterial and bacterial pyelonephritis. Immunofluorescent localisation of bacterial antigen. New England Journal of Medicine, 281, 1375–1382.

Arakawa, K., Masaki, Z., Oside, Y., Yamada, J. and Momose, S. (1973) Divided renal and peripheral venous renin as a means of predicting operative curability of renal hypertension. Clinical Science and Molecular Medicine, 45, 311s–314s.

Arrant, B.S. Edelmann, C.M. and Spitzer, A. (1971) The congruence of creatinine and inulin clearances in children: use of the Technicon AutoAnalyser. Journal of Pediatrics, 81, 559–561.

Arturson, G., Groth, T. and Grotte, G. (1971) Human glomerular membrane porosity and filtration pressure: dextran clearance analysed by theoretical models. Clinical Science, 40, 137–158.

AutoTechnicon Manual (1963) AutoAnalyzer methodology. File NIIa. (Ed. Chancey) Technicon Instrument Corporation, New York.

Bailey, R.R. (1973) The relationship of vesico-ureteric reflux to urinary tract infection and chronic pyelonephritis – reflux nephropathy. Clinical Nephrology, 1, 132–141.

Baldwin, D.S. (1977) Poststreptococcal glomerulonephritis. A progressive disease. American Journal of Medicine, 62, 1–11.

Bangham, D.R., Robertson, I., Robertson, J.I.S., Robinson, C.T. and Tree, M. (1975) An international collaborative study of renin assay; establishment of the international reference preparation of human renin. Clinical Science and Molecular Medicine, 48, Suppl. 2, 135s–159s.

Barger, A.C. and Herd, J.A. (1971) The renal circulation. New England Journal of Medicine, 284, 482–490.

Barratt, T.M. and Chantler, C. (1975) Clinical assessment of renal function. In Paediatric Nephrology (Eds. Rubin, M.I. and Barratt, T.M.) pp. 55–83. Williams and Wilkins, Baltimore.

Barratt, T.M. and Crawford, R. (1970) Lysozyme excretion as a measure of renal tubular dysfunction in children. Clinical Science, 39, 457–465.

Barzel, U.S., Sperling, O., Frank, M. and de Vries, A. (1964) Renal ammonium excretion and urinary pH in idiopathic uric acid lithiasis. Journal of Urology, 92, 1–5.

Beardwell, C.G. (1971) Radioimmunoassay of arginine vasopressin in human plasma. Journal of Clinical Endocrinology and Metabolism. 33, 254–260.

Beevers, D.G., Brosn, J.J., Fraser, R., Lever, A.F., Morton, J.J., Robertson, J.I.S., Semple, P.F. and Tree, M. (1975) The clinical value of renin and angiotensin estimations. Kidney International, Suppl., S181–201.

Bennett, W.M. and Porter, G.A. (1971) Endogenous creatinine clearance as a clinical measure of glomerular filtration rate. British Medical Journal, 4, 84–86.

Berggard, I. and Bearn, A.G. (1968) Isolation and properties of a low-molecular weight β_2-globulin occuring in human biological fluids. Journal of Biological Chemistry, 243, 4095–4103.

Berliner, R.W. and Bennett, C.M. (1967) Concentration of urine in the mammalian kidney. American Journal of Medicine, 43, 777–789.

Berlyne, G.M., Varley, H., Nilwarangkur, S. and Hoerni, M. (1965) Endogenous-creatinine clearance and glomerular-filtration rate. Lancet, ii, 874–876.

Bijvoet, O.L.M. (1969) Relationship of plasma phosphate concentration to tubular reabsorption of phosphate. Clinical Science, 37, 23–36.

Black, D.A.K. (1965) Renal rate mirabile. Lancet, ii, 1141–1151.

Black, D.A.K. (1967) Mechanisms of urinary concentration. In Renal Disease, 2nd edn. Chap. 4, Blackwell Scientific Publications, Oxford.

Black, D.A.K. (1974) Limited role of steroids in managing the nephrotic syndrome. In Controversy in Internal Medicine, 2nd edn. (Eds. F.J. Ingelfinger, R.V. Ebert, M. Finland and A.S. Relman) Saunders, Philadelphia.

Black, J.A. (1965) Detection of renal insufficiency in children. Journal of Clinical Pathology, 18, 546–549.

Bonsnes, R.W. and Taussky, K.K. (1945) On the colorimetric determination of creatinine by the Jaffé reaction. Journal of Biological Chemistry, 158, 581–591.

Boyarsky, S. and Smith, H.W. (1957) Renal concentrating operation at low urine flows. Journal of Urology, 78, 511–524.

Breckenridge, A. and Metcalfe-Gibson, A. (1965) Methods of measuring glomerular filtration rate. A comparison of inulin, vitamin B12 and creatinine clearances. Lancet, ii, 265–276.

Brenner, B.M. and Rector, F.C. (1976) The Kidney, Vol. 1. Saunders, Philadelphia.

Bricker, N.S., Klahr, S. and Lubowitz, H. (1972) The kidney in chronic renal disease. In Clinical Disorders of Fluid and Electrolyte Metabolism, 2nd edn. (Eds. M.H. Maxwell and C.R. Kleeman) McGraw-Hill,, New York.

Bricker, N.S. (1967) Obstructive nephropathy. In Renal Disease, 2nd edn. (Ed. D.A.K. Black) Blackwell Scientific Publication, Oxford.

Brod, J. and Sirota, J.H. (1948) Renal clearance of endogenous creatinine in man. Journal of Clinical Investigation, 27, 645–654.

Brodehl, J. and Bickel, H. (1973) Aminoaciduria and hyperaminoaciduria in childhood. Clinical Nephrology, 1, 149–168.

Brown, J.J., Davies, D.L., Lever, A.F. and Robertson, J.I.S. (1964) The estimation of renin in human plasma. Biochemical Journal, 93, 594–600.

Brown, J.J., Fraser, R., Lever, A.F., Morton, J.J., Robertson, J.I.S., Tree, M., Bell, P.R.F., Davidson, J.K. and Ruthven, I.S. (1973) Hypertension and secondary hyperaldosteronism associated with a renin-secreting juxta-glomerular cell tumour. Lancet, ii, 1228–1231.

Brun, C., Crone, C., Davidson, H.G., Fabricius, J., Hansen, A.T., Lassen, N.A. and Munck, O. (1955) Renal blood-flow in anuric human subjects determined by use of radioactive krypton 85. Proceedings of the Society for Experimental Biology and Medicine, N.Y., 89, 687–690.

Bunge, G. (1873) Uber die bedeutung des kochsalzes und das verhalten der kalisalze im menschlichen organismus. Zeitschrift für Biologie, 9, 104–143.

Burg, M.B. and Green, N. (1973) Function of the thick ascending limb of Henle's loop. American Journal of Physiology, 224, 659–668.

Burg, M.B. and Orloff, J. (1970) Electrical potential differences across proximal convoluted tubules. American Journal of Physiology, 219, 1714–1716.

Calcagno, P.L. and Rubin, M.I. (1963) Renal extraction of PAH in infants and children. Journal of Clinical Investigation, 42, 1632–1639.

Camara, A.A., Arn, K.D., Reimer, A. and Newburgh, L.H. (1951) The 24 hour creatinine clearance as a means of determining the state of the kidney. Journal of Laboratory and Clinical Medicine, 37, 743–763.

Cameron, J.S. (1979) Natural history of glomerulonephritis. In Renal Disease, 4th edn. (Ed. D.A.K. Black and N.F. Jones) Blackwell Scientific Publications, Oxford.

Cameron, J.S., Maisy, M.N. and Ogg, C.S. (1970) Creatinine clearance in patients with proteinuria, Lancet, i, 424–425.

Cameron, J.S. and Simmonds, H.A. (1976) Uric acid and the kidney. In 12th Conference in Advanced Medicine (Ed. D.K. Peters) Pitman Medical, London.

Chantler, C. (1971) M.D. Thesis, University of Cambridge.

Chantler, C. and Barratt, T.M. (1972) Estimation of the glomerular filtration rate from the plasma clearance of 51 chromium edetic acid. Archives of Disease in Childhood, 47, 613–617.

Chantler, C., Garnett, E.S., Parsons, V. and Veall, N. (1969) Glomerular filtration rate measurement in man by the single injection method using ^{51}Cr-EDTA. Clinical Science, 37, 169–180.

Chapman, E.M. and Halstead, J.A. (1933) The fractional phenolsulphonephthalein test in Bright's disease. American Journal of Medical Sciences, 186, 223–232.

Chopra, J.S., Mallick, N.P. and Stone, M.C. (1971) Hyperlipoproteinaemias in the nephrotic syndrome. Lancet, i, 317–320.

Clarkson, A.R., MacDonald, M.K., Cash, J.D. and Robson, J.S. (1971) Serum and urinary fibrin/fibrinogen degradation products in glomerulo-nephritis. British Medical Journal, 3, 255–260.

Cockroft, D. and Gault, M.K. (1976) Prediction of creatinine clearance from serum creatinine. Nephron, 16, 31–41.

Cohen, B.D., Stein, I.M. and Bones. J.E. (1968) Guanidinosuccinic aciduria in uraemia. A possible alternate pathway for urea synthesis. American Journal of Medicine, 45, 63–68.

Cohen, M.L., Patel, J.K. and Baxter, D.L. (1971) External monitoring and plasma disappearance for the determination of renal function: comparison of effective renal plasma flow and glomerular filtration rate. Paediatrics, 48, 377–392.

Cohen, M.L., Smith, F.G., Mindell, R.S. and Vernier, R.L. (1969) A simple reliable method of measuring glomerular filtration rate using low dose sodium iothalamate ^{131}I. Pediatrics, 43, 407–415.

Cole, B.R., Giangiacomo, J., Ingelfinger, J.R. and Robson, A.M. (1972) Measurement of renal function without urine collection. Evaluation of the constant infusion technique for determination of inulin and PAH clearances. New England Journal of Medicine, 287, 1109–1114.

Cook, J.G.H. (1975) Technical Bulletin No. 36. Factors influencing the assay of creatinine. Annals of Clinical Biochemistry, 12, 219–232.

Danovitch, G.M., Weinberger, J. and Berlyne, G.M. (1972) Uric acid in advanced renal failure. Clinical Science, 43, 331–341.

Darmady, E.M., Offer, J. and Woodhouse, M.A. (1973) The parameters of the ageing kidney. Journal of Pathology, 109, 195–207.

Davies, D.P. and Saunders, R. (1973) Blood urea: normal values in early infancy related to feeding practices. Archives of Disease in Childhood, 48, 563–565.

Davies, D.F. and Shock, N.W. (1950) The variation of measurement of inulin and diodrast tests of kidney function. Journal of Clinical Investigation, 29, 491–495.

Davison, A.M., Thorson, D., MacDonald, M.K., Rae, J.K., Uttley, W.S. and Clarkson, A.R. (1973) Identification of intrarenal fibrin deposition. Journal of Clinical Pathology, 26, 102–112.

Dawborn, J.K. (1965) Application of Hevrovsk's inulin method to automatic analysis. Clinica Chimica Acta, 12, 63–66.

Dent, C.E. (1947) The aminoaciduria of the Fanconi syndrome. A study making extensive use of techniques based on paper partition chromatography. Biochemical Journal, 41, 240–253.

DeLuca, H.F. (1974) Vitamin D – 1973. American Journal of Medicine, 57, 1–12.

Diamond, J.M. (1965) The mechanism of isotonic water absorption and secretion. Symposium of the Society for Experimental Biology, 19, 329–347.

Dicker, S.E. (1970) Mechanisms of Urine Concentration and Dilution in Animals. Arnold, London.

Ditzel, J. and Junker, K. (1972) Abnormal glomerular filtration rate, renal plasma flow, and renal protein excretion in recent and short-term diabetics. British Medical Journal, 1, 13–19.

Ditzel, J., Vestergaard, P. and Brinkløv, M. (1972) Glomerular filtration rate determined by ^{51}Cr EDTA complex. Scandinavian Journal of Urology and Nephrology, 6, 166–170.

Dodge, W.F., Travis, L.B. and Daeschner, C.W. (1967) Comparison of endogenous creatinine clearance with inulin clearance. American Journal of Disease in Childhood, 113, 683–692.

Donaldson, I.M.C. (1968) Comparison of the renal clearance of inulin and radioactive diatrizoate ("Hypaque") as measures of the glomerular filtration rate in man. Clinical Science, 35, 513–524.

Doolan, P.D., Alben, E.L. and Theil, G.B. (1962) A clinical appraisal of the plasma concentration and endogenous clearance of creatinine. American Journal of Medicine, 32, 65–79.

Dormandy, T. (1967) Osmometry. Lancet, i, 267–270.

Dossetor, J.B. (1966) Creatinemia versus uremia. Annals of Internal Medicine, 65, 1287–1299.

Dubach, U.C., Metz, I. and Schmid, P. (1967) Serum Kreatininwerte bei 2258 arbeitstatigen Personen verschiedenen Alters und Geschlechts. Klinicheskaya Meditsina (Moskva), 5, 621–629.

Edelmann, C.M. (1967) Maturation of the neonatal kidney. In Proceedings of the 3rd International Congress of Nephrology, Vol. 3, Washington, 1966. p. 1, Karger, Basel.

Edelmann, C.M. (1973) Paediatric nephrology. E. Mead Johnson Award Address, 1972. Pediatrics, 51, 854–865.

Edelmann, C.M., Barnett, H.L., Stark, H., Boichis, H. and Soriano, J.R. (1967) A standardised test of renal concentrating capacity in children. American Journal of Diseases of Children, 114, 639–644.

Edelmann, C.M., Barnett, H.L. and Stark, H. (1966) Effect of urea on concentration of urinary non-urea solute in premature infants. Journal of Applied Physiology, 21, 1021–1025.

Edelmann, C.M., Boichis, H., Soriano, J.R. and Stark, H. (1967a) The renal response of children to acute ammonium chloride acidosis. Pediatric Research, 1, 452–460.

Edelmann, C.M., Soriano, J.R., Boichis, H., Gruskin, A. and Aosta, M. (1967b) Renal bicarbonate reabsorption and hydrogen ion excretion in normal infants. Journal of Clinical Investigation, 46, 1309–1317.

Edwards, O.M., Bayliss, R.I.S. and Millen, S. (1969) Urinary creatinine excretion as an index of the completeness of 24 hour urine collections. Lancet, ii, 1165–1166.

Edwards, K.D.G. and Whyte, H.M. (1959) The measurement of creatinine in plasma and urine. Australian Journal of Experimental Biology and Medical Science, 36, 383–394.

Edwards, K.D.G. and Whyte, H.M. (1969) Plasma creatinine level and creatinine clearance as tests of renal function. Australian Annals of Medicine, 8, 218–224.

Ekert, H., Barratt, T.M., Chantler, C. and Turner, M.W. (1972) Immunologically reactive equivalent of fibrinogen in serum and urine of children with renal disease. Archives of Disease in Childhood, 47, 90–96.

Eliahou, H.E. and Bata, A. (1965) The diagnosis of acute renal failure. Nephron, 2, 287–295.

Enger, E. and Blegen, E.M. (1964) The relationship between endogenous creatinine clearance and serum creatinine in renal failure. Scandinavian Journal of Clinical Laboratory Investigation, 16, 273–280.

Fahmy, A.R., Niederwieser, A., Pataki, G. and Breener, M. (1961) Dunnschicht-Chromatographie von Aminosauren auf Kieselgel. G. Helvetica Chimica Acta, 44, 2022–2026.

Farmer, C.D., Tauxe, W.N., Maher, F.T. and Hunt, J.C. (1967) Measurement of renal function with radio-iodinated diatrizoate and *o*-iodohippurate. American Journal of Clinical Pathology, 47, 9–16.

Favré, H.R. and Wing, A.J. (1968) Simultaneous ^{51}Cr edetic acid, inulin and endogenous creatinine clearances in 20 patients with renal disease. British Medical Journal, 1, 84–86.

Ferriss, J.B., Brown, J.J., Fraser, R., Kay, A.W., Lever, A.F., Neville, A.M., O'Muircheartaigh, I.G., Robertson, J.I.S. and Symington, T. (1970) Hypertension with aldosterone excess and low plasma-renin: preoperative distinction between patients with and without adrenocortical tumour. Lancet, ii, 995–1000.

Fisher, M. and Veall, N. (1975) Glomerular filtration rate estimation based on a single blood sample. British Medical Journal, 2, 542.

Frimpter, G.W. (1973) Aminoacidurias due to inherited disorders of metabolism. New England Journal of Medicine, 289, 835–841 and 895–901.

Fressinaud, P., Corvol, P. and Menard, J. (1974) Radioimmunoassay of urinary antidiuretic hormone in man: stimulation-suppression tests. Kidney International, 6, 184–190.

Galambos, J.T., Herndon, E.G. and Reynolds, G.H. (1964) Specific gravity determination. Fact or fancy? New England Journal of Medicine, 270, 506–508.

Gardiner, K.D. (1976) Cystic Diseases of the Kidney. John Wiley, New York.

Gault, M.H., Kinsella, T.D., Gonda, A. and Gerguson, G.A. (1966) The plasma phenolsulphonaphthalein index (PSPI) of renal function. II. Correlation with other parameters of renal function and indications for use. Canadian Medical Association Journal, 94, 68–71.

Gell, P.G.H. and Coombs, R.R.A. (1968) Clinical Aspects of Immunology, 2nd edn. Blackwell Scientific Publications, Oxford.

Germuth, F.G. and Rodriguez, E. (1973) The Immunopathology of the Human Glomerulus. Little and Brown, Boston.

Giebisch, G. and Windhager, E.E. (1964) Renal tubular transfer of sodium, chloride and potassium. American Journal of Medicine, 36, 643–669.

Giovannetti, S., Balestri, P.L. and Barsotti, G. (1973) Methylguanidine in uremia. Archives of Internal Medicine, 131, 709–713.

Goldman, R. and Moss, J. (1959) Synthesis of creatine in nephrectomised rats. American Journal of Physiology, 197, 865–868.

Goldman, R., Yadley, R.A. and Nourok, D.S. (1967) Comparison of endogenous and exogenous creatinine clearances in man. Proceedings of the Society of Experimental Biology and Medicine, 125, 205–210.

Gordillo-Paniagua, G., Velasquez-Jones, L. (1976) Acute renal failure. Pediatric Clinics of North America, 23, 817–828.

Gordon, A., DePalma, J.R. and Maxwell, M.H. (1972) Water, electrolyte and acid–base disorders associated with acute and chronic dialysis. In Clinical Disorders of Fluid and Electrolyte Metabolism, 2nd edn. (Eds. M.H. Maxwell and C.R. Kleeman), McGraw-Hill, New York.

Graystone, J.E. (1968) Creatinine excretion during growth. In Human Growth (Ed. D.B. Chek) pp. 182–197, Lea and Febiger, Philadelphia.

Györy, A.Z., Edwards, K.D.G., Stewart, J.H. and Whyte, H.M. (1974) Comprehensive one day renal function testing in man. Journal of Clinical Pathology, 27, 382–391.

Hagstam, K.E., Nordenfelt, I., Svensson, L. and Svensson, S.E. (1974) Comparison of different methods for determination of glomerular filtration rate in renal disease. Scandinavian Journal of Clinical Laboratory Investigation, 34, 31–36.

Hall, C.L., Pejhan, N., Terry, J.M. and Blainey, J.D. (1975) Urinary fibrin-fibrinogen degradation products in nephrotic syndrome. British Medical Journal, 1, 419–422.

Hardwicke, J. (1970) Proteinuria. Scientific Basis of Medicine. Annual Reviews, 10, 211–229.

Hare, R.S. (1950) Endogenous creatinine in serum and urine. Proceedings of the Society for Experimental Biology and Medicine, N.Y., 74, 148–151.

Harries, J.D., Mildenberger, R.R., Malowany, A.S. and Drummond, K.N. (1972) A computerised cumulative integral method for the precise measurement of the glomerular filtration rate. Proceedings of the Society for Experimental Biology and Medicine, N.Y., 140, 1148–1155.

Harrison, J.F., Lunt, G.S., Scott, P. and Blainey, J.D. (1968) Urinary lysozyme, ribonuclease and low-molecular-weight protein in renal disease. Lancet, i, 371–374.

Harvey, A.M., Malvin, R.L. and Vander, A.J. (1966) Comparison of creatinine secretion in men and women. Nephron, 3, 201–205.

Hatfield, P.J. and Simmonds, H.A. (1974) Uric acid and the kidney-current concepts. Guy's Hospital Reports, 123, 271–297.

Haugen, H.N. and Blegen, E.M. (1953) The true endogenous creatinine clearance. Scandinavian Journal of Clinical Laboratory Medicine, 5, 67–71.

Healy, J.K. (1968) Clinical assessment of glomerular filtration rate by different forms of creatinine clearance and a modifed urinary phenolsulphonphthalein excretion test. American Journal of Medicine, 44, 348–358.

Heath, D.A., Knapp, M.S. and Walker, W.H.C. (1968) Comparison between inulin and ^{51}Cr-labelled edetic acid for the measurement of glomerular filtration rate. Lancet, ii, 1110–1112.

Heptinstall, R.H. (1967) The limitations of the pathological diagnosis of chronic pyelonephritis. In Renal Disease, 2nd edn. (Ed. D.A.K. Black) Blackwell Scientific Publications, Oxford.

Heptinstall, R.H. (1974) Pathology of the Kidney, 2nd edn. Little, Brown and Co., Boston.

Hilton, P.J., Lavender, S., Roth, Z. and Jones, N.F. (1969) Creatinine clearance in patients with proteinuria. Lancet, ii, 1215–1216.

Hopper, J., Jr. (1951) Creatinine clearance. A simple way of measuring renal function. Quoted in Wesson (1969) (see later).

Husdan, H. and Rapaport, A. (1968) Estimation of creatinine by the Jaffé reaction. Clinical Chemistry, 14, 222–238.

Isaacson, L.C. (1960) Urinary osmolarity in thirsting normal subjects. Lancet, i, 467–468.

Jones, J.D. and Burnett, P.C. (1974) Creatinine metabolism in humans with decreased renal function: creatinine deficit. Clinical Chemistry, 20, 1204–1212.

Josephson, B. (1963) The clinical value of the "apparent" serum creatinine concentration. Scandinavian Journal of Clinical Laboratory Investigation, Suppl. 69, 121–129.

Kampmann, J., Siersbaek-Nielsen, K., Kristensen, M. and Hansen, J.M. (1974) Rapid evaluation of creatinine clearance. Acta Medica Scandinavica, 196, 517–520.

Kassirer, J.P. (1971a) Clinical evaluation of kidney function – glomerular function. New England Journal of Medicine, 285, 385–389.

Kassirer, J.P. (1971b) Clinical evaluation of kidney function – tubular function. New England Journal of Medicine, 285, 499–502.

Kerr, D.N.S. (1979) Acute renal failure. In Renal Disease, 4th edn. (Eds. D.A.K. Black and N.F. Jones) Blackwell Scientific Publications, Oxford.

Kim, K.E., Onesti, G., Ramirez, O., Brest, A.N. and Swartz, C. (1969) Creatinine clearance in renal disease. A reappraisal. British Medical Journal, 4, 11–14.

Kodicek, E., Lawson, D.E.M. and Wilson, P.W. (1970) Biological activity of a polar metabolite of Vitamin D_3. Nature (London), 228, 763–764.

Kranes, S.M. (1972) Renal glycosuria. In The Metabolic Basis of Inherited Disease, 3rd edn. (Eds. J.D. Stanbury, J.B. Wyngaarden and D.B. Fredrickson), McGraw-Hill, New York.

Lant, A.F. and Wilson, G.M. (1972) Diuretics. In Renal Disease, 3rd edn. (Ed. D.A.K. Black) p. 591, Blackwell, Oxford.

Lancet Editorial (1970) Plasma-phosphate and tubular reabsorption of phosphate, Lancet, i, 820–822.

Lavender, S., Hilton, P.J. and Jones, N.R. (1969) The measurement of glomerular filtration-rate in renal disease. Lancet, ii, 1216–1219.

Lewis, W.H., Jr. and Alving, A.S. (1938) Changes with age in the renal function in adult men. American Journal of Physiology, 123, 500–515.

Luke, R.G., Briggs, J.D., Allison, M.E. and Kennedy, A.C. (1970) Factors determining response to mannitol in acute renal failure. American Journal of Medical Science, 259, 168–174.

Luke, R.G., Linton, A.L., Briggs, J.D. and Kennedy, A.C. (1965) Mannitol therapy in acute renal failure. Lancet, i, 980–982.

Mabry, C.C. and Todd, W.R. (1963) Quantitative measurement of individual and total free amino-acids in urine. Rapid method employing high voltage paper electrophoresis and direct densitometry and its application to the urinary excretions of amino-acids in normal subjects. Journal of Laboratory and Clinical Medicine, 61, 146–157.

Maisey, M.N., Ogg, C.S. and Cameron, J.S. (1969) Measuring glomerular filtration-rate, Lancet, i, 733.

Mandel, E.E., Jones, F.L., Wills, M.J. and Cargill, W.H. (1953) Renal excretion of creatinine and inulin in man. Journal of Laboratory and Clinical Medicine, 42, 621–637.

Masarei, J.R.L. (1975) Validity of corrections for creatinine excretion and creatinine clearance. New Zealand Medical Journal, 82, 197–198.

McCance, R.A. and Hatemi, N. (1961) Control of acid–base stability in the newly born. Lancet, i, 293–297.

McGiff, J.L., Crowshaw, K., Terraguo, N.A. and Lonigro, A.J. (1971) Renal prostaglandins: their biosynthesis, release, effects and fate. In Renal Pharmacology (Eds. J.W. Fisher and E.J. Cafruny) Butterworths, London.

Metcoff, J. (1975) Metabolic and enzymatic features of the kidney In Pediatric Nephrology (Eds. M.I. Rubin and T.M. Barratt) pp. 41–54, Williams and Wilkins, Baltimore.

Miles, B.E., Paton, A. and De Wardener, H.E. (1954) Maximum urine concentration. British Medical Journal, 2, 901–905.

Miller, B.F. and Dubos, R. (1937) Determination by a specific enzymatic method of the creatinine content of blood and urine from normal and nephritic individuals. Journal of Biological Chemistry, 121, 457–464.

Miller, B.F., Leaf, A. and Mamby, A.R. (1952) Validity of the endogenous creatinine clearance as a measure of glomerular filtration rate in the diseased human kidney. Journal of Clinical Investigation, 31, 309–313.

Milne, M.D., Scribner, B.H. and Crawford, M.A. (1958) Non-ionic diffusion, and the excretion of weak acids and bases. American Journal of Medicine, 24, 709–729.

Moore, S. and Stein, W.H. (1954) Procedures for the chromatographic determination of amino acids on four percent cross-linked sulfonated polystyrene resins. Journal of Biological Chemistry, 21, 893–906.

Morris, R.C. (1969) Renal tubular acidosis. Mechanisms, classification and implications. New England Journal of Medicine, 281, 1405–1413.

Morrison, R.B.I. (1979) Urinalysis and assessment of renal function. In Renal Diseases, 4th edn. (Eds. D.A. K. Black and N.F. Jones) Blackwell Scientific Publications, Oxford.

Morton, J.J., Waite, M.A., Brown, J.J., Lever, A.F. and Robertson, J.I.S. (1975) The estimation of angiotensin I and II in the human circulation by radioimmunoassay. In Hormones in Human Plasma (Ed. H.N. Antenaides) Excerpta Medica, Amsterdam.

Muldowney, F.P., Carroll, D.V., Donohoe, J.F. and Freaney, R. (1971) Correction of renal bicarbonate wastage by parathyroidectomy. Implications in acid–base homeostasis. Quarterly Journal of Medicine, 40, 487–498.

Naish, P., Evans, D.J. and Peters, D.K. (1974) Urinary fibrinogen derivative excretion and intraglomeruler fibrin deposition in glomerulonephritis. British Medical Journal, 1, 544–546.

Nanra, R.S., Clyne, D. and Kincaid-Smith, P. (1969) The use of the modified PSP excretion test in the clinical management of patients with renal allografts. Medical Journal of Australia, 1, 1083–1087.

Nordin, B.E.C. and Fraser, R. (1960) Assessment of urinary phosphate excretion. Lancet, i, 947–950.

Nordin, B.E.C. and Hodgkinson, A. (1973) Urinary tract calculi. In Renal Disease, 3rd edn. (Ed. D.A.K. Black) p. 759, Blackwell Scientific Publications, Oxford.

Pak Poy, R.K. (1965) Urinary pH in gout. Australian Annals of Medicine, 14, 35–39.

Papper, S. (1973) The effects of age in reducing renal function. Geriatrics, 28, 83–87.

Peart, W.S. (1972) Hypertension and the kidney. In Renal Disease, 3rd edn. (Ed. D.A.K. Black) Blackwell Scientific Publications, Oxford.

Penington, D.G. (1972) Haematological changes in renal disease. In Renal Disease, 3rd edn. (Ed. D.A.K. Black) Blackwell Scientific Publications, Oxford.

Peters, D.K. (1974) The immunological basis of glomerulonephritis. Proceedings of the Royal Society of Medicine, 67, 557–562.

Peters, D.K., Charlesworth, J.A., Lachmann, P.J. and Williams, D.G. (1973) Mechanisms of C3 breakdown by hypocomplementaemic serum from patients with mesangiocapillary nephritis. In Protides of the Biological Fluids (Ed. H. Peeters), Pergamon Press, Oxford.

Pierro, A. and Johnson, R.E. (1970) Creatinine excretion. Lancet, i, 784.

Pitts, R.F. (1964) Renal production and excretion of ammonia. American Journal of Medicine, 36, 720–742.

Popper, H. and Mandel, E. (1937) Filtrations und resorptionsleistrung in der nierenpathologie. Ergebnisse der Inneren Medizin, Kinderheilk, 53, 685–794.

Porter, G.A., Kloster, F.E., Herr, R.J., Starr, A., Griswold, H.E., Kimsey, J. and Lenertz, H. (1966) Relationship between alterations in renal hemodynamics during cardiopulmonary bypass and postoperative renal function. Circulation, 34, 1005–1021.

Rapaport, A. and Husdan, H. (1968) Endogenous creatinine clearance and serum creatinine in the clinical assessment of kidney function. Canadian Medical Associations Journal, 98, 149–156.

Rector, F.C. (1976) Acidification and ammonia production; chemistry of weak acids and bases; buffer mechanisms. In The Kidney (Eds. B. Brenner and F.C. Rector) pp. 318–343, W.B. Saunders, Philadelphia.

Relman, A.S. and Levinsky, N.G. (1971) Clinical examination of renal function. In Diseases of the Kidney, 2nd edn. (Eds. M.B. Strauss and L.G. West) Little Brown and Co., Boston.

Robinson, J.R. (1972a) Principles of renal physiology. In Renal Disease, 3rd edn. (Ed. D.A.K. Black), Blackwell Scientific Publications, Oxford.

Robinson, J.R. (1972b) Fundamentals of Acid–Base Balance, 4th edn. Blackwell Scientific Publications, Oxford.

Robinson, R.R. (1972) Clinical significance of proteinuria in asymptomatic patients. Proceedings of the 5th International Congress on Nephrology, 3, 27–33.

Robson, J.S., Ferguson, M.H., Olbrich, O. and Stewart, C.P. (1949) The determination of the renal clearance of inulin in man. Quarterly Journal of Experimental Physiology, 35, 111–134.

Robson, J.S. (1972) The nephrotic syndrome. In Renal Disease, 3rd edn. (Ed. D.A.K. Black) Blackwell Scientific Publications, Oxford.

Rodriguez-Soriano, J. and Edelmann, C.M. (1969) Renal tubular acidosis. Annual Review of Medicine, 20, 363–382.

Roscoe, M.H. (1958) Plasma chromogen and the endogenous creatinine clearance. Journal of Clinical Pathology, 11, 173–176.

Rose, G.A. and Durbin, H. (1967) Measuring glomerular filtration-rate. Lancet, ii, 159.

Rose, G.A. (1969) Measurement of glomerular filtration rate by inulin clearance without urine collection. British Medical Journal, 2, 91–93.

Rosenbaum, J.L. (1970) Evaluation of clearance studies in chronic kidney disease. Journal of Chronic Disease, 22, 507–514.

Rowe, J.W., Shock, N.W., DeFronzo, R.A. (1976a) The influence of age on the renal response to water deprivation in man. Nephron, 17, 270–278.

Rowe, J.W., Andres, R., Tobin, J.D., Norris, A.H., Shock, N.W. (1976b) Age-adjusted standards for creatinine clearance. Annals of Internal Medicine, 84, 567–568.

Schainuck, L.I., Striker, G.E., Cutler, R.E. and Bendit, E.P. (1970) Structural–functional correlations in renal disease. II: The correlations. Human Pathology, 1, 631–641.

Schambelan, M., Glickman, M., Stockigt, J.R. and Biglieri, E.G. (1974) Selective renal-vein renin sampling in hypertensive patients with segmented renal lesions. New England Journal of Medicine, 290, 1153–1157.

Schirmeister, J., Willmann, H., Kiefer, M. and Kallauer, W. (1964) Fur und wider die Brauchbarkeit der endogenen kreatinin-clearance in der funktionellen Nierendiagnostik. Deutsche Medizinische Wochenschrift, 89, 1640–1647.

Schoen, E.J. (1957) Minimum urine total solute concentration in response to water loading in normal men. Journal of Applied Physiology, 10, 267–270.

Scott, P.J. and Hurley, P.J. (1968) Demonstration of individual variation in constancy of 24-hour urinary creatinine excretion. Clinica Chimica Acta, 21, 411–414.

Shannon, J.A. and Smith, H.W. (1935) The excretion of inulin, xylose and urea in normal and phlorizinized man. Journal of Clinical Investigation, 14, 393–401.

Shannon, J.A. (1935) The renal excretion of creatinine in man. Journal of Clinical Investigation, 14, 403–410.

Shock, N.W. (1946) Kidney function tests in aged males. Geriatrics, 1, 232–239.

Siersbaek-Nielsen, K., Mølholm Hansen, J., Kampmann, J. and Kirstensen, M. (1971) Rapid evaluation of creatinine clearance. Lancet, i, 1133–1134.

Sigman, E.M., Elwood, C.M. and Knox, F. (1966) The measurement of glomerular filtration rate in man with sodium iothalamate ^{131}I (Conray). Journal of Nuclear Medicine, 7, 60–68.

Silkalns, G.I., Jeck, D., Earon, J., Edelmann, C.M., Chervu, L.R., Blaufox, M.D. and Spitzer, A. (1973) Simultaneous measurement of glomerular filtration rate and renal plasma flow using plasma disappearance curves. Journal of Pediatrics, 83, 749–757.

Sirota, J.H., Baldwin, D.S. and Villarreal, H. (1950) Diurnal variations in renal function in man. Journal of Clinical Investigation, 29, 187–192.

Slatopolsky, E. and Bricker, N.S. (1973) The role of phosphorus restriction in the prevention of secondary hyperparathyroidism in chronic renal disease. Kidney International, 4, 141–145.

Smart, G.A. (1973) In Price's Textbook of the Practice of Medicine, 11th edn. (Ed. R. Bodley Scott) pp. 491–493, Oxford University Press, London.

Smith, H.W. (1951) The Kidney: Structure and Function in Health and in Disease. Oxford University Press, New York.

Smith, H.W. Finkelstein, N., Aliminosa, L., Crawford, B. and Graber, M. (1945) Renal clearance of substituted hippuric acid derivatives and other aromatic acids in dog and man. Journal of Clinical Investigation, 24, 388–404.

Smith, H.W., Goldring, W. and Chasis, H. (1938) The measurement of the tubular excretory mass, effective blood flow and filtration rate in the normal human kidney. Journal of Clinical Investigation, 17, 263–278.

Smith, H.W., Goldring, W., Chasis, H., Ranger, H.A. and Bradley, S.E. (1943) The application of saturation methods to the study of glomerular and tubular function in the human kidney. Journal of Mount Sinai Hospital, 10, 59–108.

Sørensen, L.B. (1960) The elimination of uric acid in man studied by means of C14-labelled uric acid. Uricolysis. Scandinavian Journal of Clinical Laboratory Investigation, 12, Suppl. 54, 1–214.

Soriano, J.R., Boichis, H., Stark, H. and Edelmann, C.M. (1967) Proximal renal tubular acidosis. A defect in bicarbonate reabsorption with normal urinary acidification. Pediatric Research, 1, 81–98.

Stacey, B.D. and Thorburn, G.D. (1966) Chromium-51 ethylenediamine tetraacetate for estimation of glomerular filtration rate. Science, 152, 1076–1077.

Stanbury, J.B., Wyngaarden, J.B. and Fredericksen, D.S. (1972) The Metabolic Basis of Inherited Disease, 3rd edn. McGraw-Hill, New York.

Stockigt, J.R., Collins, R.D., Noakes, C.A., Schambelan, M. and Biglieri, E.G. (1972) Renal-vein renin in various forms of renal hypertension. Lancet, i, 1194–1198.

Thalassinos, N.C., Leese, B., Latham, S.C. and Joplin, G.F. (1970) Urinary excretion of phosphate in normal children. Archives of Disease in Childhood, 45, 269–272.

Tobias, G.J., McLaughlin, R.F. and Hopper, J. (1962) Endogenous creatinine clearance. A valuable clinical test of glomerular filtration and a prognostic guide in chronic renal disease. New England Journal of Medicine, 266, 317–323.

Van Es, L.A., Blok, R.P., Schoenfeld, L., Glassock, R.J. (1977) Chronic nephritis induced by antibodies reacting with glomerular-bound immune complexes. Kidney International, 11, 106–115.

Van Pilsum, J.F. and Seljeskog, E.L. (1958) Long term endogenous creatinine clearance in man. Proceedings of the Society for Experimental Biology and Medicine (N.Y.), 97, 270–272.

Verger, D., Leroux-Robert, C., Ganter, P. and Richet, G. (1967) Les tophus goutteux de la medullaire renale des uremiques chroniques. Etude de 17 cas decouvertes au cours de 62 autopsies. Nephron, 4, 356–370.

Walser, M. and Bodenlos, L.J. (1959) Urea metabolism in man. Journal of Clinical Investigation, 38, 1617–1626.

Walton, R.J., Bijvoet, O.L.M. (1975) Nomogram for derivation of renal threshold phosphate concentration. Lancet, ii, 309–310.

Wardener, H.E. de (1972) Control of sodium reabsorption. In Renal Disease, 3rd edn. (Ed. D.A.K. Black) Blackwell Scientific Publications, Oxford.

Wardener, H.E. de (1967) The Kidney. Churchill, London.

Waters, W.E., Sussman, M., Asscher, A.W. (1967) A community study of urinary pH and osmolality. British Journal of Preventive and Social Medicine, 21, 129–132.

Watkin, D.M. and Shock, N.W. (1955) Agewise standard value for C-IN, C-PAH and Tm-PAH in adult males. Journal of Clinical Investigation, 34, 969 (abstract).

Wellwood, J.M., Ellis, B.G., Hall, J.M., Robinson, D.R. and Thompson, A.E. (1973) Early warning of rejection? British Medical Journal, 2, 261–265.

Wellwood, J.M., Ellis, B.G., Price, R.G., Hammond, K., Thompson, A.E. and Jones, N.F. (1974) The excretion of urinary *N*-acetylglucosaminidase in patients with renal disease. Communication to Renal Association.

Wesson, L.G. (1969) Physiology of the Human Kidney. Grune and Stratton, New York and London.

Wibell, L. and Bjørsell–Ostling, E. (1973) Endogenous creatinine clearance in apparently healthy individuals as determined by 24 hour ambulatory urine collection. Uppsala Journal of Medical Science, 78, 43–47.

Wibell, L., Evrin, P.E. and Berggard, I. (1973) Serum β_2-microglobulin in renal disease. Nephron, 10, 320–331.

Wilson, B.W., Stacey, B.D. and Thorburn, G.D. (1969) Automated determination of inulin in the estimation of glomerular filtration rate. Australian Journal of Experimental Biology and Medical Science, 47, 113–123.

Wilson, C.B. (1972) Immune complex glomerulonephritis. Proceedings of the 5th International Congress of Nephrology, 1, 68–74.

Wilson, C.B. (1979) Immunological aspects of glomerulonephritis. In Renal Disease, 4th edn. (Eds. D.A.K. Black and N.F. Jones) Blackwell Scientific Publications, Oxford.

Wilson, C.B. and Dixon, F.J. (1974) The diagnosis of immunopathologic renal disease. Kidney International, 5, 389–401.

Winberg, J. (1959a) Determination of renal concentrating capacity in infants and children without renal disease. Acta Paediatrica (Stockholm), 48, 318–328.

Winberg, J. (1959b) The 24-hour true endogenous creatinine clearance in infants and children without renal disease. Acta Paediatrica (Stockholm), 48, 443–452.

Wolf, A.V. and Pillay, V.K.G. (1969) Renal concentration tests. Osmotic pressure, specific gravity, refraction and electrical conductivity compared. American Journal of Medicine, 46, 837–843.

Wrong, O. and Davies, H.E.F. (1959) The excretion of acid in renal disease. Quarterly Journal of Medicine, 28, 259–313.

Wrong, O. (1965) Urinary hydrogen ion excretion. Journal of Clinical Pathology, 18, 520–526.

FURTHER READING

Bauman, J.W. and Chinard, F.P. (1975) Renal Function: Physiological and Medical Aspects, C.V. Mosby, St. Louis.

Black, D.A.K. and Jones, N.F. (Eds.) (1979) Renal Disease, 4th edn., Blackwell, Oxford.

Deetjen, P., Boylan, J.W. and Kramer, K. (1975) Physiology of the Kidney and of Water Balance, Springer-Verlag, New York.

Mitchell, F.L., Veall, N. and Watts, R.W.E. (1972) Renal function tests suitable for clinical practice. Annals of Clinical Biochemistry, 9, 1–20.

Pitts. R.F. (1974) Physiology of the Kidney and Body Fluids, 3rd edn., Year Book Medical Publishers, Chicago.

Strauss, M.B. and Welt, L.G. (1963) Diseases of the Kidney, Little, Brown, Boston.

Wardener, H.E. de (1967) The Kidney, 3rd edn., Churchill, London.

ADDENDUM

Since 1975, there have been developments in the understanding of the *renin–angiotensin* system, reviewed by Brown et al. (1979).

In assessing *renal concentrating ability*, vasopressin tannate in oil is no longer available, and is replaced by desmopressin (desamino-cys-1,8-D-arginine-vasopressin) (Curtis and Donovan, 1979).

Brown, J.J., Lever, A.F. and Robertson, J.I.S. (1979) Hypertension and the kidney. In Renal Disease, 4th edn. (Eds. D.A.K. Black and N.F. Jones) Chap. 25, Blackwell Scientific Publications, Oxford.

Curtis, J.R. and Donovan, B.A. (1979) Assessment of renal concentrating ability. British Medical Journal, 1, 301–305.

Chapter 10

Liver function

E. Anthony Jones and Paul D. Berk

Section on Diseases of the Liver, Digestive Diseases Branch, National Institute of Arthritis, Metabolism and Digestive Diseases, National Institutes of Health, Bethesda, MD 20205 and Department of Medicine, Mount Sinai School of Medicine and the City University of New York, NY 10029, U.S.A.

CONTENTS

Chemical diagnosis of disease, edited by
S.S. Brown, F.L. Mitchell and D.S. Young

10.1. INTRODUCTION

The liver plays an important role in the regulation of many aspects of carbohydrate, lipid and protein metabolism, as a result of which there is bidirectional passage across the hepatocyte surface membrane of substances such as glucose, aminoacids, glycerol, free fatty acids and vitamins.

Carbohydrate is mainly stored in the liver as glycogen. Regulation of hepatic glycogenolysis is largely responsible for the maintenance of normal blood glucose concentrations. Glucose can also be produced de novo within the liver (gluconeogenesis) by hydrolysis of fats and proteins and by the metabolism of fatty acids, glycerol and aminoacids. Hepatic metabolism of glucose by means of the citric acid and Embden–Meyerhof pathways is the main source of energy (ATP) for metabolic processes. Synthesis of triglycerides from glycerol and fatty acids, and of proteins – which include both cell structural proteins and enzymes – from aminoacids also occurs within the liver cell. Aminoacids are utilized in the synthesis of melanin and haem, the latter serving as prosthetic group for several important enzymes such as cytochrome P-450. In addition, aminoacids are utilized with folic acid in the synthesis of bases, which are incorporated together with sugar and phosphate into co-enzymes, RNA and DNA. The liver cell is one of the main sites of synthesis of cholesterol, and of bile acids which are synthesized from cholesterol. Ammonia, produced in the intestine from the interaction of enteric organisms with urea and aminoacids, and delivered to the liver via the portal vein, and to a lesser extent ammonia derived from protein metabolism in peripheral tissues, is converted largely into urea by the Krebs–Henseleit cycle within the liver cell. The various metabolic pathways involved in these and many other hepatic processes, along with their complex interrelationships, have been reviewed by Holldorf et al. (1970).

The hepatocyte is responsible for the synthesis and release into the hepatic sinusoid of a number of proteins which are exported. These include most of the major plasma proteins and lipoproteins.

Certain endogenous products of metabolism such as bilirubin and many hormones, and exogenous substances such as drugs, organic anions and toxins, which find their way into the circulation, are extracted from plasma by the hepatocyte. In contrast to the excretory function of the kidney, that of the liver deals largely with materials which are protein-bound in the circulation. If these substances are insoluble in water, they are rendered water-soluble within the hepatocyte either by the process of metabolic transformation to more polar products, or by conjugation with radicals such as glucuronide, glycine, taurine and sulphate. These conjugates are subsequently secreted into bile or urine. The main organic constituents of bile, which are largely secreted by the hepatocyte, are conjugates of bilirubin, bile salts, phospholipids, and cholesterol. The bile salts undergo a physiologically important enterohepatic circulation.

Some of the normal metabolic functions of the liver are very poorly understood. This fact is illustrated by a paucity of knowledge concerning the mechanism of coma associated with hepatic insufficiency. Presumably, the liver is responsible either for synthesizing undetermined substance(s) necessary for normal cerebral metabolism or for removing from the circulation undetermined substance(s) which inhibit(s) cerebral metabolism.

This chapter is concerned with laboratory tests which are relevant to the evaluation of patients with hepatobiliary diseases and which, in most cases, can be carried out on specimens of serum or urine. Many aids to the diagnosis of hepatobiliary lesions which are available to the clinician are outside the scope of this chapter. These include radiology, liver biopsy, peritoneoscopy, bacteriology, skin tests, haematology and most tests involving the use of radioisotopes, including hepatic scintiscanning. Instances where serological tests for parasitic, bacterial and viral hepatic infections are indicated are given. However, no attempt has been made to describe these tests in detail, since they are adequately reviewed in standard textbooks and elsewhere (e.g. Miller and Brown, 1969).

In discussing individual tests, the diagnostic information that may be obtianed is presented, together with the broader inferences that can be made regarding the pathophysiology associated with the different disease states. It is felt that this approach will best enable the clinician and the scientist to assess the full implications of the overall clinical picture and the laboratory findings. A number of lists of the causes of certain specific test abnormalities are given; these lists, of necessity, are by no means comprehensive. They do, however, include the most commonly encountered causes of the particular test abnormality and, when appropriate, some other causes which are considered to illustrate points of particular interest. In discussing each individual test, or series of tests, relevant pathophysiology relating to the interpretation of results is given. Such background information has been given in a much more comprehensive form for some tests, such as the serum bilirubin concentration, than for others.

The nomenclature of hepatobiliary diseases used in this chapter conforms to that proposed by the International Symposium on the Nomenclature of Liver Diseases held in April, 1974 (Leevy et al., 1976). The reference ranges from serum biochemical tests which are quoted in this chapter are, unless specifically stated to the contrary, those of the Clinical Chemistry Service, Clinical Center, U.S. National Institutes of Health.

10.2. STATIC CHEMICAL TESTS

10.2.1. Bile pigments

The association of jaundice and of changes in the colour of the urine and faeces with disease of the liver dates to antiquity (Watson, 1976a). The biochemical basis for these changes has been considerably clarified within the past century. Five simple tests – the measurement of direct-reacting and total bilirubin concentration in plasma, a qualitative determination of the presence or absence of bilirubin in the urine, and quantitation of the urobilinogen content of urine and faeces – can, when properly interpreted, provide the clinician with a great deal of information about the status of the hepatobiliary system. Despite their simplicity and value, it seems that many clinicians rarely derive from these procedures the maximum potential information. Since the evaluation of jaundice is so important in the management of patients with hepatobiliary disease and the proper interpretation of these tests depends on an understanding of current concepts of bilirubin metabolism, these are reviewed briefly below. Readers are referred elsewhere (Schmid 1972; Berk et al. 1974a) for more detailed treatment of this subject.

10.2.1.1. Synopsis of bilirubin metabolism

10.2.1.1.1. Sources of bilirubin. Bilirubin is the normal metabolic end-product of a series of enzymatic reactions by which the haem moiety of haemoglobin and other haem proteins is catabolized (Figure 10.1). During the first step in the sequence, the haem ring is opened by an oxidative reaction in which the α bridge carbon is quantitatively split out as carbon monoxide. The resulting molecule of biliverdin is rapidly reduced to bilirubin. Hence, one molecule of bilirubin and one of carbon monoxide are formed for each molecule of haem degraded (Tenhunen et al., 1968), and measurement of either product can be used to estimate the rate of haem catabolism in man (Berk et al., 1974b).

Most of the bilirubin produced in normal man results from the catabolism of the haemoglobin of mature red blood cells by reticuloendothelial cells of the spleen, liver, and bone marrow. Hepatic parenchymal and renal tubular cells participate in the catabolism of any circulating free haemoglobin. An additional source of bilirubin, variously estimated at 10 to 25% of normal bilirubin production, was initially recognized because

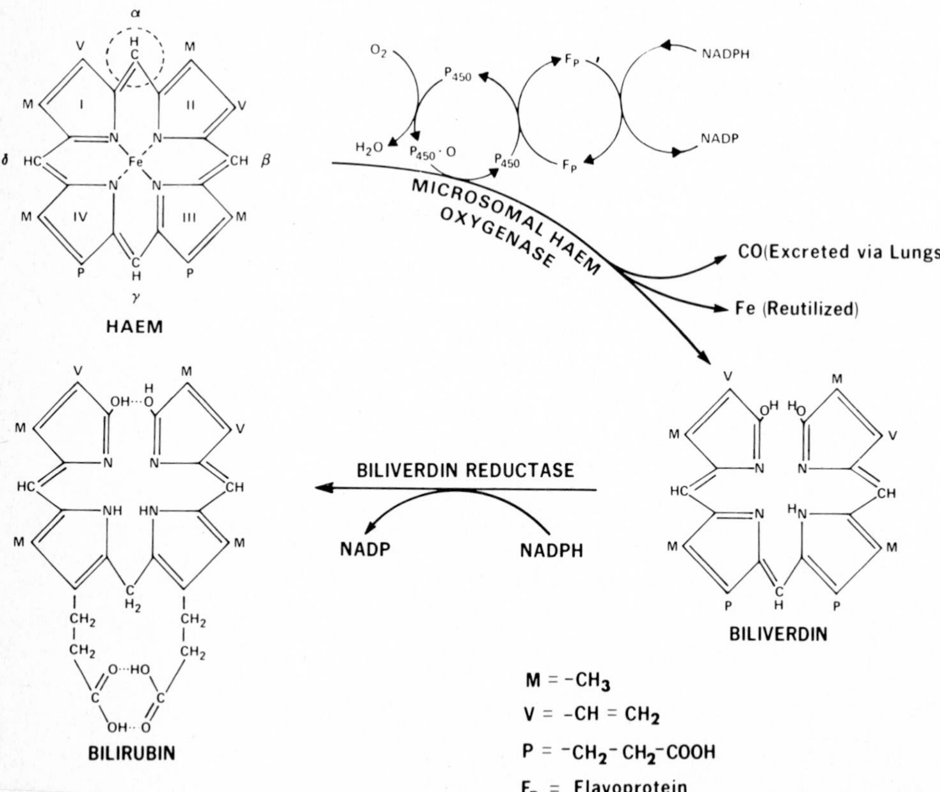

Figure 10.1. Catabolism of haem to bilirubin by microsomal haem oxygenase and soluble biliverdin reductase. Bilirubin is shown in a folded configuration believed to be stabilized by the formation of intramolecular hydrogen bonds (···). (Modified from Tenhunen et al., 1968 and reproduced, with permission, from Berk et al., 1974a)

of its association with the "early labelling" of bile pigments (Figure 10.2) following administration of isotopically labelled haem precursors (London et al., 1950; Gray et al., 1950). This component is now known to arise in part from ineffective erythropoiesis in the bone marrow, and in part from the rapid turnover of haem-containing microsomal enzymes in liver. Potential contributions from the catabolism of extra-hepatic haem proteins such as myoglobin, catalase and peroxidase have not been confirmed in man.

Increased catabolism of haemoglobin is the only documented cause of increased bilirubin production. This may occur either from the haemoglobin of circulating red blood cells (haemolysis) or, in specific situations, from an increased catabolism of the haemoglobin of red cell precursors in the bone marrow (increased ineffective erythropoiesis). Hence, either of these situations may be associated with unconjugated hyperbilirubinaemia. Increased bilirubin production arising from hepatic haem proteins has been postulated but has not been conclusively shown to occur in either animals or man.

Unconjugated bilirubin formed at peripheral sites is transported to the liver tightly complexed to albumin. When there is less than one bilirubin molecule per molecule of albumin, the dissociation constant of this complex (7×10^{-9}) assures that the quantity of unbound bilirubin is very small (Jacobsen, 1969). Although each albumin molecule can bind more than one molecule of bilirubin, additional molecules are bound appreciably less tightly than the first, so at increased serum unconjugated bilirubin concentrations there is a correspondingly higher concentration of free (non-protein-bound) bilirubin. Since it is the concentration of free bilirubin which, in the newborn period, is critical in the pathogenesis of kernicterus, it is essential to know the concentrations of both bili-

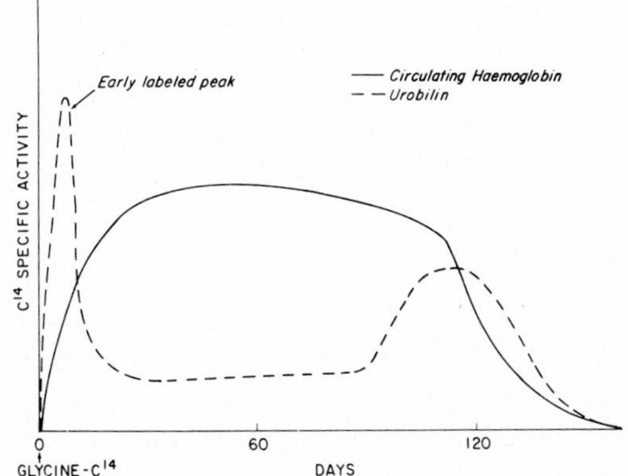

Figure 10.2. Specific activity of circulating haemoglobin haem and the appearance of labelled urobilin (stercobilin) in the faeces after administration of the haem precursor [^{14}C]glycine to a normal individual. Haem specific activity rises rapidly during the first few days after injection of the isotope as the label is incorporated into young erythrocytes. This is followed by a long plateau period, and a decline in specific activity at 100 to 120 days as the senescent erythrocytes are destroyed. Most labelled urobilin appears in the faeces in a broad peak coinciding with this breakdown of senescent cells. A smaller "early labelled peak" fraction appears during the first few days after injection of the isotope, and is thought to result from both ineffective erythropoiesis and the rapid turnover of non-haemoglobin hepatic haem. (Reproduced, with permission, from Berk et al., 1975)

rubin *and* albumin in order to estimate the risk of bilirubin encephalopathy *. Factors associated with additional risk include acidosis, increased plasma concentrations of free fatty acids, and the administration of a variety of drugs such as sulphonamides, which increase the free bilirubin concentration by competitively displacing bilirubin from its binding sites on the albumin molecule (Brodersen, 1974). It is generally believed that the binding of conjugated bilirubin to albumin is appreciably less tight than that of unconjugated bilirubin, but quantitative data are lacking.

10.2.1.1.2. Hepatic bilirubin metabolism. The hepatic transport of bilirubin can be conveniently considered in terms of the following four distinct but related stages –

(i) *Transfer of unconjugated bilirubin from plasma into the liver cell.* This process occurs by a mechanism which is, as yet, incompletely understood. It appears that bilirubin is separated from albumin prior to hepatic uptake (Bloomer et al., 1973), and that the uptake process is saturable and shows selective mutually competitive inhibition by other organic anions such as bromosulphthalein and indocyanine green (Scharschmidt et al., 1975). Although these characteristics suggest the presence within the liver cell membrane of a carrier-mediated transport process for bilirubin uptake, the binding of bilirubin to liver cell membrane fractions has not yet been demonstrated. The rate of hepatic bilirubin uptake has been shown to be normal in the presence of both severe unconjugated and conjugated hyperbilirubinaemia, indicating that uptake is independent of the subsequent metabolic fate of the molecule. Exchange of bilirubin between liver and plasma is bidirectional. The flux from liver to plasma is believed to represent principally passive diffusion down a concentration gradient.

(ii) *Intracellular binding.* The majority of the unconjugated bilirubin within the liver cells exists in the cytosol, bound to two organic-anion-binding proteins designated Y (ligandin) and Z (Levi et al., 1969; Arias et al., 1976). These proteins are responsible for the "storage" of bilirubin and other organic anions within the liver cell, and play an important, although as yet imprecisely defined, role in the subsequent transport of such molecules into the bile. Y is one of a family of related proteins which enzymatically catalyzes the conjugation of bromosulphthalein and other substrates with glutathione (Jakoby, 1976), but the relevance of this property of the protein to bilirubin metabolism is unclear. The cytoplasmic protein-bound bilirubin is in equilibrium with bilirubin bound to receptor sites on microsomal membranes.

(iii) *Conjugation.* Within the hepatic microsomes, conjugation of lipophilic unconjugated bilirubin with small polar molecules to form water-soluble conjugated bilirubin is catalyzed by the enzyme UDP-glucuronyltransferase (EC 2.4.1.17). The principal bilirubin conjugates in normal man are mono- and diglucuronides (Jansen and Billing, 1971; Gordon and Goresky, 1976). Traces of glucose, xylose, and disaccharide conjugates are also present in human bile (Heirwegh et al., 1974). Cholestasis is associated with a marked increase in the proportion of highly polar disaccharide conjugates (Fevery et al., 1972).

* Based on the relative molecular masses of albumin (about 66,000) and bilirubin (585), saturation of the first binding site, with consequent abrupt increase in the concentration of free bilirubin, occurs at a bilirubin concentration of 600 μmol/litre (35 mg/dl) in plasma having an albumin concentration of 600 μmol/litre (4 g/dl), and proportionally lower bilirubin concentrations in plasma with lower albumin concentrations.

(iv) *Biliary excretion.* Little, if any, conjugated bilirubin is ordinarily present within either the liver cell (Bernstein et al., 1966) or the plasma (Brodersen, 1966), indicating that conjugation is followed by the rapid removal of the conjugate across the canalicular membrane into the bile canaliculi. Transport across the bile canalicular membrane is a saturable, concentrative, energy-dependent process (Goresky, 1965). It appears that a common mechanism is involved in the excretion of bilirubin, bromosulphthalein, indocyanine green and certain other cholephilic anions, which is distinct from that involved in the secretion of bile acids (Alpert et al., 1969).

When unconjugated bilirubin is administered by rapid continuous infusion, both the plasma bilirubin concentration and the biliary excretion rate for bilirubin initially rise. Ultimately, a maximal rate of biliary excretion (T_{MAX}) is achieved, in spite of a continuing increase in the total plasma bilirubin concentration (Arias et al., 1961). The latter is associated with both an increase in the plasma conjugated bilirubin concentration and an elevated concentration of conjugated bilirubin in the hepatic vein which exceeds that in peripheral vessels (Raymond and Galambos, 1971). Thus, it is the biliary secretion of conjugated bilirubin, rather than the processes of hepatic uptake or conjugation, which limits the overall capacity of the liver to transport bilirubin from blood to bile.

In contrast to the enzyme system for conjugating bilirubin, which is well preserved in most lesions which produce either hepatocellular damage or cholestasis, the transport of conjugated bilirubin from hepatocyte to bile canaliculus appears to be extremely sensitive to various types of liver injury. Hence an elevation of the plasma conjugated (i.e. direct-reacting) bilirubin concentration often precedes, or occurs in the absence, of, an elevated total bilirubin concentration in acquired hepatobiliary diseases. In addition, an increase in the bilirubin production rate to values in excess of T_{MAX} may occur very rarely during acute massive haemolytic episodes, and in these unique circumstances it may be responsible for elevation of the conjugated, as well as unconjugated, plasma bilirubin concentration in patients without intrinsic hepatic dysfunction (Schalm and Weber, 1964). Finally, in patients in whom T_{MAX} is reduced from any cause, a more modest degree of haemolysis – which commonly accompanies many forms of hepatobiliary disease – may be responsible for an elevation of the conjugated, as well as the unconjugated, bilirubin concentration in plasma.

10.2.1.1.3. Fate within the gastrointestinal tract. There does not appear to be significant absorption of conjugated bilirubin from the human gastrointestinal tract. Although unconjugated bilirubin is absorbed from the upper gastrointestinal tract, little unconjugated bilirubin is normally available for absorption from this region of the gut in adults. In the neonatal period, high activity of β-glucuronidase (EC 3.2.1.31) within the gut may result in deconjugation of some conjugated bilirubin; as a consequence of this effect, an enterohepatic circulation of bilirubin has been postulated (Poland and Odell, 1971) to contribute to the physiologic hyperbilirubinaemia of the newborn (section 10.5.1.3.2).

In the adult, conjugated bilirubin is degraded by bacteria within the lower small bowel and colon. The process involves both deconjugation and reduction to a series of colourless urobilinogens and related products (Watson, 1976b). In normal subjects, only approximately 5% of the bilirubin which is initially excreted into the bile ultimately appears as bilirubin in the faeces. The remainder appears principally, but not exclusively, as one or more urobilinogens. It is important to recognize that the conversion of bilirubin into urobilinogen is not quantitative (Figure 10.3), so that even accurate quantitative measurements of faecal urobilinogen excretion may appreciably underestimate the rate of bilirubin production (Bloomer et al., 1970). It is noteworthy that, although the colour of normal faeces is often attributed to the presence of bile pigments, and the pale appearance of the stools in cholestasis to a failure of bile pigment excretion, the major faecal bile pigments – the urobilinogens and other chromogens – are colourless until their oxidation to the corresponding coloured urobilins, which occurs on prolonged standing. Hence, the usual explanation for stool colour in health and cholestatic disease does not stand close scrutiny, and a definitive explanation requires additional detailed examination of the pigments involved (With, 1968).

A proportion of the urobilinogen formed in the lower intestine is absorbed, and undergoes an enterohepatic circulation, which gives rise to small but measurable quantities of urobilinogen in the plasma (Schmidt et al., 1971). Normally, most of the urobilinogen reaching the plasma is re-excreted into the bile, but a small fraction is cleared by the kidney and appears in the urine. The hepatic capacity for urobilinogen excretion is limited and is readily reduced further by hepatocellular injury. When this occurs, or when there is increased bile pigment production (e.g. haemolysis), there is diversion of increased amounts of urobilinogen into the urine, providing that there is not appreciable associated cholestasis (Bernstein, 1971). An increased quantity of urobilinogen may also

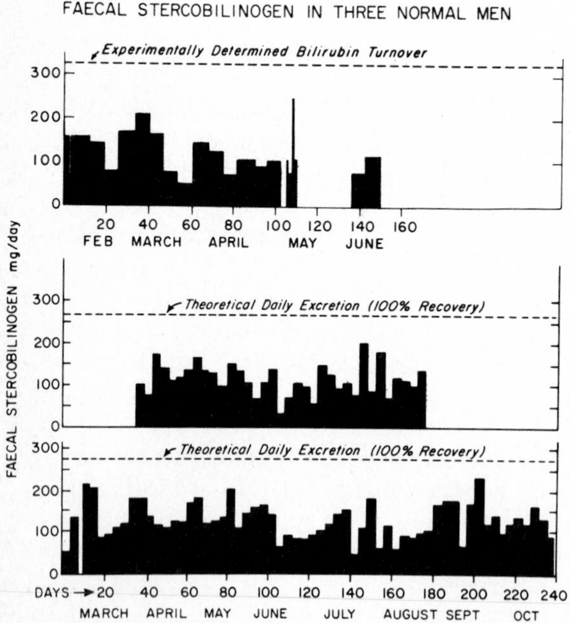

Figure 10.3. Faecal urobilinogen (stercobilinogen) excretion in three normal subjects. In all cases there were considerable but variable discrepancies between measured or estimated rates of bilirubin production and actual yields of stercobilinogen. (Reproduced, with permission, from Bloomer et al., 1970)

appear in the urine in association with prolonged intestinal transit time, as in constipation, or bacterial overgrowth of the small bowel, possibly because of augmented absorption or increased production, respectively (Lester, 1964). Urinary urobilinogen excretion, which depends on a combination of glomerular filtration, secretion by the proximal tubule, and pH-dependent re-absorption in the distal tubule, is diminished in renal insufficiency or in the presence of an acid urine (Bourke et al., 1965).

10.2.1.1.4. Renal bilirubin excretion. In healthy individuals, the kidneys play a minor role in bilirubin metabolism in that only a very small proportion of daily bilirubin production is ordinarily excreted by the renal route (Berk et al., 1969). Using routine clinical methods bilirubin is undetectable in the urine of normal subjects, or in the urine of patients with exclusively unconjugated hyperbilirubinaemia in whom serum bilirubin concentrations may be as high as 680 μmol/litre (40 mg/dl). In contrast, when the plasma concentration of conjugated bilirubin is increased, conjugated bilirubin appears in the urine. The concentration of plasma bilirubin at which bilirubinuria occurs is variable. Bilirubinuria is common at low – often sub-icteric – concentrations of plasma conjugated bilirubin during the early stages of acute viral hepatitis, a phenomenon which has been effectively used in screening for early cases during hepatitis epidemics (Neefe and Reinhold, 1946). However, bilirubin may disappear from the urine despite plasma conjugated bilirubin concentrations of up to 170 μmol/litre (10 mg/dl) during the resolving stage of this disease (Watson and Hoffbauer, 1947). The mechanism for renal bilirubin excretion is believed to be glomerular filtration of a small non-protein-bound fraction. It is possible that a change in the predominant type of bilirubin conjugate, with a concomitant change in albumin binding affinity, accounts for the differences in the degree of renal bilirubin excretion in early, compared with resolving, acute hepatitis. Others have speculated that changes in bile salt metabolism are responsible for this phenomenon (Fulop and Sandson, 1967).

10.2.1.1.5. Clearance of unconjugated bilirubin. Non-volatile metabolic wastes, such as unconjugated bilirubin, as well as exogenously administered drugs and toxins, are eliminated from the body predominantly by the liver and kidneys. If the quantity of a substance excreted per unit time (U.V) and its plasma concentration (P) are known, the volume of plasma cleared of the substance per unit time (C) may be readily calculated from the familiar clearance equation C = U.V/P. Since quantitation of materials excreted in the faeces is difficult, use of this equation has been largely restricted to calculation of renal clearances (Chapter 9). Recently, however, it has become possible to measure the rate of daily bilirubin turnover (BRT) from the plasma disappearance curve of unconjugated radiolabelled bilirubin without the need for faecal sampling (Berk et al., 1969). Since in the steady-state BRT is very nearly equivalent to the amount of bilirubin excreted in bile per unit time, the clearance equation may be re-written:

$$C_{BR}(\mathrm{ml \cdot min^{-1} \cdot kg^{-1}}) = \frac{\mathrm{BRT(mg \cdot kg^{-1} \cdot d^{-1})}}{\overline{\mathrm{BR}}(\mathrm{mg\ dl^{-1}})} \times \frac{1}{14.4} \qquad [1]$$

where C_{BR} is the hepatic bilirubin clearance, and $\overline{BR}$ is the plasma unconjugated bilirubin concentration. The constant 14.4 is derived from the number of minutes/day and the factor which converts $\overline{BR}$ from mg/dl to mg/ml. If this equation is solved for $\overline{BR}$ –

$$\overline{BR} \simeq \frac{BRT}{C_{BR}} \qquad [2]$$

Thus it is evident that the plasma unconjugated bilirubin concentration varies directly with increasing bilirubin production, as measured by BRT, and inversely with hepatic bilirubin clearance (Berk et al., 1974a). It can be further shown (Figure 10.4) that, whereas a 2-fold increase in BRT or a 50% reduction in C_{BR} will both produce a doubling of $\overline{BR}$, the actual magnitude of the increment in bilirubin concentration (in mg/dl) will be much greater in individuals in whom clearance values are initially reduced. The relationships between BRT, C_{BR}, and $\overline{BR}$ are analogous to the more familiar relationships between urine creatinine excretion, renal creatinine clearance and serum creatinine concentration. Their applicability to the assessment of hepatic function has not been generally appreciated.

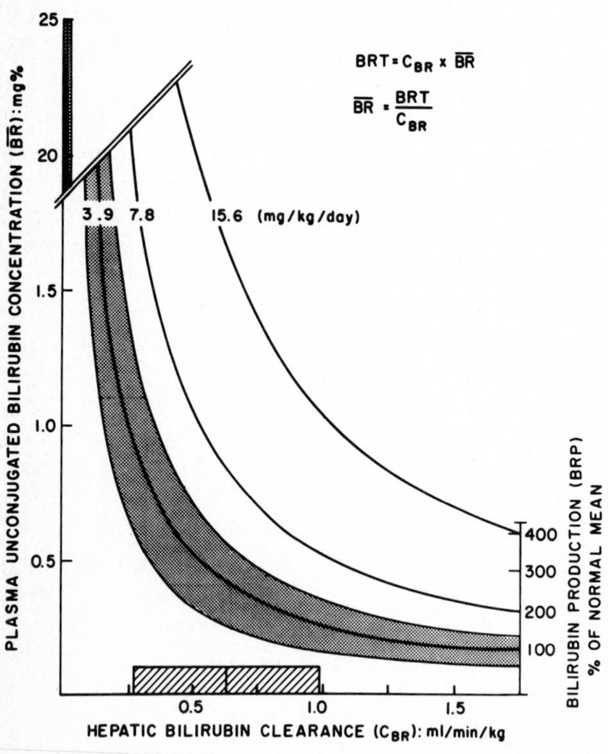

Figure 10.4. Relationship between bilirubin production, as estimated from measurements of plasma bilirubin turnover (BRT), hepatic bilirubin clearance (C_{BR}), and the plasma concentration of unconjugated bilirubin ($\overline{BR}$). Stippled area represents the normal range for bilirubin production; bar on horizontal axis is the normal range (mean ±2 S.D.) for hepatic bilirubin clearance. (Reproduced, with permission, from Berk et al., 1974a)

10.2.1.2. Plasma bilirubin

In the van den Bergh reaction, the tetrapyrrole skeleton of bilirubin and its conjugates is cleaved and diazotized to form purple dipyrrolic azo pigments, whose concentration is readily measured spectrophotometrically. The violet colour which develops immediately after a diazonium reagent (e.g. diazotized sulphanilic acid) is added to plasma is called the direct reaction. When alcohol, caffeine or other accelerators are then added, additional colour develops. The maximum colour which develops is proportional to the total bilirubin concentration. The difference between the concentrations of total and direct reacting bilirubin is designated the indirect reacting pigment.

It is often useful to the clinician to consider the direct and indirect reacting fractions as representing conjugated and unconjugated bilirubin, respectively. However, this is clearly an over-simplification as indicated by the observations that: (a) solutions made from pure, crystalline unconjugated bilirubin commonly contain as much as 10% of direct reacting bilirubin; and (b) normal human plasma contains only trace amounts of true conjugated bilirubin as determined by elaborate isotopic techniques (Brodersen, 1966) despite the presence of easily measurable quantities of direct reacting pigment.

Bilirubin is unstable on exposure to light, being rapidly degraded to products which do not give a positive diazo reaction. Hence plasma specimens should be analyzed as quickly as possible, and protected from light until the determination is carried out. Acceptable determinations can be obtained on plasma or serum samples after 48 hours of storage provided they have been kept refrigerated and in the dark.

It is apparent from equation (2) above that an increase in the plasma concentration of unconjugated bilirubin may result from either an increase in bilirubin production, or a reduction in the hepatic clearance of unconjugated bilirubin. The latter, in turn, may result from inefficient delivery of bilirubin to the liver cell (decreased or poorly distributed hepatic blood flow), or defects in the processes of hepatocellular uptake, intracellular binding, or conjugation. An increase in the plasma concentration of conjugated bilirubin results from defective excretion of conjugated bilirubin into the bile canaliculus, obstruction to biliary flow at any site in the biliary tract from the bile canaliculus to the ampulla of Vater or, rarely, from a rate of bilirubin production which exceeds the T_{MAX} for biliary excretion of conjugated bilirubin. Hence, elevation of the direct reacting plasma bilirubin concentration is almost always a highly specific indicator of hepatobiliary dysfunction, while an isolated increase in the indirect reacting fraction may have a hepatic and/or haematologic cause. Unconjugated bilirubin concentrations between 17 and 68 μmol/litre (1.0 and 4.0 mg/dl) may result either from haemolysis alone, hepatic dysfunction alone, or some combination of the two. As indicated in Figure 10.5, a plasma unconjugated bilirubin concentration in excess of 68 μmol/litre (4.0 mg/dl) invariably indicates hepatobiliary dysfunction irrespective of the presence or absence of co-existing haemolysis (Berk et al., 1974a).

Reference ranges. It can be deduced from equation (2) above that the distribution of unconjugated bilirubin concentrations within a normal population will not have a symmetrical distribution about the mean, but will be skewed toward higher values (Bloomer et al., 1971a; Berk et al., 1974a). This can be demonstrated graphically from Figure 10.4 by drawing ordinates corresponding to the normal mean and range for hepatic unconjugated bilirubin clearance so as to intersect the corresponding curves for the normal mean

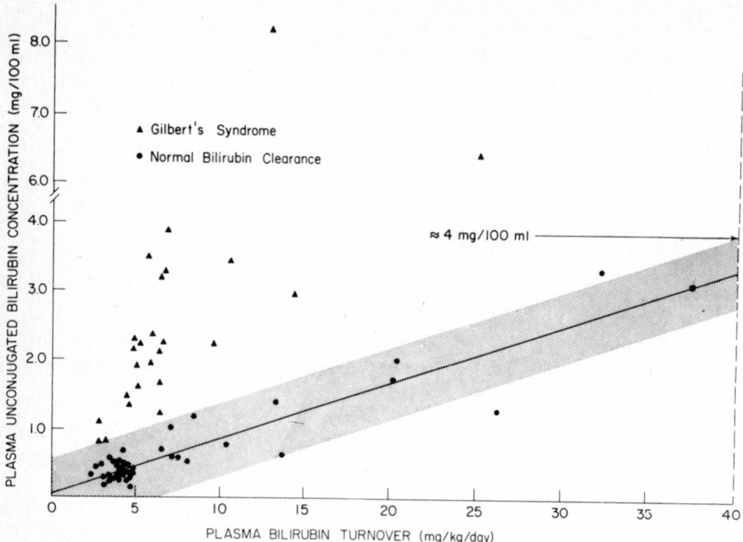

Figure 10.5. Relation between plasma bilirubin turnover and the plasma concentration of unconjugated bilirubin. When hepatic bilirubin clearance is within the relatively narrow normal range, the plasma unconjugated bilirubin concentration will increase linearly with increasing rates of bilirubin production, as indicated by the regression line. The stippled area represents two standard errors of the estimate about the regression line. Extrapolation of the regression line to the maximum achievable rate of bilirubin production, or approximately 40 mg/kg body weight per day, indicates the highest value for the plasma unconjugated bilirubin concentration that can occur as the result of sustained haemolysis in an individual with normal hepatic bilirubin clearance. This value is approximately 70 μmol/litre (4 mg/100 ml) (Reproduced, with permission, from Berk et al., 1975)

and range for bilirubin turnover. Abscissae through the appropriate points of intersection will give approximate values for the normal mean and range of the plasma unconjugated bilirubin concentration. A positive skew for the total plasma bilirubin concentration (consisting predominantly of unconjugated bilirubin) was, in fact, observed in two large series of 849 (Butt et al., 1966) and 719 (Zieve et al., 1951) healthy individuals, respectively. The skewed cumulative distribution of total plasma bilirubin concentrations in the former of these two series was found to approximate closely a log-normal function (Figure 10.6A). Application of a log-normal distribution to equation (2), using values for plasma bilirubin turnover and hepatic bilirubin clearance determined in normal subjects, indicates that the plasma concentration of unconjugated bilirubin will be between 3 and 15 μmol/litre (0.2 and 0.9 mg/dl) for 95% of a normal population, and that 99% of such a population will have a value less than 17 μmol/litre (1.0 mg/dl) (Bloomer et al., 1971a). The cumulative distribution function for unconjugated bilirubin concentrations calculated in this manner (Figure 10.6B) closely parallels that observed clinically for total bilirubin (Butt et al., 1966), while the calculated upper limit of unconjugated bilirubin concentration 17 μmol/litre (1.0 mg/dl) is identical to that determined experimentally in the Clinical Chemistry Laboratory of the U.S. National Institutes of Health.

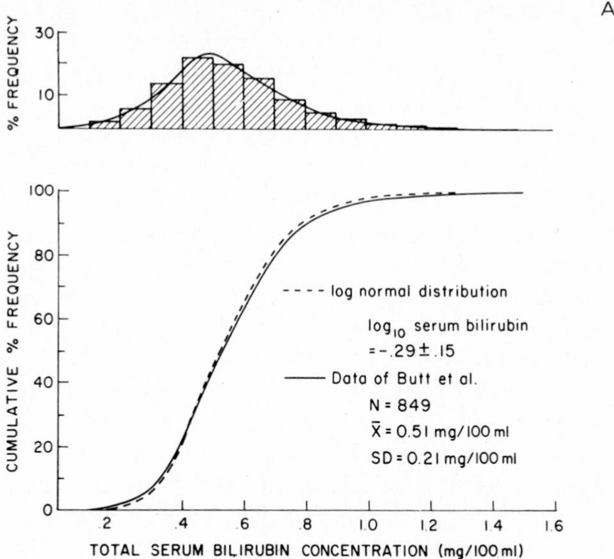

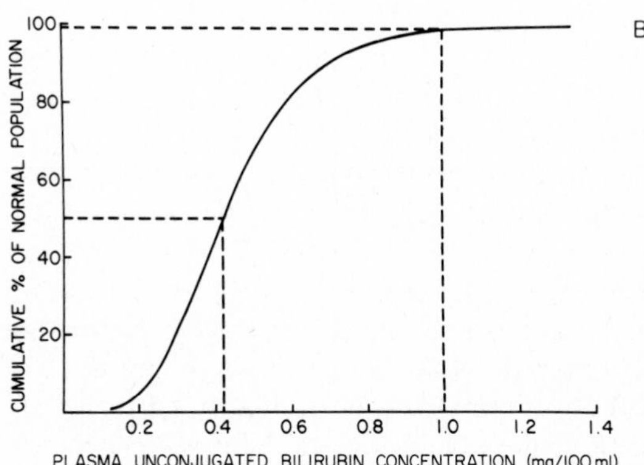

Figure 10.6. A: frequency distribution (above) and cumulative frequency (below) of total serum bilirubin concentrations measured in 849 normal subjects, plotted from published data (Butt et al., 1966). The cumulative frequency curve (below) closely approximates a log-normal function. B: theoretical cumulative distribution function for plasma unconjugated bilirubin concentration in normal individuals, calculated as a log-normal function from experimental measurements of plasma bilirubin turnover and hepatic bilirubin clearance. The curve parallels the experimentally determined data for total bilirubin concentration (Fig. 10.6A), while the upper limit of normal for unconjugated bilirubin, 1.0 mg/dl (17 μmol/litre) is identical to that determined experimentally. (Reproduced, with permission, from Bloomer et al., 1971a)

The normal range for direct reacting bilirubin is less well established, in part because this measurement reflects both the very small plasma content of conjugated bilirubin and the tendency of a small but variable proportion of unconjugated bilirubin to give a prompt direct reaction. The upper limit of normal for direct reacting bilirubin in the presence of a normal plasma bilirubin concentration, ⩽21 μmol/litre (1.2 mg/dl), has empirically been set at 3 μmol/litre (0.2 mg/dl). Values greater than 3 μmol/litre (0.2 mg/dl) are very rarely seen in normal subjects (Watson, 1956; Nosslin, 1960). In contrast, values in excess of 3 μmol/litre (0.2 mg/dl) are not uncommonly seen in patients with established hepatobiliary disease despite normal total bilirubin concentrations. In one study, such values were invariably associated with 45-minute bromosulphthalein retention in excess of 9% (section 10.4.1.1) (Gambino et al., 1967). In a reliable laboratory, an elevated value for the direct reacting bilirubin concentration is a highly sensitive and almost specific test of hepatic and/or biliary dysfunction, particularly if the total bilirubin concentration is normal. When the total bilirubin concentration is increased, precise interpretation of the direct reacting fraction is more empirical, but a useful rule of thumb is to consider any direct reacting fraction which is less than 10% of total bilirubin to be within normal limits and any value in excess of 15% of an elevated total bilirubin concentration as clearly abnormal, or at least in need of investigation. Because the value for direct reacting bilirubin varies more with the method employed than does that of the total, it is particularly important that the reference range for the former be established in the laboratory which performs the test.

10.2.1.3. Urine bilirubin

Bilirubin is not detectable by routine methods in the urine either of normal subjects or of individuals with purely unconjugated hyperbilirubinaemia, irrespective of the plasma total bilirubin concentration. However, conjugated bilirubin readily appears in the urine when the plasma conjugated bilirubin concentration is increased; hence the presence of bilirubinuria is more or less a specific indicator of hepatobiliary disease.

The presence of bilirubin in the urine is readily demonstrated qualitatively or semi-quantitatively by a number of simple procedures (With, 1968). The Harrison spot test is positive at urine bilirubin concentrations of 0.1 to 0.25 mg/dl (2 to 4 μmol/litre). Although accurate and easy to use, it has largely been superceded in North America by the use of dip-sticks or tablets impregnated with diazo reagents. Of these, the latter are the more sensitive, readily detecting bilirubin concentrations of 0.05 to 0.1 mg/dl (1 to 2 μmol/litre). It should be emphasized that not every dark urine in a jaundiced patient indicates bilirubinuria. The presence of bilirubinuria should always be confirmed by one of these simple techniques. In a jaundiced patient, dark urine which does not contain bilirubin suggests haemolysis (section 10.2.1.5).

During cholestatic jaundice, urinary excretion may become the principal route of bilirubin elimination. Because of the instability of bilirubin in urine, particularly when exposed to light, attempts to measure 24-hour urinary bilirubin excretion quantitatively often provide erratic results even in the presence of complete biliary obstruction. Therefore there is little clinical value in attempting quantitative estimates of 24-hour urine bilirubin output.

10.2.1.4. Faecal urobilinogen (stercobilinogen)

Daily excretion of urobilinogen and related urobilinoids in the faeces averages 67 to 470 μmol (40 to 280 mg) in normal individuals (Watson, 1937; Bloomer et al., 1970). Since results vary widely from day to day in a given individual, the measurement is usually performed on a pooled 3-day faecal specimen.

A marked reduction in faecal urobilinogen to less than 8 μmol (5 mg) per day occurs in severe cholestasis from any cause, and hence is of no diagnostic value. In a patient with either a T-tube in the common bile duct or a spontaneous biliary fistula, very low values for faecal urobilinogen (in the absence of antibiotic therapy) indicate almost complete diversion of bile from the intestine.

Except for the transient increase which may follow the relief of large duct biliary obstruction, an increased faecal excretion of urobilinogen is indicative of increased bilirubin production. It is, therefore, more specific in this regard than an increase in urine urobilinogen, which may also result from hepatocellular disease. Unfortunately, as noted above, the conversion of bilirubin into urobilinogen is less than complete, and varies widely from day to day and individual to individual (Figure 10.3). Of the total daily production of bilirubin only about 50% (range 18 to 98%) is recoverable in the faeces as urobilinogen, so that approximately 30% of patients with haemolysis and increased bilirubin production have faecal urobilinogen values within the normal range (Bloomer et al., 1970). Hence, although an elevated faecal urobilinogen excretion indicates bilirubin overproduction, a normal value does not rule it out. Because urobilinogen formation depends on the action of intestinal bacteria, quantitative faecal urobilinogen measurements made during, or within about 2 weeks of, administration of antibiotics, particularly orally administered broad spectrum agents, are likely to yield low values.

The method of measuring faecal urobilinogen is technically arduous, aesthetically unpleasant for the laboratory technician, and does not enable an accurate estimate of bilirubin overproduction to be made. When accurate quantitation of bilirubin production from red cells is required in the assessment of a haemolytic state it can most easily be obtain from measurements of red cell life span (Berk et al., 1976). Other accurate techniques for quantitating bilirubin metabolism, which are available only in specialized centres, are measurements of bilirubin turnover and carbon monoxide production as indicated in section 10.2.1.1.1 and 10.4.4.

10.2.1.5. Urine urobilinogen

Urine urobilinogen excretion is readily measured using Ehrlich's aldehyde reagent. Dipsticks impregnated with this reagent are widely available and permit semi-quantitative measurement of urine urobilinogen in five increments from ⩽2 μmol/litre (0.1 mg/dl) to >200 μmol/litre (12 mg/dl). Because urobilinogen is converted on standing into non-reactive products this test should be performed on freshly voided urine.

The reabsorption of urobilinogen from the distal renal tubule is highly pH dependent, increasing markedly at acid pH, so that both the absolute urobilinogen excretion and the ratio of urobilinogen clearance to creatinine clearance diminish markedly in the presence of an acid urine (Bourke et al., 1965). Urobilinogen is also unstable at acid pH. As a result of these factors, estimates of urine urobilinogen made from acid urine are of limited value.

The normal daily excretion of urobilinogen is $\leqslant 7$ μmol (4 mg). There is a well documented diurnal variation, possibly related to a corresponding variation in urine pH, with peak urobilinogen output usually occurring between 12.00 and 16.00 hours (Bourke et al., 1965). The urobilinogen content of a 2-hour specimen of urine obtained within this period normally contains less than 2 μmol (1.2 mg) urobilinogen, and this determination is widely used in lieu of one on a complete 24-hour urine collection. As with determinations in faeces, the value for urine urobilinogen excretion may be reduced if antibiotics have recently been administered.

Absence of urobilinogen from the urine of a jaundiced patient, like its absence from faeces, strongly suggests cholestasis, but gives no indication of the cause. According to Sherlock, the complete absence of urobilinogen from the urine for 7 consecutive days is suggestive of complete large duct biliary obstruction due to malignancy. Obstruction due to stone or stricture is often partial and is likely to be accompanied by the intermittent appearance of some urobilinogen in the urine (Sherlock, 1975). An increased urine urobilinogen may indicate either bilirubin overproduction (e.g. haemolysis) or hepatocellular disease. The occurrence of increased values in these conditions may be prevented by concomitant cholestasis.

On prolonged standing of urine specimens, urobilinogen may be oxidized to urobilin. In the presence of increased excretion of urobilinogen, a urine which is colourless when voided subsequently takes on a deep orange-brown colour which may be mistaken for bilirubin. If the urine is dark in a jaundiced patient it is important to determine the nature of the urinary pigment. While the presence of bilirubin suggests hepatocellular or cholestatic jaundice, the absence of bilirubin and the presence of excess urobilin, most simply established by Schlesinger's method (With, 1968), strongly suggests haemolysis.

The physiology of the faecal and urine bile pigments is well illustrated by the changes in their excretion which occur (Figure 10.7) during the course of typical acute viral hepatitis (Sherlock, 1975). The first detectable abnormality in bile pigment metabolism is the appearance of bilirubinuria early in the prodromal, pre-icteric phase. This occurred in more than 85% of one series of patients (Pollock, 1945). It usually persists into the healing phase, when it may disappear despite persisting hyperbilirubinaemia. A transient increase in urine urobilinogen excretion may occur later in the prodromal period, as the result of hepatocellular dysfunction, but this is a less constant finding. If jaundice develops, impaired bilirubin secretion into bile results in a marked decrease or absence of urobilinogen from both the urine and faeces and the development of pale stools. Re-appearance of a dark stool colour, and increasing amounts of urobilinogen in faeces and urine generally herald the onset of recovery. Increased urine urobilinogen excretion may subsequently occur and persist long after bilirubinuria has ceased. Increased urinary urobilinogen excretion may be the last abnormality of routine tests of bile pigment metabolism to return to normal.

Measurements of bile pigments in urine are probably widely underutilized. These tests are no more subject to error than most other tests which are employed in the evaluation of hepatobiliary function. The simplicity, sensitivity and low cost of measurements of urine bilirubin and urobilinogen argue strongly in their favour.

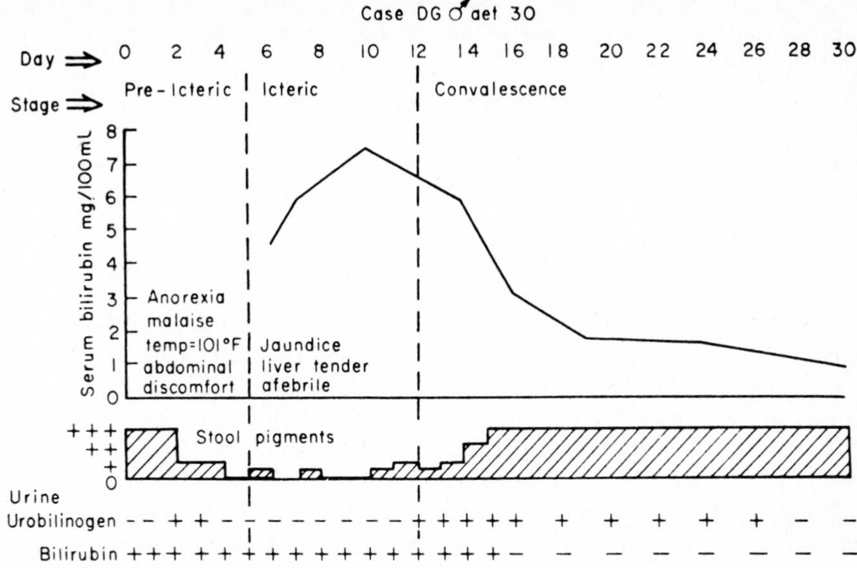

Figure 10.7. Laboratory tests reflecting bile pigment metabolism during the course of a patient with moderately severe, icteric type B viral hepatitis: see text for details. (Reproduced, with permission, from Sherlock, 1975)

10.2.2. Porphyrin metabolism

The liver contains appreciable quantities of haem-containing enzymes with rapid turnover rates, such as cytochromes P-450 and b_5, and it is a major site of the porphyrin biosynthesis required to produce the haem needed by these enzymes. Biochemical findings in a number of inherited disorders of the porphyrin biosynthetic pathway within the liver – the so-called "hepatic porphyrias" – are described in Chapter 20.

The liver is also the site of elimination of the porphyrin by-products of haem biosynthesis. Quantitatively the most significant of these is coproporphyrin. Most coproporphyrin is secreted into bile and appears in faeces; a small quantity appears in the urine. In cholestasis, biliary excretion of coproporphyrin is decreased, and there is a corresponding increase in urinary excretion of coproporphyrin.

Quantitation of both total urine coproporphyrin and the ratio of its two isomers (coproporphyrin I and III) is of diagnostic value only in patients with Dubin–Johnson and Rotor's syndromes, two hereditary disorders characterized by conjugated hyperbilirubinaemia (section 10.5.1.1.3).

10.2.3. Bile acids

10.2.3.1. Physiology

Bile acids are a class of compounds whose basic structure consists of (a) a flat, hydrophobic, fully saturated steroid nucleus; (b) a polar group at the end of the side-chain attached to the nucleus; and (c) one or more hydroxyl groups attached directly to the nucleus. In the free bile acids, the polar group on the side-chain is a carboxyl radical. The bile acids may be conjugated in a peptide linkage through this carboxyl group to the aminoacids glycine or taurine. The acidic group of the aminoacid moiety then becomes the free polar site on the side-chain. The hydroxyl groups on the steroid nucleus and the polar side-chain groups all project from one side of the planar molecule, thereby producing both a highly polar hydrophilic and a non-polar hydrophobic surface (Figure 10.8) (Haslewood, 1967; Hofmann and Small, 1967; Small, 1971; Hofmann and Kern, 1971). Although the conjugated bile acids are, technically, bile salts, the two terms are often used interchangeably.

The principal primary bile acids – cholic acid and chenodeoxycholic acid – are synthesized in the liver from cholesterol by complex pathways (Figure 10.9) involving a minimum of 14 enzymatic steps (Danielsson, 1976). These steps involve (a) the stereospecific saturation of the double bond (Δ^{5-6}) to form 5β compounds in which the A and B rings are in the *cis* orientation; (b) additional stereospecific hydroxylations of the nucleus at the 7α or 7α and 12α positions; and (c) shortening of the side-chain by three carbon atoms with oxidation of the C_{24} terminal carbon atom to a carboxyl group (Hofmann and Kern, 1971). It appears that the predominant pathways for the synthesis of both the trihydroxy (3α,7α,12α) primary bile acid (cholic acid) and the dihydroxy (3α,7α) primary bile acid (chenodeoxycholic acid) do not diverge until after the addition of the 7α-hydroxyl group. The activity of the microsomal 7α-hydroxylase system correlates with the overall rate of bile acid biosynthesis and it has been postulated that 7α-hydroxylation is rate-limiting in the biosynthetic pathway. Moreover, the rate of bile acid synthesis appears to be regulated by the quantity of bile acids being returned to the liver. Recently, however, other regulatory mechanisms have been proposed. It is becoming clear that there are alternative pathways for the biosynthesis of the bile acids, and that 7α-hydroxylation is not necessarily a control point in all of these pathways. At the moment, the regulation of bile acid synthesis is an area of intensive research activity (Mosbach, 1972; Carey, 1973; Danielsson, 1976).

The primary bile acids are conjugated with glycine and taurine prior to their active

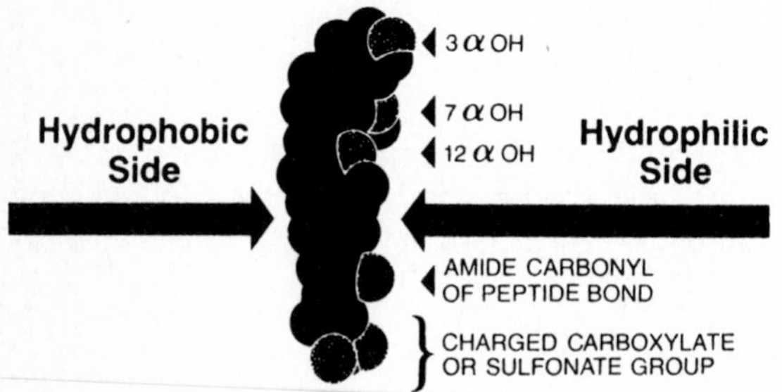

Figure 10.8. Side view of a three-dimensional model of glycine or taurine conjugate of cholic acid. Note that the molecule is nearly flat, although the *cis* juncture of the A and B rings causes it to be slightly kinked near the top. The bile salt molecule contains distinct hydrophobic and hydrophilic surfaces. (Reproduced, with permission, from Hofmann and Kern, 1971)

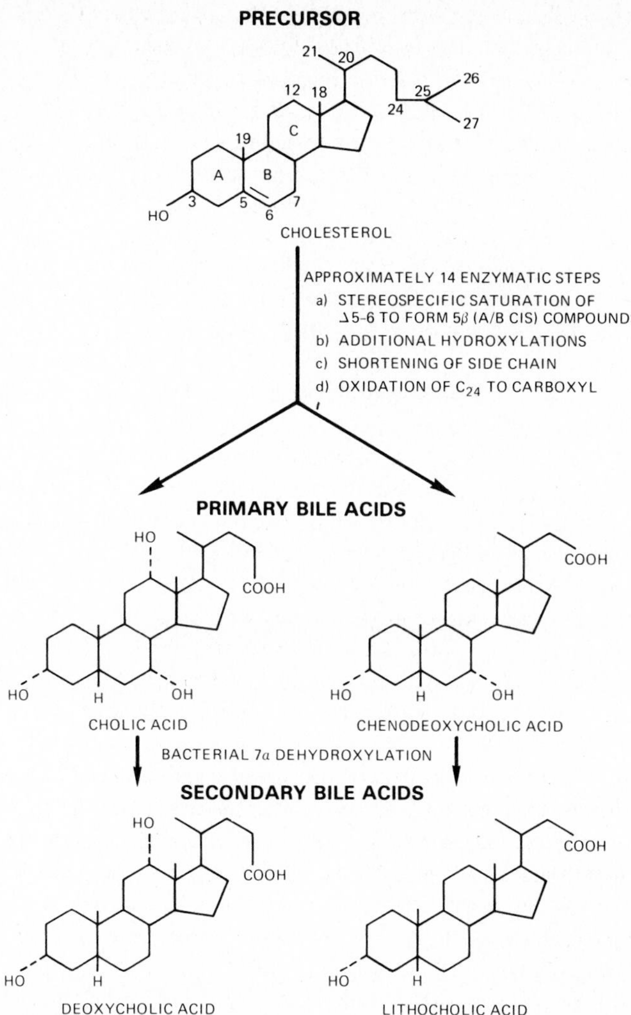

Figure 10.9. Schematic pathway for synthesis of the principal human primary and secondary bile acids from cholesterol.

transport into the bile. The ratio of glycine to taurine bile salts in normal man averages about 3:1, and is largely determined by the available supply of taurine, which is used preferentially for conjugation (Sjovall, 1959). Following the initial biliary secretion of the conjugated primary bile acids, they are stored in the gall bladder during the fasting state. It should be noted that almost all of the bile acid pool exists within the gall bladder during fasting, and within the intestinal lumen during digestion. The amount of primary bile acids in portal blood at any time is relatively small. Because of the virtually complete hepatic extraction of bile acids from the hepatic blood supply, and their rapid re-excretion into the bile, the quantity of bile acids present in peripheral blood or within the liver normally represents a very small fraction of the total bile acid pool (Hofmann, 1976).

The hepatic uptake of bile salts from the circulation represents a concentrative, saturable carrier-mediated process (Erlinger et al., 1976) which is different from that involved in the uptake of bilirubin, or the synthetic test dyes bromosulphthalein and indocyanine green (Scharschmidt et al., 1975). Binding to Y and Z proteins (section 10.2.1.1.2) does not appear to play a major role in bile acid transport (Kamisaka et al., 1975), and the concentrative transport system for the biliary excretion of bile acids is also different from that involved in bilirubin excretion (Alpert et al., 1969). Hence, while the hepatic transport of bile acids and bilirubin involves analogous mechanisms for uptake, conjugation and biliary excretion, these two principal endogenous cholephils do not share any major transport processes.

The hepatic uptake of bile salts is much more efficient than that of bilirubin. Almost 100% of the bile salts present in plasma are removed by one passage through the liver (Hofmann, 1976). The corresponding figure for bilirubin is only about 5%, while those for bromosulphthalein (section 10.4.1) and indocyanine green (section 10.4.2) are intermediate between these values (Martin et al., 1975). As a result of this highly efficient extraction process, bile salt uptake by the liver in normal individuals is limited only by the quantities delivered by hepatic blood flow. Hence, hepatic bile salt uptake and, consequently, peripheral serum bile salt concentrations, would be expected to be highly sensitive indicators of disorders involving impaired hepatocellular function and/or decreased or poorly distributed hepatic blood flow (as can occur in cirrhosis). Measurements of serum bile salt concentrations in various disease states tend to confirm this expectation (section 10.2.3.2).

Infusion studies have determined values for hepatic storage capacity (S) and biliary transport maximum (T_{MAX}) (see section 10.4.1.4 for further explanation of these parameters), for certain bile acids in animals (Erlinger et al., 1976). As yet, such studies have had no clinical application. The bile acids undergo a highly efficient enterohepatic circulation, which involves three discrete pathways (Figure 10.10A) following contraction of the gall bladder (Hofmann, 1976). These are: (a) passive jejunal reabsorption of the glycine conjugate of chenodeoxycholic acid; (b) active ileal reabsorption of all conjugated bile salts; and (c) passive colonic reabsorption of free bile acids, which are formed by bacterial deconjugation of conjugated bile salts within the gut. The action of enteric bacteria is also responsible for chemical alterations of the bile acid molecules which result in the formation of the secondary bile acids. Although more than 20 secondary bile acids have been isolated from human faeces, the most important quantitatively are deoxycholic acid and lithocholic acid (Carey, 1973). These are di- and monohydroxy bile acids formed from cholic acid and chenodeoxycholic acid, respectively, by the action of bacterial 7α-dehydroxylase (Figure 10.9). Following colonic reabsorption, the secondary bile acids are also conjugated in the liver. In addition, a high proportion of the conjugates of lithocholic acid are sulphated. While the conjugates of deoxycholic acid are efficiently reabsorbed, and therefore continue to participate in the enterohepatic circulation, the sulphated glycine and taurine conjugates of lithocholic acid are poorly reabsorbed. Hence, lithocholate normally makes only a single pass through the liver prior to its loss in the faeces (Hofmann, 1976). It has now been recognized that sulphation of the other primary and sec-

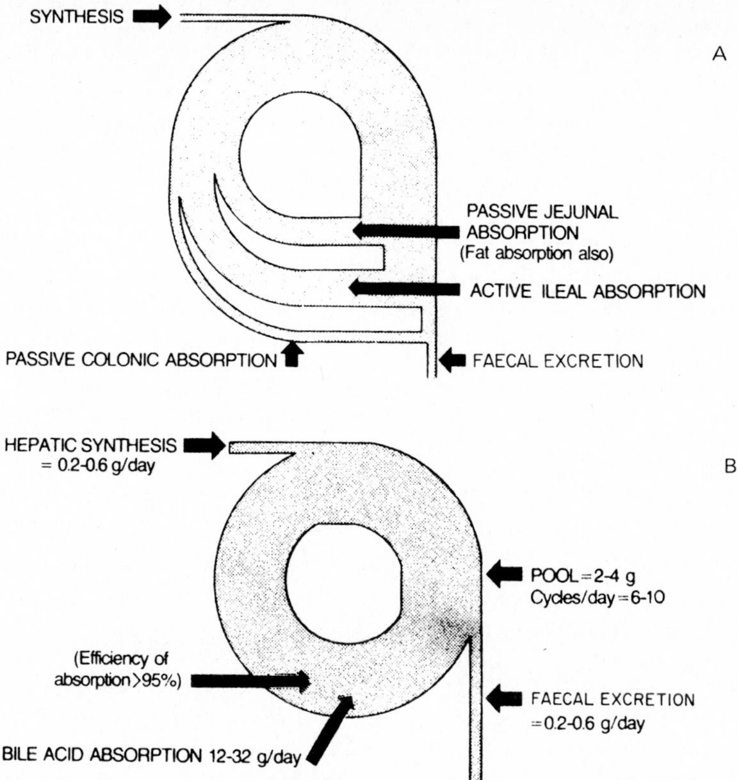

Figure 10.10. A: multiple enterohepatic circulations are responsible for efficient conservation of the bile acid pool. The importance of passive jejunal and colonic absorption in healthy man has not been determined. (Reproduced, with permission, from Hofmann and Kern, 1971) B: schematic representation of the actual quantitative aspects of the circulation of bile acids in man. Bile acid pool sizes may be determined by isotope dilution. In the steady state, faecal excretion is equivalent to hepatic synthesis. (Reproduced, with permission, from Hofmann and Kern, 1971)

ondary bile acids also occurs, and that urinary excretion of bile acid sulphates is a major route of bile acid elimination during cholestasis (Stiehl et al., 1976). Its importance in healthy man has yet to be established.

The dynamics of the enterohepatic circulation of bile acids are summarized schematically in Figure 10.10B, and the effect of enterohepatic recycling on serum bile acid concentrations is given in Figure 10.11. Values for steady-state bile acid synthesis derived from analysis of faecal metabolites are only about 50% of values derived from isotopic turnover studies; the reason for this discrepancy is unclear. Isotopic techniques suggest de novo synthesis in adults of 400 to 600 mg/day of cholic acid, and 200 to 300 mg/day of chenodeoxycholic acid. Turnover rates of deoxycholic and lithocholic acids amount to 30 to 50% of the rates of synthesis of the primary bile acids from which each is derived (Hofmann, 1976).

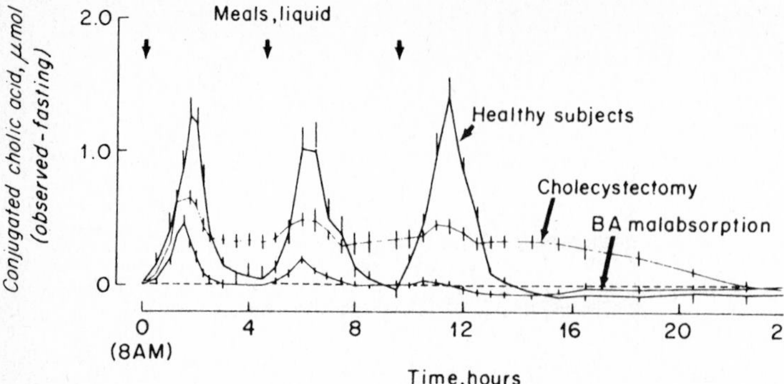

Figure 10.11. Serum concentrations of conjugates of cholic acid (plotted as observed minus fasting values) during three equicaloric liquid meals and on overnight fast in eight healthy subjects, six previously cholecystectomized individuals, and five patients with bile acid malabsorption secondary to ileal resection. In the latter group, the post-prandial serum increase became progressively smaller through the day, due to depletion of the bile acid pool by faecal loss. (Reproduced, with permission, from La Russo et al., 1974)

The bile acids have many physiologic roles. These include (a) regulation of the hepatic synthesis of cholesterol and new bile acids; (b) solubilization of lipids, notably cholesterol, during biliary lipid excretion, thereby tending to prevent formation of calculi within the biliary tract; (c) formation, within the intestinal lumen, of micelles that promote absorption of various lipids and fat-soluble compounds; (d) regulation of the rate of bile flow and biliary electrolyte excretion; and (e) regulation of salt and water balance within the colon. Intestinal bile salt physiology is considered in Chapter 12 of this book and hepatic bile salt physiology has been extensively reviewed elsewhere (Carey, 1973; Javitt, 1975; Erlinger et al., 1976).

10.2.3.2. Clinical applications

To date, the only measurements of bile acids which have proved clinically useful are measurements of serum bile acid concentrations. In the course of hepatobiliary disease, serum bile acids are altered in two principal ways: the bile acid concentrations tend to be increased, and the ratio of cholic acid to chenodeoxycholic acid in plasma may be altered. Both phenomena may be diagnostically helpful.

10.2.3.2.1. Fasting serum bile acid concentrations. Measurement of serum bile acids is technically difficult. Currently three main approaches, with numerous modifications, are being employed. These are (a) assays involving the enzyme 3-hydroxysteroid dehydrogenase; (b) gas chromatography; and (c) radioimmunoassay. Values obtained with the steroid dehydrogenase assay are often appreciably higher than those obtained by gas chromatography or radioimmunoassay. The upper limit of normal for fasting bile acid concentrations, measured by the steroid dehydrogenase technique, has been reported to be as high as 15 μmol/litre (Barnes et al., 1975) or almost five times that obtained from radioimmunoassay of conjugates of cholic and chenodeoxycholic acids (Simmonds et al.,

1973; Schalm et al., 1975). Values obtained by chromatographic methods tend to agree fairly well with those obtained by radioimmunoassay, and the former remains the technique against which radioimmunoassays are standardized (Simmonds et al., 1973). However, different authors report an appreciable variation in the upper limit of normal for total fasting serum bile acids by gas chromatography. It is apparent, therefore, that the interpretation of serum bile acid concentrations is critically dependent on the method employed and the individual laboratory where the test is set up.

Regardless of the method employed and the corresponding reference range, the numerous reports of elevated fasting serum bile acid concentrations in a large proportion of patients with acute or chronic hepatitis, alcoholic liver disease, cirrhosis, large duct biliary obstruction or intrahepatic cholestasis of various aetiologies indicate that this single static determination is a highly sensitive indicator of hepatobiliary dysfunction (Neale et al., 1971; Kaplowitz et al., 1973a; Korman et al., 1974; Barnes et al., 1975). It appears to be at least as sensitive an indicator of hepatocellular damage as the serum aminotransferases (section 10.2.4.1.1), but marginally less sensitive in this respect than bromosulphthalein retention at 45 minutes (Kaplowitz et al., 1973a) as shown in Figure 10.12. In one study, serum concentrations of conjugates of cholic acid were determined by radioimmunoassay in a group of patients with chronic active hepatitis who were in remission, as judged by routine serum biochemical tests and hepatic histology following administration of corticosteroids. Abnormal values for the cholic acid conjugates were found in the majority of the group of patients whose disease subsequently relapsed on withdrawal of treatment, whereas normal values predominated in the group of patients whose remissions were sustained after withdrawal of treatment (Korman et al., 1974).

10.2.3.2.2. Post-prandial serum bile acid concentrations

As a result of gall bladder contraction and efficient enterohepatic recirculation, the intestinal absorption of bile acids increases over the 2 h after a meal so that measurement in serum at this time constitutes, in effect, an endogenous bile acid loading test. Thus, a 2-hour post-prandial measurement of serum bile acids would be expected to be an even more sensitive measure of hepatobiliary disease than a measurement in the fasting state: this prediction has been confirmed in several studies (Kaplowitz et al., 1973a; Barnes et al., 1975). In healthy individuals, serum bile acid concentrations return to normal baseline values by 2 hours after a meal. In contrast, elevated values at this time are almost invariably found in patients with hepatobiliary disease (Figure 10.12), even when values in the fasting state are normal (Kaplowitz et al., 1973a). It is likely that the simple 2-hour post-prandial measurement of the serum concentration of bile acids will ultimately prove to be one of the most sensitive static tests of hepatobiliary function. It remains to be seen whether more complex procedures, such as those involving intraduodenal bile salt infusions or measurement of bile acid disappearance rates from plasma, (section 10.4.3) will have any advantage.

10.2.3.2.3. Ratio of trihydroxy- to dihydroxy-bile acids in serum

Determination of the ratio of trihydroxy- to dihydroxy-bile acids (or of cholic acid to chenodeoxycholic acid) may be of some diagnostic and prognostic value in patients with hepatobiliary disease (Carey, 1973; Javitt, 1975). For instance, the majority (~80%) of patients with cirrhosis or other types of hepatocellular lesion have a trihydroxy/dihydroxy concentration ratio of less than 1, whereas the majority (again ~80%) of patients

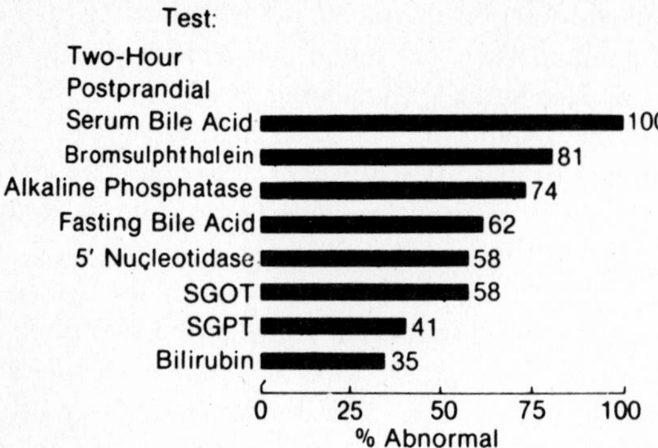

Figure 10.12. Frequency of abnormal serum biochemical tests in a series of patients with various hepatobiliary diseases. The 2 hour post-prandial serum bile acid measurement (2 h pp BA) was the most sensitive indicator of hepatic dysfunction. (Reproduced, with permission, from Kaplowitz et al., 1973a)

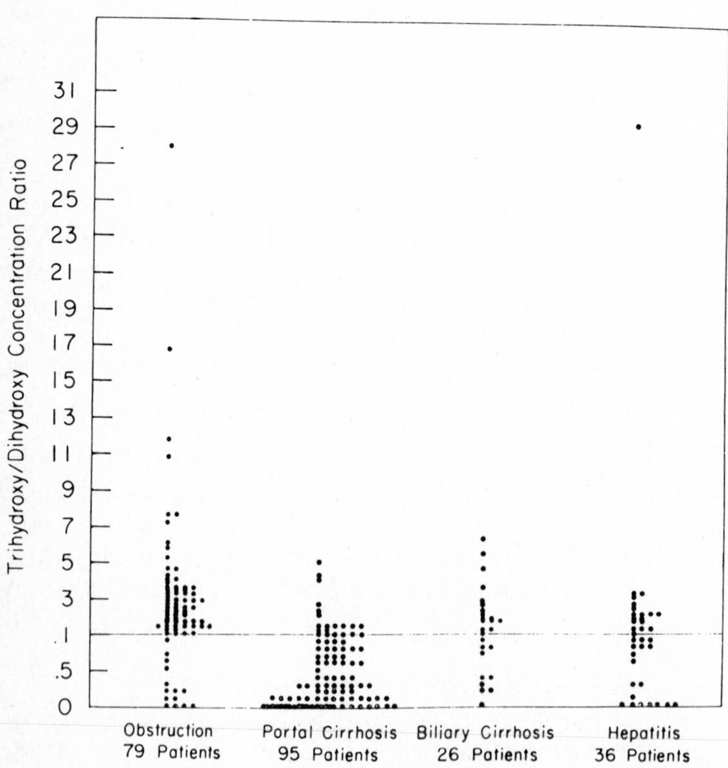

Figure 10.13. Distribution of values for the trihydroxy-/dihydroxy-bile salt concentration ratios in serum for four major groups of hepatobiliary disease. (Reproduced, with permission, from Carey, 1973)

with predominantly cholestatic disease have ratios in excess of 1 (Figure 10.13). The ratio is of no value in distinguishing intrahepatic cholestasis from obstruction of the large biliary ducts. Because the ratio cannot be determined accurately in normal individuals by gas chromatography, clinical interpretation of changes in this ratio are useful only in patients with appreciably elevated serum bile salt concentrations, who are usually clinically jaundiced.

Although serum bile acid measurements have much to recommended them, current methodology, which is general is fairly complex, will for the time being markedly restrict their availability. It is likely that in the near future improved radioimmunoassay procedures, involving the use of simple kits, will make such tests available to more laboratories.

10.2.4. Serum enzymes

The activities of a number of enzymes in serum are used as an aid to the evaluation of patients with hepatobiliary diseases, as outlined in Chapter 12. Their interpretation is often largely empirical (Wilkinson, 1970a; Skrede et al., 1973). Serum enzymes have an intracellular origin. Presumably they gain access to plasma principally from injured cells, but possibly also from intact cells. In a large number of conditions involving different extra-hepatic tissues, many of which are associated with cellular damage, increased activities of a number of intracellular enzymes, which are also present in the hepatocyte, are found in serum.

Factors relevant to the use of measurements of the activity of a serum enzyme in the diagnosis of hepatobiliary diseases include :the distribution of the enzyme in different tissues; its intracellular localization; the location of the enzyme within the hepatobiliary system; whether the enzyme is released in appreciable amounts from damaged cells and/or from cells with increased permeability of their surface membrane; whether activators, inhibitors or co-enzymes of the enzyme are present in plasma; the rate of synthesis of the enzyme and its rate of clearance from the plasma; the duration and pattern of elevated activities of the enzyme in serum in specific disease states, and the relationship of these activities to the results of non-enzyme tests (Wilkinson, 1970a; Zimmerman and Seeff, 1970; Skrede et al., 1973).

Whilst all of this information is desirable, only a small proportion of it is available for most serum enzyme tests. In reversible inflammatory processes, increased membrane permeability may be responsible for increased leakage of soluble cytoplasmic enzymes from cells. This phenomenon may also be the explanation for the increased serum activities of alanine aminotransferase and isocitrate dehydrogenase during recovery from severe malnutrition (McLean, 1962), when hepatocytes are presumably intact. However, in lesions associated with cell necrosis, mitochondrial and microsomal enzymes may be found in plasma (Wilkinson, 1970b) in addition to those of cytoplasmic origin. There may be increased serum activity of an enzyme if there is an increase in the amount of enzyme available for release, as occurs for instance, in large duct biliary obstruction which is associated with increased synthesis of alkaline phosphatase (Kaplan and Righetti, 1970). It is generally assumed that the marked elevation of serum activities of aminotransferases in the acute hepatitic syndrome is due to increased release of intracellular enzymes, but the possibility that there is also increased synthesis of these enzymes has not been excluded

(Wilkinson, 1970a). Increased serum activity of an enzyme may also occur if its rate of disappearance from the plasma is decreased. With regard to this possibility, it is clear that the rates of disappearance of different enzymes from plasma vary (Wilkinson, 1970a), possibly due to a selective effect of intravascular inhibitors, such as urea, or to different rates of endogenous catabolism. However, there is at present no convincing evidence that a decreased rate of clearance contributes to any appreciable extent to high serum enzyme activities in any hepatobiliary disease. In contrast, a decreased serum activity of an enzyme may occur if a disease interferes with the synthesis of an enzyme (e.g. cholinesterase in most hepatobiliary diseases and cholesterol esterase in hepatocellular disease) (Zimmerman and Seeff, 1970).

Very few enzymes are localized so exclusively in the liver that an elevation of their activity in serum unequivocally indicates hepatic injury. Examples of enzymes which are almost exclusively found in hepatocytes are iditol dehydrogenase, ornithine carbamoyltransferase and glutamate dehydrogenase. The most probable origin of a high serum enzyme activity can often be determined on clinical grounds. For instance, there is usually no difficulty in determining whether a high aspartate transaminase activity is due to acute hepatitis or to a recent myocardial infarct. As the contribution of various enzymes from different tissues to plasma varies, the source of abnormal serum enzyme values can often be assessed by measuring the activities of an appropriate combination of enzymes, an approach which increases the overall diagnostic value of enzyme determinations. Selection of which enzymes to measure should also take into account the different subcellular localizations of enzymes. The significance of enzyme tests can be further increased by correlating the results of these tests with the results of other liver function tests and indices of disease. It must be emphasized that normal values for serum enzymes do not exclude hepatobiliary diseases; for instance, serum enzyme activities may be normal in the presence of cirrhosis or hepatic neoplasia.

Most of the enzymes which are commonly measured in sera of patients with hepatobiliary diseases fall into two large groups based on the usual significance of a raised serum activity. In one group, increased activities predominantly reflect lesions affecting the parenchymal liver cell (hepatocyte); in the other, they predominantly reflect lesions affecting the biliary tract. In the discussion which follows, the adjectives "mild", "moderate" and "marked" or the corresponding adverbs, refer to an elevated serum enzyme activity from 1 to 3 times, from 3 to 10 times and over 10 times the upper limit of normal, respectively.

10.2.4.1. Hepatic parenchymal cell enzymes

10.2.4.1.1. Aspartate aminotransferase (EC 2.6.1.1), alanine aminotransferase (EC 2.6.1.2). Aspartate aminotransferase (formerly called glutamic oxaloacetic transaminase) and alanine aminotransferase (formerly called glutamic pyruvate transaminase) activities in serum are commonly measured in the evaluation of patients with hepatobiliary diseases. These enzymes catalyze respectively the following reactions –

aspartate + α-ketoglutarate ⇌ oxaloacetate + glutamate
alanine + α-ketoglutarate ⇌ pyruvate + glutamate

Aspartate aminotransferase, of which separate cytoplasmic and mitochondrial isoenzymes can be distinguished by electrophoresis, is found particularly in hepatocytes, skeletal muscle, myocardium, kidney, pancreas and red cells. Alanine aminotransferase exists largely in cytoplasm and most of this enzyme is found in hepatocytes (Zimmerman and Seeff, 1970). These enzymes, which are distributed in interstitial fluid, are not excreted to any appreciable extent in bile or urine and presumably undergo a process of protein catabolism. As aspartate aminotransferase is appreciably less specific for liver than alanine aminotransferase, more care is required in interpreting raised serum activities of the former enzyme than the latter. A raised activity of aspartate transaminase usually implies recent or continuing damage to the liver, heart or skeletal muscle, or haemolysis, while a raised activity of alanine aminotransferase suggests that there is probably a hepatic lesion. Only rarely is the probable origin of a raised serum aminotransferase activity unclear. In this context, the demonstration of abnormal bromosulphthalein retention (section 10.4.1.1) would suggest impaired hepatic function and would point to a hepatic source for the increased serum activity of the enzyme. Activities of both of these enzymes in serum are normally higher in neonates than adults and may be increased as a result of leakage through abnormally permeable hepatocyte cell membranes, without necessarily implying the death of cells. Serum aspartate aminotransferase activity may be spuriously low in azotaemia (Cohen et al., 1974) which may complicate acute or chronic liver failure.

In acute viral hepatitis, the serum alanine aminotransferase activity usually rises more rapidly, and reaches a higher value than that of aspartate aminotransferase and remains abnormal for a longer time. Values for both of these enzymes tend to be higher in icteric than non-icteric acute hepatitis (Clermont and Chalmers, 1967). In this disease, measurement of only one of the aminotransferases is usually adequate (Salkie, 1971). In contrast, in alcoholic liver disease serum aspartate aminotransferase activity is usually higher than the serum alanine aminotransferase, which tends to be only moderately elevated (Zimmerman and Seeff, 1970). In alcoholism, raised serum activities of enzymes derived from skeletal muscle, such as creatine kinase, are often present and aspartate aminotransferase derived from skeletal muscle may contribute to the raised serum activities of this enzyme (Konttinen et al., 1970). Marked elevation of serum aspartate aminotransferase activity can occur in delerium tremens (Zimmerman and Seeff, 1970). However, if any hepatic lesion is associated with appreciable liver cell necrosis, the increased release of mitochondrial enzymes from cells may result in a relatively greater increase in aspartate than alanine aminotransferase activity due to an increased contribution of the mitochondrial isoenzyme of aspartate aminotransferase (Zimmerman and Seeff, 1970; Wilkinson, 1970b; Skrede et al., 1973). The clinical significance of aspartate/alanine aminotransferase ratios is comprehensively discussed by Zimmerman and Seeff (1970). Apart from acute hepatitis, serum aspartate aminotransferase tends to be a more sensitive but less specific test for the detection of hepatobiliary disease than alanine aminotransferase.

Raised serum aminotransferase activities occur early (Figures 10.14 and 10.15) during the course of acute viral hepatitis (Clermont and Chalmers, 1967) or of drug-induced hepatocellular necrosis – i.e, a few days to a few weeks before the onset of jaundice – while the finding of normal serum aminotransferase activities early on in the course of an episode of jaundice virtually excludes acute hepatitis. Serum activities of the aminotrans-

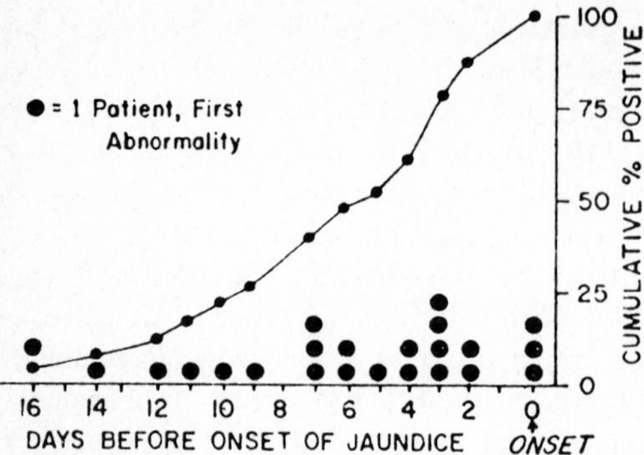

Figure 10.14. Incidence of abnormal values for serum aspartate aminotransferase in 23 subjects being followed during the preicteric stages of acute viral hepatitis. (Reproduced, with permission, from Clermont and Chalmers, 1967)

ferases are valuable in screening for inapparent (anicteric) viral hepatitis during epidemics, for relapsing acute hepatitis and for acute hepatitis in drug addicts or after blood transfusion. Markedly elevated values for serum aminotransferases (especially when greater than 20 times the upper limit of normal) nearly always imply injury to the liver and sug-

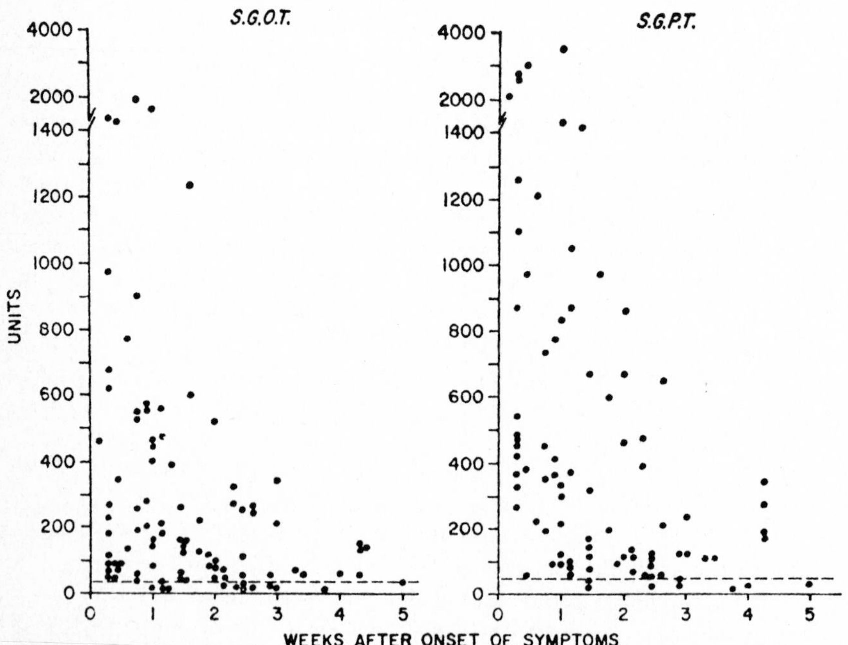

Figure 10.15. Relationship of the serum aspartate (SGOT) and alanine (SGPT) aminotransferases on admission to hospital to the onset of symptoms in acute viral hepatitis. Markedly elevated values (>400 units) occur in an appreciable proportion of cases during the first 3 weeks of symptoms. (Reproduced, with permission, from Clermont and Chalmers, 1967)

gest acute necrosis of hepatocytes due to viral hepatitis (Figure 10.16), drugs or toxins (Breen and Schenker, 1971). However, marked elevation of the activities of the aminotransferases in serum can also occur in association with a low cardiac output with or without shock, hypoxia, or severe congestive cardiac failure (Breen and Schenker, 1971), and also very rarely in chronic active hepatitis and large duct biliary obstruction (Mossberg and Ross, 1963; Stern et al., 1973). When ascending cholangitis complicates an obstructive lesion of the biliary tract, such as a gall stone, marked elevation of serum activities of

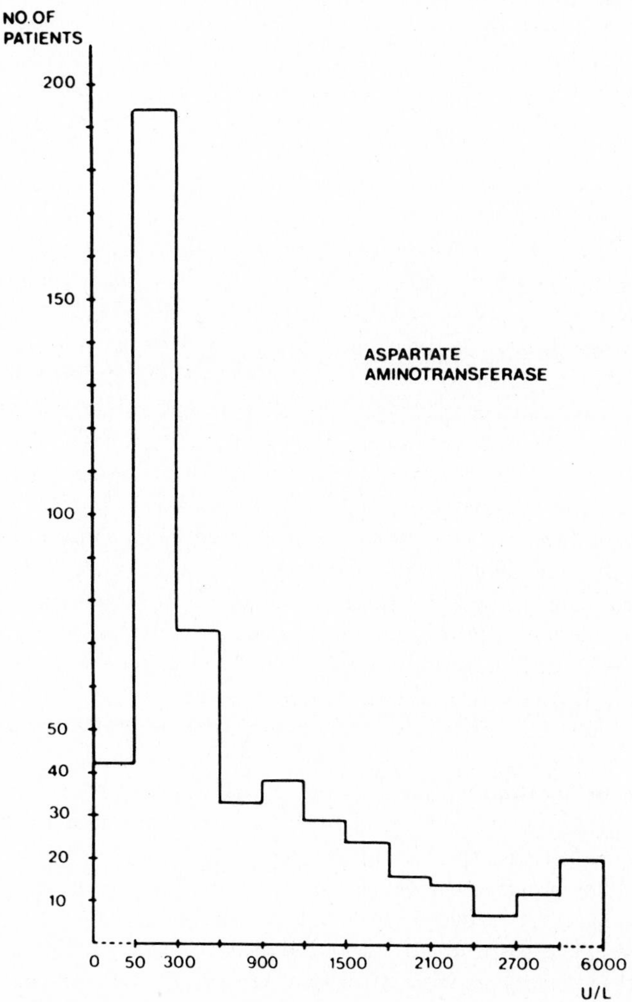

Figure 10.16. Distribution of serum aspartate aminotransferase (AST) values in 500 patients with biopsy-verified acute hepatitis at the time of biopsy. The diagnosis in each case was presumed to be acute viral hepatitis. The upper limit of normal for AST is 34 U/litre. Note that in many patients enzyme activities were not markedly raised. (Reproduced, with permission, from Petersen et al., 1974)

aminotransferases may occur. In acute hepatitis an appreciable fall in the activity of aminotransferases in serum may have taken place as early as the second week of jaundice, in which case values are far less useful diagnostically (Petersen et al., 1974). The rise and fall of serum aminotransferase values tend to take longer in type B than in type A hepatitis (Krugman et al., 1967). These tests generally remain abnormal after other laboratory indices of the disease such as serum bilirubin concentration, alkaline phosphatase and ornithine carbamoyltransferase activities have returned to normal (Wacker et al., 1972). Marked elevations of serum activities of the aminotransferases tend to be more often found in pre-cirrhotic than cirrhotic chronic active hepatitis and may, in this context, be due to the activity of the disease process, to complicating acute hepatitis, or to the effects of drugs. Marked elevations in cirrhosis may be due to complications such as drug toxicity, delerium tremens, pancreatitis or post-transfusion hepatitis. Mildly or moderately elevated activities may be due to non-hepatic lesions and are not of value in differentiating between lesions which predominantly affect hepatocytes and those which predominantly affect the biliary tract. For example, within a few dys of the onset of acute large duct biliary obstruction, there is usually a moderate elevation of serum activities of aminotransferases presumably due to the effect of cholestasis on the hepatocyte (Mossberg and Ross, 1963). The abnormal values tend to persist until after relief of the obstruction. Moderate elevations of activities may also be due to primary biliary cirrhosis and other causes of intrahepatic cholestasis; chronic persistent and chronic active hepatitis; drugs such as oxyphenisatin, isoniazid, sulphonamides, α-methyldopa and aspirin; cirrhosis of various aetiologies; the Budd Chiari syndrome; alcoholic hepatitis; secondary carcinoma or lymphoma involving the liver; liver cell carcinoma; acute pancreatitis; acute cholecystitis; the hepatic lesion occurring after jejunoileal by-pass; infectious mononucleosis; opiates given after cholecystectomy; congestive cardiac failure; intrahepatic infections including abscesses; extrahepatic infections associated with disturbed hepatic function (Neale et al., 1966); and hepatic granulomas. In uncomplicated fatty infiltration of the liver, it is very rare for serum alanine and aspartate aminotransferase activities to be more than mildly elevated. In cardiac disease, a raised serum alanine aminotransferase activity is most often secondary to the hepatic congestion of right-sided heart failure. The incidental finding of a raised serum aspartate or alanine aminotransferase activity may be the first indication of a latent asymptomatic cirrhosis or asymptomatic precirrhotic Wilson's disease.

Serial serum aminotransferase measurements are useful in following the course of acute hepatitis. Persistence of raised serum activities of aminotransferases for more than 6 months after an attack of acute hepatitis, suggests that the hepatic lesion may be undergoing progression to a chronic lesion such as chronic persistent hepatitis or chronic active hepatitis, although values that have been raised for as long as a year may still spontaneously return to normal with complete resolution of the hepatic lesion. The actual value of the elevated serum transaminase activity in acute or chronic hepatitis is not a reliable index of the severity of the underlying lesion or of the prognosis. For instance, serum aminotransferase activities are often markedly increased in patients with acute viral hepatitis who subsequently recover rapidly. Furthermore, values for the serum aminotransferases which are normal or only mildly elevated are not a reliable indication of histological remission of disease activity in chronic active hepatitis, and the occurrence of markedly elevated values does not necessarily indicate failure of treatment of this lesion. In patients with chronic active hepatitis who are treated with corticosteroids, an increase in the dose of the drug is often associated with a decrease in the serum activities of the aminotransferases. The exact significance of such an observation is not clear. Serum aminotransferase activities can be particularly unreliable as an index of the severity of disease and/or prognosis in patients with massive hepatic necrosis. There is, however, a tendency for the activities to fall to values which are only mildly raised, or within the normal range, as a pre-terminal event in massive hepatic necrosis, possibly due to a paucity of surviving liver cells. The same phenomenon is often seen pre-terminally in cirrhosis. Thus, falling serum aminotransferase values are only reassuring when accompanied by clinical improvement.

In patients with hepatic tumours, the serum aspartate aminotransferase activity may occasionally be normal, but it is usually increased, the degree of increase being a rough index of the mass of the tumour. When aspartate and alanine aminotransferase values are used to monitor treatment of patients with hepatic neoplasia, increased values may reflect progression of the disease and/or side-effects of treatment. In spite of the well recognized problems of interpreting the significance of serum aminotransferase activities, measurements of these enzymes are extensively used in the routine assessment of patients with hepatobiliary disease and in monitoring their relapses, complications and response to therapy.

10.2.4.1.2. Other hepatic parenchymal cell enzymes. The serum activities of a number of other enzymes tend to increase when hepatocytes are damaged or undergo necrosis. Some of these enzymes, like aspartate aminotransferase, have low specificity for liver diseases; these include fructose-1,6-diphosphate aldolase, malate dehydrogenase, isocitrate dehydrogenase and phosphohexoseisomerase (glucose phosphate isomerase). Others, like alanine aminotransferase, have high liver specificity; these include iditol (sorbitol) dehydrogenase, ornithine carbamoyltransferase, alcohol dehydrogenase and glutamate dehydrogenase. Some of these enzymes (e.g., isocitrate dehydrogenase and ornithine carbamoyltransferase) are sensitive indicators of liver cell disease, whereas others (e.g. glutamate dehydrogenase and iditol dehydrogenase) are not. Some are located in mitochondria (e.g. glutamate dehydrogenase) and increased activities of these particular enzymes in plasma may be an index of cell necrosis (Zimmerman and Seeff, 1970). Serum ornithine carbamoyltransferase activity may be increased in association with slight liver damage when the serum alanine aminotransferase activity is not raised (Skrede et al., 1973). The times for which the activities of different enzymes in serum remain elevated in viral hepatitis differ. For instance, the serum activity of iditol dehydrogenase returns to normal much more quickly than that of the aminotransferases whereas γ-glutamyltransferase activity continues to rise after the activities of the aminotransferases have started to fall (Wieme and Demeulenaere, 1971). The serum activities of some of these enzymes (e.g. isocitrate and iditol dehydrogenases) tend to be normal, or only slightly elevated, in large duct biliary obstruction (Wilkinson, 1970a). Glutamate dehydrogenase activity may be particularly high in serum in large duct biliary obstruction for reasons which are not clear (Zimmerman and Seeff, 1970). However, measurements of this enzyme do not enable a reliable differentiation between large duct biliary obstruction and intrahepatic cholestasis to be made. It has been claimed (Mezey et al., 1968) that serum activity of alcohol dehydrogenase may be useful in differentiating intra-hepatic from extra-hepatic causes of cholestasis, but wider application of measurements of this enzyme will be necessary to confirm its usefulness to the clinician. In general, these enzymes have not been as extensively studied in hepatobiliary disorders as have the aminotransferases, and most are more difficult to assay. At present none of them appears to have any particular advantage for the evaluation of hepatobiliary disease over aspartate and alanine aminotransferases (Clermont and Chalmers, 1967).

10.2.4.2. Biliary tract enzymes

10.2.4.2.1. Alkaline phosphatase. Alkaline phosphatase (EC 3.1.3.1; orthophosphoric monoester phosphohydrolase) is an enzyme which liberates inorganic phosphate from a variety of organic orthophosphate esters. The physiological role of the protein which has alkaline phosphatase activity in vitro is unknown. It has low organ specificity and exists in serum in the form of isoenzymes derived largely from liver, bone, intestine and, in the third trimester of pregnancy, placenta. Alkaline phosphatase can be demonstrated in the brush border of the bile canaliculus, the sinusoidal surface of hepatocytes, the enterocytes of the small intestine, the renal proximal convoluted tubule, epithelial cells lining the alveoli of the lactating mammary gland and the outermost surface of the syncytial-trophoblast of the placenta (Kaplan, 1972). Alkaline phospahtase is also found in the white blood cells and may be present in some malignant tumours (Kaplan, 1972; Warnes, 1972). Its pathway of degradation is unknown. It is not excreted to any appreciable extent in bile or urine. When infused, the rate of disappearance of the enzyme from plasma is independent of the patency of the bile ducts (Clubb et al., 1965; Wilkinson, 1970a; Kaplan, 1972). It seems likely that alkaline phosphatase undergoes a process of protein catabolism.

In general, the activity of the serum alkaline phosphatase in hepatobiliary disease reflects the degree of bile stasis rather than hepatocellular necrosis. Indeed, the fact that the activity tends to be only mildly or moderately raised in cases of massive hepatic necrosis (Ritt et al., 1969) indicates that leakage of preformed enzyme from hepatocytes is not an adequate explanation for the high serum activity of this enzyme in many other hepatobiliary disorders. The raised serum activity associated with large duct biliary obstruction in the rat has been shown to be due to a selective increase in the hepatic isoenzyme, and this increase can be inhibited by cyclophosphamide, an inhibitor of protein synthesis (Kaplan and Righetti, 1970). Thus, if these observations can be extrapolated to man, it would seem that the increased serum alkaline phosphatase activity associated with bile stasis may be due largely to increased synthesis of alkaline phosphatase in the hepatocyte, while the falling values which tend to occur in terminal biliary cirrhosis and the reduced values in kwashiorkor may be due to decreased synthesis of this enzyme. There is, in general, a poor correlation between serum alkaline phosphatase activity and serum total bilirubin concentration in patients with hepatobiliary diseases. This may, in large measure, be a reflection of the fundamental differences between the metabolism of alkaline phosphatase and that of bilirubin (section 10.2.1).

Moderate or marked elevations of serum alkaline phosphatase activity occur in patients with complete large duct biliary obstruction (e.g. carcinoma of the head of the pancreas), intrahepatic cholestasis and infiltrative disorders of the liver; mild elevations of activity are usually found in patients with predominantly hepatocellular lesions such as viral hepatitis or cirrhosis. Serum alkaline phosphatase measurements do not enable differentiation of intra-hepatic and extra-hepatic causes of cholestasis. They are of limited value in differentiating lesions associated with biliary obstruction from predominantly hepatocellular diseases. However, there is an overlap between values obtained in patients with hepatocellular disease (Petersen et al., 1974) and those obtained in patients with biliary tract lesions, so that clear separation of the two types of disorder on the basis of the alkaline phosphatase activity is not possible. Nevertheless, the fact that values in cholestatic viral hepatitis (Figure 10.17) are not usually as high as those found in cholestatic drug jaundice or large duct biliary obstruction can be helpful to the clinician. In intrahepatic cholestasis, the serum alkaline phosphatase may be as high as 20 times the upper limit of normal. In complete large duct biliary obstruction the typical finding is a moderate elevation, although in patients with large duct biliary obstruction due to cholelithiasis or carcinoma of the pancreas or bile duct, values that are only mildly elevated or even normal can occur (Stern et al., 1973). Usually in fatty liver or inactive cirrhosis the alkaline phosphatase

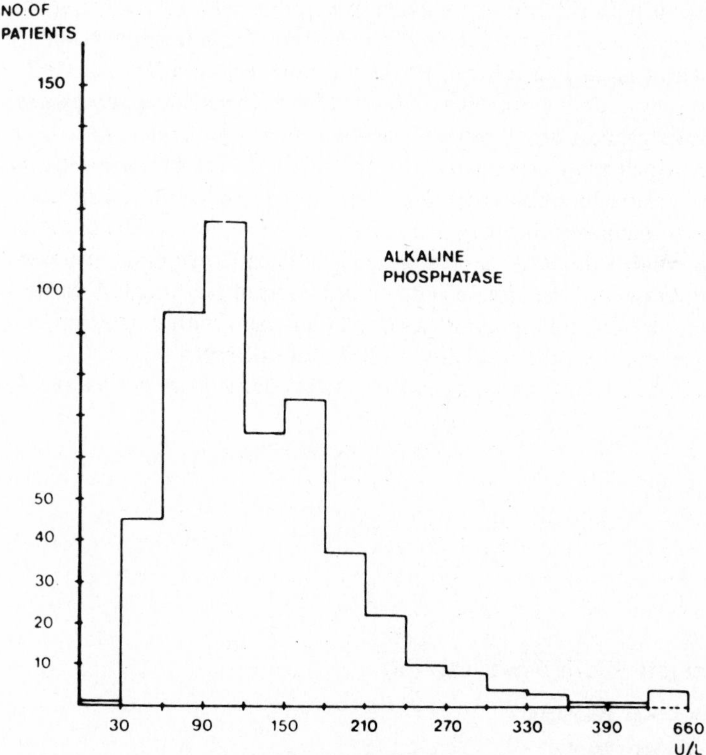

Figure 10.17. Distribution of serum alkaline phosphatase values in 500 patients with biopsy-verified acute hepatitis at the time of biopsy. The diagnosis in each case was presumed to be acute viral hepatitis. The upper limit of normal for alkaline phosphatase is 90 U/litre. Note that moderately elevated activities do occur but are uncommon. (Reproduced, with permission, from Petersen et al., 1974)

activity is only mildly increased and may be normal. However, in some patients with alcoholic cirrhosis marked elevations may occur due to severe fatty change causing intrahepatic cholestasis, or to alcoholic pancreatitis or a pancreatic pseudocyst producing large duct biliary obstruction. Large nodules of regeneration in macronodular cirrhosis may cause more bile duct compression than smaller ones in micronodular cirrhosis. This phenomenon may be responsible for higher activities of serum alkaline phosphatase in patients with the former lesion.

Causes of moderate elevation of the serum alkaline phosphatase activity *in the absence of jaundice,* include space-occupying lesions in the liver such as primary or secondary neoplasia; abscesses or cysts; hepatobiliary disease complicating cystic fibrosis; hepatic lymphoma; granulomata (such as sarcoid and TB); amyloid; a stone or tumour involving one main hepatic duct; transient or partial large duct biliary obstruction due to stones or carcinoma of the ampulla of Vater; the post-cholecystectomy cystic duct remnant syndrome (Bodvall, 1973); early primary biliary cirrhosis (Fox et al., 1973); chronic pancreatitis; carcinoma of the pancreas; and drugs which can induce cholestasis such as chlorpromazine. The finding of a raised serum alkaline phosphatase activity is a sensitive screening test for the early detection of these conditions and may be the only abnormal laboratory test result found in patients with an obstructive lesion of large bile ducts. A normal serum alkaline phosphatase activity makes most unlikely, but does not exclude, primary biliary cirrhosis (Figure 10.18), or large duct biliary obstruction (Sherlock and Scheuer, 1973; Stern et al., 1973), and can occur in extrahepatic biliary atresia. The alkaline phosphatase activity is raised in a large proportion of patients with secondary carcinoma of the liver. Virtually any lesion in which there is inflammation or infiltration of the portal tracts, including bacterial and sclerosing cholangitis, Hodgkin's disease and schistosomiasis is usually associated with an increase in activity of the enzyme. When the alkaline phosphatase activity is used to monitor the effects of treatment on hepatic neoplasia, increased values may indicate progression of the disease and/or side-effects of treatment. A particularly high or rising serum alkaline phosphatase activity in a patient with cirrhosis, other than primary biliary cirrhosis, raises the possibility of liver cell carcinoma.

Marked elevations of serum alkaline phosphatase activity occur in bone diseases in

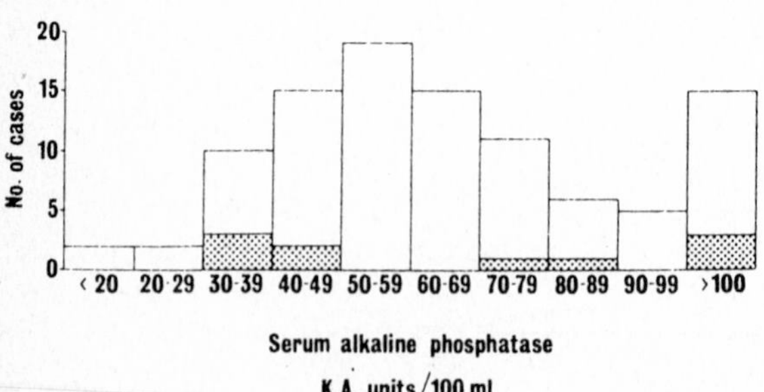

Figure 10.18. Serum alkaline phosphatase activities at the time of presentation in 100 patients with primary biliary cirrhosis. The upper limit of normal is 14 K.A. units/dl. Values exceeding 50 K.A. units/dl occurred in 71%; normal values were rare. Male patients are shown as hatched columns. (Reproduced, with permission, from Sherlock and Scheuer, 1973)

which there is increased osteoblastic activity, e.g. Paget's disease, and mild physiologic elevations occur during adolescence due to the increased osteoblastic activity associated with active growth (Sereny and McLaughlin, 1970). Increased values may also occur in a number of conditions which do not primarily involve liver or bone. The hepatic isoenzyme appears to contribute to the raised serum alkaline phosphatase activity found in some patients with Hodgkin's disease (stages I and II), myeloid metaplasia, congestive cardiac failure, inflammatory bowel disease and intra-abdominal infections (Kaplan, 1972). The serum activity of the hepatic isoenzyme of alkaline phosphatase may be increased in the absence of a hepatobiliary lesion (Brensilver and Kaplan, 1975). The intestinal isoenzyme contributes to the raised serum alkaline phosphatase in some disorders of the small bowel such as α-chain disease and in some patients with alcoholic cirrhosis and certain tumours (Fishman et al., 1965); a variant isoenzyme may contribute to an increased serum alkaline phosphatase activity which is associated with carcinoma of the bronchus and other malignancies (Kaplan, 1972; Warnes, 1972). Raised serum alkaline phosphatase activity may also occur in association with non-metastatic hypernephroma (Walsh and Kissane, 1968), renal transplants, thyrotoxicosis, rheumatoid arthritis, pulmonary infarction and infusion of albumin of placental origin (Lum and Gambino, 1972; Warnes, 1972). Because the serum alkaline phosphatase activity is raised in so many conditions, the finding of a normal value for this test is sometimes of more help diagnostically than a raised value.

In most clinical situations, the source of a raised serum alkaline phosphatase is usually obvious. However, when this is not so, as may occur when a raised value is discovered in an apparently healthy individual, it is necessary to employ further procedures to identify the likely source. Useful tests in this context are serum activities of 5′-nucleotidase, leucine aminopeptidase or γ-glutamyltransferase, all of which would, as a rule, be raised if the cause of the alkaline phosphatase elevation is a hepatobiliary lesion, but normal if the cause is an osseous lesion. Sometimes however the situation may be complex. For example, patients late in the course of primary biliary cirrhosis often have metabolic bone disease. The value of the serum alkaline phosphatase activity in these patients may be relatively greater than that predicted from the activities of 5′-nucleotidase, leucine aminopeptidase or γ-glutamyltransferase. Alternatively, specific tests may be done to determine the relative contributions of the different isoenzymes to an increase in the serum alkaline phosphatase activity. In this context, the techniques which have been employed include electrophoretic separation of isoenzymes, especially using polyacrylamide gel, and assessments of the relative sensitivity of isoenzymes to denaturation by heat or urea. The liver isoenzyme is more stable to heat and to urea than the bone isoenzyme. These techniques are not easy and the interpretation of the results is often difficult. Different methods of preparation of specimens produce variations in the electrophoretic pattern, and the electrophoretic differences between the liver and bone isoenzymes are in any case small. Often it is not possible to obtain reliable quantitation of all the isoenzymes in a given serum. In addition, there is sometimes a poor correlation between the results of isoenzyme determinations and the organs presumed to be the site of disease, so that overlap of results in different groups of patients may occur (Winkelman et al., 1972). Because of the numerous potential problems involved in the estimation and interpretation of isoenzymes of alkaline phosphatase in serum, their determination probably does not have a place in the routine evaluation of hepatobiliary disorders (Baron, 1970). However, in the rare case in which the cause of a raised alkaline phosphatase activity remains unclear after a conventional clinical and laboratory assessment, it is possible that isoenzyme studies may provide definitive diagnostic information not obtainable by other means. For instance, unusual isoenzyme patterns may occur in association with certain malignant tumours such as hepatocellular carcinoma (Higashino et al., 1975). The isoenzymes can be quantitated by immunological and chromatographic techniques, but these have not yet been applied in a clinical context (Warnes, 1972).

10.2.4.2.2. γ-Glutamyltransferase (EC 2.3.2.2). This enzyme is found particularly in the biliary tract, pancreas, intestine and kidney. It is produced along the whole biliary tract from the bile canaliculus to the common bile duct, and also in pancreatic acini and small ductules; it appears to have both a microsomal and cytoplasmic intracellular distribution. This enzyme can, in addition, be demonstrated histochemically near the luminal border of renal tubular cells, enterocytes and vascular endothelial cells. It is absent from myocardium and skeletal muscle (Naftalin et al., 1969; Rosalki and Rau, 1972; Lum and Gambino, 1972). The hepatobiliary duct system is the source of γ-glutamyltransferase activity in normal serum (Naftalin et al., 1969; Rosalki and Rau, 1972).

The serum enzyme activity tends to be markedly elevated in patients with large duct biliary obstruction, intrahepatic cholestasis and infiltrative disorders of the liver (Dragosici et al., 1976). Values are usually only moderately elevated in predominantly hepatocellular diseases. As cirrhosis progresses, the activity tends to fall and may become very low in terminal liver failure (Cushieri and Baker, 1974). Although it has been claimed that γ-glutamyltransferase may be superior to alkaline phosphatase in differentiating between predominantly biliary tract and hepatocellular lesions, it is nevertheless of limited value in this respect (Cushieri and Baker, 1974; Betro et al., 1973). In general, changes in serum γ-glutamyltransferase and alkaline phosphatase activities tend to parallel each other in hepatobiliary diseases, although rises in the former enzyme may be relatively greater than those of the latter. Measurement of serum γ-glutamyltransferase appears to be more sensitive than that of 5′-nucleotidase, alkaline phosphatase or leucine aminopeptidase as a screening test in anicteric patients for the presence of hepatobiliary disease, including hepatic neoplasia (Whitfield et al., 1972). In contrast to the situation with 5′-nucleotidase and leucine aminopeptidase, moderately raised serum activities of γ-glutamyltransferase have a relatively low specificity for hepatobiliary disease (Whitfield et al., 1972). However, markedly increased activities do suggest a lesion involving the intra- or extra-hepatic bile ducts, pancreatitis or hepatic neoplasia (Betro et al., 1973). The highest values tend to be associated with large duct biliary obstruction due to lesions in the vicinity of the ampulla of Vater (Naftalin et al., 1969). High activities in the absence of jaundice raise the possibility of malignancy. The serum γ-glutamyltransferase activity may be raised while all other serum enzyme activities are normal in patients suffering from malignancy, chronic hepatitis or alcoholism. In chronic hepatitis a raised serum γ-glutamyltransferase activity presumably indicates that the disease is not quiescent, but values do not correlate well with relapses and remissions of the disease (Cushieri and Baker, 1974). Serum activity may be raised in the presence of hepatic granulomata.

Measurement of serum γ-glutamyltransferase activity can be used as a screening test for chronic alcoholism (Figure 10.19). In alcoholics, a raised serum activity of this

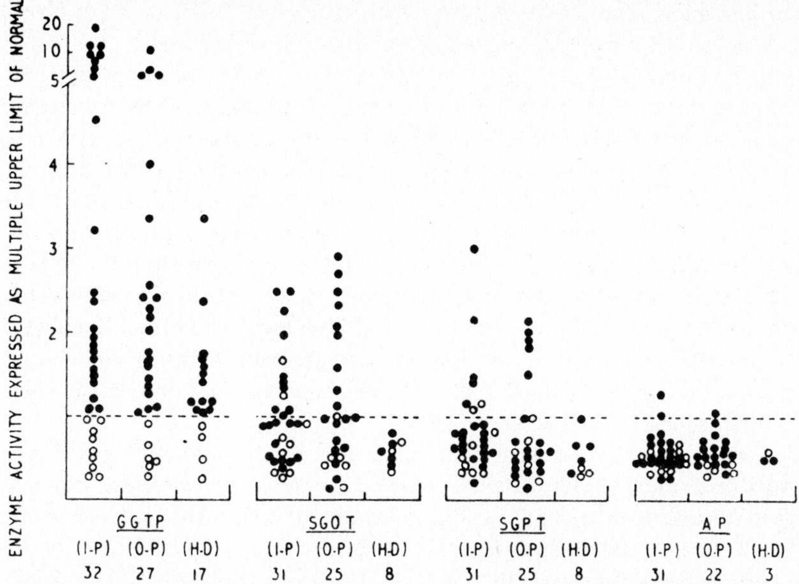

Figure 10.19. Serum enzyme activities in alcoholic in-patients (I-P), alcoholic outpatients (O-P) and outpatient heavy drinkers (H-D). GGTP = γ-glutamyltransferase; SGOT = aspartate aminotransferase; SGPT = alanine aminotransferase; AP = alkaline phosphatase. Open circles represent enzyme activities in patients with normal serum γ-glutamyltransferase activity. (Reproduced, with permission, from Rosalki and Rau, 1972).

enzyme, in the absence of elevation of the serum activity of any other enzyme, does not necessarily imply that there is significant underlying structural liver disease and is not in itself an indication for liver biopsy. A raised γ-glutamyltransferase activity is the earliest serum enzyme abnormality in the alcoholic that can readily be detected by a routine clinical chemistry laboratory. During follow-up of an alcoholic, a raised activity suggests that the patient may not be abstaining from alcohol. Elevation of the activity in an alcoholic, who does not have established structural liver disease by light microscopy, probably implies either microsomal damage or enzyme induction in the hepatocyte due to recent alcohol intake (Rosalki and Rau, 1972).

Raised activities are also found in patients who have been treated, for periods usually greater than 6 months, with certain drugs which are microsomal enzyme inducers such as phenytoin, barbiturates and aminopyrine. In such subjects, who are usually epileptics, there is typically no other evidence of liver disease. It seems probable, as with alcohol ingestion, that these drugs are either causing microsomal damage or enzyme induction, including induction of γ-glutamyltransferase, with subsequent release of the enzyme into the circulation (Whitfield et al., 1972; Bartels et al., 1975).

Serum γ-glutamyltransferase activity may be increased in patients with cholecystitis or pancreatitis in the absence of associated large duct biliary obstruction. In pancreatitis, a raised value may be due to release of the enzyme from pancreatic acini or due to a reaction in adjacent bile ducts. The activity tends to remain elevated for about 4 to 6 weeks after the relief of large duct biliary obstruction (Cushieri and Baker, 1974).

Measurement of serum γ-glutamyltransferase activity is helpful in determining which organ is responsible for a high serum alkaline phosphatase activity, since the former enzyme activity is not elevated in uncomplicated osseous disease (Betro et al., 1973). In combined hepatobiliary and osseous lesions, such as may occur in primary biliary cirrhosis, the increase in the alkaline phosphatase activity may be relatively greater than that of γ-glutamyltransferase. In contrast to the serum alkaline phosphatase, serum γ-glutamyltransferase activities are normal in pregnancy and in children after the age of 3 months. Thus, measurements of γ-glutamyltransferase may be particularly useful in the diagnosis of hepatobiliary disease in pregnancy and childhood (Lum and Gambino, 1972; Shore et al., 1975). However, in women who are pregnant or taking oral contraceptives, elevation of the enzyme activity due to viral hepatitis may be relatively less marked than in other subjects (Combes et al., 1974).

Other lesions which may be associated with raised serum γ-glutamyltransferase activities include congestive cardiac failure; diabetes mellitus; renal transplant rejection; renal tumours without hepatic involvement; nephrotic syndrome; and highly vascular brain lesions (Lum and Gambino, 1972; Whitfield et al., 1972).

10.2.4.2.3. Leucine aminopeptidase (EC 3.4.11.1). Leucine aminopeptidase (naphthylamidase) hydrolyses aminoacids from the *N*-terminal end of various proteins and polypeptides, reacting most rapidly with leucine-containing substances. The enzyme catalyzes the following reaction –

L-leucyl-β-naphthylamide $\rightarrow$ β-naphthylamine + leucine

and it is usually β-naphthylamide which is quantitated in the assay of the enzyme. The use of other substrates may yield different results, since a different peptidase may be assayed. Leucine aminopeptidase can be demonstrated in the biliary duct system, duodenum, small intestine, pancreas, testis, stromal cells of the uterus, and particularly in the renal tubules. It exists in serum in the form of several isoenzymes; in normal serum, isoenzymes of hepatobiliary origin predominate.

As with alkaline phosphatase, 5′-nucleotidase and γ-glutamyltransferase, the highest serum activities of this enzyme are found in patients with large duct biliary obstruction, intrahepatic cholestasis and infiltrative disorders of the liver. Leucine aminopeptidase is less sensitive than γ-glutamyltransferase, but approximately as sensitive as 5′-nucleotidase and alkaline phosphatase in the detection of hepatobiliary disease, including intrahepatic neoplasia. Marked elevation of serum leucine aminopeptidase activity tends to occur in the same hepatobiliary diseases in which high serum activities of alkaline phosphatase, 5′-nucleotidase and γ-glutamyltransferase occur. Raised values are found in late pregnancy. However, activities are normal in osseous disease. The enzyme has appreciable specificity for hepatobiliary lesions and has a place in the evaluation of the source of a raised serum alkaline phosphatase activity. In pancreatic neoplasia not associated with large duct biliary obstruction or hepatic secondary neoplasia, the serum leucine aminopeptidase activity is normal (Zimmerman and Seeff, 1970).

The different isoenzymes of leucine aminopeptidase can be identified by electrophoresis. However, the source of all the serum isoenzymes has not yet been established. Electrophoresis of leucine aminopeptidase has not been widely applied in clinical laboratories.

10.2.4.2.4. 5′-Nucleotidase. 5′-Nucleotidase (EC 3.1.3.5; 5′-ribonucleotide phosphohydrolase) is found principally, but not exclusively, in the plasma and canalicular membranes of hepatocytes and bile duct epithelial cells (Goldberg, 1973). The enzyme catalyzes the following reaction which is employed in its assay –

$$\text{adenosine-5'-P} + H_2O \rightleftharpoons \text{adenosine} + H_3PO_4$$

It also hydrolyzes inosine-5′-phosphate. The physiological function of this enzyme is unknown, but an elevated activity in serum is almost specific for hepatobiliary diseases and, in contrast to alkaline phosphatase, does not appear to depend on increased hepatic synthesis of the enzyme. The serum activity of 5′-nucleotidase is normal in physiological situations such as growth, in which the serum alkaline phosphatase is higher than in normal adults. However, serum 5′-nucleotidase activity is elevated in late pregnancy. It is not affected by age or sex and it is normal, or only minimally elevated, in bone disease. Hence, this enzyme is of value in indicating by non-electrophoretic means one source for a raised serum alkaline phosphatase activity (Goldberg, 1973).

As with alkaline phosphatase, leucine aminopeptidase and γ-glutamyltransferase, the serum activity of 5′-nucleotidase tends to be markedly elevated in diseases associated with large duct biliary obstruction, intra-hepatic cholestasis and infiltrative disorders of the liver. Values are usually mildly – and sometimes moderately – increased in hepatocellular disease. If primary biliary cirrhosis, secondary carcinoma of the liver and drug-induced cholestasis can be excluded, marked elevation of 5′-nucleotidase is likely to be due to large duct biliary obstruction, and acute hepatitis, chronic hepatitis or cirrhosis are unlikely.

5′-Nucleotidase appears to offer a less discriminating test in differentiating between hepatocellular and biliary tract lesions than alkaline phosphatase. Although serum 5′-nucleotidase activity is not elevated in all patients with hepatobiliary diseases (like alkaline phosphatase, leucine aminopeptidase and γ-glutamyltransferase) it is a sensitive screening test for intrahepatic space-occupying lesions, such as secondary carcinoma (Goldberg, 1973). Mild elevations of the serum alkaline phosphatase activity can occur in the presence of a normal serum 5′-nucleotidase activity in patients with hepatobiliary disease who do not have any extra-hepatic lesion responsible for the increase in serum alkaline phosphatase (Breen and Schenker, 1971). However, serum 5′-nucleotidase may be more strikingly and persistently abnormal than the serum alkaline phosphatase activity in chronic liver diseases, including primary biliary cirrhosis (Phelan et al., 1971).

10.2.4.3. Other enzymes

The serum activities of some other enzymes which fall into neither of the two major categories above have been applied to the diagnosis of hepatobiliary diseases (Zimmerman and Seeff, 1970). One of these, lactate dehydrogenase (EC 1.1.1.27), is worthy of special note. This enzyme catalyzes the following reaction –

$$\text{lactate} + \text{NAD} \rightleftharpoons \text{pyruvate} + \text{NADH} + H^+$$

In uncomplicated acute or chronic hepatocellular disease and obstructive lesions of extra- and intra-hepatic bile ducts, the serum activity of this enzyme tends to be only mildly increased. However, in patients with liver cell carcinoma or secondary carcinoma of the liver, marked elevation of the serum activity of this enzyme may be found; the degree of elevation tends to reflect the total mass of tumour. Markedly increased activities are also found in megaloblastic anaemia, shock and anoxia. Moderately increased values may be found in association with certain complications of alcoholic liver disease such as alcoholic myopathy, delerium tremens, haemolytic anaemia and pancreatitis. Other causes for moderate increases in activity include myocardial infarction, leukaemia, infectious mononucleosis and progressive muscular dystrophy (Zimmerman and Seeff, 1970).

10.2.4.4. The role of enzyme tests

The clinical application of measurements of the activities of enzymes in serum has enhanced the precision of the diagnosis and management of hepatobiliary diseases. However, none of the available enzyme tests enables a reliable distinction to be made between predominantly cholestatic and predominantly hepatocellular jaundice, or between intra-hepatic and extra-hepatic causes of cholestasis. Furthermore, the results of none of these tests are diagnostic of a specific hepatobiliary disease. Although a large number of enzyme tests can be used, only a relatively few are both necessary and adequate for routine use in the diagnosis and management of hepatobiliary diseases. Accordingly, it is recommended that the clinician become familiar with the behaviour of just a few representative and relevant enzyme tests. The panel of tests suggested by Zimmerman and Seeff (1970), comprising aspartate aminotransferase, alanine aminotransferase, alkaline phosphatase and lactate dehydrogenase, is highly appropriate.

10.2.5. Plasma proteins *

Proteins produced by the liver cell which are exported from the cell are synthesized on polyribosomes bound to the rough endoplasmic reticulum, from which they are discharged into the plasma (Tavill, 1972). Changes in the concentration of an individual protein in the plasma may be due to an altered rate of either synthesis or catabolism of the protein, change in plasma volume, altered distribution between vascular and extravascular pools, or abnormal losses into the gut, urinary tract, or other sites. Many plasma proteins, including albumin, fibrinogen, α_1-antitrypsin, haptoglobin, caeruloplasmin, transferrin and prothrombin, are synthesized by parenchymal liver cells. In hepatocellular diseases, there is often a tendency for the concentrations of these proteins in plasma to fall. It is usually assumed that a diminished synthetic rate of these proteins by the liver is a major factor which contributes to this phenomenon. However, in chronic hepatocellular disease another factor which tends to lower the concentration of all proteins in plasma is an increased plasma volume (Lieberman and Reynolds, 1967). Several liver-produced plasma

* The proteins circulating in the plasma (see Chapter 6) are usually referred to as the "plasma proteins". However, as the concentrations of all of them, except fibrinogen, are usually measured in serum, these proteins other than fibrinogen, are also known as "serum proteins". Except when fibrinogen is implicated, the terms "plasma proteins" and "serum proteins" are used synonymously in this chapter.

proteins are acute phase proteins, the serum concentrations of which tend to rise in response to certain phenomena associated with tissue injury, such as inflammation. These proteins include fibrinogen, haptoglobin, α_1-antitrypsin, C3 and caeruloplasmin (Koj, 1974). An acute phase response may contribute to well maintained, or increased, serum concentrations of these proteins in hepatocellular diseases. In general, increased catabolism and abnormal losses do not appear to be important factors contributing to the hypoproteinaemia which is associated with hepatocellular disease alone. In gastrointestinal lesions, such as the stagnant loop syndrome and pancreatic exocrine insufficiency (see Chapter 12), which may be associated with the ineffective utilization of dietary protein nitrogen for anabolism, and in kwashiorkor and malnutrition, the supply of amino-acids reaching the liver cell may be inadequate to sustain normal rates of protein synthesis. This is probably the main factor contributing to the decreased plasma concentration of many liver cell-produced plasma proteins, including albumin, commonly found in these syndromes. Among plasma proteins which are not synthesized by the liver cell are the five known classes of immunoglobulins, which are synthesized by B cells of the lymphoid system. Changes in the serum concentrations of IgG, IgM, and IgA tend to occur independently of changes in the serum concentrations of liver cell-produced plasma proteins in patients with hepatobiliary diseases. The concentration of many plasma proteins can be readily and fairly accurately measured using the radial immunodiffusion technique (Mancini et al., 1965) with commercially available reagents.

10.2.5.1. Total plasma protein concentration

Total plasma protein concentration is usually little changed in hepatobiliary lesions associated with cholestasis and acute hepatocellular disease. In chronic hepatocellular disease, there is a tendency for the serum concentration of albumin to fall and that of γ-globulin to rise. The former phenomenon may predominate in advanced hepatocellular disease, so resulting in a decrease in the total plasma protein concentration, whereas the latter phenomenon may predominate in some patients with chronic active (usually HB_sAg-negative) hepatitis, so resulting in an increase in the total plasma protein concentration. The total plasma protein concentration per se is of little value in the evaluation of hepatobiliary disease. It is a useful measurement, principally because it permits the individual protein bands obtained by electrophoresis of serum to be expressed in terms of relative concentration of protein.

10.2.5.2. Protein electrophoresis

Electrophoresis of serum proteins (see Chapter 6) is of limited absolute diagnostic value in hepatobiliary disease. However, although the changes observed are not specific for hepatobiliary diseases, it may be a useful investigation in patients who are known to have a hepatobiliary lesion, provided that other diseases which produce changes in the concentrations of serum proteins can be excluded (Hobbs, 1967). It can also be useful in following the disease state of such patients.

The finding of a normal electrophoretic pattern in a jaundiced patient is a point against chronic liver disease, such as cirrhosis, unless the patient has recently had a massive transfusion of blood or plasma. While the pattern may be normal at the onset of jaundice due to many causes, it is useful to repeat such an examination later. The finding of a raised γ-globulin at this time is suggestive of an infectious process such as viral hepatitis, glandular fever or bacterial cholangitis, whereas a persistence of the normal pattern would be consistent with drug-induced jaundice or early large duct biliary obstruction. The incidental finding of a raised serum γ-globulin concentration in the absence of jaundice may be the first indication of a latent asymptomatic cirrhosis. The serum γ-globulin is usually normal in alcoholics who do not have cirrhosis. Persistent elevation of γ-globulin for months following an attack of acute hepatitis, with or without associated hypoalbuminaemia, may indicate progression of the lesion to chronic hepatocellular disease. However, such an abnormality is not incompatible with eventual complete recovery. Other causes of persistent elevation of the γ-globulin such as chronic infections, e.g. tuberculosis, should always be considered. In general, the maintenance of normal serum albumin and γ-globulin concentrations after acute hepatitis suggests a good prognosis. In contrast, plasma protein concentrations may be normal in acute fulminant liver failure since the duration of the illness may be short in relation to the half-lives of most of the plasma proteins. If large duct obstruction has been present for more than several weeks, elevation of α_2- and β-globulin is usually observed, due mainly to increased serum concentrations of α_2- and β-lipoproteins (section 10.2.5.4.8). Elevation of α- and β-globulins may also be found in other conditions, such as connective tissue disorders, irrespective of the presence of liver disease.

The α_2-globulin band includes haptoglobin. In haemolysis, this protein forms a complex with free haemoglobin which results in a decrease in the concentration of circulating haptoglobin. The concentration may approach zero during brisk intravascular haemolysis, but is less markedly reduced in extravascular haemolytic states. In jaundice associated with haemolysis, the concentration of α_2-globulin is therefore usually reduced. If the haemolysis has an autoimmune basis, an increase in γ-globulin may also occur. An increase in α_2-globulin is a common finding (e.g. in hepatic neoplasia) and is usually due, at least in part, to an increased serum concentration of haptoglobin, which behaves as an acute phase protein. An increase in α_2-globulin makes an appreciable degree of haemolysis unlikely.

The classical electrophoretic pattern which is seen in established cirrhosis is a decrease in albumin and a variable increase in γ-globulin. The latter tends to be greatest in chronic active hepatitis and less marked in inactive cirrhosis. In cirrhosis, the increase in γ-globulin includes fast γ-globulin (mainly IgA), and this results in filling in of the gap which is normally present between β- and γ-globulins (β–γ fusion or bridging). A similar pattern may be found in other conditions, including non-metastatic hypernephroma (Walsh and Kissane, 1968) and chronic infection. However, in chronic infection a raised α_2-globulin is usual, whereas α_2-globulin tends to be relatively normal in most cirrhotics. In pre-cirrhotic chronic active hepatitis, the albumin concentration may be either well maintained or reduced, but particularly in HB_sAg-negative cases, γ-globulin is usually markedly elevated at an early stage of the disease (globulin concentration >30 g/litre) and β–γ fusion tends to be absent. The serum γ-globulin usually falls toward normal in chronic active hepatitis if corticosteroid therapy is given (Cook et al., 1971). In primary biliary cirrhosis the protein electrophoretic pattern may be normal in early cases, but subsequently raised α_2-, β- and γ-globulin bands are usually found. A markedly reduced serum albumin concentration associated with a true cirrhosis is not usually found in this disease until late in the clinical course. The protein electrophoretic changes in primary biliary cirrhosis are essentially a combination of those found in chronic large duct biliary obstruction and chronic hepatocellular disease.

A particularly low concentration of α_1-globulin (<2 g/litre) raises the possibility that a hepatic lesion may be that of α_1-antitrypsin deficiency (section 10.2.5.4.2).

The ratio of the concentration of albumin to that of total globulin should not be used, as it is not a satisfactory substitute for individual measurements of the serum concentrations of albumin and globulins.

10.2.5.3. Quantitative immunoelectrophoresis

By the technique of crossed immunoelectrophoresis (Laurell, 1965) many different proteins can be recognized in human serum (Figure 10.20); by using appropriate pure standards, the concentrations of many of these proteins can be measured (Minchin-Clarke and Freeman, 1968). This elegant technique has been used to examine sera from patients with

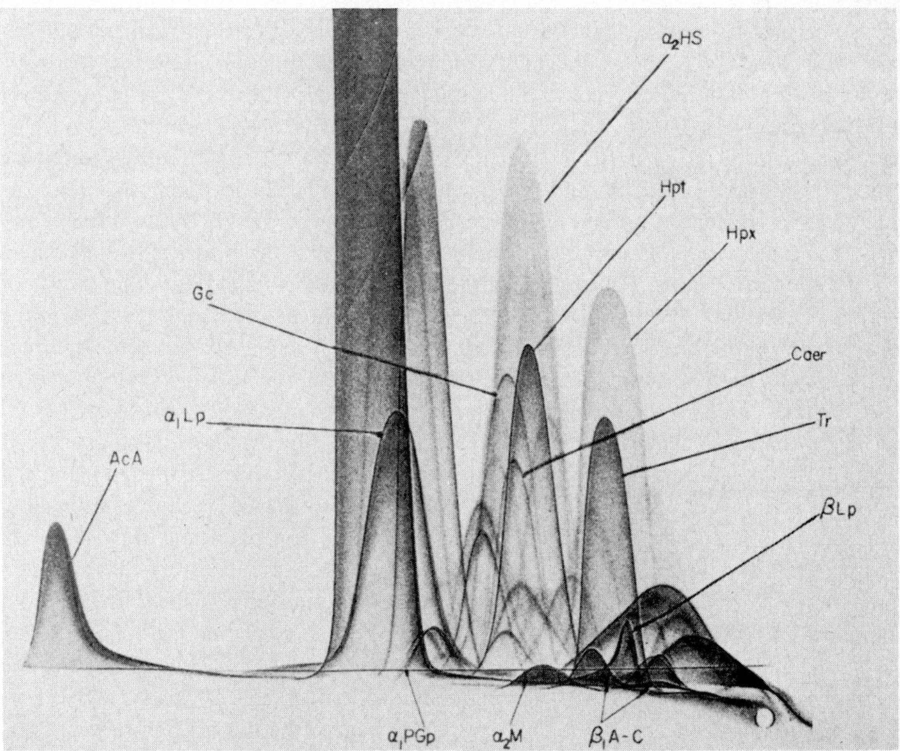

Figure 10.20. Laurell's antigen–antibody crossed electrophoresis of serum from a normal subject. AcA = acetylated albumin control; α_1 Lp = α_1-lipoprotein; Gc = group component; α_2 Hs = α_2-glycoprotein; Hpt = haptoglobin; Hpx = haemopexin; Caer = caeruloplasmin; Tr = transferrin; βLp = β-lipoprotein; β_1 A–C = β_1 A–C globulin; α_2M = α_2-macroglobulin; α_1 PGp = α_1-easily-precipitable glycoprotein. The largest peak which overlaps the α_1 Lp peak is albumin. (Reproduced, with permission, from Minchin-Clarke and Freeman, 1968)

various acute and chronic hepatocellular diseases and lesions associated with cholestasis, and changes in the relative concentrations of one or more proteins in association with specific disease entities have been reported (Amin et al., 1970; Murray-Lyon et al., 1972, 1974). The abnormalities described so far, while of interest, do not appear to be sufficiently specific or consistent to be of appreciable value in the evaluation of individual patients with hepatobiliary diseases. However, it seems unlikely that the full potential clinical application of this powerful technique has yet been realized.

10.2.5.4. Individual plasma proteins

10.2.5.4.1. Albumin. Albumin is synthesized by the liver cell and is the protein secreted by this cell in the largest quantity, about 15 g/day in adults (Rothschild et al., 1973). In patients with chronic hepatocellular disease, particularly chronic active hepatitis and cirrhosis from any cause, the serum concentration of albumin tends to be subnormal. A low serum concentration of albumin in these conditions is commonly attributed to a low synthetic rate of this protein. Indeed, the serum albumin concentration has been used as an index of liver cell function in the assessment of cirrhotic patients for elective portacaval shunts, a low concentration (less than 30 g/litre) in a patient with cirrhosis often being regarded as an index of poor liver cell function. However, there is a poor correlation between the rate of albumin synthesis and the severity of chronic liver disease (Hasch et al., 1967). An increased plasma volume often contributes to hypoalbuminaemia in cirrhotic patients (Lieberman and Reynolds, 1967), as a consequence of which the intravascular albumin pool tends to be relatively less abnormal than the serum albumin concentration and may even be in the normal range (Dykes, 1968). Conversely, a normal serum albumin concentration can occur in the presence of decompensated chronic liver disease. For instance, although a fall in the colloid osmotic pressure of plasma is considered to be a factor which contributes to the development of ascites in the cirrhotic patient, the serum albumin concentration is occasionally normal in the presence of ascites which complicates chronic liver disease. The synthetic rate of albumin may even be supranormal in some patients with ascites secondary to alcoholic cirrhosis even when there is hypoalbuminaemia (Rothschild et al., 1969). Finally, particular caution is required in interpreting values for serum albumin concentration determined in jaundiced sera by the certain dye-binding methods. Bilirubin tends to displace such dyes from albumin, resulting in spuriously low values for serum albumin concentrations (Miyada et al., 1972). In summary, the serum albumin concentration per se is not a very reliable index of the functional capacity of the liver in patients with chronic hepatocellular disease.

In acute liver disease, the serum albumin concentration is an even less reliable index of liver cell function than in chronic liver disease. A patient with acute massive hepatic necrosis may die of fulminant liver failure, after only a few days of illness, with a normal serum albumin concentration. This can occur because the normal half-time for survival of albumin in the circulation is about 18 days (Cohen et al., 1961). Thus, if albumin synthesis were suddenly to cease completely, it would take a few weeks for an appreciable fall in the serum albumin concentration to occur, in the absence of abnormal losses or increased catabolism. It follows that the finding of a low serum albumin concentration early on during an illness, which initially appears to be an acute hepatitic episode, would raise the possibility that the patient is suffering from either an acute exacerbation of a pre-existing chronic hepatic lesion, such as chronic active hepatitis, or co-existent acute and chronic hepatocellular lesions. If the serum albumin concentration is initially normal during an acute hepatitic episode, but tends to fall progressively during the subsequent several weeks or few months, the possibility of progression of an acute hepatitis to massive hepatic necrosis or to chronic active hepatitis should be considered. However, a low serum albumin concentration in this context is not incompatible with subsequent complete recovery. The serum albumin concentration tends to be well maintained for long periods in cholestatic viral hepatitis, drug-induced cholestasis, large duct biliary obstruction and early primary biliary cirrhosis.

In a patient with hypoalbuminaemia associated with chronic hepatocellular disease, a rise in the serum concentration of albumin is sometimes regarded as an index of improving liver cell function. This may be so if it occurs spontaneously, or in a malnourished alcoholic patient who is deprived of alcohol and given a nutritious diet. It is not necessarily so if it occurs as a result of an unphysiological stimulus to albumin synthesis, as may occur when corticosteroid drugs are given. These drugs induce complex disturbances of nitrogen and protein metabolism, which include increased catabolism of proteins in peripheral tissues and the accumulation of aminoacids in the liver. In chronic hepatocellular disease, corticosteroid therapy is usually associated with an increased synthetic rate of albumin. This phenomenon may well be secondary to corticosteroid-induced changes in nitrogen metabolism and may not necessarily be a reflection of a general improvement in liver cell function (Cain et al., 1970). In contrast, in alcoholic liver disease a falling serum albumin concentration, despite adequate diet and abstinence from alcohol, is a bad prognostic index (Combes and Schenker, 1975).

If the serum albumin concentration seems inappropriate in relation to the clinical picture, and an adequate explanation is not apparent, specific investigations of albumin metabolism may occasionally be necessary to evaluate the hypoalbuminaemia adequately. In particular, a turnover study of radioiodinated albumin would enable the synthetic rate, distribution, and total rate of degradation due to catabolism and/or abnormal losses to be quantitated; the plasma disappearance curve and the faecal excretion of the label of $[^{51}Cr]$albumin given intravenously would permit an assessment of the magnitude of enteric loss of albumin (Waldmann, 1966).

Extreme hypoalbuminaemia occurs in analbuminaemia, an inborn error of hepatic albumin synthesis (Benhold and Kallee, 1959).

10.2.5.4.2. α_1-Antitrypsin. A marked decrease in the serum concentration of α_1-antitrypsin relative to other plasma proteins is found in the disease entity, α_1-antitrypsin deficiency. In this disorder, there appears to be an abnormality in the assembly of the α_1-antitrypsin molecule which includes impaired sialylation and an associated defect in the release of the molecule from the hepatocyte. The low serum concentration of this protein, which could be due to decreased synthesis and/or increased catabolism, is responsible for a low serum α_1-globulin concentration. This condition may be associated with neonatal hepatitis; neonatal cholestasis; cirrhosis in infancy, childhood or adult life; hepatocellular carcinoma; or the development of pulmonary emphysema at an unusually early age (Brunt, 1974; Sharp, 1976). The antitryptic activity of serum, which is usually measured spectrophotometrically with trypsin and a synthetic substrate, is usually low when the serum concentration of α_1-globulin is reduced (Lieberman et al., 1969). The antitryptic activity of serum is largely, but not entirely, due to α_1-antitrypsin, the remainder being due to a few other proteins which have electrophoretic mobilities which are different from α_1-antitrypsin. Measurement of the serum concentration of α_1-antitrypsin is indicated in any infant with unexplained cholestasis, or any patient with evidence of chronic liver disease, the cause of which is not obvious.

If a low serum concentration of α_1-antitrypsin is found, it is desirable to determine the patient's phenotype with respect to the isoenzymes of α_1-antitrypsin, i.e. the protease inhibitor or Pi phenotype. This is done by examining the pattern of the isoenzymes of α_1-antitrypsin after acid starch gel electrophoresis (Figure 10.21), preferably followed by crossed immunoelectrophoresis (Fagerhol and Laurell, 1967). Isoenzymes of α_1-antitrypsin revealed by this technique have been designated F (fast), M (medium), S (slow) and Z (ultra-slow) according to their relative electrophoretic mobilities; the patterns of isoenzymes specific for particular Pi phenotypes are designated by two of these letters. Most normal people are of the Pi phenotype MM. Patients with hepatic lesions characteristic of α_1-antitrypsin deficiency usually have the rare Pi phenotype ZZ. Occasionally individuals with other rare Pi phenotypes (MZ, FZ and SZ), which are usually associated with only moderately decreased serum concentrations of α_1-antitrypsin, may have hepatic lesions which are similar to, but usually less severe than, those characteristically associated with the Pi ZZ phenotype. The exceedingly rare phenotype PiOO is associated with no detectable α_1-antitrypsin (Talamo et al., 1973).

Diastase-resistant periodic acid Schiff-positive inclusion bodies in periportal hepatocytes are the characteristic histological hallmark of α_1-antitrypsin deficiency. Whenever

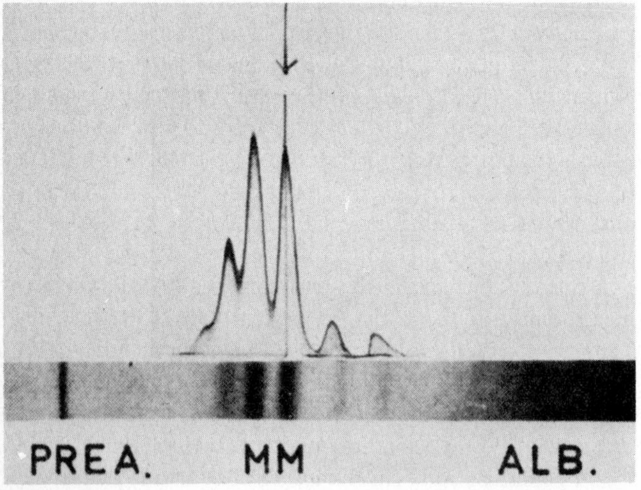

Figure 10.21. The prealbumin zone after discontinuous starch gel electrophoresis of serum from a normal (PiMM) individual (below) and the immunoprecipitation line developed after subsequent antigen–antibody (anti-α_1-antitrypsin) crossed electrophoresis (above). The arrow indicates band 4 of the PiMM phenotype. PREA = prealbumin orosomucoid; MM = α_1-antitrypsin bands of PiMM; ALB = albumin. (Reproduced, with permission, from Fagerhol and Laurell, 1967)

they are found in liver biopsies, determinations of serum α_1-antitrypsin concentration and Pi phenotype are indicated.

Determination of the Pi phenotypes of members of the family of a patient with α_1-antitrypsin deficiency may identify asymptomatic Pi ZZ, FZ, MZ and SZ individuals. Serum α_1-antitrypsin is usually normal, or somewhat increased, in cirrhosis due to causes other than α_1-antitrypsin deficiency. A well maintained or increased value in fulminant liver failure has been interpreted as suggesting the presence of some hepatic regeneration and hence possibly a favourable prognosis.

10.2.5.4.3. Caeruloplasmin. Caeruloplasmin is the only copper-containing protein in plasma and it is responsible for the oxidase activity of plasma. The latter property is utilized in one of the common methods of measuring the concentration of this protein. Its main function is presumed to be the transport of copper. A low serum concentration of caeruloplasmin ($<$0.2 g/litre) occurs in about 95% of patients who are homozygous and about 10% of subjects who are heterozygous for Wilson's disease (Scheinberg, 1973) (section 10.5.5). A low serum concentration of caeruloplasmin in these individuals presumably reflects a selective defect in the synthesis of this protein in the liver cell. Since a normal serum caeruloplasmin concentration can occur in overt clinical Wilson's disease (Scheinberg and Sternlieb, 1963) a deficiency of this protein in plasma is presumably not of fundamental importance to the development of the manifestations of the disease. A consideration of the relative frequencies of homozygotes and heterozygotes for Wilson's disease in the general population indicates that of subjects with low serum caeruloplasmin concentrations, only about one in 100 will be homozygous for Wilson's disease (Scheinberg, 1973). Nevertheless, the serum caeruloplasmin concentration (Figure 10.22) remains one of the most useful investigations in the evaluation of a patient suspected of having the disease (Strickland and Leu, 1975), and it is a useful screening test for identifying asymptomatic homozygotes in relatives of a known case of the disease. The serum caeruloplasmin in Wilson's disease may increase during episodes of the disease associated with considerable hepatic necrosis and inflammation, and it may increase from low to normal values if a patient with Wilson's disease is a recipient of a liver transplant (Groth and Starzl, 1975). In compensated cirrhosis which is not due to Wilson's disease, the serum caeruloplasmin concentration is almost invariably greater than 0.2 g/litre and may be higher than the upper limit of the reference range. High values may also occur in pregnancy, when oestrogen therapy is given, and in association with large duct biliary obstruction (Gault et al., 1966). Low values may occur in the presence of very severe decompensated hepatocellular disease which is not due to Wilson's disease (Walshe and Briggs, 1962; Gault et al., 1966). Since a patient who has clinical, biochemical, serological, and hepatic histological abnormalities which are indistinguishable from chronic active hepatitis may have Wilson's disease, and hence require copper chelation therapy, the serum caeruloplasmin should be measured (Figure 10.23) in all patients with the picture of chronic hepatitis (Sternlieb and Scheinberg, 1972).

10.2.5.4.4. Complement components. In addition to several plasma inhibitors, all nine components of the complement system are plasma proteins. These components interact in a sequential manner, analogous to the interaction of the plasma clotting factors in blood coagulation. They are responsible for mediating immune cytolysis, chemotaxis, opsonization and anaphylaxis (Ruddy et al., 1972). At least some of the complement

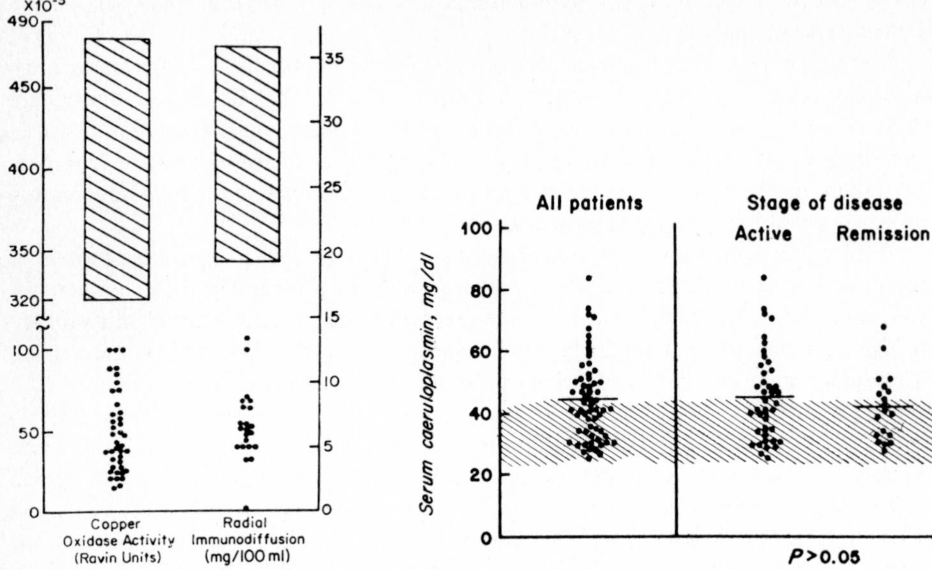

Figure 10.22. Serum caeruloplasmin in patients with Wilson's disease measured by two different methods. The shaded areas represent normal ranges. Normal values of serum caeruloplasmin can occur in Wilson's disease (see text). (Reproduced, with permission, from Strickland and Leu, 1975)

Figure 10.23. Serum caeruloplasmin concentrations in patients with chronic active hepatitis. Left panel = all patients; right panel = patients divided according to the stage of their disease (active or remission); horizontal band = range in normal subjects. (Reproduced, with permission, from LaRusso et al., 1976)

components appear to behave as acute phase proteins. Individual components can be quantitated in terms both of their concentration in serum and of their biological (haemolytic) activity. The complement component which is normally present in the highest concentration in serum is the third component, C3. The serum total haemolytic complement activity (CH_{50}) and the concentrations of C3, C4 and a few of the other components, have been measured in a variety of hepatobiliary disorders. The serum CH_{50} and the concentration of C3 tend to be reduced in cirrhosis, normal in chronic active hepatitis, and increased in compensated primary biliary cirrhosis, whereas the serum concentration of C4 tends to be reduced in all three of these conditions. Low serum concentrations of C3 have been found in massive hepatic necrosis, an observation consistent with reduced hepatic synthesis of C3 and/or increased consumption due to activation of the complement system (Potter et al., 1973). Changes in serum complement occur in the syndrome of polyarthritis and urticaria that sometimes immediately precedes the icteric phase of HB_sAg-positive acute hepatitis. In this syndrome, transient reductions of the serum CH_{50} and concentrations of C4, and to a lesser extent of C3, occur. These changes are presumed to reflect consumption of complement by circulating immune complexes (Alpert et al., 1971). Serum CH_{50} may also be reduced during the rejection of a hepatic graft

(Williams and Smith, 1972). However, normal serum concentrations of complement components do not exclude increased utilization of complement by an immune process. In general, ranges of values for complement components in serum during the course of acute hepatitis and in various chronic hepatocellular diseases and lesions associated with cholestasis tend to be wide, with considerable overlap of values between different groups of patients. The factors contributing to abnormal values of serum complement components in hepatobiliary lesions have not yet been adequately evaluated, and in most patients the values themselves are not particularly useful to the clinician.

10.2.5.4.5. Clotting factors. The blood clotting factors comprise a group of plasma proteins, the sequential interaction of which is responsible for initiating blood coagulation. Those synthesized by the hepatic parenchymal cell include factors I (fibrinogen), II (prothrombin), V, VII, IX and X, but not factor VIII. An adequate supply of vitamin K to the liver is necessary for optimal synthesis of factors II, VII, IX and X. Individual plasma clotting factors are not usually measured routinely, but tests which depend on the presence of several liver cell-synthesized factors are used widely in the assessment of hepatobiliary disease. These tests include the one-stage prothrombin time (which tests the extrinsic coagulation pathway and depends on factors I, II, V, VII and X), the partial thromboplastin time (which tests the intrinsic clotting system), the Normotest (which depends on factors II, VII and X) and the Thrombotest (which is sensitive to factor IX, assays the integrity of the intrinsic as well as the extrinsic coagulation pathway and is also sensitive to endogenous inhibition of prothrombin synthesis). Results of these tests are abnormal if any of the factors contributing to these tests are deficient in plasma. In evaluating results of these tests in patients with hepatobiliary diseases, care must be taken to check whether the patient is receiving any drug, such as phenindione, which interferes with hepatic synthesis of clotting factors. Congenital deficiencies of clotting factors, and deficiency of vitamin K_1 due to dietary deficiency or malabsorption, must also be excluded.

Two phenomena associated with hepatobiliary disease markedly affect the plasma concentrations of liver cell-synthesized clotting factors. These are, irrespective of the cause, the severity of a hepatocellular lesion and the degree of cholestasis. In hepatocellular disease, there is often an element of bile salt secretory failure, while in cholestasis there is impaired delivery of conjugated bile salts into the intestine. These phenomena can lead to inadequate emulsification of dietary lipids with the result that there tends to be malabsorption of fat and fat-soluble vitamins, including vitamin K (Chapter 12). In addition, broad spectrum antibiotics which are commonly given for hepatic encephalopathy may diminish the synthesis of vitamin K by intestinal bacteria. Inadequate vitamin K in the liver leads to impaired synthesis of factors II, VII, IX, and X and hence to prolonged prothrombin and partial thromboplastin times. An element of cholestasis is very common in most hepatobiliary disorders, even in those considered to be due primarily to hepatocellular lesions. Thus, after the initial evaluation of a patient it is often not possible to assess to what extent a prolonged prothrombin time may be secondary to cholestasis or due to hepatocellular disease per se. This problem can usually be resolved by administering vitamin K_1 (10 mg) intramuscularly. A single injection should be adequate, but most physicians give daily injections for 3 days. This treatment effectively corrects the defect in plasma clotting factors due to malabsorption of vitamin K. A return to normal, or an appreciable improvement in the prothrombin time, within 24 hours of giving vitamin K suggests good liver cell function. A prolonged prothrombin time in any patient with a hepatobiliary lesion is as an indication for parenteral vitamin K therapy. The degree to which the prothrombin time remains prolonged after this therapy reflects in most cases the degree to which the synthesis of liver cell-produced clotting factors is depressed due to intrinsic hepatic disease, and can be regarded as an index of hepatocellular insufficiency (Roberts and Cederbaum, 1972). In chronic hepatocellular disease, values more than 4 seconds prolonged indicate extensive severe parenchymal disease and usually a poor prognosis. Values in this range are relative, but not absolute, contraindications to surgery. Portal-systemic shunts, in particular, are associated with a high mortality rate from liver cell failure if the prothrombin time is prolonged. Hepatocellular necrosis secondary to shock or hypoxaemia may be associated with marked prolongation of the prothrombin time. If, in a patient with presumed large duct biliary obstruction, vitamin K_1 fails to correct a prolonged prothrombin time rapidly, the diagnosis should be questioned.

The survival half-times in plasma of two of the clotting factors which are assessed by the prothrombin time are very short – less than 1 day (Koller, 1973) – while those of most other plasma proteins are much longer, e.g. 18 days for albumin (Cohen et al., 1961). This fact explains why the prothrombin time becomes prolonged rapidly, and before any appreciable fall in serum albumin concentration, when a severe acute hepatocellular lesion develops (Figure 10.24). Of the widely used tests employed in the assessment of patients with hepatocellular disease, a test of the function of plasma clotting fac-

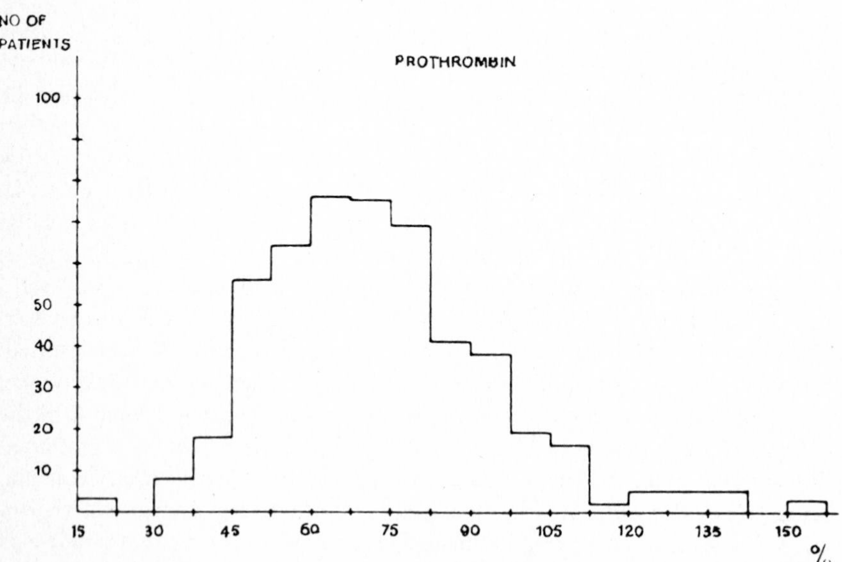

Figure 10.24. Distribution of the ratio of the prothrombin time in a patient to that in the control expressed as a percentage in 500 patients with biopsy-verified acute hepatitis. The diagnosis in each case was presumed to be acute viral hepatitis. Values below 75% are abnormal. A small proportion of the patients had a severe coagulation defect. (Reproduced, with permission, from Petersen et al., 1974)

tors, such as the post-parenteral vitamin K prothrombin time, appears to give the most reliable indication of the protein synthetic capacity of the liver. A prolonged prothrombin time may precede clinical deterioration and has been related to poor prognosis and the development of coma in acute hepatocellular disease, including alcoholic steatonecrosis (Colombi, 1970; Clark et al., 1973; Hillenbrand et al., 1974). It has been used as an indication for hospitalization of patients with acute hepatitis, since there is then an increased likelihood of the development of fulminant hepatic failure. However, the prothrombin time does not enable one to predict whether an individual patient in hepatic coma will survive or die (Ritt et al., 1969; Koller, 1973). Normalization of the prothrombin time precedes or accompanies clinical improvement in massive hepatic necrosis. In acute hepatocellular disease, normal values for plasma clotting factors do not exclude the possibility of progression to chronic hepatocellular disease. An increasing prothrombin time which is not corrected by vitamin K indicates failure of treatment and deteriorating liver cell function in chronic liver disease. The prothrombin time is not a sensitive test for minor hepatocellular dysfunction, and normal or only slightly abnormal results are found in many patients with compensated cirrhosis.

Of the clotting factors which contribute to the prothrombin time, factor VII has the shortest survival half-time in the circulation – about 2 hours (Koller, 1973). In severe acute hepatocellular disease, the plasma concentration of factor VII decreases earlier, to a greater extent and more consistently than that of other clotting factors. In acute liver failure, the plasma concentration of factor VII, and to a lesser extent that of total fibrinogen (determined by the clot opacity technique), appear to correlate well (Figure 10.25) with survival in patients exhibiting variable degrees of hepatic encephalopathy (Dymock et al., 1975), but the factor VII concentration correlates poorly with survival in patients with the most severe (grade IV) hepatic encephalopathy (Gazzard et al., 1976).

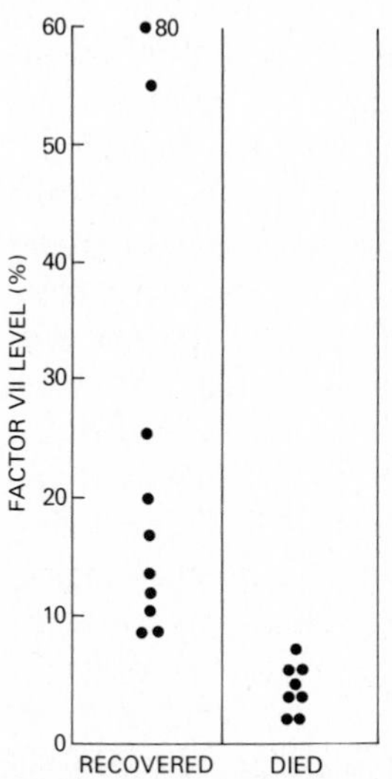

Figure 10.25. Relationship between factor VII levels and survival in fulminant liver failure. The plasma half-life of factor VII is about 2 hours (Reproduced, with permission, from Dymock, 1975)

An assessment of the adequacy of plasma clotting factors, the bleeding time and the number of circulating platelets is essential before embarking on invasive investigations such as needle biopsy of the liver, splenic venography and percutaneous cholangiography. A value for the prothrombin time which makes these investigations permissible is difficult to define, since the risk of bleeding seems to correlate only roughly with the result of this test. This is particularly so because of the inherent variability of the tests for plasma clotting factors both in a single laboratory and between different laboratories. A clinical assessment of bleeding tendency is at least as important as laboratory tests in evaluating whether it is safe to proceed with an invasive manoeuvre.

In severe hepatocellular disease, particularly acute massive hepatic necrosis, a prolonged prothrombin time is often present in association with thrombocytopoenia, increased fibrin/fibrinogen degradation products, increased quantities of plasminogen activator and decreased quantities of plasminogen in plasma. In acute liver failure, these findings do not necessarily imply a poor prognosis. The degree of these abnormalities is usually consistent with mild intravascular coagulation with secondary fibrinolysis. Thus, in this context, it is possible that increased consumption of clotting factors may contribute to their low plasma concentrations. The severity of bleeding in patients with this syndrome appears to correlate best with the plasma plasminogen concentration (Hillenbrand et al., 1974). Evidence which lends some support to the existence of intravascular coagulation in (chronic) hepatocellular disease is the observation that, in patients with cirrhosis, the survival half-life of radioiodinated fibrinogen in the circulation is significantly decreased and that it increases when heparin is administered (Tytgat et al., 1971). The possibility of disseminated intravascular coagulation should be considered in any patient with hepatocellular disease which is complicated by a coagulation defect. At the present time, many aspects of the possible relationship between intravascular coagulation and liver disease are very controversial and await definitive resolution (Bloom, 1975).

10.2.5.4.6. α-Foetoprotein. α-Foetoprotein is a plasma protein which is synthesized by liver cells. It is the protein present in highest concentration in the serum of the human foetus early in gestation (Abelev, 1971), its concentration reaching a peak value of about 3 g/litre at about the 12th week of gestation. Subsequently, the concentration decreases until after the age of one year, when it is normally less than 30 μg/litre. The concentration of α-foetoprotein in the serum of a normal adult can be measured in concentrations as low as 5 μg/litre using a double antibody radioimmunoassay. During pregnancy a physiological rise and fall in the serum concentration of α-foetoprotein occurs in the maternal circulation due to passage of foetal α-foetoprotein to the maternal circulation.

An appreciable proportion of patients with hepatocellular carcinoma (Chapter 25) has a raised serum concentration of α-foetoprotein. However, even a normal serum α-foetoprotein concentration, as determined by radioimmunoassay, does not exclude a diagnosis of heptocellular carcinoma. In one large series (Figure 10.26) in which a radioimmunoassay was used, 72% of patients with this disease had an increased serum α-foetoprotein concentration, and 51% of the patients had a concentration greater than 3000 μg/litre (Waldmann and McIntyre, 1974).

A raised serum concentration of α-foetoprotein, usually in the range of 40 to 500 μg/litre, has also been found in an appreciable proportion of patients with non-neoplastic chronic hepatocellular diseases (Figure 10.26), particularly HB_sAg-negative chronic active

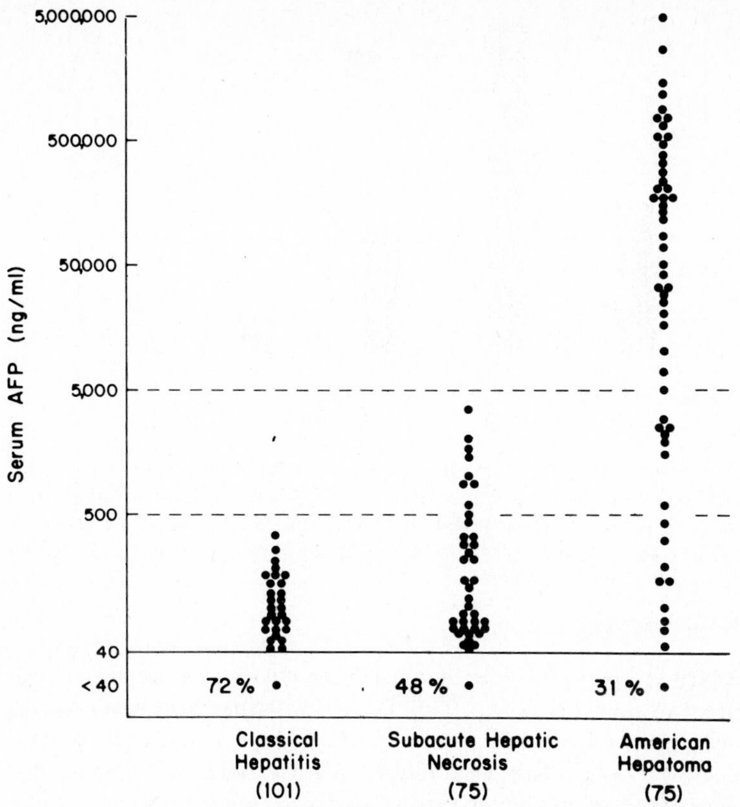

Figure 10.26. Serum levels of α-foetoprotein (AFP) in 75 patients with subacute hepatic necrosis with bridging lesions, 101 patients with classical acute hepatitis without bridging lesions and 75 American patients with hepatocellular carcinoma. (Reproduced with permission, from Bloomer et al., 1975)

hepatitis (Silver et al., 1974b), but also including alcoholic liver disease. This observation limits the usefulness of a slightly raised serum α-foetoprotein concentration in the diagnosis of hepatocellular carcinoma. The serum α-foetoprotein concentration is often raised during the course of acute viral hepatitis. The concentration usually reaches its highest value as the serum aspartate aminotransferase activity is falling, and the highest values (Figures 10.26 and 10.27) tend to occur in patients with bridging necrosis between adjacent central veins or portal triads (Silver et al., 1974a; Bloomer et al., 1975). It may also rise after withdrawal of alcohol in liver disease of the alcoholic. These findings are consistent with the notion that an increased serum concentration of α-foetoprotein in non-neoplastic hepatocellular diseases may reflect hepatic regeneration after parenchymal damage. If this is so, it would appear that the serum α-foetoprotein concentration measures a unique aspect of liver function which is not assessed by other tests used in the evaluation of hepatobiliary disease. However, in some patients with acute viral hepatitis the serum α-foetoprotein concentration appears to parallel the serum aspartate aminotransferase activity fairly closely, raising the possibility that, in some cases, it may be

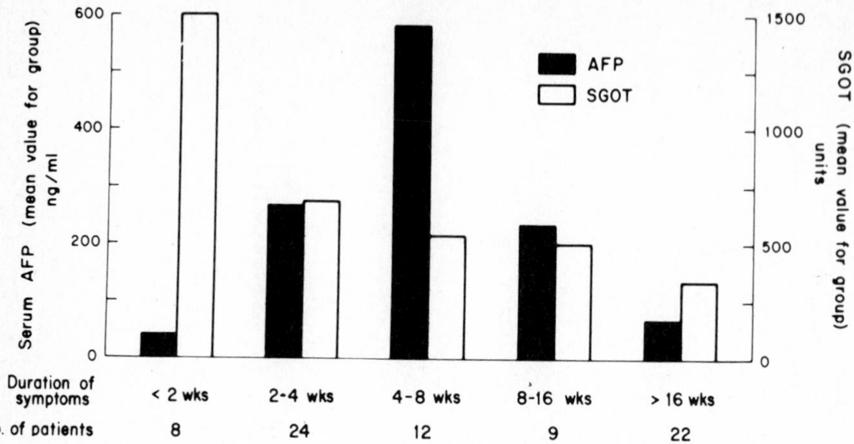

Figure 10.27. Serum α-foetoprotein (AFP) concentrations and aspartate aminotransferase (SGOT) levels in patients with viral subacute hepatic necrosis related to time of initial symptoms. Patients have been grouped according to duration of symptoms and mean values for AFP and SGOT are shown for each group. The highest concentrations of AFP tend to occur after the highest levels of SGOT. (Reproduced, with permission, from Bloomer et al., 1975)

reflecting the acute phase response to liver injury or alternatively a phenomenon associated with the presence of the virus (Kew, 1974). Patients with fulminant viral hepatitis may develop a raised serum α-foetoprotein concentration (Karvountzis and Redeker, 1974; Murray-Lyon et al., 1976). This may indicate the occurrence of some hepatic regeneration but it does not necessarily imply that recovery will ensue.

Serum α-foetoprotein concentrations are not markedly different in patients with HB_sAg-positive or -negative disease, including liver cell carcinoma.

The mean serum α-foetoprotein concentration in infants with neonatal hepatitis has been reported to be significantly greater than that in infants with congenital biliary atresia (Zeltzer et al., 1974), suggesting that the measurement of this protein may be of value in differentiating these two causes of neonatal jaundice. However, more data are required to evaluate the clinical usefulness of this observation. Increased concentrations also occur in Indian childhood cirrhosis (Nayak et al., 1972). The serum α-foetoprotein concentration which is associated with any particular hepatic lesion tends to be higher in children than adults.

The finding of high serum concentrations of α-foetoprotein in patients with the immunodeficiency disease ataxia telangiectasia is of considerable interest. This finding probably implies a defect in the differentiation of hepatocytes in this condition (Waldmann and McIntyre, 1972).

10.2.5.4.7. Immunoglobulins. IgM, IgA, and IgG in particular, account for most of serum γ-globulin, Markedly raised serum concentrations of IgG, IgM, and IgA are found in a large proportion of patients with chronic hepatocellular diseases. The high serum concentrations of at least IgG and IgM appear to be associated with high synthetic rates of these proteins, phenomena which usually reflect a response of the reticuloendothelial system to increased antigenic stimulation. Such antigen stimulation may arise in chronic liver disease, at least in part, as a result of inefficient clearance of enteric bacterial antigens by the diseased liver. In interpreting the possible significance of raised serum concentrations of immunoglobulins, consideration should be given to the fact that IgM, IgA and IgG concentrations are usually elevated for a limited period after many intercurrent infections, which do not involve the liver or biliary system.

Serum IgG is most commonly raised in chronic active hepatitis and cryptogenic cirrhosis, IgA in cirrhosis of the alcoholic and IgM in primary biliary cirrhosis and cirrhosis of the alcoholic. The range of values for the serum concentrations of all three of these immunoglobulins in chronic liver diseases tends to be wide and overlaps the reference ranges so that no single pattern of serum immunoglobulin concentrations appears to be specific for any particular chronic liver disease. Corticosteroid therapy in patients with chronic active hepatitis is usually associated with normal serum IgM and IgA concentrations, but the serum IgG, although generally lower than pretreatment values, tends to remain elevated in an appreciable proportion of cases (Feizi, 1968). In alcoholics who do not have liver disease, the serum IgA is usually normal (Hobbs, 1967). Serum IgG may be raised in conditions associated with hepatic granulomata, such as sarcoidosis.

Serum immunoglobulin concentrations are of some limited use in the differential diagnosis of cholestasis. While the serum IgM concentration is of little value in distinguishing between different chronic liver diseases, it is elevated in more than 80% of patients with cholestasis, due to primary biliary cirrhosis (Figure 10.28); however it is normal in most patients with cholestasis due to large duct biliary obstruction (Feizi, 1968; Bevan et al., 1969; MacSween et al., 1972) (Figure 10.29). This measurement is not as discriminating in this context as the mitochondrial antibody test (section 10.3.1.1). In cholestasis due to drugs, such as chlorpromazine, the serum concentrations of IgG, IgM, and IgA tend to be normal in early cases (Hobbs, 1967; Bevan et al., 1969).

Serum immunoglobulin concentrations may also be of some help in determining whether an acute hepatitic episode is due to acute viral hepatitis or to hitherto unrecognized chronic active hepatitis. At the onset of jaundice in acute viral hepatitis, serum immunoglobulin concentrations are usually normal, but subsequently the serum IgM usually rises and only later may the serum IgG become elevated. Changes in serum immunoglobulins tend to occur later in HB_sAg-positive than HB_sAg-negative cases. In HB_sAg-positive patients, anti-HB_s of both IgM and IgG classes is found. These changes are usually transient and subside with resolution of the acute illness (Ajdukiewicz et al., 1972). Persistent elevation of serum IgG raises the possibility of progression of the acute lesion to chronic hepatitis. If a clinically acute hepatitic episode is due to an exacerbation of chronic active hepatitis, the serum IgG concentration is usually elevated from the outset.

The increase in serum γ-globulin which is present in most patients with chronic hepatocellular disease, and in some patients with acute hepatitis, is typically polyclonal, but occasionally monoclonal bands are found. Such a finding in this context does not usually imply the presence of myelomatosis or other malignant disease of the lymphoid system. In acute viral hepatitis, there may be a transient IgM or IgG paraprotein which may have antibody activity directed against IgG or α-foetoprotein. In chronic active hepatitis and/or cirrhosis, there may be persistent IgG, IgM or IgA paraproteins which may have antibody activity directed against smooth muscle. In primary biliary cirrhosis, there may

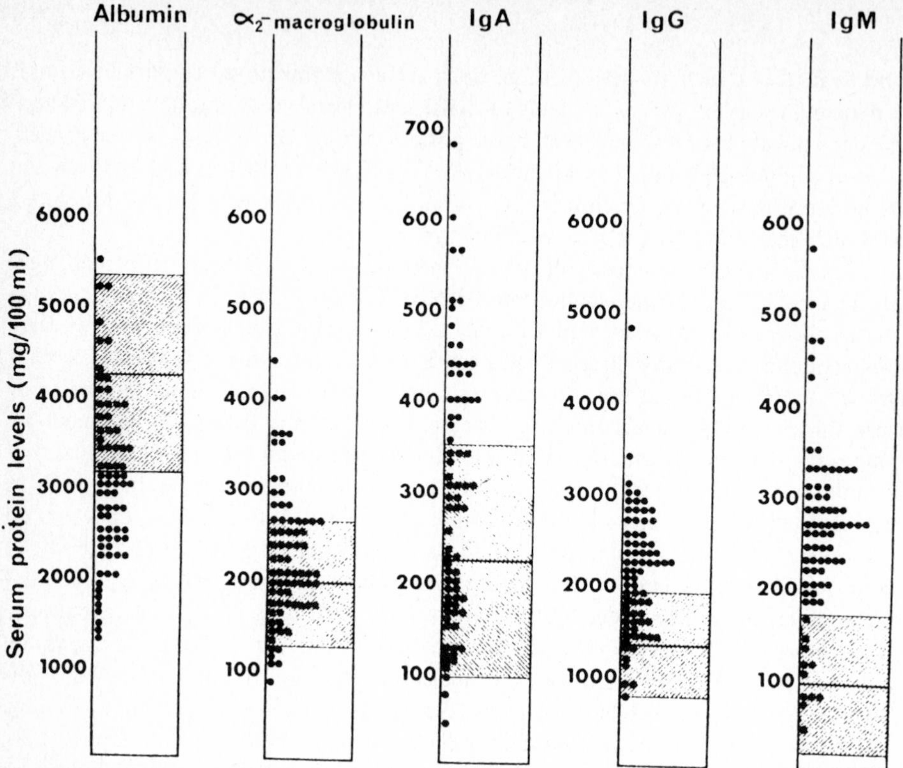

Figure 10.28. Serum albumin, α_2-macroglobulin, IgA, IgG and IgM in primary biliary cirrhosis patients. Shaded area = range for controls (mean ±1 S.D.). (Reproduced, with permission, from MacSween et al., 1972)

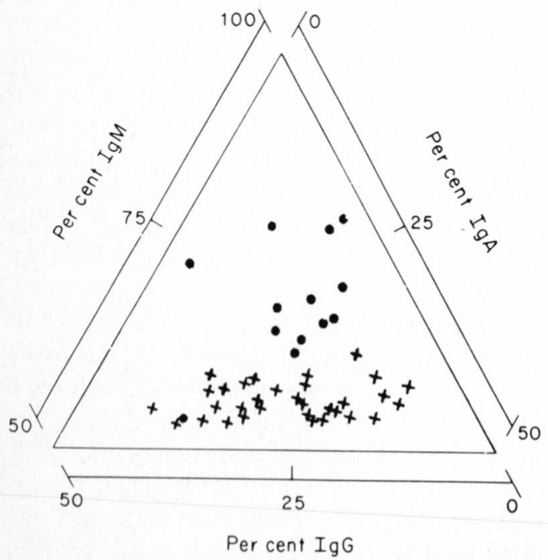

Figure 10.29. Serum immunoglobulin concentrations expressed as a percentage of total immunoglobulin concentration (IgG + IgM + IgA) plotted on triangular coordinates. Cases of primary biliary cirrhosis (•) are clearly separated from cases of large duct biliary obstruction (X) except in one instance. (Reproduced, with permission, from Bevan et al., 1969)

be a persistent IgM paraprotein which may have antibody activity against mitochondria. The other paraproteins which are occasionally found in association with hepatocellular diseases include cryoglobulins (Eliakim et al., 1972; Roux et al., 1974).

There is a paucity of data on the serum concentrations in hepatobiliary diseases of the other two classes of immunoglobulins, IgD and IgE, which are normally present in serum in very low concentrations.

10.2.5.4.8. Lipoproteins. The liver is the site of synthesis of high-density lipoproteins and very low-density lipoproteins. It is involved in the catabolism of chylomicrons and possibly of low-density lipoproteins. It also produces enzymes which affect the metabolic conversions of all the plasma lipoprotein subclasses (Chapter 5). Complex and poorly understood changes in plasma lipoproteins occur in patients with different hepatobiliary diseases. Conventional electrophoresis of serum from patients with chronic cholestasis reveals larger β bands than are seen in healthy individuals. Using agarose gel electrophoresis one pre-β-, one β- and two α-lipoprotein bands may be seen in serum from normal individuals. An absence of pre-β-lipoprotein has been noted in non-biliary cirrhosis, while pre-β-lipoprotein has been detected in primary biliary cirrhosis. Lack of both α- and pre-β-lipoproteins has been found during the first week of jaundice in acute viral hepatitis (Papadopoulos and Charles, 1970). With significant impairment of hepatic function, regardless of cause, the α and pre-β bands disappear and only a broad β band remains, which may, nevertheless, be associated with an increased heterogeneity of lipoprotein structure (McIntyre et al., 1975). A broad densely staining β-lipoprotein band is found not only in cholestasis but also in type II or type III hyperlipoproteinaemia. It is important to determine whether the observed changes are due to cholestasis or to primary hyperlipoproteinaemia, since the therapeutic implications are different.

Preparative ultracentrifugation which is too complex to use on a routine basis, has been employed to investigate in detail the plasma lipoprotein abnormalities which occur in cholestasis (Seidel et al., 1969). These changes include an increase in low-density lipoproteins and the appearance of an immunologically unique and chemically distinct β-lipoprotein (lipoprotein X, LP-X) which has a high content of unesterified cholesterol and phospholipids. This lipoprotein makes a major contribution to the increased plasma free cholesterol in cholestasis (McIntyre et al., 1975). It is not detectable in normal serum (Seidel et al., 1969). While quantitation of LP-X is not a routine laboratory procedure, if a monospecific antiserum to LP-X is available, a qualitative immunoelectrophoretic technique can readily be used to screen sera for its presence. Apart from deficiency of the enzyme lecithin:cholesterol acyltransferase, or when serum activity of this enzyme is appreciably increased, the presence of LP-X appears to be a highly specific and sensitive index of cholestasis, irrespective of whether there is concomitant hyperbilirubinaemia (Seidel et al., 1973; Ritland et al., 1973). However, the detection of LP-X does not assist the clinician in differentiating between extra-hepatic and intra-hepatic causes of cholestasis or in determining any particular cause of cholestasis (McIntyre et al., 1975). LP-X may be detected in the serum of patients with acute or chronic hepatocellular diseases with cholestatic features. The presence of LP-X does not correlate closely with the serum alkaline phosphatase activity; it may be present when the activity of this enzyme is normal, or it may be undetectable when the activity is raised. Apart from lecithin:cholesterol acyltransferase deficiency, LP-X has not been detected in non-hepatobiliary diseases (Seidel et al., 1973; Ritland, 1976).

The pattern of changes in plasma lipoproteins which occur in cholestasis is similar to that in patients with lecithin:cholesterol acyltransferase deficiency. However, the activity of this enzyme per se appears to be of little or no value in the differential diagnosis of hepatobiliary disease (McIntyre et al., 1975). Measurements of lipoproteins have yet to be shown to be of appreciable value in assessing hepatic function or in evaluating a patient with a hepatobiliary disease.

10.2.5.4.9. Other plasma proteins. Plasma concentrations of a number of other proteins, including fibrinogen, orosomucoid, C-reactive protein, prealbumin, β_2-glycoprotein, haemopexin, haptoglobin and α_2-macroglobulin, have been measured in patients with hepatobiliary diseases. The ranges of values obtained in individual diseases tend to overlap with the ranges both in other diseases and in healthy individuals. Hence the measurement of the serum concentrations of these proteins appears to be of little use in the evaluation of hepatobiliary diseases (Braun and Aly, 1971; Hallen and Laurell, 1972).

10.2.5.5. Tests depending on plasma proteins

A number of rather empirical tests appear to reflect changes in the concentrations of plasma proteins, particularly increased concentrations of immunoglobulins, and in some instances phospholipids (Combes and Schenker, 1975). These tests include the thymol turbidity, zinc sulphate turbidity and cephalin cholesterol flocculation tests. Results tend to be normal in uncomplicated cholestatic syndromes and abnormal in hepatocellular diseases. The cephalin cholesterol flocculation test is the most discriminating in this respect. However, in general these tests are not specific and do not provide information which cannot readily be obtained from other tests which are used routinely in the evaluation of hepatobiliary diseases, such as serum protein electrophoresis and measurement of immunoglobulins. The occasional disparities between the results of turbidity and flocculation tests and other liver tests facilitates neither the diagnosis of individual hepatobiliary diseases nor the exclusion of hepatobiliary disease. These tests should be abandoned.

10.2.5.6. Plasma proteins in ascitic fluid

In patients with ascites, it is usual to measure the total protein concentration in the fluid obtained from a diagnostic ascitic fluid tap. Values below 20 g/litre indicate a transudate, and those above 20 g/litre are consistent with an exudate (Chapter 2). Concentrations well above 20 g/litre are usually found in patients with peritoneal infections such as tuberculous peritonitis, but a wide range of values consistent with a transudate or exudate is found in patients with cirrhosis, the Budd–Chiari syndrome, congestive cardiac failure and malignancies.

10.2.5.7. Proteinuria

Proteinuria occurs in certain neonatal cholestatic syndromes due to inborn errors of metabolism, notably hereditary fructose intolerance, tyrosinaemia and galactosaemia, and in certain infections which cause an acute hepatitic syndrome (e.g. Weil's disease and yellow fever).

10.2.6. Lipids

Cholesterol synthesis by the liver is probably increased in cholestasis, possibly secondary to regurgitation of biliary phospholipids (Quarfordt et al., 1973). This phenomenon appears to be the most important factor contributing to the increased serum concentration of cholesterol which is found in association with hepatobiliary diseases. In these diseases, an increased serum cholesterol concentration is almost always associated with a raised serum alkaline phosphatase. The serum cholesterol concentration usually rises within a few days of the onset of acute cholestasis. Values in the range of 7.7 to 10 mmol/litre (300 to 400 mg/dl) are common during the course of acute cholestasis due to large duct biliary obstruction, drugs or cholestatic viral hepatitis, while values greater than 26 mmol/litre (1 g/dl) may occur with lesions which cause chronic cholestasis such as primary biliary cirrhosis or unrelieved large duct biliary obstruction. In such patients, the serum cholesterol is usually appreciably elevated when xanthomas are evident. If the degree and/or duration of cholestasis appears to be insufficient to account for the actual concentration of the serum cholesterol, then other diseases which may be associated with high values should be considered, such as diabetes mellitus, the nephrotic syndrome, hypothyroidism, and certain congenital hyperlipidaemias (Chapter 5). The serum cholesterol concentration may be transiently depressed early on and transiently elevated later on in the course of typical acute viral hepatitis (Wacker et al., 1972). Values for serum cholesterol are usually elevated in Nieman–Pick disease and types I and III glycogenosis, but normal in Gaucher's disease. The serum cholesterol concentration tends to be reduced in malnutrition and severe hepatocellular disease, and may fall to a very low value preterminally in cirrhosis and massive hepatic necrosis.

Administration of the drug clofibrate to a patient with hypercholesterolaemia secondary to cholestasis may be associated with a paradoxical rise in the serum cholesterol concentration (Schaffner, 1969).

The ratio of esterified to free cholesterol tends to be low in jaundiced patients with normal or increased serum total cholesterol concentrations, whether the jaundice be due primarily to cholestasis or to hepatocellular disease. In cholestasis this phenomenon is due to a rise in free cholesterol, and in hepatocellular lesions to a fall in esterified cholesterol. Serum cholesterol ester concentration tends to be increased during recovery from acute hepatitis and in association with fatty liver and cholelithiasis. The role of reduced activity of lecithin–cholesterol acyltransferase in the genesis of the changes in serum lipids in cholestasis has not been clarified (McIntyre et al., 1975).

In addition to cholesterol, fasting serum concentrations of triglycerides, free fatty acids, phospholipids such as lecithin, and total lipids are usually elevated in cholestasis and may be elevated in predominantly hepatocellular diseases. Serum lipids are increased in types I and III glycogenoses. In kwashiorkor, which is associated with marked fatty metamorphosis of the liver, elevation of the serum free fatty acid concentration occurs. Increased serum concentrations of lipids, including cholesterol, are found in Zieve's syndrome, which occurs in severe alcoholics (Zieve, 1966).

Cholesterol inhibits the haemolytic effect of streptolysin O (Badin and Barillec, 1968) so that the hypercholesterolaemia associated with hepatobiliary disease may give rise to falsely high antistreptolysin O titres. A true measurement of the titre can be made following pretreatment of serum with isoamyl alcohol (Badin and Barillec, 1969).

Although changes in various aspects of lipid metabolism, as reflected by measurements of serum lipids, are common in all forms of hepatobiliary disease, investigations of serum lipids in this context are of very limited value.

10.2.7. Low molecular weight nitrogenous compounds

10.2.7.1. Ammonia

Ammonia chiefly arises in the lumen of the intestine as a result of the interaction between enteric organisms and nitrogenous substances including aminoacids, and to a lesser extent from the turnover of nitrogenous compounds in peripheral tissues. Ammonia is readily absorbed from the intestine and the concentration of ammonia in portal vein blood is normally appreciable. However, as a result of the hepatic uptake of ammonia and its subsequent incorporation into urea and aminoacids, such as arginine in the Krebs–Hensleit urea cycle, and glutamine via amination of glutamate, the concentration of ammonia in arterial blood is normally much less than that in the portal vein. The concentration is higher in systemic venous than arterial blood because of the contribution from peripheral tissues, including deamination of glutamine in the kidney. Thus, the ammonia concentration in arterial blood gives a better index of the efficacy of hepatic extraction of ammonia than does the ammonia concentration of peripheral venous blood.

The ammonia concentration in arterial blood tends to rise in patients with severe acute or chronic hepatocellular disease. It is usually raised in fulminant liver failure; in hepatic encephalopathy complicating chronic hepatocellular disease; and, whether or not there is encephalopathy, in the presence of marked portal-systemic shunting of blood through collaterals or surgically induced shunts. It is generally assumed that factors responsible for this effect include diminished activities of enzymes involved in the hepatic extraction of ammonia (Reichle et al., 1973; Maier et al., 1974), and, in cirrhotics, reduced hepatic blood flow and intra- and extra-hepatic portal-systemic shunting of blood. An increased concentration of ammonia in arterial blood may be an important factor contributing to the pathogenesis of hepatic encephalopathy, particularly when it complicates chronic liver disease (Schenker et al., 1974). However, the correlation between the arterial blood ammonia concentration and the clinical degree of encephalopathy is not close (Record et al., 1975), although the correlation tends to be improved if the mean of several estimations of arterial blood ammonia is used. In a patient with undiagnosed coma, the finding of a raised arterial blood ammonia concentration would raise the possibility of hepatic coma; however, it should be kept in mind that non-hepatic causes of coma may occur in patients with liver disease in whom the arterial blood ammonia concentration is elevated. Furthermore, a normal concentration does not exclude hepatic encephalopathy.

The concentration of ammonia in cerebrospinal fluid tends to be increased in hepatic pre-coma or coma, but it is sometimes also elevated in liver disease which is not associated with encephalopathy.

In the ammonia tolerance test, the pattern of rise and fall of arterial blood ammonia is determined after the oral administration of a dose of an ammonium salt. The magnitude of the increase in arterial blood ammonia concentration in this test has been used as an index of the magnitude of portal-systemic collateral circulation or the patency of a portacaval shunt (Castell and Johnson, 1966).

The blood ammonia concentration is increased not only in the presence of hepatocellular disease but also in certain inborn errors of metabolism which involve deficiencies of specific enzymes in the urea cycle. Patients with these hereditary hyperammonaemia syndromes suffer from encephalopathy, particularly if augmentation of the blood ammonia concentration occurs secondary to precipitating factors such as constipation or the ingestion of a protein-containing meal. Blood ammonia concentrations in these syndromes tend to be higher than in acquired liver diseases, while routine serum biochemical tests are normal (Hsia, 1974).

10.2.7.2. Urea

The liver has a large reserve capacity for synthesis of urea, which is the main product arising from hepatic extraction and metabolism of ammonia. This process may be impaired in acute or chronic hepatocellular diseases. The serum concentration of urea tends to be reduced in chronic hepatocellular diseases (Jones et al., 1972) and very low concentrations are occasionally found in patients with massive hepatic necrosis. A low protein intake and broad spectrum antibiotics (which serve to reduce intestinal ammonia formation) and over-hydration also tend to lower the blood urea concentration in patients with hepatic disease. Factors which tend to increase the concentration in such patients include dehydration; a high protein intake; gastrointestinal haemorrhage; massive paracentesis; loss of bile from a biliary fistula; renal failure from any cause, including that associated with hepatic failure and with severe prolonged cholestasis, particularly following surgery (Dawson, 1965); and corticosteroid therapy (Jones et al., 1972). Hepatic insufficiency due to causes which also induce renal damage, such as Weils disease and poisoning with carbon tetrachloride or *Amanita phalloides*, tend to be associated with elevated blood urea concentrations early in the clinical course.

Endogenous urea which passes from the blood to the intestinal lumen is the main source of ammonia. Any rise in blood urea concentration results in more urea becoming available as substrate for hydrolysis by bacterial urease in the intestine; hence, in the absence of factors which suppress this metabolic pathway, this leads to increased intestinal synthesis of ammonia (Jones et al., 1969). Consequently, any rise in blood urea concentration in a patient with hepatocellular disease is potentially undesirable.

Blood urea concentration is normal in the hereditary hyperammonaemia syndromes.

10.2.7.3. Aminoacids

Aminoacids arise in the body from digestion of protein in the gut and the catabolism of body proteins. Various metabolic pathways are available for their deamination, including the Krebs–Hensleit cycle in the liver (Hsia, 1974). They are utilized for protein synthesis both in the liver and in other tissues. Massive necrosis of liver cells results in release of appreciable quantities of aminoacids into the circulation. In severe chronic hepatocellular disease and portal-systemic enceophalopathy, abnormalities of plasma aminoacids include increased concentrations of methionine, phenylalanine, aspartic acid, glutamic acid, tyrosine, ornithine (Fischer et al., 1974) and octopamine (Manghani et al., 1975). In cerebrospinal fluid, the concentrations of certain aminoacids such as glutamine, and α-ketoglutarate are elevated in most patients with hepatic coma, but normal in coma due to other causes (Hourani et al., 1971; Duffy et al., 1974). Minor changes in the pattern of excretion of aminoacids in urine are detectable in acute hepatitis and cirrhosis, while heavy aminoaciduria occurs in massive hepatic necrosis. Increased urinary excretion of octopamine occurs in portal-systemic encephalopathy (Manghani et al., 1975). Urinary excretion of aminoacids may be increased in certain inborn errors of metabolism which are associated with neonatal cholestasis and cirrhosis, notably tyrosinaemia, glactosaemia and hereditary fructose intolerance, and also in some hereditary hyperammonaemia syndromes (Hsia, 1974).

10.2.7.4. Uric acid

Increased concentrations of uric acid in serum may be found in liver disease of the alcoholic (section 10.5.3), the acute hepatitic syndrome associated with fatty infiltration of the liver (Alvira and Forman, 1974) and type I glycogenosis. Low concentrations of uric acid in serum may be found in Wilson's disease.

10.2.8. Electrolytes, blood gases and pH

Measurements of plasma electrolytes in patients with hepatobiliary disease are of particular importance in the management of cirrhotic ascites, hepatic encephalopathy and biliary fistula.

In patients with untreated ascites, there is marked retention of sodium and the urinary sodium excretion is usually exceedingly low (less than 5 mmol/day). Plasma sodium concentrations are often reduced in these patients, but when low are usually a reflection of maldistribution of sodium, a relative excess being in the intracellular compartment. Whether the plasma sodium concentration is normal or low in cirrhosis with ascites, the total body sodium is almost invariably increased. Sodium chloride supplementation is only very rarely indicated in patients with chronic liver disease. Examples of such indications are when there is dilutional hyponatraemia after intravenous adminstration of inappropriate quantities of sodium-free fluids, and when the intravascular volume is contracted after massive paracentesis or overzealous diuretic therapy. A rise in plasma sodium concentration and/or an increase in the excretion of sodium in the urine may indicate improving liver cell function or a favourable response to treatment for ascites such as dietary sodium restriction and/or diuretics.

The plasma potassium concentration also is often reduced in cirrhosis, with or without ascites, and in fulminant liver failure. Hypokalaemia is often associated with an increase in plasma bicarbonate concentration and hence a metabolic alkalosis. Hypokalaemia almost invariably reflects potassium depletion. These patients may be deficient in potassium even if the plasma potassium concentration is normal, irrespective of whether diuretics have been administered in the recent past (Soler et al., 1976). Hence, potassium chloride supplements are often indicated except when an increased plasma potassium concentration has been found.

The plasma potassium concentration may not correlate closely with the degree of hepatic encephalopathy. Even so, it should be determined frequently in patients with chronic portal-systemic encepahopathy, acute hepatic coma associated with chronic hepatocellular disease and fulminant hepatic failure, so that the maintenance of normal values can be facilitated.

The most common electrolyte disturbances which occur during the treatment of ascites with diuretics are hypokalaemia, hyponatraemia, and hypochloraemia (Sherlock et al., 1966). The development of any of these electrolyte disturbances may be associated with the precipitation of hepatic precoma; the presence of a severe electrolyte abnormality is an indication to stop diuretic therapy, at least temporarily.

If appropriate fluid and electrolyte replacement is not given, loss of bile via a biliary fistula can lead to hyponatraemia, hypochloraemic acidosis and prerenal azotaemia.

A wide spectrum of disturbances of acid–base balance may occur in patients with liver failure. Patients in hepatic coma often hyperventilate and develop a respiratory alkalosis, while hypokalaemia, often present in patients with decompensated liver disease, may be associated with a metabolic alkalosis. In addition, extensive tissue necrosis may occur in patients with massive hepatic necrosis, particularly in the presence of hypotension; this may result in the accumulation of lactic acid and other acidic metabolites in the blood and hence a metabolic acidosis, as occurs for example in Reye's syndrome (Alvira and Forman, 1974). Finally, a complicating severe pulmonary infection can lead to a respiratory acidosis. Thus, in patients in liver failure – particularly if the underlying lesion is massive hepatic necrosis – complex changes in acid–base balance may occur (Record et al., 1975). As in the management of critically ill patients in general, arterial blood gases and pH should be determined frequently in patients with fulminant liver failure or those who have just received a hepatic transplant. Precise therapy for acid–base disturbances depends on accurately determining the type of disturbance present and the factors contributing to it (Chapter 3).

10.2.9. Plasma glucose

Although the liver plays a central role in the complex processes of carbohydrate homeostasis, the only laboratory test of carbohydrate metabolism which is ordinarily of clinical value in the management of liver disease is the plasma glucose concentration.

A raised fasting plasma glucose concentration, or impaired glucose tolerance, may be found in patients with hepatobiliary disease as a consequence of hepatogenous diabetes (Megyesi et al., 1967); alcoholic pancreatitis; tumours or stones responsible for large duct biliary obstruction also causing obstruction to the pancreatic duct system; iron deposition in the pancreas in primary haemochromatosis; portacaval shunts; and co-existing diabetes mellitus. Diabetes mellitus per se, if uncontrolled, may be associated with hyperbilirubinaemia, increased serum alkaline phosphatase activity and globulin concentration and increased bromosulphthalein retention. The mechanism of these abnormalities in diabetes mellitus is unknown.

Hypoglycaemia can occur after portacaval anastomosis, after appreciable alcohol ingestion, in liver cell carcinoma (section 10.5.2), massive hepatic secondary carcinoma, hepatic sarcoma and in types I, III and VI glycogenosis. The plasma glucose concentration falls after fructose administration in hereditary fructose intolerance. Severe hypoglycaemia can occur, particularly in children, with massive hepatic necrosis and acute liver failure associated with hepatic steatosis, such as Reye's syndrome (Alvira and Forman, 1974). The hypoglycaemia in fulminant liver failure may be due in large measure to impaired hepatic glucose release (glycogen depletion). In this clinical syndrome, frequent estimates of plasma glucose are necessary to facilitate maintenance of normal blood sugar, as the hypoglycaemia of acute liver failure may be very resistant to treatment (Samson et al., 1967). In a patient suspected of having hepatic encephalopathy, estimation of the plasma glucose concentration is mandatory as hepatic and hypoglycaemic encephalopathies are similar clinically and electroencephalographically.

The disturbances of glucose homeostasis in hepatocellular disease are associated with changes in the serum concentrations of hormones which play an important role in the regulation of glucose metabolism, such as insulin, glucagon and growth hormone. Techniques such as radioimmunoassay are available for measurements of these hormones, but have not been widely applied in the routine clinical assessment of patients with hepatobiliary diseases.

10.2.10. Vitamin B_{12}

Serum concentrations of vitamin B_{12} are usually increased in patients with acute hepatitis, cholangitis and intrahepatic space-occupying lesions such as secondary neoplasia, while values tend to be normal in large duct biliary obstruction and intrahepatic cholestasis which is not due to space-occupying lesions (Rachmilewitz and Eliakim, 1968). In a patient with a fever of unknown origin associated with increased values for serum aminotransferase and alkaline phosphatase activities and bromosulphthalein retention, a raised serum B_{12} suggests an intrahepatic infection (Neale et al., 1966). A raised value may also be found in patients with myeloproliferative disorders. In active hepatocellular diseases and liver cell carcinoma, a raised serum vitamin B_{12} concentration may be due to its release from hepatocytes and/or to an increased serum concentration of a B_{12}-binding protein (Rachmilewitz et al., 1972; Waxman and Gilbert, 1973). It follows that in patients with active hepatocellular disease or hepatic tumours, the serum B_{12} concentration could be normal or increased in the presence of vitamin B_{12} deficiency.

10.3. IMMUNOLOGIC TESTS

10.3.1. Non-organ-specific antibodies

Some antibodies present in the serum of most normal subjects are found in abnormally high titre in patients with certain hepatobiliary diseases, particularly chronic active hepatitis and cirrhosis. Transient increases in titre of some of these antibodies may occur during the course of acute hepatitis. These antibodies include those to several intestinal bacterial antigens and those to measles and rubella. It would appear that a wide variety of antigenic stimuli may contribute to the hyper-γ-globulinaemia of chronic liver disease. Failure of Kupffer cells of the diseased liver to sequester antigens, may contribute to the hyperglobulinaemia (Triger and Wright, 1973). Measurement of the titres of antibodies against intestinal bacterial antigens and virus, other than hepatitis B virus, has not been applied to routine clinical evaluation of patients with hepatobiliary disease.

In contrast, a number of antibodies, other than those related to hepatitis viruses, which are often detected in sera of patients with certain hepatobiliary diseases are only rarely detected in sera of normal subjects. The detection of some of these antibodies has been found to be of some value in the assesment of patients with hepatobiliary diseases. Those which have been most widely applied and found to be most useful in this context are certain autoantibodies, in particular mitochondrial antibody, smooth muscle antibody and antinuclear antibody. These antibodies are non-organ- and non-species-specific. They are found most commonly in the hepatobiliary disorders which are associated with other evidence of disturbed immunity, notably chronic active hepatitis, primary biliary cirrhosis and cryptogenic cirrhosis; they are not usually detectable in other types of chronic liver disease of equal severity such as alcoholic cirrhosis. The titres of these antibodies do not correlate with the severity of liver cell or bile duct destruction. The presence of these antibodies in apparently healthy relatives of patients with these diseases may indicate a familial predisposition to hepatobiliary disease (Galbraith et al., 1974). Other autoantibodies, such as rheumatoid factor, which are more typically found in non-hepatic autoimmune disorders may also be found in these three hepatobiliary diseases, and there is a marked serological overlap between "autoimmune" hepatobiliary disease and a number of non-hepatic autoimmune disorders. Other autoantibodies which have been detected in hepatobiliary diseases include antibodies against bile ducts, bile canaliculi, renal glomerular endothelium and reticulin (Doniach and Walker, 1972). None of these antibodies has been shown to be of any pathogenic significance and only mitochondrial antibody, smooth muscle antibody and antinuclear antibody are usually regarded as being of sufficient diagnostic value to be included with routine tests used in the evaluation of hepatobiliary disease. When present these antibodies persists after hepatic transplantation (Smith et al., 1971).

Mitochondrial, smooth muscle and antinuclear antibodies are usually detected by immunofluorescence or by complement fixation. Storage of sera at temperatures as low as −20 °C may be associated with a decrease in titre. Hence, the use of fresh sera for antibody testing is recommended. To avoid false positive results or prozone effects, it is usually necessary to dilute the test serum; to avoid detecting non-specific immunofluorescence, great care should be taken in the selection of an appropriate tissue to demonstrate fluorescence due to a particular antibody (Doniach and Walker, 1972).

10.3.1.1. Mitochondrial antibody

Mitochondrial antibody is directed against a lipoprotein on the inner membrane of mitochondrial christae. It may be of IgM, IgG, or IgA class. It is particularly important to distinguish immunofluorescence due to this antibody from that due to microsomal antibodies. Mitochondrial antibody reacts preferentially with distal renal tubules, the renal medulla, and stomach, whereas microsomal antibody reacts preferentially with the third part of the proximal renal tubule and liver. Mitochondrial antibody must also be distinguished from brush border heterophile antibody, heterogenous reticulin antibody, vascular endothelial antibody, and antibody against cardiolipin (Doniach and Walker, 1974).

The detection of mitochondrial antibody is particularly useful in the diagnosis of primary biliary cirrhosis. It can be detected in the serum of the majority of patients with this disease (Doniach et al., 1966; Goudie et al., 1966; Klatskin and Kantor, 1972; Doniach and Walker, 1974) as summarized in Table 10.1. The mitochondrial antibody titre does not correlate with the stage of the disease or with the serum IgM concentration (section 10.2.5.4.9), which is often raised in this condition (Doniach et al., 1966). The titre of mitochondrial antibody tends to remain constant for long periods. Patients with primary biliary cirrhosis who have detectable mitochondria antibody have similar clinical, serum biochemical and hepatic histologic findings to those in whom this antibody cannot be detected (Klatskin and Kantor, 1972). Other autoantibodies such as smooth muscle antibody and antinuclear antibody are not found as often as mitochondrial antibody in primary biliary cirrhosis (Table 10.1).

The widest application of the mitochondrial antibody test is as an aid to diagnosis of cholestatic jaundice since, in contrast to its high incidence in primary biliary cirrhosis this antibody is present in only a small proportion of cases with cholestatic jaundice due to acute large duct obstruction (Doniach et al., 1966; Klatskin and Kantor, 1973). Furthermore, there is some doubt about whether the pattern of immunofluorescence detected in cases of uncomplicated large duct biliary obstruction in some reports was specific for mitochondrial antibody, as other antibodies can produce a similar pattern (Doniach and Walker, 1974). Since primary biliary cirrhosis and acute large duct biliary obstruction are unlikely to be confused on clinical grounds, the main potential value of this test lies in helping to distinguish primary biliary cirrhosis from other causes of chronic cholestasis and particularly from other causes of intrahepatic cholestasis. If it were certain that chronic cholestasis were due to primary biliary cirrhosis alone, then a laparotomy would be unnecessary. Unfortunately, the mitochondrial antibody test may be positive occasionally in patients with uncomplicated chronic large duct biliary obstruction (Lam et al., 1972). Thus, when cholestatic jaundice does not resolve spontaneously and the diagnosis is not certain, irrespective of the result of the mitochondrial antibody

TABLE 10.1.

SERUM NON-ORGAN-SPECIFIC ANTIBODIES IN HEPATOBILIARY DISEASES

(Based on the data of Doniach et al., 1966; Goudie et al., 1966; Doniach, 1972; Doniach and Walker, 1972, 1974; Klatskin and Kantor, 1972).

	Per cent positive						
	Primary biliary cirrhosis	Chronic active hepatitis [1]	Cryptogenic cirrhosis [2]	Other cirrhotics	Large duct biliary obstruction	Acute hepatitis	Control subjects [3]
Mitochondrial	84–98	11–28	6–31	0–7	0–7	0–4 [4]	0.5–2
Smooth muscle	49–50	67	28–40	0	0	8–60	⩽3
Nuclear	24–46	70–80	38	–	–	–	⩽2

[1] HB_sAg-negative.

[2] With other evidence of disturbed immunity.

[3] Includes normal subjects and hospital patients without hepatobiliary disease.

[4] Transient and low titre.

test, cholangiography (e.g. retrograde or transhepatic) is indicated and if unsuccessful, laparotomy should in most cases be performed. The mitochondrial antibody test has been reported to be positive in a primary biliary cirrhosis-like syndrome co-existing with large duct biliary obstruction (Kaplowitz et al., 1973b). Furthermore, there is an increased prevalence of gall stones in primary biliary cirrhosis; an exacerbation of cholestasis due to occlusion of a major duct by a gall stone, although rare, can occur in this disease. A sudden increase in the intensity of jaundice in a patient with primary biliary cirrhosis, if not associated with an obvious precipitating factor, is an indication for retrograde or transhepatic cholangiography. The mitochondrial antibody test may occasionally be positive in cholestatic jaundice due to chlorpromazine (Rodriquez et al., 1969). Although both cholestasis and the mitochondrial antibody usually disappear after withdrawal of the drug, a syndrome of chronic cholestasis resembling primary biliary cirrhosis may occasionally be precipitated by this agent. The mitochondrial antibody test is rarely positive in cholestatic drug jaundice due to other agents (Doniach et al., 1966; Goudie et al., 1966).

Two cholestatic syndromes in which clinical and hepatic histological features may closely resemble those found in primary biliary cirrhosis are pericholangitis and primary sclerosing cholangitis, both of which occur in association with ulcerative colitis. In these two syndromes the mitochondrial antibody test is usually negative. It is clear that the value of the mitochondrial antibody test is not absolute as an aid to the diagnosis of cholestatic jaundice. It should be noted that, since large duct biliary obstruction is so much more common a cause of cholestasis than primary biliary cirrhosis, of all the patients with cholestasis due to either large duct biliary obstruction or primary biliary cirrhosis who are positive for this test, less then 70% may have primary biliary cirrhosis (Sturdevant, 1973). Nevertheless, the serum titre of this antibody should probably be determined routinely in any patient with cholestasis lasting longer than 3 months, the cause of which is not clear, or in any patient who presents with cholestasis of insidious onset or is found in routine screening to have a raised serum alkaline phosphatase activity.

The mitochondrial antibody test is often positive in patients with cryptogenic cirrhosis and chronic active hepatitis, though less frequently so than in patients with primary biliary cirrhosis (Table 10.1). There is a tendency for the patients with these other types of chronic liver disease who are mitochondrial antibody-positive to be middle-aged females with cholestatic features, having raised serum IgM concentration and hepatic histology with some similarity to that found in primary biliary cirrhosis (Doniach et al., 1966; Klatskin and Kantor, 1972). The precise frequency with which the mitochondrial antibody test is positive in cryptogenic cirrhosis and chronic active hepatitis depends to a large extent on the criteria used for diagnosis and the geographic region. The mitochondrial antibody test is only occasionally positive in other types of chronic liver disease of comparable severity. For instance, the test may be positive in a case of Wilson's disease in whom there is evidence of active hepatocellular disease (e.g. chronic active hepatitis) (Sternlieb, 1972). The mitochondrial antibody test is sometimes positive in acute HB_sAg-positive or -negative viral hepatitis, infectious mononucleosis, and acute hepatitis following halothane anaesthesia (Rodriquez et al., 1969). In these situations, the positive test is transient and the titre of the antibody is low.

The mitochondrial antibody test is positive in a small proportion of patients with various collagenoses, especially Sjogren's syndrome and scleroderma, idiopathic autoimmune haemolytic anaemia, thyroiditis, gastritis, adrenalitis, and myasthenia gravis. Some of these patients may have subclinical liver disease, but in others the test may remain positive for years without liver disease becoming manifest.

The mitochondrial antibody test is sometimes found to be positive in entirely asymptomatic apparently healthy individuals. Some of these subjects are found to have no evidence of hepatobiliary disease at all, the test being positive in a very small proportion (less than 1%) of the general population (Doniach, 1972). Others may be shown to have subclinical primary biliary cirrhosis, in which case the serum alkaline phosphatase activity will almost certainly be raised (Fox et al., 1973; Sherlock and Scheuer, 1973). Alternatively, a chronic hepatitis with aggressive features, also associated with a raised serum alkaline phosphatase activity, may be found (Walker et al., 1970).

10.3.1.2. Smooth muscle antibody

Smooth muscle antibody is directed against the actomyosin component of the smooth muscle cell. Satisfactory tissues for the detection of this antibody by immunofluorescence are rat stomach and human cervix. It is often found, in high titre, in serum of patients with HB_sAg-negative chronic active hepatitis (Table 10.1). It appears transiently, and usually in low titre, in the majority of patients with acute hepatitis (Figure 10.30), possibly as a consequence of liver cell damage (Holborrow et al., 1971; Ajdukiewicz et al., 1972). The antibody is usually of IgG or IgM class, the IgM class predominating in early viral hepatitis (Holborrow et al., 1971). Smooth muscle antibody may occasionally be found in viral diseases other than viral hepatitis, such as infectious mononucleosis, and it has been detected in association with tumours. Low titres of this antibody are found in an appreciable proportion of patients with primary biliary cirrhosis and cryptogenic cir-

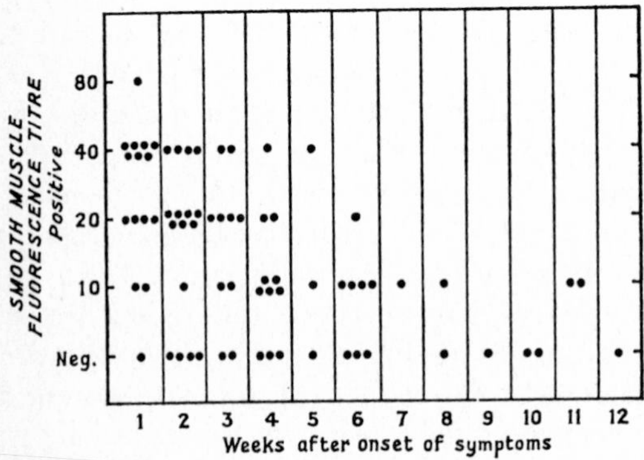

Figure 10.30. Relation between the presence and titre of smooth muscle antibody in serum and time of onset of symptoms in acute viral hepatitis. (Reproduced, with permission, from Ajdukiewicz et al., 1972)

rhosis associated with other evidence of disturbed immunity (Table 10.1). The presence of smooth muscle antibody in serum is not a feature of systemic lupus erythematosus (Doniach, 1972; Doniach and Walker, 1972).

10.3.1.3. Antinuclear antibody

Antinuclear antibody is detected satisfactorily by immunofluorescence using fresh sections of rat liver. The antibody is usually of IgG class. There is a high incidence of this antibody in serum from patients with HB_sAg-negative chronic active hepatitis, whether or not the LE cell test (section 10.3.1.5) is positive. This antibody is also detectable in an appreciable proportion of patients with primary biliary cirrhosis and cryptogenic cirrhosis associated with other evidence of disturbed immunity (Table 10.1). In patients with active hepatocellular disease, a persistent and strongly positive antinuclear antibody test would suggest chronic active hepatitis. In viral hepatitis, if this test is positive, the antibody usually appears only transiently, and in low titre, and only rarely in HB_sAg-positive cases. Antinuclear antibody is often found in connective tissue disorders such as systemic lupus erythematosus and non-hepatic autoimmune diseases. It occurs in low titre in some elderly subjects who appear to be in normal health. In assessing the possible significance of antinuclear antibody, particular attention should be paid to a patient's drug therapy. A number of drugs including procaineamide, hydralazine, isoniazid, methyldopa, hydantoins, penicillin and oxyphenisatin may provoke the appearance of this antibody, and it may be present in patients with chronic active hepatitis following ingestion of oxyphenisatin.

10.3.1.4. Microsomal antibody

Microsomal antibody can be detected by immunofluorescence using liver tissue. If renal tissue is used, care must be taken in distinguishing immunofluorescence due to this antibody from that due to mitochondrial antibody (section 10.3.1.1). Microsomal antibody has been found in an appreciable number of patients with HB_sAg-negative chronic active hepatitis but only in a few patients with other hepatobiliary diseases. The subgroup of patients with chronic active hepatitis who are positive for this test has an approximately equal sex distribution, a younger average age than that of patients who are positive for mitochondrial antibody, and absence of appreciable cholestasis and HB_sAg (Smith et al., 1974). No diagnostic or prognostic value for this antibody test has yet been defined.

10.3.1.5. LE cells

The LE cell test is not one which is usually done in the routine evaluation of patients with hepatobiliary diseases. This test may be positive in patients with active hepatocellular disease, in particular patients with chronic active hepatitis in whom the test for smooth muscle antibody is positive. The precise frequency with which the LE cell test is positive in these patients may depend on how diligently LE cells are sought. It seems probable that a positive test in this context is essentially a non-specific manifestation of active liver cell disease; in general, patients who are positive for this test tend to have more active and severe disease than those who are negative for the test (Soloway et al.,

1972). In some classifications of chronic active hepatitis, patients with a positive LE cell test are regarded as a distinct subgroup. The term lupoid hepatitis has been applied to such patients. This is an unfortunate term as it might be taken as implying the existence of a close pathophysiologic relationship between chronic active hepatitis and connective tissue disorders, such as systemic lupus erythematosus, in which hepatic lesions are usually insignificant.

10.3.2. Hepatitis-related tests

The hepatitis B virus particle (Dane particle) consists of an internal core surrounded by a clearly defined external coat. Both the surface coat and the internal core have readily identifiable antigenic determinants which are known respectively as the hepatitis B surface antigen (HB_sAg) and the hepatitis B core antigen (HB_cAg). The core of the Dane particle has been shown to contain a virus-specific DNA-polymerase and double stranded DNA, so providing substantive evidence that this particle, which is epidemiologically associated with type B hepatitis, is indeed a true virus. The core is probably produced in the nucleus of liver cells and then released into the cytoplasm where it is enveloped by coat material containing HB_sAg to form the complete hepatitis B virus particle. In addition, a great excess of viral coat material is syntheiszed and released into the circulation unassociated with core component. By electron microscopy, unassembled viral coat material appears as 20 nm spheres or as tubular forms of similar diameter but varying lengths (Figure 10.31). The vast majority of HB_sAg, when present in serum, represents unassembled virus. Nevertheless, when HB_sAg is detected in serum some complete virus particles are almost always present and the patient must be regarded as being infected with the hepatitis B virus and having potentially infective blood (Holland and Alter, 1975).

10.3.2.1. Antigens

10.3.2.1.1. Hepatitis B surface antigen. The presence of HB_sAg in serum can be detected by a number of methods of which radioimmunoassay is the method of choice because of its superior sensitivity, objectivity and specificity. However, as false positive results are possible with the radioimmunoassay, positive results should be confirmed by an independent method (Table 10.2) or by specificity testing (McIntyre and Heathcote, 1974; Holland and Alter, 1975).

HB_sAg is specific for hepatitis virus B infection which may or may not have been transmitted by parenteral inoculation. Detection of HB_sAg is of considerable help in distinguishing type B hepatitis from other forms of viral hepatitis and from non-viral hepatitis such as that due to drugs. In acute anicteric or icteric type B hepatitis, the appearance of HB_sAg in serum is the first abnormality that can be detected (Figure 10.32). This antigen appears in serum between 12 days and 24 weeks (usually 4 to 8 weeks) after known exposure. Thus, it appears during the incubation period of the disease, before the serum aminotransferases rise and prior to the onset of clinical hepatitis (Giles et al., 1969). In uncomplicated infections, the titre may begin to fall from a peak value before the onset of symptoms. HB_sAg is usually cleared completely from serum within 3 months of the onset of symptoms (Figure 10.32). It follows that it is desirable to test for HB_sAg

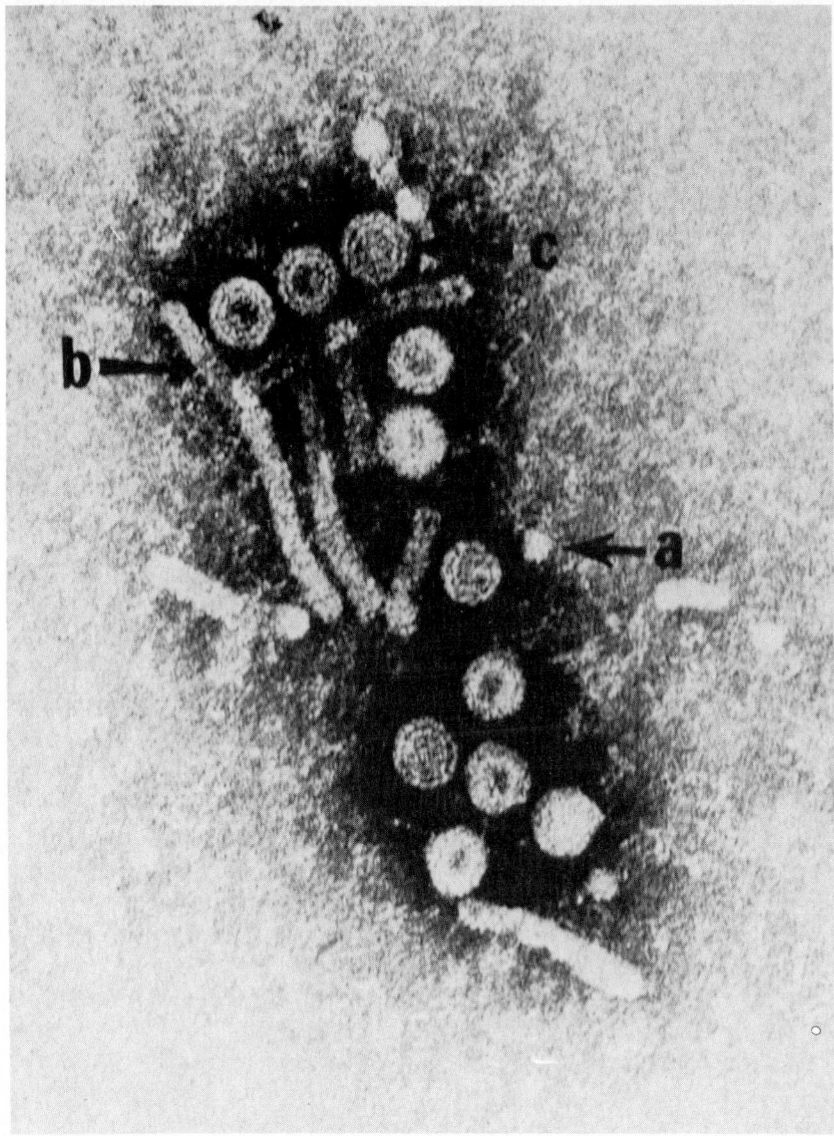

Figure 10.31. Electron microscopic appearance (× 150,000) of particles associated with hepatitis B surface antigen (HB_sAg). a = 20 nm spherical form; b = tubular or filamentous form; c = 42 nm Dane particle consisting of a 28 nm internal core and an outer membrane which contains HB_sAg. (Reproduced, with permission, from Holland and Alter, 1976)

as soon as a diagnosis of viral hepatitis is suspected and that a single negative result does not exclude hepatitis B infection (Table 10.3). HB_sAg-positive acute hepatitis may be associated with a syndrome of arthritis, urticaria and low serum complement concentration immediately prior to the elevation of the serum aminotransferases (Alpert et al.,

TABLE 10.2.

SENSITIVITY OF METHODS OF DETECTING HEPATITIS B SURFACE ANTIGEN

Generation of sensitivity	Method	Relative sensitivity	Particles per ml
First	Agar gel diffusion	1	10^{13}
Second	Counterelectrophoresis Rheophoresis Complement fixation Latex agglutination	2–10	10^{12}
Third	Reversed passive haemag-glutination Radioimmunoassay	10^2–10^4	10^9
	Infectivity	10^6–10^7	10^6

1971). This syndrome may be due to immune complexes of HB_sAg and antiHB_s (section 10.3.2.1.4).

Of particular importance in assessing the clinical significance of the presence of HB_sAg in serum is an attempt to determine the approximate time when the antigen first appeared in the serum. It is possible for acute non-B hepatitis to occur in a patient who is a chronic carrier of HB_sAg. In this context, the screening of an old, deep frozen specimen of serum for the antigen may be of considerable diagnostic value. The characteristic rise

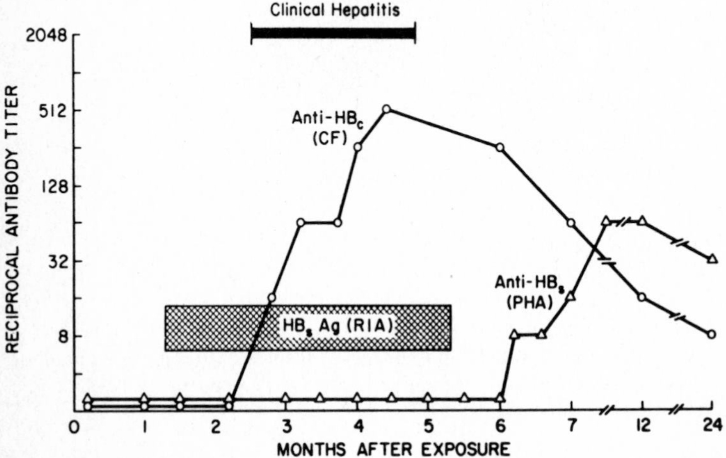

Figure 10.32. Serological responses in a moderately severe case of type B hepatitis. Hepatitis B surface antigen (HB_sAg) was determined in radioimmunoassay (RIA); antibody to hepatitis B surface antigen (antiHB_s) by passive haemagglutination (PHA) and antibody to hepatitis B core antigen (antiHB_c) by complement fixation (CF). (Reproduced, with permission, from Hoofnagle et al., 1975)

TABLE 10.3.

INTERPRETATION OF PATTERNS OF REACTIVITY FOR HB_sAg, ANTI-HB_s AND ANTI-HB_c (From Hoofnagle et al., 1975)

HB_sAg	Anti-HB_s	Anti-HB_c	Interpretation
+	–	–	Acute HBV [1] hepatitis, early in course
+	–	+	(1) Acute HBV hepatitis, late in course (2) Chronic HB_sAg carrier state
–	+	+	Late convalescence from HBV hepatitis
–	+	–	(1) Late convalescence from HBV hepatitis (2) Seroconversion (3) Repeat antigenic stimulation by HB_sAg without reinfection
–	–	+	(1) Early convalescence from HBV hepatitis (2) Chronic carrier state with subdetectable levels of HB_sAg

[1] HBV = hepatitis B virus.

and fall of the serum titre of HB_sAg in association with an attack of acute hepatitis, or the de novo appearance of antiHB_s (section 10.3.2.2.1), is diagnostic of infection with hepatitis B virus. Thus it may be possible to distinguish a second de novo attack of acute viral hepatitis from a recurrence of a previous infection if, for instance, in the former circumstance one attack was due to hepatitis virus B and the other to hepatitis virus A. It is not possible to distinguish between acute type B hepatitis and other forms of acute hepatitis on the basis of biochemical tests of serum.

Persistence of HB_sAg in serum for more than 3 months after an attack of acute hepatitis, like persistence of elevated serum aminotransferase activities, raises the possibility that the patient's hepatic lesion may be undergoing progression to a chronic lesion, such as chronic persistent hepatitis or chronic active hepatitis (Nielsen et al., 1971), as illustrated in Figure 10.33. Thus, it is important to check that HB_sAg is cleared from serum following HB_sAg-positive acute hepatitis. The finding of HB_sAg in some patients with chronic active hepatitis has led to the HB_sAg-positive cases being regarded as a distinct entity, or subgroup of chronic active hepatitis. Results of most of the routine laboratory tests in HB_sAg-positive and -negative chronic hepatitis are in general similar, although there is the impression that HB_sAg-positive cases tend to have milder abnormalities of serum biochemical tests such as serum aminotransferase activities and γ-globulin concentration, and a lower frequency and titre of serum non-organ-specific autoantibodies (Dudley et al., 1972; Finlayson et al., 1972). The serum IgG concentration and smooth muscle antibody titre tend to be higher in HB_sAg-negative cases, while antinuclear factor and mitochondrial antibody are rarely found in HB_sAg-positive cases (Dudley et al., 1973). This distinction between HB_sAg-positive and -negative patients with chronic active hepatitis may have important therapeutic implications, – for instance, the responses of patients in the two groups to corticosteroid therapy may be different.

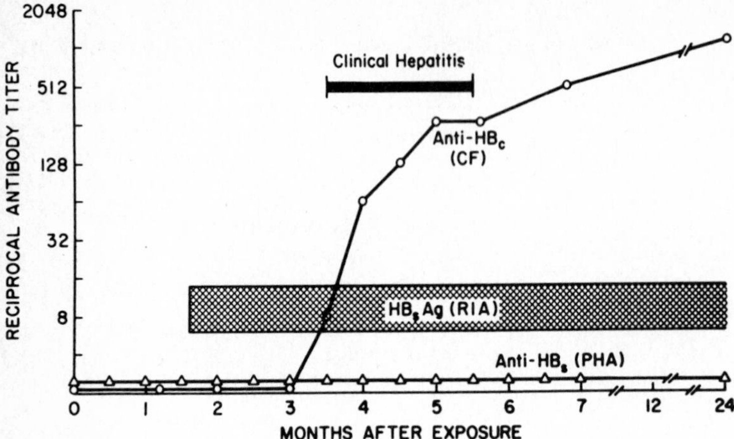

Figure 10.33. The chronic HB$_s$Ag carrier state developing in a patient exposed to hepatitis B virus. See legend to Figure 10.32. (Reproduced, with permission, from Hoofnagle et al., 1975)

HB$_s$Ag has been found in the serum not only in cases of acute and chronic hepatitis but also in cases of cirrhosis and liver cell carcinoma. These observations have led to the suggestion that infection with hepatitis B virus may in some cases trigger a sequence of pathological events which progresses from acute to chronic hepatitis, then to cirrhosis and ultimately, if the patient survives long enough, to liver cell carcinoma (Dudley et al., 1972). In all of these conditions, the finding of HB$_s$Ag in serum may imply that hepatitis virus B infection is causally related to the hepatic lesion. However, the possibility must always be considered that the patient may be a carrier of the antigen and that its presence may be unrelated to a particular underlying hepatic lesion. For instance, HB$_s$Ag is sometimes found in patients with liver disease associated with, and characteristic of, alcoholism. Sometimes it is possible to resolve the problem of the significance of the presence of HB$_s$Ag by finding hepatic histological features which are diagnostic of hepatitis B virus infection (e.g. "ground glass" hepatocytes or hepatocytes which stain selectively with aldehyde–fuchsin–Shikata or orcein stains). The absence of detectable HB$_s$Ag in the serum of a patient with chronic liver disease does not exclude the possibility that this antigen might have been detectable at an earlier stage of the disease, and that the disease may have been initiated by hepatitis B virus infection. HB$_s$Ag has been found in patients with primary biliary cirrhosis, but this association is rare and may be due to coincidental factors such as previous blood transfusion (Maddrey et al., 1972; MacSween et al., 1973).

Subjects who are found as a result of screening procedures to be chronic carriers of HB$_s$Ag may have no evidence of liver disease as assessed by a routine clinical, biochemical, serological and hepatic histological evaluations. However, some chronic carriers do have hepatic histological changes of chronic persistent hepatitis or chronic active hepatitis (Woolf et al., 1974). These lesions may or may not be associated with raised values for the serum aminotransferases and γ-globulin. Needle biopsy of the liver should be considered in the asymptomatic carrier of HB$_s$Ag even if the results of all other laboratory tests are normal. However, significant structural liver disease is rare in the presence of normal routine serum biochemical tests, and the very small likelihood that a treatable lesion will be detected must be carefully weighed against the small but inherent risks of liver biopsy.

In undiagnosed cholestatic jaundice, the recent acute appearance of HB_sAg would raise the possibility of cholestatic type B viral hepatitis. However, most cases of cholestatic viral hepatitis appear to be due to non-B disease; thus the presence of the antigen would not obviate the necessity for further investigations such as percutaneous or retrograde cholangiography if the cholestasis persisted.

HB_sAg-positive liver disease and the HB_sAg carrier state appear to be more common in subjects from certain geographic areas, such as Mediterranean, Far Eastern and African countries. Because the presence of HB_sAg in serum implies that the patient's blood is potentially infective, the finding of HB_sAg has important implications in addition to those which relate to diagnosis. The epidemiologic implications of HB_sAg are compounded by the fact that HB_sAg may also be found in body secretions such as saliva and semen.

A number of subtypes of HB_sAg can be demonstrated. The antigen has a common determinant "a" and two sets of subdeterminants "d" or "y", and "w" or "r", which behave as allelic pairs. Thus, HB_sAg-positive sera can be divided into four major subtypes (adw, adr, ayw, ayr), each of which reflects a certain strain of hepatitis B virus. In a particular patient, the subtype remains constant during the clinical course of the hepatitis B related disease or carrier state. Determinations of the subtypes of the antigen are useful in epidemiologic studies of hepatitis B infection but do not contribute to the clinical evaluation of an individual patient.

10.3.2.1.2. Hepatitis A antigen. There is as yet no readily detectable marker antigen for hepatitis A infection which is analogous to HB_sAg. However, it is possible to confirm a diagnosis of acute type A hepatitis virus infection by demonstrating specific antibody seroconversion (section 10.3.2.2.3).

10.3.2.1.3. "Non-A, non-B" disease. It has recently been recognized that, after a latent period following blood transfusion – which could correspond to the incubation period of a viral infection – there is a rather high incidence of acute hepatitis which, serologically, is unrelated to hepatitis B, hepatitis A, cytomegalo or Epstein–Barr viruses. These cases have been designated "non-A, non-B" hepatitis. Evidence suggesting that these cases are of viral origin stems from the observations that they occur approximately 10 times more frequently following transfusion of commercial, rather than voluntarily donated, blood and that routine hepatic histology is indistinguishable from that of other forms of viral hepatitis with the exception that ground-glass cells, and cells which stain preferentially with Shikata or orcein stains indicative of HB_sAg-positive disease, are not found. No marker or antibody test which is specific for this presumed viral disease has yet been discovered (Feinstone et al., 1975).

10.3.2.1.4. Immune complexes. In some disorders, such as polyarteritis nodosa and glomerulonephritis, the clinical picture is suggestive of immune complex disease. In addition, serum complement levels may be depressed and the serum may exhibit anticomplementary activity. In some cases HB_sAg, antiHB_s and complement have been demonstrated in the pathologic lesion suggesting that hepatitis B virus infection may bear a pathogenic relation to extrahepatic lesions.

10.3.2.1.5. "e" Antigen. This antigen is a newly discovered soluble antigen which does not appear to be associated with any particle. It appears to be antigenically and physically distinct from HB_sAg, but has so far been found only in HB_sAg-positive sera, particularly from patients with active and continuing liver disease (Eleftheriou et al., 1975; Feinman et al., 1975). e Antigen appears to be a marker for infectivity, and HB_sAg-positive mothers who are e antigen-positive are likely to give birth to HB_sAg-positive babies (Okada et al., 1976).

10.3.2.2. Antibodies

10.3.2.2.1. Anti-hepatitis B surface antigen (antiHB_s). Detection of antiHB_s can be diagnostically helpful in patients who are HB_sAg-negative. After an attack of acute type B hepatitis, only some patients have detectable antiHB_s in their serum weeks or months after HB_sAg disappears, and the titre of this antibody is usually low. This observation contrasts with the marked antibody response which is found in association with most common viral diseases such as measles. The detection of rising titres of antiHB_s implies recent infection with the hepatitis B virus (Figure 10.32), and the detection of a stable titre of this antibody implies past infection with the B virus, which may or may not have been clinically overt. The presence of the antibody probably also implies recovery from hepatitis B infection and immunity to re-challenge with the hepatitis B virus. AntiHB_s may not be detected in acute hepatitis until after HB_sAg has been cleared (Figure 10.32). This antibody is absent from the serum of chronic carriers of HB_sAg (Table 10.3 and Figure 10.33). Sensitive haemagglutination and radioimmunoassay techniques are used to detect antiHB_s (Barker et al., 1975).

10.3.2.2.2. Anti-hepatitis B core antigen (antiHB_c). The detection of antiHB_c in serum is possible using a commercially available radioimmunoassay. The significance of the presence of this antibody is not yet certain. It becomes detectable during the course of hepatitis B virus infections while HB_sAg is still present and before the appearance of anti-HB_s. The detection of rising titres of this antibody appears to be diagnostic of recent infection with the hepatitis B virus (Figure 10.32). AntiHB_c appears to correlate with the degree and duration of hepatitis B viral replication and may become a valuable method of diagnosing infection with this virus, especially when the HB_sAg status is not helpful (Barker et al., 1975; Hoofnagle et al., 1975). This antibody is present in chronic carriers of HB_sAg (Fig. 10.33 and Table 10.3). In contrast to antiHB_s, it does not appear to play a protective role in preventing type B hepatitis reinfection.

10.3.2.2.3. Antibodies to hepatitis A virus. Antibodies to the hepatitis A virus can be detected by means of a specific immune adherence assay (Krugman et al., 1975; Miller et al., 1975) or a blocking radioimmunoassay which uses antigen derived from stool or liver of marmosets infected with the hepatitis A virus. An appreciable rise in titre appears to be diagnostic of hepatitis virus A infection. A radioimmunoassay is currently available for routine clinical use.

10.3.2.2.4. Antibody to "e" antigen (anti-e). Anti-e appears in HB_sAg-positive acute hepatitis before the clearance of HB_sAg and before the appearance of antiHB_s. It tends to be associated with mild or inactive liver disease and asymptomatic carriage of HB_sAg Eleftheriou et al., 1975; Feinman et al., 1975). HB_sAg-positive mothers who are positive for anti-e are unlikely to give birth to HB_sAg-positive babies (Okada et al., 1976).

10.4. DYNAMIC TESTS

For the most part, the tests described above involve one measurement of the amount of some metabolite, antigen, antibody, or enzyme in blood, urine or faeces at a single point in time. While these tests are performed because experience shows them to correlate in some useful way with the condition of the liver and/or biliary system, most of them are, at best, indirect measurements of hepatic function. In the following section, several procedures are described which permit quantitative assessment of the capacity of the liver to perform specific metabolic or excretory functions. Some of these procedures can provide the clinician with useful information which is not obtainable by other means.

Methods are available for measuring the rates of synthesis and catabolism of various proteins which are exported from the liver cell such as albumin (Dykes, 1968) and fibrinogen (Tytgat et al., 1971); the maximal capacity of the liver to synthesize urea (Rudman et al., 1973), or to metabolize specific nutrients such as galactose (Tygstrup, 1964a); the rates at which the liver clears either exogenous compounds (e.g. bromosulphthalein and indocyanine green; sections 10.4.1 and 10.4.2) or endogenous metabolites (e.g. bile acids and bilirubin; sections 10.4.3 and 10.4.4), and the rates of metabolism of various drugs (e.g. aminopyrine; Hepner and Vesell, 1975). Laboratory methods are also available for estimating the total hepatic activity of a number of liver enzymes. For instance, the urinary excretion of hippuric acid after oral administration of sodium benzoate is a measure of the activity of the hepatic glycine conjugating enzyme (glycine-*N*-acylase) (Quick, 1933). Alternatively, the urinary excretion of urocanic acid after oral administration of histidine is a measure of the activity of the hepatic enzyme urocanase (EC 4.2.1.49), which is reduced in severe malnutrition and chronic hepatocellular disease; while the urinary excretion of formiminoglutamic acid (FIGLU) after oral histidine is a measure of the activity of the hepatic enzyme FIGLU transferase and/or the subject's folic acid status (Hoffbrand et al., 1966). Furthermore, urinary D-glucaric acid excretion has been used as an indicator of the degree of hepatic microsomal enzyme induction (Hunter et al., 1971). While all of these tests are of considerable theoretical interest, only a few of them have been widely applied clinically. These procedures are of value principally in determining the functional state of the liver, rather than in arriving at specific diagnosis, and many are currently available only in specialized research institutes. A few of them, however, have undergone sufficient clinical evaluation to warrant inclusion in this section and are therefore discussed below.

10.4.1. Bromosulphthalein (phenoltetrabromophthalein disulfonate) disappearance

Although the removal of bromosulphthalein from plasma was proposed as a test of liver function more than 50 years ago (Rosenthal and White, 1925) it remains one of the most sensitive tests available. Following the intravenous administration of the dye, it binds tightly to albumin (Baker and Bradley, 1966) and, to a lesser extent, to α_1-lipoprotein (Baker, 1966) within the circulation, from which it is removed principally by the parenchymal cells of the liver (Krebs and Brauer, 1949). It exhibits minimal extra-hepatic uptake (principally in skeletal muscle; Cohn et al., 1947), some renal excretion (roughly 2% of the administered dose in normal subjects, but up to 20% in those with impaired hepatic excretion; Ingelfinger et al., 1948), and a small degree of enterohepatic recirculation. Its overall transfer from blood to bile involves (a) hepatic uptake, (b) intracellular binding to glutathione-*S*-transferase such as ligandin and to Z protein (Levi et al., 1969), (c) conjugation with the tripeptide glutathione (cysteine–glycine–glutamic acid) and (d) biliary excretion (Jablonski and Owen, 1975). Both its hepatic uptake and biliary excretion appear to be carrier-mediated processes shared with indocyanine green and bilirubin (sections 10.4.2 and 10.4.4), but distinct from those involved in bile acid transport (Gorensky, 1965; Scharschmidt et al., 1975). In contrast to bilirubin, up to 30% of the bromosulphthalein excreted in bile may be unconjugated, even in normal subjects. The remaining 70% is excreted principally as the glutathione conjugate, with small quantities conjugated to components of glutathione (e.g. bromosulphthalein–cysteine–glycine or bromosulphthalein–cysteine) (Combes and Stakelum, 1960; Javitt et al., 1960). Since both hepatic uptake and biliary excretion are saturable processes, the results of bromosulphthalein removal tests are dependent on the dose employed.

The widespread use of these tests is based on the recognition that dye removal from the circulation is delayed when there is impairment of liver cell function or cholestasis, irrespective of the cause of these phenomena (Combes and Schenker, 1975; Jablonski and Owen, 1975). In the simplest of these tests, the bromosulphthalein content of plasma is determined at a particular time after the intravenous administration of a standard dose. Using this simple test, abnormal retention of the dye in plasma is found in a high proportion of patients with all types of hepatobiliary disease. It is therefore a highly sensitive but non-specific diagnostic aid. It offers no information, however, concerning the mechanism(s) responsible for delayed removal of the dye. The test can be refined by obtaining multiple blood specimens during either the first 20, or 60, or more minutes after injection, in order to define either the initial plasma disappearance rate (Ingelfinger et al., 1948) or the complete plasma disappearance curve. The latter, which usually corresponds to the sum of two exponential functions, can be analyzed mathematically to obtain information about the fractional rate of (a) hepatic uptake; (b) reflux from liver to plasma; and (c) biliary excretion (Barber-Riley et al., 1961). The storage capacity of the liver for bromosulphthalein may also be calculated from the curve. However, storage capacity is most often determined by analysis of plasma concentrations during continuous infusion of bromosulphthalein (section 10.4.1.4), a technique which also permits calculation of the transport maximum (T_{MAX}) for biliary excretion. Although these expanded tests may be even more sensitive than the single specimen test, their greater cost, complexity and inconvenience have largely restricted their use to the detailed evaluation of well defined hepatic lesions, particularly certain discrete physiologic defects.

10.4.1.1. Conventional bromosulphthalein test

In the conventional test, 5 mg/kg body mass of dye is injected intravenously during a 30-second interval, with great care taken to avoid extravasation. A single blood specimen is obtained 45 minutes later from the opposite arm. A minority of clinicians prefer a 30- or 60-minute sampling time. After separation of plasma and alkalinization to convert the dye to a characteristic magenta color, its plasma concentration is determined spectrophotometrically. It is assumed that the dye has been initially distributed within a plasma volume of 50 ml/kg body mass, at an initial concentration of 10.0 mg/dl. Hence, BSP retention at 45 minutes [R_{45}] in per cent, is calculated as:

$$R_{45}(\%) = \frac{\text{plasma concentration at 45 min (mg/dl)}}{10.0} \times 100 = \text{plasma concentration at 45 min} \times 10 \quad [3]$$

The upper limit of normal is usually taken as 5%, although some authors consider 7% to be within normal limits (Combes and Schenker, 1975; Jablonski and Owen, 1975) and Zieve and Hill (1955) reported an even wider normal range. Earlier reports that bromosulphthalein retention in normal adult subjects increases with ageing have not been confirmed (Koff et al., 1973). Elevated values are not uncommon in obese subjects without liver disease when the dose is calculated on the basis of total body mass (Zelman, 1952; Zieve and Hill, 1955). None of the various recommendations for correcting the dose in such individuals has proved entirely satisfactory.

Abnormal values for R_{45} occur in a large proportion of cases of structural liver and biliary tract disease of all types, including fatty liver, hepatitis, cirrhosis, lesions resulting in cholestasis and drug-induced hepatocellular necrosis (Combes and Schenker, 1975; Jablonski and Owen, 1975). It is therefore of greatest value as a screening test for patients with hepatobiliary disease. Because hepatic bromosulphthalein uptake depends on hepatic blood flow, the test may be abnormal in patients with congestive heart failure even in the absence of intrinsic liver damage. Other causes of increased retention in the absence of a hepatobiliary lesion include fever (Blaschke et al., 1973), extra-hepatic infection (Neale et al., 1966), recent surgery, prolonged fasting, the recent administration of rifamycin or cholecystographic media, both of which compete with bromosulphthalein for biliary excretion, and non-metastatic hypernephroma (Walsh and Kissane, 1968). Natural or synthetic oestrogens and anabolic steroids decrease hepatic excretory function and may cause increased retention. Slightly abnormal bromosulphthalein retention, presumably on the same physiological basis, occurs in some women during the third trimester of normal pregnancy, and in some women taking contraceptive steroid drugs (Combes and Schenker, 1975; Jablonski and Owen, 1975).

Bromosulphthalein retention may be normal in the presence of increased plasma concentrations of unconjugated bilirubin due either to haemolysis or to certain inherited metabolic disorders of bilirubin metabolism (Crigler–Najjar syndrome, most patients with Gilbert's syndrome). A normal test result may therefore be reassuring in patients in whom unconjugated hyperbilirubinaemia is the sole abnormality of routine serum biochemical tests (Berk et al., 1974a). A small proportion of patients with Gilbert's syndrome will, however, have abnormal retention due to a constitutional metabolic defect (Berk et al., 1972; Martin et al., 1976), and may require liver biopsy to rule out structural disease.

Normal bromosulphthalein tests may be encountered with discrete neoplastic lesions of the liver which do not interfere with biliary drainage, or have not replaced an extensive portion of the liver parenchyma, with hepatic fibrosis due to methotrexate therapy or exposure to vinyl chloride, and with granulomatous disease of the liver. Very occasionally, retention tests may be normal in patients with cirrhosis. A factor which sometimes tends to reduce the apparent degree of retention in cirrhosis is dilution of bromosulphthalein due to a markedly expanded plasma volume (Lieberman and Reynolds, 1967). In most of these cirrhotic patients, however, more detailed studies of bromosulphthalein kinetics will be clearly abnormal (Mendenhall and Leevy, 1961; Schoenfield et al., 1970). Profound hypoalbuminaemia, such as is seen in the nephrotic syndrome, may accelerate removal of the dye from plasma and could, at least in theory, lead to a falsely negative test (Grausz and Schmid, 1971).

Bromosulphthalein occasionally produces local thrombophlebitis; injection outside the vein is intensely irritating, and may causes severe tissue necrosis and sloughing, which requires subsequent skin grafting. Accordingly, poorly accessible veins represent a relative contraindication to its use. The most serious complication of the test is anaphylaxis, of which at least 20 instances – 9 fatal – have been reported (Landau et al., 1967). This represents an incidence of roughly one reaction per million doses injected. For this reason, availability of epinephrine and steroids at the bedside is routine at the U.S. National Institutes of Health during the test, and the risk is considered excessive in any patient with a history of previous reaction to bromosulphthalein or of multiple allergic reactions to other agents.

Although bromosulphthalein retention is a highly sensitive test, it *is* non-specific and therefore of little help in establishing either a diagnosis or prognosis. Accordingly, it is of little value in patients in whom the presence of hepatobiliary disease has been established by other means.

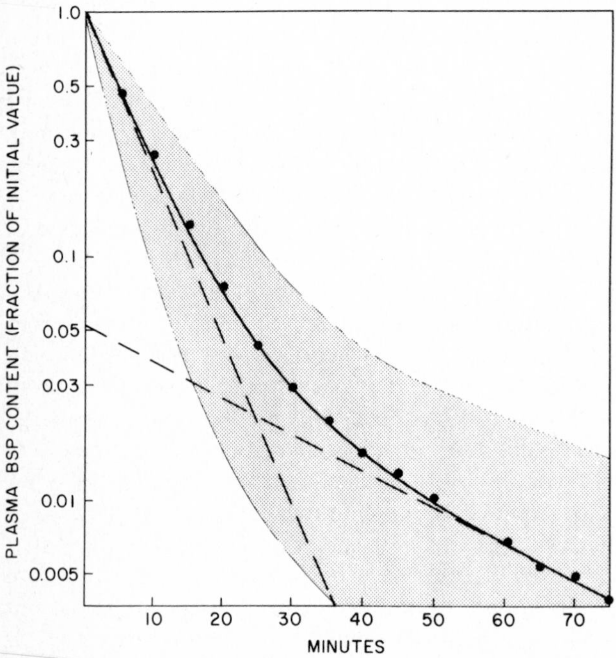

Figure 10.34. Typical plasma bromosulphthalein (BSP) disappearance curve in a normal individual. Solid line represents computer fit of the data to a sum of two exponential functions, dashed lines are the individual exponentials with half lives of 4.7 and 20.3 minutes, and shaded area represents the observed normal range. (Reproduced, with permission, from Berk et al., 1972)

10.4.1.2. Bromosulphthalein percentage disappearance rate

In this procedure, multiple blood samples are obtained between 5 and 15 minutes after injection of the usual dose (5 mg/kg body mass), and plasma bromosulphthalein concentrations are plotted semi-logarithmically against time. The data are usually consistent with a single exponential disappearance, whose rate constant, K_{BSP}, is determined by the method of least squares. The normal range for K is 0.09 to 0.16 min^{-1}, or, when expressed as a percentage disappearance rate 9 to 16% per minute (Ingelfinger et al., 1948). The rapid plasma disappearance which is found by this technique reflects both hepatic blood flow and hepatocellular uptake of dye. Determination of the plasma disappearance rate appears to be more sensitive than the conventional 45-minute retention test in detecting disease associated with abnormalities of these two processes.

10.4.1.3. Plasma bromosulphthalein disappearance curve

If blood sampling is continued for 60 or more minutes following injection, a complete plasma bromosulphthalein disappearance curve is obtained (Richards et al., 1959; Barber-Riley et al., 1961). This usually corresponds to the sum of two exponential functions (Figure 10.34) of the form $X(t) = X_0(Ae^{-k_1t} + Be^{-k_2t})$, where $X(t)$ = plasma bromosulphthalein concentration at t minutes after injection; X_0 is the concentration extrapolated to zero time; k_1 and k_2 are the two exponential rate constants; and A and B are the coefficients of the two exponential terms, normalized so that $A + B = 1$. The volume of distribution (VD_{BSP}) is determined from the equation VD_{BSP} (ml/kg) = [injected dose (5 mg/kg)/X_0 (mg/dl)] $\times$ 100, and corresponds closely to independent measurements of plasma volume. The fraction of the plasma bromosulphthalein pool which is irreversibly removed per minute (k_e $minute^{-1}$) is given by the relationship:

$$k_e = \frac{1}{\int_0^\infty \frac{X(t)}{X_0}\,dt} = \frac{1}{\frac{A}{k_1} + \frac{B}{k_2}} \qquad [4]$$

while the clearance (C_{BSP}), the volume of plasma cleared of BSP per minute, is calculated as C_{BSP} (ml/min per kg) = $k_e \times VD_{BSP}$ (Fauvert, 1959; Berk et al., 1972; Blaschke et al., 1973). The data may also be analyzed in terms of a simple two compartment model of bromosulphthalein metabolism, illustrated in Figure 10.35, which enables numerical values for the fractional transfer rates and pool sizes of the model to be derived (Richards et al , 1959; Barber-Riley et al., 1961). Reference values for k_e, C_{BSP} and the model transfer rates are presented in Table 10.4 (Berk et al., 1972; Martin et al., 1976). Relative hepatic bromosulphthalein storage capacity (section 10.4.1.4) can also be estimated by means of the model (Quarfordt et al., 1971).

The model which is commonly used for this analysis (Figure 10.35) is clearly an oversimplification of the metabolic process. Measurements of the plasma bromosulphthalein concentration which are used in the construction of the disappearance curve reflect *total* plasma concentration and therefore give no indication of the relative quantities of conjugated and unconjugated bromosulphthalein present; in other words, the model makes no provision for bromosulphthalein conjugation or its physiological consequences. Hence,

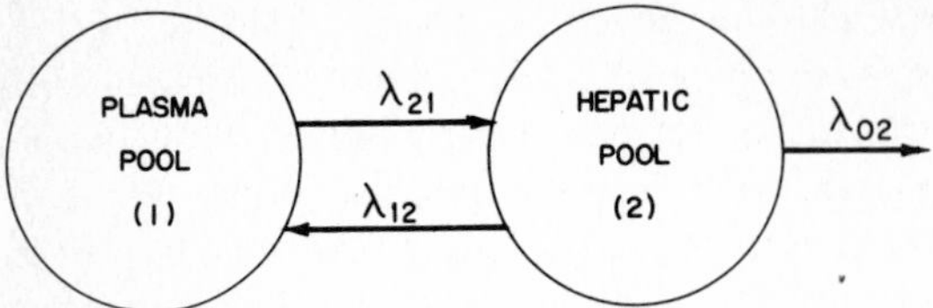

Figure 10.35. A widely used two-compartmental model of bromosulphthalein (BSP) metabolism. Values for the λ's, which are the fractional transfer rates between compartments, are calculated from the experimental plasma BSP disappearance curves. The fractional rate of hepatic BSP uptake is denoted by λ_{21}, of reflux from liver to plasma by λ_{12}, and of irreversible removal of BSP from the hepatic compartment by λ_{02}. (Reproduced, with permission, from Blaschke et al., 1973)

while reduction in the uptake parameter strongly suggests defective hepatic uptake of the dye a decrease in the biliary excretion parameter may reflect impaired conjugation as well as defective biliary secretion, and an increase in the reflux parameter may result from numerous factors, including defective intracellular binding or, paradoxically, impaired biliary excretion (Berk et al., 1972; Blaschke et al., 1973). Accordingly, compartmental analysis of bromosulphthalein disappearance curves is of relatively little value in most patients with established hepatobiliary disease. It has, however, proved helpful in the evaluation of patients with selective defects in bromosulphthalein transport such as are seen in certain variants of Gilbert's syndrome (Berk et al., 1972; Martin et al., 1976).

Extending a plasma disappearance curve to 90 minutes is of particular value in the diagnosis of the Dubin–Johnson syndrome. The early portions of the curve, including 45 minute retention, are either normal or only mildly abnormal, but a reflux of conjugated dye from liver to plasma, such that the plasma total bromosulphthalein content at 90 minutes is greater than that at 45 minutes, is virtually diagnostic of this condition (Shani et al., 1970a; Wolkoff et al., 1976). This "secondary rise" may persist for hours, and is not seen in Rotor's syndrome (section 10.5.1.1.3) in which the early portions of the curve

TABLE 10.4.

PHYSIOLOGIC VARIABLES CALCULATED FROM PLASMA BROMOSULPHTHALEIN DISAPPEARANCE CURVES: VALUES IN NORMAL INDIVIDUALS

k_e = Fraction of plasma bromosulphthalein pool irreversibly removed per minute; C_{BSP} = bromosulphthalein clearance; λ_{21} = fraction of plasma bromosulphthalein pool entering liver per minute; λ_{12} = fraction of hepatic bromosulphthalein pool refluxing to plasma per minute; λ_{02} = fraction of hepatic bromosulphthalein pool transferred into bile per minute.

Variable	Normal mean ± S.D.	Units
k_e	0.12 ± 0.02	min^{-1}
C_{BSP}	4.5 ± 0.7	ml/min per kg
λ_{21}	0.14 ± 0.02	min^{-1}
λ_{12}	0.004 ± 0.002	min^{-1}
λ_{02}	0.029 ± 0.018	min^{-1}

and the 45 minute retention are usually quite abnormal (Schiff et al., 1959; Wolkoff et al., 1976).

10.4.1.4. Bromosulphthalein infusion test

If the dye is infused at a rapid rate for 60 minutes, the plasma concentration will rise, the rise being linear with time over the second half of the infusion (Figure 10.36A). If the infusion rate is appreciably reduced for an additional hour, a linear decline in plasma bromosulphthalein concentration is observed. If it is assumed that there is neither extravascular sequestration nor extrahepatic excretion of bromosulphthalein during the infusions, and that at the concentrations achieved during the study the saturable process of biliary excretion of the dye is proceeding at its maximal rate, then the infusion rate I (mg/min) must equal the excretion rate T_M (mg/min) plus the rate of change in the combined BSP content of plasma (Q_p) and liver (Q_1) –

$$I = T_M + \frac{dQ_p}{dt} + \frac{dQ_1}{dt} \qquad [5]$$

The plasma content of bromosulphthalein is equal to the plasma volume (PV) times the plasma concentration c. If it is further assumed that the liver content increases linearly as the plasma concentration increases, so that S mg of bromosulphthalein are stored in

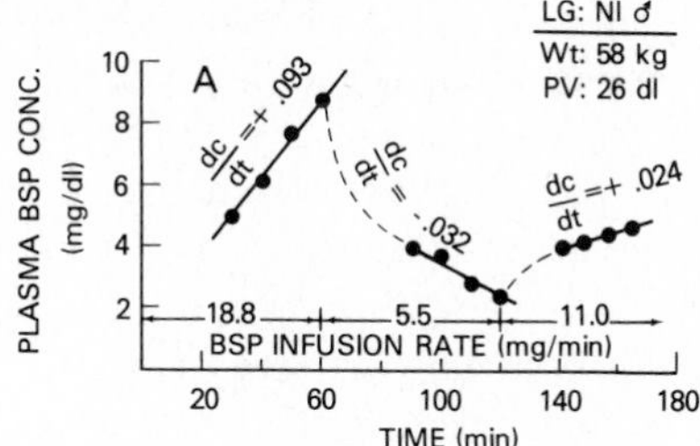

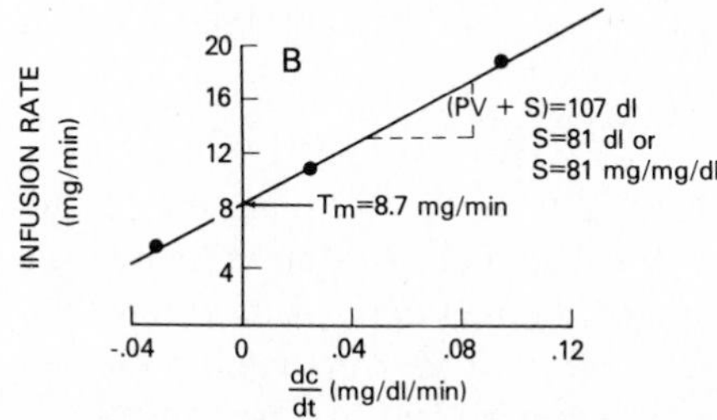

Figure 10.36. Estimation of bromosulphthalein (BSP), T_m and S in normal man. A: typical plasma BSP concentration–time curve during 3 different infusion rates in a normal subject (section 10.4.1.4). Note that the slope of the curve is approximately linear during the second half of each infusion. B: determination of T_m and S, by the method of least squares, from the three paired values for infusion rate and corresponding slope. (Redrawn, with permission, from Wheeler et al., 1960)

the liver for every mg/dl increase in plasma concentration, the above equation can be expressed as follows –

$$I = T_M + (PV + S)\frac{dc}{dt} \qquad [6]$$

In this equation S, the relative hepatic storage capacity for bromosulphthalein, represents the number of mg of dye retained in the liver for each mg/dl plasma bromosulphthalein concentration (mg per mg/dl), and dc/dt represents the slope of the linear portion of the plot of the plasma concentration with time at a given infusion rate. Note that the commonly employed units for S (mg per mg/dl) correspond to units of volume (dl). If PV is determined experimentally or estimated from tables, then equation [6] contains two unknowns, T_m and S. Hence, if two infusion rates (I_1, I_2) are utilized and two corresponding slopes $(dc/dt)_1$ and $(dc/dt)_2$, are determined, then T_M and S can be calculated by simultaneous equations. In fact, the most common protocol employs three infusion rates: 0.3 mg/min per kg for 1 hour, and 30 and 60% of the initial rate during the second and third hours, respectively (Figure 10.36A, B). Infusion rates are halved in patients who are expected to have appreciable hepatic dysfunction (Wheeler et al., 1960; Combes and Schenker, 1975; Jablonski and Owen, 1975).

In normal individuals, T_M averages 8.2 ± 1.5 (S.D.) mg/min, and S = 61 ± 14 mg bromosulphthalein stored per mg/dl of plasma concentration.

In general, T_M and S are both reduced in patients with diffuse hepatic disorders such as cirrhosis and viral hepatitis. The reduction of T_M persists during the healing phase of viral hepatitis long after S has returned to normal. A reduction in T_M may be the sole abnormality which is found in certain cholestatic states associated with the administration of particular steroid hormones or during the last trimester of pregnancy (Combes and Schenker, 1975; Jablonski and Owen, 1975).

Determination of T_M and S for bromosulphthalein has been a useful research tool for investigation of numerous altered physiologic states. The combination of normal values for S with a markedly reduced T_M (<2 mg/min) is virtually diagnostic of the Dubin–Johnson syndrome. Apart from the diagnosis of this condition, such studies are rarely indicated in the evaluation of individual patients. This is particularly true, since the infusion test may be associated with a higher complication rate than the single injection test.

10.4.1.5. Dibromosulphthalein test

Dibromosulphthalein (phenol-3,6-dibromosulphthalein disulfonate) was introduced as a compound for liver function testing in 1964 (Javitt, 1964), and has been in limited use since that time. Its hepatic transport is similar to that of bromosulphthalein with the important exception that it is *not* conjugated with glutathione, but is excreted in the bile unaltered. In normal subjects, its plasma disappearance rate is 21 to 25% per minute and S is 125 ± 56 (S.D.) mg per mg/dl, values that are greater than the corresponding values for bromosulphthalein. T_M is similar for both compounds. Both appear to be equally sensitive in detecting impaired liver cell function and cholestasis (Dhumeaux et al., 1974).

10.4.2. Indocyanine green disappearance

Indocyanine green, a water soluble tricarbocyanine dye, is rapidly removed from the circulation by the liver and excreted into the bile without conjugation (Wheeler et al., 1958; Cherrick et al., 1960; Caesar et al., 1961). As with bromosulphthalein, it is virtually completely protein-bound within the vascular space, albumin being the principal carrier (Cherrick et al., 1960; Baker, 1966). Currently, its major medical use is for indicator dilution studies during cardiac catheterization. However, its rapid excretion via the liver without significant extrahepatic removal or enterohepatic circulation (Wheeler et al., 1958; Cherrick et al., 1960; Hunton et al., 1960; Caesar et al., 1961), and its complete freedom from the problems of tissue necrosis or anaphylaxis, which may occur occasionally with bromosulphthalein (section 10.4.1.1), have prompted the increasing use of plasma indocyanine green disappearance curves as a test of liver function. The most commonly used protocol for this purpose involves determination of the plasma fractional disappearance rate (k_{ICG}) or half-life, or plasma retention at 20 minutes, following the rapid intravenous injection of dye at a dose of 0.5 mg/kg body mass. The plasma concentration is readily determined spectrophotometrically. Although no serious allergic reactions to the dye itself have been reported, the usual preparation contains small amounts of sodium iodide. Therefore, it should be used with caution in patients having a history of iodide sensitivity, and radioactive iodine uptake studies should not be performed for at least 7 days after administration.

10.4.2.1. Plasma indocyanine green disappearance curves and percentage retention

At the U.S. National Institutes of Health, plasma dye concentrations are usually determined during the first 30 minutes after injection of a 0.5 mg/kg body mass dose, and k_{ICG} (min^{-1}) is determined from specimens obtained between 5 and 12 minutes. During this period, the curve in normal subjects invariably corresponds to a single exponential function. Usually a slower second component to the plasma curve becomes apparent at some time after 12 minutes. In most instances, plasma concentrations are too low at this stage to permit reliable determination of this second exponential.

In normal subjects, the plasma indocyanine green disappearance rate is appreciably faster than that of bromosulphthalein. Furthermore, a significant difference has been found for k_{ICG} in normal men and in normal women (men: 0.205 ± 0.005 (S.E.) min^{-1}; women: 0.243 ± 0.006 min^{-1}; $P < 0.01$) (Martin et al., 1975).

Some authors use plasma dye retention at 20 minutes as a simple test of liver function, analogous to the conventional bromosulphthalein test. When employing a dose of 0.5 mg/kg, retention of less than 4% is considered within normal limits (Cherrick et al., 1960). This test is less sensitive than determination of the plasma indocyanine green disappearance rate. Others have estimated the volume of distribution (VD_{ICG}) by extrapolation of the disappearance curve to zero time, and calculated the clearance as: C_{ICG} (ml/min per kg) = $k_{ICG} \times VD_{ICG}$. The normal value for C_{ICG} is 8.9 ± 0.3 (S.E.) ml/min per kg following a dose of 0.5 mg/kg (Martin et al., 1975). Because the half-life of injected ICG is short relative to the intravascular mixing time, calculation of VD_{ICG}, and hence C_{ICG}, may be subject to errors resulting from non-uniform mixing. Accordingly, analysis of the plasma disappearance curve in terms of the fractional disappearance rate is more reliable than analysis in terms of clearance, although the latter may be intellectually more appealing.

Determination of k_{ICG} following a dose of 0.5 mg/kg has been reported to provide an accurate index of the functional status of the liver in patients with severe liver disease, and, in view of its safety, this test may be suitable for serial assessments in such patients. In general, the test is less sensitive than the corresponding bromosulphthalein test for detecting minimal hepatobiliary dysfunction. However, Leevy and co-workers report that determination of k_{ICG} following intravenous administration of 5.0 mg/kg is of equivalent sensitivity to bromosulphthalein testing (Leevy et al., 1967). The normal range of k_{ICG} at this dose is 0.179 ± 0.006 (S.E.) min^{-1} (Martin et al., 1975). To date, the U.S. Food and Drug Administration has not approved the administration of this dose except as an experimental procedure. Furthermore, the cost of indocyanine green is such that, at a dose of 5.0 mg/kg, dye for the test will cost approximately 50 times more than the corresponding amount of bromosulphthalein, making the former test prohibitively expensive as a routine investigation.

The hepatic uptake mechanism for indocyanine green can be saturated, and the rate of hepatic dye uptake with increasing dose has been shown to follow Michaelis–Menten kinetics (Paumgartner et al., 1970; Martin et al., 1976). A dose of up to 10.0 mg/kg is required to determine V_{MAX} and K_m adequately in normal subjects (Paumgartner et al., 1970) but there is relatively little experience in terms of safety with some of the higher doses employed. In patients with liver disease, V_{MAX} and K_m are frequently defined with doses no higher than 5.0 mg/kg. While useful as a research technique, for clinical purposes the requirement for multiple injections is cumbersome and provides little information which is not obtainable with a single 5 mg/kg disappearance curve employing either indocyanine green or, much more economically, bromosulphthalein.

10.4.2.2. Indocyanine green infusion test

T_M and S values for indocyanine green have been determined by means of continuous infusion studies analogous to those employed with bromosulphthalein (section 10.4.1.4). In normal subjects reported mean values vary widely, T_M from 0.95 to 7.9 mg/min, and S from 70 to 129 mg per mg/dl (Howard et al., 1965; Kanai, 1972). The reason for this variability is not clear, but may be related to the anticholeretic effect of indocyanine green in large doses. Since measurement of T_M is meaningless in the absence of adequate bile flow, use of the infusion test for determination of T_M and S is of dubious value.

10.4.2.3. Use of ear densitometry

An electronic dichromatic ear densitometer has been used to determine indocyanine green kinetics without the need for blood sampling. Although data obtained in this way were reported to agree with values obtained by direct blood sampling (Leevy, 1965; Leevy et al., 1967), such agreement has not been consistently obtained. Blood sampling for determination of plasma concentrations is therefore recommended.

10.4.3. Bile acid disappearance

As a result of methodologic advances which permit increasingly accurate measurements of bile acids in various body fluids, a great deal of work has been devoted to the diagnostic value of such measurements. Measurements of fasting and/or post-prandial concentrations of either individual or total serum bile acids have been found to be an extremely sensitive indication of hepatobiliary dysfunction (sections 10.2.3.2.1 and 10.2.3.2.2).

It has recently been suggested that determination of the plasma disappearance rate of an intravenously injected dose of either unlabelled cholylglycine or various radiolabelled bile acids may be an even more sensitive indicator of hepatic disease. Using a radioimmunoassay which is specific for conjugates of cholic acid, the plasma half-life in normal subjects of an intravenously injected dose of 5 μmol/kg unlabelled cholylglycine was found to be 2.6 ± 0.1 (S.E.) minutes, and the plasma concentration of cholic acid had returned to the normal fasting level (<1.0 μmol/litre) by 10 minutes (Korman et al., 1975). The fractional disappearance rate, 0.27 ± 0.01 min^{-1} (27% per minute), if due entirely to hepatic removal, would imply essentially 100% hepatic extraction in a single passage through the liver, since it is virtually identical to reported values for fractional hepatic blood flow (Martin et al., 1975). However, the mean calculated volume of distribution of 1200 ml/kg body mass is clearly implausible, suggesting both significant removal before uniform mixing within the plasma and, possibly, appreciable extraheptic removal. The initial disappearance rates of [^{14}C]cholic acid were even faster, with half-lives of 1.7 ± 0.1 minutes for both cholylglycine and cholyltaurine (Cowen et al., 1975). This corresponds to a mean fractional clearance rate of 0.41 min^{-1}, or almost 150% of fractional hepatic blood flow. Further work is needed to clarify the physiologic interpretation of these data.

The cholylglycine tolerance test, expressed as either a fractional disappearance rate or 10 minute retention, has been reported to be a more sensitive indicator of impaired hepatic function than the serum bilirubin concentration, aspartate aminotransferase or alkaline phosphatase activity, 60 minute bromosulphthalein retention or fasting plasma cholylglycine concentration (LaRusso et al., 1975). The 60 minute bromosulphthalein retention is probably the least sensitive of the various tests in use with this dye, and fasting bile acid concentrations are less sensitive indicators of hepatobiliary dysfunction than those measured 2 hours post-prandially. Hence, the real value of bile acid clearance studies as liver function tests in clinical medicine remains to be established. In addition, the development of the sensitive radioimmunoassays for various bile acids, which are essential if such tests are to be conducted without the need for injection of radiolabelled bile acids, has been subject to numerous technical problems not yet completely resolved.

10.4.4. Disappearance of unconjugated bilirubin

The application of radiolabelled unconjugated bilirubin to the study of the kinetics of unconjugated bilirubin in normal subjects (Berk et al., 1969) and in patients with disorders of bilirubin metabolism (Berk et al., 1974a, 1975) has proved to be a *most* valuable research tool in the investigation of the pathophysiology of bilirubin metabolism. The use of radiolabelled bilirubin has largely supplemented earlier tests which involved the injection of large quantities of non-radioactive bilirubin (Billing et al., 1964; With, 1968). Such studies provide useful information about the pathophysiology responsible for individual cases of unconjugated hyperbilirubinaemia, in particular permitting quantitation of both bilirubin production and hepatic bilirubin clearance (section 10.2.1.1.5). However, their value in diagnosis is limited. The plasma disappearance curve of radiolabelled unconjugated bilirubin is similar in Gilbert's syndrome and in cirrhosis (Barrett et al., 1968; Berk et al., 1970; Owens et al., 1977). For methodological reasons, this technique cannot be utilized in the evaluation of patients with conjugated hyperbilirubinaemia; it is too expensive and complicated for routine clinical application, but it remains a valuable research tool.

10.4.5. Galactose elimination capacity

D-Galactose is a common physiologic nutrient, derived principally from the hydrolysis of lactose (milk sugar) to glucose and galactose by the intestinal mucosal enzyme lactase. It is removed from the circulation principally by the liver. There is, in addition, a small but readily measurable rate of renal elimination but, apparently, only trivial uptake by other sites.

Net removal by the liver involves (a) stereospecific carrier-mediated entry of D-galactose into the liver cell, a process which involves a bidirectional flux of the free sugar; and (b) phosphorylation of D-galactose to galactose-1-phosphate by the intracellular enzyme galactokinase. Galactose-1-phosphate does not readily pass through cell membranes, and the effect of phosphorylation is 2-fold: it prevents return of the hexose moiety to the circulation, and also prevents the accumulation of any significant intracellular pool of free galactose (Goresky et al., 1973). The further metabolism of galactose-1-phosphate involves its conversion into UDP-galactose, and thence to UDP-glucose by the enzymes galactose-1-phosphate uridylyl transferase and epimerase, respectively. Although the former enzyme is deficient in subjects with galactosaemia (Isselbacher et al., 1956) in virtually all other circumstances the conversion of galactose to galactose-1-phosphate is the rate-limiting step in galactose metabolism (Keiding, 1973). In the dog, for example, the capacity of the transport system which is responsible for initial liver cell uptake is 40 times that for phosphorylation, and the K_m values for these two processes are <15 mg/dl, and ~ 500 mg/dl, respectively (Goresky et al., 1973).

When the plasma galactose concentration is low (<30 mg/dl), hepatic extraction of galactose averages 88% in normal man. Measurements of galactose removal have been used as the basis for estimates of hepatic blood flow during both constant infusion and single injection studies (Tygstrup and Winkler, 1954, 1958). In contrast, when the plasma galactose concentration is high (>40 mg/dl), a constant hepatic artery/hepatic vein concentration difference occurs which is indicative of a constant maximal rate of hepatic galactose sequestration (Tygstryp and Winkler, 1954; Waldstein et al., 1960).

During the past four decades, a variety of studies of galactose metabolism, involving oral administration, single injection or continuous infusion techniques, have been proposed as tests of hepatic function. Although little used in the United States or United Kingdom, such procedures are employed in Western Europe, particularly in Scandinavia.

The procedure currently in widest use is the single injection test described by Tygstrup (1961, 1963). After the intravenous injection of 0.5 grams of galactose per kg body mass over approximately 5 minutes, plasma galactose concentrations are determined at 5 minute intervals from 20 to 60 minutes after the start of the injection. The quantity of galactose excreted in the urine over this time period is also determined. A typical plasma galactose curve in a normal subject is illustrated in Figure 10.37. It consists of 3 distinct segments: the first segment (Figure 10.37, t_0–t_1) consists of a rapid rise in galactose concentration which reaches a maximum of 200 to 300 mg/dl just after conclusion of the injection; this is followed by a rapid decrease over the subsequent 10 to 15 minutes due to a combination of extravascular distribution, hepatic uptake and renal excretion, but this portion of the curve has not been found useful for further analysis; after this initial period, the plasma galactose content declines in a more regular fashion for an average of approximately 20 minutes (Figure 10.37, t_1–t_2), until the plasma galactose concentration falls below 30 to 50 mg/dl; at this point the third portion, characterized by a flattening out of the disappearance curve, supervenes. Hepatic vein catheterization studies indicate that the second portion of the curve corresponds to a period during which hepatic extraction of galactose is incomplete, but is characterized by a constant hepatic arteriovenous gradient. In contrast, the onset of the third portion (Figure 10.37, t_2) corresponds to the initial disappearance of galactose from hepatic venous blood, indicating almost complete hepatic extraction (Tystrup and Winkler, 1954).

The second portion of the curve (t_1–t_2) has usually been analyzed in terms of an exponential disappearance which gives a $T_{1/2}$ of 12.0 ± 2.6 (S.D.) min^{-1} in normal subjects (Tengstrom, 1968). However, Tygstrup and Winkler (1954) have shown that a statistically superior fit to this portion of the curve can be obtained with a simple linear function, implying a constant rate of hepatic galactose removal independent of plasma concentration during this time period. This is also more consistent with the hepatic vein catheterization studies which indicate saturation of hepatic uptake during this interval (Tygstrup and Winkler, 1954). Starting 20 minutes after injection, they fit those concentrations >40 mg/dl (>2.5 μmol/litre) to a straight line, which is then extrapolated to the time at

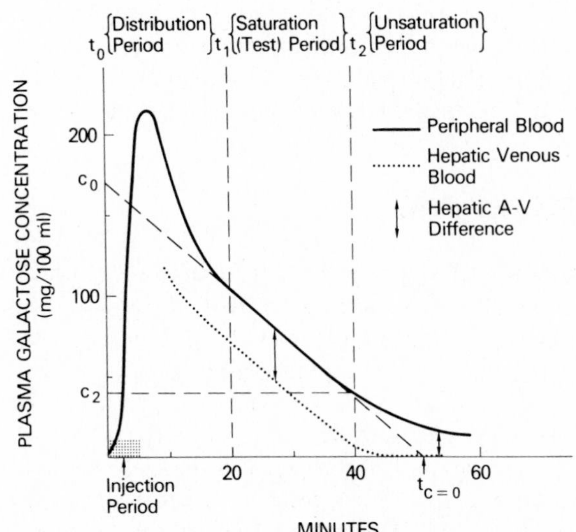

Figure 10.37. Schematic representation of plasma galactose concentration–time curve following the intravenous injection of a single dose of 0.5 g/kg body mass. See text (section 10.4.5) for details.

which the blood galactose concentration is zero (Figure 10.37, $t_c = 0$). The galactose elimination capacity (GEC) is defined as follows:

$$GEC = \frac{I - U}{t_c = 0 + 7}, \qquad [7]$$

where I is the dose of galactose injected, U is the amount excreted in the urine during the 60 minutes of the test, and 7 is a correction factor to account for the fact that the mean galactose concentration–time curve throughout the total volume of distribution lags approximately 7 minutes behind the curve measured in peripheral blood. The GEC corresponds to the maximal rate of hepatic galactose extraction, and has a range in normal individuals of 270 ± 40 (S.D.) mg/min per m^2 of body surface or 6.7 ± 1.0 mg/min per kg body mass (Tygstrup, 1964a).

The GEC represents a measure of the metabolic capacity of the liver, and is relatively little influenced by biliary secretory capacity. As such, it is reduced either when the number of metabolically active liver cells is diminished or, presumably, if the metabolic activity (e.g. ATP content) of individual cells is decreased. GEC correlates well with other measures of metabolic activity such as serum albumin concentration (section 10.2.5.4.1), prothrombin time (section 10.2.5.4.5), and antipyrine clearance (section 10.4.6) in patients with chronic liver disease (Tygstrup, 1964a; Andreasen et al., 1974). The correlation between GEC and bromosulphthalein retention in an unselected population of patients with hepatobiliary dysfunction is only fair. This is probably due, in large measure, to the fact that the latter is highly dependent not only on hepatic metabolic activity but also on biliary secretory function (Tygstrup, 1964b; den Blaauwen and Thijs, 1973; Nilsson and Hultman, 1974).

GEC appears to be more sensitive than any of the routine static tests in the detection of hepatic dysfunction, but is somewhat less sensitive than the routine bromosulphthalein test. Its principal advantages over the latter are the complete absence of complications or reactions resulting from administration of galactose and its greater specificity as an index of hepatocellular dysfunction. Hence it is particularly appropriate for sequential evaluation of patients with chronic disease.

10.4.6. Tests depending on hepatic drug metabolism

A major function of the liver is the biotransformation of drugs to metabolites which, depending on their structure and physicochemical properties, are subsequently excreted either by the liver into bile, or via the kidneys. Increased intensity or duration of the effects of certain drugs in patients with liver disease has long been recognized clinically (Sherlock, 1975), and is now known to be associated in part with the impairment of various hepatic drug-metabolizing pathways. The activities of such pathways may be assessed in various ways, including determination of the plasma half-life of an administered drug (Kunin et al., 1959; Andreasen et al., 1974), the rate of excretion of its metabolites in the urine (Barniville and Misk, 1959; Kunin et al., 1959) or the determination of the activities of certain drug-metabolizing enzymes in needle biopsy specimens of hepatic tissue (Remmer et al., 1973). For practical and methodological reasons, none of these approaches has proved to be generally useful as a clinical test of hepatic function.

It is becoming increasingly apparent that certain specific drug-metabolizing pathways are more sensitive to hepatocellular injury than others. Thus, *N*-demethylation tends to be reduced in minimal hepatic injury while glucuronidation appears to be preserved until extensive damage has supervened. This explains why the metabolism of diazepam may be markedly slowed in patients with liver disease (Klotz et al., 1975), while that of the related sedative, oxazepam, is not (Shull et al., 1976). Diazepam is converted by *N*-demethylation and hydroxylation into oxazepam, while oxazepam's principal metabolism is via glucuronidation.

Based on an original suggestion by Lauterberg and Bircher (1973), several groups have now established that the rate of *N*-demethylation can be assessed in vivo from the rate of excretion of $^{14}CO_2$ in the breath following the administration of [^{14}C]dimethylamino-antipyrine ([^{14}C]aminopyrine) (Hepner and Vesell, 1974; Preisig et al., 1976). The test is, in principle, equally applicable to studying the metabolism of any other drug whose principal metabolic pathway involves *N*-demethylation, and preliminary results with a diazepam breath test have been reported (Hepner and Vesell, 1976).

For the [^{14}C]aminopyrine breath test, 1.5 μCi [^{14}C]aminopyrine, containing only a minute tracer quantity of drug, is administered by mouth to a non-ambulant patient. Two hours later, breath samples are passed directly into scintillation vials containing an absorbant with indicator until the entrapment of precisely 2 μmol of CO_2 is denoted by the appropriate colour change. From the specific activity of the collected $^{14}CO_2$ and an assumed CO_2 excretion rate of 9 μmol/kg per hour, the total $^{14}CO_2$ output over 2 hours can be determined and expressed as a proportion of the dose. The 2 hour test appears to be just as sensitive as the original 12 hour test (Hepner and Vesell, 1974, 1975).

Normal individuals excrete 7.0 ± 1.3% of administered ^{14}C in 2 hours following oral administration of [^{14}C]aminopyrine (Hepner and Vesell, 1975). Markedly reduced values are seen in patients with hepatocellular disease (cirrhosis, hepatitis) and in many patients with hepatic neoplasia. Values tend to be either normal or only minimally reduced in patients with lesions causing predominantly cholestasis. Results of the 2 hour breath $^{14}CO_2$ output correlate well with those of the aminopyrine metabolic clearance rate in patients with cirrhosis, results of this test also correlate well with both serum albumin concentration and 45 minute bromosulphthalein retention. The breath test was abnormal in several cirrhotic patients without abnormalities of routine serum biochemical tests (including bromosulphthalein retention), and has been reported to be of equal sensitivity to measurement of serum bile acids in detecting hepatocellular dysfunction (Hepner and Demers, 1976).

While experience with this test is still very limited, its sound rationale and methodologic simplicity suggest that it has a useful role as a screening procedure, provided that future studies confirm the preliminary enthusiastic reports.

10.5. LABORATORY TESTS IN SELECTED CLINICAL SITUATIONS

10.5.1. Hyperbilirubinaemia and jaundice

The immediate problem posed by a patient manifesting either subclinical hyperbilirubinaemia or frank jaundice is whether or not the condition is associated with a structural lesion of the hepatobiliary system. The following routine tests should be carried out: (a) a direct reacting and total bilirubin concentration; (b) serum aspartate and alanine aminotransferases; (c) alkaline phosphatase; and (d) plasma protein electrophoresis. If, of these tests, an elevated serum bilirubin concentration is the only abnormality, the presence of "structural" hepatobiliary disease can be excluded with a very high degree of probability. It is then probable that the cause of the hyperbilirubinaemia is a specific metabolic defect in one of the steps in the hepatic transport of bilirubin from blood to bile and/or is outside the hepatobiliary system and is related to bilirubin overproduction (Schmid, 1972; Berk et al., 1974a). The latter situation gives rise to a predominantly unconjugated hyperbilirubinaemia, while the former may produce either unconjugated or conjugated hyperbilirubinaemia, depending on the nature of the metabolic defect. A classification of these "pure bilirubinopathies" without abnormalities of other routine serum biochemical tests is presented in Table 10.5. Included in this group are several inherited causes of hyperbilirubinaemia of which Gilbert's syndrome is extremely common, although frequently unrecognized. With the exception of the Crigler–Najjar syndrome (section 10.5.1.1.2), which is usually associated with early death due to kernicterus, the remaining inherited hyperbilirubinaemias appear to be without influence on

TABLE 10.5.

HEREDITARY CAUSES OF "PURE" HYPERBILIRUBINAEMIA

(I) Unconjugated hyperbilirubinaemia due to increased bilirubin production
- (A) Hereditary haemolytic anaemias
  - (1) Erythrocyte membrane disorders
    - (a) hereditary spherocytosis
    - (b) hereditary elliptocytosis
    - (c) hereditary stomatocytosis
  - (2) Disorders of erythrocyte metabolism
    - (a) deficiencies of glycolytic enzymes
    - (b) deficiencies of other glucose-metabolizing enzymes
    - (c) deficiencies of oxidation–reduction systems
  - (3) Haemoglobin abnormalities
    - (a) disorders of synthesis (thalassaemias)
    - (b) structural variants
- (B) Shunt hyperbilirubinaemia

(II) Unconjugated hyperbilirubinaemia due to decreased hepatic bilirubin clearance
- (A) Clearly related to glucuronyltransferase deficiency
  - (1) Congenital non-haemolytic jaundice: type I (Crigler–Najjar syndrome)
  - (2) Congenital non-haemolytic jaundice: type II
- (B) Mechanism uncertain
  - (1) Gilbert's syndrome

(III) Conjugated hyperbilirubinaemias
- (A) Dubin–Johnson syndrome
- (B) Rotor's syndrome
- (C) Hepatic storage disease

longevity. Accurate diagnosis in these conditions is nevertheless highly important in order that the patient can be reassured as to the benign nature of his condition, so as to avoid unwarranted medical or surgical intervention and unfair penalties with regard to employment opportunities or eligibility for life insurance. The detailed characterization of the defects in these conditions have led to major advances in knowledge of the physiology and pathophysiology of bilirubin metabolism.

Jaundice due to structural lesions of the hepatobiliary system is associated with abnormalities of other routine serum biochemical tests. There may be a predominantly unconjugated hyperbilirubinaemia (Levine and Klatskin, 1964), but conjugated or mixed hyperbilirubinaemia is more usual.

10.5.1.1. Hyperbilirubinaemia as the sole serum biochemical abnormality

10.5.1.1.1. Unconjugated hyperbilirubinaemia due to increased bilirubin production. Increased bilirubin production resulting from either haemolysis or excessive ineffective erythropoiesis is a common cause of mild to moderate unconjugated hyperbilirubinaemia. A broad classification of haemolytic anaemias may be found in any standard textbook of haematology. The causes of increased ineffective erythropoiesis (Table 10.6) are, with the exception of shunt hyperbilirubinaemia, readily recognized disorders of haem or haemoglobin biosynthesis.

Shunt hyperbilirubinaemia is a rare, usually familial, disorder characterized by a haemolytic anaemia which is mild in relation to the associated extreme erythroid hyperplasia of the bone marrow (Israels et al., 1959). Faecal urobilinogen excretion is markedly increased and isotopic "early labelled peak" studies (section 10.2.1.1.1) have suggested that at least 75% of bile pigment production is derived from ineffective erythropoiesis in the bone marrow (Israels and Zipursky, 1962). Splenectomy is associated with prolongation of the red cell life span but normoblastic hyperplasia and high faecal urobilinogen excretion persist. In some patients, the serum bilirubin has been in the range of 70 to 140 μmol/litre (4 to 8 mg/dl) implying an associated defect in hepatic bilirubin handling (section 10.2.1.2) (Israels et al., 1959), but in others the serum bilirubin has been in the range of 35 to 43 μmol/litre (2.0 to 2.5 mg/dl), which is consistent with normal hepatic function (Verwilghen et al., 1969).

10.5.1.1.2. Unconjugated hyperbilirubinaemia due to decreased hepatic bilirubin clearance. (i) *Congenital non-haemolytic jaundice (types I and II).* In 1952 Crigler and Najjar described six related infants in whom severe jaundice appeared within the first 3 days

TABLE 10.6.

RECOGNIZED CAUSES OF INCREASED INEFFECTIVE ERYTHROPOIESIS

Pernicious anaemia and (presumably) other megaloblastic anaemias
Erythropoietic porphyria and protoporphyria
"Shunt" hyperbilirubinaemia syndromes
Thalassaemia syndromes
Refractory (sideroblastic) anaemias
Lead poisoning

after birth, and persisted throughout life (Crigler and Najjar, 1952). This recessive inborn error of bilirubin metabolism, now designated type I congenital non-haemolytic jaundice, is characterized by the perinatal onset of severe unconjugated hyperbilirubinaemia, usually in excess of 340 μmol/litre (20 mg/dl) (Table 10.7). Bilirubin production is normal. The hyperbilirubinaemia has been shown to result from a virtually complete inability to conjugate bilirubin (Axelrod et al., 1957; Arias et al., 1969). Bilirubin clearance is consequently reduced to approximately 1% of normal (Bloomer et al., 1971b; Blaschke et al., 1974b). As a result of the severe hyperbilirubinaemia, kernicteric brain damage is almost inevitable, and the majority of these patients die in infancy or early childhood with severe neurologic disease. Failure of the plasma bilirubin concentration in these patients to decrease in response to phenobarbitone therapy (Table 10.7) is a useful diagnostic feature (Arias et al., 1969).

In contrast to the patients described above, those with a phenotypically similar syndrome, now classified as type II congenital non-haemolytic jaundice, characteristically have a somewhat lower bilirubin concentration which usually does not exceed 340 μmol/litre (20 mg/dl). Although hepatic bilirubin-UDP-glucuronyltransferase cannot be detected by assay, it is presumably present in small amounts since glucuronides of bilirubin are demonstrable in the bile (Arias et al., 1969). Perhaps because of the lower bilirubin concentrations – most often 100 to 340 μmol/litre (6 to 20 mg/dl) – kernicterus in this syndrome is uncommon and survival appears to be normal (Arias et al., 1969;

TABLE 10.7.

PRINCIPAL DIFFERENTIAL CHARACTERISTICS OF TYPE I AND TYPE II CONGENITAL NON-HAEMOLYTIC JAUNDICE

Feature or value	Type I (Crigler–Najjar)	Type II
Onset of jaundice	Birth	Usually at birth; occasionally not until adulthood
Serum bilirubin concentration	18–50 mg/100 ml, usually >20 mg/100 ml	6–22 mg/100 ml, usually <20 mg/100 ml
Bilirubin UDP-glucuronyl-transferase	Absent	Not detectable
Bile	Frequently colourless, contains no bilirubin glucuronide. May contain non-glucuronide conjugates	Deeply pigmented. Contains bilirubin glucuronide
Kernicterus	Almost inevitable	Uncommon
Survival	Usually die in infancy or early childhood with severe neurologic defects	Probably normal. No intellectual impairment
Inheritance	Autosomal recessive	Autosomal dominant (?)
Response to phenobarbitone	None	Lowers plasma bilirubin concentration

Gollan et al., 1975). Thus, in contrast to type I congenital non-haemolytic jaundice, patients with the type II syndrome are likely to be encountered in adult practice. These patients respond to phenobarbitone with a striking reduction in the plasma bilirubin concentration, as do patients with Gilbert's syndrome (Arias et al., 1969).

(ii) *Constitutional hepatic dysfunction (Gilbert's syndrome).* The term Gilbert's syndrome has traditionally been applied to patients with mild chronic unconjugated hyperbilirubinaemia which is associated with normal values for other routine serum biochemical tests and essentially normal hepatic histology, overt haemolysis having been excluded as a cause of the hyperbilirubinaemia (Schmid, 1972; Berk et al., 1974a, 1975). While once considered a rarity, increasing use of serum bilirubin measurements as a screening test has led to the recognition that Gilbert's syndrome is, in fact, quite common. The prevalence is approximately 5% in healthy college students admitted to the U.S. National Institutes of Health to serve as normal volunteers. Although most often detected among adolescents and young adults, cases in somewhat older age groups are being recognized.

In one large series (Foulk et al., 1959), more than 80% of cases had a total bilirubin concentration of less than 50 μmol/litre (3 mg/dl) when initially evaluated; a mean unconjugated bilirubin concentration of 27 μmol/litre (1.6 mg/dl) was found in the U.S. National Institutes of Health series (Berk et al., 1975). Values fluctuate with time, and at least one patient in four will have some normal values during prolonged follow-up (Foulk et al., 1959). Other routine serum biochemical tests are normal in the absence of coincidental disease. The gall bladder is usually visualized on oral cholecystography despite the elevated bilirubin concentration.

Patients with classical Gilbert's syndrome have a decrease in hepatic bilirubin clearance to about one-third of normal (Berk et al., 1970). Both a partial deficiency of hepatic bilirubin-UDP-glucuronyltransferase (Arias and London, 1957; Black and Billing, 1969) and defective hepatic bilirubin uptake (Schmid and Hammaker, 1959; Berk et al., 1970) have been proposed as the underlying mechanism for the reduced bilirubin clearance. In addition, a subgroup has been identified in which hepatic aspects of bilirubin metabolism are identical to those of classical Gilbert's syndrome, but the degree of hyperbilirubinaemia is much greater than usual as a result of the concurrent presence of haemolysis, and hence increased bilirubin production (Berk et al., 1970; 1972).

Therapy with phenobarbitone or glutethimide has been shown to normalize the plasma bilirubin concentration and increase hepatic bilirubin clearance (Black and Sherlock, 1970; Black et al., 1974; Blaschke et al., 1974a). This effect is not specific or of diagnostic value.

Although bromosulphthalein tests are usually described as giving normal results in Gilbert's syndrome, mild retention at 45 minutes of up to 20% has been observed in 20% of cases at the U.S. National Institutes of Health. Detailed studies of bromosulphthalein and indocyanine green kinetics have documented a constitutional defect in hepatic organic anion uptake in this particular subpopulation (Berk et al., 1972; Martin et al., 1976). Hence, an abnormal bromosulphthalein test does not necessarily indicate the presence of structural liver disease in the presence of unconjugated hyperbilirubinaemia.

Although chronic unconjugated hyperbilirubinaemia has been postulated as a sequel to viral hepatitis, the prevalence of antiHB_s among sporadic cases of Gilbert's syndrome seen at the U.S. National Institutes of Health has been less than that in a control population. Many instances of "post-hepatitic hyperbilirubinaemia" undoubtedly represent previously unrecognized cases of Gilbert's syndrome.

In the evaluation of patients with chronic unconjugated hyperbilirubinaemia, in whom serum enzyme tests are normal, values for red cell volume and half-life (determined using ^{51}Cr-labelled red cells) are extremely useful both for ruling out haemolysis, and for the indirect estimation of hepatic bilirubin clearance (Berk et al., 1974c) as shown in Figure 10.38. Liver biopsy, while helpful, is not essential for diagnosis if all other routine serum biochemical tests, including 45 minute bromosulphthalein retention are normal. In cases with abnormal retention of the dye, percutaneous liver biopsy is required to rule out structural liver disease. At the U.S. National Institutes of Health, the "fasting test" (Felsher et al., 1970) has been of little value in confirming the diagnosis of this condition. Equivalent proportional increases in bilirubin concentration in response to a 48-hour fast have been observed both in normal subjects and in subjects with Gilbert's syndrome (Bloomer et al., 1971c). The observation that fasting does not augment unconjugated

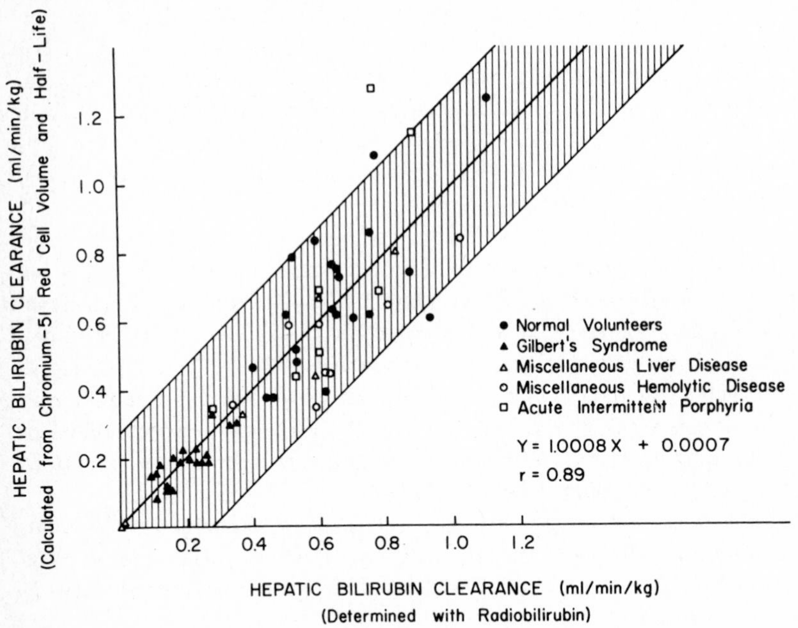

Figure 10.38. Comparison of estimated hepatic bilirubin clearance, on the ordinate, with values determined directly from the plasma disappearance curves of unconjugated bilirubin, on the abscissa, in 61 patients and normal volunteers. The estimated value for bilirubin clearance, C^*_{BR}, was calculated from the theoretical relationship:

$$C^*_{BR} = 2.9575 \times \frac{TRCV \times MCHC}{\overline{BR} \times (3.8 \times T_{1/2} - 11.8)}$$

TRCV and $T_{1/2}$ are the total red cell volume and half-life, measured with ^{51}Cr, $\overline{BR}$ is the plasma unconjugated bilirubin concentration, and MCHC, the mean corpuscular haemoglobin concentration (g/ml). (Reproduced, with permission, from Berk et al., 1974c) hyperbilirubinaemia associated with structural liver disease could be diagnostically useful but requires further confirmation (Owens and Sherlock, 1973). Administration of nicotinic acid also augments the hyperbilirubinaemia of Gilbert's syndrome (Fromke and Miller, 1972), but the diagnostic specificity of this test also requires validation.

10.5.1.1.3. Conjugated hyperbilirubinaemia. (i) *The Dubin–Johnson syndrome* is a rare, benign disorder characterized by chronic non-haemolytic predominantly conjugated hyperbilirubinaemia with bilirubinuria, and macroscopically visible black pigmentation of the liver (Sprinz and Nelson, 1954; Dubin, 1958). Its recognition is important in that it has been confused with more serious disorders such as chronic hepatitis or cholestasis. The hyperbilirubinaemia results from a specific defect of the biliary transport system for conjugated bilirubin (Gutstein et al., 1968; Alpert et al., 1969; Shani et al., 1970a) and, hence, other routine serum biochemical tests and serum bile acid concentrations are normal (Javitt, 1975). The degree of icterus may be increased by intercurrent illness, pregnancy, or drugs such as oral contraceptives which decrease the hepatic excretion of organic anions. Often the disorder is not noted until a woman becomes pregnant or is started on an oral contraceptive drug, when subclinical hyperbilirubinaemia may be exacerbated (Cohen et al., 1972).

Serum bilirubin is usually in the range of 34 to 85 μmol/litre (2 to 5 mg/dl) but may occasionally be as high as 340 μmol/litre (20 mg/dl). Approximately 50% or more is in the direct fraction, and bilirubinuria may be found. The degree of jaundice may fluctuate, and in any given individual with the Dubin–Johnson syndrome, occasional bilirubin determinations may be in the normal range. Oral cholecystography usually does not visualize the gall bladder. Plasma bromosulphthalein concentration 45 minutes after intravenous administration of a 5 mg/kg dose may be normal or may show mild retention (Berk et al., 1975). Of diagnostic significance, however, is the fact that in approximately 90% of patients, plasma bromosulphthalein concentration is higher 90 minutes after its intravenous administration than at 45 minutes (Mandema et al., 1960; Schoenfield et al., 1963; Shani et al., 1970a). This has been attributed to reflux of conjugated dye from the liver cell into the circulation (section 10.4.1.3). In the Dubin–Johnson syndrome, the maximal hepatic secretory rate of bromosulphthalein (T_M (=T_{MAX})) is markedly reduced (0.9 ± 0.4 mg/min compared with 8.3 ± 0.9 mg/min in healthy individuals) while relative hepatic storage capacity (S) is normal (82 ± 16 mg per mg/dl) (Cohen et al., 1972). This constellation of findings is virtually diagnostic of the condition.

Recent work has shown that there is a diagnostic abnormality of urinary coproporphyrin excretion in the Dubin–Johnson syndrome (Ben-Ezzer et al., 1971; Wolkoff et al., 1973). Two isomers of coproporphyrin, coproporphyrins I and III, are normally found in urine, with a mean of 75% of urinary coproporphyrin normally in the isomer III form. In the Dubin–Johnson syndrome urinary total coproporphyrin excretion is normal, but over 80% is coproporphyrin I (Figure 10.39). An intermediate abnormality is seen in heterozygotes for this disorder, in whom urinary total coproporphyrin is decreased by about 40%, and the proportion of coproporphyrin I averages 32%. The reason for the alteration in urinary coproporphyrin excretion in these individuals is unclear.

A suspected diagnosis of Dubin–Johnson syndrome can be confirmed by a bromosulphthalein infusion test or a 90-minute plasma disappearance curve, or by urinary coproporphyrin isomer analysis (Table 10.8).

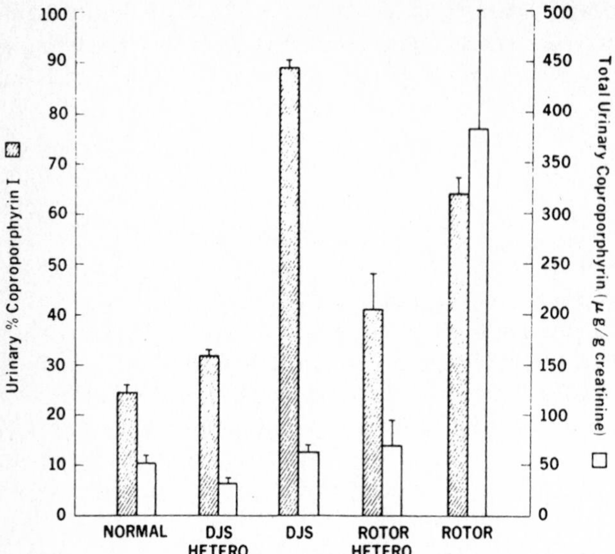

Figure 10.39. Urinary coproporphyrin excretion in Dubin–Johnson and Rotor's syndromes. The shaded bars represent the percentage of total urinary coproporphyrin excreted as coproporphyrin I. The open bars represent total urinary coproporphyrin excretion. Vertical bars represent S.E.M. Total urinary coproporphyrin excretion is normal in the Dubin–Johnson syndrome (DJS) but the coproporphyrin I is markedly elevated (>80%). Both variables are elevated in Rotor's syndrome. Thus the two disorders are distinct with respect to urinary coproporphyrin excretion. Results in obligate heterozygotes for each of these disorders (DJS Hetero, Rotor Hetero) lie intermediate between results in normal individuals and in individuals manifesting the respective disorder. (Reproduced, with permission, from Berk et al., 1975)

(ii) *Rotor's syndrome.* Rotor's syndrome is a rare benign disorder which is characterized by chronic non-haemolytic predominantly conjugated hyperbilirubinaemia without excess hepatic pigmentation (Rotor et al., 1948). It is seen much less frequently than the Dubin–Johnson syndrome. As in the Dubin–Johnson syndrome, other routine serum biochemical tests are normal. The concentration of serum bilirubin may fluctuate in a given individual and bilirubinuria may be present. Fifty per cent or more of the serum bilirubin is direct reacting. The degree of icterus may be increased by intercurrent infection. Oral cholecystography usually visualizes the gall bladder in Rotor's syndrome – in contrast to Dubin–Johnson syndrome – and there is markedly abnormal retention of bromosulphthalein in plasma 45 minutes after the intravenous administration of a 5 mg/kg dose, retention at this time usually being between 30 and 50%. A secondary rise in plasma bromosulphthalein concentration at 90 minutes has not been described in Rotor's syndrome (Schiff et al., 1959; Okolicsanyi et al., 1969).

Analysis of urinary coproporphyrin excretion in subjects with Rotor's syndrome reveals an approximately 5-fold increase in total urinary coproporphyrin, of which an average of 64% is coproporhyrin I (Fig. 10.39). This pattern is distinctly different from that seen in the Dubin–Johnson syndrome, and the two disorders can be differentiated

TABLE 10.8.

PRINCIPAL DIFFERENTIAL CHARACTERISTICS OF DUBIN–JOHNSON AND ROTOR'S SYNDROMES

	Dubin–Johnson Syndrome	Rotor's Syndrome
Appearance of liver	Grossly black	Normal
Histology of liver	Dark pigmentation, predominantly in centrilobular areas; otherwise, normal	Normal. No increase in pigmentation
Serum bilirubin	Elevated – usually from 34 to 85 μmol/litre (2 to 5 mg/dl), occasionally as high as 340 μmol/litre (20 mg/dl); predominantly direct-reacting	Elevated – usually from 2 to 5 mg/dl; occasionally as high as 20 mg/dl: predominantly direct-reacting
Routine liver tests	Normal except for bilirubin	Normal except for bilirubin
45-Minute plasma bromosulphthalein retention	Normal or elevated – secondary rise by 90 minutes	Elevated – no secondary rise by 90 minutes
Oral cholecystogram	Usually does not visualize the gall bladder	Usually visualizes the gall bladder
Urinary coproporphyrin	Normal total: >80% as coproporphyrin I	Elevated total. Elevated proportion of coproporphyrin I but <80%
Mode of inheritance	Autosomal recessive	Autosomal recessive

on this basis (Wolkoff et al., 1976). Heterozygotes for Rotor's syndrome have an abnormality in urinary coproporphyrin excretion which is intermediate between that in normal individuals and subjects with the syndrome, i.e. a normal total urinary coproporphyrin excretion of which a mean of 41% is coproporphyrin I.

Thus, while Rotor's syndrome is clinically similar to the Dubin–Johnson syndrome, these two syndromes can be differentiated by tests of bromosulphthalein metabolism and urinary coproporphyrins (Table 10.8).

(iii) *Hepatic storage disease.* Recently, a third disorder manifested by conjugated hyperbilirubinaemia has been described in several individuals and has been termed "hepatic storage disease". Bromosulphthalein excretion rate (T_M) is normal or mildly decreased, while the hepatic storage capacity (S) is very low (Hadchouel et al., 1971). The differentiation of this disorder from Rotor's syndrome is not clear at this time (Dhumeaux and Berthelot, 1975).

10.5.1.2. Hyperbilirubinaemia associated with abnormalities of other serum biochemical tests

When unconjugated and/or conjugated hyperbilirubinaemia is associated with abnormalities of any of the other routine serum biochemical tests, a structural lesion of the hepatobiliary system is suggested. It has been traditional to attempt to classify such lesions into those which are "hepatocellular" and those which are "cholestatic". In practice most diseases which cause primary hepatocellular damage are associated with an element of cholestasis, and most lesions which affect primarily the intra- or extra-hepatic bile ducts are associated with an element of hepatocellular damage in addition to cholestasis. Thus, the results of laboratory tests in most hepatobiliary lesions are consistent with an hepatocellular lesion and/or an obstructive lesion of the biliary tract. Often, results of laboratory tests exhibit a particularly non-specific pattern in that the activities of both the serum aminotransferases and alkaline phosphatase are moderately elevated and the plasma protein electrophoresis pattern is equivocal. This pattern is of very limited diagnostic value since its causes include inter alia, viral hepatitis, cirrhosis, large duct biliary obstruction, drug-induced hepatic injury, primary biliary cirrhosis, the Budd–Chiari syndrome, veno-occlusive disease, Weil's disease, hepatic granulomata, congestive cardiac failure, porphyria cutanea tarda and Gaucher's disease. More helpful diagnostically are those patterns of results which suggest a predominantly hepatocellular lesion and those which suggest a lesion causing predominantly cholestasis (Table 10.9); such patterns alert the physician to the problems posed by the acute hepatitic syndrome and its sequelae, and those posed by cholestasis, respectively. When results of the routine tests, including HB_sAg, suggest a predominantly hepatocellular lesion, then, depending on all the clinical information available, management of the patient may not require any more elaborate investigations (McIntyre and Heathcote, 1974). However, when results of the routine tests show a non-specific pattern, or suggest a lesion that causes predominantly cholestasis, then, if the abnormalities persist, management of the patient usually requires additional investigations such as liver biopsy and/or cholangiography to make a definitive diagnosis. Different drugs can cause different patterns of abnormalities in routine serum biochemical tests, either non-specific or suggestive of a predominantly hepatocellular or predominantly cholestatic lesion; these have been comprehensively reviewed (Zimmerman, 1974).

10.5.1.2.1. Acute hepatitic syndrome and fulminant liver failure. The acute hepatitic syndrome is the term applied to the condition which is associated with evidence of acute severe liver cell necrosis and/or acute hepatic insufficiency, usually in a subject without previous evidence of liver disease. Serial laboratory tests, including at least serum bilirubin, aspartate or alanine aminotransferase and prothrombin time in uncomplicated cases, are desirable in following the course of this potentially fatal syndrome (Figures 10.14–10.16, 10.24 and 10.40). Causes of the syndrome can be divided into two main types. In type I acute hepatitic syndrome, there is acute necrosis of liver cells, and the most useful laboratory finding is very high serum aspartate aminotransferase activity (Figure 10.16) which is almost invariably present early in the clinical course. It should be emphasized that the activity of this enzyme may rapidly fall to values that are diagnostically far less helpful, and that this may occur in association with the development of hepatic encephalopathy. Causes of this syndrome include infection with hepatitis virus A, B or "non-A, non-B" (section 10.3.2.1); ingestion of potentially hepatotoxic drugs such as paracetamol (acetaminophen), monoamine oxidase inhibitors, methyldopa, oxyphenisatin, isoniazid or aspirin; exposure to halothane; carbon tetrachloride poisoning; ingestion of poisonous mushrooms (*Amanita phalloides*); occlusion of the hepatic artery; and radiation injury to the liver. Results of routine serum biochemical tests do not allow the clinician to distinguish between these various causes. In type II acute hepatitic syndrome, there is acute hepatic insufficiency which is often manifest clinically by signs of hepatic

TABLE 10.9.

TYPICAL PATTERNS OF RESULTS FOR ROUTINE LABORATORY TESTS IN SEVEN HEPATOBILIARY LESIONS WHICH CAUSE CONJUGATED HYPERBILIRUBINAEMIA [1]

↑ Increased; ↓ decreased; N = normal; 0 = absent; number of arrows: 1 = mild; 2 = moderate; 3 = marked.

	Amino-transferases	Alkaline phosphatase	Lactate dehydrogenase	γ-Glutamyl-transferase	Albumin	Cholesterol	IgG	IgM	Vitamin B_{12}	Frequency of mitochondrial antibody
Acute viral hepatitis	↑↑↑ [2]	↑	↑	↑	N	↑ or ↓ [3]	↑ [4]	↑ [5]	↑↑↑	↑ [6]
Chronic active hepatitis	↑↑	↑	↑	↑	N or ↓	N or ↓	↑↑↑	↑↑	↑↑	↑↑
Primary biliary cirrhosis	↑	↑↑↑	↑	↑↑↑	N or ↓	↑↑↑	↑	↑↑↑	↑↑	↑↑↑
Drug cholestasis	↑	↑↑↑	↑	↑↑↑	N	↑↑ [7]	N or ↑	N or ↑	↑	0 or ↑
Large duct biliary obstruction	↑	↑↑↑	↑	↑↑↑	N	↑↑↑ [7]	N or ↑	N or ↑	N [8]	0 or ↑
Secondary carcinoma	↑	↑↑↑	↑↑↑	↑↑↑	N or ↓	↑ or ↓	N or ↑	N or ↑	↑	0
Alcoholic liver disease	↑ or ↑↑ [9]	↑	↑	↑↑↑ [10]	N or ↓	↑ or ↓ [11]	↑	↑↑	↑↑↑ [12]	0

[1] Exceptions to these patterns occur, many of which are indicated in the text.
[2] Alanine higher than aspartate aminotransferase; highest values early in clinical course; [3] transiently abnormal values; [4] late; [5] early; [6] occasionally transient positive test: HB_sAg-positive if due to hepatitis B virus.
[7] If jaundice prolonged.
[8] In absence of cholangitis and secondary carcinoma.
[9] Aspartate higher than alanine aminotransferase; [10] also increased when alcohol intake is high in absence of structural liver disease.
[11] Occasional high values associated with haemolysis (Zieve's syndrome).
[12] Alcoholic hepatitis or cirrhosis.

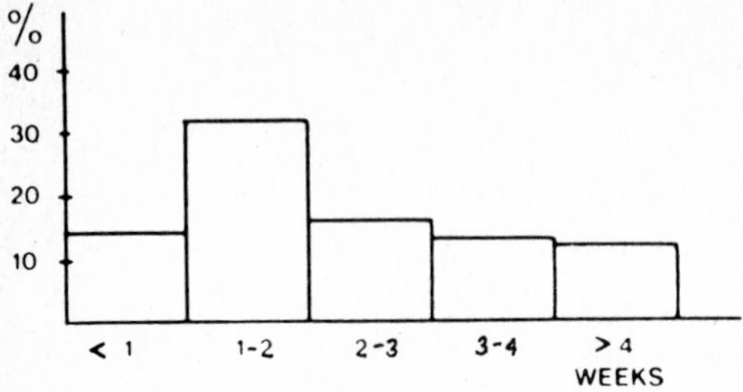

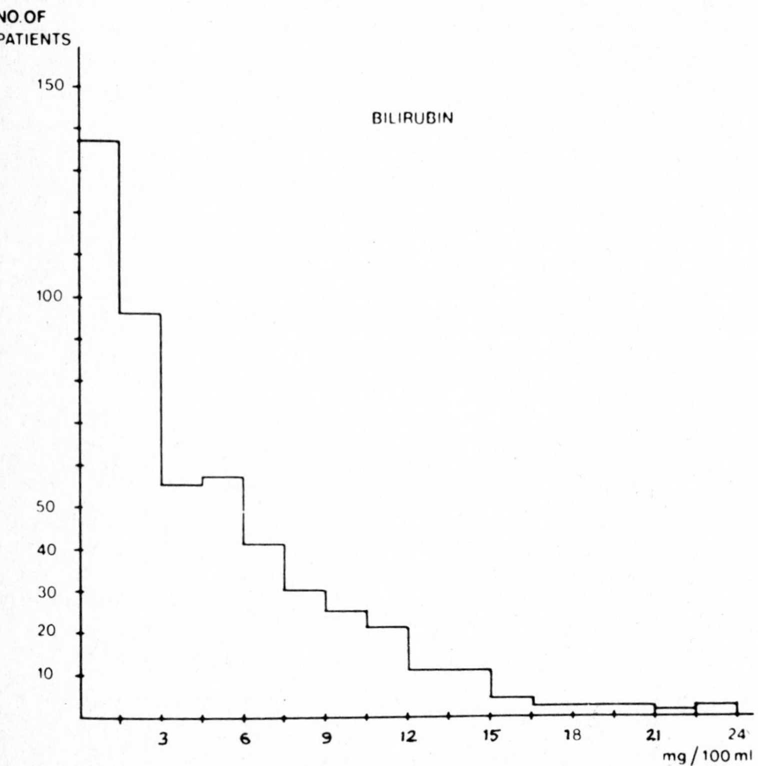

Figure 10.40. Duration of hyperbilirubinaemia (above) and distribution of serum total bilirubin concentration in 500 patients with biopsy-verified acute hepatitis at the time of biopsy. The diagnosis in each case was presumed to be acute viral hepatitis. (Reproduced, with permission, from Petersen et al., 1974)

encephalopathy, while the serum aminotransferase activities are usually only moderately increased. Infiltration of hepatocytes with small fat droplets, rather than marked liver cell necrosis, is a characteristic histologic finding in these patients. The type II syndrome occurs in fatty liver of pregnancy, Reye's syndrome and tetracycline overdosage, each of which is associated with a similar pattern of results of routine serum biochemical tests. A raised serum uric acid concentration is a common finding in type II, but not type I, patients. Results of laboratory tests in acute alcoholic hepatitis, which is usually classified separately from the acute hepatitic syndrome, resemble those found in patients in group II. Testing of serum for the presence of HB_sAg is mandatory in all patients with the acute hepatitic syndrome. In some cases, tests for hepatitis virus A infection and serum drug or toxin measurements may be helpful. Laboratory monitoring of a patient with this syndrome may be important in determining the management of the case, even in the absence of encephalopathy. An increasing prothrombin time which is not corrected by parenteral vitamin K_1 indicates that the patient should be under observation in hospital.

Certain infections other than viral hepatitis may be associated with a syndrome which can resemble an acute hepatitic syndrome (McIntyre and Heathcote, 1974). These include Weil's disease, glandular fever (infectious mononucleosis), Q fever, yellow fever, herpes simplex, visceral cryptococcus and cytomegalovirus infection. Laboratory tests which are of value in diagnosing these conditions include urine testing for protein and appropriate serological tests in Weil's disease and yellow fever, the heterophile antibody test (Paul Bunnel test) in glandular fever, and appropriate serological tests in Q fever, herpes simplex, cryptococcus and cytomegalovirus infection.

In the absence of very high serum aminotransferase activity abnormal values for most of the routine serum biochemical tests in the acute hepatitic syndrome may be similar to those found in association with large duct biliary obstruction and drug-induced cholestasis. However, measurement of serum alkaline phosphatase may be helpful. It is rare for the serum activity of this enzyme to be more than mildly elevated in the acute hepatitic syndrome (Figure 10.17). Any one of the patterns of values of routine biochemical tests which are found in the acute hepatitic syndrome may be found in severe congestive cardiac failure, the diagnosis of which depends on physical rather than laboratory findings.

Raised serum concentrations of protein-bound iodine, vitamin B_{12} and transferrin iron (Rachmilewitz et al., 1972) are non-specific findings associated with liver cell necrosis. In acute hepatitis, the peak for serum iron occurs after peak values for bilirubin, and alanine and aspartate aminotransferases are reached.

The term "fulminant liver failure" is used when the mental changes of hepatic encephalopathy occur in a patient with an acute hepatitic syndrome (Williams, 1972). The occurrence of this dreaded complication may be predicted by a progressive increase of the prothrombin time that cannot be corrected by parenteral vitamin K. Results of other laboratory tests in the acute hepatitic syndrome which suggest a poor prognosis, and may be associated with hepatic encephalopathy, include decreasing subnormal concentrations of serum cholesterol and plasma sodium and glucose, and increasing supranormal concentrations of plasma ammonia and urea. Azotaemia may reflect the presence of the renal failure which may occur as a complication of acute liver failure. Alternatively, it may be attributable to the agent causing the syndrome also being toxic to the kidney, as occurs in poisoning with *Amanita phalloides* or carbon tetrachloride, and in Weil's disease. Occasionally, the acute hepatitic syndrome is associated with very low values for blood urea concentration, an observation which may be due inter alia to the hepatic lesion being responsible for a depression of hepatic urea synthesis (section 10.2.7.2). There is a tendency for the serum bilirubin concentration to fall pre-terminally in the acute hepatitic syndrome. In acute alcoholic hepatitis, but not in the acute hepatitic syndrome per se, a serum bilirubin concentration greater than 85 μmol/litre (5 mg/dl) is considered a bad prognostic finding (Combes and Schenker, 1975). Serum alanine and aspartate aminotransferases are of no prognostic value in fulminant liver failure. It has been suggested that well maintained or increased serum levels of α_1-antitrypsin and α-foetoprotein (Murray-Lyon et al., 1976) may be associated with a favourable prognosis in this syndrome.

When following up a patient after an acute hepatitic episode, the finding of normal routine serum biochemical tests, including the aminotransferases, is reassuring and usually implies ultimate return to normal of hepatic function and structure. On the other hand, persistent elevation of serum aminotransferase activities raises the possibility of progression of the acute lesion to chronic hepatitis. The precise diagnosis of chronic hepatitis can only be made by liver biopsy, which should be considered if the serum aminotransferases remain elevated 6 months after an acute hepatitic episode. Other abnormal results of routine tests following an acute hepatitic episode which would necessitate consideration of liver biopsy include hypoalbuminaemia, hyper-γ-globulinaemia and the presence (section 10.3) of smooth muscle antibody, mitochondrial antibody, antinuclear antibody or HB_sAg. Persistent unconjugated hyperbilirubinaemia in the absence of abnormal results of other routine tests following an acute hepatitic episode may be due to Gilbert's syndrome. An acute hepatitic episode with markedly increased serum aminotransferase activities may occur during the course of chronic active hepatitis, when it may represent the mode of presentation of this form of chronic liver disease, or be due to coincidental viral hepatitis. One of the most helpful laboratory tests in such cases is the serum IgG concentration which is frequently elevated in HB_sAg-negative chronic hepatitis.

10.5.1.2.2. Cholestasis. The term cholestasis implies impaired secretion of bile or partial or complete impairment of bile flow into the duodenum. When cholestasis occurs, irrespective of the cause, routine serum biochemical tests usually show conjugated hyperbilirubinaemia, moderate or marked elevation of the alkaline phosphatase activity, increased serum cholesterol concentration and mildly or moderately elevated aminotransferase activities. The serum cholesterol concentration may be only slightly elevated early in the course of an episode of acute cholestasis, while exceedingly high values – greater than 26 mmol/litre (10 g/litre) – may occur in chronic cholestasis (e.g. primary or secondary biliary cirrhosis). Serum LP-X is usually detectable in the presence of cholestasis (section 10.2.5.4.8). The causes of cholestasis which have to be considered most often are large duct biliary obstruction, certain drugs such as chlorpromazine and erythromycin estolate, primary biliary cirrhosis and viral hepatitis with cholestatic features. Causes of large duct biliary obstruction include gall stones in the common hepatic or common bile ducts; carcinoma of the head of the pancreas, ampulla of Vater or the bile ducts near the junction of the left and right main hepatic ducts; chronic pancreatitis; biliary stricture; choledochal cyst; aneurysm of the hepatic artery; duodenal diverticulum; primary extrahepatic sclerosing cholangitis; ascariasis in the bile ducts; duodenal ulcer with involvement of the common bile duct; haematobilia; enlarged lymph glands at the porta hepatis; and benign tumours of the bile ducts. Other intra-hepatic causes of cholestasis include space-occupying lesions; severe infections (with or without direct hepatic involvement); Hodgkin's disease (with or without demonstrable Hodgkin's tissue in the liver); ulcerative colitis; primary intrahepatic sclerosing cholangitis; congestive cardiac failure; cholestatic jaundice of pregnancy; secondary syphilis; other drugs such as oral contraceptives and 17-α-alkylated steroids; and benign recurrent cholestasis. Women taking oral contraceptive drugs who contract viral hepatitis are likely to develop cholestasis (cholestatic viral hepatitis). Cholestasis may be associated with bacterial cholangitis in lesions such as choledocholithiasis, cholecystocolic fistula, congenital dilation of intrahepatic bile ducts, tumour of the bile ducts and liver fluke infestation. Cholestatic episodes may occur during the course of chronic liver disease including chronic active hepatitis and particularly in alcoholic liver disease. The serum vitamin B_{12} concentration is usually normal when cholestasis is not associated with intrahepatic space-occupying lesions, intra-hepatic infections or hepatocellular disease.

Mild degrees of cholestasis may be associated with normal serum conjugated and unconjugated bilirubin concentrations, or with normal serum total but increased conjugated bilirubin concentrations (section 10.2.1.2) as shown in Figure 10.41. In general, the value of the serum alkaline phosphatase activity reflects the degree of organic obstruction of the bile ducts.

Routine serum biochemical tests are rarely of value in determining the cause of cholestasis. Laboratory tests which are of some value in this respect include mitochondrial antibody (section 10.3.1.1), HB_sAg (section 10.3.2.1.1), the specific immune adherence assay for antibodies to hepatitis virus A (section 10.3.2.2.3), serum amylase and lipase (elevated in some patients with alcoholic liver disease with pancreatitis or with occlusion of pancreatic ducts by tumour or stone), serological tests for syphilis, and serum IgG concentration (section 10.2.5.4.7). In carcinoma of the head of the pancreas or chronic pancreatitis, a raised fasting plasma glucose concentration or a diabetic type of glucose tolerance test may be found.

When corticosteroids (e.g. prednisolone 30 mg daily) are administered to patients with conjugated hyperbilirubinaemia due to cholestasis, a marked fall in the degree of hyperbilirubinaemia may be induced, e.g. a greater than 40% fall in serum total bilirubin concentration in 5 days; the mechanism of this effect is unknown. Because this phenomenon appears to occur more commonly in patients with cholestasis due to causes other than large duct biliary obstruction, the effect of corticosteroids on the serum bilirubin con-

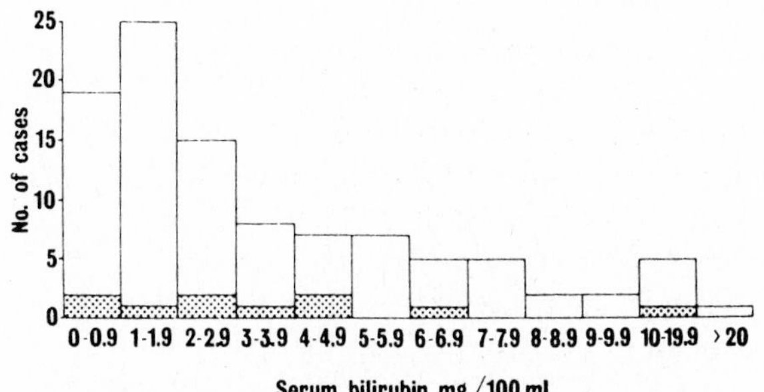

Figure 10.41. Serum total bilirubin concentrations at time of presentation of 100 patients with primary biliary cirrhosis. Values were less than 2 mg/100 ml in 41%. Male patients are shown in hatched columns. (Reproduced, with permission, from Sherlock and Scheuer, 1973)

centration has been used as a test to determine whether cholestasis is due to large duct biliary obstruction and hence whether surgical intervention is necessary. However, false positive and false negative results of this test are not uncommon. No laboratory tests, including the effect of corticosteroids on the serum bilirubin concentration, are as useful in determining the cause of cholestasis as needle biopsy of the liver and/or adequate cholangiography.

10.5.1.3. Unique situations

10.5.1.3.1. Jaundice in pregnancy. Certain physiological changes in serum biochemical test values occur in pregnancy. These include raised serum alkaline phosphatase, leucine aminopeptidase and 5′-nucleotidase activities and, in the third trimester, a mild rise in serum total cholesterol concentration without increase in the cholesterol ester concentration. Retention of bromosulphthalein may be slightly increased during pregnancy. Women taking oral contraceptive drugs have a hormonal status resembling that of early pregnancy and may exhibit a slight and reversible increase in bromosulphthalein retention. The results of laboratory tests in cholestatic jaundice of pregnancy are similar to those that may occur in association with other causes of cholestasis in pregnancy, such as large duct biliary obstruction due to gall stones, and also to those that occur in cholestasis associated with the taking of oral contraceptive drugs. In contrast to viral hepatitis in pregnancy, laboratory tests in acute fatty liver of pregnancy reveal only moderately increased values of the serum aminotransferase activities and often a raised serum uric acid concentration (section 10.2.7.4). In toxaemia of pregnancy, the serum activities of alkaline phosphatase and the aminotransferases may be elevated and there may be unconjugated hyperbilirubinaemia due to haemolysis, but the diagnosis of this syndrome does not depend on the results of these tests.

10.5.1.3.2. Neonatal jaundice. (i) *Unconjugated hyperbilirubinaemia.* A moderate degree of unconjugated hyperbilirubinaemia ("physiological jaundice") is extremely common in the newborn period. This results from a complex set of causes, including a true increase in bilirubin production, a further augmentation of the bilirubin load on the liver resulting from intestinal bilirubin deconjugation, reabsorption and enterophepatic circulation, defective hepatic uptake, and suboptimal hepatic levels of Y protein and glucuronyltransferase. Delayed closure of the ductus venosus with diversion of some portal blood around the liver may also contribute (Berk et al., 1974a).

In addition to haemolytic disease due to blood group incompatibility, and severe pyogenic infections, several distinct neonatal syndromes have been described in which there is a marked unconjugated hyperbilirubinaemia due to faulty hepatic bilirubin clearance. One of these is associated with an inhibitor of bilirubin conjugation in mother's milk. These conditions have been reviewed elsewhere (Berk et al., 1974a). Routine laboratory tests are of limited value in distinguishing between these syndromes.

(ii) *Conjugated hyperbilirubinaemia.* Infantile pyogenic infections may induce conjugated hyperbilirubinaemia with a cholestatic or hepatitic picture. Routine laboratory tests do not enable a reliable distinction to be made between neonatal hepatitis and biliary atresia, the diagnoses of which depend on hepatic histology and cholangiography. However, serum aminotransferase activities greater than 20 times the upper limit of normal would favour neonatal hepatitis, while values less than 5 times the upper limit of normal would favour biliary atresia. Appreciably increased values for serum cholesterol concentration would also favour biliary atresia. Serum α-foetoprotein concentration tends to be higher, and serum 5′-nucleotidase tends to be lower, in neonatal hepatitis than in biliary atresia (Yeung, 1972; Zeltzer et al., 1974) and serum LP-X is detected more frequently in biliary atresia than in neonatal hepatitis (Poley et al., 1973). However, there is insufficient experience of the use of these three tests in this context to determine how useful they are as an aid to diagnosis.

Several laboratory tests can be helpful in the diagnosis of neonatal cholestasis. These include HB_sAg (section 10.3.2.1.1) the specific immune adherence assay for hepatitis A antibodies (section 10.3.2.2.3), serum α_1-antitrypsin concentration (section 10.2.5.4.2), the sweat test, and serological tests for syphilis, toxoplasma, cytomegalovirus, EB virus and herpes simplex. Proteinuria and aminoaciduria may be found if cholestasis is secondary to galactosaemia, hereditary fructose intolerance or tyrosinaemia.

When well recognized causes of cholestasis have been excluded, it is possible that detailed investigations using techniques which are only available in research laboratories may reveal an inborn error of metabolism, e.g. a defect in cholic acid synthesis (Hanson et al., 1975).

10.5.1.3.3. Postoperative jaundice. If jaundice, occurring in the immediate postoperative period (and also after severe burns), is associated with routine serum biochemical tests which are consistent with an acute hepatitic syndrome, the causes may include viral hepatitis (possibly post-transfusion), halothane-associated hepatitis, drug-induced acute hepatic necrosis (e.g. antibiotics), hypotension, hypoxaemia and surgical interference with the hepatic blood supply. The results of routine biochemical tests do not enable the clinician to distinguish between these possibilities. Testing for HB_sAg (section 10.3.2.1.1) is mandatory, and the specific immune adherence tests for hepatitis A antibodies should be considered (section 10.3.2.2.3).

If, on the other hand, postoperative jaundice is associated with routine serum biochemical tests which are indicative of cholestasis, the possibilities include cholestatic drug reactions, a gall stone in the common bile duct, a surgical error resulting in stricture of the common hepatic or common bile duct, hepatic or extra-hepatic infection (including intra-abdominal abscess), benign postoperative intra-hepatic cholestasis, hypotension and hypoxaemia. Again, the results of routine biochemical tests do not enable the clinician to distinguish between these various possibilities. In benign postoperative intra-hepatic cholestasis (Schmid et al., 1965), unconjugated and conjugated hyperbilirubinaemia is marked, possibly in part due to blood transfusions during surgery, while serum activities of alanine and aspartate aminotransferases and alkaline phosphatase are either normal or only mildly increased. However, intra-hepatic cholestasis with moderately increased serum alkaline phosphatase activity may follow major surgery which was associated with haematoma formation, blood transfusions and hypotension (Kantrowitz et al., 1967).

Postoperative jaundice in which there is an increase in the serum concentration of unconjugated bilirubin raises the possibility of haemolysis, or resorption of large haematomas. Haemolysis after surgery can be due to a wide variety of different causes, which include transfusion of stored blood, artificial heart valves and clostridial infection. If haemolysis in the postoperative period is associated with impaired liver function, e.g. as a consequence of hypotension or hypoxaemia, there may be an increase in the serum concentration of conjugated bilirubin (LaMont and Isselbacher, 1973; Morgenstern, 1974) (section 10.2.1.1.2).

10.5.2. Intra-hepatic space-occupying lesions

Intra-hepatic space-occupying lesions include primary and secondary neoplasia, cysts and abscesses. The most widely used screening test for these lesions is the serum alkaline phosphatase. Serum γ-glutamyltransferase, 5′-nucleotidase and leucine aminopeptidase can also be used for this purpose; the first of these enzymes appears to be the most sensitive test. Serum lactate dehydrogenase activity may be particularly high in the presence of primary or secondary hepatic tumours.

The considerable value of the serum α-foetoprotein concentration, preferably measured by radioimmunoassay, in diagnosing liver cell carcinoma has been described (section 10.2.5.4.6). It is possible that the combination of assays of serum α-foetoprotein and other oncofoetal proteins such as carcinoembryonic antigen may be superior to the use of α-foetoprotein alone in the diagnosis of liver cell carcinoma. A leucocyte adherence inhibition test for the immunodiagnosis of liver cell carcinoma has been described (Halliday et al., 1974). This is an in vitro test of the cell mediated immunity exhibited by leucocytes of sensitized individuals in the presence of an appropriate antigen; the serum from a subject who responds positively to the test blocks the phenomenon. Pooled extracts containing antigens from several hepatocellular carcinomata are required as a source of antigen for the application of this test to the detection of hepatocellular carcinoma. False positive results may be obtained in other hepatic diseases such as haemochromatosis and acute alcoholic hepatitis. The leucocyte adherence inhibition test, like α-foetoprotein, may yield a positive result long before symptoms or signs attributable to tumour are apparent. Liver cell carcinoma should be considered when values for serum biochemical tests in a cirrhotic patient become markedly more abnormal without an obvious precipitating factor being evident. HB_sAg status is not helpful. Several abnormal laboratory test results may be found in patients with liver cell carcinoma which are not usually found in patients with uncomplicated cirrhosis or other intrahepatic space-occupying lesions. These abnormalities include hypoglycaemia, hypercalcaemia, elevated serum vitamin B_{12} concentration, elevated serum mucoprotein concentration, hyperlipidaemia, dysfibrinogenaemia and cryofibrinogenaemia (Margolis and Homcy, 1972). Elevation of vitamin B_{12} appears to be due to an increased serum concentration of a B_{12} binding protein (Waxman and Gilbert, 1973). In patients with liver cell carcinoma, the gradual development of fasting hypoglycaemia occurs as a preterminal phenomenon in patients whose tumours are rapidly growing and poorly differentiated, while a more precipitous fall in fasting plasma glucose concentration, which may be difficult to correct, tends to occur with better differentiated lesions and may be due to acquired glycogenosis (McFadzean and Yeung, 1969). Hypoglycaemia may also occur with hepatic sarcomas.

In patients presenting with fever of unknown origin without hyperbilirubinaemia, the serum alkaline phosphatase and alanine and aspartate aminotransferase activities may be mildly elevated as a consequence of infections or abscesses not directly involving the hepatobiliary system. Similar results of laboratory tests may be obtained in patients with pyogenic liver abscess or other intra-hepatic infections. As the bromosulphthalein test may be mildly abnormal as a non-specific response to fever due to any cause (Blaschke et al., 1973), this test is not helpful in establishing a hepatic lesion as the cause of an unexplained fever. Of particular help in differentiating between intra-hepatic and extra-hepatic infection is the serum vitamin B_{12} concentration which tends to be elevated only if the infection is intra-hepatic (Neale et al., 1966). Serum biochemical tests do not enable a pyogenic liver abscess to be differentiated from an amoebic liver abscess.

Several serological tests may aid in the diagnosis of amoebic liver disease. All occasionally yield false positive or false negative results, and accordingly none is ultimately definitive in making a diagnosis of amoebic liver disease. Similarly, serological tests are of limited value in the diagnosis of intrahepatic hydatid cysts.

10.5.3. Alcoholism

Appreciable alcohol consumption may be associated with the development of fatty liver, hepatitis, hepatic fibrosis and/or cirrhosis (Chapter 23).

The metabolism of alcohol in the liver results in the formation of acetaldehyde and an increased ratio of NADH to NAD. The latter causes hyperlactic acidaemia which predisposes to acidosis, decreased renal excretion of uric acid and elevation of the serum uric acid concentration. Hyperlipidaemia and ketosis may arise as a consequence of the potentiation by alcohol of underlying abnormalities of the metabolism of carbohydrate and lipids, e.g. type IV hyperlipoproteinaemia. Elevation of serum lipids secondary to alcohol consumption depends on the integrity of the hepatocyte, and the magnitude of this effect diminishes with progression of hepatocellular disease. Hypoglycaemia is a rare complication of alcoholism which may arise from an alcohol-induced block of hepatic gluconeogenesis and glycogen depletion. More often, alcoholics may have increased fasting plasma glucose concentrations or impaired glucose tolerance, which may be a reflection of enhanced gluconeogenesis or pancreatitis. Appreciable serum concentrations of the metabolite of alcohol, acetaldehyde, and the product of its mitochondrial metabolism, acetate, may be found. Elevation of serum acetaldehyde concentration tends to be potentiated by the impaired hepatic mitochondrial oxidizing capacity which occurs in the presence of a severe hepatocellular lesion (Lieber, 1975). Figure 10.42 summarizes the relevant metabolic pathways.

Alcohol ingestion readily induces a rise in serum γ-glutamyltransferase. It somewhat less readily induces a rise in serum aspartate aminotransferase. If raised serum activities of these enzymes are found after alcohol consumption, they do not necessarily imply underlying structural alcoholic liver disease and abnormal values may return to normal if no alcohol is taken for a short period. However, if abnormal enzyme values persist when alcohol is not being consumed, the possibility of underlying structural liver disease is suggested. If no significant structural liver disease is present, serum γ-glutamyl transferase values can be used as a sensitive index of whether an alcoholic subject is continuing to drink alcohol. A more specific test in this context, and one that does not depend on whether or not there is underlying structural liver disease, is determination of the ethanol concentration in a random plasma specimen (Hamlyn et al., 1975).

The results of laboratory tests in patients with alcoholic hepatitis are not specific. The picture is often similar to that of a type II acute hepatitic syndrome (section 10.5.1.2.1).

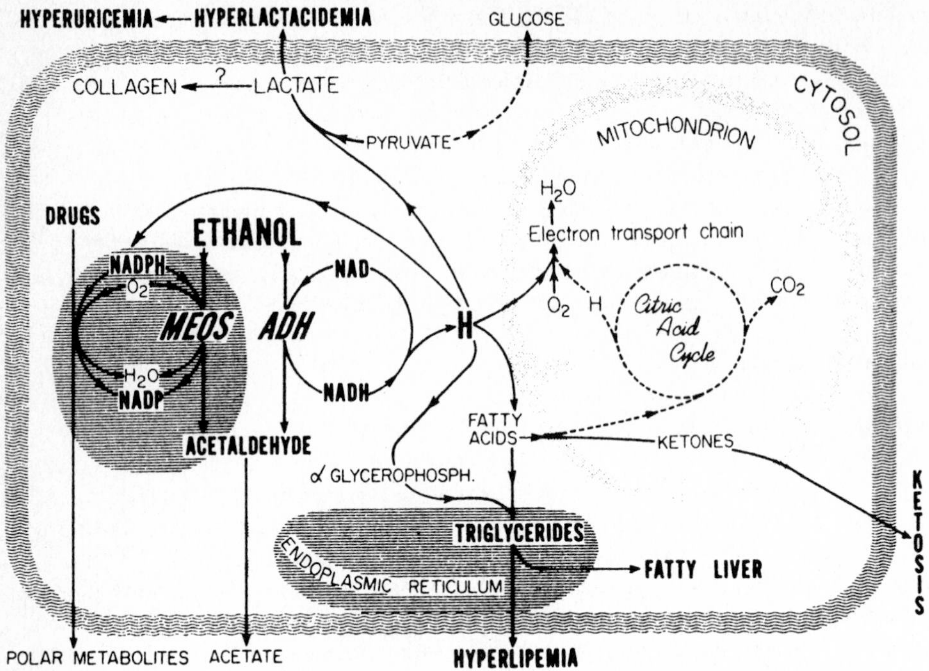

Figure 10.42. Metabolism of ethanol in the hepatocyte and schematic representation of its link to fatty liver, hyperlipaemia, hyperlactacidaemia, ketosis and hypoglycaemia. Pathways that are decreased by ethanol are presented as dashed lines. ADH = alcohol dehydrogenase; MEOS = microsomal ethanol-oxidizing system; NAD = nicotinamide adenine dinucleotide; NADH = nicotinamide adenine dinucleotide, reduced form; NADP = nicotinamide adenine dinucleotide phosphate; NADPH = nicotinamide adenine dinucleotide phosphate, reduced form. (Reproduced, with permission, from Lieber, 1975)

Worthy of particular note is the very modest increase in serum alanine aminotransferase activity, the value for which is usually less than that of serum aspartate aminotransferase (Zimmerman and Seeff, 1970). There may, in addition, be cholestatic features due to the hepatocellular lesion itself or to large duct biliary obstruction secondary to alcoholic pancreatitis or pseudocyst. Hypoalbuminaemia and hyper-γ-globulinaemia may be present. Marked elevations of serum cholesterol concentration and other lipids are sometimes found (Zieve's syndrome).

Reduced serum concentrations of folic acid, thiamine and vitamin B_6 and a positive FIGLU test (Hoffbrand et al., 1966) are commonly found in alcoholics with and without liver disease whose nutritional status is poor.

10.5.4. Iron overload states

Iron overload states include primary haemochromatosis, secondary haemochromatosis in the alcoholic, transfusion siderosis and siderosis secondary to haemolytic states and to cirrhosis with a large portacaval shunt (Barry, 1974). Currently available tests of iron metabolism do not enable these conditions to be differentiated.

10.5.4.1. Serum iron and total iron-binding capacity

The liver is the main site of iron storage in the body and the plasma iron pool normally accounts for only about 0.1% of the total body iron. The serum iron concentration represents the net effect of a dynamic equilibrium between iron entering the plasma from intestinal absorption, the reticuloendothelial system and storage sites, and iron leaving the plasma for haemoglobin synthesis, storage and excretion. Exchange between plasma and storage sites is usually small compared with turnover for haemoglobin synthesis and catabolism. The serum iron concentration correlates poorly with tissue storage levels. However, when storage iron is increased, the serum iron concentration is usually raised.

Serum total iron-binding capacity reflects the concentration of the plasma protein transferrin and has been traditionally more readily measured than transferrin. Total iron-binding capacity is inversely related to iron stores when these are reduced, but is usually within the normal range when iron stores are normal or increased.

Serum iron is often expressed as a percentage (normally 20 to 25%) of the total iron-binding capacity, and values greater than 75% (when the total iron-binding capacity is normal) suggest iron excess. Saturation is high in idiopathic haemochromatosis largely due to a raised serum iron concentration, whereas a similar value in other forms of cirrhosis is often due mainly to a lowered total iron-binding capacity (Barry, 1973). This index has no intrinsic value and separate assessment of serum iron and total iron-binding capacity values is recommended.

The pattern of increased serum iron concentration and normal total iron-binding capacity which is typically found in idiopathic haemochromatosis, is also found in other states of iron overload. However, this pattern may be modified by the presence of severe hepatocellular disease which tends to be associated with low values for total iron-binding capacity, possibly due to impaired hepatic synthesis of transferrin. The extent to which the serum iron concentration can rise is less when the total iron-binding capacity is reduced. Thus, patients with advanced iron overload and cirrhosis, in whom the total iron-binding capacity is low, may have normal serum iron concentrations. It is also evident that in patients with a low serum total iron-binding capacity, the percentage of iron saturation may be increased in the absence of iron overload. In many diverse neoplastic, inflammatory or infective disorders, which are associated with altered reticuloendothelial activity, both serum iron concentration and total iron-binding capacity may be low.

In hepatic lesions associated with active liver cell necrosis, such as the acute hepatitic syndrome, a raised serum iron concentration is often found and does not imply increased iron stores, but rather increased liberation of iron from damaged liver cells and failure to utilize absorbed iron.

Although intestinal absorption of iron must have been excessive at some time in patients with idiopathic haemochromatosis, iron absorption tests may give normal results and do not have a place in the routine laboratory evaluation of these patients. Measurements of serum iron concentration and total iron-binding capacity are used in screening for iron overload in apparently healthy relatives of patients with idiopathic haemochromatosis.

10.5.4.2. Chelation tests

Diethylenetriamine pentaacetic acid and desferrioxamine are used in chelation tests to determine the total body iron store. The former is a synthetic chelating agent reactive for many metals and is eliminated in the urine within 6 hours of its administration. The latter can be derived from actinomycetes; it has a specific affinity for iron, and it is eliminated in both bile and urine, mostly during the first 24 hours after its administration. These substances may act by competing with transferrin for ferritin iron across cell membranes (Barry, 1973).

Chelation tests involve measuring iron in urine and necessitate particular care with regard to the use of iron-free containers for urine collections and iron-free apparatus and reagents. The simplest type of chelation test involves administration of a standard dose of a chelating agent and subsequently measuring the amount of iron excreted in an appropriately timed urine collection. The magnitude of iron excretion in such a test is only a semi-quantitative index of body iron stores, as the amount of iron appearing in the urine does not include all that was chelated. This problem has to a large extent been resolved by giving ^{59}Fe-labelled diethylenetriamine pentaacetic acid or desferrioxamine along with the corresponding unlabelled chelating agent and measuring the proportion of the administered ^{59}Fe which is recovered bound to chelate in the urine. This enables the total amount of iron chelated to be calculated, and forms the basis of more accurate and clini-

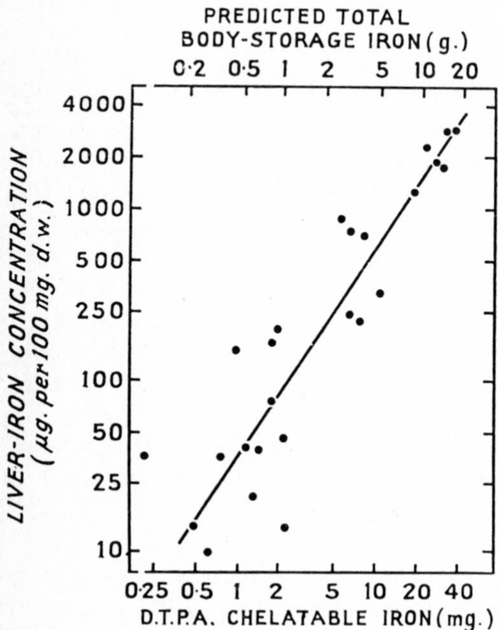

Figure 10.43. Relationship between liver iron concentration (Y), iron chelatable by diethylenetriamine pentaacetic acid (DTPA) (X) and predicted total body storage iron. Y = 76.2 X −36.0. Predicted total body-storage iron (g) = DPTA-chelatable iron (mg) ×0.46. (Reproduced, with permission, from Barry and Sherlock, 1971)

cally useful measurements of total chelatable body iron (Barry et al., 1970).

In idiopathic haemochromatosis, measurements of chelatable body iron obtained using either chelating agent correlate equally well with mobilizeable storage iron, as determined by repeated phlebotomy; the measurements enable body iron stores, and hence the required amount of venesection treatment, to be predicted. Diethylenetriamine pentaacetic acid-chelatable iron also correlates closely with liver iron concentration and with mobilizeable storage iron in iron-overload states other than idiopathic haemochromatosis (Figure 10.43). Results using desferrioxamine in disorders other than idiopathic haemochromatosis do not correlate so well with estimates of storage iron based on other techniques, and it has been suggested that desferrioxamine chelates a highly reactive labile iron source which is not accessible to diethylenetriamine pentaacetic acid. However, diethylenetriamine pentaacetic acid-chelatable iron appears to give a more reliable index of pathological iron overload (Barry, 1973).

10.5.4.3. Serum ferritin

Ferritin is normally a predominantly intracellular iron-binding protein. An immunoradiometric assay has been developed for measuring the concentration of the protein in serum, but is not yet widely available. Increased concentrations have been found in patients with

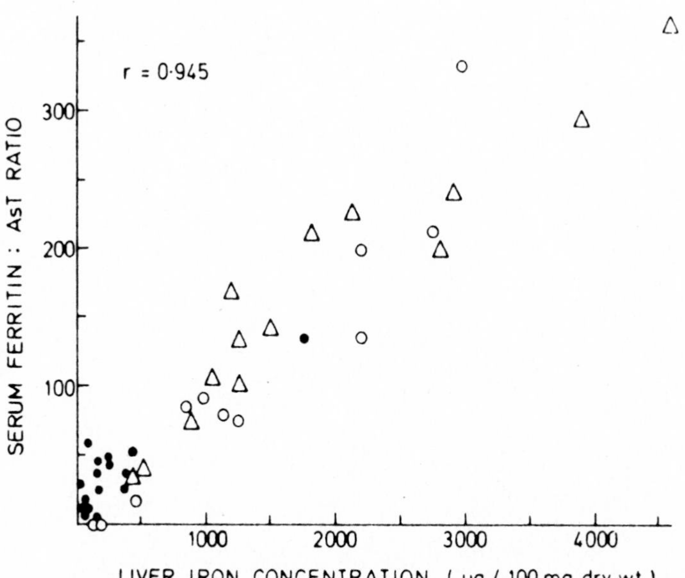

Figure 10.44. Relationship between serum ferritin/aspartate aminotransferase (AsT) ratio and liver iron concentration. (Reproduced, with permission, from Prieto et al., 1975)

a variety of acute and chronic hepatobiliary diseases. The circulating concentration of ferritin in disease appears to depend on the degree of liver cell damage and the magnitude of hepatic iron stores. It is assumed that increased amounts of ferritin present in serum have been released from damaged hepatocytes. Serum ferritin/serum aspartate aminotransferase ratios (the numerical values of which depend on enzyme measurement conditions) have been found to correlate well with liver iron concentration (Figure 10.44), and may be useful in monitoring treatment in idiopathic haemochromatosis. High values of this ratio appear to indicate marked iron excess (Prieto et al., 1975; Jacobs and Worwood, 1975). Serum ferritin may be normal in latent haemochromatosis.

10.5.5. Copper overload states

Particular care is necessary when measuring serum and urinary copper concentrations that appropriate containers and laboratory apparatus and reagents are not contaminated with copper. The concentrations of copper in the liver and certain other tissues are increased in Wilson's disease and in conditions associated with prolonged cholestasis such as primary biliary cirrhosis. In these various conditions, certain tests for abnormal copper metabolism are likely to show a similar pattern. There is usually an increased serum concentration of non-caeruloplasmin-bound copper, increased urinary excretion of copper, and appreciable augmentation of the urinary excretion of copper after giving the copper

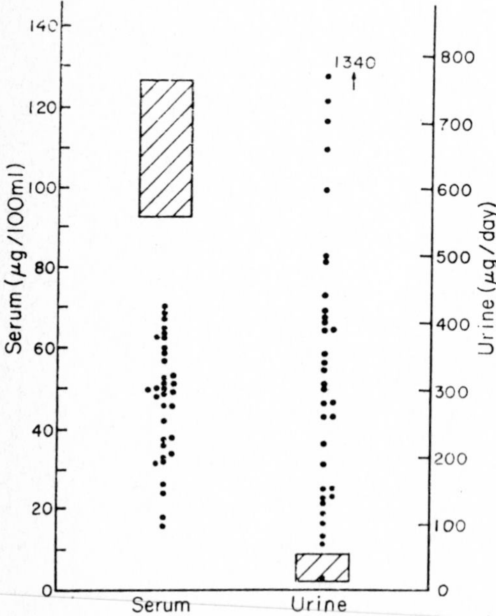

Figure 10.45. Serum total copper and urine copper in patients with Wilson's disease. Shaded bars represent the ranges of values for normal subjects. (Reproduced, with permission, from Strickland and Leu, 1975)

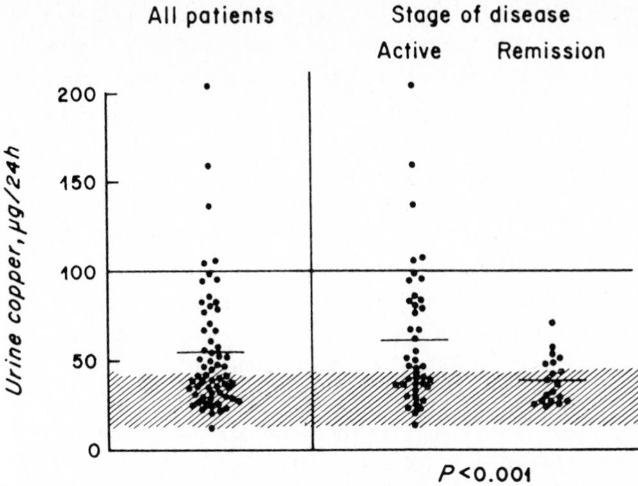

Figure 10.46. Daily urinary copper excretion in patients with chronic active hepatitis. Left panel = all patients; right panel = patients divided according to the stage of their disease (active or remission); horizontal band = range in normal subjects; solid horizontal line = value for daily urinary copper excretion typical of Wilson's disease. (Reproduced, with permission from La Russo et al., 1976)

chelating drug penicillamine (Deering et al., 1975; Strickland and Leu, 1975). Although measurement of these variables of copper metabolism do not enable a distinction to be made between chronic cholestasis and Wilson's disease, there are usually clear-cut differences between these two syndromes in terms of their clinical picture and the serum total copper and caeruloplasmin concentrations (section 10.2.5.4.3; Figures 10.22, 10.23, 10.45 and 10.46). Particularly high values for serum non-caeruloplasmin-bound copper and urinary copper may occur spontaneously in Wilson's disease due to an abnormally large flux of copper from the tissues. When this occurs, haemolysis and hence an increase in the serum unconjugated bilirubin concentration may occur (McIntyre et al., 1967). A fairly late development in syndromes of copper overload is renal tubular insufficiency secondary to deposition of copper in the renal tubules. This can result in uricosuria, aminoaciduria, glycosuria, and a reduced serum uric acid concentration. Wilson's disease sometimes presents with a syndrome resembling chronic active hepatitis (Sternlieb and Scheinberg, 1972). Urinary copper excretion may be moderately increased in chronic active hepatitis (La Russo et al., 1976) and hence its measurement is not a reliable method of distinguishing Wilson's disease from chronic active hepatitis. Abnormal laboratory indices of copper metabolism tend to revert to normal after liver transplantation in patients with Wilson's disease (Groth and Starzl, 1975).

10.5.6. Evaluation of the post-liver transplant patient

After liver transplantation, routine serum biochemical tests do not enable jaundice due to rejection of the graft to be distinguished from jaundice due to other causes such as cholangitis or large duct biliary obstruction related to the biliary tract reconstruction, azathioprine hepatotoxicity, hepatic artery thrombosis or viral hepatitis. More than one of these causes of jaundice may co-exist. In acute severe rejection, the picture may resemble that of a type I acute hepatitic syndrome with marked elevation of serum aspartate and alanine aminotransferase activities and marked prolongation of the prothrombin time. When rejection is less severe, and more chronic, the picture may be predominantly one of cholestasis, with appreciable elevation of the serum alkaline phosphatase activity (Williams et al., 1973). Laboratory tests which might reflect the immunologic process causing rejection have been used in an attempt to differentiate rejection from other causes of jaundice. The leucocyte migration test, a test of cell mediated immunity, may enable the presence of lymphocytes in peripheral blood which are sensitized to the graft to be detected. This test has given abnormal results in the presence of jaundice due to rejection, and normal results when jaundice was due to other causes after hepatic transplantation. In addition, serum CH_{50} (a measure of total haemolytic complement activity – section 10.2.5.4.4), which tends to be normal or increased when jaundice is due to large duct biliary obstruction or cholangitis, may be reduced in association with hepatic rejection (Williams and Smith, 1972), but it may also be reduced in association with a coincidental HB_sAg-positive acute hepatitis or massive hepatic necrosis.

After transplantation of an inadequately preserved ischaemic liver, hypoalbuminaemia, hypoprothrombinaemia, hypoglycaemia and electrolyte and acid–base disturbances complicate the typical picture of an acute hepatitic syndrome (Groth and Starzl, 1975).

10.6. AIDS TO THE INTERPRETATION OF LABORATORY TESTS

Because of the low specificity of most laboratory tests in the diagnosis of individual hepatobiliary diseases, approaches have been sought to maximize the diagnostic usefulness of the results of a given set of laboratory tests. A sequential Bayesian model has been developed so as to predict, from a set of variables which include routine serum biochemical tests, the probability that a jaundiced patient has one of 11 common causes of jaundice, and the probability that surgical or medical treatment is required (Knill-Jones et al., 1973). Also, an iterative graphic system has been developed to facilitate interpretation of laboratory data from patients with hepatobiliary diseases (Strandjord et al., 1973). By the use of canonical or discriminant function analysis, it has been shown that measurements of serum alkaline phosphatase, albumin, aspartate aminotransferase, α_2-, β- and γ-globulins and cholesterol are of more value in differentiating between six liver diseases than measurements of serum total bilirubin, unconjugated bilirubin, total globulin, α_1-globulin and urea (Baron, 1970). A computer has been used in the evaluation of patients who have had serum biochemical evidence of a hepatobiliary lesion for at least one month, without a definitive diagnosis becoming apparent. Diseases which can conform to this pattern and which can resemble each other closely include large duct biliary obstruction due to gall stones or tumour, chronic active hepatitis, primary biliary cirrhosis, drug-induced cholestasis and cholestatic viral hepatitis. Predictions based on computer analysis were more accurate than those based on clinical judgement in determining whether surgical or medical management was required. However, in general, clinical data tend to feature more prominently than serum biochemical tests in the predictions (Burbank, 1969). Analyses of this type may be more useful in suggesting the most appropriate further investigation, such as cholangiography or liver biopsy, rather than the definitive diagnosis. It is apparent that the full potential of computer analysis in the interpretation of laboratory tests in the diagnosis and management of patients with hepatobiliary diseases has not yet been determined.

Finally, an algorithm has been proposed for the monitoring of aminotransferase activities in patients ingesting hepatotoxic drugs. Such a scheme, in conjunction with other data such as alkaline phosphatase activity and results of a liver biopsy, can be used to facilitate decisions whether to discontinue a drug or maintain or increase its dose (Hofmann and Thistle, 1974).

10.7. CONCLUDING REMARKS

The initial routine laboratory evaluation of a patient with a hepatobiliary lesion should include at least the following "static" tests: serum total and direct reacting bilirubin concentrations; alkaline phosphatase, alanine and aspartate aminotransferase activities; total protein and protein electrophoresis; prothrombin time; and HB_sAg. All of these tests should be available at the local hospital. Urine tests for bilirubin and urobilinogen, while not essential, are very easily carried out, and complement the routine blood tests. Elevation of serum conjugated bilirubin and the presence of bilirubinuria are highly specific indicators of a hepatobiliary lesion, particularly if the serum alkaline phosphatase and alanine aminotransferase activities are raised also. Testing for bilirubin in urine can be used as a screening test for preicteric or anicteric hepatitis. The serum alkaline phosphatase activity is of particular help in the detection of intra- or extra-hepatic obstructive lesions of the biliary tract, intra-hepatic space-occupying lesions and infiltrative lesions of the liver. Other serum enzyme tests can be useful in the interpretation of alkaline phosphatase activities. When the serum alkaline phosphatase activity is elevated in the presence of normal values for serum total and conjugated bilirubin, serum leucine aminopeptidase, 5′-nucleotidase or γ-glutamyltransferase measurements can be helpful in determining whether a hepatobiliary or osseous lesion is present. Very high values for serum lactate dehydrogenase suggest that a raised serum alkaline phosphatase activity is due to intra-hepatic neoplasia. Serum alanine and aspartate aminotransferase activities are most helpful as sensitive indicators of hepatocellular injury. Aspartate aminotransferase is sometimes more sensitive, but is less liver-specific than alanine aminotransferase. A protein electrophoretic pattern which shows a decrease in serum albumin and/or increase in serum γ-globulin concantration raises the possibility of chronic hepatocellular disease. The prothrombin time, after the parenteral administration of vitamin K_1, is a sensitive index of the protein synthetic capacity of the liver; as such, it is particularly useful in assessing the severity of both acute and chronic hepatocellular diseases. As HB_sAg is found in a wide spectrum of hepatobiliary syndromes other than acute hepatitis, the testing for this antigen should be a routine procedure in patients with evidence suggesting a lesion of the hepatobiliary system.

Of the "dynamic" tests, the bromosulphthalein test, which has been widely applied, is probably the one of choice. Its only disadvantages are occasional local and systemic complications but the incidence of these is very low. In general, the test is most useful when the serum conjugated bilirubin concentration is normal. In this situation the conventional 45 minute bromosulphthalein test is a very sensitive screening test for a hepatobiliary lesion.

Other tests which should be available, at least on a regional basis, are those for serum mitochondrial antibody, α-foetoprotein, α_1-antitrypsin, caeruloplasmin and copper, and urinary copper. Of the non-organ-specific antibody tests, only the mitochondrial antibody test is of appreciable help in making a specific diagnosis, primarily in the evaluation of a patient with chronic cholestasis. The usefulness of high serum concentrations of α-foetoprotein in the diagnosis and treatment of patients with hepatocellular carcinoma has been widely confirmed. α_1-Antitrypsin deficiency enters into the differential diagnosis of neonatal hepatitis and cholestasis, chronic liver disease in childhood or adult life, and liver cell carcinoma, while Wilson's disease enters into the differential diagnosis of chronic liver disease in a young person: thus the physician should be familiar with the specific laboratory tests which help in the diagnosis of these two diseases.

Of the newer, less widely applied, tests the 2 hour post-prandial serum bile acid concentration appears to be a particularly sensitive test of hepatobiliary dysfunction. It is, of course, most important that if a new test is being applied, a reference range of values for the test must be established in the laboratory where the test is being conducted.

Usually, it is desirable to perform laboratory tests as soon as possible after appropriate specimens have been received, so as to avoid adverse effects of storage of specimens on the accuracy of assays. This applies in particular to serum bilirubin and alkaline phosphatase. Storage of about 10 ml of serum at –20 °C is, however, often useful, particularly if the diagnosis is not immediately clear and an emergency treatment is about to be instituted which may affect the results of laboratory tests. The availability of stored serum may enable additional tests to be requested at a later data as indications for them become apparent.

The laboratory tests available for the evaluation of hepatobiliary diseases can be of value in making a diagnosis; in monitoring progress and the effects of therapy; and in defining associated pathophysiologic disturbances. When interpreting values of aspartate aminotransferase, alkaline phosphatase and γ-glutamyltransferase activities, account must be taken of the patient's age (Kattwinkel et al., 1973). If results of laboratory tests are obtained which appear to be at variance with the patient's clinical status, it may be necessary to repeat the relevant tests and confirm the validity of the unexpected values. Interpretation of atypical results is facilitated if, prior to their occurrence, the patient's course was well documented both in terms of clinical and laboratory data. A careful history of all drug therapy must never be omitted. It is important to emphasize that there are numerous limitations to all of the tests discussed. For instance: (i) routine serum biochemical tests may be normal in compensated inactive macronodular cirrhosis, methotrexate- and vinyl chloride-induced hepatic injury, congenital hepatic fibrosis, polycystic disease of the liver, cholelithiasis, type I glycogenosis, hepatic amyloidosis, hepatic tumours, and even chronic active hepatitis; (ii) laboratory tests do not enable extra-hepatic causes of cholestasis to be distinguished from intra-hepatic causes; (iii) corticosteroid therapy is often associated with falls in serum aminotransferase activity and bilirubin and γ-globulin concentrations and a rise in serum albumin, but the relationships of these changes to possible effects of therapy on an underlying disease process are far from clear. Nevertheless, while the significance of the result of a particular test taken in isolation may be quite non-specific or equivocal, its value to the physician may be much more definitive if it is interpreted in the light of all the available clinical and laboratory data.

While laboratory tests sometimes enable the diagnosis of a hepatobiliary lesion to be made with a reasonable degree of certainty, more often the information derived from them is limited to an indication of the probable nature of the lesion and of the most appropriate further investigations such as cholangiography and/or liver biopsy, which are most likely to yield a definitive diagnosis. It is possible that the further application of computer analysis may help the clinician to obtain the maximum amount of information from the results of a given set of laboratory tests.

Finally, although the emphasis in this chapter has been on biochemical and immunologic laboratory tests, these tests, although of considerable importance, should, nevertheless, consitute only a small portion of the overall data base which is used in the diagnosis and management of a particular patient. A carefully taken history can be of very considerable help in diagnosis, and for certain conditions, such as drug-induced liver injury, it may be indispensible. Similarly, the detection of a palpable gall bladder or of an intrahepatic arterial bruit during a meticulous physical examination will be of more value in arriving at a diagnosis than an extensive – and expensive – battery of laboratory tests. The application of "tincture of time" in certain cases of hepatobiliary disease will often make clear the mysterious, without the necessity of substantial diagnostic phlebotomy.

To the extent that diagnostic procedures are indicated, those described above represent only a fraction of the available armamentarium. In skilled hands, the "1 second" aspiration liver biopsy technique of Menghini can provide hepatic tissue for examination at an extremely low risk to the patient. The interpretation of such small specimens requires special skill on the part of the pathologist, but in experienced hands it can provide extraordinarily valuable information relating to a clinical problem. Radiographic techniques are also of help in a variety of settings. In particular, the use of "skinny needle" percutaneous transhepatic cholangiography and endoscopic retrograde pancreaticocholangiography and pancreatography may provide precise diagnostic information about the lesion responsible for a cholestatic illness. Lastly, the role of arteriography and radioisotope scanning in the detection and evaluation of hepatic neoplasms and other intra-hepatic space-occupying lesions is considerable.

Many of the procedures just enumerated are invasive and will provide, rapidly, information which may ultimately become available from less aggressive measures. The increasingly wide-spread application of such invasive procedures is an example of "Sutton's Law" *. Since, in skilled hands, the complication rate from such procedures is small and since both the medical and cost benefits from shortening hospitalization may be considerable, the aggressive approach is not without merit. However, every physician must evalu-

* Willie Sutton, a notorious American bank robber, was repeatedly jailed for his exploits, but promptly returned to a life of crime after each of several dramatic escapes from prison. On one such occasion, while on his way back to prison, he was asked by a reporter why he kept on robbing banks. "Because that's where the money is" was his reply.

ate the experience with, and the complication rate of, such procedures at his own institution, as well as the skill of those interpreting the results, in deciding on his own diagnostic approach in specific patients. The usefulness of the results obtained from any test or diagnostic procedure depends to a large extent on the quality of the questions being asked by the clinician.

REFERENCES

Abelev, G.I. (1971) Alpha-fetoprotein in ontogenesis and its association with malignant tumours. Advances in Cancer Research, 14, 295–358.

Ajdukiewicz, A.B., Dudley, F.J., Fox, R.A., Doniach, D. and Sherlock, S. (1972) Immunological studies in an epidemic of infective short-incubation hepatitis. Lancet, i, 803–806.

Alpert, E., Isselbacher, K.J. and Schur, P.H. (1971) The pathogenesis of arthritis associated with viral hepatitis: complement–component studies. New England Journal of Medicine, 285, 185–189.

Alpert, S., Mosher, M., Shanske, A. and Arias, I.M. (1969) Multiplicity of hepatic excretory mechanisms for organic anions. Journal of General Physiology, 53, 238–247.

Alvira, M.M. and Forman, D.T. (1974) Biochemical abnormalities in Reye's syndrome. Annals of Clinical Laboratory Science, 4, 477–483.

Amin, A.H., Clarke, H.G., Freeman, T., Murray-Lyon, I.M., Smith, P.M. and Williams, R. (1970) Studies by quantitative immunoelectrophoresis on iron binding proteins in haemochromatosis. Clinical Science, 38, 613–616.

Andreasen, P.B., Ranek, L., Statland, B.E.E. and Tygstrup, N. (1974) Clearance of antipyrine: dependence of quantitative liver function. European Journal of Clinical Investigation, 4, 129–134.

Arias, I.M., Gartner, L.M., Cohen, M., Ben-Ezzer, J. and Levi, A.J. (1969) Chronic nonhemolytic unconjugated hyperbilirubinemia with glucuronyl transferase deficiency. Clinical biochemical, pharmacologic and genetic evidence for heterogeneity. American Journal of Medicine, 47, 395, 409.

Arias, I.M. and London, I.M. (1957) Bilirubin glucuronide formation in vitro; demonstration of a defect in Gilbert's disease. Science, 126, 563–564.

Arias, I.M., Johnson, L. and Wolfson, S. (1961) Biliary excretion of injected conjugated and unconjugated bilirubin by normal and Gunn rats. American Journal of Physiology, 200, 1091–1084.

Arias, I.M., Fleischner, G., Listowsky, I., Kamisaka, K., Mishkin, S. and Gatmaitan, Z. (1976) On the structure and function of ligandin and Z protein. In The Hepatobiliary System (Ed. W. Taylor) pp. 81–103, Plenum Press, New York.

Axelrod, J., Schmid, R. and Hammaker, L. (1957) Biochemical lesion in congenital non-obstructive, non-haemolytic jaundice. Nature (London), 180, 1426–1427.

Badin, J. and Barillec, A. (1968) Effet des lipides de la beta-lipoprotéine humaine normale sur le pouvoir hémolytique de la streptolysine O et de la digitonine. Annales de Biologie Clinique, 26, 213–229.

Badin, J. and Barillec, A. (1969) Dosage specifique de l'antistreptolysine O sérique après élemination des lipopotéines par l'alcool isoamylique. Annales de Biologie Clinique, 27, 395–402.

Baker, K.J. (1966) Binding of sulfobromophthalein (BSP) sodium and indocyanine green (ICG) by plasma α_1 lipoproteins. Proceedings of the Society for Experimental Biology and Medicine, 122, 957–963.

Baker, K.J. and Bradley, S.E. (1966) Binding of sulfobromophthalein (BSP) sodium by plasma albumin: its role in hepatic BSP extraction. Journal of Clinical Investigation, 45, 281–287.

Barber-Riley, G., Goetzee, A.E., Richards, T.G. and Thomson, J.Y. (1961) The transfer of bromsulphthalein from the plasma to bile in man. Clinical Science, 20, 149–159.

Barker, L.E., Gerety, R.J., Hoofnagle, J.H. and Nortman, D.F. (1975) Viral hepatitis B: detection and prophylaxis. In Transmissible Disease and Blood Transfusion (Eds. T.J. Greenwald and G.A. Jamieson) pp. 81–111, Grune and Stratton, New York.

Barnes, S., Gallo, G.A., Trash, D.B. and Morris, J.S. (1975) Diagnostic value of serum bile acid estimations in liver disease. Journal of Clinical Pathology, 28, 506–509.

Barniville, H.T.F. and Misk, R. (1959) Urinary glucuronic acid excretion in liver disease and the effect of a salicylamide load. British Medical Journal, 1, 337–340.

Baron, D.N. (1970) A critical look at the value of biochemical liver function tests with special reference to discriminant function analysis. Annals of Clinical Biochemistry, 7, 100–103.

Barrett, P.V.D., Berk, P.D., Menken, M. and Berlin, N.I. (1968) Bilirubin turnover studies in normal and pathologic states using bilirubin-^{14}C. Annals of Internal Medicine, 68, 355–377.

Barry, M. (1973) Iron overload: clinical aspects, evaluation and treatment. Clinics in Haematology, 2, 405–426.

Barry, M. (1974) Progress report: iron and the liver. Gut, 15, 324–334.

Barry, M., Cartei, G.C. and Sherlock, S. (1969) Differential ferrioxamine test in haemochromatosis and liver disease. Gut, 10, 697–704.

Barry, M., Cartei, G.C. and Sherlock, S. (1970) Quantitative measurement of iron stores with diethylenetriaminepenta-acetic acid. Gut. 11, 891–898.

Barry, M. and Sherlock, S. (1971) Measurement of liver-iron concentration in needle biopsy specimens. Lancet, i, 100–103.

Bartels, H., Hauck, W. and Vogel, I. (1975) Aminopyrine – an effective modifier of liver and serum gamma glutamyl transpeptidase. Journal of Pediatrics, 86, 298–301.

Ben-Ezzer, J., Rimington, C., Shani, M., Seligsohn, U., Sheba, C. and Szeinberg, A. (1971) Abnormal excretion of the isomers of urinary coproporphyrin by patients with Dubin–Johnson syndrome in Israel. Clinical Science, 40, 17–30.

Berk, P.D., Howe, R.B., Bloomer, J.R. and Berlin, N.I. (1969) Studies of bilirubin kinetics in normal adults. Journal of Clinical Investigation, 48, 2176–2190.

Berk, P.D., Bloomer, J.R., Howe, R.B. and Berlin, N.I. (1970) Constitutional hepatic dysfunction (Gilbert's syndrome). American Journal of Medicine, 49, 296–305.

Berk, P.D., Blaschke, T.F. and Waggoner, J.G. (1972) Defective bromosulfphthalein clearance in patients with constitutional hepatic dysfunction (Gilbert's syndrome). Gastroenterology, 63, 472–481.

Berk, P.D., Berlin, N.I. and Howe, R.B. (1974a) Disorders of bilirubin metabolism. In Duncan's Diseases of Metabolism, 7th edn. (Eds. P.K. Bondy and L. Rosenberg) pp. 825–880, Saunders Publishing Company, Philadelphia.

Berk, P.D., Rodkey, F.L., Blaschke, T.F., Collison, H.A. and Waggoner, J.G. (1974b) Comparison of plasma bilirubin turnover and carbon monoxide production in man. Journal of Laboratory and Clinical Medicine, 83, 29–37.

Berk, P.D., Berlin, N.I., Scharschmidt, B.F. and Blaschke, T.F. (1974c) Clearance (C_{BR}) della bilirubina epatica nella diagnosi differenziale della iper-bilirubinemia non coniugata: valutazione della C_{BR} in base a studi con cromo radioattivo. Epatologia, 20, 245–256.

Berk, P.D., Wolkoff, A.W. and Berlin, N.I. (1975) Inborn errors of bilirubin metabolism. Medical Clinics of North America, 59, 803–816.

Berk, P.D., Blaschke, T.F., Scharschmidt, B.F., Waggoner, J.G. and Berlin, N.I. (1976) A new approach to quantitation of the various sources of bilirubin in man. Journal of Laboratory and Clinical Medicine, 87, 767–780.

Bernstein, R.B. (1971) Comparison of serum clearance and urinary excretion of mesobilirubinogen-H^3 in control subjects and patients with liver disease. Gasterenterology, 61, 733–738.

Bernstein, L.H., Ben-Ezzer, J., Gartner, L. and Arias, I.M. (1966) Hepatic intracellular distribution of tritium-labelled unconjugated and conjugated bilirubin in normal and Gunn rats. Journal of Clinical Investigation, 45, 1194–1201.

Betro, M.G., Oon, R.C.S. and Edwards, J.B. (1973) Gamma-glutamyl transpeptidase in diseases of the liver and bone. American Journal of Clinical Pathology, 60, 672–678.

Bevan, G., Baldus, W.B. and Gleich, G.J. (1969) Serum immunoglobulin levels in cholestasis. Gastroenterology, 56, 1040–1046.

Billing, B.H., Williams, R. and Richards T.G. (1964) Defects in hepatic transport of bilirubin in congenital hyperbilirubinaemia and analysis of plasma bilirubin disappearance curves. Clinical Science, 27, 245–257.

den Blaauwen, D.H. and Thijs, L.G. (1973) The bromsulphalein and galactose tolerance tests in patients with various liver diseases: a comparative study. Gastro-enterologia Belgica, 36, 345–375.

Black, M. and Billing, B.H. (1969) Hepatic bilirubin UDP-glucuronyl transferase activity in liver disease and Gilbert's syndrome. New England Journal of Medicine, 280, 1266–1271.

Black, M. and Sherlock, S. (1970) Treatment of Gilbert's syndrome with phenobarbitone. Lancet, i, 1359–1362.

Black, M., Fevery, J., Parker, D., Jacobson, J., Billing, B.H. and Carson, E.R. (1974) Effect of phenobarbitone on plasma [^{14}C]bilirubin clearance in patients with unconjugated hyperbilirubinaemia. Clinical Science and Molecular Medicine, 46, 1–17.

Blaschke, T.F., Berk, P.D., Rodkey, F.L., Scharschmidt, B.F., Collison, H.A. and Waggoner, J.G. (1974a) Drugs and the liver. 1. Effects of glutethimide and phenobarbital on hepatic bilirubin clearance, plasma bilirubin turnover and carbon monoxide production in man. Biochemical Pharmacology, 23, 2795–2806.

Blaschke, T.F., Berk, P.D., Scharschmidt, B.F., Guyther, J.R., Vergalla, J. and Waggoner, J.G. (1974b) Crigler–Najjar syndrome: an unusual course with development of neurologic damage at age eighteen. Pediatric Research, 8, 573–590.

Blaschke, T.F., Elin, R.J., Berk, P.D., Song, C.S. and Wolff, S.M. (1973) Effect of induced fever on sulfobromophthalein kinetics in man. Annals of Internal Medicine, 78, 221–226.

Bloom, A.L. (1975) Intravascular coagulation and the liver. British Journal of Haematology, 30, 1–7.

Bloomer, J.R., Berk, P.D., Howe, R.B., Waggoner, J.G. and Berlin, N.I. (1970) Comparison of fecal urobilinogen excretion with bilirubin production in normal volunteers and patients with increased bilirubin production. Clinica Chimica Acta, 29, 463–471.

Bloomer, J.R., Berk, P.D., Howe, R.B. and Berlin, N.I. (1971a) Interpretation of plasma bilirubin levels based on studies with radioactive bilirubin. Journal of the American Medical Association, 218, 216–220.

Bloomer, J.R., Berk, P.D., Howe, R.B. and Berlin, N.I. (1971b) Bilirubin metabolism in congenital nonhemolytic jaundice. Pediatric Research, 5, 256–274.

Bloomer, J.R., Barrett, P.V., Rodkey, F.L. and Berlin, N.I. (1971c) Studies on the mechanism of fasting hyperbilirubinemia. Gastroenterology, 61, 479–487.

Bloomer, J.R., Waldmann, T.A., McIntire, K.R. and Klatskin, G. (1975) Relationship of serum α-fetoprotein to the severity and duration of illness in patients with viral hepatitis. Gastroenterology, 68, 342–350.

Bloomer, J.R., Berk, P.D., Vergalla, J. and Berlin, N.I. (1973) Influence of albumin on the hepatic uptake of unconjugated bilirubin. Clinical Science, 45, 505–516.

Bodvall, B. (1973) The polycholecystectomy syndromes. Clinics in Gastroenterology, 2, 103–126.

Bourke, E., Milne, M.D. and Stokes, G.S. (1965) Mechanisms of renal excretion of urobilinogen. British Medical Journal, 2, 1510–1514.

Braun, H.J. and Aly, F.W. (1971) Die Klinische Bedeutung der quantitativen Serum-hemopexinbestimmung im vergleich zum Haptoglobin. Klinische Wochenschrift, 49, 451–458.

Breen, K.J. and Schenker, S. (1971) Liver function tests. Critical Reviews in Clinical Laboratory Science, 2, 573–599.

Brensilver, H.L. and Kaplan, M.M. (1975) Significance of elevated liver alkaline phosphatase in serum. Gastroenterology, 68, 1556–1562.

Brodersen, R. (1966) Bilirubin diglucuronide in normal human blood serum. Scandinavian Journal of Clinical and Laboratory Investigation, 18, 361–370.

Brodersen, R. (1974) Competitive binding of bilirubin and drugs to human serum albumin studied by enzymatic oxidation. Journal of Clinical Investigation, 54, 1353–1364.

Brunt, P.W. (1974) Progress report: antitrypsin and the liver. Gut, 15, 573–580.

Burbank, F. (1969) A computer diagnostic system for the diagnosis of prolonged undifferentiating liver disease. American Journal of Medicine, 46, 401–415.

Butt, H.R., Anderson, V.E., Foulk, W.T., Baggenstoss, A.H., Schoenfield, L.J. and Dickson, E.R. (1966) Studies of chronic idiopathic jaundice (Dubin–Johnson syndrome) II. Evaluation of a large family with the trait. Gastroenterology, 51, 619–630.

Caesar, J., Shaldon, S., Chiandussi, L., Guevara, L. and Sherlock, S. (1961) The use of indocyanine green in the measurement of hepatic blood flow and as a test of hepatic function. Clinical Science, 21, 43–57.

Cain, G.D., Mayer, G. and Jones, E.A. (1970) Augmentation of albumin but not fibrinogen synthesis by corticosteroids in patients with hepatocellular disease. Journal of Clinical Investigation, 49, 2198–2204.

Castell, D.O. and Johnson, R.B. (1966) An index of portal-systemic collateral circulation in chronic liver disease. New England Journal of Medicine, 275, 188–192.

Cherrick, G.R., Stein, S.W., Leevy, C.M. and Davidson, C.S. (1960) Indocyanine green: observations on its physical properties, plasma decay and hepatic extraction. Journal of Clinical Investigation, 39, 592–600.

Clark, R., Borirakchanyavat, V., Gazzard, B.G., Rake, M.O., Shilkin, K.B., Flute, P.T. and Williams, R. (1973) Disordered hemostasis in liver damage from paracetamol overdose. Gastroenterology, 65, 788–795.

Clermont, R.J. and Chalmers, T.C. (1967) The transaminase tests in liver disease. Medicine, 46, 197–207.

Cohn, C., Levine, R. and Streicher, D. (1947) The rate of removal of intravenously injected bromsulphalein by the liver and extra-hepatic tissue of the dog. American Journal of Physiology, 150, 299–303.

Clubb, J.S., Neale, F.C. and Posen, S. (1965) The behaviour of infused human placental alkaline phosphatase in human subjects. Journal of Laboratory Clinical Medicine, 66, 493–507.

Cohen, G.A., Donabedian, R.K., Goffinct, J.A., Lerner, E. and Conn, H.O. (1974) Low glutamic oxalacetic transaminase (GOT) levels in azotemia. Gastroenterology, 67, 783 (abstract).

Cohen, L., Lewis, C. and Arias, I.M. (1972) Pregnancy, oral contraceptives and chronic familial jaundice with predominantly conjugated hyperbilirubinemia (Dubin–Johnson syndrome). Gastroenterology, 62, 1182–1190.

Cohen, S., Freeman, T. and McFarlane, A.S. (1961) Metabolism of ^{131}I-labelled human albumin. Clinical Science, 20, 161–170.

Colombi, A. (1970) Early diagnosis of fatal hepatitis. Digestion, 3, 129–145.

Combes, B., Shore, G.M., Cunningham, F.G., Walker, F.B., Shorey, J. and Ware, A. (1974) Suppression by pregnancy and birth control pills (BCP) of the rise in serum gamma glutamyl transpeptidase (GGT) in viral hepatitis. Gastroenterology, 67, 784 (abstract).

Combes, B. and Stakelum, G.S. (1960) Conjugation of sulfobromophthalein sodium with glutathione in thioether linkage by the rat. Journal of Clinical Investigation, 39, 1214–1222.

Cook, G.C., Mulligan, R. and Sherlock, S. (1971) Controlled prospective trial of corticosteroid therapy in active chronic hepatitis. Quarterly Journal of Medicine, 40, 159–185.

Cowen, A.E., Korman, M.G., Hofmann, A.F. and Thomas, P.J. (1975) Plasma disappearance of radioactivity after intravenous injection of labelled bile acids in man. Gastroenterology, 68, 1567–1573.

Crigler, J.F. and Najjar, V.A. (1952) Congenital familial non-hemolytic jaundice with kernicterus. Pediatrics, 10, 169–180.

Cushieri, A. and Baker, P.B. (1974) Gamma-glutamyl-transpeptidase in hepato-bilary disease: value as an enzymatic liver function test. British Journal of Experimental Pathology, 55, 110–115.

Davidson, D.C., McIntosh, W.B. and Ford, J.A. (1974) Assessment of plasma glutamyl transpeptidase activity and urinary D-gluconic acid excretion as indices of enzyme induction. Clinical Science and Molecular Medicine, 47, 279–283.

Dawson, J.L. (1965) The incidence of postoperative renal failure in obstructive jaundice. British Journal of Surgery, 52, 663.

Deering, T.B., Dickson, E.R., Geall, M.G., Fleming, C.R., McCall, J.T. and Goldstein, N.P. (1975) The effect of D-penicillamine on urinary copper excretion in primary bilary cirrhosis. Gastroentrology, 69, 816 (abstract).

Dhumeaux, D. and Berthelot, P. (1975) Chronic hyperbilirubinemia associated with hepatic uptake and storage impairment. Gastroenterology, 69, 988–993.

Dhumeaux, D., Berthelot, P. and Javitt, N.B. (1974) Dibromsulphalein (DBSP) estimation of hepatic transport function in man. European Journal of Clinical Investigation, 4, 181–185.

Doniach, D., Roitt, I.M., Walker, J.G. and Sherlock, S. (1966) Tissue antibodies in primary biliary cirrhosis, active chronic (lupoid) hepatitis, cryptogenic cirrhosis and other liver diseases and their clinical applications. Clinical and Experimental Immunology, 1, 237–262.

Doniach, D. and Walker, G. (1972) Immunopathology of liver disease. Progress in Liver Diseases, 4, 381–402.

Doniach, D. and Walker, J.G. (1974) Progress Report. Mitochondrial antibodies (AMA). Gut, 15, 664–668.

Dragosici, B., Ferenci, P., Pesendorfer, F. and Wewalka, F.G. (1976) Gamma-glutamyltranspeptidase (GGTP): relationship to other enzymes for diagnosis of liver disease. Progress in Liver Diseases, 5, 436–449.

Dubin, I.N. (1958) Chronic idiopathic jaundice: a review of 50 cases. American Journal of Medicine, 24, 268–292.

Dudley, F.J., O'Shea, M.J., Ajdukiewicz, A. and Sherlock, S. (1973) Serum autoantibodies and immunoglobulins in hepatitis associated antigen (HAA)-positive and -negative liver diseases. Gut, 14, 360–364.

Dudley, F.J., Scheuer, P.J. and Sherlock, S. (1972) Natural history of hepatitis associated antigen: positive chronic liver disease. Lancet, ii, 1388–1393.

Duffy, T., Vergara, F. and Plum, F. (1974) α-ketoglutaramate in hepatic encephalopathy. In Brain Dysfunction and Metabolic Disorders, Research Publications: Association for Research in Nervous and Mental Disease, Vol. 53 (Ed. F. Plum) pp. 39–52, Raven Press, New York.

Dykes, P.W. (1968) The rates of distribution and catabolism of albumin in normal subjects and in patients with cirrhosis of the liver. Clinical Science, 34, 161–183.

Dymock, I.W. (1975) Assessment of survival prospects in acute hepatic failure – The value of a coagulation screen. In Artificial Liver Support (Eds. R. Williams and I.M. Murray-Lyon) pp. 290–297, Pitman Medical, London.

Dymock, I.W., Tucker, J.S., Woolf, I.L., Potter, L. and Thomson, J.M. (1975) Coagulation studies as a prognostic index in acute liver failure. British Journal of Haematology, 29, 385–395.

Eleftheriou, N., Thomas, H.C., Heathcote, J. and Sherlock, S. (1975) Incidence and clinical significance of e antigen and antibody in acute and chronic liver disease. Lancet, ii, 1171–1173.

Eliakim, M., Zlotnick, A. and Slavin, S. (1972) Gammopathy in liver disease. Progress in Liver Diseases, 4, 403–417.

Fagerhol, M.K. and Laurell, C.-B. (1967) The polymorphism of "prealbumins" and α_1-antitrypsin in human sera. Clinica Chimica Acta, 16, 199–203.

Fauvert, R.E. (1959) The concept of hepatic clearance. Gastroenterology, 37, 603–616.

Feinman, S.V., Berris, B. and Sinclair, J.C. (1975) e-Antigen and anti-e in HBsAg carriers. Lancet, ii, 1173–1174.

Feinstone, S.M., Zapikian, A.Z., Purcell, R.H., Alter, H.J. and Holland, P.V. (1975) Transfusion-associated hepatitis not due to viral hepatitis type A or B. New England Journal of Medicine, 292, 767–770.

Feizi, T. (1968) Immunoglobulins in chronic liver disease. Gut, 9, 193–198.

Felsher, B.F., Rickard, D. and Redeker, A.G. (1970) The reciprocal relation between caloric intake and the degree of hyperbilirubinemia in Gilbert's syndrome. New England Journal of Medicine, 283, 170–172.

Fevery, J., Van Damme, B., Michiels, R., De Groote, J. and Heirwegh, K.P.M. (1972) Bilirubin conjugates in bile of man and rat in the normal state and in liver disease. Journal of Clinical Investigation, 51, 2482–2492.

Finlayson, N.D.C., Krohn, K., Anderson, K.E., Jokelainen, P.T. and Prince, A.M. (1972) Inter-relations of hepatitis B antigen and autoantibodies in chronic idiopathic liver disease. Gastroenterology, 63, 646–652.

Fischer, J.E., Yoshimura, N., Aquirre, A., James, J.H., Cummings, M.G., Abel, R.M. and Deindoerfer, F. (1974) Plasma amino acids in patients with hepatic encephalopathy: effects of amino acid infusions. American Journal of Surgery, 127, 40–47.

Fishman, W.H., Inglis, N.I. and Kraut, M.J. (1965) Serum alkaline phosphatase of intestinal origin in patients with cancer and with cirrhosis of the liver. Clinica Chimica Acta, 12, 298–303.

Foulk, W.T., Butt, H.R., Owen, C.A. and Whitcomb, F.F. (1959) Constitutional hepatic dysfunction (Gilbert's disease): its natural history and related syndromes. Medicine, 38, 25–46.

Fox, R.A., Scheuer, P.J. and Sherlock, S. (1973) Asymptomatic primary biliary cirrhosis. Gut, 14, 444–447.

Fromke, V.L. and Miller, D. (1972) Constitutional hepatic dysfunction (CHD; Gilbert's disease): a review with special reference to a characteristic increase and prolongation of the hyperbilirubinemia response to nicotinic acid. Medicine, 51, 451–464.

Fulop, M. and Sandson, J. (1967) The effect of bile salts on the binding of bilirubin by plasma proteins. Clinical Science, 33, 459–469.

Galbraith, R.M., Smith, M., MacKenzie, R.M., Dudley, E.T., Doniach, D. and Williams, R. (1974) High prevalence of seroimmunologic abnormalities in relatives of patients with active chronic hepatitis or primary biliary cirrhosis. New England Journal of Medicine, 290, 63–69.

Gambino, S.R., Other, A. and Burns, W. (1967) Direct serum bilirubin and the sulfobromophthalein test in occult liver disease. Journal of the American Medical Association, 201, 1047–1049.

Gault, M.H., Stein, J. and Aronoff, A. (1966) Serum ceruloplasmin in hepatobiliary and other disorders: significance of abnormal values. Gastroenterology, 50, 8–18.

Gazzard, B.G., Henderson, J.M. and Williams, R. (1976) Factor VII levels as a guide to prognosis in fulminant hepatic failure. Gut, 17, 489–491.

Giles, J.P., McCollum, R.W., Berndtson, L.W. and Krugman, S. (1969) Relation of Australian-SH antigen to the Willowbrook MS-2 strain. New England Journal of Medicine, 281, 119–122.

Goldberg, D.M. (1973) 5′-Nucleotidase: recent advances in cell biology, methodology and clinical significance. Digestion, 8, 87–99.

Gollan, J.L., Huang, S.N., Billing, B.H. and Sherlock, S. (1975) Prolonged survival in three brothers with severe type 2 Crigler–Najjar syndrome: ultrastructural and metabolic studies. Gastroenterology, 68, 1543–1555.

Gordon, E.R. and Goresky, C.A. (1976) Separation and elucidation of the structure of the bilirubin tetrapyrroles secreted in human and dog bile. Gastroenterology, 70, 889 (abstract).

Goresky, C.A. (1965) The hepatic uptake and excretion of sulfobromophthalein and bilirubin. Canadian Medical Association Journal, 92, 851–857.

Goresky, C.A., Bach, G.G. and Nadeau, B.E. (1973) On the uptake of materials by the intact liver. Journal of Clinical Investigation, 52, 991–1009.

Goudie, R.B., MacSween, R.N.M. and Goldberg, D.M. (1966) Serological and histological diagnosis of primary biliary cirrhosis. Journal of Clinical Pathology, 19, 527–538.

Grausz, H. and Schmid, R. (1971) Reciprocal relation between plasma albumin level and hepatic sulfobromophthalein removal. New England Journal of Medicine, 284, 1403–1406.

Gray, C.H., Neuberger, A. and Sneath, P.H.A. (1950) Studies in congenital porphyria. Biochemical Journal, 47, 87–92.

Groth, C.G. and Starzl, T.E. (1975) Transplantation of the liver. In The Liver (Ed. F.F. Becker) pp. 885–908, Marcel Dekker, Inc., New York.

Gutstein, S., Alpert, S. and Arias, I.M. (1968) Studies of hepatic excretory function IV. Biliary excretion of sulfobomophthalein sodium in a patient with Dubin–Johnson syndrome and a biliary fistula. Israel Journal of Medical Sciences, 4, 36–40.

Hallen, J. and Laurell, C.B. (1972) Plasma protein pattern in cirrhosis of the liver. Scandanavian Journal of Clinical and Laboratory Investigation, 29, Suppl. 124, 97–103.

Halliday, W.J., Halliday, J.W., Cambell, C.B., Maluish, A.E. and Powell, L.W. (1974) Specific immunodiagnosis of hepatocellular carcinoma by leucocyte adherence inhibition. British Medical Journal, 2, 349–352.

Hamlyn, A.N., Brown, A.J., Sherlock, S. and Baron, D.N. (1975) Casual blood-ethanol estimations in patients with chronic liver disease. Lancet, ii, 345–347.

Hanson, R.F., Isenberg, J.N., Williams, G.C., Hachey, D., Szczepanik, P., Klein, P.D. and Sharp, H.L. (1975) The metabolism of 3α,7α,12α-trihydroxy-5β-cholestan-26-oic acid in two siblings with cholestasis. Journal of Clinical Investigation, 56, 577–587.

Hasch, E., Jarnum, S. and Tygstrup, N. (1967) Albumin synthesis rate as a measure of liver function in a patient with cirrhosis. Acta Medica Scandinavica, 182, 83–92.

Haslewood, G.A.D. (1967) Bile Salts. Methuen, London.

Heirwegh, K.P.M., Fevery, J., Meuwissen, J., De Groote, J., Compernolle, F., Desmet, V. and Van Roy, F.P. (1974) Recent advances in the separation and analysis of diazo-positive bile pigments. Methods of Biochemical Analysis, 22, 205–250.

Hepner, G.W. and Vesell, E.S. (1976) Variability of hepatic microsomal response to liver disease and diphenylhydantoin. Gastroenterology, 70, 985 (abstract).

Hepner, G.W. and Vesell, E.S. (1974) Assessment of aminopyrine metabolism in man by breath analysis after oral administration of ^{14}C-aminopyrine: effects of phenobarbital, disulfiram and portal cirrhosis. New England Journal of Medicine, 291, 1384–1388.

Hepner, G.W. and Vesell, E.S. (1975) Quantitative assessment of hepatic function by breath analysis after oral administration of (^{14}C)aminopyrine. Annals of Internal Medicine, 83, 632–638.

Higashino, K., Ohtani, R., Kudo, S., Hashinotsuma, M., Hada, T., Kang, K.Y., Ohkochi, T., Takahashi, Y. and Yamamura, Y. (1975) Hepatocellular carcinoma and a variant alkaline phosphotase. Annals of Internal Medicine, 83, 74–78.

Hillenbrand, P., Parbhoo, S.P., Jedrychowski, A. and Sherlock, S. (1974) Significance of intravascular coagulation and fibrinolysis in acute hepatic failure. Gut, 15, 83–88.

Hobbs, J.R. (1967) Serum Proteins in liver disease. Proceedings of the Royal Society of Medicine, 60, 1250–1254.

Hoffbrand, A.V., Neale, G., Hines, J.D. and Mollin, D.L. (1966) The excretion of forminoglutamic acid and urocanic acid after partial gastrectomy. Lancet, i, 1231–1236.

Hofmann, A.F. (1976) The enterohepatic circulation of bile acids in man. Advances in Internal Medicine, 21, 501–534.

Hofmann, A.F. and Small, D.M. (1967) Detergent properties of bile salts: correlation with physiological function. Annual Review of Medicine, 18, 333–376.

Hofmann, A.F. and Thistle, J.L. (1974) An algorithm for monitoring and managing drug hepatotoxicity. Gastroenterology, 67, 309–313.

Holborrow, E.J., Johnson, G.D., Farrow, L.J., Zuckerman, A.J. and Taylor, P.E. (1971) Immunofluorescent detection of autoantibodies in the sera of acute infective hepatitis patients. Annals of the New York Academy of Sciences, 177, 214–217.

Holland, P.V. and Alter, A.J. (1975) The clinical significance of hepatitis B virus antigens and antibodies. Medical Clinics of North America, 59, 849–855.

Holland, P.V. and Alter, H.J. (1976) Current concepts of viral hepatitis. In Viral Infections: A clinical Approach (Ed. W.L. Drew) pp. 189–211, F.A. Davis, Philadelphia.

Holldorf, A.W., Forster, E. and Falk, H. (1970) Pathways of liver metabolism in schematic illustrations. Progress in Liver Diseases, 3, 29–48.

Hoofnagle, J.H., Gerety, R.J. and Barker, L.F. (1975) Antibody to hepatitis-B core antigen. In Transmissible Disease and Blood Transfusion. (Eds. T.J. Greenwalt and G.A. Jamieson) pp. 43–55, Grune and Stratton, New York.

Hourani, B.T., Hamlin, E.M. and Reynolds, T.B. (1971) Cerebrospinal fluid glutamine as a measure of hepatic encephalopathy. Archives of Internal Medicine, 127, 1033–1036.

Hsia, D.Y.Y. (1967) Clinical variants of galactosemia. Metabolism, 16, 419–437.

Hsia, Y.E. (1974) Inherited hyperammonemic syndromes. Gastroenterology, 67, 347–374.

Hunter, J., Carrella, M., Maxwell, J.D., Stewart, D.A. and Williams, R. (1971) Urinary D-gluconic-acid excretion as a test for hepatic enzyme induction in man. Lancet, i, 572–575.

Howard, M.M., Senyszyn, J. and Leevy, C.M. (1965) Use of dichromatic ear densitometry to evaluate kinetics of indocyanine green (ICG) removal in liver disease. Gastroenterology, 48, 501–502.

Hunton, D.B., Bollman, J.L. and Hoffman, H.N. II (1960) Studies of hepatic function with indocyanine green. Gastroenterology, 39, 713–724.

Ingelfinger, F.J., Bradley, S.E., Mendeloff, A.I. and Kramer, P. (1948) Studies with bromosulphalein. Part 1. Disappearance from the blood after a single intravenous injection. Gastroenterology, 11, 646–657.

Israels, L.G., Suderman, H.J. and Ritzmann, S.E. (1959) Hyperbilirubinemia due to an alternate path of bilirubin production. American Journal of Medicine, 27, 693–702.

Israels, L.G. and Zipursky, A. (1962) Primary shunt hyperbilirubinaemia. Nature (London), 193, 73–74.

Isselbacher, K.J., Anderson, E.P., Kurahashi, K. and Kalckar, H.M. (1956) Congenital galactosemia: a single enzymatic block in galactose metabolism. Science, 123, 635–636.

Jacobs, A. and Worwood, M. (1975) Ferritin in serum: clinical and biochemical implications. New England Journal of Medicine, 292, 951–956.

Jacobsen, J. (1969) Binding of bilirubin to human serum albumin: determination of the dissociation constants. Federations of European Biochemical Societies Letters, 5, 112–114.

Jakoby, W.B. (1976) In The Chemistry and Physiology of Bile Pigments, (Eds. P.D. Berk and N.I. Berlin) U.S. Department of Health, Education and Welfare Publication, U.S. Government Printing Office, Washington, D.C.

Jansen, F.H. and Billing, B.H. (1971) The identification of monoconjugates of bilirubin in bile as amide derivatives. Biochemical Journal, 125, 917–919.

Javitt, N.B. (1964) Phenol-3,6-dibromphthalein disulphonate: a new compound for the study of liver disease. Proceedings of the Society for Experimental Biology and Medicine, 117, 254–257.

Javitt, N.B., Wheeler, H.O., Baker, K.J., Ramos, O.L. and Bradley, S.E. (1960) The intrahepatic conjugation of sulfobromopthalein and glutathione in the dog. Journal of Clinical Investigation, 39, 1570–1577.

Joblonski, P. and Owen, J.A. (1969) The clinical chemistry of bromsulfopthalein and other cholephilic dyes. Advances in Clinical Chemistry, 12, 309–386.

Jones, E.A., Cain, G.D. and Dickinson, R. (1972) Corticosteroid-induced changes in urea metabolism in patients with hepatocellular diseases. Gastroenterology, 62, 612–617.

Jones, E.A., Smallwood, R.A., Craigie, A. and Rosenoer, V.M. (1969) The enterohepatic circulation of urea nitrogen. Clinical Science, 37, 825–836.

Kamisaka, K., Listowsky, I., Gataitan, Z. and Arias, I.M. (1975) Interactions of bilirubin and other ligands with ligandin. Biochemistry, 14, 2175–2180.

Kanai, T. (1972) Clinical study on the transport of indocyanine green in the liver. Japanese Journal of Gastroenterology, 69, 228–243.

Kantrowitz, P.A., Jones, W.A., Greenberger, N.J. and Isselbacher, K.J. (1967) Severe postoperative hyperbilirubinemia simulating obstructive jaundice. New England Journal of Medicine, 276, 591–598.

Kaplan, M.M. (1972) Alkaline phosphatase. Gastroenterology, 62, 452–468.

Kaplan, M.M. and Righetti, A. (1970) Induction of rat liver alkaline phosphatase: the mechanism of the serum elevation in bile duct obstruction. Journal of Clinical Investigation, 49, 508–516.

Kaplowitz, N., Kok, E. and Javitt, N.B. (1973a) Postprandial serum bile acid for the detection of hepatobilary disease. Journal of the American Medical Association, 225, 292–293.

Kaplowitz, N., Finlayson, N.D.C., Walmsley, P., Thurnher, N. and Javitt, N.B. (1973b) Hepatobiliary disease associated with serum antimitochondrial antibody. American Journal of Medicine, 54, 725–730.

Karvountzis, G.G. and Redeker, A.G. (1974) Relation of alpha-fetoprotein in acute hepatitis to severity and prognosis. Annals of Internal Medicine, 80, 156–160.

Kattwinkel, J., Taussig, L.M., Statland, B.E. and Verter, J.I. (1973) The effects of age on alkaline phosphatase and other serologic liver function tests in normal subjects and patients with cystic fibrosis. Journal of Pediatrics, 82, 234–242.

Keiding, S. (1973) Galactose elimination capacity in the rat. Scandinavian Journal of Clinical and Laboratory Investigation, 31, 319–325.

Kew, M.C. (1974) Progress Report. Alpha-fetoprotein in primary liver cancer and other diseases. Gut, 15, 814–821.

Kunin, C.M., Glazko, A.J. and Finland, M. (1959) Persistance of antibiotics in blood of patients with acute renal failure. II Chloramphenicol and its metabolic products in the blood of patients with severe renal disease or hepatic cirrhosis. Journal of Clinical Investigation, 38, 1498–1508.

Klatskin, G. and Kantor, F.S. (1972) Mitochondrial antibody in primary biliary cirrhosis and other diseases. Annals of Internal Medicine, 77, 533–541.

Klotz, U., Avant, G.R., Hoyumpa, A., Schenker, S. and Wilkinson, G.R. (1975) The effect of age and liver disease on the disposition and elimination of diazepam in adult man. Journal of Clinical Investigation, 55, 347–359.

Knill-Jones, R.P., Stern, R.B., Girmes, D.H., Maxwell, J.D., Thompson, R.P.H. and Williams, R. (1973) Use of sequential Bayesian model in diagnosis of jaundice by computer. British Medical Journal, 1, 530–533.

Koff, R.S., Garvey, A.J., Burney, S.W. and Bell, B. (1973) Absence of an age effect on sulfobromophthalein retention in healthy men Gastroenterology, 65, 300–302.

Koj, A. (1974) Acute phase reactants; their synthesis, turnover and biological significance. In Structure and Function of Plasma Proteins, Vol. 1 (Ed. A.C. Allison) pp. 73–125, Plenum Press, London.

Koller, F. (1973) Theory and experience behind the use of coagulation tests in diagnosis and prognosis of liver disease. Scandinavian Journal of Gastroenterology, 8, Suppl. 19, 51–61.

Korman, M.G., Hofmann, A.F. and Summerskill, W.H.J. (1974) Assessment of activity in chronic active liver disease: serum bile acids compared with conventional tests and histology. New England Journal of Medicine, 290, 1399–1402.

Korman, M.G., LaRusso, N.F., Hoffman, N.E., Hofmann, A.F. (1975) Development of an intravenous bile acid tolerance test: plasma disappearance of cholylglycine in health. New England Journal of Medicine, 292, 1205–1209.

Krebs, J. and Brauer, R.W. (1949) Uptake of bromsulphthalein by the liver of the rat: studies with radioactive bromsulphthalein (BSP). Federation Proceedings, 8, 310.

Krugman, S., Friedman, H. and Lattimer, C. (1975) Viral hepatitis, type A: identification by specific complement fixation and immune adherence tests. New England Journal of Medicine, 292, 1141–1143.

Krugman, S., Giles, J.P. and Hammond, J. (1967) Infectious hepatitis: evidence for two distinctive clinical, epidemological and immunological types of infection. Journal of the American Medical Association, 200, 365–373.

Lam, K.C., Mistilis, S.P. and Perrott, M. (1972) Positive tissue antibody tests in patients with prolonged extra-hepatic biliary obstruction. New England Journal of Medicine, 286, 1400–1401.

LaMont, J.T. and Isselbacher, K.J. (1973) Postoperative jaundice. New England Journal of Medicine, 288, 305–307.

Landau, S., Salwen, M., Posner, A. and Silverberg, S.G. (1967) Anaphylactoid reaction to sodium sulfobromophthalein. Journal of the American Medical Association, 202, 238–239.

LaRusso, N.F., Hoffman, N.E., Hofmann, A.F. and Korman, M.G. (1975) Validity and sensitivity of an intravenous bile acid tolerance test in patients with liver disease. New England Journal of Medicine, 292, 1209–1214.

LaRusso, N.F., Korman, M.G., Hoffman, N.E. and Hoffmann, A.F. (1974) Dynamics of the enterohepatic circulation of bile acids. New England Journal of Medicine, 291, 689–692.

LaRusso, N.F., Summerskill, W.H.J. and McCall, J.T. (1976) Abnormalities of chemical tests for copper metabolism in chronic active liver disease: differentiation from Wilson's disease. Gastroenterology, 70, 653–655.

Laurell, C.-B. (1965) Antigen antibody crossed electrophoresis. Analytical Biochemistry, 10, 358–361.

Lauterberg, B. and Bircher, J. (1973) Hepatic microsomal drug metabolizing capacity measured in vivo by breath analysis. Gastroenterology, 65, 556 (abstract).

Leevy, C.M. (1965) Clinical aspects of the hepatic circulation. Gastroenterology, 48, 790–804.

Leevy, C.M., Smith, F., Longueville, J., Paumgartner, G. and Howard, M.M. (1967) Indocyanine green clearance as a test for hepatic function: evaluation by dichromatic ear densitometry. Journal of the American Medical Association, 200, 236–240.

Lester, R. (1964) The intestinal phase of bile pigment excretion. Gastroenterology, 47, 424–427.

Levi, A.J., Gatmaitan, Z. and Arias, I.M. (1969) Two hepatic cytoplasmic protein fractions, Y and Z and their possible role in the hepatic uptake of bilirubin, of sulfobromophthalein and other anions. Journal of Clinical Investigation, 48, 2156–2167.

Levine, R.A. and Klatskin, G. (1964) Unconjugated hyperbilirubinemia in the absence of overt hemolysis: importance of acquired disease as an etiologic factor in 366 adolescent and adult subjects. American Journal of Medicine, 36, 541–552.

Lieber, C.S. (1975) Interference of ethanol in hepatic cellular metabolism. Annals of the New York Academy of Sciences, 252, 24–50.

Lieberman, F.L. and Reynolds, T.B. (1967) Plasma volume in cirrhosis of the liver: its relation to portal hypertension, ascites and renal failure. Journal of Clinical Investigation, 46, 1297–1308.

Lieberman, J., Mittman, C. and Schneider, A.S. (1969) Screening for homozygous and heterozygous α_1-antitrypsin deficiency. Journal of the American Medical Association, 210, 2055–2060.

London, I.M., West, R., Shemin, D. and Rittenberg, D. (1950) On the origin of bile pigment in normal man. Journal of Biological Chemistry, 184, 351–358.

Lum, G. and Gambino, S.R. (1972) Serum gamma-glutamyl transpeptidase activity as an indicator of disease of liver, pancreas or bone. Clinical Chemistry, 18, 358–362.

McFadzean, A.J.S. and Yeung, R.T.T. (1969) Further observations on hypoglycaemia in hepatocellular carcinoma. American Journal of Medicine, 47, 220–235.

McIntyre, N., Clink, H.M., Levi, A.J., Cummings, J.N. and Sherlock, S. (1967) Hemolytic anaemia in Wilson's disease. New England Journal of Medicine, 276, 439–444.

McIntyre, N., Harry, D.S. and Pearson, A.J.G. (1975) The hypercholesterolaemia of obstructive jaundice. Gut, 16, 379–391.

McIntyre, N. and Heathcote, J. (1974) The laboratory in the diagnosis and management of viral hepatitis. Clinics in Gastroenterology, 3, 317–336.

MacSween, R.N.M., Yeung Laiwah, A.A.C., Busuttil, A.A., Thomas, M.A., Ross, S.K., Watkinson, G., Millman, I. and Blumberg, B.S. (1973) Australia antigen and primary biliary cirrhosis. Journal of Clinical Pathology, 26, 335–339.

MacSween, R.N.M., Horne, C.H.W., Moffat, A.J. and Hughes, H.M. (1972) Serum protein levels in primary biliary cirrhosis. Journal of Clinical Pathology, 25, 789–792.

McLean, A.E.M. (1962) Serum enzymes during recovery from malnutrition. Lancet, ii, 1294–1295.

Maddrey, W.C., Saito, S., Shulman, N.R. and Klatskin, G. (1972) Coincidental Australia antigenemia in primary biliary cirrhosis. Annals of Internal Medicine, 76, 705–709.

Mancini, G., Carbonara, A.O. and Heremans, J.F. (1965) Immunochemical quantitation of antigens by single radial immunodiffusion. International Journal of Immunochemistry, 2, 235–254.

Mandema, E., De Fraiture, W.H., Nieweg, H.O. and Arends, A. (1960) Familial chronic idiopathic jaundice (Dubin–Sprinz disease), with a note on brom-sulphalein metabolism in this disease. American Journal of Medicine, 28, 42–50.

Manghani, K.K., Lunzer, M.R., Billing, B.H. and Sherlock, S. (1975) Urinary and serum octopamine in patients with portal-systemic encephalopathy. Lancet, ii, 943–946.

Margolis, S. and Homcy, C. (1972) Systemic manifestations of hepatoma. Medicine, 51, 381–391.

Martin, J.F., Mikulecky, M., Blaschke, T.F., Waggoner, J.G., Vergalla, J. and Berk, P.D. (1975) Differences between the plasma indocyanine green disappearance rates of normal men and women (39090) Proceedings of the Society for Experimental Biology and Medicine, 150, 612–617.

Martin, J.F., Vierling, J.M., Wolkoff, A.W., Scharschmidt, B.F., Vergalla, J., Waggoner, J.G. and Berk, P.D. (1976) Abnormal hepatic transport of indocyanine green in Gilbert's syndrome. Gastroenterology, 70, 385–391.

Megyesi, C., Samols, E. and Marks, V. (1967) Glucose tolerance and diabetes in chronic liver disease. Lancet, ii, 1051–1056.

Mendenhall, C.L. and Leevy, C.M. (1961) False-negative bromsulfalein tests. New England Journal of Medicine, 264, 431–433.

Mezey, E., Cherrick, G.R. and Holt, P.R. (1968) Serum alcohol dehydrogenase, an indication of intrahepatic cholestasis. New England Journal of Medicine, 279, 241–248.

Miller, L.H. and Brown, H.W. (1969) The serologic diagnosis of parasitic infections in medical practice. Annals of Internal Medicine, 71, 983–991.

Miller, W.J., Provost, P.J., McAleer, W.J., Ittensohn, O.L., Villarejos, V.M. and Hilleman, M.R. (1975) Specific immunoadherence assay for human hepatitis A antibody: application to diagnostic and epidemiologic investigations. Proceedings of the Society for Experimental Biology and Medicine, 149, 254–261.

Minchin-Clarke, H.G. and Freeman, T. (1968) Quantitative immunoelectrophoresis of human serum proteins. Clinical Sciences, 35, 403–413.

Miyada, D.S., Baysinger, V., Notrice, S. and Nakamura, R.M. (1972) Albumin quantitation by dye binding and salt fractionation techniques. Clinical Chemistry, 18, 52–56.

Morgenstern, L. (1974) Postoperative jaundice: an approach to a diagnostic dilemma. American Journal of Surgery, 128, 255–261.

Mosbach, E.H. (1972) Hepatic synthesis of bile acids: biochemical steps and mechanisms of rate control. Archieves of Internal Medicine, 130, 478–487.

Mossberg, S.M. and Ross, G. (1963) High serum transaminase activity associated with extrahepatic biliary disease: a clinical and pathologic study of sixty patients with serum glutamic-oxalacetic transaminase levels of 300 units or greater. Gastroenterology, 45, 345–353.

Murray-Lyon, I.M., Minchin-Clarke, H.G., McPherson, K. and Williams, R. (1972) Quantitative immunoelectrophoresis of serum proteins in cryptogenic cirrhosis, alcoholic cirrhosis and active chronic hepatitis. Clinica Chimica Acta, 39, 215–220.

Murray-Lyon, I.M., Orr, A.H., Gazzard, B., Kohn, J. and Williams, R. (1976) Prognostic value of serum alpha-fetoprotein in fulminant hepatic failure including patients treated by charcoal haemoperfusion. Gut, 17, 576–580.

Murray-Lyon, I.M. and Williams, R. (1974) Quantitative immunoelectrophoresis of plasma proteins in acute viral hepatitis, extrahepatic biliary obstruction, primary biliary cirrhosis and idiopathic haemochromatosis. Clinica Chimica Acta, 51, 303–308.

Naftalin, L., Child, V.J., Morley, D.A. and Smith, D.A. (1969) Observations on the site of origin of serum gamma-glutamyltranspeptidase. Clinica Chimica Acta, 26, 297–300.

Nayak, N.C., Chawla, V., Malaviya, A.N. and Chandra, R.K. (1972) α-Fetoprotein in Indian childhood cirrhosis. Lancet, i, 68–69.

Neale, G., Caughey, D.E., Mollin, D.L. and Booth, C.C. (1966) Effects of intrahepatic and extrahepatic infection on liver function. British Medical Journal, 1, 382–387.

Neale, G., Lewis, B., Weaver, V. and Panveliwalla, D. (1971) Serum bile acids in liver diseases. Gut, 12, 145–152.

Neefe, J.R. and Reinhold, J.G. (1946) Laboratory aids in diagnosis and management of infectious (epidemic) hepatitis; analysis of results obtained by studies on 34 volunteers during early convalescent stages of induced hepatitis. Gastroenterology, 7, 393–413.

Nielsen, J.O., Dietrichson, O., Elling, P. and Christoffersen, P. (1971) Incidence and meaning of persistence of Australia antigen in patients with acute viral hepatitis: development of chronic hepatitis. New England Journal of Medicine, 285, 1157–1160.

Nilsson, L.H. and Hultman, E. (1974) A comparison of the bromsulphalein and galactose elimination test in patients with either chronic bowel inflammation or alcoholic liver disease. Scandinavian Journal of Gastroenterology, 9, 319–323.

Nosslin, B. (1960) The direct diazo reaction of bile pigments in serum: experimental and clinical studies. Scandinavian Journal of Clinical and Laboratory Investigation, 12, Suppl. 49, 1–176.

Okada, K., Kamiyama, I., Inomata, M., Imai, M., Miyakawa, Y. and Mayumi, M. (1976) e-Antigen and anti-e in the serum of asymptomatic carrier mothers as indicators of positive and negative transmission of hepatitis B virus to their infants. New England Journal of Medicine, 294, 746–749.

Okolicsanyi, L., Torrado, A., Nussle, D., Gardiol, D. and Gautier, A. (1969) Etude clinique et ultrastructurale d'un cas de syndrome de Rotor. Revue Internationale de Hepatologie, 19, 393–406.

Owens, D. and Sherlock, S. (1973) Diagnosis of Gilbert's syndrome: role of reduced caloric intake test. British Medical Journal, 3, 559–563.

Papadopoulos, N.M. and Charles, M.A. (1970) Serum lipprotein patterns in liver disease. Proceedings of the Society for Experimental Biology and Medicine, 134, 797–799.

Paumgartner, G., Probst, Kraines, R. and Leevy, C.M. (1970) Kinetics of indocyanine green removal from the blood. Annals of the New York Academy of Sciences, 170, 134–147.

Petersen, P., Christoffersen, P., Elling, P., Juhl, E., Dietrichson, O., Faber, V., Iversen, K., Nielsen, J.O. and Poulsen, H. (1974) Acute viral hepatitis: a survey of 500 patients. Clinical biochemical, immunological and morphological features at time of diagnosis. Scandinavian Journal of Gastroenterology, 9, 607–613.

Phelan, M.B., Neale, G. and Moss, D.W. (1971) Serial studies of serum alkaline phosphatase and 5'-nucleotidase levels in hepatobiliary disease. Clinica Chimica Acta, 32, 95–102.

Poland, R.L. and Odell, G.B. (1971) Physiologic jaundice: the enterohepatic circulation of bilirubin. New England Journal of Medicine, 284, 1–6.

Poley, J.R., Alaupovic, P., McConathy, W.J., Seidel, D., Roy, C.C. and Weber, A. (1973) Diagnosis of extrahepatic biliary obstruction in infants by immunochemical detection of LP-X and modified ^{131}I-Rose Bengal excretion test. Journal of Laboratory and Clinical Medicine, 81, 325–341.

Pollock, M.R. (1945) Pre-icteric stage of infectious hepatitis: value of biochemical findings in diagnosis. Lancet, ii, 626–630.

Potter, B.J., Trueman, A.M. and Jones, E.A. (1973) Serum complement in chronic liver disease. Gut, 14, 451–456.

Prieto, J., Barry, M. and Sherlock, S. (1975) Serum ferritin in patients with iron overload and with acute and chronic liver diseases. Gastroenterology, 68, 525–533.

Quarfordt, S.H., Hilderman, H.L., Valle, D. and Waddel, E. (1971) Compartmental analysis of sulfobromophthalein transport in normal patients and patients with hepatic dysfunction. Gastroenterology, 60, 246–255.

Quarfordt, S.H., Oelschlager, H., Krigbaum, W.R., Jakoi, L. and Davis, R. (1973) Effect of biliary obstruction on canine plasma and biliary lipids. Lipids, 8, 522–530.

Quick, A.J. (1933) The synthesis of hippuric acid: a new test of liver function. American Journal of Medical Sciences, 185, 630–635.

Rachmilewitz, M. and Eliakim, M. (1968) Serum B_{12}: a diagnostic test in liver disease. Israel Journal of Medical Sciences, 4, 47–54.

Rachmilewitz, M., Moshkowitz, B., Rachmilewitz, B., Gosswicz, N. and Gross, J. (1972) Serum vitamin B_{12} protein in viral hepatitis. European Journal of Clinical Investigation, 2, 239–242.

Raymond, G.D. and Galambos, J.T. (1971) Hepatic storage and excretion of bilirubin in the dog. American Journal of Gastroenterology, 55, 119–134.

Record, C.O., Iles, R.A., Cohen, R.D. and Williams, R. (1975) Acid–base and metabolic disturbances in fulminant hepatic failure. Gut, 16, 144–149.

Reichle. F.A., Bernstein, M.R., Hower, R.D., Reichle, R.M., Shuman, L.S. and Rosemond, G.P. (1973) Urea cycle enzyme activity in human hepatic cirrhosis after experimental portocaval shunt. Surgical Forum, 24, 246–248.

Remmer, H., Schoene, B., Fleischmann, R. and Held, H. (1973) Induction of the unspecific microsomal hydroxylase in the human liver. In The Liver: Quantitative Aspects of Structure and Function (Eds. G. Paumgartner and R. Preisig) pp. 232–240, Karger, Basel.

Richárds, T.G., Tindall, V.R. and Young, A. (1959) A modification of the bromsulphthalein liver function test to predict the dye content of the liver and bile. Clinical Sciences, 18, 499–511.

Ritland, S. (1976) The abnormal "lipoprotein of cholestasis", lipoprotein-X. Scandinavian Journal of Gastroenterology, 10, 785–789.

Ritland, S., Blomhoff, J.P., Elgjo, K. and Gjone, E. (1973) Lipoprotein-X (LP-X) in liver disease. Scandinavian Journal of Gastroenterology, 8, 155–160.

Ritt, D.J., Whelan, G., Werner, D.J., Eigenbrodt, E.H., Schenker, S. and Combes, B. (1969) Acute hepatic necrosis with stupor or coma. An analysis of thrity-one patients. Medicine, 48, 151–172.

Roberts, H.R. and Cederbaum, A.I. (1972) The liver and blood coagulation: physiology and pathology. Gastroenterology, 63, 297–320.

Rodriquez, M., Paronetto, F., Schaffner, F. and Popper, H. (1969) Antimitochondrial antibodies in jaundice following drug administration. Journal of the American Medical Association, 208, 148–150.

Rosalki, S.B. and Rau, D. (1972) Serum-glutamyl transpeptidase activity in alcoholism. Clinica Chimica Acta, 39, 41–47.

Rosenthal, S.M. and White, E.C. (1925) Clinical application of the bromsulphalein test for hepatic function. Journal of the American Medical Association, 84, 1112–1114.

Rothschild, M.A., Oratz, M. and Schreiber, S.S. (1973) Albumin metabolism. Gastroenterology, 64, 324–337.

Rothschild, M.A., Oratz, M., Zimmon, D., Schrieber, S.S., Weiner, I. and Van Caneghan, A. (1969) Albumin synthesis in cirrhotic subjects with ascites studied with carbonate-^{14}C. Journal of Clinical Investigation, 48, 344–350.

Rotor, A.B., Manahan, L. and Florentin, A. (1948) Familial non-hemolytic jaundice with direct Vandenberg reaction. Acta Medica Philippina, 5, 37–49.

Roux, M.E.B., Florin-Christensen, A., Arana, R.M. and Doniach, D. (1974) Paraproteins with antibody activity in acute viral hepatitis and chronic autoimmune liver diseases. Gut, 15, 396–400.

Ruddy, S., Gigli, I. and Austen, K.F. (1972) The complement system of man I and II. New England Journal of Medicine, 287, 489–495 and 545–549.

Rudman, D., DiFulco, T.J., Galambos, J.T., Smith, R.B. III, Salam, A.F. and Warren, W.D. (1973) Maximal rates of excretion and synthesis of urea in normal and cirrhotic subjects. Journal of Clinical Investigation, 52, 2241–2249.

Salkie, M.L. (1971) Too many tests? Lancet, ii, 915–916.

Samson, R.I., Trey, C., Timme, A.H. and Saunders, S.H. (1967) Fulminating hepatitis with recurrent hypoglycaemia and hemorrhage. Gastroenterology, 53, 291–300.

Schaffner, F. (1969) Paradoxical elevation of serum cholesterol by clofibrate in patients with primary biliary cirrhosis. Gastroenterology, 57, 253–255.

Schalm, L. and Weber, A.P. (1964) Jaundice with conjugated bilirubin in hyperhaemolysis. Acta Medica Scandinavica, 176, 549–553.

Schalm, S.W., Turcotte, J., Hofmann, A.F. and Cowen, A.E. (1975) A new bile acid radioimmunoassay: development, validation and preliminary application of an assay for chenodeoxycholyl conjugates. Gastroenterology, 68, 913.

Scharschmidt, B.F., Waggoner, J.G. and Berk, P.D. (1975) Hepatic organic anion uptake in the rat. Journal of Clinical Investigation, 56, 1280–1292.

Scheinberg, I.H. (1973) Doubt Wilson disease (letter). Archives of Neurology, 29, 449.

Scheinberg, I.H. and Sternlieb, I. (1963) Wilson's disease and the concentration of caeruloplasmin in serum. Lancet, i, 1420–1421.

Schenker, S., Breen, K.J. and Hoyumpa, A.M., Jr. (1974) Hepatic encephalopathy: current status. Gastroenterology, 66, 121–151.

Schiff, L., Billing, B.H. and Oikawa, V. (1959) Familial nonhemolytic jaundice with conjugated bilirubin in the serum: a case study. New England Journal of Medicine, 260, 1315–1318.

Schmid, M., Hefti, M.L., Gattiker, R., Kistler, H.J. and Senning, A. (1965) Benign postoperative intrahepatic cholestasis. New England Journal of Medicine, 272, 545–550.

Schmid, R. (1972) Hyperbilirubinemia. In The Metabolic Basis of Inherited Disease, 3rd edn. (Eds. J.B. Stanbury, J.B., Wyngaarden and D.S. Fredrickson) pp. 1141–1178, McGraw Hill, New York.

Schmid, R. and Hammaker, L. (1959) Glucuronide formation in patients with constitutional hepatic dysfunction (Gilbert's disease). New England Journal of Medicine, 260, 1310–1314.

Schmidt, M., Frohlich, G., Schmidt, D. and Stich, W. (1971) Der Urobilinkorperstoffwechsel des Menschen. I. Eine neue Methode zur Bestimmung der Urobilinkörper im menschlichen serum und Harn. Blut, 22, 120–124.

Schoenfield, L.J., Onstad, G.R. and Goldstein, N.P. (1970) Normal sulfobromophthalein retention in established liver disease. American Journal of Digestive Diseases, 15, 337–342.

Schoenfield, L.J., McGill, D.B., Hunton, D.B., Foulk, W.T. and Butt, H.R. (1963) Studies of chronic idiopathic jaundice (Dubin–Johnson syndrome) 1. Demonstration of hepatic excretory defect. Gastroenterology, 44, 101–111.

Seidel, D., Alaupovic, P. and Furman, R.H. (1969) A lipoprotein characterizing obstructive jaundice. I. Method for quantitative separation and identification of lipoproteins in jaundiced subjects. Journal of Clinical Investigations, 48, 1211–1223.

Seidel, D., Gretz, H. and Ruppert, C. (1973) Significance of the LP-X test in differential diagnosis of jaundice. Clinical Chemistry, 19, 86–91.

Sereny, G. and McLaughlin, L. (1970) Serum alkaline phosphatase values in normal adolescents. Canadian Medical Association Journal, 102, 1400–1401.

Shani, M., Gilon, E., Ben-Ezzer, J. and Sheba, C. (1970a) Sulfobromophthalein tolerance test in patients with Dubin–Johnson syndrome and their relatives. Gastroenterology, 59, 842–847.

Shani, M., Seligsohn, U., Gilon, E., Sheba, C. and Adam, A. (1970b) Dubin–Johnson syndrome in Israel. I Clinical, laboratory and genetic aspects of 101 cases. Quarterly Journal of Medicine, 39, 549–567.

Sharp, H.L. (1976) The current status of α-1-antitrypsin, a protease inhibitor, in gastrointestinal disease. Gastroenterology, 70, 611–621.

Sherlock, S. (1975) Diseases of the Liver and Biliary System, 5th edn. Blackwell, Oxford.

Sherlock, S. and Scheuer, P.J. (1973) The presentation and diagnosis of 100 patients with primary biliary cirrhosis. New England Journal of Medicine, 289, 674–678.

Sherlock, S., Senewiratne, B., Scott, A. and Walker, J.G. (1966) Complications of diuretic therapy in hepatic cirrhosis. Lancet, i, 1049–1052.

Shore, G.M., Hoberman, L., Dowdey, A.B.C. and Combes, B. (1975) Serum gamma-glutamyl transpeptidase activity in normal children. American Journal of Clinical Pathology, 63, 245–250.

Shull, H.J., Wilkinson, G.R., Johnson, R. and Schenker, S. (1976) Normal disposition of oxazepam in acute viral hepatitis and cirrhosis. Annals of Internal Medicine, 84, 420–425.

Silver, H.K.B., Denault, J., Gold, P., Thompson, W.G., Shuster, J. and Freedman, S.O. (1974a) The detection of α_1-fetoprotein in patients with viral hepatitis. Cancer Research, 34, 244–247.

Silver, H.K.B., Gold, P., Shuster, J., Javitt, N.B., Freedman, S.O. and Finlayson, N.D.C. (1974b) α_1-Fetoprotein in chronic liver disease. New England Journal of Medicine, 291, 506–508.

Simmonds, W.J., Korman, M.G. Go VLW and Hoffman, A.F. (1973) Radioimmunoassay of conjugated cholyl bile acids in serum. Gastroenterology, 65, 705–711.

Sjovall, J. (1959) Dietary glycine and taurine on bile acid conjugation in man; bile acids and steroids 75. Proceedings of the Society for Experimental Biology and Medicine, 100, 676–678.

Skrede, S., Blomhoff, J.P., Elgjo, K., Gjone, E. (1973) Biochemical tests in evaluation of liver function. Scandinavian Journal of Gastroenterology, Suppl. 19, 37–46.

Small, D.M. (1971) The physical chemistry of cholanic acids. In The Bile Acids (Eds. P.P. Nair and D. Kritchevsky) pp. 249–355, Plenum, New York.

Smith, M.G.M., Williams, R., Doniach, D. and Calne, R.Y. (1971) Effect of orthotopic liver transplantation on serum autoantibodies. Lancet, ii, 1006–1009.

Smith, M.G.M., Williams, R., Walker, J.G., Rizzetto, M. and Doniach, D. (1974) Hepatic disorders associated with liver–kidney microsomal antibodies. British Medical Journal, 2, 80–84.

Soler, N.G., Jain, S., James, H. and Paton, A. (1976) Potassium status of patients with cirrhosis. Gut, 17, 152–157.

Soloway, R.D., Summerskill, W.H.J., Baggenstoss, A.H. and Schoenfeld, L. (1972) "Lupoid" hepatitis a nonentity in the spectrum of chronic active liver disease. Gastroenterology, 63, 458–465.

Sprinz, J. and Nelson, R.S. (1954) Persistant nonhemolytic hyperbilirubinemia associated with lipochrome-like pigment in liver cells: Report of four cases. Annals of Internal Medicine, 41, 952–962.

Stern, R.B., Knill-Jones, R.P. and Williams, R. (1973) Pitfalls in the diagnosis of jaundice due to carcinoma of the pancreas or biliary tree. British Medical Journal, 1, 533–534.

Sternlieb, I. (1972) Evolution of the hepatic lesion in Wilson's disease (hepatolenticular degeneration). Progress in Liver Diseases, 4, 511–525.

Sternlieb, I. and Scheinberg, I.H. (1972) Chronic hepatitis as a first manifestation of Wilson's disease. Annals of Internal Medicine, 76, 59–64.

Stiehl, A., Ast, E., Czygan, P. and Liersch, M. (1976) Formation, metabolism, and excretion of bile salt sulfates in man. In The Hepatobiliary System: Fundamental and Pathological Mechanisms (Ed. W. Taylor), pp. 453–468, Plenum, New York.

Strandjord, P.E., Clayson, K.J. and Roby, R.J. (1973) Computer assisted pattern recognition and the diagnosis of liver disease. Human Pathology, 4, 67–77.

Strickland, G.T. and Leu, M.-L. (1975) Wilson's disease. Clinical and laboratory manifestations in 40 patients. Medicine, 54, 113–137.

Sturdevant, R.A.L. (1973) Antimitochondrial antibody in diagnosis of liver disease. Annals of Internal Medicine, 78, 313–314.

Talamo, R.C., Langley, C.E., Reed, C.E. and Makino, S. (1973) α_1-Antitrypsin deficiency: a variant with no detectable α_1-antitrypsin. Science, 181, 70–71.

Tavill, A.S. (1972) The synthesis and degradation of liver produced proteins. Gut, 13, 225–241.

Tengström, B. (1968) An intravenous galactose tolerance test and its use in hepatobiliary diseases. Acta Medica Scandinavica, 183, 31–40.

Tenhunen, R., Marver, H.S. and Schmid, R. (1968) The enzymatic conversion of heme to bilirubin by microsomal heme oxygenase. Proceedings of the National Academy of Sciences of the U.S.A., 61, 748–755.

Triger, D.R. and Wright, R. (1973) Hyperglobulinaemia in liver disease. Lancet, i, 1494–1496.

Tygstrup, N. (1961) The urinary excretion of galactose and its significance in clinical intravenous galactose tolerance tests. Acta Physiologica Scandinavica, 51, 263–274.

Tygstrup, N. (1963) Determination of the hepatic galactose capacity after a single intravenous injection in man: the reproducibility and the influence of uneven distribution. Acta Physiologica Scandinavica, 58, 162–172.

Tygstrup, N. (1964a) The galactose elimination capacity in control subjects and in patients with cirrhosis of the liver. Acta Medica Scandinavica, 175, 281–289.

Tygstrup, N. (1964b) The galactose elimination capacity in relation to clinical and laboratory findings in patients with cirrhosis. Acta Medica Scandinavica, 175, 291–300.

Tygstrup, N. and Winkler, K. (1954) Kinetics of galactose elimination. Acta Physiologica Scandinavica, 32, 354–362.

Tygstrup, N. and Winkler, K. (1958) Galactose blood clearance as a measure of hepatic blood flow. Clinical Science, 17, 1–9.

Tytgat, G.N., Collen, D. and Verstraete, M. (1971) Metabolism of fibrogen in cirrhosis of the liver. Journal of Clinical Investigation, 50, 1690–1701.

Verwilghen, R., Verhaegen, H., Waumans, P. and Beert, J. (1969) Ineffective erythropoiesis with morphologically abnormal erythroblasts and unconjugated hyperbilirubinaemia. British Journal of Haematology, 17, 27–33.

Wacker, W.E.C., Riorden, J.F., Snodgrass, P.J., Chang, L.W., Morse, L.J., O'Brien, T.F. and Reddy, W.J. (1972) The Holy Cross hepatitis outbreak: clinical and chemical abnormalities. Archives of Internal Medicine, 130, 357–360.

Waldmann, T.A. (1966) Protein-losing enteropathy. Gastroenterology, 50, 422–443.

Waldmann, T.A. and McIntire, K.R. (1974) The use of radioimmunoassay for alpha-fetoprotein in the diagnosis of malignancy. Cancer, 34, 1510–1515.

Waldstein, S.S., Greenburg, L.A., Biggs, A.D. Jr. and Coin, L. (1960) Demonstration of hepatic maximum removal capacity (L_m) for galactose in humans. Journal of Laboratory and Clinical Medicine, 55, 462–475.

Walker, J.G., Doniach, D. and Doniach, L. (1970) Mitochondrial antibodies and subclinical liver disease. Quarterly Journal of Medicine, 39, 31–48.

Walsh, P.N. and Kissane, J.M. (1968) Non-metastic hypernephroma with reversible hepatic dysfunction. Archives of Internal Medicine, 122, 214–222.

Walshe, J.M. and Briggs, J. (1962) Caeruloplasmin in liver disease. A diagnostic pitfall. Lancet, ii, 263–265.

Warnes, T.W. (1972) Alkaline phosphatase. Gut, 13, 926–929.

Watson, C.J. (1937) Studies of urobilinogen: urobilinogen in urine and faeces of subjects without evidence of disease of liver or biliary tract. Archives of Internal Medicine, 59, 196–205.

Watson, C.J. (1956) The importance of the fractional serum bilirubin determination in clinical medicine. Annals of Internal Medicine, 45, 351–368.

Watson, C.J. (1976a) In The Chemistry and Physiology of Bile Pigments (Eds. P.D. Berk and N.I. Berlin) U.S. Department of Health Education and Welfare Publication, U.S. Government Printing Office, Washington, D.C., pp. 3–16.

Watson, C.J. and Hoffbauer, F.W. (1947) Liver function in hepatitis. Annals of Internal Medicine, 26, 813–842.

Waxman, S. and Gilbert, H.S. (1973) A tumor related vitamin B_{12} binding protein in adolescent hepatoma. New England Journal of Medicine, 289, 1053–1056.

Wheeler, H.O., Cranston, W.I. and Meltzer, J.I. (1958) Hepatic uptake and biliary excretion of indocyanine green in the dog. Proceedings of the Society for Experimental Biology and Medicine, 99, 11–14.

Wheeler, H.O., Meltzer, J.I. and Bradley, S.E. (1960) Biliary transport and hepatic storage of sulfobromophthalein sodium in the unanaesthetized dog, in normal man and in patients with hepatic disease. Journal of Clinical Investigation, 39, 1131–1144.

Whitfield, J.B., Pounder, R.E., Neale, G. and Moss, D.W. (1972) Serum γ-glutamyl transpedtidase activity in liver disease. Gut, 13, 702–708.

Wieme, R.J. and Demeulenaere, L. (1971) Enzyme assays in liver disease. Journal of Clinical Pathology, 24, Suppl. 4, 51–59.

Wilkinson, J.H. (1970a) Clinical significance of enzyme activity measurements. Clinical Chemistry, 16, 882–890.

Wilkinson, J.H. (1970b) Clinical applications of isoenzymes. Clinical Chemistry, 16, 733–739.

Williams, R. (1972) Problems of fulminant hepatic failure. British Medical Bulletin, 28, 114–119.

Williams, R. and Smith, M.G.M. (1972) Liver transplantation: a clinical and immunological appraisal. Progress in Liver Disease, 4, 433–446.

Williams, R., Smith, M., Shilkin, K.B., Herbertson, B., Joysey, V. and Calne, R.Y. (1973) Liver transplantation in man: the frequency of rejection, biliary tract complications and recurrence of malignancy based on an analysis of 26 cases. Gastroenterology, 64, 1026–1048.

Winkelman, J., Nedler, S., Demetriou, J. and Pileggi, V.J. (1972) The clinical usefulness of alkaline phosphatase isoenzyme determinations. American Journal of Clinical Pathology, 57, 625–634.

With, T.K. (1968) The bile pigments in urine. The bile pigments in faeces. In The Bile Pigments. pp. 491–557, 585–613, Academic Press, New York.

Wolkoff, A.W., Cohen, L.F. and Arias, I.M. (1973) Inheritance of the Dubin–Johnson syndrome. New England Journal of Medicine, 288, 113–117.

Wolkoff, A.W., Wolpert, E., Pascasio, F.N. and Arias, I.M. (1976) Rotor's syndrome: a distant inheritable pathophysiologic entity. American Journal of Medicine, 60, 173–179.

Woolf, I.L., Boyes, B.E., Jones, D.M., Whittaker, J.G., Tapp, E., MacSween, R.N.M., Renbon, P.H., Stratton, F. and Dymock, I.W. (1974) Asymptomatic liver disease in hepatitis-B antigen carriers. Journal of Clinical Pathology, 27, 348–352.

Yeung, C.Y. (1972) Serum 5′-nucleotidase in neonatal hepatitis and biliary atresia: preliminary observations. Pediatrics, 50, 812–814.

Zelman, S. (1952) The liver in obesity. Archives of Internal Medicine, 90, 141–156.

Zeltzer, P.M., Neerhout, R.C., Foukalsrud, E.W. and Stienhm, E.R. (1974) Differentiation between neonatal hepatitis and biliary atresia by measuring serum alpha-fetoprotein. Lancet, i, 373–375.

Zieve, L. (1966) Hemolytic anemia in liver disease. Medicine, 45, 497–505.

Zieve, L. and Hill, E. (1955) An evaluation of factors influencing the discriminative effectiveness of a group of liver function tests. I. Normal limits of eleven representative hepatic tests. Gastroenterology, 28, 766–784.

Zieve, L., Hill, E., Hanson, M., Falcone, A.B. and Watson, C.J. (1951) Normal and abnormal variation and clinical significance of the one-minute and total serum bilirubin determinations. Journal of Laboratory and Clinical Medicine, 38, 446–469.

Zimmerman, H.J. (1974) Hepatic injury caused by therapeutic agents. In The Liver, Normal and Abnormal Function (Ed. F.F. Becker) pp. 225–302, Marcel Dekker, New York.

Zimmerman, H.J. and Seeff, L.B. (1970) Enzymes in hepatic disease. In Diagnostic Enzymology (Ed. E.L. Coodley) pp. 1–38, Lea and Febiger, Philadelphia.

ADDITIONAL REFERENCES

Bennhold, H. and Kallee, E. (1959) Comparative studies on the half-life of ^{131}I-labelled albumins and nonradioactive human serum albumin in a case of analbuminemia. Journal of Clinical Investigation, 38, 363–372.

Carey, J.B., Jr. (1973) In The Bile Acids, Vol. 2 (Eds. P.B. Nair and D. Kritchevsky) pp. 55–82, Plenum Press, New York.

Combes, B. and Schenker, S. (1975) Laboratory tests. In Diseases of the Liver, 4th edn. (Ed. L. Schiff) pp. 204–246, J.B. Lippincott Co., Philadelphia.

Danielsson, H. (1976) Bile acid metabolism and its control. In The Hepatobiliary System (Ed. W. Taylor) pp. 389–407, Plenum Press, New York.

Doniach, D. (1972) Autoimmunity in liver diseases. Progress in Clinical Immunology, 1, 45–70.

Erlanger, S., Glasinovic, J.C., Poupon, R. and Dumont, M. (1976) Hepatic transport of bile acids. In The Hepatobiliary System (Ed. W. Taylor) pp. 433–452, Plenum Press, New York.

Hadchouel, P., Charbonnier, A., Lageron, A., Lemonnier, F., Rautureau, M., Scott, J. et Caroli, J. (1971) A propos d'une nouvelle forme d'ictère chronique idiopathique. Hypothèse physiopatholigique. Revue Medico-Chirugicale des Maladies du Foie, 46, 61–68.

Hepner, G.W. and Demers, L.M. (1976) Aminopyrine metabolism and serum bile acids in patients with liver disease. In The Liver: Quantitative Aspects of Structure and Function, Vol. 2 (Eds. R. Preisig, J. Bircher and G. Paumgartner) pp. 309–314, Cantor, Aulendorf.

Hofmann, A.F. and Kern, F., Jr. (1971) Bile acids. Disease a Month, November, 1971.

Jarvitt, N.B. (1975) Bile acids and hepatobiliary disease. In Diseases of the Liver, 4th edn. (Ed. L. Schiff) pp. 111–145, J.B. Lippincott Co., Philadelphia.

Konttinen, A., Härtell, G. and Lonhija, A. (1970) Multiple serum enzyme analyses in chronic alcoholics. Acta Medica Scandinavica, 188, 257–264.

Leevy, C.M., Popper, H. and Sherlock, S. (1976) Diseases of the liver and biliary tract; standardization of nomenclature, diagnostic criteria and diagnostic methodology. Fogarty International Center Proceeding No. 22, DHEW Publication No. (NIH)76-725, U.S. Government Printing Office, Washington, D.C.

McIntyre, N., Agorastos, J. and Harry, D.S. (1975) Plasma lipid and lipoprotein determination as an index of liver function. In The Liver: Quantitative Aspects of Structure and Function (Eds. R. Preisig, J. Bircher and G. Paumgartner) pp. 408–412, Cantor, Aulendorf.

Maier, K.P., Volk, B., Hoppe-Seyler, G. and Gerok, W. (1974). Urea cycle enzymes in normal liver and in patients with alcoholic hepatitis. European Journal of Clinical Investigation, 4, 193–195.

Owens, D., Jones, E.A. and Carson, E.R. (1977) Studies of the kinetics of unconjugated [^{14}C]bilirubin metabolism in normal subjects and patients with compensated cirrhosis. Clinical Science and Molecular Medicine, 52, 555–570.

Preisig, R., Küpfer, A., Gikalov, I. and Bircher, J. (1976) Breath analysis of hepatic microsomal function in man. In The Liver: Quantitative Aspects of Structure and Function (Eds. R. Preisig, J. Bircher and G. Paumgartner) pp. 324–331, Cantor, Aulendorf.

Waldmann, T.A. and McIntire, K.R. (1972) Serum-α-foetoprotein levels in patients with ataxia telengiectasia, Lancet, ii, 1112–1115.

Watson, C.J. (1976b) The urobilinoids: milestones in their history and some recent developments. In The Chemistry and Physiology of Bile Pigments (Eds. P.D. Berk and N.I. Berlin) pp. 469–482, U.S. Department of Health Education and Welfare Publication, U.S. Government Printing Office, Washington, D.C.

Chapter 11

Gastric function

James B. Elder and Provash C. Ganguli

Department of Surgery, The Royal Infirmary, Manchester M13 9WL, England

CONTENTS

Chemical diagnosis of disease, edited by
S.S. Brown, F.L. Mitchell and D.S. Young

11.1. SALIVA

11.1.1. Physiology of salivary secretion

Saliva is the mixed serous and mucous secretion of the large and multiple small salivary glands of the mouth which aids in the tasting, chewing, lubricating and swallowing of food. Although very small amounts of saliva are secreted during rest, the rate of secretion varies widely and the total output in 24 hours is of the order of 800 ml. Primary salivary secretion takes place in the serous and mucous acini but this is modified by the duct epithelium during transport of saliva to the buccal cavity (Davenport, 1961). Most of these processes are under the influence of the autonomic nervous system and endocrine glands (Petersen, 1972). Mixed saliva aspirated from the mouth contains water, electrolytes, vitamins, enzymes, blood group substances, immunoglobulins and many other proteins. The age and sex of the subject, the typical diet, time of day, size of the glands, duration and nature of the stimuli, the flow rate of saliva from the glands, corticosteroids, gastrointestinal hormones and a variety of drugs, *all* affect the composition of the saliva (Mason and Chisholm, 1975). Salivary mucus, lysozyme, lactoferrin and thiocyanate-dependent factors appear to have an antibacterial function; they contribute to the maintenance of oral hygiene in addition to the mechanical washing action of the saliva and the subsequent removal of bacteria through the act of swallowing. The salivary glands have secretory IgA, as well as IgM and IgG, and these comprise a local immunological system. Anything, therefore, which promotes chewing stimulates salivary flow, strengthens the teeth and activates the above set of mechanisms. Particles of food remaining between the teeth, however, act as foci for bacterial proliferation and deposition of plaque.

11.1.2. Methods of investigation

The usual methods of investigation of salivary gland function comprise measurement of salivary flow rate and of alterations in composition of saliva, radioisotope scanning of the glands using ^{99m}technetium-labelled sodium pertechnetate, radiology and sialography, and tissue biopsy, as well as microbiological, serological, immunochemical and virological studies. Only the first two of these topics will be discussed here as they lend themselves to biochemical investigation.

11.1.3. Measurement of salivary flow rate

Secretion can be collected from the larger glands either in pure form by cannulation of the duct, or as mixed saliva. The techniques which have been employed for collecting parotid or submandibular gland secretions have involved the use of either a suction cup over the duct orifices or a polyethylene catheter within the specific ducts. Collection of mixed saliva can be achieved by spitting, by a suction cannula in the gingival sulcus or by the use of cotton rolls which soak up the secretion. Salivary flow rate may vary from being barely perceptible to as high as 4 ml/min. It may be studied under basal or stimulated conditions; a parasympathomimetic drug, such as pilocarpine, or a gustatory stimulus, like citric acid, is often used in the investigation. For a suitable test, stagnant secretions should be flushed out by a stimulant. This is followed by a period of 30 to 60 minutes during which the basal salivary secretory rate is studied; finally, the same or another stimulant is applied, and the maximum rate of flow studied for a further 5 minutes. General clinical states can influence the salivary flow; for example, stress, anxiety, dehydration or infection may decrease salivary secretion, while cigarette smoking may initially increase it. A very large number of drugs can alter salivary secretion (Mason and Chisholm, 1975).

Chronic dryness of the mouth (xerostomia) is fairly common and is not in itself a specific disease. This condition may be confirmed by measuring the flow rate of mixed salivary secretion by any of the methods outlined above. The commonest causes of xerostomia are Sjogren's disease, candiosis, systemic infections and endocrine disorders such as diabetes mellitus; in addition, it can result from the effects of drugs. It should not be confused with thirst, although patients with xerostomia may complain of thirst rather than dryness of the mouth as their chief or presenting complaint.

11.1.4. Alterations in the composition of saliva

In fibrocystic disease, the concentrations of sodium, calcium, phosphorus, urea and uric acid are all increased in salivary secretion. In infants, a salivary sodium secretion above 10 mmol/litre may be used as a screening test for this disorder (Lawson et al., 1969). However, the measurement of sodium and chloride in sweat after local stimulation by pilocarpine iontophoresis is more accurate as a diagnostic procedure in fibrocystic disease (Di Sant' Agnese et al., 1953; Gibson and Cooke, 1959). Together with the thyroid and the gastric mucosa, the salivary glands share the ability to concentrate iodine and bromine; these appear in the saliva and they may be used as markers of salivary gland function. The normal plasma/salivary iodide ratio is about 1:10 and this is altered in thyroid disease. Such measurements, however, have found favour only in the investigation of rare conditions such as dyshormonogenesis and congenital iodide trapping defects (Mason and Chisholm, 1975).

11.2. HYDROCHLORIC ACID

11.2.1. Physiology of gastric acid secretion

The stomach allows a relatively large quantity of food to be ingested, sterilized, mixed and then delivered in a co-ordinated fashion to the absorptive millieu of the small intestine. It thus functions as a "hopper and a mill". The storage of food in the proximal part of the stomach is accompanied by a receptive relaxation of the muscle wall and this is dependent upon the integrity of the vagal nerve supply. Hydrochloric acid, enzymes, electrolytes and intrinsic factor are secreted by the stomach in a total volume which is of the order of 1.5 litres per 24 hours. Mixing and churning of the food and gastric secretions takes place in the antrum resulting in the formation of chyme. During this process, the osmolarity of the meal is adjusted to about 300 to 350 mOsm/kg. Peristaltic waves begin in the fundus at a site known as the "pacemaker" and move distally through the antrum to the proximal duodenum. By this mechanism, gastric chyme is discharged intermittently into the duodenum. The so-called "pyloric sphincter' is, in fact, usually open for most of the inter-digestive periods, closing only intermittently during the time following ingestion of a meal.

Traditionally, gastric secretion is divided into three phases: "cephalic", "gastric" and "intestinal". However, these phases do not always occur sequentially and often overlap. The sight and smell of food initiate the "cephalic" phase of gastric secretion and the efferent impulses are carried by the vagus nerves. During this phase, hydrochloric acid, pepsin, mucus, intrinsic factor and gastrin are secreted. The magnitude of the cephalic phase in man is difficult to quantify, but probably amounts to no more than 20% of the maximal secretory capacity.

Both physical and chemical factors are responsible for the production of the "gastric" phase. Distension of the body of the stomach stimulates acid and pepsin secretion directly, and distension of the pyloric gland area also stimulates acid secretion by means of a pyloro-oxyntic reflex. Distension, together with amino acids or protein in the food, release gastrin from the endocrine cells in the pyloric gland area, provided that the antral pH is greater than 3. Gastrin is secreted into the portal circulation and traverses the liver, eventually reaching the acid-bearing area of the stomach via the systemic circulation. Here it stimulates hydrochloric acid secretion, but it is not known whether this action is mediated directly by gastrin or indirectly by histamine (Black et al., 1972) or acetylcholine. All the gastric secretions which are produced in the "cephalic" or "gastric" phases, whether of exocrine or endocrine origin, are under the control of short and long vagal nerve reflexes and are mediated by cholinergic mechanisms.

By means of a humoral mechanism, as yet not fully characterized, food in the upper small intestine also stimulates acid secretion from the stomach; it is likely that "intestinal gastrin" may be partly responsible for the "intestinal" phase of gastric secretion. However, some of the other gastrointestinal hormones may also stimulate the parietal cells as well as play a part in the control of gastric emptying.

Powerful inhibition of acid secretion occurs when acid or fat enters the duodenum and jejunum, and this is mediated by both neural and humoral mechanisms. Hyperosmolar solutions in the duodenum also inhibit acid and pepsin secretion from the stomach and osmoreceptors in the duodenum play a large part in the control of gastric emptying. In addition, there are many polypeptides in the intestinal mucosa which, under physiological conditions, may act as inhibitors of gastric secretion. Secretin, glucagon, gastric inhibitory polypeptide, vasoactive-intestinal polypeptide and urogastrone have been identified as possible candidates for this role; however, the precise effects and interactions of these substances await further elucidation. It is evident that the interplay of excitatory and inhibitory mechanisms acting simultaneously are responsible for the control of gastric secretion and some of these are summarized in Figure 11.1. This subject has been reviewed critically by Scratcherd (1973).

Acid in the stomach acts as a barrier to bacterial contamination of the upper small intestine, and it also activates pepsin, allowing some preliminary digestion of protein within the stomach. Fat digestion under the influence of gastric lipase may be initiated in the stomach but takes place largely in the small intestine. Water, alcohol and certain

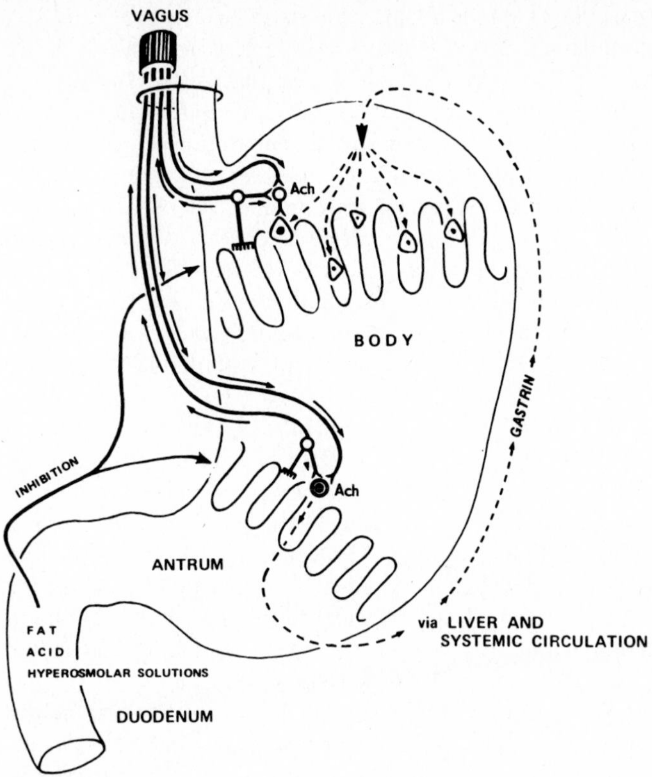

Figure 11.1. Schematic representation of stimulatory and inhibitory factors which regulate gastric secretion.

lipid-soluble drugs such as aspirin are absorbed directly from the stomach (Davenport, 1969).

Normally, bile and small intestinal contents do not reflux to any great extent into the stomach. However, increased duodenogastric reflux has been reported in patients with gastric ulcer (Rhodes et al., 1969); in particular, lysolecithin concentrations have been found to be high in the gastric juice of such patients (Johnson and McDermott, 1974).

The electrolytes of gastric juice are a variable mixture of water, anions and cations. The chief anion is chloride, but lesser amounts of bicarbonate, sulphate, phosphate and certain organic substances are also secreted into the stomach. Hydrogen and potassium are the most important cations and these are present in gastric secretion in far higher concentrations than in other body fluids; thus loss of large quantities of gastric juice usually leads to alkalosis and hypokalaemia. Calcium and magnesium are the other cations which are secreted by the stomach. There is an inverse relationship between hydrogen ion and sodium ion concentrations in gastric juice; at high rates of secretion the concentration of H^+ increases and that of Na^+ decreases, but the total outputs of both ions increase. No direct measurements have been made of the concentrations of these ions in the parietal and non-parietal cells of the gastric glands. However, Makhlouf et al. (1966) have extrapolated from data obtained during gastric secretion tests and calculated the concentration of these ions as follows: in the parietal component, H^+, 149; K^+, 17; Cl^-, 166 mmol/litre; in the non-parietal component, Na^+, 137; K^+, 6; Cl^-, 117; HCO_3^-, 25 mmol/litre. There are two main theories relating to the composition of gastric juice. Firstly, in the two-component hypothesis of Pavlov and Hollander, the parietal cells are assumed to secrete H^+ and Cl^- and the non-parietal cells produce Na^+, K^+, HCO_3^- and other ions; thus the final composition of gastric juice will be dependent on the proportion of these two components in the mixture. Secondly, the back-diffusion theory of Teorell postulates that the parietal cells secrete an iso-osmotic solution of HCl and KCl and that H^+ is exchanged for Na^+ by the duct cells of the parietal and gastric glands. Although controversy rages, it is probable that these two hypotheses are not mutually exclusive (Makhlouf et al., 1966).

Back-diffusion of hydrogen ions into the mucosa undoubtedly takes place but the amounts involved are small. While contact with bile increases back-diffusion, both in the antrum and fundus, recent studies suggest that the secretory state of mucosa, and hence its acid–base status, are important determinants of the tolerance of gastric mucosa to back diffusion of hydrogen ions (O'Brien and Silen, 1976). Neutralization of gastric acid secretions normally takes place in the duodenum, but in patients with duodenal ulcer, the basal bicarbonate content of the duodenum has been found to be only one-half of that in control subjects (Guttierrez and Baron, 1976). Defective neutralization of acid in the duodenum may be a factor in the aetiology of diseases such as duodenal ulcer.

Many drugs affect the stomach, increasing its susceptibility to gastritis and gastric erosions, or exacerbating existing peptic ulcer disease. Foremost among these compounds are corticosteroids and drugs of the anti-inflammatory group such as aspirin, indomethacin and phenylbutazone. Some investigators have suggested that the use of such drugs should be combined with routine antacid therapy in order to maintain gastric pH at a relatively high level and thus render activation of pepsin unlikely.

11.2.2. Methods of investigation

Diagnex blue (Squibb), which is the blue dye azure A combined with a carboxylic cation exchange resin, has been used to develop a tubeless gastric secretion test, the main application of which has been for screening patients who may have achlorhydria, especially those with cancer of the stomach. However, this method is not reliable and has a high incidence of false negative results; thus it is not often used (Christiansen, 1966).

Nasogastric intubation is essential for performing a gastric secretion test. Many substances stimulate gastric acid secretion but the main drugs which are used nowadays for clinical investigation are histamine, Histalog, pentagastrin and insulin. Recently some workers have stimulated gastric secretion by food or the meat extract Oxo; in both types of test the acid secretory response is measured by intragastric titration using sodium bicarbonate (Fordtran and Walsh, 1973; Taylor et al., 1977).

11.2.3. Gastric secretion test

The patient should not take any drug which affects gastric secretion for at least 24 hours before the procedure. The test is usually carried out in the morning after a 12-hour overnight fast. Nasogastric intubation is performed, and the tip of the tube placed in the most dependent portion of the stomach, preferably under fluoroscopic control. Some workers prefer to establish that the tube is draining the stomach adequately by performing a water recovery test (Hassan and Hobsley, 1970). The fasting gastric contents are removed and continuous aspiration continued using an electric vacuum pump. It is important to interrupt the suction at frequent intervals; insufflating air to clear blockage of the tube by mucus or by the mucosa is also essential. Unstimulated spontaneous gastric secretion is collected as four successive 15-minute aspirates during the first hour. A stimulant of gastric secretion is then administered parenterally, and the aspiration is continued for another four or eight 15-minute periods, depending on which gastric stimulant is administered to the patient.

The volume and titratable acidity are measured and the total acid output is calculated and expressed as mmol/15 minute period. The acid content of the gastric juice should be measured by electrometric titration to pH 7 or pH 7.4. Titration using Topfer's reagent, phenopthalein, or another indicator should now be abandoned (Moore, 1967). The pepsin content of the samples may also be assayed, but for pepsin assays to be meaningful it is essential that the gastric juice be collected over ice and the specimens should be stored at 4 °C and not in a deep freeze. If the intrinsic factor content of the acid gastric juice is to be measured, the pH of the sample should be raised to 11 and maintained for 20 minutes; the pH may then be lowered to between 7 and 8 prior to storage at –25 °C for subsequent assay. This procedure is necessary to prevent the peptic digestion of intrinsic factor.

11.2.4. Basal acid secretion

Spontaneous gastric secretion from a resting untrained subject cannot be considered to have been collected under truly "basal" conditions on the first occasion that the test is performed; thus for this measurement to be really meaningful a 2-hour basal collection is required (Gillespie et al., 1972). However, this is hardly practical and is not performed for routine clinical investigation but rather for research purposes. This is possibly the reason for the poor reproducibility of the 1-hour basal secretion – the coefficient of variation of this measurement is often 50%. The hydrochloric acid concentration of basal secretion is usually between 40 and 60 mmol/litre, with a pH of 0.9 to 1.2. A 12-hour nocturnal basal secretion test was formerly popular but it is exceedingly uncomfortable; in addition, the results obtained are often unreliable as it is seldom practical to ensure patency of the nasogastric tube and completeness of the collections for the whole 12-hour period. Even when these precautions have been taken, the information obtained from this test is seldom of great diagnostic value. An acid output of 100 mmol or more for the 12-hour period is strongly indicative of a Zollinger–Ellison Syndrome, but the diagnosis of this condition may be made with equal or greater certainty by measuring circulating serum gastrin concentration (section 11.5.2.). A 2-hour basal secretion test will often yield as much or more information than a 12-hour nocturnal secretion test.

11.2.5. Augmented histamine test

Histamine acid phosphate (40 μg/kg body weight given subcutaneously) produces maximal acid secretory response within 1 hour after the injection in white Caucasians (Kay, 1953): the dose needed for thin Indians is about 50 to 55 μg/kg (Desai et al., 1970). The extra-gastric effects of histamine may be reduced by an injection of an antihistamine drug like mepyramine maleate (100 mg intramuscularly) 30 minutes before the administration of histamine, without affecting gastric secretion. However, mepyramine maleate produces drowsiness and headache, and certain side-effects of histamine, including pain at the site of injection, nausea, alterations in pulse rate and even circulatory collapse, may also rarely occur. Thus, the augmented histamine test is not without some danger and it has largely been superceded by other gastric secretory tests.

11.2.6. Histalog stimulation test

Betazole hydrochloride (Histalog, Lilly) is a synthetic analogue of histamine; when it is used in a dose of 1.5 mg/kg body weight, it stimulates gastric secretion to the same extent as histamine. Histalog does not have the same side-effects as histamine and so no prior injection of an antihistamine is required. This drug takes longer to produce maximal acid stimulation than histamine so that gastric secretions need to be collected for eight 15-minute periods instead of for 1 hour, as is the case with histamine. Even Histalog occasionally produces side-effects, and bleeding from the gastric mucosa during this test has been reported. Nevertheless, this test is still performed in the United States (Sun and Roth, 1974).

11.2.7. Pentagastrin stimulation test

Pentagastrin (Peptavlon, Imperial Chemical Industries) contains the biologically active C-terminal tetrapeptide fragment of gastrin; a dose of 6 μg/kg body weight, given subcutaneously or intramuscularly, has been shown to produce a maximal acid secretory response within 1 hour of the injection. Pentagastrin is practically free of side-effects although very rarely it may produce transient nausea, abdominal discomfort or faintness (Multicentre Study, 1969).

11.2.8. Maximum acid output

The acid secretory response to histamine, Histalog or pentagastrin is quite reproducible and the coefficients of variation for these tests are usually less than 10%. Maximum acid output after histamine or pentagastrin may be calculated as the "peak 30-minute gastric acid output", "mid-half hour acid output" or the "hour after the injection of the stimulant". Excellent correlation exists between all three methods of expressing the results (Table 11.1), and this, combined with the good reproducibility of these tests, makes it possible to compare data from various centres (Multicentre Study, 1969).

There is also a good correlation between the maximum acid output and body weight or lean body mass (Baron, 1969). Card and Marks (1960) have shown that in patients

TABLE 11.1

CORRELATION COEFFICIENTS (r) BETWEEN RESULTS IN 100 CASES OF THE AUGMENTED HISTAMINE TEST EXPRESSED IN THREE DIFFERENT WAYS (after Kay, 1967)

All correlation coefficients are statistically significant ($P < 0.001$).

Period	Peak half-hour vs mid half-hour	Mid half-hour vs one hour	One hour vs peak half-hour
r	0.925	0.909	0.942

with duodenal ulcer, there is a good correlation between maximum acid output and the total parietal cell mass. However, after vagotomy the parietal cells are less sensitive to these gastric acid stimulants and larger doses may be required to produce "maximal" acid secretory responses post-operatively (Multicentre Study, 1967).

For the clinical diagnosis of achlorhydria, it is essential to establish that even after maximal doses of histamine, Histalog or pentagastrin, the pH of the gastric juice is not less than 7.0.

The basal and maximum acid outputs of normal subjects and of patients with duodenal ulcer, recurrent duodenal ulcer after surgery and recurrent peptic ulcer are shown in Table 11.2. The basal acid secretion of normal subjects and patients with gastric ulcer and gastric carcinoma are statistically indistinguishable; the upper limit of "normal" is usually taken to be 5 mmol/h for males or females. Similarly, the maximum

TABLE 11.2

BASAL OUTPUT AND STIMULATED ACID OUTPUT TO PENTAGASTRIN (6 μg/kg BODY WEIGHT) IN NORMAL SUBJECTS AND THREE GROUPS OF PATIENTS (data from Elder and Smith, 1975)

Normal subjects (mean ± S.D., mmol/h)		Patients with duodenal ulcer (mean ± S.D., mmol/h)		Patients with recurrent duodenal ulcer after surgery (mean ± S.D., mmol/h)		Patients with gastric ulcer (mean ± S.D., mmol/h)	
B.A.O. *	M.A.O. **	B.A.O.	M.A.O.	B.A.O.	M.A.O.	B.A.O.	M.A.O
Males							
3.3 ± 2.9	29 ± 10	5.1 ± 3.8	40 ± 14	3.4 ± 3.8	28 ± 22	1.7 ± 2.1	15 ± 8.2
(n = 21)		(n = 72)		(n = 27)		(n = 17)	
Females							
0.9 ± 0.7	16 ± 2.6	3.0 ± 2.7	29 ± 12	1.5 ± 0.9	13 ± 8.2	–	–
(n = 6)		(n = 38)		(n = 5)			

* Basal acid output (B.A.O.) = sum of four 15-minute outputs (mmol/h).

** Maximal acid output (M.A.O.) = peak 30-minute output (i.e. sum of the two highest successive 15-minute outputs after stimulation).

acid outputs of these groups of subjects are statistically similar. However, about 20% of patients with cancer of the stomach have true achlorhydria (Fischerman and Koster, 1962). In normal subjects, the maximum acid output is usually taken to be less than 40 mmol/h for males and 30 mmol/h for females.

Only about one-quarter of the patients with duodenal ulcer have a basal acid output greater than 5 mmol/h, while in patients with recurrent peptic ulcer the findings are very variable and dependent on the nature and extent of previous surgery. In the Zollinger–Ellison Syndrome, a basal acid secretion of greater than 15 mmol/h in the unoperated patient, and greater than 5 mmol/h in patients who have had previous surgery, is a usual, although not invariable, finding (Baron, 1970).

One-third to one-half of patients with dudodenal ulcer have a maximum acid output greater than 40 mmol/h for males and 30 mmol/h for females, and Baron (1963) has drawn attention to the interesting observation that patients with duodenal ulcer very rarely have an output below 15 mmol/h. In patients with recurrent peptic ulcer and those with Zollinger–Ellison Syndrome, the maximum acid output is very variable and dependent on the extent of previous gastric surgery. In the Zollinger–Ellison syndrome the basal acid secretion is often greater than 60% of the maximum acid output, while in recurrent ulceration due to other causes this is not the usual finding (Baron and Williams, 1973).

There are two unusual conditions associated with coarse, hypertrophied or "giant" gastric mucosal folds – hypertrophic, hypersecretory gastropathy and hypertrophic, exudative gastrophy (Menetrier's disease). Although these two conditions appear similar on radiological or endoscopic examination of the stomach, they are very different in their natural history and gastric secretory responses, and especially in their histological appearances (Baron, 1970). In the former condition there is hypersecretion of acid and pepsin, and histologically the gastric glands appear hypertrophied; this condition is usually associated with gastric ulcer, duodenal ulcer or the Zollinger–Ellison syndrome. In contrast, in Menetrier's disease, hyposecretion of acid and pepsin is the usual finding, but in addition there is a high concentration of protein in the gastric juice. Histologically the gastric glands are enlarged but the parietal and peptic cells are replaced by mucin-containing cells and the mucosa is markedly oedematous and infiltrated by chronic inflammatory cells. Menetrier's disease often produces hypoproteinaemia, and the mucosal changes may lead to atrophic gastritis or even carcinoma (Chusid et al., 1964). A combined syndrome consisting of acid hypersecretion, gastric mucosal hypertrophy and protein-losing gastropathy has now been described (Brooks et al., 1970).

11.2.9. Insulin stimulation test

Insulin hypoglycaemia stimulates the vagal centre in the hypothalamus and this produces gastric acid and endogenous gastrin secretion via cholinergic mechanisms. The insulin stimulation test is performed in a manner similar to other acid secretion tests except that gastric juice is collected for eight 15-minute periods after the administration of soluble insulin in a dose of 0.2 units/kg body weight, as a bolus intravenous injection. In addition, blood samples should be taken at the time of injection and at 30 and 45 minutes thereafter, so that the degree of hypoglycaemia may be assessed. This is necessary as there is a dose–response relationship between insulin dosage, blood glucose concentration and acid secretory response. It has been shown that there are direct correlations between peak acid output after insulin, and the rate of fall of blood glucose and the lowest blood glucose concentration. Insulin in the above dosage should lower blood glucose concentration below 40 mg/dl for the test to be considered satisfactory. Precautions should be taken to make it possible to reverse the hypoglycaemia rapidly should symptoms occur. The test should not be performed in patients with angina pectoris or after recent myocardial infarction. Hypoglycaemic symptoms are reduced if insulin is administered as an intravenous infusion in a dose of 0.04 units/kg per h; the resulting test is both effective and reproducible (Carter et al., 1972).

Hollander (1946, 1948) described the insulin stimulation test as a method for assessing the integrity of the vagal nerve pathways after vagotomy. His criteria for a *positive* response are as follows: firstly, considering the eight 15-minute gastric juice collections after insulin, an increase in free acid concentration of 20 mmol/litre or more in at least two consecutive samples, when compared to the mean acidity of two 15-minute basal periods; secondly, if there is no free acid in the basal gastric juice, an increase of 10 mmol/litre or more in at least two consecutive samples after administration of insulin is considered to be a positive response. In Hollander's view, a truly negative test should fulfil two additional criteria: a blood sugar concentration of less than 50 mg/dl after the insulin injection, and the patient should be capable of secreting hydrochloric acid after histamine.

During the 30 years since the insulin stimulation test was described, many workers have suggested additional or different qualitative or quantitative criteria for the interpretation of this test; these have been discussed critically by Baron and Williams (1973). Only one group of workers has subjected their criteria to appropriate statistical analysis. These state that firstly, after insulin, an acid output in any 15-minute period of more than three times the mean basal value is indicative of a positive response ($P = 0.01$) and secondly, if the basal gastric juice is an acid, an acid output of 0.3 mmol after insulin in any 15-minute collection is also taken as a positive test and indicative of incomplete vagotomy (Gillespie et al., 1972). The original criteria of Hollander still remain the most widely used basis for interpreting the response obtained after insulin for deducing the completeness or otherwise of vagotomy (Bachrach and Bachrach, 1967).

The insulin stimulation test is reproducible in normal subjects and in patients with duodenal ulcer. A negative test performed soon after surgery (whether truncal, selective or highly selective vagotomy) may subsequently convert to a positive response, and it has been suggested that this occurs within 6 months after vagotomy. Thus many workers prefer not to perform an insulin stimulation test for at least 6 months after surgery for peptic ulcer disease (Gillespie et al., 1970; Smith et al., 1972).

11.3. PEPSIN

11.3.1. Chemistry and physiology of pepsin secretion

Considerable attention has been focussed on hydrochloric acid secretion but this alone will not achieve digestion – only sterilization. The enzymes of gastric juice are pepsin, renin, lipase, gelatinase, lysozyme, urease, carbonic anhydrase and β-glucuronidase. The main proteolytic enzyme is pepsin, which is not a single entity but a group of enzymes which originate from, and are stored in, the chief cells of the acid and pyloric gland areas; the precursor substances are called pepsinogens. Seven or eight different pepsinogens and pepsins have been described by workers using electrophoretic mobility as the method for the separation of these enzymes and their precursors. Others who have employed column chromatography have described fewer substances (Samloff, 1969). Pepsinogens have molecular masses of the order of 40,000 daltons and are stable at a neutral pH. At a pH below 4.5, acid activates pepsinogens by splitting off the inhibitor portion of the molecules (which has a molecular mass of about 7000 daltons) to yield active pepsins. Pepsin also activates pepsinogen by an autocatalytic process.

Human pepsinogens are divided into two unrelated immunological groups; group I is made up of pepsinogens 1 to 5 and group II of pepsinogens 6 and 7. Samloff has shown that both groups of pepsinogens are present in serum but he was able to identify only group I pepsinogens in the urine (uropepsin). Group I pepsinogens are more sensitive to an alkaline pH, have lower pH optima and hydrolyze the synthetic polypeptide *N*-acetyl-L-phenylalanyl-L-diiodotyrosine, while group II pepsinogens have properties which are the converse. Some workers have suggested that these biochemical characteristics may be used as the basis for the separate determination of pepsinogens of groups I and II.

Cholinergic stimuli like carbachol, insulin hypoglycaemia, sham feeding and instillation of acetylcholine solution into the stomach, are the most powerful methods for the stimulation of pepsin secretion. Although parenteral administration of gastrin, pentagastrin or histamine is effective, they are more potent as stimulants of gastric acid rather than pepsin (Hirschowitz, 1967). Secretin and the chemically related hormone glucagon, which are inhibitors of basal and pentagastrin-stimulated gastric acid output, have anomalous actions on pepsin secretion: secretin stimulates while glucagon does not affect pepsin secretion. Gastric inhibitory polypeptide and vasoactive intestinal polypeptide are also chemically related to glucagon; the former inhibits both acid and pepsin secretion while the latter stimulates pepsin output (Grossman, 1974). It would not be surprising if the interplay of both nervous and humoral mechanisms which are known to influence other gastrointestinal secretions were also found to be involved in the physiological control of pepsin secretion.

11.3.2. Methods of investigation

There is a close correlation between gastric acid and pepsin secretion in man. Thus pepsin secretion tests are usually performed at the same time as the insulin stimulation test. However, 0.2 units of insulin per kg body weight does not produce "maximal" pepsin secretion (Isenberg et al., 1969).

11.3.3. Measurement of pepsin in gastric juice

Pepsin output has been less well documented than acid output, and this is doubtless due to the difficulties in estimation. The usual methods of estimating pepsin activity depend on the colorimetric measurement of the tyrosine products of digestion which react with the Folin phenol reagent (Anson and Mirsky, 1932). Since no purified human material is available, comparison is made with a porcine pepsin reference material. Nephelometry and synthetic or radiolabelled substrates have also been used in the estimation of pepsin activity (Piper, 1960). Serial dilutions of gastric juice samples give a non-linear response with respect to their peptic activity and it was suggested that this was due to the presence of an inhibitor. However, Samloff and Dadufalza (1977) have shown that linear results may be obtained for the sample dilution–peptic activity curves if attention is paid to the final chloride concentrations of the gastric juice samples. Freezing leads to 40 or 50% loss of peptic activity in gastric juice. Again, the presence of bile in gastric juice will interfere with the measurement of peptic activity if the end point is determined by a colorimetric technique.

Pepsinogen appears in the blood and uropepsin in the urine, but measurement of the latter is nowadays seldom used clinically. Human gastrectomy specimens have been used as starting material for extraction of fundic and pyloric pepsinogens and for raising antibodies, with the result that serum pepsinogen I can now be measured by radioimmunoassay (Samloff et al., 1975).

11.3.4. Clinical usefulness

In man, pentagastrin is a less powerful stimulus to pepsin secretion than insulin-induced hypoglycaemia. In general, the pattern of pepsin output follows acid output, but the dose–response curve for acid output plateaus much earlier than that for pepsin.

Pepsin values for normal subjects, patients with primary duodenal ulceration and patients with recurrent ulceration after surgery for duodenal ulcer are shown in Table 11.3. No significant differences can be found in the basal levels between the two

TABLE 11.3

BASAL OUTPUT AND STIMULATED PEPSIN OUTPUT TO INSULIN (0.2 units/kg body weight) IN NORMAL SUBJECTS AND TWO GROUPS OF PATIENTS (data from Elder and Smith, 1975)

Normal subjects (mean ± S.D., mg/h) ***		Patients with primary duodenal ulcer (mean ± S.D., mg/h)		Patients with recurrent duodenal ulcer after surgery (mean ± S.D., mg/h)	
B.P.O. *	M.P.O. **	B.P.O.	M.P.O.	B.P.O.	M.P.O
Males					
32 ± 29	320 ± 170	42 ± 34	1600 ± 600	42 ± 58	230 ± 370
(n = 21)		(n = 29)		(n = 24)	
Females					
60 ± 81	170 ± 150	25 ± 17	290 ± 120	17 ± 5.9	59 ± 46
(n = 5)		(n = 21)		(n = 3)	

* Basal pepsin output (B.P.O.) = sum of four 15-minute outputs.
** Maximal pepsin output (M.P.O.) = sum of four 15-minute outputs.
*** 1 mg = 2340 International Units.

patient groups in males. It is interesting to note that in males with recurrent ulceration, basal pepsin secretion is comparable to that seen in the group not operated upon, whereas the maximal pepsin response is normal. These data suggest that the tendency for recurrent ulceration may be associated with a sustained basal pepsin secretion rather than with a large maximal response. Because of small numbers, the data for females are difficult to analyze.

Clinically, the ratio of basal pepsin output to basal acid output is low in patients with the Zollinger–Ellison syndrome compared to those with duodenal or gastric ulcer. A relationship between active duodenal ulceration and peak pepsin output to insulin has been suggested; values for the latter finding correlate with peak acid output to pentagastrin, and therefore probably reflect the peptic cell mass (Elder and Smith, 1975).

Increase in *serum* pepsinogen following an injection of Histalog has been suggested as a good discriminant for patients with recurrent peptic ulceration after vagotomy (Samloff et al., 1975). This is interesting and likely to be helpful, since the measurement of pepsin activity in *gastric juice* in such patients is often inaccurate owing to reflux of bile and alkaline pancreatic juice.

As yet no safe antipepsin is available for clinical use. Preliminary reports of such a naturally occurring substance – "pepstatin" – are encouraging and the results of prospective double-blind clinical trials in patients with peptic ulcer are eagerly awaited.

11.4. GASTRIC MUCUS

11.4.1. Chemistry and physiology of mucus secretion

Mucus is secreted by specialized cells of the gastric glands and appears as a highly hydrated polymeric material which forms a selective, semi-permeable, macromolecular barrier to the proteolytic and hydrolytic gastric luminal contents. The molecular mass of mucus is of the order of 2×10^6 daltons, but whether it is secreted as smaller units which subsequently polymerize is not known (Allen and Snary, 1972). The thin layer of mucus provides a protective covering for the epithelial cells by virtue of its adhesive, cohesive, viscous and lubricating properties. These properties result from an unusual chemical structure consisting principally of a polypeptide core of threonine, serine, proline, glycine and alanine, with oligosaccharide side chains of variable length (Hough and Jones, 1972). Using the molar ratio of each carbohydrate in the side chains to the amount of glucosamine present, a characteristic pattern emerges in the quantitative relationship of these carbohydrates within each side chain; these patterns are the same both for the visible, relatively insoluble mucus and for the spent soluble mucus, suggesting that breakdown of polymers may have occurred. Similar carbohydrate patterns are found in salivary and biliary mucus (Schrager et al., 1972). In healthy gastric mucosa, the side chains of the surface mucus confer a strong resemblance to the specific blood group substances. Stimulation of gastric mucus secretion follows mechanical irritation or chemical irritants such as chincophen and eugenol. Carbenoxolone also stimulates mucus secretion, whereas alcohol precipitates mucus (Parke, 1976). Gastric mucus absorbs water and binds pepsin, but only has a weakly neutralizing effect upon acid.

11.4.2. Methods of investigation

Gastric mucus, as for all other mucus secretions of the gastrointestinal tract, is difficult to investigate, since even the technique of sampling by suction via a nasogastric tube can alter the chemical configuration of the substances present. No standard test has been defined for clinical use. True gastric mucus from healthy human mucosa probably contains no sulphated or sialic acid-containing mucins, but since gastric secretions may contain contaminant mucins from salivary, bronchial, pharyngeal, oesophageal, biliary and small intestinal secretions, mucus substances containing sulphate and sialic acid have often erroneously been reported in gastric mucus (Lambert, 1974). Measurement of mucus secretion for clinical investigations is usually limited to departments with extensive research facilities, as many of the laboratory techniques are difficult and time consuming. Some centres, however, have used the estimation of *N*-acetylneuraminic acid in gastric juice as a measure of total mucus production by the stomach (Parke, 1976).

In human duodenal mucosa, no differences have been found in the amounts of sulphated glycoproteins in mucosal biopsies from patients with duodenal ulcer compared to biopsies taken from non-ulcer control subjects (Andre et al., 1974). On the other hand, in gastric ulcer patients, examination of the mucosa with the naked eye often reveals mucus secretions as coagulated masses adherent to the mucosa, in contrast to the normal glistening appearance of the healthy stomach.

11.4.3. Alterations in disease

In disease states such as intestinal metaplasia of the stomach and gastric carcinoma, abnormal mucus substances are often secreted which result in "foreign blood group characteristics" in the carbohydrate side chains of mucus; these are different from those of the host (Schrager and Oates, 1973).

Alteration of mucus synthesis following the continued ingestion of aspirin, indomethacin, spironolactone or steroids is brought about by the inhibition of glycosylation of the polypeptide core (Parke, 1976). It has been suggested that these drugs result in the production of a "defective" mucus and that this is responsible for the mucosal damage and ulceration which are associated with the use of these therapeutic agents. Experimentally, in rats, exposure to cold and restraint in combination, inhibits mucus synthesis and leads to gastric erosions (Parke, 1976).

11.5. GASTRIN

11.5.1. Chemistry and physiology of gastrin

Gastrin is a polypeptide hormone which is present in the G-cells of the pyloric gland area of the stomach. Gregory and Tracy (1975) have prepared pure gastrin from the antral extracts of many mammalian species. They and their colleagues have established the amino acid sequences of these hormones. Porcine, bovine, canine and human gastrin have been synthesized (Gregory, 1968). Natural gastrin prepared from antral mucosa was shown to be composed of 17 aminoacids and have a molecular mass of 2100 daltons. In tissue extracts and serum, the hormone gastrin is present as gastrin I and gastrin II; gastrin II differs from gastrin I in having a sulphate group in place of the hydroxyl radical on the single tyrosyl residue in position 12. There are no differences between the biological actions of gastrin I and II. The C-terminal tetrapeptide of gastrin is composed of Try–Met–Asp–Phe–NH_2; this fragment possesses the full spectrum of actions of the hormone but is only one-seventh as potent as the heptadecapeptide hormone.

Recent studies have shown that gastrin is present both in antral extracts and in serum in a number of molecular sizes. The large molecule of gastrin is known as "big" gastrin and has 34 aminoacids and a molecular mass of 3900 daltons; this has been designated as G-34. The original heptadecapeptide gastrin is called "little" gastrin, G-17; "big" gastrin is made up of "little" gastrin and an additional heptadecapeptide at the *N*-terminal end; they are linked by a Lys–Lys bond (Scheme 11.1). Another, smaller gastrin called "mini" gastrin is also present in antral mucosa and serum; this molecule contains the terminal 13 aminoacids of the original heptadecapeptide gastrin and has been designated as G-13. "Big", "little" and "mini" gastrins are all present as the sulphated (form II) and non-sulphated (form I) varieties (Gregory and Tracy, 1975). Separation of the members of this family of gastrins can be performed using conventional column gel permeation chromatography (Yalow, 1974). In the antral mucosa there is far more G-17 than G-34 gastrin, while the converse is true in the duodenum and upper small intestine. The potency ratios of these gastrins are G-13: G-17: G-34 as 8:2:1. Two other gastrins have been reported but they have not been characterized completely and are not biologically active; these are "big-big" gastrin and component I (Rehfeld et al., 1974; Yalow, 1974). Some gastrin-containing tumours contain a tridecapeptide which is structurally similar to the first 13 *N*-terminal aminoacids of G-17; this gastrin has not been named specifically and is biologically inactive (Dochray and Walsh, 1975).

Human big gastrin (HG-34), molecular mass 3839 daltons

```
1    2   3   4  -5   6   7   8   9   10  11  12  13  14  15  16  17  18  19  20  21  22  23  24
Pyro-Leu-Gly-Pro-Gln-Gly-His-Pro-Ser-Leu-Val-Ala-Asp-Pro-Ser-Lys-Lys-Gln-Gly-Pro-Trp-Leu-Glu-Glu-

25  26  27  28  29  30  31  32  33  34
Glu-Glu-Glu-Ala-Tyr-Gly-Trp-Met-Asp-Phe-NH2
                 |
                 R
```

Human heptadecapeptide (little) gastrin (HG-17), molecular mass 2098 daltons

```
1    2   3   4   5   6   7   8   9   10  11  12  13  14  15  16  17
Pyro-Gly-Pro-Trp-Leu-Glu-Glu-Glu-Glu-Glu-Ala-Tyr-Gly-Trp-Met-Asp-Phe-NH2
                                             |
                                             R
```

Human minigastrin (HG-14), molecular mass 1851 daltons

```
1   2   3   4   5   6   7   8   9   10  11  12  13  14
Trp-Leu-Glu-Glu-Glu-Glu-Glu-Ala-Tyr-Gly-Trp-Met-Asp-Phe-NH2
                                 |
                                 R
```

Scheme 11.1. Aminoacid sequences of chemically characterized human gastrins. Pyro, pyroglutamyl; gastrin I, R = OH; gastrin II, R = SO_3H.

Gastrin is a very potent stimulant of gastric acid secretion. This action is produced both by endogenously released hormone and by parenterally administered gastrin or pentagastrin. In addition, gastrin is a weak stimulant of gastric pepsin, and pancreatic, biliary and intestinal gland electrolyte and enzyme secretions as well as gastric, intestinal and biliary motilities. The main sites of degradation of gastrin and pentagastrin are in the small intestine, stomach, kidneys and liver (Walsh and Grossman, 1975).

The stimulation and inhibition of gastrin release is under an autoregulatory mechanism. Vagal stimulation during the cephalic phase of gastric secretion initiates endogenous gastrin release. The presence of food in the stomach buffers the residual gastric juice and raises intragastric pH, and this probably augments gastrin release. Antral distension by food and the presence of proteins, polypeptides, peptones and aminoacids in the food, or after initial digestion of food in the stomach, prolongs the release of the hormone. As the stomach empties, antral distension decreases. This, along with the gradual fall in intragastric pH due to the presence of hydrochloric acid which has been secreted as a response to the elevated concentrations of circulating gastrin, initiates the process responsible for the "switching off" of endogenous gastrin release. Inhibition of gastrin secretion commences at pH 3 and is probably complete by pH 1.

11.5.2. Measurement of gastrin in serum

Gastrin in serum is best measured by radioimmunoassay since bioassays of gastrin are exceedingly insensitive. Because of the large variety of molecular forms of gastrin in serum, serum gastrin concentration, as measured by radioimmunoassay, will depend on whether the antiserum in use cross-reacts with all or some of the species of gastrin. In the fasting subject, the main forms of gastrin in the serum are "big-big" gastrin and G-34 while, after a meal, G-17 and G-13 are present in the serum in higher concentrations. Thus, if an antiserum with a poor affinity for the larger molecular forms is used in the gastrin assay the fasting serum gastrin concentration will be reported as being exceedingly low while the post-prandial concentration will reflect the more correct value. Obviously the converse will be the finding if an antiserum with a low affinity for the smaller molecular species is used for the radioimmunoassay of gastrin. This is one of the main reasons for the variability in the reported values of serum gastrin concentration in health and disease. However, if a recognized reference preparation is used and the gastrin assay is performed in a manner similar to those of other hormone assays, the within- and between-batch variabilities are not dissimilar to those found with insulin or growth hormone (Ganguli and Hunter, 1972; Stadil and Rehfeld, 1973).

11.5.3. Fasting serum gastrin concentration

Fasting serum gastrin concentrations in normal subjects and in patients with duodenal or gastric ulceration are shown in Table 11.4. There is considerable variation in the reported literature, which may be accounted for on the basis of the different antisera, gastrin standards and assay methods which have been employed. Ganguli and Hunter (1972), Hansky and Korman (1973) and Wesdorp and Fischer (1974) found that fasting serum gastrin concentrations in gastric ulcer patients were much greater than in normal sub-

TABLE 11.4

FASTING SERUM GASTRIN CONCENTRATIONS (MEANS ± S.E.) IN NORMAL SUBJECTS AND IN TWO GROUPS OF PATIENTS

Reference	Normal subjects		Duodenal ulcer		Gastric ulcer	
	n	Gastrin (pg/ml)	n	Gastrin (pg/ml)	n	Gastrin (pg/ml)
Trudeau and McGuigan (1970)	102	165 ± 28	42	82 ± 12	9	126 ± 4
Ganguli and Hunter (1972)	113	105 ± 7	27	91 ± 6	14	285 ± 31
Hansky and Korman (1973)	252	36 ± 4	206	13 ± 1	75	99 ± 6
Stadil and Rehfeld (1973)	120	52 ± 5	103	50 ± 2	–	–
Wesdorp and Fischer (1974)	30	54 ± 9	101	61 ± 7	31	93 ± 17
Lamers (1976)	100	66 ± 2	80	70 ± 2	17	92 ± 28

jects, but this was not the case in the observations of Trudeau and McGuigan (1970) or Lamers (1976) in their series of patients. Similar variant findings have been reported in patients with carcinoma of the stomach.

Duodenal ulcer patients have been reported as having higher, similar, or lower fasting serum gastrin concentrations than normal subjects, but the reasons for these different findings are not obvious. The present authors agree with Hansky and Korman (1973) that fasting serum gastrin concentration is related to intragastric pH at the time that the specimens for the serum gastrin measurements are taken, and thus support their observation and suggestion that duodenal ulcer patients have lower fasting intragastric pH than normal subjects, and that their serum gastrin concentrations are usually lower. In contrast to normal subjects, patients with gastric ulcer have raised intragastric pH and elevated serum gastrin concentrations. However, it should be emphasized that fasting serum gastrin concentration is a poor discriminant in patients with duodenal ulcer. Similarly, it should be stated that the correlation between basal acid output and fasting serum gastrin concentration is also poor in these patients.

In achlorhydria, serum gastrin concentration is markedly raised, and this is due to the absence of acid inhibition of endogenous gastrin release. In addition, in some of these patients, there is an excess of gastrin production due to an increase in the number of gastrin cells either in the antrum or in ectopic sites such as the acid-bearing area of the stomach. Some achlorhydrics have diffuse atrophic gastritis and antritis, and in these patients serum gastrin concentration may be only marginally elevated or within the normal range (Korman et al., 1971). Many patients with the Zollinger–Ellison syndrome have hypergastrinaemia and their serum gastrin concentrations are often 10 to 1000 times the normal value. However some patients with gastrinomas may be normogastrinaemic, especially if single, random, serum samples are examined; it has been claimed that this finding may be encountered in 20 to 40% of these cases (Walsh and Roth, 1976).

In the Zollinger–Ellison syndrome, the serum gastrin concentration may fluctuate from day to day and probably during different times of the same day. Thus the diagnostic value of these measurements may be greatly increased by examining multiple blood samples, and especially by performing gastrin stimulation tests (section 11.5.4.).

Fasting hypergastrinaemia has also been reported in some patients with uncomplicated duodenal ulcer, duodenal ulcer with pyloric stenosis, or recurrent peptic ulceration after previous gastric surgery; some of these patients have proven or presumed antral gastrin cell hyperplasia (Ganguli et al., 1974; Straus and Yalow, 1975). Similarly, patients with an excluded retained antrum have fasting hyperglycaemia (Korman et al., 1972).

Fasting hypergastrinaemia is present in patients with chronic renal failure, the short gut syndrome or hepatocellular decompensation; since these are the sites of inactivation of gastrin, these observations are to be expected. After renal transplantation and when renal function improves, the fasting serum gastrin concentration returns to normal (Walsh and Grossman, 1975).

Intravenous calcium infusion has been shown to stimulate gastric acid secretion and endogenous gastrin release. Thus it is not surprising that patients with hypercalcaemia, especially due to hyperparathyroidism, have elevated fasting serum gastrin concentrations. After parathyroidectomy and in the normocalcaemic state, these patients have normal serum gastrin concentrations. The hypergastrinaemia of hyperparathyroidism may be misdiagnosed as due to the Zollinger–Ellison syndrome, especially as both such groups of patients may have severe and intractable peptic ulcer disease. It must be remembered that both of these diseases may co-exist in the same individual (Walsh and Roth, 1976).

In peptic ulcer patients, fasting serum gastrin concentration is greater after gastric surgery than prior to operation. This has been documented after truncal or selective vagotomy with drainage, as well as after highly selective vagotomy. However, if the vagotomy is incomplete as defined by a positive insulin stimulation test (section 11.2.9.), the magnitude of the rise in serum gastrin concentration is less marked. After vagotomy, fasting intragastric pH is higher than in patients who have not been operated upon and this is one possible explanation for this observation. However, it is not possible to exclude the likelihood that the intact vagus may have some effect on the gastrin cell either directly or via other as yet ill-understood mechanisms (Hansky and Korman, 1973; Walsh and Grossman, 1975).

If after antrectomy and gastroduodenal anastomosis (Billroth I operation) the serum gastrin concentration is not dissimilar to the preoperative value then the likely origin of gastrin in such a patient is the duodenum. If, however, after antrectomy and gastrojejunal anastomosis (Polya operation) the serum gastrin concentration is decreased as compared to the preoperative value, then this is probably because the gastric secretions and food by-pass the duodenum (Stern and Walsh, 1973).

After head injuries or burns, stress ulceration of the stomach and duodenum are seen; these patients have been reported to have elevated serum gastrin concentrations. Less clearly understood are the observations of raised concentrations in patients with rheumatoid arthritis and vitiligo, although the intragastric pH of these patients at the time that specimens for gastrin estimation were taken has not been reported in detail (Hansky and Korman, 1973).

11.5.4. Gastrin stimulation test

Usually, this test is performed in the morning after an overnight fast. The stimulant may be administered orally by means of a "standard breakfast" (a steak meal or a meat extract solution such as Oxo) or parenterally; the latter procedure may employ a bolus or continuous intravenous infusion. Intravenous injections of soluble insulin (0.2 units/kg body weight) or secretin (1 to 3 units/kg body weight) stimulate gastrin secretion. An intravenous infusion of calcium gluconate (4 mg/kg per hour) for 4 hours or until the serum calcium concentration rises by 1 mmol/litre (4 mg/dl) above the pre-infusion level, is the other commonly used stimulant of endogenous gastrin release. If insulin hypoglycaemia is employed, blood sugar measurements should be performed before, and 30 and 45 minutes after, the injection; if a calcium infusion is given, serum calcium estimations should be performed at half hourly intervals during the test. Both of these stimulants are potentially dangerous and appropriate precautions should be taken.

The time course of the response to the stimuli vary, being most rapid after an Oxo meal or secretin injection. Thus blood specimens for measurements of serum gastrin concentration should be taken 5 minutes before, just prior to giving the stimulus, and at 5, 10, 15, 20, 30, 45, 60, 75 and 90 minutes after the stimulant. Feeding, insulin hypoglycaemia and calcium infusion take longer to produce their effect. Thus blood specimens for gastrin estimation should be taken 5 minutes before, just prior to, and at 15 minute intervals for 2 hours after insulin or feeding, and up to 4 hours after calcium gluconate stimulation.

Feeding, Oxo, insulin and calcium gluconate all stimulate endogenous gastrin release in normal subjects and duodenal ulcer patients, but there is disagreement as to whether these conditions can be differentiated by means of some of these tests. The pattern of response in gastric ulcer has been studied in too few patients and only by the occasional investigator; thus it is difficult to state categorically whether this condition can be differentiated from normal by means of a gastrin stimulation test.

An injection of atropine sulphate (0.6 mg intramuscularly) followed by feeding, has been shown to produce a more marked elevation in serum gastrin concentration in duodenal ulcer patients than in normal subjects (Walsh et al., 1971). The usual finding after feeding alone, is that duodenal ulcer patients and normal subjects produce similar responses. However, the combined test has not been used extensively.

Most investigators agree that calcium infusion stimulates gastrin release in normal subjects and in duodenal ulcer patients, the magnitude of the response in patients being about twice that in normal subjects (Reeder et al., 1974).

Continuous alkalinization of the stomach with sodium bicarbonate solution along with insulin hypoglycaemia produced endogenous gastrin release which was greatest in duodenal ulcer patients, less marked in gastric ulcer patients and least in normal subjects (Hanksy and Korman, 1973). This test, however, has been used only by these workers.

In normal subjects and in patients with duodenal ulcer, intravenous secretin decreases fasting serum gastrin concentration, and food stimulates gastrin release, but it is not possible to diagnose duodenal ulcer by this test.

Fordtran and Walsh (1973), modifying the intragastric titration test of Stavney et al. (1966), gave their patients a meal consisting of steak, buttered toast and water. Rapid intragastric titration of acid was performed every 3 minutes, using variable amounts of sodium bicarbonate solution, and the gastric contents were maintained at pH 5.5. Adequate mixing was ensured and the test continued for one hour. Blood specimens were taken for gastrin estimation throughout the procedure. This test has the advantage that it permits the simultaneous measurement of gastric acid and serum gastrin responses to the meal. Both were found to be greater in duodenal ulcer patients than in normal subjects. The test does not take into consideration the rate of gastric emptying, either of solids or liquids, nor the influence that the maintenance of intragastric pH at 5.5 may have on gastric emptying. Earlier workers have reported that duodenal ulcer patients may have a faster rate of gastric emptying than normal subjects, and although literature reports vary, this may affect the results of such a test. If other workers are able to confirm the observations of Fordtran and Walsh (1973), their test may gain greater acceptance and application.

Malagelada et al. (1976) described a method for studying gastric acid and gastrin secretory responses after the ingestion of an ordinary solid and liquid meal without the use of intragastric titration. Employing both gastric and duodenal intubation, and infusion of ^{14}C-labelled polyethylene glycol, this method also quantifies and corrects for pyloric losses, and thus obviates some of the problems inherent in the test of Fordtran and Walsh (1973). However, it is too early to know whether we yet have an "ideal" gastric function test.

To summarize, although many simple, and a few elaborate, gastrin stimulation tests have been devised, no thorough and detailed study comparing these tests has been reported; nor is there information on the most reproducible and best method of differentiating normal subjects from duodenal ulcer or gastric ulcer patients by means solely of their gastrin responses.

11.5.5. Zollinger–Ellison syndrome

The main gastrin stimulation tests which are used to diagnose gastrinomas are gastrin responses to feeding, intravenous injection of secretin or glucagon, and the calcium infusion test. Normal subjects and patients with duodenal ulcer or antral gastrin cell hyperplasia, respond to feeding with a 2- to 10-fold increase in serum gastrin concentration. Patients with gastrinomas either do not respond at all, or show a rise which is less than 100% the pre-stimulation value (Lamers, 1976).

Most patients suspected of having a Zollinger–Ellison tumour, whether with normogastrinaemia or hypergastrinaemia, respond to calcium or secretin challenge with an increase in serum gastrin concentration of 100% or more. Thompson et al. (1975) reported that 10 of 11 patients with gastrinomas had a positive secretin test; this finding is similar to those of Walsh and Roth (1976) and of the present authors. However, Creutzfeldt et al. (1975) found that this test gave a positive result in only 6 of 9 patients. None of these workers have found the glucagon stimulation test to be useful in the diagnosis of gastrinomas.

Experiences with calcium infusion tests for the diagnosis of gastrinomas are not dissimilar to the findings with the secretin test. Creutzfeldt et al. (1975) and Thompson et al. (1975) found that all their Zollinger–Ellison patients gave a positive calcium infusion test; Walsh and Roth (1976) and the present authors have similar findings.

Lamers (1976) performed gastrin stimulation tests in normal subjects and in patients with duodenal ulcer or Zollinger–Ellison syndrome, using a "standard" meal, calcium and secretin. He found that almost all of the normal subjects and duodenal ulcer patients had a positive meal-stimulated gastrin response, but this test was positive only in 1 of 9 patients with Zollinger–Ellison syndrome. Secretin or calcium infusion tests were positive in 13 of 15 proven gastrinoma cases. It is interesting that he did not find the combination of a positive calcium and a negative secretin test, or vice versa, in any of the 13 subjects in whom these tests were positive. However, 2 of 15 patients with histologically proven gastrinomas had negative results from the secretin *and* calcium infusion tests; one of the two had fasting hypergastrinaemia while the other had a normal fasting serum gastrin level. Unfortunately, neither of these last patients was investigated with the meal stimulation tests and thus it was not possible to comment on the diagnostic value of this test in patients with false negative response to calcium and secretin stimulation.

The information in the literature, together with the present authors' experience, suggests that once the diagnosis of the Zollinger–Ellison syndrome is made on clinical grounds, the results from the acid secretion tests should substantiate this diagnosis. After multiple, random, serum gastrin measurements, the diagnostic certainty is about 70 to 80%. Finally, gastrin stimulation tests may be required, and these should confirm diagnosis in another 10 to 15% of patients. Unfortunately, in a small proportion of cases, probably about 5%, all the tests may fail to establish an unequivocal laboratory diagnosis of the presence of a gastrinoma.

REFERENCES

Allen, A. and Snary, D. (1972) The structure and function of gastric mucus. Gut, 13, 666–672.

Andre, F. Bourhours, D., Andre, C., Descus, F. and Lambert, R. (1974) The carbohydrate and ester sulphate content of mucosal biopsies in health and in patients with duodenal ulcer. Clinica Chimica Acta, 56, 255–259.

Anson, M.L. and Mirsky, A.E. (1932) The estimation of pepsin with haemoglobin. Journal of General Physiology, 16, 59–63.

Bachrach, W.H. and Bachrach, L.B. (1967) Re-evaluation of the Hollander test. Annals of the New York Academy of Science, 140, 915–923.

Baron, J.H. (1963) Studies of basal and peak acid output with an augmented histamine test. Gut, 4, 136–144.

Baron, J.H. (1969) Lean body mass, gastric acid and peptic ulcer. Gut, 10, 637–642.

Baron, J.H. (1970) The clinical use of gastric function tests. Scandinavian Journal of Gastroenterology, 5, Suppl. 6, 9–46.

Baron, J.H. and Williams, A.J. (1973) Gastric secretion tests. In Recent Advances in Surgery. (Ed. Selwyn Taylor). Churchill Livingstone, Edinburgh and London.

Black, J.W., Duncan, W.A.M. and Durant, C.J. (1972). Definition and antagonism of histamine$_2$-receptors. Nature, 236, 385–390.

Brooks, A.M., Isenberg, J.I. and Goldstein, H. (1970). Giant thickening of the gastric mucosa with acid hypersecretion and protein-losing gastropathy. Gastroenterology, 58, 73–79.

Card, W.I. and Marks, I.N. (1960) The relationship between the acid output of the stomach following "maximal" histamine stimulation and the parietal cell mass. Clinical Science, 19, 147–163.

Carter, D.C., Dozois, R.R. and Kirkpatrick, J.R. (1972) The insulin infusion test of gastric secretion. British Medical Journal, 2, 202–204.

Christiansen, P.M. (1966) The azure A method as a screening test of gastric acid secretion. Scandinavian Journal of Gastroenterology, 1, 9–20.

Chusid, E.L., Hirsch, R.L. and Colcher, H. (1964) Spectrum of hypertrophic gastropathy. Archives of Internal Medicine, 114, 621–628.

Creutzfeldt, W., Arnold, R., Creutzfeldt, C. and Tracks, N.S. (1975) Pathomorphologic biochemical and diagnostic aspects of gastrinomas (Zollinger–Ellison syndrome). Human Pathology, 6, 47–76.

Davenport, H.W. (1961) Physiology of the Digestive Tract. Year Book Medical Publisher, Inc., Chicago.

Davenport, H.W. (1969) Gastric mucosal haemorrhage in dogs. Effects of acid, aspirin and alcohol. Gastroenterology, 56, 439–449.

Desai, H.G., Autia, F.P., Gupte, U.V. and Potnis, P.R. (1969) Dose of histamine for maximal stimulation of gastric acid secretion. Gastroenterology, 57, 636–640.

Di Sant' Agnese, P.A., Darling, R.C., Perera, G.A. and Shea, E. (1953) Abnormal electrolyte composition of sweat in cystic fibrosis of the pancreas. Paediatrics, 12, 549–563.

Dochray, G.J. and Walsh, J.H. (1975) Amino terminal gastrin fragment in serum of Zollinger–Ellison syndrome patients. Gastroenterology, 68, 220–230.

Elder, J.B. and Smith, I.S. (1975) Gastric acid output, pepsin and lean body mass in normal and duodenal ulcer subjects. Lancet, 1, 1000–1003.

Fischerman, K. and Koster, K.H. (1962) The augmented histamine test in the differential diagnosis between ulcer and cancer of the stomach. Gut, 3, 211–218.

Fordtran, J.S. and Walsh, J.H. (1973) Gastric acid secretion rate and buffer content of the stomach after eating. Journal of Clinical Investigation, 52, 645–657.

Ganguli, P.C. and Hunter, W.M. (1972) Radioimmunoassay of gastrin in human plasma, Journal of Physiology (London), 220, 499–510.

Ganguli, P.C., Polak, J.M., Pearse, A.G.E., Elder, J.B. and Hegarty, M. (1974) Antral gastrin cell hyperplasia in peptic ulcer disease. Lancet, 1, 583–585.

Gibson, L.E. and Cooke, R.E. (1959) A test for concentration of electrolytes in sweat in cystic fibrosis of the pancreas utilising pilocarpine by iontophoresis, Paediatrics, 23, 545–549.

Gillespie, G., Elder, J.B., Gillespie, I.E., Kay, A.W. and Campbell, E.H.G. (1970) The long term stability of the insulin test. Gastroenterology, 58, 625–632.

Gillespie, G., Elder, J.B., Smith, I.S., Kennedy, F., Gillespie, I.E., Kay, A.W. and Campbell, E.H.G. (1972) An analysis of spontaneous gastric acid secretion in normal and duodenal ulcer subjects: new criterion for the insulin test. Gastroenterology, 62, 903–911.

Gregory, R.A. (1968) Gastrin – The natural history of a peptide hormone. Harvey Lectures, 64, 121–155.

Gregory, R.A. and Tracey, H.J. (1975) The chemistry of the gastrins: some recent advances. In Gastrointestinal Hormones (Ed. J.C. Thompson) pp. 13–24, University of Texas Press, Austin.

Grossman, M.I. (1974) Gastrointestinal Hormones: spectrum of actions and structure–activity relations. In Endocrinology of the Gut (Eds. W.Y. Chey and F.P. Brooks) pp. 65–75, Charles B. Slack, Thorofare.

Guttierrez, L.V. and Baron, J.H. (1976) A comparison of basal and stimulated gastric acid and duodenal bicarbonate secretion in patients with and without duodenal ulcer disease. American Journal of Gastroenterology, 66, 270–276.

Hansky, J. and Korman, M.G. (1973) Immunoassay studies in peptic ulcer. In Clinics in Gastroenterology, Vol. 2, No. 2 (Ed. W. Sircus) pp. 275–292, W.B. Saunders.

Hassan, M.A. and Hobsley, M. (1970) Position of subject and of nasogastric tube during a gastric secretion study. British Medical Journal, 1, 458–460.

Hirschowitz, B.I. (1967) Secretion of pepsinogen. In Handbook of Physiology, Vol. 2, Section 6 (Ed. C.F. Code) pp. 889–918, American Physiological Society, Washington.

Hollander, F. (1946) The insulin test for the presence of intact nerve fibres after vagal operations for peptic ulcer. Gastroenterology, 7, 607–614.

Hollander, F. (1948) Laboratory procedures in the study of vagotomy with particular reference to the insulin test. Gastroenterology, 11, 419; 425.

Hough, L. and Jones, J.V.S. (1972) Human gastric mucosa. Part I. The preparation of a glycopolypeptide and some aspects of its structure. Carbohydrate Research, 23, 1–16.

Isenberg, J.I., Stenning, G.F., Ward, S. and Grossman, M.I. (1969) Relation of gastric secretory response in man to dose of insulin. Gastroenterology, 57, 395–398.

Johnson, A.G. and McDermott, S.G. (1974) Lysolecithin: a factor in the pathogenesis of gastric ulceration? Gut, 15, 710–713.

Kay, A.W. (1953) Effect of large doses of histamine on gastric secretion of HCL. British Medical Journal, 2, 77–80.

Kay, A.W. (1967) An evaluation of gastric secretion tests (Memorial Lecture). Gastroenterology, 53, 834–844.

Korman, M.G., Strickland, R.G. and Hansky, J. (1971) Serum gastrin in chronic gastritis. British Medical Journal, 2, 16–18.

Korman, M.G., Scott, D.F. and Hansky, J. (1972) Hypergastrinaemia due to an excluded gastric antrum: a proposed method for differentiation from Zollinger–Ellison Syndrome. Australian and New Zealand Journal of Medicine, 3, 266–268.

Lambert, R. (1974) The contamination of gastric juice by the mucous secretion of the upper digestive tract. Rendiconti di Gastro-enterologia, 6, 60–64.

Lamers, C.B.H.W. (1976) Some Aspects of the Zollinger–Ellison Syndrome and Serum Gastrin. Doctorate Thesis of the University of Nijmegen, pp. 63–86, 141–157.

Lawson, D., Westcombe, P. and Saggar, B. (1969) Pilot trial of an infant screening programme for cystic fibrosis: measurement of parotid salivary sodium at four months. Archives of Diseases of Childhood, 44, 715–718.

Makhlouf, G.M., McManus, J.P.A. and Card, W.I. (1966) A quantitative statement of the two component hypothesis of gastric secretion. Gastroenterology, 51, 149–171.

Malagelada, J.R., Longstreth, G.F., Summerskill, W.H.J. and Go, V.L.W. (1976) Measurement of gastric functions during digestion of ordinary solid meals in man. Gastroenterology, 70, 203–210.

Mason, D.K. and Chisholm, D.M. (1975) Salivary glands in health and disease. W.B. Saunders, London.

Moore, E.W. (1967) The terminology and measurement of gastric acidity. Annals of the New York Academy of Science, 140, 866–874.

Multicentre Study (1967) The effect of vagotomy on gastric secretion elicited by pentagastrin in man. Lancet, 2, 534–536.

Multicentre Study (1969) Intramuscular pentagastrin compared with other stimuli as tests of gastric secretion. Lancet, 1, 341–343.

O'Brien, P. and Silen, W. (1976) Influence of acid secretory state on the gastric mucosal tolerance to back diffusion of H^+. Gastroenterology, 71, 760–765.

Parke, D.V. (1976) Gastric mucus and carbenoxolone. In Topics in Gastroenterology-4 (Eds. S.C. Truelove and J.A. Ritchie) Blackwell Scientific Publications, London.

Petersen, O.H. (1972) Electrolyte transports involved in the formation of saliva. In Oral Physiology (Eds. N. Emmeln and Y. Zotterman) pp. 21–31, Pergamon Press, Oxford.

Piper, D.W. (1960) The estimation of peptic activity in gastric juice using radio-iodinated serum albumin as substrate. Gastroenterology, 38, 616–621.

Reeder, D.D., Becker, H.D. and Thompson, J.C. (1974) Increases in serum gastrin after calcium in duodenal ulcer patients, patients with the Zollinger–Ellison syndrome and normal man. In Endocrinology of the Gut (Eds. W.Y. Chey and F.P. Brooks) pp. 290–301, Charles B. Black, Thorofare.

Rehfeld, J.F., Stadil, F. and Vikelsoe, J. (1974) Immunoreactive gastrin components in human serum. Gut, 15, 102–111.

Rhodes, J., Barnado, D.E., Phillips, S.F., Rovelstad, R.A. and Hofmann, A.F. (1969) Increased reflux of bile into the stomach of patients with gastric ulcer. Gastroenterology, 57, 241–252.

Samloff, I.M. (1969) Slow moving protease and the seven pepsinogens. Electrophoretic demonstration of the existence of light proteolytic fractions in human gastric mucosa. Gastroenterology, 57, 659–669.

Samloff, I., Liebman, W.M. and Panitch, N.M. (1975) Serum Group I pepsinogens by radioimmunoassay in control subjects and patients with peptic ulcer. Gastroenterology, 69, 83–90.

Samloff, I.M. and Dadufalza, V. (1978) Effect of ionic strength on the proteolytic activities of human group I and group II pepsins. Gastroenterology, in press.

Schrager, J. and Oates, M.D.G. (1973) A comparative study of the major glycoprotein isolated from normal and neoplastic gastric mucosa. Gut, 14, 324–329.

Schrager, J., Oates, M.D.G. and Rosbottom, A. (1972) The isolation and partial characterisation of the principal biliary glycoprotein. Digestion, 6, 338–355.

Scratcherd, T. (1973) Gastric secretory mechanisms and peptic ulcer. In Clinics in Gastroenterology, Vol. 2, No. 2 (Ed. W. Sircus), pp. 259–274, W.B. Saunders, London.

Smith, I.S., Gillespie, G., Elder, J.B., Gillespie, I.E. and Kay, A.W. (1972) Time of conversion of insulin response after vagotomy. Gastroenterology, 62, 912–917.

Stadil, F. and Rehfeld, J.F. (1973) Determination of gastrin in serum. An evaluation of the reliability of radioimmunoassay. Scandinavian Journal of Gastroenterology, 8, 101–112.

Stavney, L.S., Hamilton, T., Sircus, W. and Smith, A.N. (1966) Evaluation of the pH sensitive telemetering capsule in the estimation of gastric secretory capacity. American Journal of Digestive Diseases, 11, 753–760.

Stern, D.H. and Walsh, J.H. (1973) Release of gastrin in post-operative duodenal ulcer patients. Gastroenterology, 64, 363–369.

Straus, E. and Yalow, R.S. (1975) Differential diagnosis of hypergastrinaemia. In Gastrointestinal Hormones (Ed. J.C. Thompson) pp. 99–114, University of Texas Press, Austin.

Sun, D.C.H. and Roth, J.L.A. (1974) Tests employed in analysis of the stomach contents and their clinical application. In Gastroenterology, Vol. 1 (Ed. H.L. Bochus) pp. 419–453, W.B. Saunders, Philadelphia.

Taylor, T.V., Elder, J.B., Ganguli, P.C. and Gillespie, I.E. (1978) A comparison of an intragastric method of estimating acid output with the pentagastrin test in normal and duodenal ulcer subjects. Gut, 19, 865–869.

Thompson, J.C., Reeder, D.D., Villar, H.V. and Fender, H.R. (1975) Natural history and experience with diagnosis and treatment of Zollinger–Ellison Syndrome. Surgery, Gynaecology and Obstetrics, 140, 721–729.

Trudeau, W.L. and McGuigan, J.E. (1970) Serum gastrin levels in patients with peptic ulcer disease. Gastroenterology, 59, 6–12.

Walsh, J.H. and Grossman, M.I. (1975) Gastrin. New England Journal of Medicine, 292, 1324–1332, 1377–1384.

Walsh, J.H., Yalow, R.S. and Berson, S.A. (1971) The effect of atropine on plasma gastrin response to feeding. Gastroenterology, 60, 16–21.

Walsh, J.H. and Roth, B.E. (1976) Hormone secreting tumours of the gastrointestinal tract. In Recent Advances in Gastroenterology (Ed. I.A.D. Bouchier) pp. 49–72, Churchill Livingstone, Edinburgh.

Wesdorp, R.I.C. and Fischer, J.E. (1974) Plasma gastrin and acid secretion in patients with peptic ulceration. Lancet, 2, 857–860.

Yalow, R.S. (1974) Heterogeneity of peptide hormones. In Recent Progress in Hormone Research, Vol. 30 (Ed. R.O. Greep) pp. 597–633, Academic Press, New York and London.

FURTHER READING

Baron, J.H. (1970) The clinical use of gastric function tests. Scandinavian Journal of Gastroenterology, 5, Suppl. 6, 9–46.

Black, J.W., Duncan, W.A.M. and Durant, C.J. (1972) Definition and antagonism of histamine$_2$-receptors. Nature, 236, 385–390.

Bockus, H.L. (1974) Gastroenterology, Vol. 1. W.B. Saunders, Philadelphia.

Bonfils, S. (Ed.) (1974) Clinics in Gastroenterology, Vol. 3, No. 3. W.B. Saunders.

Bouchier, I.A.D. (1976) Recent Advances in Gastroenterology, Vol. 3. Churchill Livingstone, Edinburgh.

Chey, W.Y. and Brooks, F.P. (Eds.) (1974) Endocrinology of the Gut. Charles B. Slack, Thorofare.

Davenport, H.W. (1977) Physiology of the Digestive Tract. Year Book Medical Publishing, Co., Chicago.

Makhlouf, G.M., McManus, J.P.A. and Card, W.I. (1966) A quantitative statement of the two component hypothesis of gastric secretion. Gastroenterology, 51, 149–171.

Mason, D.K. and Chisholm, D.M. (1975) Salivary Glands in Health and Disease. W.B. Saunders, London.

Moore, E.W. (1967) The terminology and measurement of gastric acidity. Annals of the New York Academy of Science, 140, 866–874.

Sircus, W. (Ed.) (1973) Clinics in Gastroenterology, Vol. 2, No. 2. W.B. Saunders, London.

Trulove, S.C. and Ritchie, J.A. (Eds.) (1976) Topics in Gastroenterology. Blackwell Scientific Publications, London.

Walsh, J.H. and Grossman, M.I. (1975) Gastrin. New England Journal of Medicine, 292, 1324–1332, 1377–1384.

Yalow, R.S. (1974) Recent Progress in Hormone Research (Ed. R.O. Greep) Academic Press, New York and London.

Chapter 12

Intestinal and pancreatic function

C. Derek Holdsworth

Gastrointestinal Unit, Hallamshire Hospital, Sheffield S10 2JF, England

CONTENTS

Chemical diagnosis of disease, edited by
S.S. Brown, F.L. Mitchell and D.S. Young

INTRODUCTION

Whether the laboratory plays a major or minor role in the diagnosis of intestinal disease depends upon the clinical problem. In this chapter, assessment of nutrition in gastrointestinal disorders is discussed first, both because this is often important in diagnosis and management, and because simple screening procedures for evidence of nutritional disturbance will normally be the first laboratory tests undertaken in any patient presenting with gastrointestinal symptoms. As intestinal disease frequently presents with diarrhoea or abdominal pain, the role of the laboratory in elucidating these symptoms is discussed next. Malabsorption and pancreatic disease depend almost exclusively on the laboratory for their diagnosis, and the account of these inevitably forms the largest section of this chapter. Finally there is a discussion of the small – but increasing – number of serological tests which are becoming of value in diagnosis.

12.1. NUTRITIONAL ASSESSMENT IN GASTROINTESTINAL DISEASE

A nutritional defect is often a presenting feature of gastrointestinal disease. It may be due to impaired intake, impaired absorption, or excessive loss. Assessment of nutritional status and elucidation of the mechanism may affect management, and in malabsorptive states they are also of diagnostic importance (section 12.4.1).

The commonest and most important deficiencies are of protein, the three main haematinics (iron, folate and vitamin B_{12}) and vitamin D.

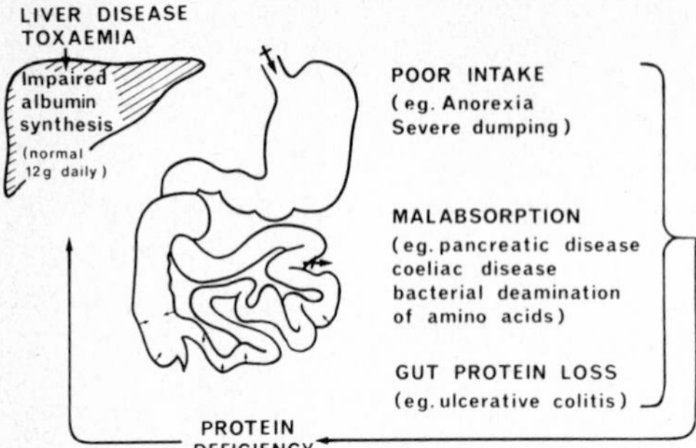

Figure 12.1. Diagram showing how gastrointestinal disease can cause hypoalbuminaemia by depressing albumin synthesis in the liver.

12.1.1. Protein nutrition

Assessment of protein nutrition is unsatisfactory (Waterlow, 1969), and in practice is limited to measurement of the serum albumin concentration. However, the wide range found in normal subjects, variations with age, and the influence of changes in distribution within the body all limit the usefulness of this test. Assessment of the significance of hypoalbuminaemia in gut disease is only satisfactory if possible mechanisms are understood; the occasional need for some special procedure to elucidate its cause can then be determined.

Hypoalbuminaemia in gut disease may be associated with decreased hepatic synthesis (Figure 12.1). In these circumstances, degradation of serum albumin as measured by the rate of disappearance of ^{131}I-labelled albumin from the circulation will usually be decreased. If the hypoproteinaemia is due to increased loss of serum proteins from the gut (protein losing enteropathy), disappearance of ^{131}I-labelled albumin from the circulation will be more rapid than normal. If the loss of albumin is from the stomach or jejunum, the protein is digested and re-absorbed so that there is no overall state of protein malnutrition, and hepatic synthesis of albumin is increased. The serum albumin concentration then only falls when the loss of serum albumin exceeds the reserve capacity of the liver for increased synthesis (Figure 12.2).

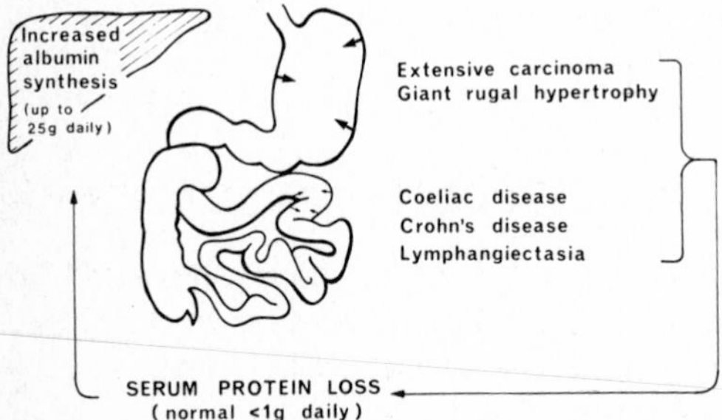

Figure 12.2. Diagram showing how protein losing enteropathy can result in hypoalbuminaemia even if hepatic synthesis of albumin is normal or increased.

In practice, the mechanisms shown in Figures 12.1 and 12.2 often operate simultaneously. The extent to which they are relevant in any individual patient can be elucidated by studies of albumin synthesis rate and albumin degradation rate (Chapter 6), but these are not applicable in routine practice. In certain circumstances, determination of the rate of albumin loss may contribute to clinical management and this is therefore discussed in more detail.

12.1.2. Protein losing enteropathy (exudative enteropathy; Waldmann, 1970)

Loss of serum protein into the bowel lumen has been demonstrated in about 70 disorders which affect the gastrointestinal tract, including most inflammatory diseases, extensive carcinoma or ulceration, infections, and coeliac disease. It may be the primary manifestation, as in intestinal lymphangiectasia, and giant rugal hypertrophy of the stomach. There are reductions in the half-lives of many serum proteins, e.g. albumin, IgG, IgA, IgM, caeruloplasmin, fibrinogen and lipoproteins. Although the loss into the bowel of each is increased to the same extent, the reduction in serum protein concentration varies according to the body's capacity to make up for the loss. The serum concentrations of proteins with longer turnover times are therefore decreased most, i.e. albumin and IgG (Table 6.2).

The rate of synthesis of the major immunoglobulins is usually normal in patients with protein losing enteropathy if there is no associated inflammatory process. A low serum concentration is not therefore a stimulus to increased immunoglobulin production, in contrast to albumin.

12.1.3. Techniques for the measurement of gastrointestinal protein loss (Waldmann, 1970)

Because of digestion and re-absorption of secreted protein, nitrogen balance techniques cannot be used. Attempts to study stool radioactivity after intravenous administration of ^{131}I-labelled serum albumin are equally inappropriate, since the iodine label is lost by metabolism, re-absorbed and excreted in the urine. Several labelled compounds have been evaluated as alternatives, but only two have been widely used.

12.1.3.1. [^{131}I]Polyvinylpyrrolidone

This is a synthetic polymer which is not absorbed by the intestine. A dose of 10 to 25 μCi is given intravenously and all stools are collected for 4 days. Normal subjects excrete in the faeces 0 to 1.5% of the dose; patients with protein loss from 3 to 30% per cent. The radiation dose is estimated at 10 to 75 mrads total to the body, 110 to 275 mrads to the gonads, and 5 to 200 mrads to the liver.

12.1.3.2. ^{51}Cr-labelled albumin, or [^{51}Cr]chromic chloride

^{51}Cr-labelled albumin has been used in the same way as [^{131}I]polyvinylpyrrolidone, but the Cr label is not re-absorbed from the gut after digestion of the labelled protein. Rather than give a labelled protein, it is simpler to inject 5 to 10 μCi of [^{51}Cr]chromic chloride intravenously. This very rapidly binds to plasma proteins in vivo. Normal subjects excrete less than 1% of the dose in a 4-day stool collection. The radiation dose is estimated as 10 to 75 mrads total to the body, and 80 to 875 mrads to the liver.

12.1.3.3. Choice of test

Both tests are completely invalidated if urine, which contains appreciable radioactivity, contaminates the stool collection; ^{59}Fe-labelled dextran has been used in children to obviate this effect as iron is not excreted significantly in urine. [^{131}I]Polyvinylpyrrolidone often contains free ^{131}I; it is a non-physiological mixture of molecular species of widely different molecular masses, and its use necessitates prior blocking of thyroid uptake by means of oral potassium iodide. [^{51}Cr]Chromic chloride has the advantage of being widely available, but there is a practical difficulty of adsorption of Cr^{3+} onto glassware, which makes accurate dispensing rather difficult. Both techniques give only qualitative information and do not enable the actual amount of protein leaking each day to be calculated.

12.1.3.4. Indications for test

There are few indications for these tests in clinical practice. Abnormal values are to be expected in severe inflammatory bowel disease, coeliac disease, etc., and measurement in these circumstances contributes little to management. However, in the diagnosis of giant rugal hypertrophy and intestinal lymphangiectasia, and in the assessment of patients presenting with idiopathic hypoalbuminaemia, the tests can be most valuable. Ideally they should be combined with studies of albumin catabolism (Chapter 6).

12.1.4. Immunoglobulins (Jones, 1972; McGuigan, 1973)

The intestinal tract contains numerous immunoglobulin-producing cells in the lamina propria. IgA-producing cells are the most common, and the majority of the IgA so produced is secreted into the gut lumen, with only a little entering the general circulation. Some IgM-producing cells are present, but relatively few producing IgG. IgA secretion is an important part of a local mucosal immune defence system.

The diagnostic value of serum immunoglobulin determinations in bowel disease is limited, as the changes secondary to bowel disease are non-specific, and bowel disease secondary to immunoglobulin deficiency is rare.

12.1.4.1. Primary immunoglobulin deficiencies

In *congenital primary agammaglobulinaemia,* plasma cells are absent from jejunal biopsies but gastrointestinal malfunction is rare. In *acquired hypogammaglobulinaemia,* diarrhoea is frequent, often with steatorrhoea. The precise cause of the steatorrhoea is unknown, but giardiasis and intestinal bacterial overgrowth are often found. In *selective IgA deficiency,* a clinical syndrome similar to coeliac disease may occur. Low serum IgA is also found in nodular *lymphoid hyperplasia* of the small intestine, which may also cause diarrhoea and malabsorption.

12.1.4.2. Immunoglobulin changes secondary to disease

In *protein losing enteropathy,* IgG is the most severely depressed immunoglobulin (section 12.1.2). In *Crohn's disease and ulcerative colitis,* the serum concentrations of immunoglobulins are similar to normal, although turnover studies show markedly increased rates of degradation and synthesis. In contrast, the serum concentrations of acute phase reactants such as α_1-antitrypsin and haptoglobulin are increased and this is reflected in increased α_2-globulin concentration on electrophoresis. In *coeliac disease,* serum IgA concentrations are often raised and IgM levels are often low on presentation, but both return to normal on a gluten-free diet. A subsequent rise in IgA may indicate the development of a complicating lymphoma, but this is certainly not always the case. In *parasitic diseases,* a raised concentration of IgE may be found.

12.1.4.3. IgA heavy chain (α-chain) disease

This is a plasma cell dyscrasia usually occurring in individuals of Mediterranean origin who present with chronic diarrhoea, malabsorption and wasting. Free α-chains can be found in serum, and on electrophoresis these migrate between the α_2- and β-globulins.

12.1.5. Assessment of folate and vitamin B_{12} status (Chanarin, 1969)

Gastrointestinal disease commonly presents with a microcytic hypochromic deficiency anaemia due to iron deficiency, with megaloblastic anaemia due to folate or vitamin B_{12} deficiency, or with a mixed deficiency anaemia. Assessment of these deficiencies is often important in diagnosis.

12.1.5.1. Folate deficiency

Folate deficiency may be the result of poor intake, poor absorption or increased demand (Figure 12.3). The measurement and significance of serum and red blood cell folate is discussed in Chapter 16. It only remains here to stress the frequency with which low serum folate concentrations occur in patients who are sufficiently ill to require hospital admission. The cause is due to poor intake and probably also an increased requirement which occurs in many diseases. Red cell folate is a much better index of true tissue depletion.

12.1.5.2. Vitamin B_{12} deficiency

In contrast to folate, body stores of vitamin B_{12} are substantial so that dietary deficiency is rare. Vitamin B_{12} deficiency therefore usually indicates B_{12} malabsorption due to the

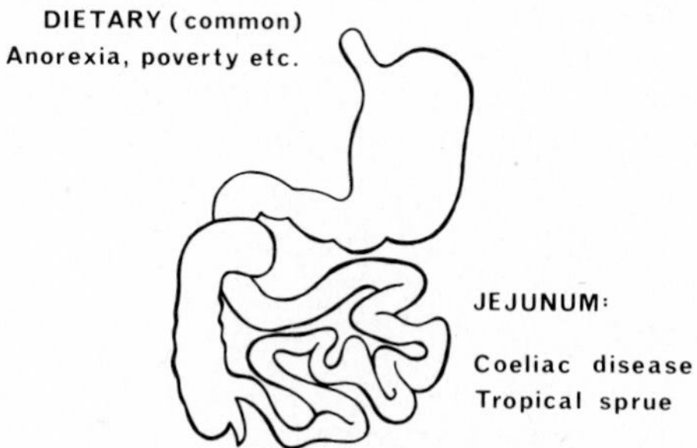

Figure 12.3. The aetiology of folate deficiency.

causes shown in Figure 12.4. However, it is important to appreciate that folate deficiency, and also severe iron deficiency, can lead to a fall in the serum B_{12} concentration which is corrected when the deficiency is repaired and does not therefore indicate true B_{12} deficiency. Vitamin B_{12} absorption tests (section 12.4.4) are often necessary to evaluate the significance of low serum concentrations.

12.1.5.3. Urinary excretion of formiminoglutamic acid and methylmalonic acid

These tests depend on assessing a metabolic pathway in which the vitamin participates. Vitamin B_{12} deficiency is usually associated with increased urinary excretion of methylmalonic acid, and folic acid deficiency with increased urinary excretion of formiminoglutamic acid after an oral dose (15 grams) of L-histidine hydrochloride. Neither test has become established in clinical practice, as the assay techniques are complex. For diagnostic purposes, a combination of serum and red cell folate measurements and vitamin B_{12} serum assays and absorption tests are usually adequate.

12.1.5.4. Significance of vitamin B_{12} and folate deficiencies in some gastrointestinal disorders

In *adult coeliac disease,* a low serum and red cell folate is so commonly found that the investigations can be used as a screening test. Megaloblastic anaemia, if present, is almost invariably due to folate deficiency. However, individuals are found occasionally, for example in screening the families of patients with coeliac disease, with unequivocally abnormal jejunal biopsies but normal serum and red cell folate. A low serum vitamin B_{12} concentration is found in rather less than half of most patients with coeliac disease. Sometimes this is secondary to severe folate deficiency, but more often it is due to vitamin B_{12} malabsorption, and indicates ileal as well as jejunal involvement. Steatorrhoea is usually more marked in such patients.

In *tropical sprue,* folate deficiency is almost invariably present, and is often the dominant clinical feature. Vitamin B_{12} malabsorption is usually present but vitamin B_{12} deficiency only occurs in chronic cases. In *pancreatic* steatorrhoea, folate and B_{12} status is

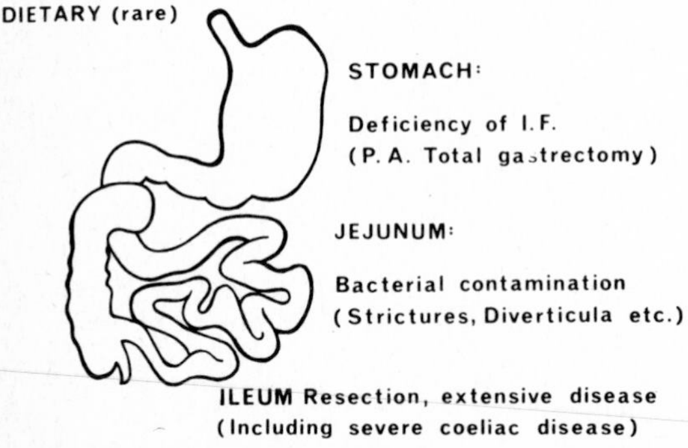

Figure 12.4. The aetiology of vitamin B_{12} deficiency: in contrast to folic acid, vitamin B_{12} malabsorption can be caused by disease of either stomach, jejunum or ileum. (I.F. = intrinsic factor; P.A. = pernicious anaemia.)

usually normal. Although vitamin B_{12} absorption is frequently low (section 12.4.4.2), megaloblastic anaemia is rare. In the *stagnant loop syndrome*, vitamin B_{12} deficiency due to malabsorption is often a prominent feature. Folate deficiency is rare and the serum folate concentration may be higher than normal.

Crohn's disease can result in vitamin B_{12} deficiency due to ileal involvement or small bowel stasis, but severe deficiency with megaloblastic anaemia is in practice confined to patients who have had resection of bowel. Low serum folate concentrations are the rule in patients who are sufficiently ill to require hospital admission, but true deficiency, with low red cell folate and anaemia, is rare. Inadequate intake and probably increased utilization are the main aetiological factors. In ulcerative colitis – and indeed in any disorder where food intake may be impaired – low serum folate values may be found, although less commonly than in Crohn's disease.

After *total gastrectomy,* vitamin B_{12} absorption is of course grossly defective and replacement therapy is mandatory. After *partial gastrectomy,* folate deficiency is rare, but clinically significant vitamin B_{12} deficiency eventually occurs in 5 to 10% of patients. The incidence of reduced serum B_{12} concentrations increases steadily from less than 5% after 2 years to over 20% after 10 years. Vitamin B_{12} malabsorption, as determined by the standard Schilling test, is present earlier and in a higher proportion of patients, especially if no food or other stimulus to intrinsic factor secretion is given. The cause of the vitamin B_{12} malabsorption after partial gastrectomy is probably multifactorial. It includes atrophic gastritis of the gastric remnant; perhaps failure to secrete intrinsic factor due to decreased gastric secretion; diminished pancreatic secretion; and occasionally stasis in a long afferent loop. Evaluation of a slightly low serum B_{12} concentration found in a patient after partial gastrectomy is therefore not always straightforward, as it may be secondary to severe iron deficiency, and a Schilling test may not give an indication of vitamin B_{12} absorption from food.

12.1.6. Iron deficiency

This differs from folate and B_{12} deficiency because, in addition to deficient intake and malabsorption, iron deficiency is often secondary to blood loss. The investigation of iron deficiency can therefore be a complicated problem involving clinical and radiological as well as laboratory assessment. The significance of serum iron and iron binding capacity determinations are discussed in Chapter 16. Serum ferritin concentrations afford a valuable indication of iron deficiency or overload, but the test is not generally available (Jacobs and Worwood, 1975).

12.1.6.1. Occult blood loss

Very often, blood loss has to be inferred from the finding of a bleeding lesion, unless blood is visible in the faeces. The detection of occult blood in the faeces can, however, provide some help in the initial evaluation of an iron deficiency anaemia. Various methods are available, all of which depend upon the peroxidase-like activity of haem, linked to hydrogen peroxide–chromogen system. The tests now in use all require the patient to be on a meat- and fish-free diet (preferably for 3 days before collecting stools) and usually to have avoided oral iron. The sensitivities of the different tests vary and can never be equated to blood loss with any precision; e.g. anything from 3.5 to 20 ml of daily loss may be needed to yield a positive result, even with a well standardized test. Normal loss is up to 2.5 ml daily. This variability and the frequently intermittent nature of gastro-intestinal bleeding from any type of lesion is a marked limitation. Even so, in most laboratories, examination of three successive stools for occult blood can be of help in the initial investigation of iron deficiency anaemia.

The quantitative measurement of blood loss requires labelling of the patient's own red blood cells with [^{51}Cr]chromic chloride, re-injection, and subsequent daily counting of radioactivity in the stools. This is a practicable procedure, since in many hospitals the same labelling procedure is done for red cell survival studies.

12.1.6.2. Iron absorption and malabsorption

The measurement of iron absorption is possible using a variety of isotopic techniques, but is not of any help in clinical practice. This is partly because iron deficiency itself leads to compensatory iron hyperabsorption. In addition, dietary iron may be absorbed poorly when inorganic iron absorption is little affected, e.g. after partial gastrectomy. In practice, iron malabsorption is most commonly due to previous gastric surgery, and next most commonly to coeliac disease.

12.1.7. Vitamin deficiencies other than B_{12} and folate

Deficiency of vitamin B_{12} and folic acid have already been discussed (section 12.1.5). Deficiency of other vitamins of the B complex does occur in malabsorptive states, but assessment of deficiency is difficult and at present is of no diagnostic help. Vitamin C deficiency is rarely a clinical problem in malabsorptive disease.

Vitamin A deficiency, sometimes manifested by low plasma concentrations, does occur in malabsorptive states and measurement of plasma concentration has been used as a screening test. It cannot be recommended since exceptions are very frequent. Clinical evidence of deficiency is rare. Vitamin E concentrations are perhaps more often low in malabsorptive states, but clinical evidence of deficiency is not seen and measurement of plasma vitamin E, although possible, is rarely used in diagnosis.

Vitamin K deficiency, in contrast, is easily assessed by determination of prothrombin time, and occurs in up to 70% of patients with coeliac disease; it is rare in pancreatic disease and small bowel stasis syndromes.

Vitamin D deficiency is important, both because of its frequency and the importance of the clinical manifestations it produces. Like vitamin K deficiency, it is rare in pancreatic disease and small bowel stasis syndromes, but common in coeliac disease. Determinations of serum calcium and phosphate concentrations and alkaline phosphatase activity are therefore routine in the assessment of possible malabsorptive disease. Pitfalls in interpretation, however are, common. The serum calcium concentration may be low secondary to depressed serum albumin concentration. The serum phosphate concentration may be normal in the presence of definite osteomalacia. Alkaline phosphatase activity may be raised for many reasons other than osteomalacia, particularly in the liver disease which frequently accompanies ulcerative colitis and Crohn's disease, and in the presence of non-clinically apparent Paget's disease. Improved routine methods for the clinical diagnosis of osteomalacia are becoming available (Chapter 22), but have not yet been extensively applied to problems of gastrointestinal disease.

12.1.8. Mineral deficiencies other than iron (see also Chapter 8)

Calcium deficiency is only seen as a manifestation of vitamin D deficiency when it can be severe, with tetany as a presenting feature. Calcium absorption in man, its relationship to vitamin D, and the mechanisms of calcium malabsorption are discussed in detail elsewhere (Holdsworth, 1975). It can be studied by both chemical balance and isotopic techniques, but these are not of diagnostic help in routine practice.

Magnesium deficiency is occasionally found to accompany hypocalcaemia in severe malabsorptive states, and may contribute to the tetany (Booth et al., 1963). In these circumstances, the serum calcium concentration may not rise until magnesium supplements are given. The serum magnesium concentration should therefore be estimated in malabsorptive states if there is tetany, or if the serum calcium concentration does not rise quickly after adequate vitamin D replacement therapy.

12.1.9. Nutritional screening in gastrointestinal disease

It is suggested that in the routine assessment of patients presenting with gastrointestinal symptoms, any laboratory screening should include the following estimations: blood haemoglobin; blood film; serum albumin, calcium, phosphate, alkaline phosphatase, and serum potassium (if diarrhoea is a symptom).

If malabsorption is suspected, it would be reasonable to include the following additional tests: prothrombin time; serum B_{12}; serum and red blood cell folate; serum iron and iron binding capacity.

Other clinical indications mentioned in the foregoing discussion of gastrointestinal disease may suggest determination of the following: plasma immunoglobulins or serum protein; electrophoresis; occult blood in stools.

Efficient use of in-patient facilities requires that the results of all such investigations should be available before a patient is admitted for any planned in-patient studies. The need for the other tests discussed in this section would then be assessed in the light of the results of these initial investigations.

12.2. DIARRHOEA (Fordtran, 1973)

12.2.1. Pathophysiological classification

It is useful to classify the causes of diarrhoea under the four headings shown in Table 12.1. This is grossly oversimplified, and in most diseases more than one of these mechanisms may be operating.

TABLE 12.1.

PATHOPHYSIOLOGICAL CLASSIFICATION OF DIARRHOEA

Type	Mechanism	Examples
Osmotic	Non-absorbed solute retaining fluid within the lumen by osmotic activity	Alactasia Magnesium sulphate purgation
Secretory	Increased secretion due to increased hormonal/chemical stimulation or an abnormal mucosa or gland	Zollinger-Ellison syndrome and W.D.H.H. syndrome (watery diarrhoea, hypokalaemia and hypochlorhydria). Cholera Ulcerative colitis Bile salt- and prostaglandin-induced
Diminished absorption	Ion transport defects, and mucosal damage by disease	Chloridorrhoea Ulcerative colitis Bile salt diarrhoea
Abnormal motility	Rapid transit which reduces contact time for absorption of fluid	Thyrotoxicosis Prostaglandin-induced

12.2.2. Normal water and electrolyte movement

A complete account of normal water and electrolyte movement is not possible here, and reference should be made to the review of Fordtran (1973). Suffice it to emphasize that considerable 2-way fluxes occur throughout the length of the intestine, and that in addition to ingested fluid, all glandular secretions such as those of stomach and pancreas have to be absorbed. All water transport is passive, secondary to osmotic pressure gradients. Water absorption is therefore dependent on the active transport systems for ions and organic solutes which are present in mucosal cells throughout the small intestine and colon. Of particular importance are the active transport systems for sodium, glucose, aminoacids and peptides in the small intestine, and for sodium in the large intestine.

TABLE 12.2.

DAILY WATER AND ELECTROLYTE EXCRETION IN ILEOSTOMY EFFLUENT AND IN NORMAL STOOL

	Fluid delivered by an ileostomy		Fluid delivered in normal stool	
	Quantity	Concentration mmol/litre	Quantity	Concentration mmol/litre
Water	1500 ml	–	100 ml	–
Sodium	75 mmol	125	4 mmol	40
Potassium	5 mmol	9	9 mmol	90
Chloride	6 mmol	60	2 mmol	20
Bicarbonate	44 mmol	74	3 mmol	30

Recent studies have shown that the normal colon absorbs about 1350 ml of water, 200 mmol of sodium, 150 mmol of chloride, and 60 mmol of bicarbonate each day. Previous estimates, based on the volume of ileostomy effluent, were lower since in these circumstances the ileum adapts and delivers less fluid (Table 12.2). The amounts of potassium entering and leaving the normal colon each day are about equal, although of course the concentration in stool water is much higher than in ileal effluent.

12.2.3. Water and electrolyte changes due to diarrhoea

As stool volume increases, stool electrolyte composition gradually approaches that normally found in the ileum, probably due simply to rapid transit and relatively decreased colonic function. Stool sodium loss is thus directly proportional to stool volume. Potassium loss rises much less steeply with increasing stool volume.

Severe diarrhoea is therefore accompanied inevitably by sodium and water depletion, and to a lesser extent by potassium depletion. Isolated potassium depletion is often seen in chronic mild diarrhoea, because stool potassium concentration is then relatively high, and renal conservation of potassium is less effective than that for sodium.

Acid-base disturbances in patients with diarrhoea are very variable. The most common is acidosis – resulting primarily from increased faecal loss of bicarbonate but sometimes aggravated by ketoacidosis due to starvation, the acidosis of a pre-renal uraemia, or lactic acidosis secondary to shock. In chronic mild diarrhoea, hypokalaemic alkalosis may be found, due to partial replacement of intracellular potassium by hydrogen ion derived from extracellular fluid.

12.2.4. Laboratory assessment of diarrhoea

In the majority of patients with diarrhoea, laboratory tests other than the simple screening suggested earlier (section 12.1.9) will be unnecessary. History, including current medication, examination of stools by the naked eye, sigmoidoscopy and bacteriological and radiological studies, will enable a diagnosis to be made in many patients. The presence of nutritional defects or of pale, bulky, frothy and malodorous stools will, however, necessitate determination of faecal fat and other tests to exclude malabsorption (section 12.4).

Chronic diarrhoea in which all of these investigations prove negative will very often be due to the irritable colon syndrome; associated pain, personality features, the passage of "rabbity" stools and sometimes mucus, will support this diagnosis. If diarrhoea is troublesome, persistent, or associated with any degree of systemic disturbance it may be necessary to admit the patient for more searching studies. A collection of stools for fat determination, if not already done, will then be mandatory. Daily record of stool frequency is made, and the nature and weight of each stool is recorded. The behaviour and personality of the patient are assessed carefully, as this may be relevant to both the irritable colon syndrome and to the concealed taking of purgatives; and previous investigations should be reviewed.

Only then should additional laboratory studies be performed, and in planning these a pathophysiological approach is appropriate. The following possibilities should be considered.

12.2.4.1. Osmotic diarrhoea

The diarrhoea should cease with a 24-hour fast. In infants, an acid pH of the stool and the presence of reducing sugar in the stool is readily detected, but in adults, other tests may be necessary to exclude lactase deficiency (section 12.4.3.8). In neonates, other disaccharidase deficiencies and glucose–galactose malabsorption must be excluded (section 12.4.3.10).

12.2.4.2. Bile salt diarrhoea

The escape of increased amounts of bile salts into the colon provokes diarrhoea due both to inhibition of sodium and water absorption, and to stimulation of secretion. Classically this is associated with moderate ileal resection of up to 100 cm, steatorrhoea being more prominent with larger resections. Usually there is a history of abdominal surgery, or radiological evidence of ileal disease. The [^{14}C]bile acid test may be abnormal (section 12.4.5), as may the Schilling test (section 12.4.4). A diminution in diarrhoea when cholestyramine is taken orally will support the diagnosis of bile salt diarrhoea, this substance being an ion exchange resin which binds bile acids.

12.2.4.3. Hormonal diarrhoeas

These may be secretory (Zollinger–Ellison and the Verner–Morrison syndrome) or due to abnormal motility (thyrotoxicosis). The diagnosis of thyrotoxicosis is discussed in Chapter 13 and of Zollinger–Ellison syndrome in Chapter 11. The Verner–Morrison syndrome (pancreatic cholera) is rare. Watery diarrhoea of up to 7 litres daily occurs, with hypokalaemia and often hypochlorhydria, hence the alternative name, the W.D.H.H. syndrome (watery diarrhoea, hypokalaemia and hypochlorhydria). The cause, as in the Zollinger–Ellison syndrome, is in most cases an islet cell tumour of the pancreas. A similar syndrome can occur due to ganglioneuroma of the adrenal gland, and to pancreatic islet cell hyperplasia. Diagnosis is generally by exclusion of any other cause for such a severe diarrhoea. However, vasoactive intestinal peptide has now been found in patients with this syndrome if it is due to pancreatic adenoma, and in one case of a ganglioneuroma, and it should therefore be looked for in possible cases before undertaking surgery (Bloom et al., 1973). The cause of the watery diarrhoea which is seen in one-third of patients with medullary carcinoma of the thyroid is uncertain, but it may be due to secretion of prostaglandins. Serum calcitonin (Chapter 8) is raised in about one-third of such patients. The role of individual hormones in the pathogenesis of these syndromes remains to be worked out, as any of these tumours may secrete many hormones.

12.2.4.4. Other chemically mediated diarrhoeas

Purgatives are the most common cause of chemically mediated diarrhoeas. Patients may go to considerable lengths to conceal their taking of purgatives and may present with severe hypokalaemia and even renal failure. An examination of urine and faeces for evidence of phenolphthalein, and of urine for evidence of anthracene purgatives, is essential in any persistent unexplained diarrhoea. If possible, faecal excretion of magnesium should also be determined (normal faecal magnesium excretion is approximately 15 mmol daily).

In the carcinoid syndrome (Kowlessar, 1973), diarrhoea is usually intermittent and associated with other factors such as episodic flushing and wheezing. In classical metastatic carcinoid, the urinary excretion of 5-hydroxyindoleacetic acid is very high, from 60 to 1000 mg (0.3 to 5.2 mmol) per 24 hours, and a qualitative urine test is invariably positive. Some carcinoids, e.g. gastric, only produce slight elevation above the normal of 2 to 8 mg (11 to 43 μmol) per 24 hours, but these are rarely associated with diarrhoea. Either false-positive or false-negative reactions can occur if the patient is taking certain drugs; foods such as bananas, pineapple, walnuts and avocados, which are rich in serotonin, must be discontinued. Slight increases in 5-hydroxyindoleacetic acid excretion also occur in untreated coeliac disease, tropical sprue, and Whipple's disease.

12.2.4.5. Congenital chloridorrhoea

This rare disorder is caused by impaired chloride absorption in the ileum and perhaps colon, and is characterized by watery diarrhoea beginning soon after birth. The possibility of chloridorrhoea is the only firm diagnostic reason for the determination of stool electrolytes. The chloride concentration of diarrhoeal fluid is greater than the sum of the sodium and potassium concentrations. There is also a systemic alkalosis.

12.3. ABDOMINAL PAIN

12.3.1. Role of the laboratory

Often the laboratory plays a minor role in the diagnosis of abdominal pain, but some causes of this symptom can only be diagnosed by laboratory examination (Table 12.3).

Some of these conditions (diabetes, hypercalcaemia, uraemia) will be recognized early in clinics which conduct biochemical screening on all patients. Others will only be found if they are considered in the diagnosis of any patient with persistent or recurrent abdominal pain for which no cause has been found on clinical and radiological examination. Many are described in other chapters of this book or are outside its scope (e.g. sickling) and will be referred to briefly or not at all.

TABLE 12.3.

SOME CAUSES OF ABDOMINAL PAIN WHICH MAY BE DIAGNOSED BY LABORATORY EXAMINATION

Abdominal disorders	Acute pancreatitis (section 12.5.4)
Metabolic disorders	Hyperlipidaemia (Chapter 5)
	Hypercalcaemia (Chapter 8)
	Porphyria (Chapter 20)
	C'1 esterase inhibitor deficiency (section 12.3.4)
Poisoning	Lead (Chapter 19)
Haematological disordes	Sickling
Other disorders	Uraemia
	Diabetes
	Syphilis

12.3.2. Hyperlipoproteinaemia (Fredrickson and Levy, 1972)

The cause of the recurrent abdominal pain seen in some patients is not always clear, as evidence of pancreatic disease (section 12.5.8) is not always present. Clinical clues such as a family history or xanthomata may not be present. Recurrent epigastric pain of any severity is therefore an indication for determination of blood lipids on a fasting specimen. The commonest type associated with attacks of severe abdominal pain is type V, but it also occurs in the less common type I, and less severe attacks of pain occur in patients with type IV. The serum amylase activity is normal, even in the presence of acute pancreatitis, more frequently than in non-hyperlipoproteinaemic patients. The reason for this is not certain.

12.3.3. Hypercalcaemia

Hypercalcaemia is a rare cause of acute pancreatitis, and persistent hypercalcaemia is also associated with an increased incidence of duodenal ulcer, perhaps due to the increased gastric acid secretion (Chapter 11). Hypercalcaemia can also cause abdominal pain in the absence of duodenal and pancreatic disease, although nausea and vomiting are common.

12.3.4. Hereditary angioneurotic oedema (Beck et al., 1973)

This rare disorder may lead to acute attacks of abdominal pain with associated vomiting and sometimes diarrhoea. A careful family history, especially of recurrent localized swelling of skin, subcutaneous tissues and mucous membranes, should suggest the diagnosis and may avoid unnecessary laparotomy.

The condition is due to deficiency of the inhibitor of the activated first component of complement (C′1 esterase inhibitor). Most patients have a reduced total complement concentration but definitive diagnosis depends on demonstration of reduced functional C′1 esterase inhibitor levels by an enzymatic assay.

Attacks can be satisfactorily terminated by an infusion of fresh frozen plasma, and in many patients attacks can be prevented by using the antifibrinolytic agent ϵ-aminocaproic acid.

12.3.5. Diabetes

This condition is only mentioned because of the variety of ways in which abdominal pain can be caused. A raised serum amylase activity is frequently found in diabetic ketosis and its significance is not clear in relationship to the epigastric pain which is sometimes observed. In long standing diabetes, autonomic neuropathy can be associated with bizarre abdominal pain in addition to the bowel disturbances more generally recognized. Finally, carcinoma of the pancreas may be the cause of pain, as it is more common in diabetic than in non-diabetic subjects.

12.4. MALABSORPTION

Malabsorption may present either with bowel symptoms, particularly diarrhoea, or as a nutritional defect. Steatorrhoea – the presence of excessive fat in the stools – is frequent, and determination of faecal fat remains the single most useful chemical test. However, it must be appreciated that the finding of normal faecal fat excretion does not exclude the diagnosis of malabsorption.

A classification of malabsorption on the basis of pathophysiology is shown in Table 12.4.

12.4.1. Place of chemical tests in diagnosis

Laboratory help is sought either to determine the presence or absence of malabsorption or to elucidate its cause. In establishing the presence of malabsorption, the determination of faecal fat is of considerable value, as steatorrhoea will often be a feature of any of the "generalized defects" shown in Table 12.4. The xylose absorption test, on the other hand, is usually abnormal only in the "malabsorption" defects shown in Table 12.4; thus it is of limited use as a screening test, but of some value in differential diagnosis. Further differential diagnosis is achieved by the use of more specific tests. The finding of complete villous atrophy in a jejunal biopsy will, for example, usually render further chemical tests for diagnosis superfluous, although estimation of faecal fat and of xylose absorption may still be undertaken so that the response to treatment may be monitored. In general, the disorders listed in Table 12.4 under "malabsorption" will be diagnosed largely by a combination of radiology and histology. Specific tests of pancreatic secretion, of bile salt metabolism, or of vitamin B_{12} absorption, are more likely to be necessary to diagnose disorders of digestion or the presence of specific defects.

The investigation of malabsorption is not however solely a matter of choosing the appropriate tests of absorptive function. The assessment of nutritional defects is important both in confirming a clinical suspicion of malabsorption and in assessing the severity of, and the need for, replacement therapy. Nutritional assessment is also often the most vital initial stage in differential diagnosis, determining the choice of absorption tests, radiological procedure, or biopsy procedure to be used for more specific diagnosis. For example, anaemia, which in malabsorptive states may be due to deficiency of vitamin B_{12}, folate, or iron, is not normally found in pancreatic insufficiency, and osteomalacia due to vitamin D deficiency is also most unusual in pancreatic insufficiency. The presence of severe steatorrhoea in a non-anaemic patient is therefore an indication for specific tests of pancreatic function. In contrast, megaloblastic anaemia due to folate deficiency would not be expected in pancreatic insufficiency, but is often a presenting feature in malabsorption due to an abnormal jejunal mucosa; and vitamin B_{12} malabsorption is an expected feature of malabsorption due to ileal resection, or to small bowel stasis with intraluminal bacterial over-growth.

It should already be apparent that the intelligent use of chemical tests in the diagnosis of malabsorptive states is not possible without some knowledge of normal absorptive mechanisms, and of the way in which these can be altered by disease. A short, but more general, account of the physiology and pathology of absorption is available (Holdsworth,

TABLE 12.4.

MALABSORPTION: CLASSIFICATION ON BASIS OF PATHOPHYSIOLOGY

Generalized defects		
Maldigestion	Chronic pancreatitis Fibrocystic disease Carcinoma of pancreas	→ Pancreatic insufficiency
	Bile duct obstruction Intrahepatic cholestasis	→ Low intraluminal bile salts
	Gastric surgery	→ Poor mixing of food with enzymes and bile salts
	Ileal resection/infiltration	→ Depleted bile salt pool
	Small bowel stasis	→ Bile salt de-conjugation Aminoacid de-amination
Malabsorption	Small bowel stasis	→ Mucosal damage
	Jejunal resection/infiltration	→ Mucosal loss
	Childhood coeliac disease Adult coeliac disease (idiopathic steatorrhoea)	→ Mucosal damage
	Tropical sprue	→ Mucosal damage

Specific defects	
Defects of specific enterocyte transport systems	Glucose/galactose malabsorption Cystinuria: Hartnup disease Congenital B_{12} malabsorption
Enzyme deficiencies	Disaccharidase deficiencies Enterokinase deficiency, etc.
Secretory deficiencies	Defective production of intrinsic factor
Other biochemical defects	Abetalipoproteinaemia

1974), with fuller accounts in McColl and Sladen, (1975), and Duthie and Wormsley (1978).

In this section, descriptions of normal absorptive mechanisms will be restricted to nutrients whose absorption is frequently measured in clinical practice, e.g. fat, vitamin B_{12}. The absorption of calcium, protein, etc. is equally important nutritionally, but determination of their absorption does not for various reasons contribute to either diagnosis or management.

12.4.2. Fat absorption

12.4.2.1. The physiology of fat absorption

The physiology of fat digestion is summarised in Figure 12.5. The importance of pancreatic lipase is self-evident: that of bile salts requires emphasis. Bile salts are necessary

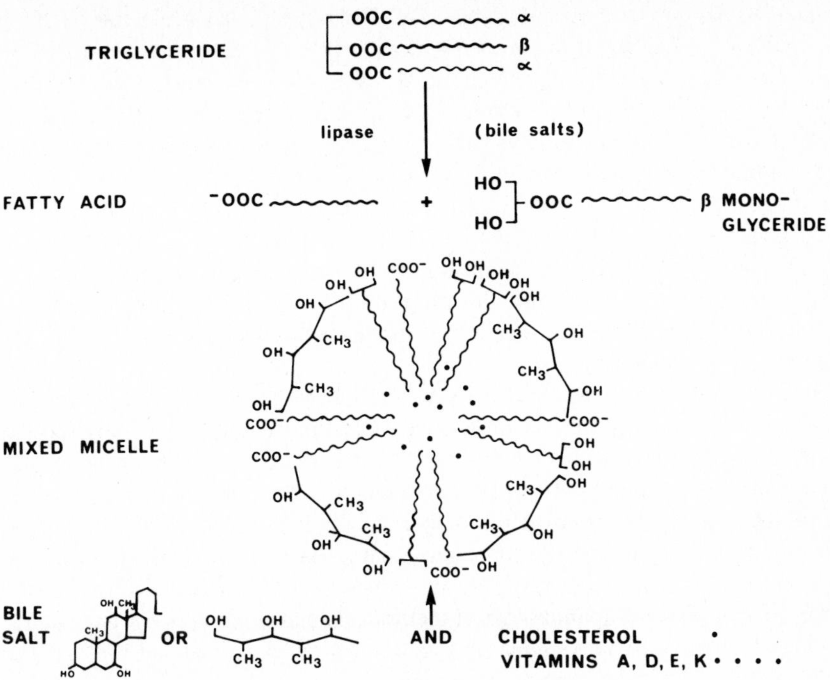

Figure 12.5. Diagrammatic representation of fat digestion and micelle formation, emphasizing the critical detergent-like role of bile salts.

for initial emulsification of fat before hydrolysis by lipase. It is also essential that they are present in an adequate concentration to form micelles, which are spherical polymolecular aggregates with the hydrophobic methyl groups of the bile salt molecule directed towards the centre and the hydrophilic hydroxyl groups directed outwards. The fatty acids and monoglycerides produced by the action of lipase also contribute to these micelles, their polar groups being directed outwards into the aqueous phase, and the non-polar groups inwards. Fat-soluble vitamins and cholesterol are incorporated in the lipid phase within the micelle. Micellar solution achieves a fine dispersion of lipid material which, without the detergent action of bile salts, would be a coarse emulsion, but which in the micelle can penetrate the intermicrovillous spaces of the enterocytes. Fatty acids and monoglycerides then enter the cells where re-synthesis to triglyceride takes place, followed by transfer to the lymphatics in chylomicrons, which contain triglyceride, cholesterol ester and free cholesterol with a coating of phospholipid and protein.

Medium chain triglycerides, in which the fatty acid chain length varies from 6 to 12 carbon atoms, instead of the 16 to 18 of normal dietary (long chain) triglycerides, are sometimes used in the dietary management of patients with defective fat absorption. Bile salts are not necessary for their absorption, and significant absorption can also take place if pancreatic lipase is absent.

Some understanding of bile salt metabolism is also necessary since maldigestion is more often due to bile salt deficiency than to lipase deficiency (Table 12.4); the essentials are shown in Figure 12.6. Bile salts are very effectively absorbed in the ileum and are re-utilized several times each day by uptake in the liver and re-secretion into bile. Any interruption of the enterohepatic circulation rapidly reduces the bile salt pool, as the capacity of the liver for bile salt synthesis is limited. The concentration of bile salts falls below that essential for micelle formation, and malabsorption of lipid results.

Interruption of the enterohepatic circulation of bile salts can occur at three points (Figure 12.6), due to (a) biliary obstruction, either intra-hepatic or extra-hepatic; (b) metabolism by organisms in the small intestine (which is normally sterile), largely by deconjugation to free bile acids which do not form effective micelles, and which are absorbed by passive non-ionic diffusion in both jejunum and ileum; or (c) resection of the ileum or extensive ileal disease.

Absorption of fat occurs largely in the jejunum in normal subjects. If the jejunal mucosa is abnormal, fat malabsorption occurs although digestion is normal. The only specific enterocyte defect which causes fat malabsorption (Table 12.4) is abetalipoproteinaemia. The defect appears to be an inability to transport chylomicrons out of the mucosal cell. The cholesterol content of plasma is therefore low, usually in the range of 30 to 80 mg/dl (0.8 to 2.1 mmol/litre), plasma triglycerides are usually less than 15 mg/dl, (0.17 mmol/litre) and betalipoprotein is either very low or undetectable by either electrophoresis, ultracentrifugation or specific immunological methods. In addition, there is a characteristic morphological abnormality on jejunal biopsy, and of red blood cells on wet preparations of fresh blood.

12.4.2.2. Determination of fat absorption (Losowsky et al., 1974)

Determination of the amount of faecal fat which is excreted per day is the only way of diagnosing steatorrhoea with confidence. As the output of fat in the faeces varies considerably from day to day, a minimum collection period of 3 days is required for diagnosis, and 5 days is better. For patients with very irregular bowel habit, longer collection periods, or the use of faecal markers, may be necessary. A diet containing 100 grams of fat daily is preferable, but for out-patient assessment it is usually unnecessary to do more

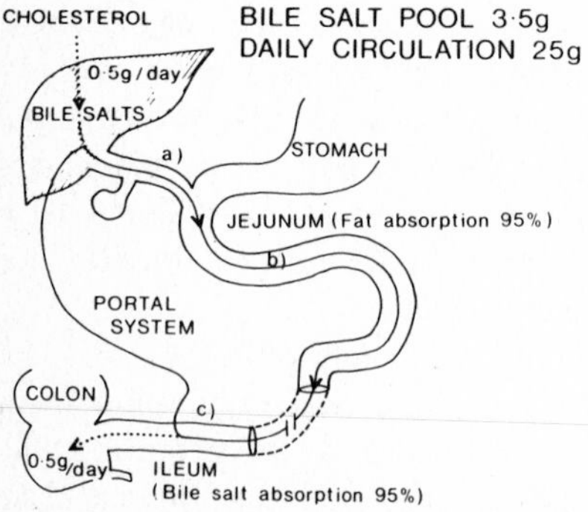

Figure 12.6. Diagram showing the normal enterohepatic circulation of bile salts, with an indication of three points (a, b and c) where gastrointestinal disease can result in abnormal bile salt metabolism.

than ensure that the patient is not anorexic and that fat restriction has not been advised. A metal pail which can be placed in a light frame and suspended within the pan of a normal toilet and subsequently fitted with a sealed lid, is suitable for domiciliary and normal ward use. Complete accuracy can only be attained on a metabolic ward.

The most accurate results are achieved by the use of continuous faecal marking. A constant amount of a non-absorbable substance is given in divided doses three times daily. After an equilibration period of 6 days, the amount of marker in any stool collection, be it only one specimen, indicates the number of days or fraction of a day to which the fat content of the stool is to be referred. Chromic oxide has been most widely used as a continuous marker, but [^{131}Ba]barium sulphate and cuprous thiocyanate have both proved satisfactory.

12.4.2.3. Chemical estimation

The most widely used method is that of van de Kamer et al. (1949). The fatty acid content of a petroleum ether extract of a saponified aliquot of homogenized stool sample is determined by titration. This is usually converted to grams of fatty acid by assuming an arbitrary equivalent weight of 284. The extraction method may need to be altered if the patient is taking medium chain triglyceride supplements. Gravimetric methods such as those of Sobel (Henry, 1966) give satisfactory but slightly higher results. The separate determination of "split" and "unsplit" fat in an attempt to differentiate pancreatic from other types of steatorrhoea is no longer used, since bacterial action invalidates the method.

12.4.2.4. Interpretation of abnormal results

A daily fat excretion of more than 6 grams indicates steatorrhoea unless the patient has ingested large amounts of indigestible fat, either as castor oil or by way of a large number of brazil nuts. In normal individuals, dietary fat intake has little effect on faecal fat excretion, and even on a fat-free diet, 1 to 3 grams of fat is excreted daily. In patients with steatorrhoea, the endogenous fat output is similar to that of normal subjects, so that if fat intake is very restricted, as in an anorexic subject, total fat output may be normal. Increasing the intake, if possible to 150 grams daily, can be useful in doubtful cases, since a borderline result may then become clearly abnormal. In infants and young children, the upper normal limit of faecal fat excretion is usually taken as 4 grams but in some laboratories is as low as 3 grams (section 12.5.9.1).

12.4.2.5. Appearance and weight of stool in steatorrhoea

Stools containing an excess of fat are typically pale, bulky, greasy and offensive, although stools with only a moderate increase in fat content may appear quite normal. There is very little factual basis for the oft-repeated statement that only steatorrhoea stools float in water and that this observation is of diagnostic help. Loose stools from any cause may float, as stool density is related to the content of gas (hydrogen and methane) rather than fat (Levitt and Duane, 1973).

The recording of stool weight is valuable in the management of patients with diarrhoea, and in individual patients, variations in stool weight can give some indication of response to treatment. In general, however, the correlation between stool weight and stool fat content is very poor.

12.4.2.6. Alternative methods of assessing steatorrhoea

A considerable variety of alternative methods of assessing steatorrhoea have been tried and found wanting: microscopic examination of faeces, serum carotene concentration, vitamin A tolerance tests and determination of blood lipids after a fatty meal. The usual pattern is an initial favourable report, followed by a more critical assessment and then the test falls into disuse. Almost any of these tests will be abnormal in patients with severe steatorrhoea, but they have a poor discrimination in the large number of patients with only minor abnormalities of fat absorption.

The use of ^{131}I-labelled fat has been extensively explored but with rather disappointing results, all methods having proved unsatisfactory when assessed critically against faecal fat excretion. Determination of $^{14}CO_2$ in the breath after ingestion of ^{14}C-labelled fat appears to be more satisfactory. The maximum specific activity of CO_2 in the breath correlates well with fat absorption, and discrimination between patients with or without steatorrhoea is satisfactory. By comparing maximum breath $^{14}CO_2$ specific activity after ingestion of ^{14}C-labelled glyceryl tripalmitate or ^{14}C-labelled palmitic acid, patients with pancreatic insufficiency can be distinguished from most other patients with steatorrhoea (Burrows et al., 1974).

12.4.2.7. Diagnostic significance of steatorrhoea

The value of faecal fat estimation is that impaired absorption of dietary fat is found in the majority of patients with a generalized malabsorption syndrome, whatever the cause, be it impaired enzyme secretion, bile salt metabolism, or mucosal damage. It is therefore the most widely applicable screening procedure.

The finding of even a slightly increased faecal fat excretion usually means that further investigations should be conducted to find the cause. But it should be remembered that the majority of patients after gastric surgery show mild steatorrhoea. Extensive investigation into the possible mechanism is unnecessary in such patients unless the steatorrhoea is gross and malnutrition obvious. If this is so, then the mechanism must be investigated fully as it may be due to a stagnant loop, coincidental coeliac disease or pancreatic insufficiency, all conditions with different specific treatment. Mild steatorrhoea can also be a feature of thyrotoxicosis, untreated pernicious anaemia, Addison's disease, cirrhosis of the liver and intestinal hurry from any cause. Mild steatorrhoea in such patients is only worth investigating if it fails to respond to treatment of the underlying condition.

The approach to differential diagnosis of steatorrhoea was indicated in the introduction to this section. Clinical findings and nutritional defects may make it obvious whether jejunal biopsy, radiology, pancreatic secretion tests, or other chemical tests should be the next investigation.

12.4.2.8. Value of faecal fat determination in differential diagnosis and management

After the initial demonstration of increased fat excretion, it is unnecessary to repeat the test in the majority of patients. Repetition after treatment may be useful in the following circumstances – and when done for these indications, a constant dietary fat intake is essential.

(a) Confirmation of diagnosis. A fall in fat excretion following oral tetracycline or another appropriate antibiotic, may confirm that steatorrhoea was due to bacterial prolif-

eration in a stagnant loop of small intestine. This is particularly useful confirmation if a patient has several bowel abnormalities, for example ileal resection for previous Crohn's disease, and a stricture causing stasis. A therapeutic trial was, in the past, also used in diagnosis of adult coeliac disease and pancreatic insufficiency. This is no longer acceptable as definitive diagnostic tests are available. A therapeutic trial or oral pancreatic supplements may be positively misleading as secondary pancreatic insufficiency can occur in any patient with severe malabsorption if there is malnutrition; the response to oral pancreatic extract is very variable, even in adults with proven pancreatic disease. Some cases of malabsorption following partial gastrectomy may be an exception to this rule. Intubation studies of pancreatic function may be impossible to interpret since, if a gastrojejunal anastomosis has been performed, complete collection of pancreatic secretion is not possible and contamination with gastric juice is inevitable.

(b) Management. In any type of malabsorptive state, it may prove useful on occasion to follow faecal fat excretion as an index of response to treatment. In pancreatic disease this should be normal practice, as the response to pancreatic supplements is subject to large individual variations. Some patients respond to adequate doses taken with meals, whereas others respond better to hourly administration. Optimal size and timing of dose is best determined by serial faecal fat determinations on a variety of therapeutic regimes.

If, in any patient with steatorrhoea, faecal fat output continues to be high in spite of treatment, it may be necessary to restrict fat intake in order to reduce excessive stool volume; this results in secondary loss of fluid, electrolytes and nitrogen. Restriction of fat intake is most often necessary after extensive bowel resection. Determination of faecal fat output on a diet restricted in the first instance to 50 grams of fat daily, and then if necessary to 30 grams of fat daily, will make possible a rational decision on the degree of fat restriction necessary. If such a patient is given medium chain triglycerides as a dietary supplement, the laboratory method used for faecal fat estimation may need modification (section 12.4.2.3).

12.4.3. Determination of carbohydrate absorption

Any carbohydrate which is not absorbed in the small intestine passes into the colon where it is metabolized by bacteria. Measurements of faecal excretion are therefore not appropriate to studies of carbohydrate absorption, although small amounts of individual sugars can often be found by chromatography of faecal extracts if sugar absorption is defective; e.g. lactose is usually found in the faeces of patients with alactasia.

For research purposes the absorption of individual sugars is best assessed by intubation of the small intestine with multilumen tubes so that disappearance from the intestinal lumen can be measured directly; diagnostic investigations are often restricted to measuring the concentration in blood or amount in urine after ingestion of the appropriate sugar. Starch tolerance tests have been found unhelpful in clinical practice, and glucose tolerance tests are of very limited value in gastrointestinal disease, so that discussion will largely be restricted to the use of xylose and lactose tolerance tests.

12.4.3.1. Carbohydrate digestion and absorption (Dawson, 1970)

The principal metabolic pathways of dietary carbohydrate are summarized in Figure 12.7.

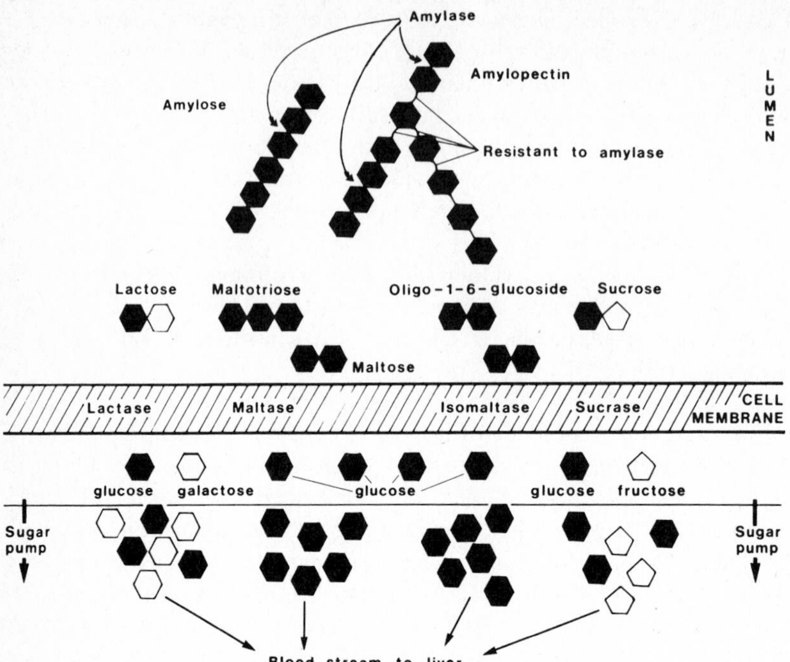

Figure 12.7. The digestion and absorption of dietary carbohydrate (Reproduced, by permission, from Dawson, 1970).

Starch, the main dietary carbohydrate, is digested by salivary and pancreatic amylase to oligosaccharides containing either two (maltose and isomaltose) or three (maltotriose) glucose molecules. Some "α-limit" dextrins with an average of eight glucose molecules remain because the 1–6 glycoside bonds at the branch points of amylopectin, and the adjacent 1 : 4α bonds, are resistant to amylase. These are all hydrolyzed by brush border enzymes to glucose, which is absorbed by a very efficient carrier-mediated active transport system.

The disaccharide lactose, which is present only in milk and milk products, is digested by the brush border enzyme lactase to its constituent monosaccharides glucose and galactose. Galactose shares the same active transport system as glucose, and is rapidly absorbed.

The disaccharide sucrose is the only other carbohydrate which is ingested in significant quantities. It is digested by a brush border enzyme to its constituent monosaccharides glucose and fructose. Fructose is absorbed by a separate transport system which is less efficient than that shared by glucose and galactose. Each of these three monosaccharides is absorbed unchanged into portal blood.

Carbohydrate absorption is normally very efficient and is probably completed in the jejunum. Generalized carbohydrate malabsorption only occurs after extensive resection of small bowel, in inflammatory disease of the gut, and with severe villous atrophy as in coeliac disease. The only specific defect of monosaccharide transport is congenital glucose–galactose malabsorption – a very rare condition. Of the disaccharidase deficiencies, only alactasia (absence of mucosal lactase) is at all common and this is discussed in section 12.4.3.7. Sucrase deficiency is always associated with isomaltase deficiency; it is much rarer, and is an inherited disorder transmitted as an autosomal recessive.

12.4.3.2. Physiology of xylose absorption

The very efficiency of absorption of glucose and galactose, and of synthetic sugars such as 3-O-methylglucose which share the same transport system, limits their value in absorption tests. 3-O-Methylglucose is a monosaccharide which is not metabolized after absorption, and can therefore be recovered completely in the urine. It would be ideal as a test for jejunal function were it not for the fact that jejunal function has to be grossly impaired before its absorption is affected.

D-Xylose is a pentose monosaccharide which is not normally present in the diet. It is actively absorbed, like glucose and galactose, but much less efficiently; its transport system has not been clearly defined, but it may share the glucose–galactose carrier with relatively poor affinity. A dose of 25 grams is absorbed to the extent of about 50% in the upper 100 cm of small intestine, and only a further 10% in the remaining 200 cm, so that tests of xylose absorption measure jejunal and not ileal function (Fordtran et al., 1962).

About half of an absorbed dose of xylose is metabolized, largely in the liver, and the remainder appears in the urine. Its metabolism may be affected by liver disease (especially if portal-systemic anastomoses are present) and its excretion by renal disease. The amount excreted in the urine after an oral dose is therefore affected by many factors in addition to jejunal function, and this limits the value of the xylose absorption test.

12.4.3.3. D-Xylose absorption test (Losowsky et al., 1974; Sladen and Kumar, 1973)

It is usual to give 25 grams of xylose dissolved in 500 ml of tap water to the fasting subject. An additional 250 ml of water is drunk after 1.5 hours. All urine passed during the 5 hours after ingestion is collected. The volume is noted and the xylose content measured either by a method specific for pentoses, or, with appropriate standards, by a non-specific method for reducing sugars. An excretion of more than 5 grams in 5 hours is usually taken as normal. A single blood specimen may be taken 1.5 hours after the dose and should contain more than 33 mg/dl (2.2 mmol/litre) of xylose. In children, it is usual to give a dose of 5 grams, and the lower limit of normal is then 25% of the administered dose, with values from 15 to 25% probably abnormal and less than 15% definitively abnormal. An alternative in children is to give 500 mg of xylose per kg body weight, the expected xylose excretion over 5 hours as a percentage of the oral dose being given by the formula (0.2 × age in months + 12)%. A blood sample at 1 hour increases diagnostic discrimination in children, as in adults, and normally contains more than 23 mg/dl (1.5 mmol/litre).

Some authors advocate a 5 gram dose in adults, but in normal subjects this is probably completely absorbed, so that the test is less sensitive using this small dose. It does avoid the nausea and diarrhoea that may follow the 25 gram dose, and it is claimed that determination of xylose in an initial 2 hour and subsequent 3 hour urine collection improves diagnostic discrimination (Sammons et al., 1967) as xylose absorption is delayed in adult coeliac disease.

12.4.3.4. Interpretation of abnormal xylose absorption test

As D-xylose is largely absorbed in the jejunum, and being a monosaccharide does not require any digestion before absorption, it is used as a test of jejunal function. In malabsorption due solely to impaired digestion, the response to the test in theory should be quite normal (Table 12.4). It would be abnormal if the jejunal mucosa had impaired function, as in coeliac disease and to a lesser degree in tropical sprue. In general this is the case, but as there are exceptions, it can only be used as a screening test. Some clinicians with extensive experience of the test claim that as jejunal biopsy is diagnostic of coeliac disease and should be done whenever small bowel disease is suspected, the xylose test should be abandoned. This is overstating the case against the test, but it must be emphasized that in both adults and children, complete villous atrophy in the upper jejunum is sometimes found when the xylose absorption test is normal by the usual criteria. Taking the more stringent criteria that both urine and blood concentrations of xylose must be low, almost all adult patients with coeliac disease will have an abnormal test (Sladen and Kumar, 1973). In infants, urinary xylose estimations are very unreliable due to the difficulty of obtaining timed urine collections, and some authorities now recommend that the urinary xylose test should be abandoned in the paediatric population. As a normal blood xylose concentration can also occur in children with coeliac disease, the xylose test cannot be used in this age group to exclude coeliac disease (Lamabadusuriya et al., 1975).

A diminished urinary xylose excretion can be due to many factors in addition to a damaged jejunal mucosa. They include the following possibilities:

(a) Intestinal hurry. Rapid transit through jejunum, as in many patients after gastric surgery, results in poor absorption. Slow transit, induced for example by atropine, does the reverse.

(b) Bacteria in the intestinal lumen. In small gut stasis this can result in diminished absorption, partly due to metabolism of the sugar by bacteria, and partly probably due to mucosal damage also caused by the bacteria.

(c) Anoxia and severe anaemia. The cause is uncertain, although in severe vitamin B_{12} deficiency impaired mucosal function is likely to be a factor.

(d) Some drugs – neomycin by damaging the jejunum; aspirin by impairing renal excretion; indomethacin by affecting absorption in some way. Obviously, all drugs should be avoided on the day of a test.

(e) Oedema and ascites. Since, after absorption, the xylose is distributed in the excess fluid, excretion is delayed.

(f) Systemic bacterial infections, severe eczema, hypothyroidism; the precise cause in these situations is uncertain.

(g) Crohn's disease with no macroscopic evidence of jejunal involvement.

(h) Impaired renal function. This is a most important factor. With increasing age, the 5-hour excretion falls, due almost entirely to impaired renal excretion. Determining xylose concentration in a 1.5 hour blood specimen is particularly useful in these circumstances.

(i) Incomplete urine collection, and failing to ensure adequate urine flow rate (60 ml/h).

12.4.3.5. Indications for use of xylose absorption test

The main use of the test is in screening for coeliac disease. When this diagnosis was considered only in wasted patients with obvious steatorrhoea the test was invariably abnormal, but in less severely affected patients it can be normal. The numerous non-specific causes of low excretion listed in the preceding section further limit its value, and as a research tool it should only be used if metabolism and excretion are also assessed by measuring excretion of an intraveous dose. A normal xylose absorption test in the presence of marked steatorrhoea usually indicates "maldigestion" (Table 12.4), and if for some reason jejunal biopsy is not possible, the test can exclude coeliac disease in these circumstances. The toxicities of various gluten fractions have been assessed by measuring the 2-hour excretion after a 5 gram oral dose given to patients in remission on a gluten-free diet, and subsequently after the gluten fraction. Serial xylose absorption tests can also be used to monitor the response to a gluten-free diet.

12.4.3.6. Glucose tolerance test (Holdsworth, 1969)

This test is rarely worth performing, either as a screening test for malabsorption or in differential diagnosis, since a flat curve is frequently found in healthy young subjects. Impaired glucose tolerance in a patient with steatorrhoea suggests pancreatic disease, and the possibility of this diagnosis is the only remaining indication for carrying out the test in patients with malabsorption.

12.4.3.7. Lactase deficiency (alactasia)

Primary alactasia. In the majority of mammals lactase activity in the small bowel mucosa declines steeply at an age which corresponds roughly to that of weaning. In man, this also occurs in many ethnic groups, so that in adults alactasia is not necessarily abnormal and is often asymptomatic. It can also be congenital, but it is then serious since lactose in milk is the sole dietary carbohydrate. These two types of primary alactasia can be called constitutional and congenital respectively.

Secondary alactasia. Whenever the small bowel mucosa is damaged, disaccharidase activity generally is depressed, but lactase activity is always depressed to a greater extent than that of other disaccharidases. This "secondary alactasia" has been well described in coeliac disease, tropical sprue, giardiasis, gastroenteritis, and malnutrition.

Familial lactose intolerance is only mentioned here to emphasize that it is not the same as congenital alactasia. There are constitutional symptoms, perhaps due to lactose entering the circulation, with mucosal lactase probably normal.

12.4.3.8. Assessment of alactasia (Dawson, 1970; Newcomer et al., 1975)

Faecal pH, sugars and organic acids. In any carbohydrate malabsorption syndrome, the unabsorbed sugars cause diarrhoea; in infants this can be dramatic and life threatening, until the offending carbohydrate is eliminated from the diet. In infants, stools are frothy, bulky (100 to 300 grams daily, compared with less than 50 grams in the normal), and have a low pH (5 or 6, instead of 7 or 8 in the normal) due to the presence of lactic acid and short chain volatile fatty acids produced by bacterial fermentation. A simple screening test on the stool can be performed with Clinitest tablets (Anderson and Burke, 1975). The results are graded 1 to 4+, with values greater than 1+ in older children abnormal.

Nearly half of normal neonates give gradings greater than 1+ with some up to 4+. The disaccharide lactulose is present in small amounts in some prepacked liquid milks and also gives a positive Clinitest. Chromatography will distinguish this from lactose. An alternative is to substitute a reconstituted powdered milk, as this does not contain lactulose.

In adults, determination of stool pH is unhelpful. The presence of lactose in the urine at any age is not specific for alactasia and is not of diagnostic help.

Lactose tolerance test. A rise in blood glucose concentration of less than 20 mg/dl (1.1 mmol/litre) following an oral dose of 50 to 100 grams of lactose dissolved in water provides suggestive evidence of lactose deficiency. It is desirable to use capillary rather than venous blood, and to take blood specimens fasting and subsequently at 15, 30, 60 and 90 minutes. In children, 2 grams of lactose per kg body weight is a suitable dose. The reference range varies somewhat with the dose of lactose used and the method of blood sugar estimation – many of the results in the literature are for total reducing sugar, so that galactose as well as glucose is measured. One study, however, showed little difference between the results of glucose oxidase and total reducing sugar methods (Cuatrecasas et al., 1965).

Any abnormal test must be followed by a control test in which amounts of glucose and galactose are given equivalent to that of the lactose, to ensure that the individual has normal tolerance to the constituent monosaccharides.

Any abdominal symptoms which develop during the test must be recorded. Of alactasic subjects, 60% develop abdominal pain, borborygmi and diarrhoea after 50 grams of lactose, and almost all after 100 grams.

Assay of small gut lactase activity. This is easily done on material obtained by per oral biopsy, and is the most reliable way of establishing the diagnosis. Results can be expressed satisfactorily per unit wet weight of mucosa, and each laboratory must establish its reference range.

Breath hydrogen. Hydrogen is one of the products of bacterial breakdown of carbohydrate in the colon. In patients with alactasia, ingestion of lactose is followed within 2 hours by an increase in breath hydrogen, whereas normal subjects have a very low or undetectable breath hydrogen unless their diet contains large amounts of undigestable sugars such as are found in beans. The test is very sensitive, and yet false-positives are rare. In adults it is, if available, preferable to any other test except direct assay of mucosal lactase, and it is ideal for population screening (Newcomer et al., 1975).

If a sugar is given which is not absorbed, even in the normal human small intestine, e.g. the disaccharide lactulose, the length of time which elapses between ingestion and the appearance of hydrogen in the breath provides a convenient measure of the transit time from mouth to caecum.

12.4.3.9. Significance of alactasia

In the infant, there is rarely doubt about the clinical significance of alactasia when it has been established. When milk, the sole source of lactose, is removed from the diet, the rapid resolution of symptoms usually removes any doubt. As lactase is the last disaccharidase to develop in the foetus, its activity is low in the mucosa of premature infants but appears to be induced therein at birth and rises rapidly within the first 3 days of life. Lactase deficiency in childhood is most commonly secondary and has been frequently demonstrated after gastroenteritis and as a feature of coeliac disease, malnutrition and pancreatic insufficiency including cystic fibrosis.

In adults, constitutional alactasia and secondary alactasia (section 12.4.3.7) are possible and it must be remembered that 10% of any Caucasian population (and a much higher proportion in many other races) is deficient in lactase. Diarrhoea or other symptoms must therefore not be attributed to this cause unless they resolve when milk and milk products are withdrawn from the diet, and recur when it is re-introduced. The amount of dietary lactose which is required to produce symptoms in alactasic subjects varies considerably. Half a litre of milk, a common daily intake in adults, contains 20 grams of lactose and is tolerated by some alactasic subjects without symptoms, whereas others are sensitive to much smaller amounts.

12.4.3.10. Assessment of other defects in sugar absorption

Sucrase–isomaltase deficiency. Symptoms occur similar to, but milder than those found in primary alactasia, but not until sucrose, dextrins or starch are introduced into the diet. Tolerance tests for sucrose are abnormal, but for maltose and lactose are usually normal. The diagnosis can be confirmed by mucosal enzyme assay, and the condition responds to the appropriate diet.

Trehalase intolerance is excessively rare. This disaccharide only occurs in mushrooms.

Glucose–galactose malabsorption causes congenital severe diarrhoea with watery acid stools. It has also been described after enteric infection in infancy. A Clinistix test, specific for glucose, on the stools is strongly positive. Blood sugar concentrations are low, and blood sugar curves are flat after oral glucose or galactose but not after fructose. Response to a synthetic formula with fructose as the sole dietary carbohydrate confirms the diagnosis.

12.4.4. Vitamin B_{12} absorption test (Toskes and Deren, 1973)

There are many possible causes of vitamin B_{12} deficiency (Figure 12.4), and measurement of serum B_{12} concentration is often important in the nutritional assessment of a patient with malabsorption (section 12.1.5). Because of the considerable body stores of the vitamin, malabsorption has to be present for several years before deficiency develops and it is therefore often useful to measure B_{12} absorption, even if the serum B_{12} concentration is normal. Vitamin B_{12} absorption tests are therefore used both to determine the cause of the deficiency in patients presenting with it (e.g. with megaloblastic anaemia and subacute combined degeneration of the cord) and as a screening test for some types of malabsorptive disease, particularly small intestinal bacterial overgrowth and ileal resection.

12.4.4.1. Methods of assessing vitamin B_{12} absorption in man

The nutritional requirement is about 2 μg daily. Vitamin B_{12} absorption in man can be assessed by giving from 0.5 to 2.0 μg of ^{57}Co- or ^{60}Co-labelled vitamin B_{12} and measuring the amount of radioactivity appearing in the urine, liver, stool, plasma, or retained in the whole body. Each of these five approaches has advantages and disadvantages, and the choice between them is usually dictated by familiarity with a particular procedure and the availability of appropriate counting apparatus.

Urinary excretion test (Schilling test). This is the most widely used test of absorption. After an oral dose of labelled vitamin B_{12} taken by the fasting subject, a "flushing" dose of 1 mg of unlabelled vitamin B_{12} is given; this blocks potential binding sites within the body so that absorbed vitamin is excreted in the urine. The flushing dose can be given at any time up to 6 hours after the oral dose, for convenience often simultaneously. Urine is collected for 24 hours and complete urine collection must be ensured. Normal subjects excrete more than 15% of the oral dose. Vitamin B_{12} is not re-absorbed by the renal tubule and excretion is directly dependent on glomerular filtration rate. The test is unreliable in the presence of renal impairment, due to either disease or old age. In intestinal disease, reproducibility of the test is not very good. Radiation dose is estimated at 20 to 120 mrads to the total body, 280 mrads to the gonads, and 370 to 660 mrads to the liver.

Hepatic uptake test. No flushing dose is required; this can be an advantage since the serum B_{12} concentration is not affected and any megaloblastic bone marrow remains abnormal. After an oral dose of labelled vitamin B_{12}, external counting is performed over the liver after 1 week, when unabsorbed vitamin B_{12} remaining in the colon will usually have been excreted. The test is ideal for out-patient work since no collection of excreta is required and the result is valid even in the presence of renal disease.

Faecal excretion test. Stools are collected until less than 1% of the oral dose appears in two consecutive days of faecal collection.

Plasma level absorption test. Radioactivity is determined in a plasma specimen 8 hours after the oral dose.

Whole body counting. If the apparatus is available, accurate quantitation of absorption is possible. A count made shortly after ingestion is compared with one a week or more later, when excretion of unabsorbed vitamin is complete.

12.4.4.2. Significance of diminished vitamin B_{12} absorption

(a) Lack of intrinsic factor. If vitamin B_{12} malabsorption is demonstrated in a patient with normal renal function, the test must be repeated giving hog intrinsic factor. Correction of the vitamin B_{12} malabsorption indicates failure of adequate intrinsic factor secretion. This is mostly usually due to pernicious anaemia, and is a manifestation of generalized gastric mucosal atrophy. Rarely, selective intrinsic factor deficiency occurs as one cause of "juvenile pernicious anaemia".

In certain conditions results can be more difficult to interpret, for example, after gastric surgery. Some such patients, and also patients with idiopathic gastric atrophy, may show depressed B_{12} absorption unless a stimulus to secretion of intrinsic factor is given, either as a meal or an intramuscular injection of carbaminocholine. After gastric resection, a Schilling test may also show apparently normal B_{12} absorption even in a patient with definite B_{12} deficiency, probably because of an inability to absorb the vitamin from foodstuffs. This has been confirmed by the inability to absorb vitamin B_{12} when it has been incorporated into egg protein.

Such is the value of measuring the absorption of vitamin B_{12} with and without intrinsic factor that it is perhaps worthwhile routinely to use a modification of the test in which [^{57}Co]vitamin B_{12} and [^{60}Co]vitamin B_{12}–intrinsic factor are administered simultaneously and the absorption of both determined.

(b) Interference with intrinsic factor–vitamin B_{12} complex. Any condition causing stasis

within the small intestine may be complicated by bacterial proliferation within the normally sterile small intestine. The bacteria involved may either take up or in some way interfere with the intrinsic factor–vitamin B_{12} complex, and cause vitamin B_{12} deficiency. In such patients, a repeat Schilling test after a 5 day course of oral tetracycline shows significantly greater absorption.

Recently it has been appreciated that pancreatic insufficiency in both children and adults can cause subnormal absorption of intrinsic factor–vitamin B_{12} complex. Simultaneous administration of pancreatic extract may improve absorption. In contrast to the small bowel stasis syndrome, it is very rare for vitamin B_{12} deficiency to develop in pancreatic disease.

(c) Ileal disease or resection. As the intrinsic factor–vitamin B_{12} complex is only absorbed in the ileum, vitamin B_{12} malabsorption is a useful index of ileal function. In Crohn's disease affecting the ileum, vitamin B_{12} malabsorption is common, but significant deficiency causing megaloblastic anaemia is unusual unless ileum has been resected. In coeliac disease, mucosal damage – although always maximal in the jejunum – may extend to the ileum and cause impaired vitamin B_{12} absorption. Severe folate or vitamin B_{12} deficiency can itself lead to mucosal damage and aggravate an already existing absorptive defect. Finally, there is a rare familial selective vitamin B_{12} malabsorption due to some abnormality of ileal mucosal cells.

(d) Drugs. p-Aminobenzoic acid, colchicine, alcohol, metformin and neomycin can also cause vitamin B_{12} malabsorption in some patients.

12.4.4.3. Value of vitamin B_{12} absorption tests in differential diagnosis

In determining the cause of vitamin B_{12} deficiency, these tests have an obvious role. The large number of malabsorptive states in which vitamin B_{12} absorption is affected gives the test some value in screening for these conditions, although it must be remembered that severe folate or vitamin B_{12} deficiency itself can lead to vitamin B_{12} malabsorption.

In differential diagnosis, the particular advantages of the Schilling test are its ease of performance and general availability. It must be remembered that the 1 mg flushing dose is an effective treatment dose; thus if the bone marrow is to be examined for megaloblastic changes this must be done first, and if the patient is anaemic, the reticulocyte response must be followed in the usual way. If the ^{14}C-labelled bile acid breath test (section 12.4.5) is not available, determination of vitamin B_{12} absorption is valuable as a test of ileal integrity or in confirming radiological or other evidence that small intestinal stasis is the cause of a malabsorptive syndrome.

12.4.5. Bile acid $^{14}CO_2$ breath test (Fromm and Hofmann, 1971; James et al., 1973)

The frequency with which disturbed bile salt metabolism occurs in malabsorptive states has already been stressed, and normal bile acid metabolism was summarized in Figure 12.6. This information has been derived by a variety of techniques not suitable for routine diagnostic use, but it is now possible to obtain some useful information about bile salt metabolism in any hospital with scintillation counting facilities for measuring ^{14}C.

The bile acid $^{14}CO_2$ breath test is done by oral administration of 5 μCi of [1-^{14}C]-glycine–glycocholic acid. Under normal conditions, almost all of the ingested dose is absorbed intact in the ileum and recirculates back to the liver for re-excretion in bile (Figure 12.6). A little escapes into the colon where the amide bond is split by bacterial action. The [1-^{14}C]glycine thus released is rapidly converted into $^{14}CO_2$ either by intestinal bacterial enzymes or by tissue enzymes after absorption, and the $^{14}CO_2$ is exhaled. As the amide bond can only be broken by the action of bacterial enzymes, the amount of $^{14}CO_2$ appearing in the breath is a direct reflection of the amount of bacterial deconjugation of bile salt that has occurred. Results are expressed as percentage of administered dose of radioactivity per mmol expired CO_2.

The test is abnormal under two circumstances. Firstly when small intestinal bacterial overgrowth results in deconjugation and metabolism before the bile acid is re-absorbed in the ileum (point b in Figure 12.6). Secondly when ileal resection or disease results in unabsorbed bile salt reaching the colon, where it is rapidly metabolized (point c in Figure 12.6).

Radiation dose is low, being 1 mrad to the total body, and approximately 6 mrad to the liver.

Interpretation. In normal subjects, very little $^{14}CO_2$ is exhaled during the first 4 hours; during the next 3 hours the amount rises, but not to more than 0.3% of dose/mmol CO_2. Most patients with ileal resection or small bowel contamination have raised excretion between 3 and 6 hours. Abnormal results are also found in patients with cholangitis.

Occasional patients with jejunal diverticula have normal $^{14}CO_2$ excretion, probably because the particular bacteria which are present lack the capacity to deconjugate the bile salt. Normal values are found in patients with ileal resection if transit through the colon is so rapid that there is insufficient time for deconjugation of the unabsorbed bile salt and subsequent absorption of the [^{14}C]glycine into blood. In all patients with watery stools which exceed 200 grams in weight daily, the stool ^{14}C should also be estimated.

Indications for test. The breath test is probably the most sensitive indirect test for establishing small bowel bacterial colonization, providing that co-existing ileal disease can be excluded. Serial tests can be useful in assessing the response to antibiotic therapy. In the assessment of ileal integrity, it can be more sensitive than the Schilling test, but the need to estimate stool ^{14}C in patients with diarrhoea makes the test less practicable both for the patient and for the routine laboratory.

12.4.6. Other tests for small bowel bacterial contamination (Hamilton et al., 1970)

12.4.6.1. Direct examination of bacterial flora

The upper small intestine is almost sterile. Aspiration of small intestinal contents for culture through a fine flexible tube swallowed by the patient is simple, but the techniques necessary for adequate bacterial analysis are time consuming. Aerobic and anaerobic culture has to be carried out on a variety of culture media and this is not practicable as a routine procedure.

12.4.6.2. Estimation of intraluminal bile salts

Bacteria within the small intestine cause deconjugation and dehydroxylation of bile acids to products which are less effective in micelle formation and may be toxic to the intestinal mucosa. One or other (or both) of these mechanisms is probably the main cause of fat malabsorption in the bacterial stasis syndromes.

Thin layer chromatography of aspirated intestinal contents enables qualitative analysis of intraluminal bile salts to be carried out easily. Visual examination of the plates is adequate for the detection of the deconjugated and dehydroxylated bile acids which are usually present if bacteria are causing significant malabsorption. Aspiration at different points within jejunum and ileum give some indication at the site of contamination if this is localized, e.g. jejunal diverticula, or an ileocolic fistula.

Determination of the actual concentrations of both normal and abnormal bile salts is possible on the same samples, but gives little information of practical value.

Thin layer chromatographic separation of intraluminal bile salts is eminently practical as a routine procedure and will usually enable abnormal results of a $^{14}CO_2$ bile acid breath test due to ileal resection to be distinguished from those due to small intestinal bacterial overgrowth. In practice, it can be combined with a Lundh test (section 12.5.5.2) although interpretation may then be complicated by the presence in the proximal jejunum of freshly secreted gall bladder bile containing re-conjugated secondary bile acids.

12.4.6.3. Urinary indican

Some intestinal bacteria, particularly *Escherichia coli* and *bacterioides,* contain the enzyme tryptophanase which can metabolize dietary tryptophan to indole. This is absorbed, converted into indican in the liver and excreted in this form in the urine.

Bacteria within the small intestine may be associated with a high urinary indican excretion due to their metabolism of dietary tryptophan. Estimation of indican in a 24-hour specimen of urine has therefore been suggested in the diagnosis of small bowel bacterial contamination. Increased urinary indican is not always found, however, since the predominant bacteria may not contain tryptophanase, and then urinary indican excretion may be normal. Furthermore, in other small bowel diseases causing malabsorption, urinary indican excretion may be increased due to unabsorbed dietary tryptophan reaching the colon and being metabolised by colonic bacteria. In pancreatic steatorrhoea, urinary indican excretion is usually very low, but there are better ways of making this diagnosis.

Estimation of urinary indican is therefore not recommended for practical use in the diagnosis of malabsorptive states. It is of historical interest, however, in that increased urinary indican was the finding which led to impaired intestinal aminoacid absorption being recognized in Hartnup disease.

12.4.7. Folic acid absorption tests (Chanarin, 1969; Rosenberg and Godwin, 1970)

Studies of folate absorption in malabsorptive states have largely been carried out using synthetic folic acid (pteroylmonoglutamic acid). The amount in urine and blood has been followed either by microbiological assay after ingestion of unlabelled folic acid, or by scintillation counting after ingestion of tritiated folic acid. Peak serum concentrations are achieved after 1 to 2 hours. Patients with tropical sprue and adult coeliac disease generally absorb less than normal individuals, but there is some overlap.

Uncertainties in interpretation make the test unsuitable for general clinical application. The degree of tissue saturation significantly affects results, and this variable is not completely abolished by prior use of saturating doses even for some days. Only a trace amount of dietary folate is actually folic acid, the majority being polyglutamate conjugates which need to be hydrolyzed within the intestinal lumen or enterocyte before absorption, so that tests of folic acid absorption may not reflect absorption of food folate. A few studies of folate polyglutamate absorption have been reported, but a practical clinical test remains to be devised.

12.4.8. Haematological response to oral folic acid

In most megaloblastic anaemias which are due to malabsorption a good haematological response will follow oral administration of physiological (100 to 200 μg) doses of folic acid, as in nutritional folate deficiency. In those megaloblastic anaemias which are due to increased folate requirement, haematological response only occurs with larger doses. Absence of response to small doses cannot therefore be used as an indication of folate malabsorption.

12.4.9. Choice of test in diagnosis of malabsorption syndromes

In the introduction to this section, it was stressed that the choice of a chemical test will be determined initially by the clinical circumstances. Measurement of faecal fat excretion remains the most widely applicable test. The finding of steatorrhoea, or a sufficiently suggestive clinical picture in its absence, should almost invariably lead to jejunal biopsy, the xylose test being used mainly as a screening test for jejunal malfunction as it can never, in itself, provide an unequivocal final diagnosis. If the jejunal biopsy is histologically normal, coeliac disease is excluded and pancreatic disease or an anatomical defect in the small intestine should be sought both by radiological means and by functional examination – e.g. bile acid breath test, vitamin B_{12} absorption test, or a test of pancreatic secretion.

These tests in the majority of patients should yield both a functional and anatomical diagnosis. The response to appropriate treatment may require monitoring by repetition of an appropriate test of absorption as well as by monitoring both the patient's subjective response and nutritional status. If response is slow or incomplete, the diagnosis may need review and the possibility of dual pathology considered.

12.5. ASSESSMENT OF PANCREATIC FUNCTION

12.5.1. Physiology of the pancreas

12.5.1.1. Enzyme secretion

The proteolytic enzymes of the pancreas, produced in the acinar cells, are all secreted into the duodenum as inactive zymogens. Trypsinogen is there converted into trypsin by enterokinase, which is itself an enzyme secreted from the brush border of duodenal mucosa. Trypsin then activates the other proteolytic enzymes, e.g. chymotrypsinogens, procollagenase, the procarboxypeptidases and proelastase. Pancreatic amylase needs no activation. Pancreatic lipase requires bile salts for full activity.

12.5.1.2. Fluid and electrolyte secretion

Pancreatic secretion of fluid and electrolytes is quite considerable; with maximal stimulation, flow rates of almost 5 ml/min can be achieved. Sodium and potassium concentrations are approximately those of plasma. The unique feature is the high concentration of bicarbonate. Under varying degrees of hormonal stimulation, bicarbonate concentration increases with increasing flow rate from 25 to 150 mmol/litre. As chloride is the other main anion, and the sum of the chloride and bicarbonate concentrations remains constant, the chloride concentration falls as flow rate increases.

12.5.1.3. Control of pancreatic secretion

There is undoubtedly some degree of vagal control of pancreatic secretion, but the importance of this is still uncertain. Hormonal control by secretin and pancreozymin secreted by small intestinal mucosa has, however, been extensively investigated. Secretin is released in response to acid entering the duodenum, and is probably the main stimulus to water and electrolyte secretion although gastrin and pancreatic polypeptide also have this action. Pancreozymin acts primarily on enzyme secretion.

There are considerable structural similarities between many of the polypeptide intestinal hormones, accompanied by much overlap of activity – sometimes synergism, sometimes antagonism. Secretin, in addition to stimulating the pancreas, also stimulates the biliary tree to secrete bicarbonate, but it inhibits secretion of gastric acid. Pancreozymin is an important stimulus to gall bladder contraction (hence its alternative name cholecystokinin) and in man it is as potent as gastrin in stimulating acid secretion. Gastrin itself is synergistic with both secretin and pancreozymin.

Secretin is now available as a synthetic chemically pure preparation (G.I.H. Laboratories). Fairly pure (about 16%) pancreozymin is available from the same source, but impurities include small amounts of G.I.P. and vasoactive intestinal peptide (section 12.2.4.3). Some commercially produced preparations of secretin and pancreozymin are very impure; moreover, biological standardization is not necessarily precise. A variety of units are used to express the potencies of hormones from different sources and this adds to the confusion; e.g. Ivy Units, Clinical Units, Crick Harper and Raper Units (Wormsley, 1972).

12.5.2. Serum and urinary amylase (Goldberg and Spooner, 1975)

α-Amylases are present in a number of tissues other than the pancreas, including salivary gland, intestinal mucosa, and Fallopian tubes. Although these can be differentiated to some extent, assay methods in routine use only measure total activity. Activities are not usually expressed in international units, since the substrates and products of various assay methods differ, but one commerically available test is stated to give a reference range of 70 to 300 IU/litre. The Somogyi unit is still in most general use, with reference values in most laboratories lying between 50 and 150 units/ml for serum.

In normal subjects, the serum amylase so measured is derived from a number of sources, probably in the main the pancreatic and salivary glands, but the elevation of activity which occurs in pancreatic necrosis is largely due to pancreatic amylase. This first reaches the circulation through venous routes, and later through lymphatics and by absorption from the peritoneum. Some of this amylase is excreted in the urine, but the fate of the remainder is unknown; this ignorance of normal metabolism is accompanied by difficulties in interpretation of the changes which occur in disease.

It is possible to determine pancreatic and salivary isoamylases separately in blood, but the value of this determination in clinical practice may prove to be limited, as a significant rise of salivary as well as pancreatic isoenzyme can occur in pancreatic disease.

A few patients have been described with an amylase of large molecular mass in the serum, in addition to normal amylase. Serum amylase activity is elevated due to this "macroamylase", but urine amylase activity is normal. The macroamylase can be separated from normal amylase by gel filtration; it is a 19S protein, in contrast to normal amylase which is a 7S protein.

12.5.3. Pancreatic disease – nomenclature

It is important to appreciate the distinction between acute and chronic pancreatitis.

Acute pancreatitis arises in a previously normal gland, and complete anatomical and functional recovery is the rule.

Chronic pancreatitis is characterized by persistent abnormality of structure and/or function.

From these definitions, it follows that the procedures necessary for diagnosis are different in the two conditions. Clinically it may at times be difficult to distinguish between a *relapsing acute pancreatitis* and a *relapsing chronic pancreatitis* since intermittent pain is the main feature of both, but observation and tests of function usually enable the two to be differentiated.

12.5.4. Acute pancreatitis

12.5.4.1. Serum amylase

Determination of amylase activity in serum remains the most widely available and useful test. Usually it is elevated 2 to 12 hours after onset, and returns to normal within 3 or 4 days: the magnitude of the rise is no index of severity and the rate of fall is no guide to speed of resolution. Two problems arise in the use of the test. First, other conditions cause elevation of serum amylase: some, e.g. mumps, hypothyroidism, renal failure and diabetic ketoacidosis, are unlikely to prove a diagnostic problem; others, such as ruptured ectopic pregnancy, acute cholecystitis, perforated peptic ulcer, intestinal strangulation, mesenteric arterial occlusion, and ruptured or dissecting aortic aneurysm, can cause a similar clinical picture. Secondly, in perhaps 5% of patients with acute pancreatitis, the serum amylase activity is not raised on presentation. In some patients even repeated tests are normal. Occasionally this will prove to be due to raised serum triglycerides which interfere with the assay.

In most conditions other than acute pancreatitis, the serum activity does not rise above twice the upper limit of normal, but in afferent loop obstruction after gastro-enterostomy or Polya gastrectomy, and in ruptured ectopic pregnancy, it can be very high.

Rarely, an elevated amylase activity will prove to be due to macroamylase (section 12.5.2).

12.5.4.2. Urine amylase and renal amylase clearance

In acute pancreatitis, the renal clearance of amylase is greater than in normal subjects and this persists even after serum amylase activity returns to normal. Urinary amylase is therefore claimed to be more valuable than serum amylase for diagnosis, and this is certainly true if the patient presents late. In the patient who presents early serum amylase is usually the preferred determination, often because an early differentiation has to be made from conditions requiring immediate laparotomy, and the surgeon cannot wait for a 24-hour urine collection. The ratio of urinary amylase activity to urinary creatinine concentration, or determination of amylase clearance on short timed urine collections can overcome this problem (Levitt et al., 1969). It may be preferable to measure the renal clearance of amylase expressed as a proportion of the simultaneously determined creatinine clearance, as this requires only the collection of a single urine specimen in addition to the usual blood sample. In normal individuals the clearance ratio is consistent within a narrow range (3 ± 1% (S.D.)); in acute pancreatitis, the ratio is significantly raised, whereas it is claimed that in other causes of hyperamylasaemia this is rarely the case (Warshaw and Fuller, 1975). This test is practicable and merits trial in routine practice. Serum lipase is a much less widely used test. It is elevated in up to 90% of patients, but interpretation is subject to most of the difficulties already described for amylase, and its determination takes up to 24 hours. Serum tryptic activity determinations have not been found diagnostically useful.

12.5.4.3. Other laboratory findings

Transient jaundice, hyperglycaemia and glycosuria may occur. Methaemalbumin is present in haemorrhagic pancreatitis and tends to indicate a poor prognosis. A fall in serum calcium concentration may be appreciable in severe cases; this is usually maximal between the fifth and eighth day of the illness, but sometimes persists for 2 weeks. Occasionally the serum magnesium concentration is low and can account for tetany which does not respond to intravenous administration of calcium.

Hyperlipoproteinaemia may be detected after an attack of acute pancreatitis but usually settles completely. Hyperlipoproteinaemia may rarely in itself be a cause of acute pancreatitis (sections 12.3.2 and 12.5.8).

Section 12.5.6 reviews the application of pancreatic function tests in differentiating acute from chronic pancreatitis.

12.5.5. Chronic pancreatitis

As the definition of this condition implies, diagnosis depends on the demonstration of functional impairment of the gland. The following tests are available for this purpose.

Direct measurement of exocrine secretion into the duodenum:

(a) after stimulation by a standard meal (Lundh test);

(b) after stimulation by intravenous secretin and pancreozymin.

Measurement of the enzyme content of faeces.

Assessing response to replacement therapy.

Assessment of endocrine function (insulin and pancreozymin secretion).

Pancreatic scanning.

Whenever possible, direct measurements of pancreatic secretion are preferred.

12.5.5.1. The secretin/pancreozymin test (Wormsley, 1972)

Intubation. Two tubes are necessary, introduced under radiological control. The tip of one tube is located in the gastric antrum and continuous suction is applied to prevent passage of gastric secretion into the duodenum. The aspirate is discarded unless the presence of bile or the finding of a non-acid pH indicates pyloric reflux, in which case it is assayed (as indicated below) and the results added to those obtained on assay of duodenal aspirate. The tip of the second tube is located in the fourth part of the duodenum and pancreatic secretion is collected by continuous aspiration.

Stimulation. Secretin may be used either alone, or with pancreozymin, or followed by pancreozymin. The two hormones may be given by rapid intravenous injection of submaximal dose, or by continuous intravenous infusion of a dose which elicits almost a maximal secretory response. Duodenal contents are then collected, commonly in 10-minute portions. Volume, bicarbonate and (after pancreozymin) one or more enzymes are measured in each aliquot.

Interpretation. Variations between techniques are so considerable that each laboratory must establish its own normal range. The possibility of variable biological potency in commercially available hormones has to be appreciated; unexpectedly low secretion values may require repetition of testing with another batch of hormone. Comparisons of data on volume and maximum bicarbonate concentration are more easily made, since at least the units of measurement are the same. Lower limits of normal for these values after intravenous secretin vary for different centres from 1.1 to 2.2 mg/kg body weight over 60 minutes for volume and from 65 to 94 mmol/litre for maximum bicarbonate concentration.

Bicarbonate concentration and output. Bicarbonate concentration alone has poor discriminatory value, in part because of its dependence on flow rate (section 12.5.1.2).

Bicarbonate output is more useful, providing that care is taken to ensure complete collection; even so, there is considerable difficulty in defining the lower limit of normal, one problem being the unknown contribution of the biliary system and the duodenal mucosa. Wormsley (1972) has suggested that after continuous infusion of secretin (section 12.5.1.3) (2 CU/kg · hour) the normal rate of collection may be considered to be greater than 15 mmol/30 min; less than 10 mmol/30 min is abnormal, and intermediate values are equivocal.

Enzyme output. Similar difficulties exist in defining the lower limit of normal for enzyme output, but most authors agree that enzyme measurements increase the diagnostic value. Although multiple enzyme determinations are the ideal, for most purposes it is sufficient to measure amylase and one proteolytic enzyme, usually trypsin. This will also enable the rare isolated deficiencies of trypsinogen or of enterokinase to be detected.

There is some controversy over the necessity for the use of pancreozymin and the determination of enzyme activities. Variations in biological potency, unpleasant flushing and colic after injection, legal restrictions on its use by some governments, and doubt about the diagnostic usefulness of the information compared with that derived from secretin alone, are arguments invoked against the use of pancreozymin.

Measurement of serum enzymes after secretin and pancreozymin. During the secretin/pancreozymin tests, serum amylase and lipase activities often rise in pancreatic disease, but remain low in normal subjects and in patients with severe pancreatic damage. Diagnostic value is very limited.

Analysis of uncontaminated pancreatic secretion. This is now possible, using fluid collected from a cannula introduced into the pancreatic duct endoscopically, followed by intravenous injection of secretin. Experience is very limited, but combined chemical and cytological examination of pancreatic juice appears promising.

12.5.5.2. The Lundh test (James 1973)

Intubation. This is simpler than the secretin/pancreozymin test and more comfortable for the patient. A thin radio-opaque tube weighted at the end by a mercury bag is swallowed and positioned under fluoroscopy in the middle or distal duodenum.

Meal and collection. A commonly used standard meal consists of 19 grams of corn oil, 15 grams of Casilan and 40 grams of glucose in 300 ml of water. Duodenal contents are collected into a cooled container by siphonage for four successive 30-minute periods. No attempt is made at quantitative recovery. Trypsin activity is determined on each specimen and the mean calculated. A simple method of assay using a synthetic substrate is available.

12.5.5.3. Measurement of the enzyme content of faeces

If for some reason intubation cannot be carried out, it may be worth assaying chymotrypsin activity in the stool, as this is low in most patients with severe pancreatic insufficiency. In adults, intubation studies are always preferable, and in children, although faecal studies have been used extensively in the past it is likely that they will soon be replaced by a modification of the Lundh test as described in section 12.5.9.1. The diagnosis of pancreatic insufficiency solely on the basis of low faecal enzyme output can only be tentative, and should always be confirmed by a more direct method.

12.5.5.4. Assessment of response to replacement therapy

Serial faecal fat estimations before and after oral replacement therapy can be of diagnostic use if no other method is available. Such a study is of value in tailoring a regime of oral enzyme replacement to a patient's needs, as the dose and frequency of administration necessary for relief of steatorrhoea varies considerably from patient to patient.

12.5.5.5. Assessment of endocrine function

Glucose tolerance test. Impaired glucose tolerance in association with steatorrhoea is very suggestive of pancreatic disease, but confirmation by more direct evidence is always necessary.

Insulin secretion. Diminished secretion can be shown in response to intensive stimulation by intravenous glucagon and tolbutamide (Joffe et al., 1968), but the test has not been extensively applied.

Pancreozymin. The serum concentration of pancreozymin is very high in most patients with exocrine pancreatic insufficiency (Harvey, 1976) but assay is difficult.

12.5.5.6. Pancreatic scanning

After intravenous administration of methionine labelled with ^{75}Se, the normal pancreas can be visualized by gamma camera or scintiscanner within 30 minutes. Uptake by the liver is considerable, but subtraction of the liver image after giving Te sulphur colloid usually resolves the problem. The pancreas is only rarely visualized in chronic pancreatitis. Defective visualization is also found often in obesity, diabetes, after gastric surgery and in some normal individuals; but a normal pancreatic image makes chronic pancreatitis unlikely, so justifying the use of scanning as a screening procedure. Radiation dose from the 200 μCi used is very high (1.3 to 1.7 rad per whole body, 0.06 to 1.4 rad to pancreas, 0.06 to 1.2 rad to liver, 11 rad to kidney). Use is inadvisable below the age of 45.

12.5.6. Pancreatic function tests in other diseases

12.5.6.1. Acute pancreatitis

Most experience is with the secretin/pancreozymin test. In 50% of patients, normal function is restored within a few days. Enzyme secretion is the last function to return to normal, and does so within 1 or 2 months. Persistent abnormality is rare and implies by definition that chronic pancreatitis is present. Surprisingly, there appears to be no risk of the test inducing a relapse.

The rate of secretion may be unusually high during the recovery phase. This also occurs in some patients with cirrhosis of the liver, haemochromatosis, biliary ductal ectasia and the Zollinger–Ellison syndrome.

Experience with the Lundh test is less extensive. In practice, the only reason for secretion tests is the differentiation of a recurrent acute pancreatitis from chronic pancreatitis. The claimed greater sensitivity of the secretin/pancreozymin test should make it the procedure of choice in this situation, but this is not yet firmly established.

12.5.6.2. Carcinoma of the pancreas

In carcinoma of the pancreas the secretin/pancreozymin test characteristically shows a low volume of secretion of normal composition. Normal secretion may be found in about 30% of patients, so that outside of specialist centres the test is little used. Skilled cytological examination of the collected fluid may by itself yield positive diagnostic information in 50% of cases; if this facility is available, the test is of much greater value.

The Lundh test has been found to be abnormal in about 70% of patients in published series, and as for the secretin/pancreozymin test, the proportion of abnormal findings was higher in carcinoma of the head rather than of the tail of the gland.

12.5.6.3. Obstructive jaundice

Both the Lundh test and secretin/pancreozymin test are abnormal in the majority of patients in whom obstructive jaundice is due to carcinoma of the pancreas, and normal if it is due to carcinoma of the biliary tree. If obstructive jaundice is due to malignant disease, there is more likely to be total absence of bile on visual inspection of the aspirate than in benign causes.

These tests now have to compete with direct anatomical demonstration of a lesion by endoscopic retrograde cholangiography or percutaneous transhepatic cholangiography. If available, one of these techniques is much to be preferred.

12.5.7. Choice of pancreatic function test in suspected chronic pancreatitis

Indirect evidence, such as impaired glucose tolerance and response to replacement therapy, are not acceptable for final diagnosis. Pancreatic scanning (section 12.5.5.6) is a useful screening test for chronic pancreatitis but frequent false positives make it unsuitable for firm diagnosis. Organ visualization by endoscopic retrograde pancreatography remains to be fully assessed, and examination by arteriography or even at surgery leaves much to be desired. With all their defects, the secretin/pancreozymin and Lundh tests are therefore often indicated in the diagnosis of suspected chronic pancreatic disease.

12.5.7.1. Chronic pancreatitis associated with steatorrhoea

Since this condition implies at least a 90% loss of pancreatic exocrine secretion, diagnosis by either of the two intubation tests is rarely a problem. The Lundh test is recommended in view of its simplicity, mean tryptic activities of less than 2 IU/litre often being found. Fears that values would be very low in coeliac disease – because of impaired hormone production by the damaged intestinal mucosa – are not justified in practice, and in any case jejunal biopsy will normally have been carried out to exclude coeliac disease before performing a Lundh test.

Severe malnutrition due to any cause will depress pancreatic function. It is possible for this to confuse diagnosis of a malabsorptive state, particularly if reliance is placed on the response to replacement therapy.

12.5.7.2. Chronic pancreatitis associated with abdominal pain

Pancreatic exocrine secretion is likely to be less impaired in this than in the previous condition, and diagnosis is therefore more difficult. In the absence of steatorrhoea, the Lundh test is probably abnormal only in 60 to 70% of patients. Much higher figures are claimed for the secretin/pancreozymin test but extensive comparative studies have not so far been carried out and in most centres the Lundh test is now preferred.

12.5.8. Other conditions associated with pancreatitis

Hypercalcaemia from any cause may result in acute or chronic pancreatitis and repeated serum calcium estimations are always worthwhile in pancreatic disease.

Recurrent acute pancreatitis and, rarely, chronic pancreatitis also occur in association with type I and type V hyperlipoproteinaemia (section 12.3.2). The relationship is obscure, but as dietary or other treatment may be helpful, investigation of fasting blood lipids should be carried out in patients with repeated attacks of severe abdominal pain. Hyperlipoproteinaemia may also develop after an attack of acute pancreatitis and may last for some days, but it must not be confused with a primary lipid disorder.

In children, the possible occurrence of neutropenia, aminoaciduria, and abnormalities of sweat electrolytes should also be sought.

12.5.9. Diagnosis of pancreatic disease in childhood (Hadorn, 1975)

Acute pancreatitis is rare in childhood, but mumps is then the most likely cause. Elevation of serum amylase activity is little help in the diagnosis of mumps pancreatitis as it may be caused by the associated parotitis; the diagnosis usually, therefore, relies solely on clinical evidence. In other types of acute pancreatitis the determination of serum amylase is a valuable test, as in adults (section 12.5.4.1).

Pancreatic insufficiency in childhood can be classified under two headings.

Generalised:
Cystic fibrosis (autosomal recessive)
Congenital hypoplasia with neutropenia
Familial chronic pancreatitis (with or without aminoaciduria)
Secondary to severe malnutrition

Isolated enzyme defects (all rare):
Lipase deficiency (autosomal recessive)
Amylase deficiency } genetic inheritance uncertain
Trypsinogen deficiency }

Enterokinase deficiency can mimic pancreatic insufficiency, and may be responsible for many cases of apparent trypsinogen deficiency.

12.5.9.1. Assessment of pancreatic insufficiency

Faecal trypsin and chymotrypsin measurement. In infants and young children these determinations are more reliable than in adults, probably because there is less colonic degradation of pancreatic enzymes. A simple gelatin film test can be used as a side-room procedure, and quantitative assays for both enzymes are readily done using synthetic substrates. These tests will be abnormal in all patients with significant pancreatic insufficiency except in cases of extremely rare isolated defects of amylase and lipase. Trypsin and chymotrypsin, however, are sometimes absent from the stools of normal infants, and this occurrence of false-positives confuses interpretation.

Faecal fat excretion. Measurement of fat excretion is practicable and abnormal values have the same significance as in adults. Serial studies can usefully corroborate clinical assessment of replacement therapy. Up to the age of 1 year, 80% fat absorption is accepted as normal; after 1 year, the value rises to 90% as in adults (section 12.4.2.4).

The secretin/pancreozymin test. As in adults, this test will always be very abnormal if pancreatic function is so poor that steatorrhoea is present (section 12.5.7). In the 20% or so of children with cystic fibrosis but no steatorrhoea, enzyme output may be normal but the volume of secretion and bicarbonate concentration very low. The sweat test, however, is so reliable in cystic fibrosis that other studies, such as the secretin/pancreozymin test, are only necessary if it gives equivocal results.

Pancreatic insufficiency with normal sweat electrolytes and no pulmonary manifestations will most often be due to congenital hypoplasia with neutropenia (Swachman syndrome).

The Lundh test. Published experience of this test in childhood is not yet available. Unpublished experience suggests that it may prove as useful as in adults, and to be preferred to studies of faecal enzymes (J.P.K. McCollum, personal communication).

Examination for isolated enzyme deficiencies (Hadorn, 1975). Isolated enzyme deficiencies are rare, but diagnosis is an interesting exercise in applied enzymology. Isolated amylase deficiency causes a fermentative diarrhoea and has been diagnosed by a starch loading test. Assay of duodenal juice will diagnose lipase deficiency. Trypsinogen deficiency and enterokinase deficiency both result in the absence of proteolytic activity in duodenal juice, but can be differentiated by activation studies. It must be added that the existence of isolated amylase deficiency and isolated trypsinogen deficiency is still disputed due to methodological problems.

12.5.9.2. Abnormalities associated with pancreatic insufficiency

Sweat electrolyte test (Swachman and Grand, 1973). Sweat is collected on weighed gauze pads attached to the forearm, sweating being induced by pilocarpine iontophoresis. At least 100 mg of sweat should be obtained, and after elution the sodium and chloride content is determined so as to estimate the concentrations of sodium and chloride in the sweat specimen. In cystic fibrosis, the concentration of both is approximately four to five times normal, the range in control infants being from 7 to 52 mmol/litre (higher in children with some allergic conditions) and in cystic fibrosis from 72 to 175 mmol/litre. Administration of the antibiotic cloxacillin may depress the sweat chloride concentration into the normal range, while that of sodium remains elevated.

Carefully carried out, this test is abnormal in 99% of patients with cystic fibrosis. Borderline results are uncommon in childhood. After adolescence, results are difficult to interpret as the normal concentrations in adults may be twice as high as in children.

Screening tests are available, including the hand plate test and direct application of a chloride electrode to the skin. They are useful but in themselves are not accurate enough for firm diagnosis. Determination of salivary electrolytes is not helpful, as even resting values show much variation, and there is even greater variability at high rates of secretion.

Neutropenia. If the sweat test is normal, the most likely cause of pancreatic insufficiency is the Swachman syndrome. The neutropenia is usually continuous but may be cyclic. Hypoplastic anaemia, bony abnormalities and thrombocytopenia are also commonly present.

12.6. IMMUNOLOGICAL TESTS IN DIAGNOSIS

Discussion will be limited to a few serological tests which have already proved of some value, or have potential diagnostic importance. Immunoglobulin changes have been mentioned previously (section 12.1.4).

12.6.1. Coeliac disease

Antibodies to milk protein do occur, but they are not specific, and their presence is not an indication of milk intolerance. If this condition is present, it is likely to be due to secondary alactasia (section 12.4.3.7). Circulating antibodies to gluten have been reported to occur in 23 to 90% of untreated coeliac patients in different published series, but are uncommon in patients maintained on a gluten-free diet. It has therefore been suggested that detection of gluten antibodies may provide a useful indication of the patients who continue to ingest gluten (Baker et al., 1975). Antireticulin antibodies, which react with reticulin or basement membrane, are uncommon in normal individuals but are found in the plasma of about 40% of adult and 90% or more of children with coeliac disease; they tend to disappear on dietary treatment.

12.6.2. Ulcerative colitis and Crohn's disease

In these disorders, serum antibodies to milk protein can be detected, but their presence does not correlate with clinical response to milk exclusion and their detection is of no help, either in diagnosis or in management. Anticolon antibodies have been found in the serum mainly of children with ulcerative colitis, but their detection is too difficult and inconsistent to be of diagnostic help. Antireticulin antibody is found in about 20% of patients with Crohn's disease, but this frequency is too low for diagnostic application.

12.6.3. Carcinoma of the gastrointestinal tract

Carcinoembryonic antigen has been found in the serum of up to 90% of patients with carcinoma of the colon. Clinical specificity has proved to be too low for the assay to be of diagnostic use, since it has been detected in a significant proportion of patients with carcinomas elsewhere in the gastrointestinal tract, and in non-malignant conditions including ulcerative colitis and alcoholic disease.

12.6.4. HL-A histocompatibility antigens

Data are still accumulating on the extent to which certain diseases occur more commonly in individuals with particular HL-A antigens. In no gastrointestinal disease so far studied does any association even approach that found between B27 and ankylosing spondylitis. In both coeliac disease and dermatitis herpetiformis, about 70% of all patients have HL-A8 antigen, but as this occurs in 25% of a control population assessment of HL-A status is not of diagnostic help.

ACKNOWLEDGEMENTS

I am most grateful to the following who have read parts of the manuscript and made suggestions and corrections which have been incorporated in the text: Dr. D.M. Goldberg (Pancreatic Function), Dr. J.T. Harries (Malabsorption and Pancreatic Disease in Infancy), Dr. N. McIntyre (Fat Absorption) and Dr. G.E. Sladen (Malabsorption).

REFERENCES

Anderson, C.M. and Burke, V. (1975) Disorders of carbohydrate digestion and absorption. In Paediatric Gastroenterology (Eds. C.M. Anderson and V. Burke) pp. 199–217, Blackwell Scientific Publications, Oxford.

Baker, P.G., Barry, R.E. and Read, A.E. (1975) Detection of continuing gluten ingestion in treated coeliac patients. British Medical Journal, 1, 486–488.

Beck, P., Wills, D., Davies, G.T., Lachman, P.J. and Sussman, M. (1973) A family study of hereditary angioneurotic oedema. Quarterly Journal of Medicine, 42, 317–334.

Bloom, S.R., Polak, J.M. and Pearse, A.G.E. (1973) Vasoactive intestinal peptide and watery-diarrhoea syndrome. Lancet, ii, 14–16.

Booth, C.C., Hanna, S., Babouris, N. and MacIntyre, I. (1963) Incidence of hypomagnesaemia in intestinal malabsorption. British Medical Journal, 2, 141–144.

Burrows, P.J., Fleming, J.S., Garnett, E.S., Ackery, D.M., Colin-Jones, D.G. and Bamforth, J. (1974) Clinical evaluation of the ^{14}C fat absorption test. Gut, 15, 147–150.

Chanarin, I. (1969) The Megaloblastic Anaemias. Blackwell Scientific Publications, Oxford and Edinburgh.

Cuatrecasas, P., Lockwood, D.H. and Caldwell, J.R. (1965) Lactase deficiency in the adult. Lancet, i, 14–18.

Dawson, A.M. (1970) The absorption of disaccharides. In Modern Trends in Gastroenterology, Vol 4 (Eds. W.I. Card and B. Creamer) pp. 105–124, Butterworths, London.

Duthie, H.L. and Wormsley, K.W. (Eds.) (1978) The Scientific Basis of Gastroenterology. Churchill-Livingstone, Edinburgh.

Fordtran, J.S. (1973) Diarrhoea. In Gastrointestinal Disease (Eds. M.H. Sleisenger and J.S. Fordtran) pp. 291–319, W.B. Saunders Co. Ltd., Philadelphia, London and Toronto.

Fordtran, J.S., Clodi, P.H., Soergel, K.H. and Ingelfinger, F.J. (1962) Sugar absorption tests, with special reference to 3-O-methyl-D-glucose and D-xylose. Annals of Internal Medicine, 57, 883–891.

Fredrickson, D.S. and Levy, R.I. (1972) Familial hyperlipoproteinemia. In The Metabolic Basis of Inherited Disease (Eds. J.B. Stanbury, J.B. Wyngaarden and D.S. Fredrickson) pp. 545–614, McGraw-Hill, New York.

Fromm, H. and Hofmann, A.F. (1971) Breath test for altered bile-acid metabolism. Lancet, ii, 621–625.

Goldberg, D.M. and Spooner, R.J. (1975) Amylase, isoamylase and macroamylase. Digestion, 13, 56–75.

Hadorn, B. (1975) The exocrine pancreas. In Paediatric Gastroenterology (Eds. C.M. Anderson and V. Burke) pp. 289–327, Blackwell Scientific Publications, Oxford.

Hamilton, J.D., Dyer, N.H., Dawson, A.M., O'Grady, F.W., Vince, A., Fenton, J.C.B. and Mollin, D.L. (1970) Assessment and significance of bacterial overgrowth in the small bowel. Quarterly Journal of Medicine, 39, 265–285.

Harvey, R.F. (1976) Radioimmunoassay. In Topics in Gastroenterology 4 (Eds. S.C. Truelove and J.A. Ritchie) pp. 231–261, Blackwell, Oxford.

Henry, R.J. (1966) Clinical Chemistry. Harper and Row, New York.

Holdsworth, C.D. (1969) The gut and oral glucose tolerance. Gut, 10, 422–427.

Holdsworth, C.D. (1974) The Gut. In Clinical Physiology (Eds. E.J.M. Campbell, C.J. Dickenson and J.D.H. Slater) pp. 488–541, Blackwell Scientific Publications, Oxford.

Holdsworth, C.D. (1975) Calcium absorption in man. In Intestinal Absorption in Man (Eds. I. McColl and G.E.G. Sladen) pp. 223–262, Academic Press, London.

Jacobs, A. and Worwood, M. (1975) Ferritin in serum: clinical and biochemical implications. New England Journal of Medicine, 292, 951–956.

James, O. (1973) The Lundh test. Gut, 14, 582–591.

James, O.F.W., Agnew, J.E. and Bouchier, I.A.D. (1973) Assessment of the ^{14}C-glycocholic acid breath test. British Medical Journal, 3, 191–195.

Joffe, B.I., Bank, S., Jackson, W.P.U., Keller, P., O'Reilly, I.G. and Vinik, A.I. (1968) Insulin reserve in patients with chronic pancreatitis. Lancet, ii, 890–892.

Jones, E.A. (1972) Immunoglobulins and the gut. Gut, 13, 825–835.

Kamer, J.H. Van de, Huinink, H. Ten Bokkel and Weyers, H.A. (1949) Rapid method for the determination of fat in faeces. Journal of Biological Chemistry, 177, 347–355.

Kowlessar, O.D. (1973) Carcinoid tumors and the carcinoid syndrome. In Gastrointestinal Disease (Eds. M.H. Sleisenger and J.S. Fordtran) pp. 1031–1041, W.B. Saunders Co. Ltd., Philadelphia, London and Toronto.

Lamabadusuriya, S.P., Packer, S. and Harries, J.T. (1975) Limitations of xylose tolerance test as a screening test in childhood coeliac disease. Archives of Disease in Childhood, 50, 34–39.

Levitt, M.D. and Duane, W.C. (1973) Floating stools – flatus versus fat. New England Journal of Medicine, 286, 973–975.

Levitt, M.D., Rapoport, M. and Cooperband, S.R. (1969) The renal clearance of amylase in renal insufficiency, acute pancreatitis and macroamylasemia. Annals of Internal Medicine, 71, 919–925.

Losowsky, M.S., Walker, B.E. and Kelleher, J. (1974) Malabsorption in Clinical Practice. Churchill Livingstone, Edinburgh and London.

McColl, I. and Sladen, G.E.G. (Eds.) (1975) Intestinal Absorption in Man. Academic Press, London.

McGuigan, J.E. (1973) Immunology and disease of the gastrointestinal tract. In Gastrointestinal Disease (Eds. M.H. Sleisenger and J.S. Fordtran) pp. 51–67, W.B. Saunders Co. Ltd., Philadelphia, London and Toronto.

Newcomer, A.D., McGill, D.B., Thomas, P.J. and Hofmann, A.F. (1975) Prospective comparison of indirect methods for detecting lactase deficiency. New England Journal of Medicine, 293, 1232–1235.

Rosenberg, I.H. and Godwin, H.A. (1970) The digestion and absorption of dietary folate. Gastroenterology, 60, 445–463.

Sammons, H.G., Morgan, D.B., Frazer, A.C., Montgomery, R.D., Philip, W.M. and Phillips, M.J. (1967) Modification of the xylose absorption test as an index of intestinal function. Gut, 8, 348–353.

Sladen, G.E.G. and Kumar, P.J. (1973) Is the xylose test still a worthwhile investigation? British Medical Journal, 3, 223–226.

Swachman, H. and Grand, R.J. (1973) Cystic fibrosis – diagnostic tests. In Gastrointestinal Disease (Eds. M.H. Sleisenger and J.S. Fordtran) pp. 1219–1220, W.B. Saunders Co. Ltd., Philadelphia, London and Toronto.

Toskes, P.T. and Deren, J.J. (1973) Vitamin B_{12} absorption and malabsorption. Gastroenterology, 65, 662–683.

Waldmann, T.A. (1970) Protein losing enteropathy. In Modern Trends in Gastroenterology, Vol. 4 (Eds. W.E. Card and B. Creamer) pp. 125–142, Butterworths, London.

Warshaw, A.L. and Fuller, A.F. (1975) Specificity of increased renal clearance of amylase in diagnosis of acute pancreatitis. New England Journal of Medicine, 292, 325–328.

Waterlow, J.C. (1969) The assessment of protein nutrition and metabolism in the whole animal, with special reference to man. In Mammalian Protein Metabolism, Vol. III (Ed. H.N. Munro) pp. 326–390, Academic Press, New York and London.

Wormsley, K.G. (1972) Pancreatic function tests. In The Exocrine Pancreas, Clinics in Gastroenterology, 1, 1 (Ed. H.T. Howat) pp. 27–51, W.B. Saunders and Co. Ltd., London, Philadelphia and Toronto.

FURTHER READING

Holdsworth, C.D., The Gut. In Clinical Physiology, 4th edn. (Eds. E.J.M. Campbell, C.J. Dickenson and J.D.H. Slater) pp. 488–541, Blackwell Scientific Publications, Oxford, 1974.

Intestinal Absorption in Man (Eds. I. McColl and G.E.G. Sladen) Academic Press, London, 1975.

The Exocrine Pancreas. Clinics in Gastroenterology, 1, 1 (Ed. H.T. Howat) W.R. Saunders Co. Ltd., London, Philadelphia and Toronto, 1972.

Gastrointestinal Disease (Eds. M.H. Sleisenger and J.S. Fordtran) W.B. Saunders Co. Ltd., Philadelphia, London and Toronto, 1973.

Modern Trends in Gastroenterology 4 (Eds. W.I. Card and B. Creamer) Butterworths, London, 1970.

Paediatric Gastorenterology (Eds. C.M. Anderson and V. Burke) Blackwell Scientific Publications, Oxford, 1975.

The Scientific Basis of Gastroenterology (Eds. H.L. Duthie and K.W. Wormsley) Churchill-Livingstone, Edinburgh and London, 1978.

Chapter 13

Thyroid function

Raymond Hoffenberg

Department of Medicine, University of Birmingham, Queen Elizabeth Hospital, Edgbaston, Birmingham B15 2TH, England

CONTENTS

Chemical diagnosis of disease, edited by
S.S. Brown, F.L. Mitchell and D.S. Young

13.1. THYROID PHYSIOLOGY

13.1.1. Synthesis of thyroid hormones

Two major hormones, thyroxine (T4) and 3,5,3′-triiodothyronine (T3), are secreted by the thyroid gland. Their synthetic pathways have largely been defined, although some steps must still be regarded as tentative. Iodine, which is an essential component of thyroid hormone molecules, is concentrated in the gland by an active transport system so as to achieve a thyroid : serum ratio of about 20 : 1. This concentration step depends on oxidative phosphorylation, is augmented by the action of pituitary thyroid-stimulating hormone (thyrotrophin; TSH) and is blocked by actinomycin D, puromycin or cycloheximide, providing evidence of its mediation through protein synthesis. Occasional defects in iodide-concentrating ability are attributed to faulty cell surface proteins ("permeases"); in such cases iodide diffuses passively into the thyroid cell.

Within thyroid cells, iodide is rapidly oxidized by a peroxidase to form iodine which immediately becomes covalently bound to free tyrosine residues of the large thyroglobulin molecule (Scheme 13.1). This tetrameric protein, of approximately 660,000 molecular mass, contains about 5650 aminoacid residues of which 120 to 125 are tyrosine; only 25 to 30 of these are converted into iodotyrosines – monoiodotyrosine (MIT) and diiodotyrosine (DIT) – and those which are in sterically favourable sites undergo oxidative coupling to form the iodothyronines T4 and T3 (Scheme 13.2).

It is basic to this whole sequence that there should be initial oxidation of iodide to iodine, without which tyrosine-iodination (or "organification") will not proceed. Absence of the essential peroxidase in certain individuals leads to defective synthesis of thyroid hormones and the accumulation of free iodide within the thyroid gland. In such individuals, this iodide may be displaced from the thyroid gland by administration of ionic perchlorate or thiocyanate.

Iodinated thyroglobulin molecules are secreted into the lumen of the thyroid gland follicles and stored there as "colloid" until required. When more hormone is needed, the thyroid cell ingests thyroglobulin from the follicular colloid by endocytosis; the engulfed protein is transported in so-called "colloid vesicles" which then appear to fuse with primary lysosomes to form phagolysosomes; proteolytic enzymes break down the thyroglobulin, and iodinated tyrosines or thyronines are released within the cell. In the

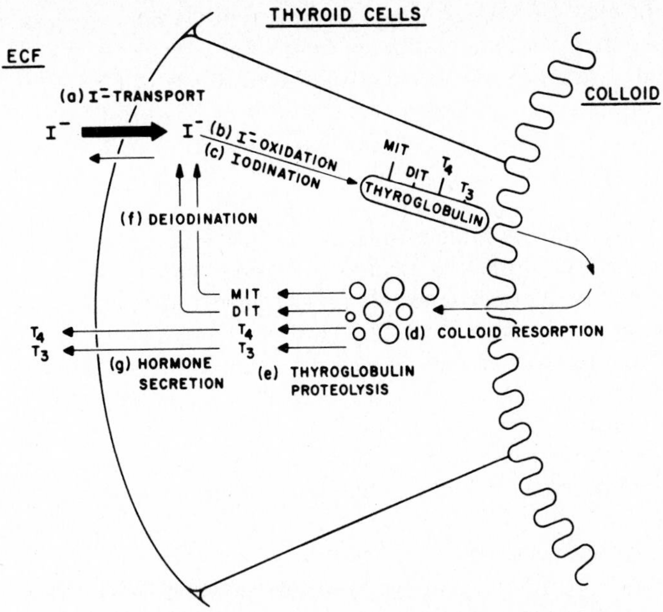

Scheme 13.1. Representation of intracellular iodine metabolism, and the formation, storage and secretion of thyroid hormones. (Reproduced, by permission, from Werner, S.C. and Ingbar, S.H. (Eds.) The Thyroid, 3rd edn, Harper and Row, New York, 1971)

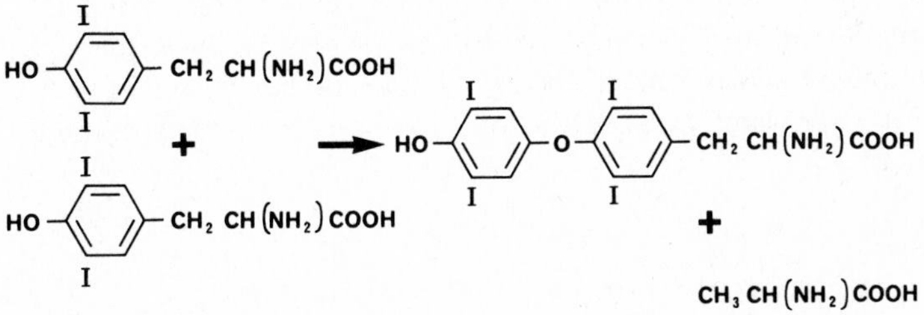

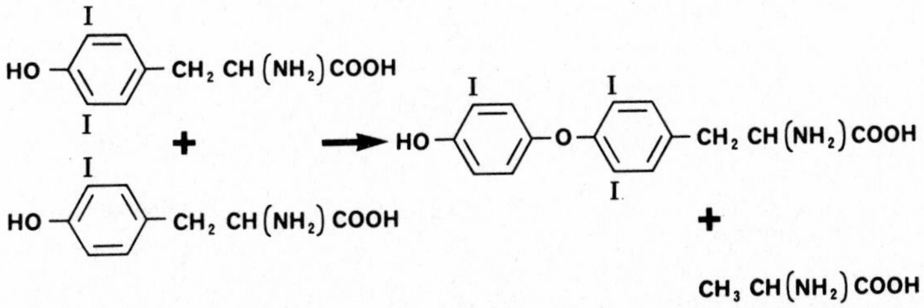

HO–C$_6$H$_2$I$_2$–CH$_2$ CH (NH$_2$) COOH + HO–C$_6$H$_2$I$_2$–CH$_2$ CH (NH$_2$) COOH → HO–C$_6$H$_2$I$_2$–O–C$_6$H$_2$I$_2$–CH$_2$ CH (NH$_2$) COOH + CH$_3$ CH (NH$_2$) COOH

HO–C$_6$H$_2$I$_2$–CH$_2$ CH (NH$_2$) COOH + HO–C$_6$H$_3$I–CH$_2$ CH (NH$_2$) COOH → HO–C$_6$H$_3$I–O–C$_6$H$_2$I$_2$–CH$_2$ CH (NH$_2$) COOH + CH$_3$ CH (NH$_2$) COOH

Scheme 13.2. Top: coupling of two diiodotyrosine molecules to form thyroxine (tetraiodothyronine) with loss of an alanine side chain. Bottom: coupling of diiodotyrosine with monoiodotyrosine to form 3,3′,5-triiodothyronine with loss of an alanine side chain.

presence of a great excess of iodotyrosine deiodinase, iodine is split off from free iodotyrosines and may be re-used by the cell for further synthesis of new hormones. T4 and T3 released by thyroglobulin proteolysis are secreted via the basal pole of the thyroid cell into the circulation.

13.1.2. Circulating thyroid hormones

In plasma, T4 and T3 are almost entirely protein-bound – to thyroxine-binding globulin (TBG), prealbumin, and albumin. In artificial conditions of hypersaturation, T4 and T3 can be shown to bind to other plasma proteins, notably α_1- and β-lipoprotein. Some characteristics of the three major binding proteins are outlined in Table 13.1. The distribution of hormone between the three proteins appears to vary according to the technique of study: for T4, about 75% is bound to TBG, 15 to 20% to prealbumin and 10% to albumin. It was previously believed that prealbumin did not bind T3 but it now seems clear that 7 to 10% of the circulating hormone is bound by this protein; the overall distribution of T3 binding is not known with certainty, but the pattern is roughly similar to that of T4.

The bonds between the thyroid hormones and proteins are not covalent; the low binding energy (5 to 8 kcals/mol, about 1/10th of the energy of covalent bonds) allows ready dissociation of the hormone, particularly of T3 for which the proteins exhibit lower binding affinity.

A small fraction of circulating hormone exists in non-protein-bound or "free" form. For T4 this is about 0.03 to 0.04% of the total circulating hormone (3 to 6 $\times 10^{-11}$ mol/litre or 20 to 30 ng/litre); for T3 it is 0.2 to 0.5% of the total (4 to 16 $\times 10^{-12}$ mol/litre or 2 to 8 ng/litre). TBG has a greater binding affinity for T4 than prealbumin, and albumin acts as a less specific low-affinity "sponge" soaking up T4 molecules which are not bound by TBG or prealbumin. Thus TBG has a limited capacity, but high affinity, for binding T4; albumin has a very large capacity but low affinity, and prealbumin is intermediate between the two.

TABLE 13.1.

SOME CHARACTERISTICS OF THYROID HORMONE BINDING PROTEINS

	Thyroxine-binding globulin (TBG)	Thyroxine-binding prealbumin (TBPA)	Albumin
Distribution of bound T4(%)	75	15–20	10
Distribution of bound T3(%)	75	7–10	10–15
Concentration (mg/litre)	15	250–350	35–50,000
Molecular mass	58,000	75,000 *	69,000
Binding capacity for T4 (mg/litre)	0.25–0.30	15–30	>450
Association constant for T4	2–4 $\times 10^{10}$	1 $\times 10^8$	1 $\times 10^6$
Association constant for T3	2 $\times 10^9$	Uncertain	3 $\times 10^5$

* TBPA complex with retinol-binding protein (molecular mass 21,000).

TBG is a glycoprotein which migrates electrophoretically as an α-globulin; it occurs in plasma at a concentration of about 250 nmol/litre (1.5 mg/dl), has a molecular mass of approximately 58,000, a single binding site for T4 per molecule, and a binding capacity for T4 of about 25 to 30 μg/dl plasma. Since the normal concentration of T4 in plasma is about 100 nmol/litre (8 μg/dl) TBG is only about 25 to 30% "saturated".

Prealbumin consists of four subunits each of about 13,500 molecular mass. One molecule of T4 may be bound to each tetramer, and the whole forms a protein–protein link with one molecule of retinol-binding protein (RBP). The complex has a molecular mass above 75,000 (prealbumin 54,000 and RBP 21,000). It should be noted that only about 1% of prealbumin molecules actually bind T4. The protein has a finite capacity of about 380 nmol (300 μg) of T4 per dl of plasma and its normal concentration in plasma is about 6 μmol/litre or 30 mg/dl.

13.1.3. Free T4 and T3

Despite their relatively low concentrations in plasma, the non-protein-bound or free moieties of T4 (or T3) are regarded as biologically important and are thought to diffuse from the circulation to enter the cells on which they act. Since there are equilibria between protein-bound and free T4 or T3, the concentrations of the free hormones will depend on: (a) the total amount of binding proteins in the plasma pool; (b) the relative amounts of each protein and the number of high-affinity and low-affinity binding sites on each; and (c) the total amount of hormone in the circulation. If the TBG concentration is increased (usually due to genetic factors or to high circulating oestrogens, as in pregnancy or after ingestion of oral contraceptive pills) or decreased (due to genetic factors, nephrotic syndrome or the action of androgens), homoeostatic adjustment keeps the free hormone concentration stable (Figure 13.1). Some drugs are bound by TBG and may displace both T4 and T3 from the protein. This reduces the concentration of protein-bound hormone, but the free hormone concentration is adjusted to normal by similar homoeostatic mechanisms.

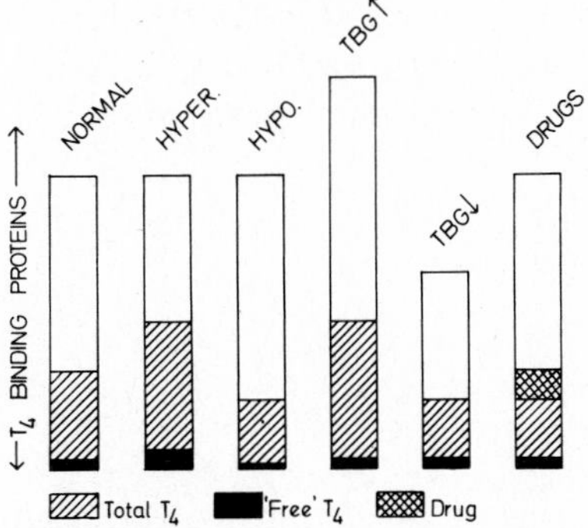

Figure 13.1. Histogram of thyroxine-binding proteins to show variations in total and free hormone concentrations in hyperthyroidism and hypothyroidism, and maintenance of normal free thyroxine concentrations with alteration of TBG concentration or displacement of hormone by drugs bound by this protein.

13.1.4. Triiodothyronine

In plasma the concentration of T4 normally ranges from 40 to 110 μg/litre (about 50 to 150 nmol/litre), and of T3 from 0.3 to 2 μg/litre (about 0.8 to 3.2 nmol/litre) according to various reports (see reviews by Sterling, 1970; Hoffenberg, 1973 and Utiger, 1974). Despite its relatively low concentration, T3 is thought to be at least as important as T4 in total metabolic activity. On the basis of kinetic studies using radio-active tracers, it has been calculated that a significant fraction of the total body T3 is derived from peripheral mono-deiodination of T4 (Hoffenberg, 1973; Utiger, 1974). Among tissues shown to be capable of deiodinating T4 to form T3 are liver cells, myocardium, kidney, anterior pituitary gland, lymphocytes and fibroblasts. Direct proof of this peripheral conversion is found in athyroidal subjects being treated with T4 substitution therapy whose circulating T3 concentration is usually within the normal range. In these subjects, the presence of T3 could only be explained by peripheral conversion of T4. On the other hand, thyroid vein samples show that both T4 and T3 are normally secreted by the gland. The relative contributions of thyroidal secretion and peripheral deiodination of T4 towards the total production of T3 have not been finally established, but it seems likely that a little less than 100 μg of T4 is produced per day, and 20 to 40 μg of T3 per day, of which between 40 and 80% is derived from peripheral conversion of T4. T3 is thought to be three to five times more active than T4 – depending on the type of response studied – which suggests that 60 to 80% of total thyroid hormone activity may be mediated through T3. Some authorities believe that T4 acts simply as a precursor or prohormone for the active hormone T3. Support for the concept that T3 is the active form of hormone arises from the demonstration of both cytosol and nuclear intracellular receptor proteins for T3 (de Groot and Strausser, 1974; de Groot and Torresani, 1975; Surks et al., 1975), but this does not preclude a role for other metabolites or analogues.

13.1.5. Metabolic pathways of T4 and T3

Apart from deiodination to T3, T4 may undergo other metabolic changes (Figure 13.2). It is not yet certain to what extent deiodination occurs at the 5 position rather than at 5′ to give 3,3′,5′-triiodothyronine or reverse T3 (rT3) – a metabolically inert product. After acute medical or surgical stress, during starvation, in some severe systemic diseases

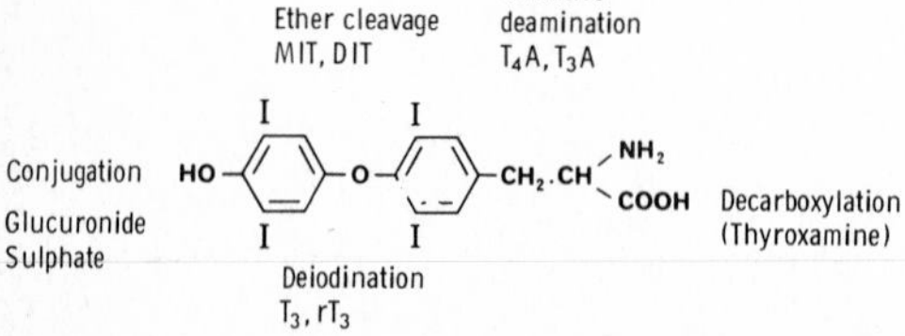

Figure 13.2. Major metabolic pathways of T4, including conjugation, ether cleavage, oxidative deamination, deiodination and decarboxylation. The products of each step are indicated, but thyroxamine has not been demonstrated with certainty in biological material.

and in hepatic disease, diversion of T4 metabolism takes place along this pathway so that the T3: reverse T3 ratio falls.

In the liver, conjugation of T4 and T3 (to glucuronic, sulphuric and some aminoacids) is known to occur and the conjugates are secreted into the gut via the bile, there to be degraded and reabsorbed by way of the enterohepatic cycle. Water-soluble conjugated hormones are also excreted into the urine, in association with small amounts of unconjugated non-protein-bound hormone (Burke and Eastman, 1974). Studies of renal handling of T4 and T3 suggest that some reabsorption of T4, but secretion of T3, takes place in the kidney; this organ also demonstrates a great capacity for deiodination of T4 to form T3. Deamination and decarboxylation of T4 and T3 may also be shown to occur – largely in the liver – and tetraiodothyroacetic acid (T4A or tetrac), triiodothyroacetic acid (T3A or triac), pyruvic and formic analogues have all been identified in man or experimental animals. Little is known about the relative rates or the metabolic significance of these alternate pathways of T4 and T3 metabolism, but circulating analogues and metabolites may possess substantial activity and may contribute materially to standard hormone assays.

13.1.6. Actions of thyroid hormones

Little definite is known about the mechanism of action of T4 or T3. Uncoupling of oxidative phosphorylation – long held to be the primary cause of the energy wastage of hyperthyroidism – is now thought to be a pharmacological rather than a physiological effect of thyroid hormones. Cytoplasmic ribosomal protein synthesis, perhaps mediated through an as yet unknown mitochondrial factor, has recently been demonstrated. Whether these effects are mediated by T3, T4 or both is still uncertain, but cytosol and nuclear receptors have been identified for T3 in most body tissues. The binding capacity for T3 appears to be greatest in the nuclei of those tissues which are most sensitive to the hormone: liver, kidney, heart and anterior pituitary gland. Tissues which respond poorly to thyroid hormones appear to have little capacity for binding T3. The subject of nuclear receptors and the initiation of thyroid hormone action is fully discussed by Oppenheimer et al. (1976).

13.1.7. Control of thyroid function

Thyroid gland function is controlled by a homoeostatic negative feed-back mechanism (Scheme 13.3) via hypothalamic thyrotrophin releasing factor (TRF) and anterior pituitary thyroid-stimulating hormone (TSH). TSH interacts with a specific thyroid cell membrane receptor to activate the adenyl cyclase system, with increase of cyclic AMP and release of thyroid hormones. These hormones are thought to cause formation of an intrapituitary protein capable of inhibiting TRF release and so achieving negative feed-back control. Several details are still obscure. Is feed-back exerted through the action of T4, T3 or both? Does it act directly on the pituitary gland or hypothalamus or both? Fairly sound evidence supports a role for T3 and an action directly on the anterior pituitary gland. Evidence of an action of T4 in feed-back control has not so far excluded the possibility of its prior conversion into T3.

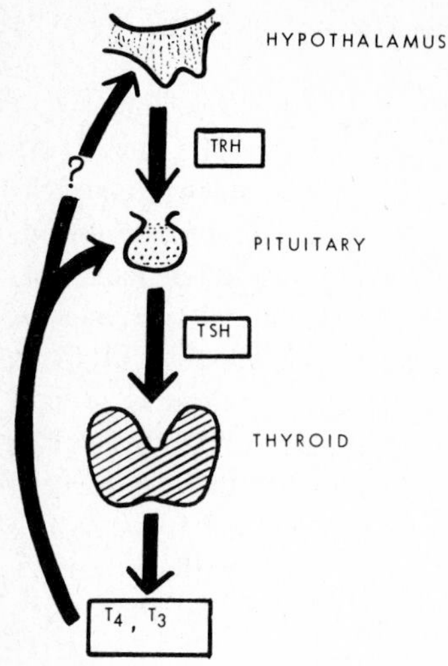

Scheme 13.3. Representation of thyroid control mechanisms with negative feed-back of thyroxine and/or triiodothyronine on the pituitary gland and possibly also on the hypothalamus.

The administration of synthetic TRH in man (section 13.3.7.1.) produces a rise in plasma TSH concentration and, unexpectedly, a similar increase in plasma prolactin concentration. In post-thyroidectomy hypothyroidism, hyperprolactinaemia is also found, which indicates responsiveness to high circulating TSH of endogenous, as well as exogenous, origin. These two actions of TRH on the pituitary gland may be divorced under experimental conditions, which raises intriguing questions about the nature and adaptability of cellular receptor sites or of the TRF molecule itself.

13.2. DISEASES OF THE THYROID GLAND

Thyroid diseases will be considered under the headings of enlargement (goitre), hyperfunction, and hypofunction.

13.2.1. Goitre

With the exception of thyroid cancer and hyperthyroidism, enlargement of the thyroid gland may be considered as a compensatory response to a decrease in the concentration of circulating thyroid hormone. This removes the inhibition of TSH secretion (Scheme 13.4) so that the thyroid gland is stimulated to hyperplasia in an attempt to compensate for the deficiency of circulating hormone. If this stimulation successfully enhances hormone production, as in the case of a partial enzyme block, the patient may be euthyroid at the expense of a goitre; if stimulation fails to effect a normal hormone output, goitrous hypothyrodism will result. In broad terms, deficient hormone production may result from (a) iodine lack, which may be absolute or relative; (b) enzyme defects of hor-

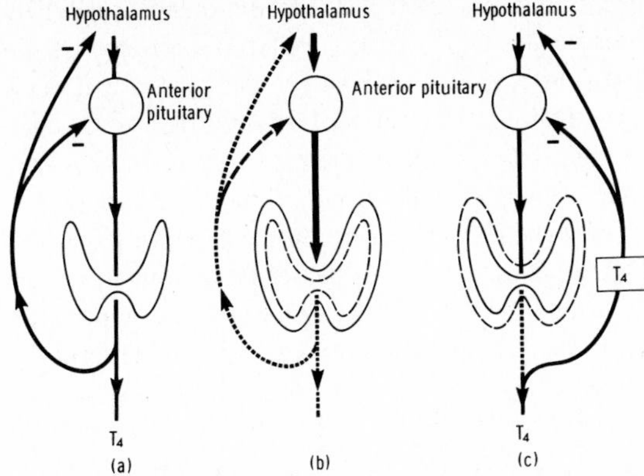

Scheme 13.4. a: representation of normal feed-back control. b: deficient thyroid hormone production removes inhibition of secretion of TSH which causes thyroid gland enlargement. c: replacement thyroxine therapy should inhibit TSH with regression of goitre.

mone synthesis, usually genetically determined; (c) antithyroid drugs of various types and modes of action; or (d) autoimmune or other varieties of thyroiditis.

Dietary iodine deficiency still exists in many parts of the world and is thought to be responsible for so-called endemic goitre. It has been estimated that about 200 million people suffer from this disorder. Programmes of iodine supplementation, including the ingenious use of injections of organic iodide-containing oily radiological contrast media (Hetzel, 1970), have done much to reduce if not eradicate the condition. The poorly documented thyroid enlargement of puberty, pregnancy, or the menopause is often attributed to a relative increase in demand for iodine but this must be regarded as speculative.

Many different enzyme defects affecting T4 synthesis have been described (Table 13.2), but absolute proof of most of these is lacking. A failure of iodide trapping may rarely occur, perhaps due to faulty cell membrane proteins, and may be overcome by a high intake of iodine; this raises the plasma iodide concentration and allows passive diffusion in sufficient quantity for adequate hormone synthesis. A failure to oxidize iodide to

TABLE 13.2.

POSTULATED DEFECTS IN SYNTHESIS OF T4 (OR T3)

Defective step	Postulated abnormality
Iodide trapping	Absence of carrier protein
"Organification"	Absence of peroxidase or deficient peroxidase activity
Iodotyrosyl coupling	Uncertain; possible deficiency of coupling enzyme but more likely unfavourable steric arrangement
Iodotyrosine deiodination	Absent or defective deiodinase
Thyroglobulin synthesis	Uncertain

iodine (peroxidase lack?) leads to deficient iodination of tyrosine ("non-organification"); several variants of this syndrome are recognized, one of which – Pendred's syndrome – is associated with nerve deafness, goitre (often nodular) and autosomal recessive inheritance. Iodothyronine formation may be impaired by failure of an enzyme responsible for coupling two tyrosine molecules but the existence of this enzyme is speculative and the disorder is more likely to result either from sparse iodination of the tyrosine residues of thyroglobulin or from some structural abnormality of the protein, leading to sterically unfavourable siting of iodotyrosines. Defective action of iodotyrosine deiodinases may lead to failure of intrathyroidal deiodination of mono- and di-iodotyrosine which are released by thyroglobulin proteolysis, and hence non-availability of their iodine residues for further hormone synthesis. This deficiency may also be overcome by dietary iodine supplementation. Finally, various types of defect in the synthesis of thyroglobulin have been proposed which may adversely influence the synthesis or release of hormone.

Antithyroid drugs may act at various levels. For example, perchlorate competitively inhibits iodide uptake, while thionamides (carbimazole, methimazole and thiouracil derivatives) interfere with organification. At least 1000 different substances are known to have goitrogenic action, almost always due to interference with the synthesis of thyroid hormones or by blocking the uptake of iodide by the gland. In autoimmune thyroiditis, gradual destruction of thyroid tissue is accompanied by compensatory hyperplasia of residual responsive parts of the gland. This, together with the accumulated cellular products of the autoimmune process, leads to increased gland size. In all the cases referred to above, decreased hormone synthesis or release results in low circulating concentrations of T4 and T3; increased TSH activity is thought to account for thyroid gland hyperplasia. It should be made clear that despite the soundness of the logic underlying this explanation of "compensatory" goitres, current techniques have generally failed to demonstrate the anticipated rise in plasma TSH level in the common varieties of simple or endemic goitre.

13.2.2. Hyperthyroidism

Hyperthyroidism has many causes (Table 13.3) only two of which are common. Graves's disease, or primary hyperthyroidism, results from diffuse hyperplastic enlargement of the gland and is currently attributed to the action of abnormal circulating thyroid-stimulating immunoglobulins (section 13.3.8.). Secondary hyperthyroidism, or Plummer's disease, is due to excess production of hormone by hyperactive thyroid nodules, either solitary or multiple. A single hyperactive or "hot" nodule may secrete enough hormone to suppress the activity of the rest of the thyroid gland, but insufficient to cause clinical or biochemical hyperthyroidism. In some cases of multinodular enlargement of the thyroid gland, hyperthyroidism is thought to be due to Graves's disease affecting the internodular tissue, not overactivity of the nodules themselves. Extremely rare causes of hyperthyroidism include abnormal TSH production by pituitary tumours, hydatidiform mole, choriocarcinoma and testicular tumours, or excessive production of thyroid hormone by functioning thyroid carcinoma or struma ovarii. "Jod Basedow" is the term used to describe hyperthyroidism in endemic goitrous areas after overenthusiastic iodide supplementation (Vidor et al., 1973), or even after administration of small doses of iodide given

TABLE 13.3.
CAUSES OF HYPERTHYROIDISM

Graves's disease (diffuse toxic goitre)

Toxic nodular goitre
  Multinodular (Plummer's disease)
  Uninodular (toxic adenoma)
  Nodular goitre with Graves's disease

Excess thyroid stimulating hormone
  Pituitary tumour
  Choriocarcinoma and hydatidiform mole
  Embryonal testicular carcinoma
  Other malignancy (?)

Extraneous thyroid hormone
  Exogenous: intentional factitious
    overenthusiastic therapy
    during T3 suppression test
    thyroid hormone induced
  Endogeneous: metastatic thyroid carcinoma
    struma ovarii

Jod-Basedow (exogenous iodide)

Transient, associated with thyroiditis
  Subacute
  Hashimoto's
  Irradiation (deep X-ray therapy or ^{131}I)
  TSH administration

Hypothalamic (?)

to block thyroid gland uptake during [^{131}I]-fibrinogen studies for the diagnosis of deep venous thrombosis.

In almost all types of hyperthyroidism, the high concentration of circulating hormone suppresses pituitary TSH secretion as well as its responsiveness to exogenous TRF. An exception to this rule is the variety due to thyrotrophin overproduction, e.g. by a pituitary tumour.

In the overwhelming majority of cases, the concentrations of both T4 and T3 in plasma are elevated. In a variable minority, hyperthyroidism is due to high concentrations of circulating T3, not T4, so-called T3-toxicosis (section 13.3.4.).

13.2.3. Hypothyroidism

This may result from failure of pituitary TSH stimulation or primary failure of the thyroid gland. The former is most commonly due to a tumour compressing the anterior pituitary gland (usually a chromophobe adenoma) or follows infarction of the gland after post-partum or other perinatal haemorrhage. In both cases other pituitary trophic hormones are usually deficient, e.g. gonadotrophins, corticotrophin or growth hormone, but isolated thyrotrophin deficiency may occur.

Primary hypothyroidism may result from idiopathic agenesis or atrophy of the gland, or from the other causes of deficient production of hormone as discussed above (section 13.2.1.). A common cause of primary hypothyroidism, with or without goitre, is autoimmune disease (usually Hashimoto's thyroiditis) or subacute thyroiditis leading to destruction of the gland. Most cases of hypothyroidism today are iatrogenic – after surgery or therapy with radioactive iodine. The prevalence after treatment with ^{131}I reaches 25% in the first year in some series, and 60% or more after prolonged follow-up (10 years or more); this prevalence may have been lessened by new techniques of administration of ^{131}I using smaller doses.

Distinction between primary and secondary hypothyroidism may clearly be based on measurement of plasma TSH, which should be absent in pituitary disease but abnormally high in primary thyroidal failure. In the latter, exaggerated and prolonged TSH response to TRF is the rule (section 13.7.1.).

13.3. THYROID FUNCTION TESTS

13.3.1. The background to current tests

It is interesting to note that thyroid function tests barely existed before World War II. Measurement of basal metabolic rate (BMR), though widely performed, was crude, imprecise, technically demanding – if true basal rates were to be recorded – and laborious. Attempts to measure thyroid hormones in blood proved unsuccessful until the description of the iodide-catalyzed reduction of Ce^{4+} by arsenite (Sandell and Kolthoff, 1937) which paved the way for introduction of the assay of serum protein-bound iodine (PBI) and its development and fuller application in the post-war years (Barker et al., 1951; Zak et al., 1952). At about the same time, as a spin-off of wartime atomic bomb research, came the identification of new radioactive isotopes with characteristics which would allow their exploitation in biological research. One of the first and most abundant was ^{131}I, and its applicability to the study of thyroid gland function was rapidly appreciated. During the years up to about 1965, thyroid function was usually tested "dynamically" with ^{131}I or other radioactive isotopes of iodine, and "statically" by assaying serum PBI. Neither test was completely satisfactory. The most popular of the radioactive iodine tests throughout this period determined thyroidal uptake at various times after the oral administration of ^{131}I. But many variants were described which measured blood or urine radioactivity or "immediate" thyroid uptake after intravenous administration of the isotope. All in vivo tests have proved imprecise, with large overlap between normal and abnormal reference ranges; idiosyncrasies of technique generally preclude inter-laboratory comparisons; and many drugs, iodine-containing or not, interfere with valid interpretation.

In this Chapter, which is concerned primarily with the clinical chemistry aspects of thyroid disease, emphasis will be placed on in vitro tests; only brief mention will be made of in vivo tests that require administration of radioactive iodine (or technetium) to the patient. There are several reasons why in vitro tests of thyroid function are today preferred to in vivo. First, the administration of a radioactive isotope to the patient is avoided; while the use of short-lived isotopes such as ^{132}I or ^{99m}Tc partially overcomes this objection, there is some resistance even to their use in pregnancy or in lactating mothers and young infants or children. In vitro tests also mean that a blood specimen – instead of the patient – can be sent to the laboratory. Most in vivo tests require repeated visits for timed determinations of thyroid uptake or blood radioactivity after administration of the isotope. Immediate uptake studies which can be performed at a single visit provide rapid results, but lack discrimination and are of little use in the diagnosis of suspect hypothyroidism. Total or partial automation of in vitro tests has greatly reduced technician involvement and allows rapid and precise assay of large numbers of samples, so leading to better diagnostic criteria. It is hardly surprising that the pendulum has swung so strongly away from in vivo tests in recent years.

Serum PBI measurement, however, has also had its problems: manual methods of ashing to destroy thyroid hormone-binding proteins and liberate iodine are tedious and unreliable; small amounts of contaminating iodine of exogenous or endogenous origin readily cause artefactual increases in the final colorimetric assay (section 13.3.2.). Automation of the PBI method reduced these difficulties and offered better precision, but did not overcome contamination problems. The introduction of a specific T4 assay heralded the swing away from in vivo tests to in vitro, although the early method described by Ekins (1960) based on electrophoresis was too elaborate for routine use. The competitive protein-binding assay of Murphy and her colleagues (1964, 1965) provided a simple approach and has largely resulted in the placing of thyroid function tests on a sounder and more scientific footing. Despite its drawbacks, PBI assay is still used by laboratories in some parts of the world and discussion of its usefulness will therefore be included in the following section.

Before considering thyroid function tests in detail, it is as well to consider the nature and quality of the iodinated comounds in serum; what it is we want to measure; and to what extent specificity is achieved. Table 13.4 lists the most common iodinated com-

TABLE 13.4.

IODINE IN SERUM

		Per decilitre	Per litre
Inorganic iodide		200–1000 ng	
Iodothyronines:	T4	4–11 μg	50–140 nmol
	T3	65–200 ng	1–3 nmol
	Reverse T3	~40 ng	~0.6 nmol
Iodotyrosines	mono(=MIT)	Uncertain	
	di(=DIT)	150 ng	3.5 nmol
Iodinated proteins:			
Thyroglobulin		510 ng	5.1 μg
Iodoalbumin		Uncertain	
Hormone metabolites:			
Tetrac		100–800 ng	1.3–11 nmol
Triac		<10 ng	<0.16 nmol
Exogenous iodocompounds			

pounds found in serum. Thyroxine forms the most prominent iodinated compound but tetrac, triac, T3 and reverse T3 are present in substantial quantities. PBI assay measures any iodine-containing material that is associated with protein and includes a small amount of non-protein-bound iodine that may be trapped in the plasma. Usually not less than 90% of PBI represents T4. Competitive protein-binding assays for T4 measure those compounds that will displace radioactive T4 from TBG, and radioimmunoassay those that compete for antibody. In both cases, the preponderance of T4 in serum and its preferential binding by TBG or by a specific antibody, minimize the contributions of other compounds.

13.3.2. Serum PBI

There is little point in reviewing earlier methods of measuring PBI since manual techniques have been almost entirely superseded by use of the AutoAnalyzer method and, as mentioned above, PBI itself is currently being replaced by more specific assays for T4.

The main advantage of PBI assay is that it is at present the best automated in vitro test of thyroid function, and many hundreds of specimens per week can be run cheaply and with relative ease in a central laboratory. The main disadvantage is its lack of specificity. Iodine in all its forms may influence the test and Acland (1971), in his excellent review of PBI assays, has appended a long list of those compounds most likely to interfere. Thus, radiographic contrast media may cause elevation of serum PBI for up to 30 years after their use. Furthermore, in the automated system, falsely high readings are likely to be found in the samples succeeding an iodine-contaminated specimen; this introduces a problem of considerable dimension as 10 to 20% of specimens sent for PBI assay may be subject to such carry-over. To circumvent this difficulty, several techniques have been devised to extract thyroxine from plasma by use of an ion-exchange resin or by an organic solvent, such as butanol, before the assay of iodine by one of the standard methods.

Thyroxine constitutes the major part of serum PBI and its concentration, expressed as T4 iodine, is normally only 5 to 10 μg/litre less than that of PBI. In general, serum PBI concentration faithfully reflects changes in that of serum T4 due to a physiological or pathological cause. In some circumstances, especially in the higher ranges of PBI, the discrepancy between PBI and T4 is inordinately large, due possibly to the presence in serum of non-thyroxine protein-bound iodine compounds. In some genetic disorders of thyroid gland metabolism, thyroglobulin leaks into the serum and high PBI values may be recorded, with normal or low T4 concentrations; the same discrepancy may be found in some forms of thyroiditis.

13.3.3. Serum T4

Ekins (1960) first pointed out that the extent of displacement of radioactive T4 from serum binding proteins was directly related to the total amount of T4 in the system; he applied this concept to the direct assay of serum T4 by "saturation analysis". A simpler procedure described as a "competitive protein binding" assay was introduced by

Murphy and her colleagues (1964, 1965). The principle is identical to that underlying radioimmunoassay:

$$T4^* + T4 + TBP \leftrightharpoons (T4^* \text{ bound to TBP}) + (T4 \text{ bound to TBP})$$

where $T4^*$ = radioactive T4 tracer; T4 = total T4;

TBP = T4-binding proteins

The technique requires the initial extraction of thyroid hormones from serum to remove the competition of their own binding proteins. This may be achieved with organic solvents, of which acid ethanol (95%) or methanol is most popular, or by use of ion exchange or gel filtration. Standardized amounts of TBP (or TBG) are added, after which protein-bound and non-protein-bound hormone are separated and determined to give the bound:free ratio. Addition of radioactive tracer T4 to the serum initially allows correction for losses during the extraction procedure, as well as determination of the bound: free ratio. Many variants have been described, differing mainly in the methods of extraction, absorption or separation, and several "kits" are commercially available. In general, these techniques are simple and quick, but reproducibility is poor without meticulous attention to detail, particularly in the timing and conditions of the final separation step. Coefficients of variation for replicability are seldom better than 10% and may be far worse (Spierto et al., 1974). The commercially available kits are generally expensive, and independent purchase of materials can lead to substantial savings in laboratories that perform many such tests.

Mean values for T4 vary from laboratory to laboratory, but a normal range of 40 to 110 ng/litre of serum (50 to 140 nmol/litre) usually applies. Occasionally, results are expressed in terms of T4-iodine (to bring them into line with PBI), in which case the normal range is about 35 to 80 ng/litre. The use of SI units to express PBI as nmol of iodine and T4 in terms of its actual molecular mass may lead to confusion; in view of the phasing out of PBI, it is suggested that use of the term "T4-iodine" should now be avoided.

Following the development of a radioimmunoassay for T3 (section 13.3.4.), most laboratories have now introduced a similar assay for T4. This has many advantages – larger numbers of specimens may be processed in a single batch; improved replication and specificity are achieved; extraction steps may be obviated and the assay is cheaper. But most techniques still have problems – high titre antibodies against T4 seem harder to raise than those against T3; non-specific protein-binding needs to be blocked by substances such as 8-anilinonaphthalene sulphonic acid or salicylate. The final separation of bound from free antigen (T4) remains a critically important step. The use of second antibody (anti-IgG) is expensive but efficient; alternative agents such as dextran-coated charcoal, ammonium sulphate or polyethylene glycol have been used. In general, good correlation is found between T4 as assayed by competitive protein binding and by radioimmunoassay techniques, and the latter is now generally adopted. Combined radioimmunoassay of T3 and T4 may be possible on the same sample by using alternate isotopes of radioactive iodine and appropriate specific antisera.

13.3.4. Serum T3

T3 was first identified in human plasma by Gross and Pitt-Rivers (1952). Its metabolic potency was shown to be high but its physiological significance was largely overlooked, primarily because of its low concentration in plasma (about 1/70th that of T4), but also because of the difficulties inherent in its accurate measurement. Interest in T3 was rekindled by reports of a new chemical assay (Naumann et al., 1967; Sterling et al., 1969), and the emergence of kinetic data which indicated that, despite its low concentration, T3 could account for 50 to 80% of total thyroid hormone metabolic activity. Relatively specific antisera were raised against polylysine-T3 (Brown et al., 1970) and later against T3-albumin conjugates (Gharib et al., 1971), so that the radioimmunoassay for T3 has now become an almost routine laboratory procedure. Many variants of the radioimmunoassay for T3 now exist (Black et al., 1975). These differ from one another in several respects: (i) some systems still require preliminary extraction using either organic solvents or resin or gel absorbents, but the majority of assays are now performed on unextracted serum; (ii) the blocking of competitive binding by serum proteins in the system needs to be achieved, by partial heat denaturation or by using substances such as 8-anilinonaphthalene sulphonic acid, tetrachlorothyronine, salicylate, merthiolate or phenytoin; (iii) the duration of incubation may vary from 40 minutes to several days, and the temperature at which this is carried out from 4 to 60°C; (iv) final separation of antibody-bound and "free" hormone is carried out by double antibody techniques, or with non-specific protein precipitants such as dextran-charcoal, ammonium sulphate or polyethylene glycol. The main technical problems now appear to have been overcome and a reference range has been agreed by most laboratories (650 to 2000 ng/litre; or 1.0 to 3.0 nmol/litre). Cross-reactions with T4 and other biologically occurring iodo-aminoacids do not significantly affect the results in most assays. High values (2 to 10 μg/litre) are almost always found in hyperthyroidism, and low values in hypothyroidism.

The syndrome of T3-toxicosis (hyperthyroidism due to a high concentration of circulating T3, with normal concentration of T4) has now been recognized and has led to the successful identification of many cases of hyperthyroidism that might otherwise have been missed. The salient features of this syndrome are outlined in Table 13.5; reports from New York suggest that it accounts for about 4% of all cases of hyperthyroidism; from Chile about 12.5% (Hollander et al., 1972); and from a personal impression, perhaps 1–2% of cases in England. Selection of case material makes it difficult to provide reliable prevalence figures but geographical variation is likely, because of the influence of dietary intake of iodine.

Other instances of divergence of T4 and T3 values are beginning to emerge. After treatment of hyperthyroidism with radioactive iodine or antithyroid drugs, or by means of surgery, patients may pass through a phase of "compensated hypothyroidism", in which serum T4 concentration is low, that of serum T3 high or normal, and that of serum TSH is high. These patients are clinically euthyroid, presumably because they have normal or high serum T3 concentrations. As yet, their natural history has not become clear; some might progress to hypothyroidism and some might revert to hyperthyroidism, but a majority seems to remain for years without alteration of clinical or biochemical status. A similar set of laboratory data (low T4, high T3, high TSH concentrations) may be

TABLE 13.5.

CHARACTERISTICS OF THE SYNDROME OF T3-TOXICOSIS – HYPERTHYROIDISM WITH NORMAL SERUM T4 BUT ELEVATED SERUM T3 CONCENTRATION

Clinical hyperthyroidisn
Normal serum PBI, total T4, free T4
Normal T4-binding proteins
Normal or raised thyroid uptake not suppressible by T3
TRF produces no rise in TSH secretion
Raised serum total or free T3
Occurrence higher in incipient or early hyperthyroidism; in recurrent hyperthyroidism; in association with toxic thyroid nodules; and in areas of relatively low iodine intake

---

found in some cases of endemic goitre and in Pendred's syndrome (section 13.2.1.).

A more obvious instance of discrepant T3 and T4 values is found in patients being treated with T3, in whom endogenous T4 secretion is suppressed; such individuals have high serum T3 concentrations, but low or immeasurable serum T4 or PBI. By contrast, if T4 replacement therapy is being given, plasma T4 and T3 concentrations are normal – the latter resulting from peripheral conversion of T4 into T3.

A new and highly significant group of conditions is also being identified in which there is probably failure of peripheral mono-deiodination of T4 to T3 (Table 13.6). In the elderly, serum T3 concentrations tend to fall (Rubenstein et al., 1973) but T4 levels are maintained. In stressed individuals, after surgery, myocardial infarction or cerebrovascular accident, the ratio of serum T3:T4 concentrations is likewise reduced. This change cannot easily be related to the simultaneous reduction in concentration of prealbumin which is found under the same conditions, and it appears to be due to independent decrease in deiodination of T4. In liver disease and in the treatment of obesity by starvation, a similar change in the T3:T4 ratio is found. In almost all cases, the concentration of serum reverse T3 is shown to increase, suggesting that mono-deiodination of T4 has been diverted along the pathway that produces this inert metabolite (section 13.1.5.) in preference to the highly active T3. It is interesting to speculate about the importance of such changes. If T3 is the predominant metabolic hormone, is hypothyroidism present when the serum T3:T4 ratio falls? Clinically this would not appear to be the case, but the

TABLE 13.6.

CONDITIONS ASSOCIATED PROBABLE DECREASED MONO-DEIODINATION OF T4 TO FORM 3,3′,5-T3

Advancing age, probably explained by associated illness
Acute stress (surgery, myocardial infarction)
Liver disease
Starvation
Propyl- or methylthiouracil treatment
Chronic illness
Glucocorticoid administration

---

abnormalities are usually short-lived and might lead to overt hypothyroidism if they were prolonged. Another important consequence is that the diagnosis might be wrong if it were based substantially on the assay of serum T3; substitution therapy should not be instituted without further confirmation of the diagnosis.

Finally, the possible existence of "T4-toxicosis" is emerging. If a thyrotoxic patient undergoes stress or suffers any of the other causes of reduced serum T3, the concentration of this hormone may decrease into the normal range while that of T4 remains high. Some examples of this combination of test results are beginning to appear.

13.3.5. Free T4 and free T3

13.3.5.1. Direct assays

It is generally accepted that the non-protein-bound or free moieties of the thyroid hormones are the biologically important compounds rather than the total hormones. It is clear that the total concentration of each will be influenced by the concentrations of the appropriate specific binding proteins in serum, and that the free fractions will be dependent upon the interaction of both hormones. Direct measurement of the concentrations of thyroid hormone binding proteins may be made in some cases by radioimmunoassay (for TBG) or by immunoelectrophoresis (for TBG and TBPA), but these techniques are not widely available. The relative concentrations of the different binding proteins and their binding affinities may significantly affect the fractions of T4 and T3 that are not protein-bound.

Several methods have been proposed for direct measurement of the concentrations of free hormones. Sterling and Brenner (1966) added a radioactive tracer of T4 ($T4^*$) to serum and measured the proportion of dialysable $T4^*$ after correction for contamination by radioactive iodide. In this way, values of 0.03 to 0.04% for dialysable T4 have been found in serum from normal subjects, with somewhat higher percentages in hyperthyroidism, and lower in hypothyroidism. This method is cumbersome, tedious, technically demanding and imprecise. Several variants have been described that make use of gel filtration columns to absorb free T4; these are simpler and quicker, but the precision is still poor. Similar dialysis and column techniques may also be applied to the direct measurement of free T3, which normally comprises about 0.2 to 0.5% of the total concentration of T3.

It must be stressed that all such methods give the proportion of free hormone, and that the absolute amounts must be calculated from the measured total concentrations. However, radioimmunoassay has been applied to the dialysable fractions of T3 and T4 from serum; this overcomes many of the technical difficulties of the foregoing assays and provides a direct answer in terms of actual concentrations of free hormones.

The description of a method for measuring T4 and T3 in urine (Chan and Landon, 1972) raised hopes that these estimations might reflect the concentration of the free hormones in serum. However, variations in renal clearance, with possible reabsorption of T4 and secretion of T3, deiodination of T4 and probably also T3 during passage through the kidney, and the effects of small amounts of proteinuria, have all militated against the use of urinary hormone measurements in this way, so that the test is not likely to gain support.

13.3.5.2. Indirect assays

By the Law of Mass Action, equilibrium will be established between T4 and thyroxine binding proteins in serum:

$$T4 + TBP \rightleftharpoons T4 \cdot TBP$$

where T4 represents total T4, TBP represents total T4 binding protein, and T4 · TBP represents T4 bound to protein. Hence, in terms of the concentrations:

$$\frac{[T4 \cdot TBP]}{[T4]\,[TBP]} = K \text{ , a constant ,}$$

where [T4] represents non-protein-bound or free T4, and [TBP] the unoccupied T4 binding sites on TBP.

Therefore

$$[T4] = \frac{K \times [T4 \cdot TBP]}{[TBP]} .$$

This relationship was recognized by Osorio et al. (1962) and exploited by Clark and Horn (1965) who derived a "free thyroxine index" of thyroid function. This developed out of an observation of Hamolsky et al. (1957) that when radioactive T3 (i.e. T3*) was added to whole blood, it partitioned between plasma and erythrocytes; the amount on the red cells was determined by the extent of saturation of plasma TBP. In hyperthyroidism, T4 occupied more of these binding sites, so that more T3* was taken up by the red cells; in hypothyroidism, decreased red cell uptake of T3* reflected a larger number of unsaturated TBP sites. It was soon realized that the erythrocytes acted simply as secondary binding sites for T3*; hence inert resin particles, strips or sponge were substituted in a test that has become known as the "T3 resin uptake". In this test, T3* and resin are added to patients' serum and the T3* taken up by the resin is measured and compared to that found with a control pool of normal serum (expressed as 100%). As an independent and isolated test, T3 resin uptake is not acceptable, since it correlates poorly with the concentration of T4 in serum and with the clinical status of the patient, largely because of the variability of the concentration of TBG in health and in disease. However, its combination with serum PBI or T4 assay to permit derivation of a "free thyroxine index" provides excellent correlation with thyroid status and overcomes the complicating effect of variable concentration of TBP on the total hormone levels (Figure 13.1). A radioimmunoassay for circulating TBG is now available but has not yet been fully evaluated. Direct measurement of TBG concentration by immunoelectrophoresis has been reported, and determination of a T4:TBG ratio has some advantages over the usual free thyroxine index (Burr et al., 1977). It is likely that T3 uptake tests will soon be superseded by direct assays of the concentration of circulating TBG. In Clark and Horn's original description, the index was calculated from the product of serum PBI concentration, as a measure of [T4 · TBP], and T3 resin uptake, as an index of [TBP]. Thus:

Free thyroxine index = serum PBI (μg/dl) × T3 resin uptake (% of normal control serum)

Confusion has recently arisen because variants of the T3 resin uptake test have been described in which materials other than resin are used, and the proportion of T3* remaining in the serum is measured, rather than that bound to the added substrate. In such tests, the use of Clark and Horn's formula is obviously incorrect, as the amount of T3* in serum correlates inversely with that taken up by the resin. It is acceptable, even if not entirely valid scientifically, to use an inverted formula:

$$\text{“Free thyroxine index”} = \frac{\text{Serum PBI or T4}(\mu\text{g/dl})}{\text{T3 uptake}(\%\text{ of normal control serum})}$$

but care must be taken in the use of such a formula to identify the type of T3 uptake test used. Given this information, it is possible to make allowances for alterations of concentration of TBG, e.g. in pregnant women or those on oral contraceptive pills. In such subjects, a raised concentration of serum PBI would be associated with an increased number of unoccupied binding sites on TBP, for which correction would be made by the T3 uptake test in deriving the free T4 index. It should be emphasized that the free thyroxine index is not a direct estimate of free T4 although, by relating the hormone and TBP concentrations, a factor is derived that correlates closely with it.

It is thus apparent that two separate tests may be needed to provide an accurate reflection of the status of circulating free thyroxine. Recently, another variant has been introduced which incorporates into a single test a measure of the T4 and TBP content of the patient's serum without providing a direct estimate of either; this is the "effective thyroxine ratio" (Mincey et al., 1971). In this test, an ethanolic extract of serum which contains T4 is added to a prepared reaction mixture so as to displace bound radioactive tracer, T4*; a small quantity of patient's serum is now added so as to effect correction for the endogenous TBP concentration, and a resin strip is then introduced to which the non-bound T4* is adsorbed. A comparison is made between the T4* which is bound by the resin, by the patient's serum and by a control serum. This test measures neither T4 nor TBP directly, but the final ratio which is obtained accurately reflects the free thyroxine index as derived from the use of the two separate tests previously described. This test, or a still newer variant, is now used in many laboratories as a single screening test of thyroid function. It appears to offer diagnostic discrimination at least as good as that of the combination of two separate tests. It is not cheap, requires careful performance and has the intrinsic disadvantage that it fails to tell the investigator anything about total circulating T4 or its binding protein. Built into the determination of free thyroxine index is the additional security which is provided by two cross-checking tests. If both T4 and T3 uptake indicate the same type of functional thyroid abnormality, the investigator may feel reassured; a discrepancy between the two might indicate an abnormality of binding proteins but may also draw attention to the possibility of technical error. This safeguard does not exist with the effective thyroxine ratio. Nevertheless, it offers a useful tool to the smaller laboratory which wishes to provide a reasonable diagnostic service without too deep an involvement in the investigation of thyroid function.

Tests of this sort, that reflect the concentration of free T4, are of no diagnostic use in T3-toxicosis, as both serum PBI or T4 concentration and the T3 uptake test will be normal; nor will they help in the other disorders mentioned above in which the T3:T4 ratio is disturbed. Apart from these exceptions, some combined measure of T4 concentration and T3 uptake provides the basic diagnostic test in most thyroid laboratories.

13.3.6. Serum TSH

The biochemical function of the thyroid gland is primarily controlled by pituitary secretion of TSH. TSH is a glycoprotein, molecular mass 28,000, consisting of two subunits – designated α and β. A similar, if not identical, α-subunit is common to other two-chain glycoprotein trophic hormones – luteinizing hormone (LH), follicle-stimulating hormone (FSH) and chorionic gonadotrophin (HCG). The β-chain appears to be unique to each glycoprotein and confers specificity of action. If pituitary gland function is impaired, the secretion of TSH diminishes and hypothyroidism ensues (secondary hypothyroidism). If failure of the thyroid gland is a primary event, e.g. due to thyroiditis or after surgery or radioactive iodine therapy, then the pituitary secretion of TSH would be expected to be enhanced. Measurement of circulating TSH concentration should therefore effectively distinguish between these two forms of thyroid failure, and in practice this does generally obtain.

13.3.6.1. Bioassay

Many techniques for the bioassay of TSH have been described, testing the response of different physiological functions of the thyroid gland – uptake and discharge of radioactive iodine, increase in gland weight, histological evidence of increase in cell height or colloid droplet formation, etc. The most widely exploited technique is usually known as the McKenzie test after that author's adaptation (1958) of a method previously applied to guinea-pigs by Adams and Purves (1956). Radioactive iodine is administered to mice whose thyroid glands have been made iodine-avid by previous exposure to iodine-deficient diets. The radioactive iodine is thus concentrated in the thyroid gland and thyroxine is then given to suppress the spontaneous discharge of hormone. This suppressive action of thyroxine can be overcome by injection of TSH. The amount of radioactivity released from the thyroid gland into the blood stream of the mouse is related to the dose of TSH. By use of appropriate standards, a bioassay for human serum TSH can be developed. Using this method, it has been possible to measure high concentrations of TSH in subjects with primary hypothyroidism. Unfortunately the relative insensitivity of the test precludes its use to detect values below the normal range, and its complexity and cumbersome nature has prevented its adoption as a routine technique. It continues to offer a useful biological confirmation of TSH activity, as measured by chemical means such as radioimmunoassay.

13.3.6.2. Radioimmunoassay

The development of a radioimmunoassay for serum TSH has greatly changed the approach to the diagnosis of thyroid disease. Not only does the technique offer good sensitivity and specificity, but partial automation allows the processing of large sample batches. This has facilitated the introduction of the thyrotrophin releasing factor stimulation test (section 13.3.7.1.) and has allowed widespread screening of patients, e.g. of infants for the early diagnosis of cretinism. Specific antisera may be developed against α- and β-subunits, as well as the whole TSH molecule, but there seems to be little or no advantage in measuring the concentrations of circulating subunits for diagnostic purposes. Although radioimmunoassay is far more sensitive than bioassay, it has still not proved possible to define precisely the lower limit of the normal range, which in most laboratories lies between 0 and 4 munits/litre of serum; thus serum TSH is undetectable by radioimmunoassay in about 20% of normal people. Lowest values are reported from laboratories that set up standard curves using TSH-free human serum obtained from severe cases of hypopituitarism, or thyrotoxic or T3-treated subjects. In hyperthyroidism, low TSH values are found, except in rare cases caused by endogenous hypersecretion of TSH; in hypothyroidism serum TSH is raised, to figures above 20 munits/litre, and exceeding 500 munits/litre in severe or long-standing cases, especially cretinism. However, moderately high TSH concentrations do not necessarily indicate hypothyroidism; they may be found in euthyroid subjects after treatment of hyperthyroidism and in apparently euthyroid subjects with autoimmune thyroiditis. Whether these subjects have incipient or subclinical hypothyroidism is debatable. In simple goitre without hypothyroidism, the predicted rise in serum TSH is not found, although large series may show a slight statistical increase over non-goitrous controls, but still remaining within the reference range.

13.3.6.3. Histochemical assay

An ingenious new system has been developed by Bitensky et al. (1974), who studied the rate of appearance of free thyroidal lysosomal enzymes in follicular cells. Leucyl-β-naphthylamide, a substrate for the lysosomal enzyme naphthylamidase, is released under TSH stimulation and may be detected by differential staining methods which are quantified by microdensitometry. This method is exquisitely sensitive, and capable of detecting as little as 10^{-5} μunits/ml of TSH. Limited studies so far performed indicate that the response curves parallel those obtained by other means of assaying TSH, and a high degree of specificity is likely. In this system, thyroidal lysosomal enzymes are also released by thyroid stimulating immunoglobulins (TSI; section 13.3.8.), but a slower time course of action is described. Despite its cumbersome nature, which limits assays to one or two per day at present, much is likely to be learned from the application of this technique because of its great sensitivity and ability to distinguish the effects of TSH and TSI.

13.3.7. Some dynamic tests of thyroid function

13.3.7.1. TRF stimulation (Hall, 1972)

The availability of synthetic TRF – a tripeptide, pyroglutamyl-histidylproline amide – has led to its application as a diagnostic tool in thyroid disease. Within a few minutes of intravenous injection, it stimulates the release of TSH from the anterior pituitary gland so that there is an increase in the serum TSH concentration, which reaches a peak value within 15 to 30 minutes and slowly returns to pre-test values within a few hours. A normal range of response has been established, which is proportional to the dose used (up to a maximum response with 500 μg) and deviations from the normal have been delineated. In hyperthyroidism, there is a lack of TSH response; in hypothyroidism there is a prolonged and exaggerated response (Figure 13.3). Pituitary failure of TSH secretion may also be demonstrated by lack of response to TRF in subjects who are not hyperthyroid; in hypothalamic disease, a delayed response is often found in which serum TSH concentration continues to rise for 60 minutes after injection. As hyper- or hypothyroidism is brought under control by appropriate therapy, the response to injection of TRH returns

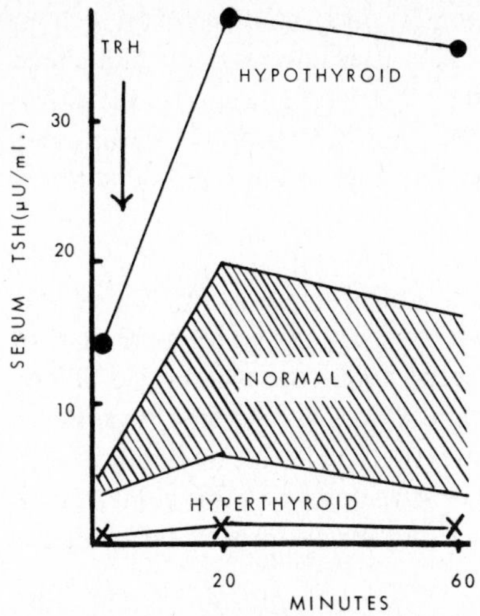

Figure 13.3. Representation of serum TSH responses to injected TRH in normal subjects (hatched area) and in hypothyroid and hyperthyroid patients.

to the normal range, and it has been suggested that the test might be used to monitor adequacy of treatment. A sex difference in response to TRF has been claimed by some workers, with greater response in women and in oestrogen-treated men; diminished response has been reported in elderly men, but not in elderly women.

Lack of response to TRH cannot be taken as absolute proof of hyperthyroidism because it may be found in some euthyroid patients with "hot" nodules or adenomas of the thyroid gland; in patients with treated Graves's disease in remission; in euthyroid exophthalmic Graves's disease; as well as in hypopituitarism as mentioned above. The demonstration or lack of response to TRF may be viewed in a negative but no less significant way – a definite response effectively rules out existing hyperthyroidism, and a lack of response excludes primary hypothyroidism. The initial enthusiasm for this test has diminished slightly, but it still has an important role to play in the diagnosis of difficult or borderline cases, especially those with suspect hypothyroidism and marginally raised TSH concentrations. In normal subjects, TRF causes release of both pituitary TSH and prolactin, but not growth hormone, FSH or corticotrophin. In hypothyroidism, exaggerated prolactin responses as well as TSH may be found. In some acromegalic patients and in some patients with chronic renal failure, a release of growth hormone has followed the administration of TRF.

It is interesting that raised concentrations of growth hormone in some acromegalic subjects impair the TSH response to TRF.

In the standard test, 200 μg of TRF is injected intravenously, but some authors have preferred to use 500 μg; serum TSH is measured in samples taken at zero time, and at 20 and 60 minutes. A response to oral TRF has been demonstrated, but a dose of 20 mg is needed for consistent response in a normal subject. The test has been used to fulfil a dual purpose by measuring both the TSH response and the slightly later consequential rise in serum T3 or T4 concentrations (Shenkman et al., 1972), thus simultaneously demonstrating pituitary and thyroidal responsiveness. Side-effects after intravenous TRF include mild nausea, a feeling of flushing, dizziness, a peculiar taste and a desire to micturate; these effects are mild, transient and may be lessened by slow injection. No serious toxicity has been reported, but effects on platelet aggregation have recently been described.

13.3.7.2. TSH stimulation

Difficulty occasionally arises in determining whether thyroidal failure is primary or secondary. In such cases, TSH may be given by intramuscular injection and response may be determined by measuring thyroidal uptake of radioactive iodine or secretion of T3 or T4. A definite response rules out primary thyroid failure; lack of response suggests its presence, although several such injections may be necessary if long-standing hypopituitarism has been present or if a patient has been given suppressive doses of a thyroid hormone for a long time. The interpretation of the response has not always proved easy and the test has largely been superseded.

13.3.7.3. T3 and T4 suppression tests

Greer and Smith (1954) suggested that thyroid hormone might be given to subjects as a test of thyroid suppressibility. In this test, thyroidal uptake of radioactive iodine was measured, and thyroid extract was then administered for 1 to 2 weeks in a dosage (180 mg/day; occasionally up to 540 mg/day) sufficient to suppress pituitary secretion of TSH in normal subjects. A repeat thyroid uptake study was then carried out to determine the extent of suppression, if any. In hyperthyroidism, suppression was found not to occur, as the gland is not subject to stimulation by TSH. This test has proved useful in distinguishing the high-uptake goitres of, for instance, iodine deficiency, from those of hyperthyroidism.

This suppression test was modified by Werner and Spooner (1955) who proposed the use of T3 instead of T4. In this variant, 120 μg of T3 in divided doses is usually given daily for 7 to 10 days. This was widely used as a test of hyperthyroidism before the advent of the TRH test, unresponsiveness to which has now been shown to correlate closely with T3 non-suppressibility. There are very few exceptions to this correlation, a rare example being hyperthyroidism due to a hyperfunctioning pituitary adenoma, in which TRF may fail to produce a rise in serum TSH, yet T3 suppression may be obtained. A few patients with possible co-existing Graves's disease and autoimmune thyroiditis have shown failure to T3-suppression, and yet a high basal level of TSH with an exaggerated response to TRH.

13.3.8. Long-acting thyroid-stimulator and thyroid-stimulating immunoglobulins

Adams (1958) reported the presence of an abnormal thyroid-stimulating substance in the sera of some patients with hyperthyroidism. This material stimulated prepared mouse thyroid glands to secrete radioactive iodine in a TSH-like response; it differed from TSH in its time course of action, with a maximum response being observed later than that produced by TSH. This unusual substance was given the name "long-acting thyroid-stimulator" (LATS) and it was soon shown definitely not to be TSH, or a related molecule, but to belong to the class of immunoglobulins, and was probably an antibody. For practical purposes, LATS has since been demonstrated only in those who are actively hyperthyroid at the time of testing or have previously been so, it has therefore seemed reasonable to attribute the functional hyperthyroid state to stimulation by LATS. A major and fundamental argument against a causative role for LATS in the pathogenesis of Graves's disease was the failure to demonstrate it in fully half of such subjects, so that many authorities dismissed it as a significant factor. The controversy was finally resolved by the further demonstration by Adams and Kennedy (1967) that another "blocking" material, which was called "LATS-protector", could be demonstrated in hyperthyroidism. By using a thyroid cell plasma membrane receptor assay, Hall and his colleagues (see Hall et al., 1975) have been able to demonstrate the presence of this LATS-protector in almost all patients with Graves's disease *. The discrepancy between its occurrence and that of LATS itself was classified by the finding that LATS-protector reacts specifically with human thyroid tissue, but not with mouse glands which form the basis of the assay for LATS. It has therefore been proposed that the terms LATS and LATS-protector should be abandoned, in favour of the more specific term "thyroid-stimulating immunoglobulins" (TSI; section 13.3.6.3.). In the receptor assay, almost all patients with untreated Graves's disease were shown to have detectable TSI, although more recent studies suggest that a significant proportion (perhaps 40%) of patients with Graves's disease may not exhibit circulating TSI.

Although it has not been finally demonstrated, it seems likely that these immunoglobulins are antibodies to the TSH receptor site on thyroid cell membranes, so that the mystery of the causation of Graves's disease seems a large step nearer solution. From a practical point of view, the receptor assay is not difficult and should provide a useful contribution to our understanding of thyroid disease. Its value as a diagnostic tool needs to be fully assessed.

13.3.9. Antibody tests

The demonstration of circulating antibodies to thyroglobulin (Roitt et al., 1956) was one of the key observations which led to the development of modern concepts of autoimmunity; in particular, to the recognition of Hashimoto's thyroiditis as a common autoimmune disorder which often presents as primary hypothyroidism or simply as a cause of goitre. It is now accepted that autoantibodies might arise to several thyroid components – thyroglobulin, colloidal material other than thyroglobulin, microsomal and nuclear intracellular constituents – and a variety of tests to detect the presence of these antibodies has now been developed. The most commonly used relate to thyroglobulin antibodies and intracellular microsomal antibodies.

Thyroglobulin antibodies are usually detected by means of a tanned red blood cell agglutination technique, but precipitin, latex agglutination and immunofluorescent systems are available.

Intracellular microsomal antibodies are popularly detected by a complement fixation test, but immunofluorescence and thyroid cell culture cytotoxicity may also be used.

In general, thyroglobulin antibody tests are too sensitive, so that weakly positive tests

* Although this claim has since been modified.

might be found in a variety of thyroid disorders apart from thyroiditis, e.g. thyroid cancer or non-toxic goitre. Positive findings in some patients with hyperthyroidism are thought to indicate a greater or lesser degree of associated thyroiditis; it is therefore considered by some to have a limited prognostic value as an indicator of potential hypothyroidism after surgery or after treatment of the disease with radioactive iodine. Complement-fixing microsomal antibodies are often not found in proved cases of thyroiditis, suggesting a lack of sensitivity of the technique. Any positive complement-fixing test should be accepted as significant, whereas minor titres of thyroglobulin antibody (less than say, 1 in 250 dilution) are of no particular diagnostic value. Recenlty, a radioimmunoassay for thyroglobulin has been developed with a high degree of positivity in sera of patients with thyroid cancer; as with so many other tumour markers, however, specificity is far from complete.

Thyroidal autoantibodies are often found in goitrous or non-goitrous cases of hypothyroidism. In the latter, they may be taken to indicate "burnt-out" atrophic or dominantly-fibrous forms of the disease. It should be pointed out that the presence of antibodies in high titre signifies autoimmune thyroiditis, but this does not rule out concomitant thyroid carcinoma or lymphoma which may be associated with this form of thyroid disease. Thyroid antibodies may commonly be found in other associated autoimmune disturbances, e.g. rheumatoid arthritis, pernicious anaemia or systemic lupus erythematosus, and in chromosomal disorders such as Turner's syndrome (gonadal dysgenesis) or Down's syndrome (trisomy 21).

13.3.10. Some "end-point" tests

A major deficiency in thyroid testing is the lack of suitable measurements of the final action of thyroid hormones at the level of the target organ or tissue.

13.3.10.1. Basal metabolic rate (BMR)

BMR is one of the oldest tests of thyroid function and is based on the determination of oxygen consumption in relation to the subject's surface area. The test result is compared to an established normal range. For many years it provided the main, if not the only, diagnostic test of thyroid dysfunction but it has almost entirely been phased out in favour of more specific biochemical assays. Reliable measurements of BMR require meticulous preparation of the patient and considerable technical skill in order to get a truly representative standardized basal reading for each subject. Overnight admission of patients is desirable, with several hours quiet rest in a post-prandial state. Any muscular exertion, anxiety or even pre-test smoking could affect the result. It is not surprising that a normal range was hard to define and that overlapping values between various thyroid states and normality were commonly found. It was usual to repeat tests until two or three results were in agreement, and the lowest was generally considered most acceptable. Because it is tedious and time consuming to perform, non-specific and poorly discriminating, the BMR has largely been abandoned. With it goes our sole measure of total body response to thyroid hormone action.

13.3.10.2. Deep tendon reflex time

It has long been recognized that deep tendon reflexes are delayed in myxoedema; methods have thus been developed over the past two decades to quantify the response, particularly of the relaxation phase of the Achilles tendon jerk. Timing of the response may be made with great accuracy by photoelectric methods, with graphical recording so as to facilitate analysis in detail. It is probably best for each operator or laboratory to establish a normal range, as techniques and instruments differ. Considerable overlap is still found, and the test has little real diagnostic value, except perhaps in the serial assessment of patients under treatment.

13.3.10.3. Red blood cell sodium content

In hyperthyroidism, the sodium content of peripheral erythrocytes is higher than normal and may be shown to diminish as the disease is brought under control (Goolden et al., 1971). Statistically significant changes in erythrocyte sodium content are not found in hypothyroidism. The test must be performed on freshly separated cells, which limits its usefulness. The test does not clearly distinguish between the different groups and is not, therefore, of much diagnostic value.

13.3.10.4. Serum cholesterol

Hyperthyroid subjects tend to have low serum cholesterol concentrations, and hypothyroid subjects high. In the diagnosis of the latter, the test has been widely used, but it is of limited value because of overlaps with the normal range and the large number of non-thyroidal disturbances that also lead to elevated concentrations, for instance diabetes mellitus, idiopathic hyperlipidaemia, and nephrotic syndrome. In hypothyroidism secondary to pituitary disease, the serum cholesterol concentration is generally not raised, but this is a minor point of distinction.

13.3.11. A place for in vivo radioactive isotope tests?

Although this Chapter is concerned primarily with in vitro tests of thyroid function, it is appropriate to consider briefly what role, if any, remains for tests requiring the administration of radioactive iodine to patients. As a routine they appear to have been largely supplanted by in vitro tests which measure the concentrations of circulating hormones. Thyroidal iodine uptake measurements lack dignostic discrimination and are inconvenient both to patients and to laboratory staff. "Immediate" uptake of radioactive iodine or technetium offers the advantage of rapid results (within 20 to 30 minutes) allowing prompt therapeutic decision making; such tests may therefore still have a place – particularly in the diagnosis of suspect hyperthyroidism, since better discrimination is found in the upper ranges of activity than in the lower. A form of thyroiditis has now been recognized in which clinical and biochemical evidence of hyperthyroidism is present, but thyroidal uptake of radioactive iodine is low or absent (Woolf and Daly, 1976; Dorfman et al., 1977); this is thought by some authors to account for as many as 15% of all cases of hyperthyroidism but this figure is probably exaggerated. Nevertheless, it is important to recognize the syndrome since the hyperthyroidism may be transient (British Medical Journal, 1977). Scanning for "hot" or "cold" thyroid nodules and for metastases from thyroid carcinoma or for ectopic thyroid tissue is still popular and is likely to remain so despite rather limited practical benefits. In thyrotoxicosis factitia, suppression of thyroidal uptake may provide a diagnostic clue, and in some centres it is customary to measure uptakes as a preliminary to ^{131}I treatment of hyperthyroidism. Long-term responses to medical treatment of hyperthyroidism have been predicted – not always successfully – by a return of suppressibility of thyroidal uptake by T3; and the perchlorate or thiocyanate discharge test (section 13.1.1.) identifies cases of failure of organification as seen in Pendred's Syndrome. With these few exceptions it seems likely that radioactive iodine tests can now be abandoned.

13.3.12. Pregnancy, the neonate and childhood

In pregnancy, the concentration of serum T4 rises in parallel with the oestrogen-induced increase in plasma TBG; this change is discernible in the first trimester and reaches peak values in the third, when the serum T4 concentration may be 50% greater than normal. Serum T3 appears to increase more gradually, although very high concentrations are found in late pregnancy. The concentration of non-protein-bound T4 probably remains normal throughout, but urinary excretion may not reflect this because of possible alterations in the renal clearance of thyroid hormones. The diagnosis of suspected hyperthyroidism in pregnancy is difficult on clinical grounds. A combined test, with derivation of the free thyroxine index, is probably most valuable.

Umbilical cord serum of neonates shows low T3 concentrations, affecting both total and free moieties. Shortly after birth, possibly within the first hour, the concentration of serum TSH rises, followed by an increase in serum T3 which reaches a peak by 24 hours, often to values greater than those found in normal adults. Thereafter serum T3 concentration gradually returns to normal. Serum T4 appears not to be affected by these changes. It has become increasingly recognized that screening of all newborn infants for hypothyroidism should be encouraged. Estimates of the prevalence of neonatal hypothyroidism range from 1 : 3000 to 1 : 7000 births (Fisher et al., 1976) and several different screening tests are advocated based on the assay of T4, TSH, T3 or rT3 in umbilical cord blood or heelprick samples taken a few days after birth. No clear decision about the best test or its timing has yet emerged.

Although there is some conflict in the literature, it is likely that circulating thyroid hormones remain normal throughout childhood and are not altered by puberty.

13.3.13. Ageing

Thyroid disease is common in the elderly, hyper- and hypothyroidism each having been found in about 2% of random hospital admissions (Jefferys, 1972). Clinically, disease in the elderly is characterized by insidiousness of onset, subtleness of presentation and masking by concomitant illness or drug therapy. The results of thyroid function tests in these patients may be quite difficult to interpret. In one series, about 20% of apparently euthyroid patients admitted to a geriatric ward showed low serum PBI or T4 concentrations, with T3 uptake values that confirmed a low TBG with normal free thyroxine index (Jefferys et al., 1972). These abnormalities were found to correlate well with the clinical status of the individuals, those who were more acutely or severely ill showing lower serum TBG concentrations and therefore lower total T4 concentrations; low serum albumin concentrations were also closely correlated. A progressive decrease in serum T3 concentration with advancing age has been demonstrated (Rubenstein et al., 1973) which is probably not related to lower TBG values *; TSH response to injected TRF has also been found to be impaired in older men but not in women (Snyder and Utiger, 1972). Thyroidal stimulation by exogenous TSH is normal in the elderly, despite some histological evidence of atrophy and fibrosis. It is difficult to account for all of these changes on the basis of a single abnormality, but the evidence points to slight impairment of hypothalamic control of anterior pituitary function, perhaps diminished peripheral mono-deiodination of T4 to T3, and a tendency to rapid and quite profound decrease in circulating TBG concentration in the presence of systemic disease.

13.3.14. Tests during or after treatment of thyroid disease

The peripheral turnover of T3 is more rapid than that of T4; it is not surprising to find that the concentration of serum T3 returns more rapidly to normal in hyperthyroid patients treated with antithyroid drugs, well in advance of T4. Once euthyroidism has been established, both T3 and T4 values generally fall within the reference ranges, but several different patterns of hormone concentrations have been observed. Worthy of mention are those cases in which high concentrations of TSH are found in association with low or low-normal serum T4 and normal or high serum T3 concentrations, i.e. where a euthyroid state is being maintained by T3. It is clear that this combination may exist for many years without clinical or biochemical supervention of hypothyroidism, particularly after treatment of hyperthyroidism by surgery or radioactive iodine. Intrathyroidal iodine deficiency in these patients may result in a preponderance of monoiodothyronines and preferential synthesis of T3. It is worth pointing out that propyl- and methylthiouracil partially block the peripheral conversion of T4 into T3 and may lead to temporary derangement of T3 production and an increase in secretion of TSH.

Circulating thyroid hormones may be measured to monitor the adequacy of replacement therapy in the treatment of hypothyroidism. Clearly, if T3 alone is used (25 to 100 μg/day) any residual thyroid function will be suppressed and low serum PBI or T4 concentrations will be found; in such cases, the serum T3 concentration may be very high (300 to 1000 ng/dl). Such values return to normal within 1 or 2 days of stopping T3 therapy. If T4 is administered, conversion into T3 takes place and "normal" values of both hormones are generally found after a few weeks of treatment. When adequate replacement therapy is given, serum TSH concentration is suppressed to normal or immeasurable levels, and an exaggerated TRF response is no longer observed.

13.3.15. Thyroid function tests in non-thyroid disease

A large number of conditions and very many drugs may affect thyroid function tests. Acute or chronic stress of surgical or "medical" origin may lead to rapid lowering of serum T3 and thyroxine binding prealbumin concentrations. In the elderly, at least, TBG is also often reduced. It is likely that the decrease in the concentrations of plasma binding

* This probably reflects associated disease rather than the ageing process itself.

proteins is due to temporary cessation of synthesis, but it is not yet clear whether the fall in T3 concentration is due to decreased synthesis (thyroidal or peripheral), to increased degradation or perhaps to sequestration into extravascular sites. Recent work suggests that mono-deiodination of T4 proceeds along a different pathway with diminished production of 3,5,3′-T3 and an increase in 3,3′,5′- or reverse-T3.

Hormone effects are multiple and varied. Of great importance is the recognition of the high circulating concentration of TBG which is induced by oestrogens during pregnancy or contained in contraceptive pills; the contrary effect is seen with androgens or anabolic agents. In liver disease, complex changes take place related to an interplay of several factors: deranged hepatic synthesis of TBG and thyroxine binding prealbumin; reduced hepatic synthesis of TBG and thyroxine binding prealbumin; reduced hepatic conversion of T4 to T3, and perhaps disturbance of other functions such as conjugation of thyroid hormones; the effect of high circulating oestrogens on serum TBG concentration; and the presence of abnormal metabolites that might displace thyroid hormones from their binding proteins or otherwise interfere with their binding characteristics. In chronic renal failure, a complex pattern of changes has also been observed: serum T4 and T3 concentrations may be lowered; there may be lack of response to TRF; renal losses of protein may affect the concentrations of binding proteins; changes of hydrogen ion concentration or accumulation of phenolic compounds or other metabolites may alter protein binding. The complexity of the changes in both liver and kidney diseases indicates the need for caution in the interpretation of thyroid function tests in these disorders, and also perhaps in other examples of systemic disease.

13.3.16. Choice of tests and a diagnostic approach

The proliferation of laboratory tests of thyroid function over the past 20 years has added precision to our diagnoses. But the physician is often embarrassed by the richness of choice, and a diagnostic approach is needed that will provide optimal information with least inconvenience to the patient and least strain and cost to the laboratory. It is the present author's view – and that perhaps of the majority of clinicians specializing in thyroid work – that thyroid function testing should preferably start with the measurement of circulating hormones. For the reasons given earlier, it is true to say that the assay of serum PBI is being phased out in favour of the more specific estimation of T4. When the measurement of PBI is abandoned, we shall regrettably lose the facility for diagnosing that interesting group of patients with abnormal circulating iodoproteins, the clue to which so often lies in a high serum PBI concentration with normal or low serum T4 concentration.

The introduction of quick, cheap, sensitive and reproducible radioimmunoassays for T3 has raised the question of whether T3 rather than T4 should be measured in plasma. In two circumstances at least, T3 assay does provide additional information of great value – T3 toxicity and "compensated hypothyroidism" (section 13.3.4.). In both conditions, the diagnosis may be suspected on other grounds but a firm ineluctable diagnosis requires the direct assay of serum T3. In almost all other problems, the assay of serum T4 provides the information needed to make a correct diagnosis, and there are several circumstances in which serum T3 alone would be misleading, e.g. where impairment of peripheral deiodination of T4 to T3 is thought to exist. This has been described in cases of inordinate reduction of serum T3 concentration, as seen after acute surgical stress, in acute or chronic illness, in liver disease, during starvation treatment of obesity, in many elderly subjects, and after cortisone or propylthiouracil therapy. In all of these situations, the concentration of serum T3 may be reduced in the face of normal serum T4 and TBG values and clinical euthyroidism; reliance on measurement of T3 alone might lead to a mistaken diagnosis of hypothyroidism. It would seem from these considerations that the assay of T4 has some advantages over the less discriminating assay of T3, but it may be necessary to measure both hormones for valid assessment of less typical cases.

It has been emphasized that the concentrations of circulating hormones are essentially influenced by the concentrations of the binding proteins, especially TBG, and that determination of the non-protein-bound fraction of T4 or T3 provides a more accurate picture of the metabolic activity of the hormones at a cellular level. Direct means of assay of the free hormones are not yet suitable for routine use so it is probably best to combine a variant of the T3 uptake test, or a direct assay of TBG, with the total hormone concentration to derive a free thyroxine index. Measurement of total serum T4 or T3 alone would suffice in most instances, particularly where the clinical diagnosis is reasonably convincing and the test is performed simply to gain supportive laboratory evidence; but such measurements may be misleading where the TBG content of serum is significantly elevated or diminished.

It is for the resolution of more difficult clinical problems that both assays are desirable. If their outcome matches the clinical diagnosis, no further tests need be made. If there is conflict between the results of the tests and the clinical impression, or between the different test results, then further steps are necessary. The possibility of gross error in specimen handling or in reporting should be investigated, and then perhaps the tests should be repeated. If the test results are normal in the face of suspected clinical hyperthyroidism, serum T3 estimation should identify possible T3-toxicosis. If hypothyroidism is suspected, serum TSH should be determined. A TRF test may provide back-up information in the negative sense referred to earlier (section 13.3.7.1.): if a response is found, hyperthyroidism may be ruled out; failure of response is incompatible with primary hypothyroidism.

A further point should be made: a clinician treats patients, not tests. Although it is highly unlikely that hyper- or hypothyroidism would exist in the face of completely normal results, benefit of the doubt should be given to the patient and a carefully conducted trial of therapeutic response should be carried out if the clinical picture is sufficiently suggestive, whatever the outcome of the tests. If the tests suggest thyroid disease but the clinical picture does not, it is reasonable just to observe the patient and to withhold treatment until a more convincing picture is seen.

13.3.17. Conclusion

The diagnostic accuracy of the currently available thyroid function tests is considerable and there must be very few cases in which they do not help to make a secure diagnosis. Occasionally, persistent borderline results are found – probably the patients themselves are on the borderline between health and disease – no test can offer greater discrimination in these circumstances but continued observation usually allows a decision to be made. The scheme outlined here, depending as it does on the performance of two separate tests, carries an element of double-check. But the tests are time consuming and expensive, and there is still a need for a quick, simple, cheap and relatively discriminatory screening test to pick out the not inconsiderable number of patients with unsuspected or obscure thyroid disease. Above all, tests must be effective in cost-benefit terms; they should reduce the time taken to make a definitive diagnosis and to embark on the correct treatment so as to minimize the patient's disability. In reviewing the tests that are, and have been available, one fact emerges strongly – the need to find some way of measuring the end-point effect of thyroid hormone activity, preferably in terms of cellular responsiveness. For it is this effect that determines the patient's symptoms and signs and which needs to be treated when it is abnormal.

REFERENCES

Acland, J.D. (1971) The interpretation of the serum protein-bound iodine: a review. Journal of Clinical Pathology, 24, 187-218.

Adams, D.D. (1958) The presence of an abnormal thyroid stimulating hormone in the serum of some thyrotoxic patients. Journal of Clinical Endocrinology and Metabolism, 18, 699–712.

Adams, D.D. and Kennedy, T.H. (1967) Occurrence in thyrotoxicosis of a gamma globulin which protects LATS from neutralization by an extract of thyroid gland. Journal of Clinical Endocrinology and Metabolism, 27, 173–177.

Adams, D.D. and Purves, H.D. (1956) Abnormal responses in the assay of thyrotrophin. Proceedings of the University of Otago Medical School. 34, 11–12.

Barker, S.B., Humphrey, M.J. and Soley, M.H. (1951) Clinical determination of protein-bound iodine. Journal of Clinical Investigation, 30, 55–62.

Bitensky, L., Alaghband-Sadeh, J. and Chayen, J. (1974) Studies on thyroid stimulating hormone and long acting thyroid stimulating hormone. Clinical Endocrinology, 3, 363–374.

Black, E.G., Griffiths, R.S., Finucane, J. and Hoffenberg, R. (1975) Radioimmunoassay of T3 and T4 in serum and urine. In Thyroid Hormone Metabolism (Eds. W.A. Harland and J.S. Orr) pp. 347–365, Academic Press, London.

British Medical Journal (1977) Leading article – Painless thyroiditis. 2, 348–349.

Brown, B.L., Ekins, R.P., Ellis, S.M. and Reith, W.S. (1970) Specific antibodies to triiodothyronine hormone. Nature, 226, 359.

Burke, C.W. and Eastman, C.J. (1974) Thyroid hormones. British Medical Bulletin, 30, 93–99.

Burr, W.A. Ramsden, D.B., Evans, S.E., Hogan, T. and Hoffenberg, R. (1977) Concentration of thyroxine-binding globulin: value of direct assay. British Medical Journal, 1, 485–488.

Chan, V. and Landon, J. (1972) Urinary thyroxine excretion as index of thyroid function. Lancet i, 4–6.

Clark, F. and Horn, D.B. (1965) Assessment of thyroid function by the combined use of the serum protein-bound iodine and resin uptake of ^{131}I-triiodothyronine. Journal of Clinical Endocrinology and Metabolism, 25, 39–45.

Dorfman, S.G., Cooperman, M.T., Nelson, R.L., Depuy, H., Peake, R.L. and Young, R.L. (1977) Painless thyroiditis and transient hyperthyroidism without goiter. Annals of Internal Medicine, 86, 24–28.

Ekins, R.P. (1960) The estimation of thyroxine in human plasma by an electrophoretic technique. Clinica Chimica Acta, 5, 453–459.

Fisher, D.A., Burrow, G.N., Dussault, J.H., Hollingsworth, D.R., Larsen, P.R., Man, E.B. and Walfish, P.G. (1976) Recommendation for screening programmes for congenital hypothyroidism. American Journal of Medicine, 61, 932–934.

Gharib, H., Ryan, R.J., Mayberry, W.E. and Hockert, T. (1971) Radioimmunoassay for triiodothyronine (T3): 1. Affinity and specificity of the antibody for T3. Journal of Clinical Endocrinology and Metabolism, 33, 509–516.

Goolden, A.W.G., Bateman, D. and Torr, S. (1971) Red cell sodium in hyperthyroidism. British Medical Journal, 2, 552–554.

Greer, M. and Smith, G.E. (1954) Method for increasing the accuracy of the radioiodine uptake as a test for thyroid function by the use of desiccated thyroid. Journal of Clinical Endocrinology and Metabolism, 14, 1374–1384.

de Groot, L.J. and Strausser, J.L. (1974) Binding of T3 in rat liver nuclei. Endocrinology, 95, 74–83.

de Groot, L.J. and Torresani, J. (1975) Triiodothyronine binding to isolated liver cell nuclei. Endocrinology, 96, 357–369.

Gross, J. and Pitt-Rivers, R. (1952) The identification of 3:5:3′-triiodothyronine in human plasma. Lancet, i, 439–441.

Hall, R. (1972) The immunoassay of thyroid-stimulating hormone and its clinical applications. Clinical Endocrinology, 1, 115–125.

Hamolsky, M.W., Stein, M. and Friedberg, A.S. (1957) The thyroid hormone-plasma protein complex in man. II. A new in vitro method for study of "uptake" of labelled hormonal components by human erythrocytes. Journal of Clinical Endocrinology and Metabolism, 17, 33–44.

Hetzel, B.S. (1970) The control of iodine deficiency. Medical Journal of Australia, 2, 615–622.

Hoffenberg, R. (1973) Triiodothyronine. Clinical Endocrinology, 2, 75–87.

Hollander, C.S., Stevenson, C., Mitsuma, T., Pineda, G., Shenkman, L. and Silva, E. (1972) T3 toxicosis in an iodine-deficient area. Lancet, ii, 1276–1278.

Jefferys, P.M. (1972) The prevalence of thyroid disease in patients admitted to a geriatric department. Age and Ageing, 1, 33–37.

Jefferys, P.M., Farran, H.E.A., Hoffenberg, R., Fraser, P.M. and Hodkinson, H.M. (1972) Thyroid-function tests in the elderly. Lancet, i, 924–927.

McKenzie, J.M. (1958) The bioassay of thyrotrophin in serum. Endocrinology, 63, 372–382.

Mincey, E.K., Thorson, S.C. and Brown, J.L. (1971) A new in vitro blood test for determining thyroid status – the effective thyroxine ratio. Clinical Biochemistry, 4, 216.

Murphy, B.E.P. (1965) The determination of thyroxine by competitive protein-binding analysis employing an anion-exchange resin and radiothyroxine. Journal of Laboratory and Clinical Medicine, 66, 161–167.

Murphy, B.E.P. and Pattee, C.J. (1964) Determination of thyroxine using the property of protein-binding. Journal of Clinical Endocrinology and Metabolism, 24, 187–196.

Naumann, J.A., Nauman, A. and Werner, S.C. (1967) Total and free triiodothyronine in human serum. Journal of Clinical Investigation, 46, 1346–1355.

Oppenheimer, J.H., Schwartz, H.L., Surks, M.I., Koerner, D. and Dillmann, W.H. (1976) Nuclear receptors and the initiation of thyroid hormone action. In Recent Progress in Hormone Research, Vol. 32, pp. 529–565.

Osorio, C., Jackson, D.J., Gartside, J.M. and Goolden, A.W.G. (1962) The assessment of free thyroxine in plasma. Clinical Science, 23, 525–530.

Roitt, I.M., Doniach, D., Campbell, P.N. and Hudson, R.V. (1956) Auto-antibodies in Hashimoto's disease (lymphadenoid goitre). Lancet, ii, 820–821.

Rubenstein, H.A., Butler, V.P. and Werner, S.C. (1973) Progressive decrease in serum triiodothyronine concentrations with human ageing: radioimmunoassay following extraction of serum. Journal of Clinical Endocrinology and Metabolism, 37, 247–253.

Sandell, E.B. and Kolthoff, I.M. (1937) Microdetermination of iodine by a catalytic method. Mikrochimica Acta, 1, 9.

Shenkman, L., Mitsuma, T., Suphavai, A. and Hollander, C.S. (1972) Triiodothyronine and thyroid stimulating hormone response to thyrotrophin-releasing hormone. Lancet, i, 111-113.

Snyder, P.J. and Utiger, R.D. (1972) Response to thyrotropin releasing hormone (TRH) in normal man, Journal of Clinical Endocrinology and Metabolism, 34, 380–385.

Spierto, F.W., Hubert, I.L. and Shaw, W. (1974) An interlaboratory and intralaboratory comparison of serum T4 methodologies. Clinica Chimica Acta, 56, 281–290.

Sterling, K. (1970) The significance of circulating triiodothyronine. Recent Progress in Hormone Research, 26, 249–286.

Sterling, K., Bellabarba, D., Newman, E.S. and Brenner, M.A. (1969) Determination of triiodothyronine concentration in human serum. Journal of Clinical Investigation, 48, 1150–1158.

Sterling, K. and Brenner, M.A. (1966) Free thyroxine in human serum. Simplified measurement with the aid of magnesium precipitation. Journal of Clinical Investigation, 45, 153–163.

Surks, M.I., Koerner, D.H. and Oppenheimer, J.H. (1975) In vitro binding of L-triiodothyronine to receptors in rat liver nuclei. Journal of Clinical Investigation, 55, 50–60.

Utiger, R.D. (1974) Serum triiodothyronine in man. In Annual Review of Medicine, Vol. 25. (Ed. W.P. Creger) pp. 289–302, Annual Reviews Inc., Palo Alto, California.

Vidor, G.I., Stewart, J.C., Wall, J.R., Wangel, A. and Hetzel, B.S. (1973) Pathogenesis of iodine-induced thyrotoxicosis: studies in northern Tasmania. Journal of Clinical Endocrinology and Metabolism, 37, 901–909.

Werner, S.C. and Spooner, M. (1955) New and simple test for hyperthyroidism employing L-triiodothyronine and the twenty-four hour I-131 uptake method. Bulletin of the New York Academy of Medicine, 31, 137–145.

Woolf, P.D. and Daly, R. (1976) Thyrotoxicosis with painless thyroiditis. American Journal of Medicine, 60, 73–79.

Zak, B., Willard, H.H., Mayers, G.B. and Boyle, A.J. (1952) Chloric acid method for determination of protein-bound iodine. Analytical Chemistry, 24, 1345–1348.

FURTHER READING

Acland, J.D. (1971) The interpretation of the serum protein-bound iodine: a review. Journal of Clinical Pathology, 24, 187–218.

Berson, S.A. (Ed.) (1972) Methods in Investigative and Diagnostic Endocrinology, Vol. 1, Part 1: The Thyroid. (Ed. J.E. Rall) North-Holland Publishing Co., Amsterdam.

Burke, C.W. and Eastman, C.J. (1974) Thyroid hormones. British Medical Bulletin, 30, 93–99.

de Groot, L.J. and Stanbury, J.B. (1976) The Thyroid and its Diseases, 4th edn. John Wiley and Sons, New York.

Evered, D.C. (1976) Diseases of the Thyroid. Pitman Medical Publishing, Tunbridge Wells, England.

Greep, R.O. and Astwood, E.B. (Eds.) (1974) Section 7: Endocrinology, Vol. III, Thyroid, Handbook of Physiology. (Eds. M.A. Greer and D.H. Solomon) American Physiological Society, Washington, D.C.

Hall, R. (1972) The immunoassay of thyroid-stimulating hormone and its clinical applications. Clinical Endocrinology, 1, 115–125.

Hall, R., Smith, B.R. and Mukhtar, E.D. (1975) Thyroid stimulators in health and disease. Clinical Endocrinology, 4, 213–230.

Harland, W.A. and Orr, J.S. (Eds.) (1975) Thyroid Hormone Metabolism. Academic Press, London.

Hershman, J.M. (1974) Clinical application of thyrotropin-releasing hormone. New England Journal of Medicine, 290, 886–890.

Hoffenberg, R. (1973) Triiodothyronine. Clinical Endocrinology, 2, 75–87.

Ingbar, S.H. and Braverman, L.E. (1975) In Annual Review of Medicine, Vol. 26. (Eds. W.P. Creger, C.H. Coggins and E.W. Hancock) pp. 443–449, Annual Reviews Inc., Palo Alto, California.

Oppenheimer, J.H., Schwartz, H.L., Surks, M.I., Koerner, D. and Dillmann, W.H. (1976) Nuclear receptors and the initiation of thyroid hormone action. Recent Progress in Hormone Research, 32, 529–565.

Ramsden, D.B. (1977) Peripheral Metabolism and Action of thyroid Hormones. Eden Press, Lancaster, England and Montreal, Canada.

Sterling, K. (1970) The significance of circulating triiodothyronine. Recent Progress in Hormone Research, 26, 249–286.

Utiger, R.D. (1974) Serum triiodothyronine in man. In Annual Review of Medicine, Vol. 25. (Ed. W.P. Creger) pp. 289–302, Annual Reviews Inc., Palo Alto, California.

Werner, S.C. and Ingbar, S.H. (eds.) (1971) The Thyroid: A Fundamental and Clinical Text, 3rd edn. Harper and Row, New York.

ADDENDUM

Much has happened in the thyroid field during the 3 years since this Chapter was written. Serum PBI measurement has now been superseded completely by T4 assay and at least one new method measures free (non-protein-bound) T4 directly by the rate of association of T4 with its antibody; this test has not been fully evaluated in clinical practice but seems to offer simplicity and ease of diagnosis in most cases of thyroid disease. Much more has been learned about the peripheral metabolism of T4 but little of clinical importance has yet emerged. Determination of "thyroid-stimulating immunoglobulins" in Graves's disease has proved far less useful than initial reports suggested, with too many negative results in undoubted cases of hyperthyroidism (probably about one-third in all) and positive results occurring in many euthyroid cases of Graves's disease. Assay of serum thyroglobulin does not distinguish thyroid cancer from other causes of goitre but seems useful in monitoring response to therapy and in detecting earlier recurrences. Big advances have been made in screening of neonates for hypothyroidism, which is available widely in North America and Europe; highest detection rates with lowest unnecessary recall rates are reported with combined assays of T4 and TSH, usually on dried filter-paper discs. We are no further in our search for tests of end-organ response to thyroid hormone action.

Chapter 14

Steroid hormones

Vivian H.T. James and Frederick L. Mitchell

Department of Chemical Pathology, St. Mary's Hospital Medical School, London W2 1PG and Division of Clinical Chemistry, Clinical Research Centre, Harrow, Middlesex HA1 3UJ, England

CONTENTS

14.1. INTRODUCTION

Although every branch of clinical chemistry has undergone considerable changes in the last few years, there have been particularly important and fundamental developments in the technology of steroid hormone assays and in the application of the assays in clinical medicine. This chapter reviews methods of steroid assay which are of significance to the clinical chemist, and discusses specific applications to diagnostic problems.

The provision of a complete range of steroid assays requires a very considerable investment in specialized laboratory staff, space and equipment, and rarely can the necessary degree of specialization be achieved. Many clinical laboratories can provide nonetheless a fairly broad range of assays, and by drawing upon more specialized resources elsewhere, offer a sufficiently wide service to cover normal clinical requirements for diagnosis and treatment. At the time of writing, the most commonly requested assays are cortisol, testosterone and progesterone in plasma and free cortisol and oestriol (or total oestrogens) in non-pregnancy and pregnancy urine. There is a lesser demand for plasma aldosterone, 17-hydroxyprogesterone and oestradiol, and for urinary aldosterone, 17-oxosteroids, 17-oxogenic steroids and for production rate measurements of aldosterone and cortisol. Less commonly, and usually for specific patients or for research studies, fairly complete "profiling" of urinary steroids may be undertaken, or studies of androgen metabolism or of steroid binding to protein may be made. The carrying out of this work requires specialized knowledge and equipment.

In this chapter, it has been found necessary to cover assay technology in rather more depth than is appropriate elsewhere in this book, since interpretation can be very dependent upon the nature – and to some extent the vagaries – of a particular assay method. Quality control in steroid measurement is much less advanced than in other areas of clinical chemistry, largely because of the major technological problems involved.

Certain parts of the field are covered in other chapters.

14.2. GROUP ASSAYS

Until comparatively recently, steroid measurements for clinical purposes were limited mainly to assays of groups of compounds since very few techniques for the routine measurement of individual steroids had been developed. In addition, few of the methods used for group measurements during the 1940s, 1950s and early 1960s were thoroughly investigated for reliability, accuracy and particularly specificity; consequently many findings in certain circumstances, especially those reported during the early part of this period, are open to question. The following group assays, however, have stood the test of time and have mostly been evaluated in depth and their limitations determined. For a comparison of some of the problems in the comparison of group and individual assays see Ernest et al. (1964).

14.2.1. Techniques

14.2.1.1. Urinary 17-oxosteroids (17-OS)

Zimmermann, in 1935, described a colour reaction which can be made reasonably specific for the 17-OS. The reaction has been applied to the assay of urinary steroids, with a preliminary hydrolysis by hot acid, followed by extraction and purification in a variety of ways (e.g. see Gray et al., 1969). Interference from non-specific chromogens, particularly in infants, is an important feature to guard against (section 14.2.2.1).

14.2.1.2. Urinary 17-hydroxycorticosteroids (17-OHCS)

In the technique described by Norymberski for this assay, destruction of the 17-OHCS during hydrolysis by hot acid is circumvented by an initial step which converts them to 17-OS. The urine is treated first with sodium borohydride to reduce all oxo groups so that they will not react with the Zimmermann reagent. The C_{21} steroids with the following side chains are then oxidized by sodium bismuthate to 17-OS which are measured, as such, as described above: 17,21-dihydroxy-20-one; 17,20,21-trihydroxy; 17,20-dihydroxy-21-deoxy; 17-hydroxy-20-one-21-deoxy. Since these are the only urinary steroids with side chains containing a 17-hydroxyl group, the assay is referred to as "total 17-OHCS". As with the 17-OS assay, interference from non-specific chromogens can occur. Gray et al. (1969) endeavoured to combine the best aspects of various published modifications, and their technique must be considered to be the method of choice for the measurement of the urinary steroid metabolites of cortisol as a group.

14.2.1.3. Urinary 17-oxogenic steroids
Norymberski and his colleagues reported an earlier technique than that for total 17-OHCS, in which 17-OS are measured by the Zimmermann reaction in the same urine specimen with and without bismuthate oxidation (Norymberski et al., 1953). The difference between the two results gives a measure of steroids with the first three of the side chains previously mentioned. The fourth is not oxidized since the 20-oxo group has not been previously reduced. Steroids with this side chain are only important in the adrenogenital syndrome with a 21-hydroxylase block, when a difference between the 17-OHCS and 17-oxogenic group assays indicates the amount of 17α-hydroxypregnanolone present in the urine and derived from 17α-hydroxyprogesterone. The method is no longer of any clinical significance.

14.2.1.4. Urinary Porter–Silber chromogens
Steroids possessing a "dihydroxyacetone side chain" develop a colour in a reaction first described by Porter and Silber (1950). The technique for urine requires mild (enzymic) hydrolysis since the corticosteroids would be destroyed by hot acid. Many modifications to the procedure were published during the 1950s, but in general it suffers from a lack of specificity, the difficulty of ensuring complete hydrolysis and its inability to measure other important metabolites. However, it has been widely used in North America.

14.2.1.5. Urinary 21-deoxyketols
Steroids with the 17-hydroxy-20-oxo-21-deoxy side chain may be converted into 17-OS by consecutive oxidation–reduction–oxidation using bismuthate and borohydride. Final measurement may then be achieved with the Zimmermann reaction (Appleby and Norymberski, 1954).

14.2.1.6. Urinary 17-deoxycorticosteroids (17-HCS)
When 17-deoxycorticosteroids are reduced with borohydride and oxidized with bismuthate, the resulting aldehyde may be measured colorimetrically (Exley and Norymberski, 1964).

14.2.1.7. Oestrogen assays
Since Kober in 1931 first described a specific colour reaction for the naturally occurring oestrogens, it has been widely used in measurement techniques which have shown remarkable evolution and continuous improvement for the last three decades. Early in the period, "total" oestrogens were measured; then a variety of chromatographic procedures was incorporated to enable the measurement of individual oestrogens. Latterly there has been a return to simpler methods, again for total oestrogens, since it was appreciated that for most clinical purposes, separation of individual steroids was not required. Such a technique, now widely used, is that of J.B. Brown et al. (1968) in which the final products of the Kober reaction may be measured either by colorimetry or by the Ittrich (1958) technique using fluorimetry after extraction, when the sensitivity is increased approximately 40-fold. Colorimetry is suitable for the large quantities of oestrogen which are present in late pregnancy urine, and fluorimetry for late and early pregnancy and non-pregnancy urines. The reliability criteria of these techniques have now been well

investigated and can be considered satisfactory. Practicability is also good since 12 analyses by the method of J.B. Borwn et al. (1968) can be completed within 4 hours. The procedures have been successfully automated for pregnancy urines (e.g. Barnard and Logan, 1971), and a careful evaluation of the automated techniques has been made (Moscrop et al., 1974).

Other techniques based on the very highly sensitive fluorescence developed by heating oestrogens with acid have been reported, but have not been widely used, largely because of their laborious nature and lack of specificity.

Attempts have been made to apply the Kober and Ittrich principles to the measurement of oestrogens in blood (Roy, 1962), but for non-pregnancy specimens the technology may be considered to be stretched beyond its limit, and blood assays are now made exclusively by radioimmunoassay methods.

14.2.1.8. Blood Porter–Silber chromogens

The Porter-Silber reaction was adapted for use on blood by Nelson and Samuels (1952) and has subsequently been widely used, particularly in North America. Its many published modifications include an ultra-micro technique (Bowman, 1967). It has largely been superseded by fluorimetric and radioimmunoassay techniques.

14.2.1.9. Blood 11-hydroxycorticosteroids (11-OHCS)

Many attempts have been made to utilize, for measurement purposes, the intense fluorescence to which the 11-OHCS can give rise, but the first successful application was that reported by Mattingly (1962). This technique was later modified and automated (Townsend and James, 1968). Both forms of the method have been thorougly investigated for accuracy and precision and are widely accepted as a practical means of measuring blood cortisol for clinical purposes. It must, however, be understood that, although they are normally present in small quantity in human blood, 11-hydroxycorticosteroids other than cortisol (e.g. corticosterone) produce fluorescence; also various compounds, both unknown and known, can interfere. The drug spironolactone produces grossly elevated values, and cyproterone acetate will also cause spurious increases.

14.2.2. Usage of group assays and reference ranges

14.2.2.1. 17-Oxosteroids (17-OS)

The urinary 17-OS in males originate from steroids secreted by the testes (approximately one-third, mainly as metabolites of testosterone) and the adrenal cortex (approximately two-thirds) by side chain removal from C_{21} steroids and by direct secretion. In females, about one-third is of ovarian origin. All the compounds are excreted as glucuronides or sulphates and some at least (e.g. dehydroepiandrosterone) are produced as sulphates. When the urinary 17-OS assay was the only practical steroid measurement available offering reasonable reliability, it was widely used for monitoring adrenal activity, but it is quite unsatisfactory for this purpose and has been superseded by the measurement of 17-OHCS and of urinary free cortisol. Figure 14.1 shows the reference ranges for 17-OS and indicates that there is a considerable variation in excretion between individuals, and that age and sex are important considerations when interpreting single measurements. There is

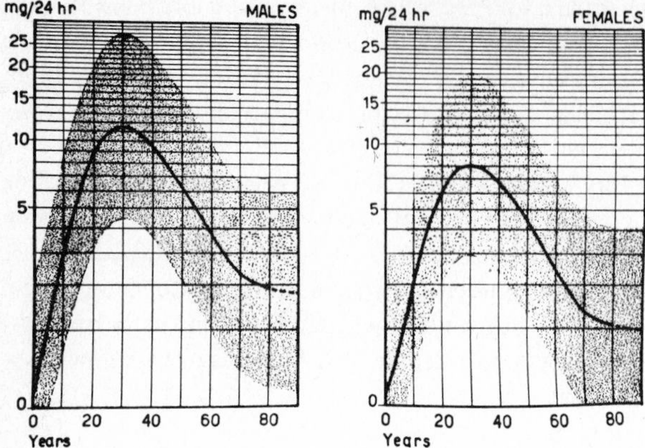

Figure 14.1. The excretion rates of 17-OS in healthy subjects of average body weight and height. Average values (full line), fiducial range ($P = 0.05$, shaded area). (Reproduced, by permission, from Borth et al., 1957)

no marked change in output in women during the menstrual cycle, but during pregnancy, the level rises slightly above that in pre-pregnancy. The concentration in blood, however, tends to fall; a feature which may be explained by the use of maternal dehydroepiandrosterone for oestrogen production. In urine, during pregnancy, a true decrease in the content of the major 17-OS (section 14.6.2) may be more than balanced by an increase in other Zimmermann-reacting compounds. Changes in the excretion of 17-OS in many pathological conditions have been sought, mostly without dramatic results. There are no marked changes in acromegaly, amenorrhoea without hirsutism, Turner's syndrome or mammary carcinoma. Increases occur in some, but not all, patients with arrhenoblastoma. In the Stein–Leventhal syndrome, the levels are often raised, but the range is such as to limit the diagnostic value. In myxoedema, the output is usually below the accepted reference range but does not always rise on treatment. Very large increases though, can occur in Cushing's syndrome caused by adrenocortical carcinoma, and sometimes in the very rare cases of virilizing adrenal tumours.

Several studies have shown that the specificity of the 17-OS assay is poor. When it is compared with the summation of individual steroid measurements, the proportion of non-specific chromogen can, exceptionally, be as high as 90% It is particularly high in infant urine when qualitatively, the make-up of the Zimmermann chromogens is very different from that found in the adult (Birchall and Mitchell, 1965). These drawbacks seriously limit the clinical value of the test.

In conclusion, there is now little use for the assay of 17-oxosteroids except when other techniques are not available for detecting excessive androgen production (particularly androgens originating other than from testosterone), and for monitoring therapy in patients with the adrenogenital syndrome. (For its use in the context of adrenal hyperfunction, see section 14.4.1.2).

14.2.2.2. Urinary adrenocorticosteroids (17-OHCS, Porter–Silber chromogens, 21-deoxyketols and 17-HCS)

The clinical value of these assays emanates from the assumption that in large part, they measure the major metabolites of cortisol or other adrenocorticosteroids, but not all the polar metabolites are quantitatively extracted with the organic solvents normally used. The normal urinary excretion patterns of the 17-OHCS are shown in Figure 14.2, and the wide ranges and variation with age, as with the 17-OS, are apparent. As would be expected from the diurnal variation of the concentration of cortisol in blood (section 14.4), the urinary excretion of cortisol metabolites is, in general, highest during the day. During pregnancy, the excretion of 17-OHCS increases gradually to approximately 5 mg/24 h above non-pregnancy values at parturition (Norymberski, 1961), but the Porter–Silber chromogens show little change. The use of the 17-OHCS assay in this assessment of adrenal function is considered in section 14.4.

The urinary 21-deoxyketols are raised in cases with the adrenogenital syndrome, when large quantities of 17-hydroxy-progesterone are produced and excreted as 17-hydroxy-pregnanolone; also during pregnancy, when they increase to a value up to 3 mg/24 h above the normal excretion of about 0.16 mg/24 h in non-pregnant women.

The 17-HCS assay has been used by Exley and Norymberski (1964) as an indication of the rate of excretion of the metabolites of corticosterone. They found the average urinary excretion in healthy adults to be 3.4 mg/24 h with a ratio of 17-OHCS:17-HCS of 2.8. During pregnancy, the excretion rose more sharply than that of the 17-OHCS and the ratio fell to 0.5 to 1.2. In infants (1 to 12 days) the predominance of 17-HCS over 17-OHCS was even more marked, with a ratio of 0.3.

During pregnancy, therefore, the production of corticosteroids in general increases, but with the contribution of the placenta and foetus, the overall pattern of excretion between different compounds is altered. Therefore in pregnancy and infant urines, group assays such as those for 17-OS and 17-OHCS must be used only with the realization that

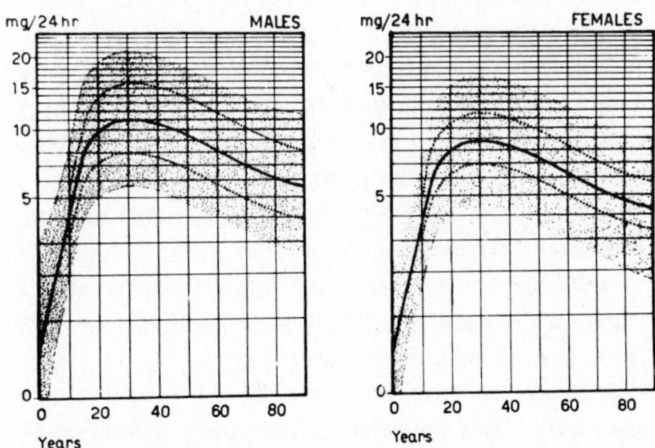

Figure 14.2. The excretion rate of 17-OHCS in healthy subjects of average body weight and height. Average values (full line), fiducial range ($P = 0.05$, shaded area), and excretion in extremely tall and heavy, and in extremely short and light, subjects (upper and lower dotted lines). (Reproduced, with permission, from Borth et al., 1957)

the steroid components of the groups are different to those normally present (sections 14.6.2 and 14.6.4).

The clinical applications of blood corticosteroid and urinary and blood oestrogen group assays cannot be considered independently from the individual steroid measurements, and they are therefore considered in the next section.

14.3. MEASUREMENTS OF INDIVIDUAL STEROIDS AND PRODUCTION RATES

For many years, a major objective in steroid endocrinology has been to produce reliable and sensitive assays for individual steroids present in biological fluids, especially for steroid hormones in blood. Problems in achieving this objective have arisen because of the relatively small concentrations present and the lack of sufficiently sensitive, selective and precise techniques for quantitation. This is the reason for the abundant literature on this subject, featuring many types of end-point including colorimetric, fluorometric, isotopic and mass-spectrometric. Most of the methods have proved highly demanding technically, and have often needed unacceptably large volumes of blood. The successful application of radioimmunoassay in this field has completely altered the situation and it is now possible to assay a very wide variety of steroids in microlitre quantities of plasma. In this section, comments will be made on individual assays which are currently of use in clinical chemistry.

Some general comments on steroid radioimmunoassay methods are pertinent, since the reader will find continuing reference to the technique in this section. General reviews dealing specifically with steroid immunoassay are available (Abraham, 1974; James and Jeffcoate, 1974; Nieschlag and Wickings, 1975) and the literature contains a large number of papers describing assay techniques. In some cases, it has proved possible to use minimal purification of the material to be assayed before submitting it to radioimmunoassay, but there is always the risk of interference by cross-reacting steroids or by unidentified substances. It is important to realise that no two samples of antisera from separate sources are identical, and also that the specificity of the antiserum may be related to the method used for separating bound and free fractions. The problem of obtaining access, either through private sources or commercially, to a good antiserum in sufficient quantity to permit continuity over a reasonable period of time, is not easily solved. It is not necessarily sufficient to know how an antiserum cross-reacts with particular steroids, since non-specific or unknown agents can reduce the specificity by interfering with the immunoassay stage. Thus, the reader who finds several papers describing rapid and specific steroid immunoassays should remember that they may only achieve their specificity because of the use of a unique antiserum, and that this reagent is unlikely to be generally available. In addition, careful appraisal of what is offered as proof of specificity is required, since this is not always convincing. These comments also apply to the use of commercial steroid kits, although manufacturers rarely offer sufficient information to enable the user to make an assessment of the specificity. The analyst and user must therefore decide what is required of the assay procedure and should be aware that analytical problems may still exist, perhaps particularly when measurements of low concentrations of steroids are being attempted.

14.3.1. Cortisol

The most widely used method for the estimation of cortisol in plasma at present is the fluorometric assay of Mattingly (1962) which is relatively simple to set up and operate and is entirely satisfactory for almost all clinical purposes. However, as discussed earlier (section 14.2.1.9), it is far from being completely specific for cortisol. The main disadvantages are the use of a strong acid reagent, and interference by spironolactone. In an endeavour to produce a more specific assay, several have been described using the protein binding principle with a plasma protein (transcortin) and tritium labelled cortisol, after the original work by Murphy (1967). However, the specificity is little better than for the fluorometric assay, with several steroids interfering, including 11-deoxycortisol, corticosterone and prednisolone. Specificity can be improved by using a preliminary extraction with carbon tetrachloride to remove 11-deoxycortisol – and incidentally providing an assay for this steroid (Spark 1971) – or by chromatography, which is inconvenient in a busy clinical laboratory. Assay kits, using transcortin are available with tritium (β)- and Se^{75} (γ)-labelled cortisol; although convenient to use, these are expensive and suffer from the foregoing limitations of specificity.

Radioimmunoassays for cortisol have been described and commercial antisera are available. If purification steps are to be avoided, it is essential to use an antiserum with high specificity for cortisol. Antisera to cortisol usually cross-react with 11-deoxycortisol, corticosterone and prednisolone. When results on individual samples using either radioimmunoassay or fluorometry were compared by Foster and Dunn (1974), little difference was found, although others have demonstrated that radioimmunoassay values are lower than those obtained with a transcortin-based assay (Farmer and Pierce, 1974; Jiang et al., 1975).

Assay by isotope dilution is very specific (Fraser and James, 1968), but is too cumbersome for the clinical laboratory.

In summary, therefore, there is still no perfect, simple measurement technique for plasma cortisol. The fluorometric assay is simple and rapid, but lacks specificity, and the use of a strong acid reagent is a disadvantage. Methods based on transcortin are a little more specific, but require special isotope counting equipment and take longer to perform. Radioimmunoassays, depending on the availability of a good antiserum, may be more specific, but take more time than the fluorometric assay. They have the significant advantage of requiring only microlitre amounts of plasma, and are therefore very suitable for paediatric work.

Urinary cortisol is best measured using a binding technique, since the simple fluorometric assay has poor specificity even though it has proved useful. A purification stage is essential if spuriously high levels are to be avoided (Ruder et al., 1972).

14.3.2. Aldosterone

Although other reliable techniques have been used, radioimmunoassay is now the procedure of choice for the measurement of plasma and urinary aldosterone. A variety of procedures has been published and although all the earlier methods used some form of chromatographic purification (e.g. paper or gel filtration chromatography) methods have recently been described which employ no purification stage and rely upon the antibody specificity. Whilst this seems adequate for urinary aldosterone, as a general rule the antisera which are at present easily available are best used in conjunction with a method employing purification. A suitable method for plasma has been published by Ito et al. (1971) and for urine (for the 18-oxo-glucosiduronate) by Langan et al. (1974).

14.3.3. Progesterone

Except for very difficult techniques using double isotope dilution and gas chromatography with electron capture, there is no real alternative to radioimmunoassay. Some authors have employed protein binding techniques using plasma protein from various species, but there are problems of specificity and protein availability. The antisera for radioimmunoassay immunogens conjugated to protein through C-11 are sufficiently specific, at least when applied to normal sera, to permit the omission of any chromatographic step, although it is prudent to include such a stage when investigating pathological sera, or sera from patients receiving drugs. Many suitable methods have been published, using the principle of selective extraction of progesterone by petroleum ether and a specific antibody (e.g. Cameron and Scarisbrick, 1973). A major application of plasma progesterone assays is in detecting ovulation, and simple and rapid techniques are available for this purpose.

14.3.4. Testosterone

Testosterone in plasma can be measured by gas chromatography and by isotope dilution techniques, but these are too complex to be generally used in the clinical laboratory, and have also been superseded, even for research purposes, by radioimmunoassay. Methods based on plasma binding proteins (sex-hormone binding globulin, testosterone-oestradiol binding globulin) can be satisfactory (André and James, 1972), but most workers now have turned to the use of antisera. No antiserum has yet been obtained which is absolutely specific for testosterone, and cross reaction occurs with dihydrotestosterone (present in sera from both males and females) and other steroids. The best antisera appear to be those derived from C-11- or C-7-conjugated antigens. To achieve complete specificity, careful preliminary chromatography is required. The method of Furuyama et al. (1970) has been found satisfactory by several workers, the interference from dihydrotestosterone normally having minimal clinical significance. By using further chromatographic separation, both steroids may be estimated (e.g. Barberia and Thorneycroft, 1974).

Techniques in which a simple extraction is made followed by radioimmunoassay, are very convenient, but depending on the method used, they will over-estimate true testosterone concentrations to some extent. This may be clinically unimportant, particularly with plasma from males, and for female samples such discrepancies are unlikely to affect the interpretation of the results.

14.3.5. Pregnanediol

For many years the chromatographic method of Klopper et al. (1955) for urinary pregnanediol was the most widely used and reliable procedure. More recently, gas chromatographic techniques have been described which are relatively simple and capable of part-mechanization. In both types of approach, an initial hydrolysis stage is required since this steroid is excreted as a glucuronoside. A typical analytical method is described by Barrett and Brown (1970). There is a decreasing requirement for urinary pregnanediol assays, now that methods for measuring plasma progesterone are available.

14.3.6. Oestradiol

It is now possible to determine oestradiol reliably in human plasma using radioimmunoassay methods. Some methods use a preliminary chromatographic separation to achieve adequate specificity, although it is apparently possible to obtain clinically satisfactory results by direct assay (Jurjens et al., 1975). As with all other immunoassays in which minimal initial purification of the sample is made, specificity is absolutely dependent upon the antibody used, and a C-6 linked antigen produces the most satisfactory antisera.

14.3.7. Paper and thin-layer chromatography

The investigation of steroid profiles in disease became practicable with the adaptation of paper chromatography to steroid analysis (Bush, 1961). The later introduction of thin-layer chromatography made it possible for profile analysis to be carried out relatively quickly without the need for any elaborate apparatus (Mitchell and Shackleton, 1969). Quantitation by reflectance scanning is adequate for diagnostic and many research purposes (relative standard deviation, approximately ±8%) but visual assessment of chromatograms is usually adequate for most purposes when a considerable excess of one or more steroids is present. Staining may be chosen so as to detect the groups of steroids of interest. The Zimmermann reagent detects 17-oxosteroids; blue tetrazolium, steroids containing a reducing group, and antimony trichloride, 3β-hydroxy-5-ene steroids.

14.3.8. Gas chromatography and mass spectrometry

Gas chromatography coupled with mass spectrometry is undoubtedly the most sophisticated technique available for the detection and measurement of steroids, both singly and in profile; however, since most steroids are unstable on the columns at the temperatures necessary, stable derivatives must first be prepared. These are usually trimethylsilyl ethers and oxime-silyl ethers. Gas chromatography alone can give excellent separation of the compounds and it is usually sufficient to identify peaks by their position. See section 14.5.2, Figure 14.5 and section 14.6.4.3, Figure 14.7. In difficult cases, however, positive identification is essential, and can best be done by passing the effluent from the chromatograph into a mass spectrometer. A computer data system is almost essential for the mass spectrometric analysis of complex steroid fractions, and with the repetitive scanning technique, the mass spectra from a steroid profile can be processed by computation in a number of ways. Identification may be either manual, or automatic from a library file. Very high sensitivity can be obtained using selected ion monitoring, and accurate quantitative assay is possible by using the mass spectrometer in peak switching mode, comparing the area of a selected peak produced by the steroid to be measured with that of a suitable epimer or other internal standard added previously. An example of this approach is shown in section 14.5.2, Figure 14.6 (Honour and Shackleton, 1977).

14.3.9. Production rates

The availability of radiolabelled steroid hormones has made possible the determination of production rates using the isotope dilution principle. The method will not distinguish the source of the hormone, therefore no distinction can be made between direct secretion and production from a peripheral precursor (e.g. testosterone from androstenedione). It is correctly described as measuring "production rates".

Either of two methods may be used. In the first, radiolabelled steroid is infused at a known, constant rate into a peripheral vein. After the infused steroid has reached equilibrium with the endogenous steroid, usually within 2 or 3 hours, a specimen of blood is withdrawn and, after careful purification, the specific activity of the steroid is determined. From the known rate of infusion and the initial and final specific activities, it is possible to calculate the rate at which new steroid is entering the plasma pool, i.e. the production rate. For a detailed discussion of the theory, the reader is referred to the papers by Tait and Burstein (1964) and Cope (1972).

The method is of general application, but there are certain specific requirements which must be met. The radiolabelled steroid should be isotopically pure and the specific activity must be known accurately. Commerically available labelled steroids may not always be satisfactory in these respects and they require special preparation before being suitable for infusion. It is essential that the infused labelled steroid has reached equilibrium with the unlabelled steroid in the plasma pool when the sample to be used for measurement is collected; to ensure this, several blood specimens are usually taken to demonstrate constant specific activity. For some steroids the method is impractical, because the time required to reach equilibrium and to ensure steady state, is too long. It is now known that many steroid hormones, e.g. cortisol, are secreted in a pulsatile fashion, and therefore anything more than a transitory steady state cannot be achieved. In these circumstances, the method cannot produce meaningful results, since it can only reflect the situation over the short period during which measurements are made; if this period is not typical, or if fluctuations in secretion are occurring, interpretation of the results is impossible. The final requirement is that the measurement of specific activity of the steroid in the plasma must be made accurately, and careful isolation of the compound is required. Since the amount present is small, this presents a major analytical problem and it is therefore best undertaken in a laboratory with considerable experience of the technique.

The second method for measuring production rates, also based on a dilution principle, requires the administration by mouth or vein of the radiolabelled steroid which is to be determined. Pure material of high specific activity is required and the amount of radioactivity administered must be known accurately. Urine is collected, and a particular metabolite of the steroid under study is isolated from the specimen and its specific activity measured. By calculation, knowing the dose administered, the specific activity of the metabolite and the period of urine collection, a production rate can be calculated. This technique is appropriate to longer term studies (24 hours or more) and allows for the possibility that secretion rates may vary over this period.

There are several criteria which have to be met. The radiolabelled steroid should be isotopically pure and the metabolite isolated must be uniquely derived from the steroid being investigated. Urine must be collected until all the radioactivity excreted in this metabolic form has appeared in the urine. The method has been employed for several steroids, including cortisol and aldosterone. Although it appears theoretically sound, it depends on the assumption that the proportion of the labelled steroid which enters the metabolite under study does not vary through the period of study, and that the labelled steroid follows precisely the same metabolic routes as the endogenous steroid. It follows that the result should be independent of the metabolite chosen, but extensive investigations have shown that this is not entirely true. It is also less easy than was thought originally to select a unique metabolite, and, for example in the case of cortisol, the secretion of cortisone has been suggested as a complicating factor. These problems, and actual comparisons of various methods for measuring cortisol production have been discussed by Zumoff et al. (1974), who concluded that true secretion rates can be measured by these isotopic methods with a maximum error of 25%.

In clinical practice, the need for measuring production rates is very limited, and although some authors have found them useful for confirming or rejecting a diagnosis in difficult cases, the alternative dynamic tests available are usually adequate.

14.4. ASSESSMENT OF ADRENOCORTICAL FUNCTION

This subject has been reviewed by Clinics in Endocrinology and Metabolism, 1972; Steinbeck and Theile, 1974; and Williams, 1974.

The major steroid hormones produced by the human adrenal cortex are aldosterone (by the zona glomerulosa) and cortisol, corticosterone, androstenedione, dehydroepiandrosterone sulphate and 11β-hydroxyandrostenedione (by the zona fasiculata and the zona reticularis). Aldosterone secretion occurs almost independently of ACTH secretion and the control mechanisms are described in section 14.5.1; it is sufficient here to state that the renin–angiotensin system and the plasma potassium concentration are probably the most important determinants. The other adrenal steroid hormones are all secreted in response to stimulation of the adrenal cortex by ACTH, and this peptide, which is synthesized in the anterior lobe of the pituitary gland, is the only agent so far recognized which will alter adrenocortical secretion of these steroids. ACTH secretion is pulsatile (Krieger et al., 1971); throughout the 24 hours (Figure 14.3), intermittent bursts of ACTH secretion occur, each followed by increases in adrenocortical steroid secretion. The effect of ACTH on the adrenal is manifested within a few minutes, and in all the studies in which estimations of peripheral concentrations of ACTH and cortisol, for example, have been made, close correspondence has almost invariably been shown. The normal pattern of ACTH secretion, and therefore of peripheral steroid levels, is now well defined with approximately 7 to 13 episodes of ACTH secretion occurring during the 24 hours, mostly during the last few hours of sleep. As much as 50% of the total cortisol produced during the 24 hour period is secreted in this relatively short period. Thus, concentrations of plasma cortisol are normally lower in the evening than in the early morning, when active pulsatile secretion is occurring.

The plasma concentration patterns of individual steroids over a period of time, depend

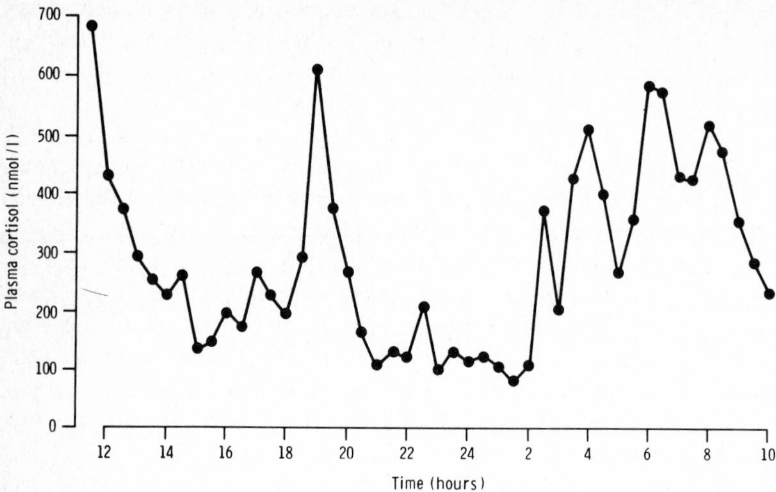

Figure 14.3. Diurnal changes in plasma cortisol in a normal subject through 24 hours.

upon their respective metabolic clearances, and when these are slow (as for dehydroepiandrosterone sulphate), the fluctuations are much smaller than, for example, with cortisol.

The release of ACTH from the anterior pituitary occurs in response to corticotrophin releasing factor (CRF), which originates in the hypothalamus and reaches the anterior pituitary via the pituitary portal circulation. Its structure has not yet been determined but it may be a polypeptide. Since release of ACTH is pulsatile, the inference is that CRF secretion is also pulsatile, but this is not necessarily so and the phenomenon may be due to other factors. ACTH release, and so presumably CRF levels, are influenced by changes in circulating cortisol concentration and by metabolic or environmental factors which are described as "stressful". It seems likely that the effect of a change in cortisol concentration is mediated at the level of the hypothalamus, and possibly the pituitary as well; high levels inhibit ACTH release and low levels permit it. Although there is some support for the view that this negative feed-back mechanism has some physiological relevance, it is mostly in evidence in pathological situations. Thus, administration of glucocorticoids therapeutically, or secretion of inappropriate amounts of cortisol by an adrenal tumour, will diminish ACTH secretion, while destruction of the adrenals (as in Addison's disease) with subsequent diminution or cessation of cortisol secretion, produces a considerable increase in ACTH secretion. It is not clear how the two mechanisms interact in normal circumstances, but it is of interest that in Addison's disease, pulsatile release of ACTH continues to occur, even though the level of plasma ACTH is elevated (Krieger and Gewirtz, 1974).

The response to "stress" has been studied extensively. Trauma, emotional disturbance, severe physical effort, hypoglycaemia and pyrexia will almost certainly initiate the discharge of CRF and cause release of ACTH, with a consequent increase in plasma cortisol levels. Again, it is not entirely clear how the negative feed-back effect and the stress response interact. It appears that release of ACTH by major stress can be blocked by glucocorticoid, but it is difficult to demonstrate this consistently, and large amounts of glucocorticoid are necessary.

This description is necessarily brief and superficial, but it is nevertheless central to any further discussion of tests of adrenocortical function which are based on the principles described above. Some comments on metabolism are also essential in this context.

About 20 mg of cortisol is produced each day by the paired adult adrenal glands. It is bound in plasma to proteins, normally 75% to the glycoprotein transcortin (or corticosteroid binding globulin, CBG), and 15% to albumin; 10% is free. Transcortin binding is relatively specific and has a fairly high association constant ($K_a = 5 \times 10^8$). Progesterone, corticosterone and the drug prednisolone will compete with cortisol for binding sites on transcortin. Albumin binding is weaker ($K_a = 1 \times 10^4$) and since many other hormones, drugs and metabolites are also bound, this binding has low specificity. The rate of synthesis of transcortin is increased by the administration of oestrogen, or during pregnancy; transcortin concentration is increased, and thus the total concentration of cortisol in plasma rises. It is only the free or unbound cortisol which is biologically active, and the changes caused by oestrogen are not usually accompanied by any marked alteration in this fraction: interpretation of cortisol levels must be made with this in mind.

Practical methods for the measurement of free cortisol in plasma have now become available and may be of considerable clinical value (Baumann et al., 1975).

Plasma cortisol concentration is determined by the rate of secretion of cortisol and the clearance:

$$\text{cortisol concentration} = \frac{\text{production rate}}{\text{metabolic clearance}}$$

Average figures for an adult subject are: plasma cortisol concentration, 150 to 600 nmol/litre (5 to 20 μg/100 ml); production rate 50 to 70 μmol/24 h (15 to 20 mg/24 h) and clearance, about 1000 litres/24 h. Since the clearance is fairly constant, changes in the secretion of cortisol are reflected rapidly and accurately by the plasma cortisol concentrations, and this is the basis for using cortisol levels in dynamic and other tests of adrenocortical function.

Cortisol is metabolized largely by the liver, and almost all of the metabolic products are excreted in the urine. Within 24 hours, more than 90% of a tracer dose of cortisol has been excreted, and thus quantitative assay of the metabolites will provide an indication of the total amount of cortisol secreted over the period of the urine collection. Since cortisol secretion is episodic, random plasma cortisol concentrations may not be easily interpreted in terms of adrenocortical activity, whereas the measurement of cortisol metabolites offers a means of integrating cortisol secretion over a period of time, normally 24 hours.

Cortisol is converted (Figure 14.4) into four major metabolites, cortol, cortolone, tetrahydrocortisol and tetrahydrocortisone. All of these compounds, which comprise about 60 to 70% of the total cortisol metabolites, are excreted as conjugates with glucu-

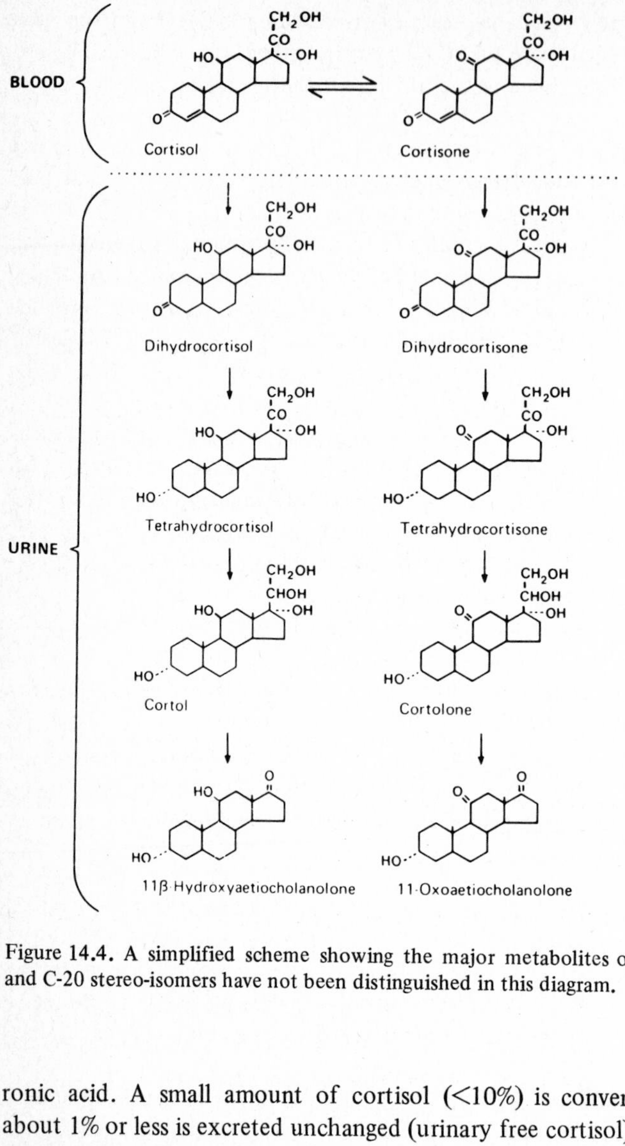

Figure 14.4. A simplified scheme showing the major metabolites of cortisol. For simplicity the C-5 and C-20 stereo-isomers have not been distinguished in this diagram.

ronic acid. A small amount of cortisol (<10%) is converted into 17-oxosteroids and about 1% or less is excreted unchanged (urinary free cortisol). This small fraction is of importance, however, since it derives from the unbound or free cortisol in plasma which passes through the glomerulus. Measurement of urinary cortisol is thus of considerable diagnostic value, indicating as it does the level of biologically active steroid in the plasma (see Cope, 1972, for a review of cortisol metabolism).

Diagnostic investigation of adrenocortical function is therefore usually based upon measurement of blood steroid concentrations, e.g. plasma cortisol, or upon the estimation of urinary steroid content, i.e. 17-oxogenic steroids or urinary free cortisol. The tests require different types of ward procedure which will be considered later. For the sake of completeness, methods have been mentioned which enable an estimate to be made, indirectly, of steroid production rates, involving the use of radiolabelled steroid tracers (section 14.3.9). In practice, there is now little clinical indication for their use.

Although it has been said earlier that in normal circumstances the secretion of ACTH and cortisol are firmly associated, and the measurement of plasma cortisol usually reveals, indirectly, the level of ACTH secretion, there are pathological situations in which dissociation occurs and the direct assay of ACTH is an invaluable diagnostic aid. It can now be measured satisfactorily by radioimmunoassay, but this is still one of the more difficult immunoassays and should ideally be carried out by an analyst with continuing experience of the method. Measurement of sub-normal levels is difficult, and in some situations the specificity of the assay is impaired. The antisera currently available will react with the ACTH molecule and also with some of its metabolic fragments. Thus in situations, e.g. surgery, in which fragmentation of the ACTH molecule occurs, these fragments cross-react and will produce an "immunoreactive" result which exceeds the concentration of biologically active ACTH present. These problems are usually of more concern in research investigations, and for diagnostic purposes the assay is adequate. When ACTH measurement is required it is important to remember that the hormone is unstable and is destroyed by excessive freezing and thawing or by allowing plasma to stand at room temperature. It is adsorbed onto glass. Laboratory advice should be sought before taking a blood sample. For a discussion of the clinical applications of ACTH assays, the reader is referred to a review by Besser (1973).

14.4.1. Investigation of pituitary–adrenal disorders

Steroid assays find their main application in this field in the investigation of primary and secondary adrenocortical hypofunction and of Cushing's syndrome. A variety of tests currently in use will be described. Only brief reference will be made to the details of the pathological disturbances in these conditions.

14.4.1.1. (a). Primary adrenocortical hypofunction (Addison's disease)
Although adrenocortical hypofunction is characterized by a number of biochemical disturbances, e.g. hyponatraemia, acidosis, hypoglycaemia, elevation of blood urea, etc., none of these is specific to this condition and none may be apparent until late in the disease process. Steroid investigations offer a definitive means of diagnosis based upon observing the response of the adrenal cortex to a challenge dose of ACTH. The response may be followed either by measuring plasma cortisol levels or urinary 17-OHCS. In practice, it is much more convenient both to the patient and to the laboratory to measure plasma cortisol. Although Addison's disease is a rare condition, the need to exclude it as a diagnosis is not uncommon and a rapid screening test is of considerable value. A convenient procedure is as follows.

No specific preparation of the patient is needed. A blood specimen is taken, followed by injection of 25 units of ACTH intramuscularly. A second blood sample is taken after 30 minutes. Both samples are analyzed for plasma cortisol for which a fluorometric assay is entirely satisfactory. When measured by fluorometry the resting level lies within the range 140 to 700 nmol/litre (5 to 24 μg/100 ml), rising at 30 minutes after stimulation to between 550 and 1100 nmol/litre (20 and 40 μg/100 ml), the increment achieved being between 200 and 700 nmol/litre (7 and 25 μg/100 ml). A response which meets these criteria is incompatible with Addison's disease. If a specific method is used for plasma cortisol, results would be expected to be about 20% lower. The results above are those expected if the test is carried out in the morning; slightly lower levels would be obtained in the afternoon. Some authors have extended the test to 1 hour instead of 30 minutes, but there does not seem to be any real advantage in doing this; only marginally higher levels are reached at this time.

It should be emphasized that this test is a screening procedure and a result which is subnormal or apparently at variance with clinical findings should be confirmed by a more prolonged test which should certainly be performed before initiating treatment. This test is made by taking a blood sample and then injecting 100 units of depot ACTH or 1 mg of depot Synacthen, followed by blood samples at 3 and 5 hours or similar convenient times. Normal subjects attain the following levels of plasma cortisol (fluorometric assay): 1 hour, 600 to 1300 nmol/litre (22 to 46 μg/100 ml); 2 hours 600 to 1500 nmol/litre (22 to 55 μg/100 ml); 3 hours 800 to 1500 nmol/litre (30 to 56 μg/100 ml); 4 hours, 1000 to 1600 nmol/litre (35 to 60 μg/100 ml); 5 hours, 1000 to 1700 nmol/litre (37 to 66 μg/100 ml).

In both the screening test and the prolonged test, patients with adrenocortical insufficiency show sub-normal responses. In Addison's disease, resting levels are usually *but not always* in the lower part of the normal range and the response to ACTH stimulation is absent. It is important to emphasise that a resting level within the normal range is not sufficient evidence on which to exclude adrenal insufficiency; some patients are able to maintain normal resting levels but are unable to respond to ACTH, and it can be disastrous to reject a diagnosis of Addison's disease because of a single, normal resting level.

It is not usually difficult to distinguish between primary and secondary adrenocortical insufficiency, but in patients with secondary insufficiency (i.e. due to lack of ACTH) adrenocortical response is usually impaired, but not absent, and in the 5-hour test a slow increase in cortisol levels occurs. If the condition is severe and long standing, then minimal responses may be seen. If there is any real problem, then measurement of plasma ACTH levels will clearly distinguish primary (high ACTH levels) from secondary (low or undetectable ACTH levels) insufficiency.

14.4.1.1. (b). Secondary adrenal hypofunction

Secondary adrenal insufficiency occurs when the adrenal cortex is deprived of ACTH stimulation; since ACTH is both steroidogenic and adrenotrophic, steroid secretion diminishes and adrenocortical atrophy occurs. This condition arises because of destruction of the pituitary (e.g. tumour) or interference with hypothalamic function causing impaired secretion of CRF. The commonest cause is corticosteroid therapy. Impairment of pituitary function may rarely be selective, but usually affects all the pituitary hormones, which show progressive and sequential failure. Gonadotrophin secretion diminishes first, followed by growth hormone, thyrotrophin and corticotrophin. It is now possible to examine selectively, in a given patient, various aspects of pituitary function (e.g. Chapter 13, section 13.3.7 for thyroid aspects). Here, pituitary–adrenal dysfunction is considered.

Two methods are used to examine the integrity of the pituitary–adrenal axis. One employs a drug, metyrapone, which exerts its action through the feed-back mechanism; the other requires the induction of a metabolic stress (hypoglycaemia), which activates the "stress" mechanism for ACTH release.

Metyrapone acts by interfering with specific stages of steroid biosynthesis within the adrenal cortex. By competing for cytochrome P_{450}, it prevents 11β-hydroxylation and thus diminishes the adrenocortical secretion of cortisol. In response to lowered cortisol concentration ACTH secretion is increased and steroid biosynthesis is accelerated, but with the production of biosynthetic precursors of cortisol, largely 11-deoxycortisol. This steroid is excreted as a tetrahydroderivative conjugated with glucuronic acid, and may be assayed as a 17-OHCS since it possesses the appropriate steroid side chain. Thus, provided that hypothalamic, pituitary and adrenal function are *all* normal, the response to administration of the drug is an increase in urinary excretion of 17-OHCS. Conversely, secondary adrenal insufficiency is manifested by an impaired excretion of 17-OHCS. An appropriate protocol is as follows – metyrapone is given every 4 hours in 6 doses of 250 mg each; urine is collected in three 24-hour periods – the day before (day 1), the day during, and the day after administering the drug. A normal response is defined as a resting level of 17-OHCS in the normal range; a value on day 2 or 3 between 23 and 46 mg/24 h and a rise of between 11 and 39 mg/24 h over day 1. A normal response can occur, rarely, in patients who by other "stress" tests show evidence of impaired pituitary function. A poor response is evidence of impaired function within the hypothalamus–pituitary–adrenal axis.

There are some disadvantages to the test. It requires complete collection of the urine specimens over a period of 3 days; some patients tolerate the drug poorly; the test is time-consuming and inconvenient on the ward; and the laboratory must have the 17-OHCS assay available. At best, it is usually several days before the clinician ordering the test is able to obtain a result from the laboratory; at worst, incomplete urine collections, failure to take the drug, drug loss by vomiting, and laboratory delays render the test less attractive than the alternative procedure which involves the production of hypoglycaemia.

To improve the efficiency of the test, several investigators have examined the possibility of using plasma assays to follow the response to metyrapone. The end-point is the level of 11-deoxycortisol achieved in the plasma, or of ACTH. Tests of this type require that maximal blocking of 11β-hydroxylation occurs, so that measurement of 11-deoxycortisol can reflect the total secretory capability of the gland. If only partial blocking occurs, measurement of only one product is misleading. Thus, although this approach is advantageous in that urine collections are unnecessary, the laboratory must be able to measure 11-deoxycortisol; but since relatively few laboratories have this capability, the test is usually performed using urinary assays.

An alternative procedure is to induce hypoglycaemia with insulin. This causes the release of ACTH and a concomitant increase in plasma cortisol which can be measured readily, with the advantage that blood samples only are required. It is quick (90 minutes), the laboratory results can usually be obtained fairly rapidly, and from the clinical point of view, the response obtained appears to be more meaningful than that given by the metyrapone test. Thus a good correlation between the response to insulin and to clinical situations, such as surgery, has been demonstrated. The disadvantages are that the test involves some degree of patient discomfort (sweating, tremor, disorientation) and some clinicians are reluctant to induce hypoglycaemia. Nevertheless, there are no reports of any untoward sequelae, and the test can always be readily terminated by intravenous glucose, if necessary. Patients with epilepsy and heart disease should not be tested in this way.

A suitable protocol is as follows – a blood sample is taken from a fasting patient using an indwelling needle; insulin is given at a dose which is appropriate to cause the blood glucose concentration to fall below 2.2 mmol/litre (40 mg/dl). This dose will depend on the tentative diagnosis, but 0.15 units/kg is sufficient in subjects with normal resistance to insulin, and 0.1 units/kg in patients with adrenal insufficiency. Blood specimens are taken at 30, 45, 60 and 90 minutes and assayed for glucose (fluoride tube) and cortisol.

Interpretation of the results is made on the basis that the blood sugar has fallen appropriately and that symptoms of hypoglycaemia have been produced. A normal response is defined as a resting cortisol concentration within the reference range, with an increment of at least 200 nmol/litre (7 μg/dl), and reaching a value of at least 550 nmol/litre (20 μg/dl). Occasionally, in an extremely apprehensive patient, or one in whom the initial venepuncture has been painful, the resting cortisol concentration may be relatively high, or even above the upper limit of normal, and the increment may then be smaller than usual. This does not present any real problem of interpretation since it clearly excludes adrenal insufficiency.

14.4.1.2. Adrenal hyperfunction – Cushing's syndrome

Cushing's syndrome occurs in patients who sustain prolonged and inappropriately high levels of glucocorticoids, which will be mainly cortisol if iatrogenic disease is excluded, since this is the only naturally occurring steroid which will cause the condition. Diagnostic tests are required to confirm the diagnosis and to indicate the underlying pathology. This may be due to excess secretion of ACTH, causing adrenal hyperplasia, or to autonomous cortisol secretion by an adrenocortical tumour. In the latter case, ACTH levels are subnormal or low. Excess ACTH secretion may occur either because of a pituitary tumour or hypothalamic lesion, or from an ectopic source, usually a carcinoma of the lung, thymus, pancreas or, less commonly, of other tissues. With regard to nomenclature, the clinical condition which arises is uniformly described as Cushing's syndrome; a pituitary or hypothalamic pathology as Cushing's disease; and if the source of ACTH is extra-pituitary, it is called the ectopic ACTH syndrome. Adrenal hyperfunction may be tested in various ways. Plasma cortisol concentration and urinary excretion of 17-OHCS and free cortisol may all be elevated in Cushing's syndrome; in severe cases, they are almost invariably abnormally high. Impaired carbohydrate tolerance and a hypokalaemic alkalosis also occur, the hypokalemia usually correlating with the severity of the condition.

Patients with severe Cushing's syndrome do not normally present any real clinical problems of diagnosis; difficulties usually arise when the clinical findings are equivocal. Plasma cortisol concentrations fluctuate, sometimes quite markedly in Cushing's syndrome, and random values are very difficult to interpret. The normal diurnal variation is lost, but this may not be easily established by occasional measurements. It must be remembered that elevated levels occur in anxious patients and also because of treatment with oestrogens (including oral contraceptive drugs), cortisol or ACTH. Spironolactone produces spurious elevation of cortisol concentrations as determined by fluorometric assay.

Conversely, low or normal values may be found by chance in patients with Cushing's syndrome because of the episodic release of cortisol which still occurs in this condition. Urinary steroid excretion, as indicated by 17-OHCS, is more consistently raised above normal, as would be expected. However, normal or only marginally raised values do occur and pose problems of interpretation. The most consistent indicator of adrenal hyperfunction involving cortisol is the urinary excretion of free cortisol. This assay, provided that it is made as specifically as possible, is without doubt the method of choice in establishing a diagnosis (Burke and Beardwell, 1973). It is particularly useful in excluding obese patients, who show normal excretion of urinary free cortisol. These findings are, of course, consistent with the postulate that urinary cortisol reflects the concentration of free cortisol in plasma. The usefulness of the assay is enhanced as an indicator of hypercortisolaemia because transcortin is saturated with cortisol when cortisol concentrations exceed the upper limit of normal; there is then an "amplification effect" when relatively large amounts of cortisol appear in the urine.

Other dynamic tests are also helpful in establishing a diagnosis. They depend upon the fact that synthetic glucocorticoids, like cortisol, will inhibit the release of ACTH through the negative feed-back mechanism and thus diminish cortisol secretion (Liddle, 1960). Either blood or urine tests may be used. For the blood test, 2 mg of dexamethasone is given orally in the evening and a blood specimen for cortisol assay is taken the next morning (08.00 to 10.00 hours). If the concentration of plasma cortisol at this time does not exceed 140 nmol/litre (5 μg/dl), a diagnosis of Cushing's syndrome is unlikely. The converse is not true, since over-anxious subjects, and some obese or psychologically disturbed patients may not show complete suppression. The urinary test requires measurement of the 24-hour excretion of 17-OHCS on a control day and then on 2 days during which dexamethasone (0.5 mg) is given every 6 hours. On the second day, less than 5 mg/day of 17-OHCS should be excreted.

It is important to distinguish between adrenocortical tumour (adenoma or carcinoma) and adrenocortical hyperplasia which is secondary to either a pituitary or an ectopic source of corticotrophin. If plasma ACTH determinations are available, then the measurement is a valuable diagnostic aid. Normal levels of ACTH range up to about 80 pg/ml. The values are low in patients with adrenal tumour, and high or in the upper part of the normal range, in patients with adrenal hyperplasia. The distinction between Cushing's disease (i.e. adrenal hyperplasia caused by a pituitary source of ACTH) and the ectopic ACTH syndrome cannot be made definitively on biochemical grounds, but in the ectopic syndrome, the plasma ACTH level is often very high (more than 300 pg/ml) and the plasma potassium concentration is often low and associated with high values for urinary 17-OHCS, urinary free cortisol, and plasma cortisol.

The estimation of urinary 17-OS is not very helpful. Values slightly higher than, or within the upper part of the reference range are found in pituitary-dependent cases; a markedly elevated level strongly suggests adrenal carcinoma, and a low normal or normal level will usually be found in adenoma (James, 1961).

McKenna et al. (1977) have shown that four out of six patients with an adrenal carcinoma had raised concentrations of plasma 17-hydroxypregnenolone, whereas values were within the normal range in patients with hypercortisolaemia due to Cushing's disease, ectopic ACTH or adrenal adenoma.

Although measurement of the plasma ACTH concentration is highly desirable if the assay is available, it is possible to obtain some indication of the pathology from dynamic tests. Administration of ACTH will not usually alter the plasma concentration or urinary steroid excretion in patients with adrenal tumour, but often does so in patients with hyperplasia. The exceptions occur in the ectopic ACTH syndrome, where maximal adrenocortical secretion may already exist. If ACTH tests are performed, they are best done on a short-term basis, so that acute response may be observed. Otherwise, the prolonged stimulation may activate atrophic tissue in patients with adrenal tumour and cause increased cortisol production.

Some investigators have used metyrapone as a diagnostic aid; in general the response is as indicated above for the administration of ACTH (Burke and Beardwell, 1973). A dexamethasone test, may also prove useful. A dose of 2 mg is given orally, every 6 hours for 2 days. Urinary 17-OHCS excretion is measured on a control day and on the second day of the test. Patients with pituitary-dependent Cushing's syndrome usually show some suppression, to values which are 50% or less of the control, whereas patients with adrenal tumour or with the ectopic ACTH syndrome show no marked change in steroid excretion.

The above tests will usually define fairly well the type of pathology involved, especially when combined with investigative procedures such as radiology of the skull and adrenal angiography. The latter technique, especially if combined with adrenal catheterization to permit the measurement of adrenal vein steroid concentrations, will often enable the clinician to localize correctly an adrenal tumour before surgery.

In summary, it is usually possible, using biochemical methods, to establish a diagnosis and the pathology in patients with Cushing's syndrome with a fair degree of confidence. The most useful measurements are those of urinary free cortisol, plasma ACTH and, where possible, adrenal vein steroid concentrations. (For general coverage see Binder and Hall, 1972).

14.5. ALDOSTERONE AND THE CONTROL OF ELECTROLYTE METABOLISM

This subject has been reviewed by Glaz and Vecsei, 1971; Ross, 1975; and Stockigt, 1976.

14.5.1. Mechanisms controlling aldosterone production

There is no evidence that aldosterone is produced in any way other than by direct secretion from the adrenal cortex. With a normal sodium intake, aldosterone is produced at a rate which ranges from 100 to 500 nmol/24 h (30 to 150 μg/24 h) in normal individuals. Through its direct effect upon the renal tubular transport of sodium, it controls extracellular volume and it is the major regulator of potassium metabolism, since hydrogen ions and potassium are exchanged for sodium in the renal tubule under the influence of aldosterone. Other mineralocorticoids are of much lower potency and are normally far less important than aldosterone (e.g. aldosterone is 25 to 100 times more active than 11-deoxycorticosterone, depending upon the test employed). However, quantitative aspects are important in this respect and although cortisol is mol for mol a relatively weak mineralocorticoid, it exerts a significant effect on electrolyte metabolism because of the relatively large amount which is secreted in comparison with aldosterone. In addition to its action on the distal convoluted tubule, aldosterone acts on sweat glands, the salivary ducts and the gastrointestinal mucosae, causing reabsorption of sodium. Enzymic defects affecting the production of aldosterone are dealt with in section 14.6.6.7.

The control of aldosterone production is complex, but is mediated mainly through the renin–angiotensin system described in Chapter 9, sections 9.1.3 and 9.4.3. Sodium retention is stimulated indirectly by a deficiency in extracellular fluid volume, and vice versa. Alterations in electrolyte balance have an effect on the secretion of aldosterone. It is likely that changes in sodium balance exert their effect through the renin–angiotensin system, whereas potassium may exert its action by a direct effect on the adrenal cortex. It has been suggested that a small increase or decrease in plasma potassium concentration is effective in increasing or decreasing aldosterone secretion so that the extracellular potassium concentration may be an important physiological regulator (Himathongkam et al., 1975; Dluhy et al., 1977). Thus, the plasma aldosterone concentration is increased by potassium loading, and potassium loss is accelerated through enhancement of the potassium–sodium distal tubular exchange. ACTH in pharmacological doses can produce an increase in aldosterone production but it seems likely that this mechanism only plays a minor role. Nevertheless, there is evidence that physiological fluctuations in plasma ACTH levels may significantly alter aldosterone secretion in normal man (Nicholls et al., 1975); indeed diurnal fluctuations in the plasma concentrations of cortisol and aldosterone are positively correlated in supine man, suggesting a common determinant (James et al., 1976). Such a clear correlation does not exist with plasma renin levels (Katz et al., 1975). Kowarski et al. (1975) found a weak, but significant correlation between aldosterone and cortisol in four out of seven subjects tested during normal activity. Ganguly et al. (1977b) have shown that 11β-hydroxylase activity appears to parallel changes in ACTH secretion, and though angiotensin stimulates steroidogenesis of corticosterone and aldosterone, it has no apparent effects on 11β-hydroxylase activity.

Since maintenance of the volume of circulating fluid is so vital for life it is scarcely surprising that more than one mechanism exists for the stimulation of aldosterone production, or indeed that aldosterone is not the only substance concerned with the regulation of body sodium.

14.5.2. Clinical investigation (see Chapter 9, section 9.4.3 for renal aspects)

The main call upon the laboratory for the investigation of aldosterone metabolism arises in the study of patients presenting with hypokalaemic hypertension, in whom a diagnosis of hyperaldosteronism may be in question. Measurements of aldosterone, its metabolites, and renin in body fluids are difficult to perform and therefore it is necessary before requesting such assays, to confirm the presence of an abnormality in electrolyte and water balance. Dysfunction of aldosterone production, however, cannot be finally diagnosed without hormone assay since electrolyte metabolism is influenced by a number of factors and organs.

Careful measurement of the plasma potassium concentration is probably the simplest and most useful initial procedure in the investigation of suspected hyperaldosteronism.

Blood specimens must be collected on several occasions with extreme care, avoiding forearm exercise. Patients with hyperaldosteronism almost invariably show at least one value below 3.7 mmol/litre (J.J. Brown et al., 1968). The urinary potassium is inappropriately high, and usually exceeds 40 mmol/24 h. The hypokalaemia is associated with an alkalosis and the plasma total carbon dioxide concentration may exceed 30 mmol/litre.

If other causes for potassium depletion are excluded (diarrhoea, purgatives, liquorice, diuretics), further biochemical investigation is indicated.

It is important that the collection of blood for the measurement of aldosterone or renin is made under strictly controlled conditions, i.e. having ensured a normal intake of sodium and potassium, and with the patient recumbent and having been lying down quietly for the previous 2 hours. The most useful procedure is to take blood after overnight bed rest before the patient achieves the upright posture. Hypokalaemia may make interpretation difficult, because it will lower the plasma aldosterone concentration; attention to the dietary intake of potassium before the test is carried out is important. Various reference ranges for total plasma aldosterone concentration have been reported, using different methods of measurement, but 14 to 400 pmol/litre (5 to 15 ng/dl) may be taken as trypical finding using modern techniques. The plasma concentration is 2 to 3 times higher during pregnancy (Smeaton et al., 1977) but the reason for this is not known; the level of aldosterone in the foetal compartment is even greater than in the maternal. Some details of assay techniques and production rate measurements have been given in section 14.3.2.

In patients with hyperaldosteronism, the plasma aldosterone concentrations are usually elevated, but it may be necessary to repeat the investigation on more than one occasion, since aldosterone secretion is episodic both in normal subjects and in patients with hyperaldosteronism. Thus values may fall within the normal range in patients with established hyperaldosteronism.

Urinary excretion of aldosterone or its metabolites is theoretically a more satisfactory investigation because it "integrates" the episodic changes which occur in aldosterone production. There is no advantage in attempting to measure the small amount – less than 3 nmol/24 h (1 μg/24 h) – of unconjugated aldosterone in urine. Unlike urinary free cortisol, it is no more useful in diagnosis than the measurement of other metabolites. The 18-oxo-glucosiduronate of aldosterone represents about 10% of the total metabolites produced and about 15 to 60 nmol (5 to 20 μg) per 24 h is excreted. It is this metabolite, together with the small amount of free aldosterone, which is commonly measured, and relatively simple radioimmunoassay methods are now available for this purpose. It is important that a fresh urine specimen should be submitted for analysis, and that it be preserved by addition of boric acid (10 ml of 10% boric acid to the 24-hour specimen); spuriously low results may be obtained on old or unbuffered urines.

Tetrahydroaldosterone is excreted in a considerably larger quantity – up to 300 nmol (100 μg) per 24 h –, but unless the expensive technique of gas chromatography-mass spectrometry (GC-MS) is used, there is a danger of interference from tetrahydro-18-hydroxy-11-dehydrocorticosterone (18-hydroxy-THA). This is a metabolite of 18-hydroxycorticosterone which appears to be secreted by the adrenal cortex in a constant relative amount to aldosterone. Figure 14.5 shows how GC-MS was used to detect a high concentration of tetrahydroaldosterone in the urine of an infant presumed to have renal-tubular

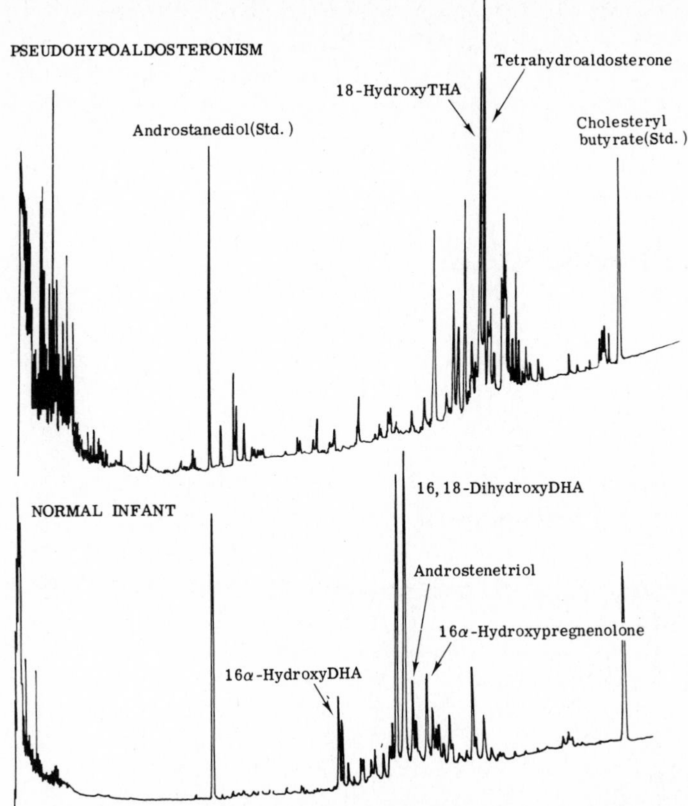

Figure 14.5. Gas chromatographic profile analysis of the urinary steroids of a normal infant 6 weeks of age and of a 4-week-old infant with renal tubule unresponsiveness to aldosterone (pseudohypoaldosteronism). The steroids were gas chromatographed as their methyloxime trimethylsilyl ethers on a glass capillary column. The major abnormalities in the patient were inappropriately low excretion of 3β-hydroxy-5-ene steroids and excessive excretion of 18-hydroxytetrahydro-Compound A (18-hydroxy-THA) and tetrahydroaldosterone. It is of particular interest to note the high excretion of 16,18-dihydroxy-DHA in the normal infant (two peaks caused by *syn-* and *anti-*forms of the oxime derivative). This compound is often the major steroid excretory product although its range of excretion is very wide. (Personal communication from Dr. C.H.L. Shackleton)

unresponsiveness to the hormone. This figure illustrates the difficulty of separating aldosterone from 18-hydroxy-THA even with capillary colums of high resolving power. Figure 14.6 shows the use of GC-MS double ion monitoring for the selective detection and measurement of tetrahydroaldosterone (by comparison with an added internal standard, 3β-5α-tetrahydroaldosterone). The two ions were selected from the mass spectrum of the methyloxime-trimethylsilyl ether for monitoring because of their masses and specificities. These techniques require special equipment and expertise and are not generally available for diagnostic purposes.

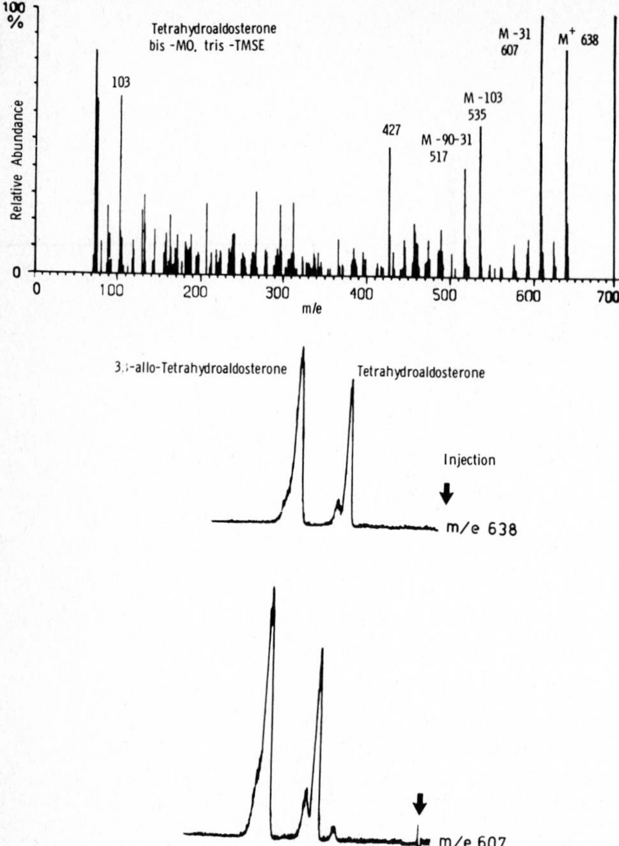

Figure 14.6. Quantitation of tetrahydroaldosterone by gas chromatography-mass spectrometry. The mass spectrometer was adjusted to switch between two ions (*m/e* 638 (parent ion) and 607) present in the mass spectrum of the methyloxime silylether of tetrahydroaldosterone. The peak area produced by tetrahydroaldosterone MO-TMSE was related to that of the internal standard 3β-5α-tetrahydro-aldosterone. (Reproduced, by permission, from Honour and Shackleton, 1977)

14.5.3. Primary aldosteronism, hypermineralocorticism and hypertension

Conn was the first to recognize the symptoms of the excessive production of aldosterone in 1956; Conn's syndrome now refers to the clinical condition which is produced by an adrenal adenoma secreting excessive amounts of aldosterone. The findings in this condition are hypokalaemia, causing muscle weakness and tiredness, and hypertension associated with headache and nocturnal polyuria caused by impairment of renal concentrating ability. The incidence of the syndrome is low (0.5 to 2% of unselected hypertensive patients).

Biglieri et al. (1972) delineated four types of hypertension as being associated with the excessive production of mineralocorticoids.

(i) Aldosterone-producing adenoma, in which plasma renin activity is subnormal and removal of the adenoma usually leads to a correction of the abnormality. This group is the largest, comprising about 75% of the patients.

(ii) Idiopathic hyperaldosteronism, in which the adrenal glands are micro- or macronodular, or may even be normal in appearance. Bilateral adrenalectomy seldom corrects the hypertension though it can correct hypokalaemia and hyperaldosteronism. This condition accounts for about 15% of the patients.

(iii) Indeterminate hyperaldosteronism, in which deoxycorticosterone administration will suppress and normalize aldosterone production.

(iv) Glucocorticoid-remediable hyperaldosteronism, in which therapy with glucocorticoids restores normality including normalization of aldosterone levels. This is a rare condition which occurs particularly in children. Some findings indicate that a steroid other than aldosterone, so far unidentified, may play a major role in ACTH-induced hypertension (New et al., 1976; Sann et al., 1976; Hoefnagels et al., 1978). Abnormalities in excretory rates, plasma concentrations and clearances of several individual adrenal steroids have been reported, but no clear primary defect which would explain the hypertension has been demonstrated (Honda et al., 1977). Glucocorticoids may be suppressing an undiscovered central system.

Surgery is usually successful in condition (i) but not in (ii), so that differential diagnosis is important. There are a number of ways in which this problem may be approached: these include direct attempts at visualization of the pathological process by angiography or venography, or by catheterization of the adrenal veins to enable the steroid levels in adrenal venous effluent to be determined; by the use of radiolabelled cholesterol to demonstrate accumulation of the isotopic material in an adenoma; or by less direct techniques which depend upon the measurement of various parameters or employ various dynamic tests. None of the techniques is ideal; they either carry some risk, or are technically demanding, or the results may be inconclusive.

Where the appropriate expertise is available, radiographic studies, isotope uptake and adrenal vein catheterization can collectively provide extremely useful information and will often indicate the pathology with some degree of certainty. The venous drainage of the adrenal gland is often complex and it is by no means simple for even an experienced operator to ensure that the appropriate vein is catheterized. It is essential that both aldosterone and cortisol are measured in the specimens obtained and due comparisons made with the concentrations in a specimen of peripheral blood taken at the same time. In a patient with an aldosterone-producing adenoma, the specimen from the affected side usually shows a high concentration of aldosterone compared with either the contralateral or peripheral values, whereas the cortisol concentrations in both adrenal vein specimens should be substantially higher than the peripheral value. Where these conditions are met, the diagnosis and localization can be made with some degree of confidence. In the case of adrenal hyperplasia, no clear-cut difference is seen between the concentrations of aldosterone in the two adrenal vein specimens although these are usually higher than the peripheral value. Again, appropriate interpretation depends upon the finding that the plasma cortisol concentrations in the adrenal vein specimens are appropriately high. If the plasma cortisol concentration is low, then interpretation should be made with great caution since findings may indicate that the catheter was not placed within the adrenal vein.

The indirect approaches depend upon the observations that patients with aldosterone-producing adenomas show more marked deviations from normality in a number of biochemical findings, than do those with hyperplasia, and that different control factors appear to be predominant in these two groups of patients. Using a so-called quadratic analysis, which combined the results of aldosterone, sodium, potassium, bicarbonate and renin measurements, Aitchison et al. (1971) were able to make a distinction between adenoma and hyperplasia; the method has not been widely used. Patients with aldosterone-producing adenoma tend to differ from those with hyperplasia in that they show a paradoxical fall of plasma aldosterone concentration on assuming the upright posture. In contrast, patients with hyperplasia, like normal subjects, show an increase in plasma aldosterone concentration (Ganguly et al., 1973). More recently, interest has focussed upon the finding that the plasma concentration of aldosterone is lowered by treatment with dexamethasone in patients with aldosterone-producing adenoma, so it appears that aldosterone production in these patients is to some extent ACTH-responsive. Acute administration of dexamethasone produces a fall in plasma aldosterone levels in patients with aldosterone producing adenoma, but there is a subsequent return to high levels of plasma aldosterone despite continued suppression of plasma cortisol. This could be due to an intrinsic alteration of aldosterone synthesis in the adenoma during prolonged ACTH suppression (Ganguly et al., 1977a).

Thus the differentiation of condition (i) from (ii) still presents difficulty, and the pathogenesis of the latter is obscure. A slightly greater degree of physiological control appears to obtain in condition (ii) since there tends to be less severe hypokalaemic alkalosis with a lower concentration of aldosterone and a higher level of renin than in (i). It is possible that the changes in the adrenal glands may be caused by, rather than the result of, the hypertension.

In condition (iii), the easy suppression of aldosterone production with deoxycorticosterone, the mild nature of the hypertension (which is easily treated with spironolactone) and the lack of evidence of potassium depletion are all deterrents to adrenal surgery.

Currently then, the approach to investigating these conditions of patients is as follows. First, to determine the electrolyte and acid–base status of the patient and ensure that adequate supplementation with potassium has been given. Second, to evaluate aldosterone production by plasma aldosterone or urinary aldosterone measurements, with subsequent confirmation that plasma renin levels are suppressed. Third, to achieve differential diagnosis by means – ideally – of a combination of expert radiography, adrenal vein catheterization and isotope studies; less satisfactorily, by studies of the effects of posture change and treatment with dexamethasone.

For the sake of completeness, mention should be made of the group of patients with hypokalaemic hypertension and with suppressed renin levels, but with normal production of aldosterone. In this condition, it is postulated that there is abnormal production of an unusual mineralocorticoid, e.g. deoxycorticosterone, and a considerable amount of work has gone into attempts to confirm this hypothesis. So far, this has not been a very successful approach and only very rarely is it possible to establish the presence of an unusual mineralocorticoid. In occasional patients, excessive production of corticosterone (Fraser et al., 1968) or deoxycorticosterone (J.J. Brown et al., 1972) occurs, but more important examples of increased secretion of deoxycorticosterone causing hypertension and hypokalaemia occur in the 11β- and 17α-hydroxylation deficiency conditions (section 14.6.6).

Recently, deficiency in steroid reductive metabolism has been implicated in the production of hypertension (Ulick et al., 1977).

Primary aldosteronism can occur with carcinoma of the adrenal cortex, but less than 20 cases have been recorded to date. A few cases have been reported of unilateral hypertrophy of the zona glomerulosa, ectopic aldosterone-secreting adenoma and malignant ovarian tumour.

In cases of Cushing's syndrome, especially those resulting from adrenal malignancy or due to ectopic corticotrophin, high levels of deoxycorticosterone and corticosterone can make a major contribution, in addition to cortisol, to the hypertension and potassium depletion.

14.5.4. Secondary aldosteronism

Conn, in 1956, used the expression "secondary aldosteronism" to describe the effects of excess secretion of aldosterone due to a stimulus outside the adrenal cortex which interfered with the normal production control mechanism. The major causative factor is the lowering of circulating volume, for which the commonest reason in modern society is diuretic therapy; this, when combined with a low salt intake, can for a few days cause a considerable rise in aldosterone production with increases in plasma renin and angiotensin concentrations. However, any reduction in plasma potassium concentration caused by therapy may later depress the aldosterone secretion rate.

The catabolism of aldosterone occurs mainly in the liver; thus in chronic liver disease, or with venous congestion of the liver due to heart failure, the clearance of aldosterone from blood is impaired. This is not necessarily compensated for by a decrease in secretion rate – indeed, an actual increase may occur and a raised plasma concentration of aldosterone may ensue.

A raised production of aldosterone is found in the nephrotic syndrome, often together with increased plasma concentrations of renin and angiotensin. Decreased plasma volume and renal blood flow are probably causative factors.

Aldosterone excretion is raised, and secretion rates have also been reported to be raised, in congestive heart failure, but it is sometimes not clear whether these effects are due to the disease or to drug treatment or other therapy. As before reduced renal blood flow is probably causative. Plasma renin and angiotensin concentrations are variable, possibly due to liver involvement interfering with the catabolism of aldosterone.

14.6. STEROID METABOLISM IN PREGNANCY, THE PERINATAL PERIOD AND IN INFANCY

Until the early 1960s, it was generally assumed that the major changes which occurred in steroid metabolism during pregnancy emanated almost entirely from the placenta. It is now known that the foetus also plays an important role and that there is a strong interrelationship and inter-dependence between the foetus, placenta, maternal endocrine glands and the mother as a whole. Each entity cannot be studied in isolation: after birth, and for many months, the infant continues to produce and excrete compounds which in utero were intended specifically for further metabolism by the placenta.

14.6.1. Physiological background

Mitchell (1967) and Mitchell and Shackleton (1969) have reviewed the general physiological background to steroid metabolism in pregnancy, the perinatal period and infancy.

During uterine life, the foetal adrenal gland grows to a considerable size. It is composed mainly of the so-called foetal zone which, until birth, is responsible for producing large quantities of C-19 steroids with the 3β-hydroxy-5-ene configuration. The total concentration of these compounds in umbilical cord blood is higher than that of any other steroid – apart from cholesterol – in human blood at any time, but the reason for their formation and presence in such large quantities is not known. The aromatization of many of these steroids to produce oestrogens may be solely a catabolic pathway which has little or no biological significance. After birth, when presumably activities necessary in utero are no longer required, the adrenal gland undergoes striking anatomical changes, involving involution of the foetal zone, as it adapts from the type of steroid production necessary in utero to that required for independent life. Many enzymes concerned with steroid metabolism are present in the foetus but not in the placenta and vice versa: thus, 3β-hydroxydehydrogenase, the aromatizing enzymes and sulphatase are all very active in the placenta, but not in the foetus; while enzymes for synthesizing the steroid nucleus, together with 16-hydroxylase and sulphokinase, are very active in the foetus and not in the placenta. Hence in steroid synthesis the foetus and placenta act together; for example, in the synthesis of oestrogens the foetus produces dehydroepiandrosterone sulphate, which in part is 16α- and 16β-hydroxylated, mainly in the foetal liver. The hydroxylated compounds then travel by the umbilical circulation to the placenta where they are aromatized to form the major source of oestrogen in the latter stage of pregnancy. Further 16-hydroxylation may later take place again in the foetus. The artierio-venous difference in the concentration of, for example, 16α-hydroxydehydroepiandrosterone and 16-oxo-androstenediol in the umbilical cord (10,700 nmol/litre (350 μg/dl) arterial and 8,200 nmol/litre (270 μg/dl) venous), indicates the considerable uptake of the placenta (Mitchell and Shackleton, 1969). Dehydroepiandrosterone from the maternal circulation can also be converted into oestrogen. The aromatizing power of the placenta increases progessively throughout pregnancy, paralleling the increase in urinary oestrogen excretion. Placental tissue up to the fifth month of gestation is capable of 16-hydroxylation, but the activity of the enzyme decreases to zero at term; this indicates a shift to a different pathway for the synthesis of oestriol, utilizing material which is already 16-hydroxylated. The activity of 16-hydroxylase is particularly striking in the foetus, but after birth its activity diminishes 10-fold over the first 10 weeks, after which it is at the same level as in adults. The importance of foetal liver 16-hydroxylase was demonstrated in the case of a pregnancy associated with cirrhosis of the foetal liver: the ratio of oestriol to oestrone plus oestradiol in the maternal urine was 1.3:1 compared with 10:1 in a previous normal pregnancy (Coyle, 1962). Enzymes for 15- and 18-hydroxylation are also very active in the foetus, producing precursors of pregnancy urine oestetrols (Taylor and Shackleton,

1977). In fact 16,18-dihydroxydehydroepiandrosterone is frequently the major neutral steroid excreted by infants, often exceeding even 16α-hydroxydehydroepiandrosterone and 16α-hydroxypregnenolone (Fig. 14.5).

Compared with its major role in the production of oestrogens, the foetus does not appear to be significantly involved in the synthesis of progesterone in pregnancy, since the concentration of pregnanediol, which is its characteristic metabolite in urine, can remain high in the mother's urine, or actually rise after the death or removal of the foetus. Progesterone is produced by the placenta almost entirely from maternal cholesterol, although foetal pregnenolone could play a minor role since there is a measurable arterio-venous difference in concentration of this steroid in umbilical cord blood.

14.6.2. Pregnancy

Various aspects of steroid metabolism in pregnancy are considered in other chapters, but it is pertinent to gather together here information relating directly to foetal activity and pregnancy.

Except in the early part of pregnancy, oestriol production roughly parallels the size of the foetus or of the foetal adrenal glands. In cases of hydatidiform mole, foetal death or anencephaly, where the foetal adrenal is of negligible size, the maternal urinary oestrogen excretion is one-tenth to one-fourth of the value found in normal pregnancy, being produced almost entirely from maternal precursors. Thus the level of oestrogen in the mother's urine may be used to monitor the well-being of the foetus. The normal pattern of excretion of oestriol in pregnancy is dealt with in Chapter 15. The ratio of urinary oestriol to oestrone and oestradiol is much higher in late pregnancy than in non-pregnant women for two reasons: firstly, the foetus actively metabolizes oestradiol to oestriol; and secondly, as explained in section 14.6.1, oestriol is produced by the placenta and foetus using synthetic pathways which do not necessarily involve other oestrogens.

When it was shown tht 15-hydroxylase was apparently active in the foetus and not in the mother, it was thought for some time that the estimation of oestetrol in maternal urine would be a more specific measure of foetal viability than oestriol, some of which is of maternal origin. However, this has not so far proved to be a fruitful approach (Taylor and Shackleton, 1977).

In pregnancy, the urinary excretion of dehydroepiandrosterone, etiocholanolone and androsterone is reduced, and, to a slightly less extent, that of 11-hydroxy-17-oxosteroids. The apparent small increase in total 17-oxosteroids, as normally measured, is almost certainly due to the presence of Zimmermann chromogens with polarities lower than that of androsterone (section 14.2.2.1).

14.6.3. Infancy

Since the experimentation which may be done on human foetuses and infants is very limited for ethical reasons, information for research has been sought and obtained in a variety of ways, no matter how indirect. Consequently, though much has been learnt, it must be stressed that current understanding of the very complex steroid picture is still incomplete and that the clinical significance of many of the aspects is not known.

Three populations of steroids may be considered to exist in infants at birth.

(i) Large amounts of oestrogen and progesterone which have been transferred from the placenta; they themselves, together with compounds arising from their metabolism, will be excreted in rapidly decreasing quantity since their source has been eliminated.

(ii) A large quantity of 3β-hydroxy-5-ene steroids which have been produced for the special requirements of uterine life, and which continue to be formed for some time after birth; their excretion in urine may actually increase during the first month, when the so-called Δ^5-steroids predominate both quantitatively and qualitatively over all others.

(iii) Cortisol and other steroids which are necessary for independent life and which must continue to be produced and metabolized.

Thus for several months after birth, there is a complex and changing pattern in the steroid content of blood and urine against which it is difficult to identify any abnormality (Cathro et al., 1963).

The types of specimens which are available for study at or shortly after birth comprise: amniotic fluid which may be collected at birth; blood, approximately 50 ml of which may be obtained from the severed umbilical vein and 15 ml from the artery; smaller quantities of blood which may be obtained from the infant itself; meconium and, later, faeces; and urine collected over 24 hour or shorter periods.

Amniotic fluid collected at birth is seldom used for routine investigations since more positive information may be obtained from the infant's urine; when obtained by amniocentesis before birth, amniotic fluid analysis can give an indication of steroid production and excretion in utero (Chapter 15). The study of arterial and venous cord blood has produced much valuable information for research, but again it has not been used to any extent for purposes of diagnosis. Blood from the infant cannot reasonably be obtained in sufficient quantity for detailed steroid fractionation except when exchange transfusions are carried out; in general, therefore, it can only be used for sensitive group steroid analysis or radioimmunoassay. Relatively large quantities of steroids are excreted in meconium but little information has been obtained from this source for research purposes and none which might be of diagnostic use. Thus, infant urine is left as the main source of information on any abnormality of steroid metabolism.

14.6.4. The investigation of infant urine

The collection of urine directly from newborn infants is not easy; for female infants it is extremely difficult. A cholostomy bag may be used with some success for males, or special attachments may be obtained. Alternatively steroids may be extracted successfully from disposable diapers provided that they contain little material which interferes with steroid measurement. Undoubtedly the use of such diapers greatly increases the practicability and accuracy of urine collection.

14.6.4.1. Oestrogens

Steroids received from the placenta in utero are largely cleared by the fifth day of life. In order, presumably, to deal with the large quantities of oestrogen received from the placenta, oestrogen catabolism in the foetus and infant is much more rapid and efficient than in the adult; oestradiol is actively hydroxylated and a much smaller proportion of oestriol received or produced, is excreted as such. Its excretion falls from about 20 μmol/24 h (7000 μg/24 h) on day 2, to 0.02 μmol/24 h (6 μg/24 h) on day 5. On the whole, measurement of the oestrogens at this time has little clinical significance.

14.6.4.2. Progesterone metabolites

Since it has been estimated that approximately the same amount of progesterone goes from the placenta to the foetus as to the mother, large quantities of its major metabolite in adults – pregnanediol – might be expected in infant urine. However, little or none is found, possibly because the infant is deficient in A-ring reducing enzymes. The relative absence of pregnanediol in the infant is perhaps fortunate since it inhibits the conjugation of bilirubin with glucuronic acid.

14.6.4.3. 3β-Hydroxy-5-ene steroids

The large quantities of these steroids which are excreted during infancy are shown in Table 14.1 in comparison with adult values. The majority of steroids are present as 3β-sulphates, and it is possible that such sulphate conjugation is important in their biosynthetic role in utero (Einarsson et al., 1976). The change with age in the excretion pattern in normal infants may be clearly seen in the results of capillary column gas chromatography (Figure 14.7). There is a steady reduction in the excretion rates of those steroids which are not normally excreted in adulthood, until they are undetectable at 9 months after birth. They can be made to fall to undetectable amounts by means of dexamethasone suppression therapy, thus indicating adrenal origin. The excretion of 21-hydroxypregnenolone must not be taken to indicate a deficiency of 17α-hydroxylase, but possibly the existence of an alternative pathway for cortisol synthesis, with 3β-hydroxy-dehydrogenase acting at a later stage. It will be important to discover whether the large quantities of the 3β-hydroxy-5-ene steroids (mostly 16-hydroxylated) excreted for many weeks after birth are produced for some purpose, or whether their presence is incidental, and due solely to degenerating enzyme systems, the activities of which are no longer required.

14.6.4.4. Corticosteroids

The excretion of 17-hydroxycorticosteroids measured as Porter–Silber chromogens (section 14.2.1.4) around day 7 is approximately 0.5 mg/24 h (2 mg/m^2 surface area per 24 h, compared with the corresponding figure of 3.1 mg for adults). By the Norymberski technique (section 14.2.1.2) the excretion is less than 4 mg/24 h. The make-up of the steroid group, however, is very different from that found in adults, and this must be borne in mind in any interpretation of group measurements.

The change in the pattern of excretion of corticosteroids in infants may be seen by studying the findings from capillary column gas chromatography, as already indicated in Figure 14.7. The comparison may also be demonstrated more simply by thin-layer chromatography (Mitchell and Shackleton, 1969).

Much less cortisol administered to infants is recovered as steroid glucosiduronate than in adults, and alternative forms of excretion, such as highly polar steroids (which are excreted in free form) and sulphate conjugates assume greater importance. Taylor et al. (1978) have identified several of the major metabolites of cortisol in infants. Quantitatively 1β- and 6α-hydroxytetrahydrocortisone and 1β- and 6α-cortolone (both α and β)

TABLE 14.1

EXAMPLES OF THE URINARY EXCRETION OF STEROIDS BY DIFFERENT INFANTS 6 WEEKS TO 9 MONTHS OF AGE, AND ADULTS (μg/24 h)

ND means that the steroid was not detected. Information, by permission, from Shackleton et al. (1973) and private communications from Drs. J. Honour and C.H.L. Shackleton. To convert approximately to μmol/24 h multiply results for pregnenes and pregnanes by 0.003 and androstenes by 0.0034.

Steroid — Age Urine volume (ml)	6 week 350	8 week 420	8 week 300	11 week 270	4 month 380	4.5 month 135	5 month 250	6 month 490	9 month 230	Adult
16α-Hydroxy-DHA	117	139	37	240	7	10	22	11	ND	580
16β-Hydroxy-DHA, 16-oxo-androstenediol	120	51	28	187	11	15	45	11	ND	315
5-Androstene-3β-16α-17β-triol	340	230	130	195	217	120	100	23	100	598
5-Androstene-3β-16β-17α-triol	52	60	18	37	ND	ND	ND	ND	ND	239
5-Pregnene-3β,20α-diol	26	16	27	24	140	48	125	29	241	407
5-Pregnene-3β,20β-diol	16	13	18	12	87	87	79	24	176	–
16α-Hydroxypregnenolone	129	207	58	250	36	15	12	11	24	55
21-Hydroxypregnenolone	25	40	ND	35	ND	ND	ND	ND	ND	104
5β-Pregnane-3α-17α-20α-triol	11	5	4	9	46	32	28	15	119	130
5-Pregnene-3β,20α-21-triol	46	73	20	46	50	25	22	15	ND	230
5-Pregnene-3β,16α-20α-21-tetrol	96	45	23	50	65	28	ND	ND	ND	–
Tetrahydrocortisone	118	320	127	300	130	400	352	258	715	3520
Tetrahydrocortisol	ND	ND	95	ND	85	120	138	87	510	1560
α-Cortolone	23	158	34	32	106	111	131	106	280	1120
β-Cortolone + β-cortol	112	156	62	107	78	61	122	79	162	1130
α-Cortol	ND	ND	15	ND	18	29	83	18	190	290
Total steroid (1)	1246	1531	717	1536	1107	1123	1319	711	2557	
Total of 16-oxygenated steroid (2)	854	732	294	959	336	188	179	56	124	
Total pregnenediols (3)	42	29	45	36	227	135	204	53	417	
Total cortisol metabolites (4)	253	634	333	439	417	721	851	548	1857	
Ratio 2/3	20.3	25.2	6.5	26.6	1.5	1.4	0.9	1.0	0.3	
Ratio 4/1	0.2	0.4	0.5	0.3	0.4	0.6	0.6	0.8	0.7	

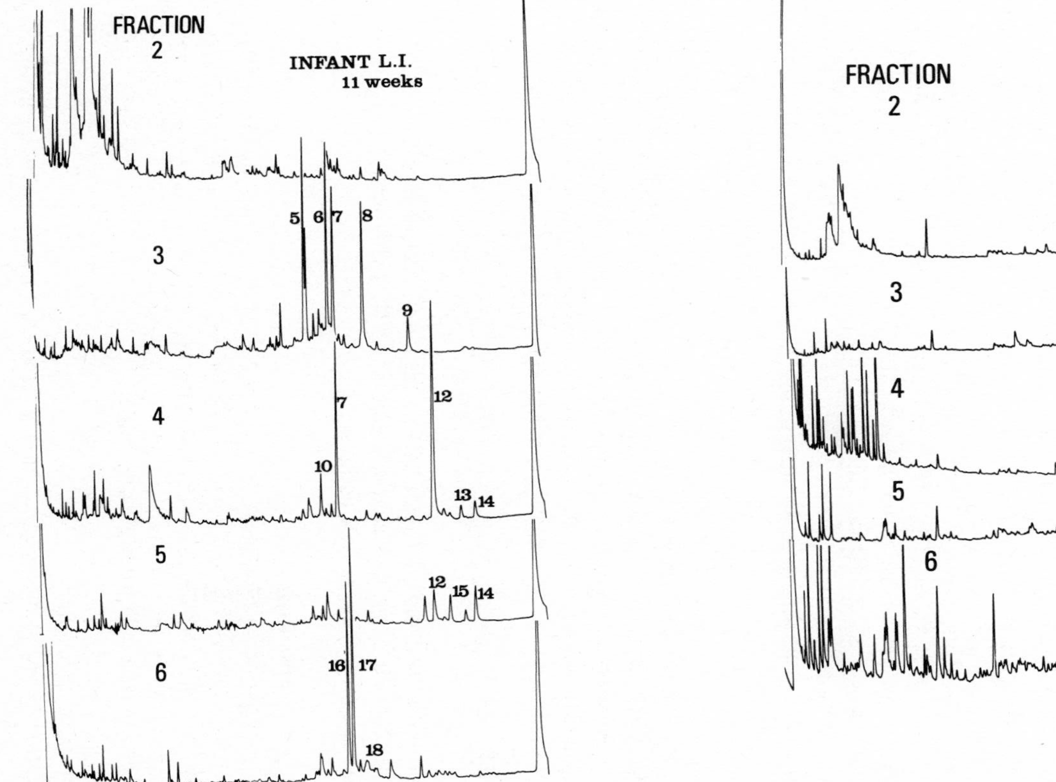

Figure 14.7 a (left) and b (right). The separation of urinary steroids (as methyloxime trimethylsilyl ethers) by capillary column gas chromatography from (a) infants aged 11 weeks, and (b) infantes aged 9 months. Prior to gas chromatography the urinary extracts were fractionated on Sephadex LH-20. The identity of each of the peaks indicated is as follows: (1) 5-pregnene-3β,20α-diol; (2) 5-pregnene-3β,20β-diol; (3) pregnanetriol; (4) 21-hydroxypregnenolone; (5) 16α-hydroxy DHA (two peaks); (6) 16-oxo-androstenediol; (7) 5-androstene-3β,16α,17β-triol; (8) 16α-hydroxy-pregnenolone; (9) 5-pregnene-3β,20α,21-triol; (10) 5-androstene-3β,16β,17α-triol; (11) tetrahydrocorticosterone; (12) tetrahydrocortisone; (13) α-cortolone; (14) β-cortolone; (15) 5-pregnene-3β,16α,20α,21-tetrol; (16 and 17) 16,18-dihydroxy-DHA (two peaks given by *syn*- and *anti*-forms of the methyloxime derivative; (18) some androstenetetrols (3, 16, 17, 18 and 3, 15, 16, 17); (19) tetrahydrocortisol and 5α-tetrahydrocortisol (broad peaks caused by underivatized 17α-hydroxyl); (20) cortols. The final peak in the chromatograms is from cholesteryl butyrate. (Reproduced, by permission, from Shackleton et al., 1973).

were the most important, apart from tetrahydrocortisone and α- and β-cortolone. In addition, many C-5 and C-20 dihydro metabolites were detected. Metabolites of cortisol retaining the 11β-hydroxyl group were noticeably reduced, compared to later life.

The increased amount of corticosterone relative to cortisol in infant urine has already been mentioned in section 14.2.2.2. It is not known whether additional corticosterone is present for a biological purpose or whether it is produced as a by-product from the different relative activities of steroid synthesizing enzymes obtaining in infancy.

14.6.5. The investigation of infant blood

The measurement of Porter–Silber chromogens in urine (section 14.2.1.4) has indicated a rapidly falling excretion pattern over the first 5 days. However, when cortisol is assayed in blood by a specific double isotope derivative dilution technique, the level is similar to that in adults, and changes little during the first 5 months. There is a low cortisol/cortisone ratio.

The cortisol production rate shows little change over the first 10 weeks when corrected for body surface area, although the values are approximately 50% higher than in adults. The corticosterone production rate during the first 2 months, when corrected for surface area, is more than 3 times that in adults. The considerable increase in transcortin binding in maternal plasma caused by oestrogen and leading to very high levels of total cortisol is not found either in the foetus or infant despite the presence of high levels of oestrogens.

The concentration of testosterone in circulating blood at birth is in the low adult range for male infants, but higher than the adult range for female infants. In both sexes, the concentration falls during the first week of life. In the male infant, there is then a sharp rise until at 30 to 60 days the values are similar to those at birth. There is no such rise in the female infant. This indicates that testicular activity is still present at birth, the transient fall probably being due to the removal of chorionic gonadotrophin followed by activation of the hypothalamic pituitary axis by negative feed-back (Forest and Cathiard, 1975).

14.6.6. Abnormalities in steroid production

Possible defects in steroid synthesis, some of which have been reviewed by Visser (1966) and Bongiovanni et al. (1967), are indicated in Figure 14.8. They will be discussed in the order in which they occur on the synthetic pathway.

14.6.6.1. Lipoid adrenal hyperplasia

In this disorder, cholesterol accumulates in the adrenal glands due to a deficiency in the side-chain splitting enzyme (desmolase) which is responsible for converting cholesterol into pregnenolone. There is adrenal insufficiency and the cortex is hyperplastic and yellow. Little or no information is available on the steroid excretion pattern. Camacho et al. (1968) have described a mild form of the disorder.

14.6.6.2. 3β-Hydroxylase deficiency

This deficiency is rare (Bongiovanni et al., 1967). It is always associated with salt loss.

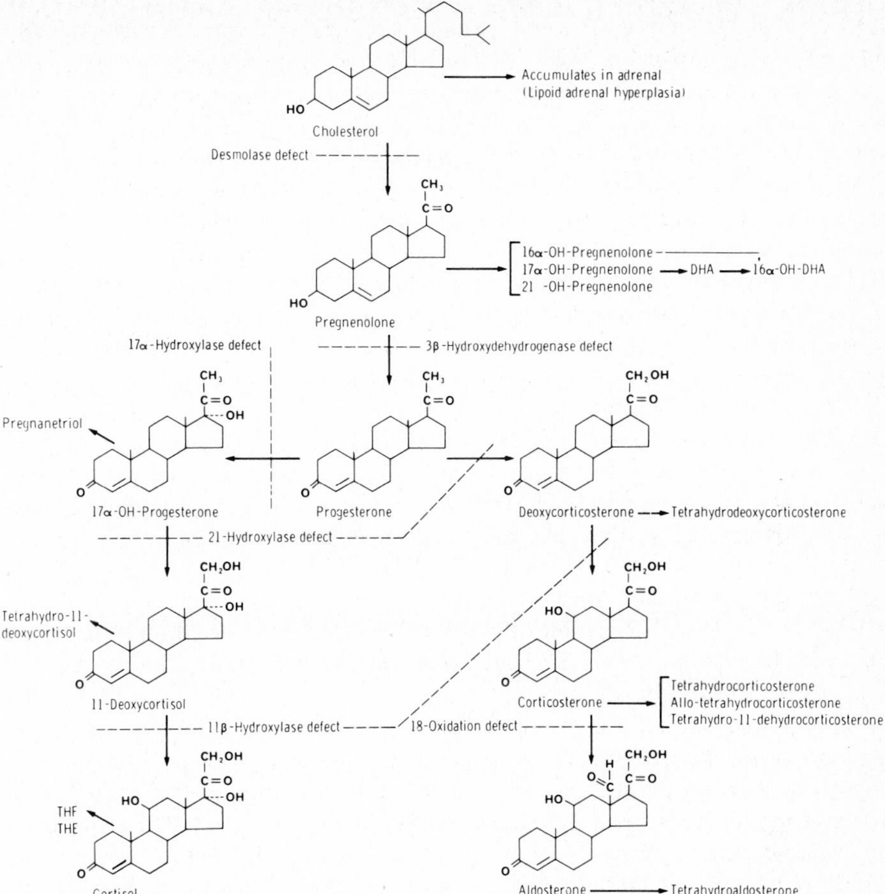

Figure 14.8. Pathways for the synthesis of cortisol, corticosterone and aldosterone showing the enzyme defects that may occur. (Redrawn from Mitchell and Shackleton, 1969)

Androgens are deficient in early embryonic life, leading to incomplete genital structures in male infants, although production of the weak androgen dehydroepiandrosterone may cause slight virilization in females. Since newborn infants normally excrete large quantities of the 3β-hydroxy-5-ene compounds which are produced before the block in the steroid synthetic chain, early diagnosis is difficult. Above normal excretions in infants of dehydroepiandrosterone and 17α-hydroxypregnenolone have been suggested as indicating the disorder. A high excretion of 5-pregnene-3β-17α-20α-triol may give the best indication of the disorder.

14.6.6.3. 17α-Hydroxylase deficiency

17-Hydroxylation is essential for the synthesis of cortisol, oestrogens and androgens, so that in cases with complete deficiency of the enzyme system (Biglieri et al., 1972), mineralocorticoids would be the only adrenal steroid hormones produced.

The syndrome may not be recognized until puberty when patients show hypertension, hypokalaemia, and primary amenorrhoea or male pseudohermaphroditism. Cortisol may be almost absent and the resulting increased production of corticotrophin leads to an increased output of those steroids which can be produced – corticosterone, deoxycorticosterone, 18-hydroxycorticosterone and progesterone. Plasma renin is reduced and aldosterone may not be detectable, probably because the increased activity of adrenal mineralocorticoids causes sodium retention and increased blood volume. Glucocorticoid treatment corrects the hypertension, hypokalaemia and abnormal production of mineralocorticoids, and promotes natriuresis. However, care must be taken in the early stages of treatment in patients with very low concentrations of aldosterone and cortisol, since a lag in increasing the production of aldosterone can lead to a hypovolaemic crisis.

A study has been made of the steroid excretion patterns of eight patients with 17α-hydroxylase deficiency (Shackleton et al., 1978) and it was interesting to find that 10 to 40% of the corticosterone metabolites present in urine had undergone 21-dehydroxylation by intestinal microflora. It was also shown, by means of highly sensitive gas chromatographic-mass spectrometric methods, that small amounts of C-19 steroids and cortisol metabolites were invariably found, indicating that the deficiency is never complete.

14.6.6.4. 21-Hydroxylase deficiency

A blockage in the 21-hydroxylation of pregnenolone (Mitchell and Shackleton, 1969) is responsible for 90% of all cases of congenital adrenal hyperplasia. The efficiency of androgen production is not affected, and because of a lack of suppression in the pituitary feed-back mechanism, virilization is a feature of the disease, with testosterone production rates in infants and children as high as 32 μmol/24 h (11,000 μg/24 h), the normal being less than 1.5 μmol/24 h (500 μg/24 h). The virilization of female patients at birth is probably due to excessive testosterone production at the time of male/female differentiation during the third month of pregnancy. Typical of the disease is the production of large quantities of 17α-hydroxyprogesterone, the compound produced immediately prior to the enzyme block. It is largely metabolized to pregnanetriol, and diagnosis is made by the detection of either or both compounds in abnormally high quantity in the urine. The excretion of 17-oxosteroids is increased, due more to overproduction of dehydroepiandrosterone and androstenedione than to the metabolism of C-21 steroids. Figure 14.9 shows a comparison of capillary column gas chromatograms of urinary extracts from a normal adult and from an adult patient with a deficiency of 21-hydroxylase. In this patient, there was a marked decrease in the metabolites of cortisol and a considerable increase in output of pregnanetriol.

One-third of patients with the disorder are termed "salt-losers"; they have an abnormally high excretion of sodium chloride with low plasma sodium and high plasma potassium concentrations. It will be seen from the pathways in Figure 14.8 that production of aldosterone can be interfered with in 21-hydroxylase deficiency and its secretion rate is indeed low in "salt-losers". If dietary sodium is reduced in normal infants and children, a 2- to 3-fold increase can be elicited in the production rate of aldosterone and in its excretion or that of its metabolites in urine: only insignificant increases can be demonstrated in "salt-losers". The reason for there being the two types of congenital adrenal hyperplasia – salt-losing and simple virilizing – is unknown.

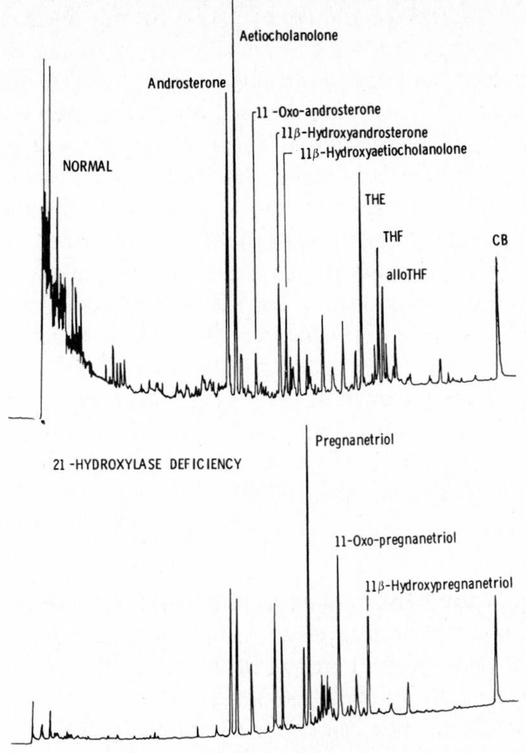

Figure 14.9. Chromatogram traces produced by capillary column gas chromatography of urinary steroids (as methyloxime trimethylsilyl ethers) from a normal adult and an adult patient with a steroidal 21-hydroxylase defect. (Personal communication from Dr. C.H.L. Shackleton)

Although pregnanetriol is the major urinary steroid metabolite in the disorder in adults and older children, it may be undetectable in infants with the defect unless highly sensitive and specific methods are used (Shackleton, 1976).

The work of Atherden et al. (1974) indicates that the estimation of 17-hydroxyprogesterone in plasma may provide a reliable method for confirming the diagnosis of 21-hydroxylase deficiency during the neonatal period: in nine infants aged 6 to 12 days with congenital adrenal hyperplasia, the concentrations ranged from 100 to 800 nmol/litre (3.4 to 25 μg/dl), compared with less than 70 nmol/litre (2.1 μg/dl) in 50 normal infants aged 10 hours to 15 days. The measurement of pregnanetriol in infant urine by many of the techniques normally used for adult urine is most unreliable because of the presence of many interfering substances. As shown in sections 14.6.4.3 and 14.6.4.4, its identification and measurement must be made against a pattern of steroid metabolism which is very different to that obtaining in adults. The production of 3β-hydroxy-5-ene steroids can be very greatly increased (more than 35 mg/24 h excreted in the urine) due to the pituitary feed-back control mechanism releasing large quantities of corticotrophin. There can be gross abnormalities, which are difficult to understand, in the excretion pattern of these steroids (Shackleton et al., 1972). If at all possible, it is preferable to delay the final diagnosis of any disorder in steroid metabolism until approximately 6 months after birth, when the production of steroids by the adrenal cortex has assumed the adult pattern. If necessary, the infant may be treated with steroid substitution therapy during this time, and for the study of urinary steroid output, placed on dexamethasone (2.5 mg daily) and fluorocortisone (0.1 mg daily), possibly with added salt by mouth – drugs which will not obscure the endogenous urinary steroid pattern – while adrenal function is stimulated by injections of long acting corticotrophin (40 units once daily). In these circumstances, it may take the adrenal 1 to 2 weeks to respond fully. It need scarcely be emphasized that since a steroid metabolic disorder requires replacement therapy for life, correct diagnosis is of the utmost importance.

21-Hydroxylase deficiency is an autosomal recessive disorder in which there are no apparent physical or biochemical abnormalities in the heterozygous carrier. They may be distinguished, though not infallibly, by measuring the concentration of plasma 17-hydroxyprogesterone after ACTH stimulation (Lee and Gareis, 1975).

14.6.6.5. 11β-Hydroxylase deficiency

This disorder is associated with virilization and hypertension, and low levels of aldosterone have been reported. 11-Deoxycortisol is present in excess in plasma, and large quantities of the tetrahydro metabolites of 11-deoxycortisol and 11-deoxycorticosterone are found in the urine, together with increased etiocholanolone and pregnanetriol.

Some findings suggest that the deficiency may be a cause of low-renin essential hypertension (Brown et al., 1972) and that 11β-hydroxylase activity may be under the influence of ACTH (Ganguly et al., 1977b).

14.6.6.6. Adrenal hypoplasia

Acute adrenal insufficiency in infancy may result from congenital adrenal hypoplasia, either isolated or in association with hypoplasia or absence of the pituitary gland. It must be suspected in a second pregnancy after a previous birth of an infant with such a disorder. Its presence in a foetus is indicated by a low maternal oestrogen excretion during the later part of pregnancy, due to a lack of oestrogen precursors produced by the foetus. It may be confirmed by finding a low concentration of cortisol in the umbilical cord blood. The urinary excretion rates for 16α-hydroxydehydroepiandrosterone, 16-oxo-androstenediol and 16α-hydroxypregnenolone have been reported to be one-tenth of the values expected in normal newborn infants. However, adrenal hypoplasia may affect only the production of mineralocorticoids and 3β-hydroxy-5-ene steroids. Thus Shackleton and his co-workers (personal communication) have studied a patient whose urinary steroid excretion pattern at 3 days of age, displayed the presence of only saturated metabolites of progesterone and cortisol (Figure 14.10), there being no detectable 3β-hydroxy-5-ene steroids or metabolites of corticosterone. The total excretion of cortisol metabolites was about 2 mg/24 h, a figure in excees of the amount normally excreted. It therefore seems probable that in normal individuals the foetal zone is responsible for synthesis of important precursors only of the mineralocorticoids.

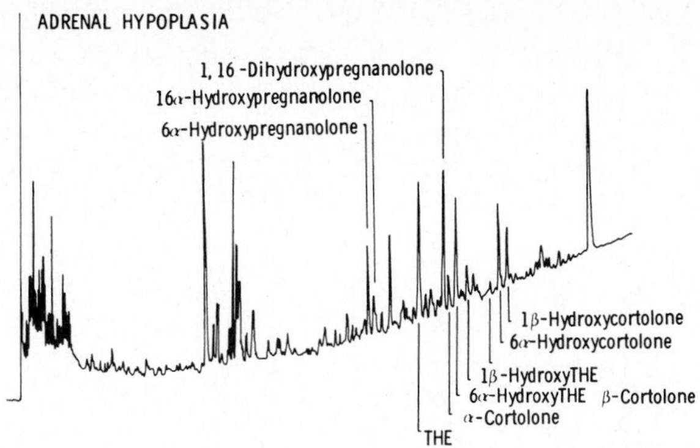

Figure 14.10. Steroid excretion by a 3-day-old infant with adrenal hypoplasia. The major steroids excreted were metabolites of progesterone (e.g. 6α-hydroxypregnanolone and 1,16-dihydroxypregnanolone) or cortisol (tetrahydrocortisone, the cortolones and 1β- or 6α-hydroxy metabolites of tetrahydrocortisone or the cortolones). Only trace amounts of 3β-hydroxy-5-ene steroids were detected. (Personal communication from Dr. C.H.L. Shackleton)

14.6.6.7. Defects in aldosterone production

A congential 18-hydroxylation defect gives rise to the salt-losing syndrome. Adrenal hyperplasia does not take place since cortisol production and the pituitary feed-back mechanism are not affected. The excretions of 17-oxosteroids and cortisol metabolites are normal, but the urine contains abnormally large quantities of 17-deoxy C-21 steroids (corticosterone and its metabolites) as shown in Figure 14.11. The excretion of 18-hydroxycorticosterone in an infant studied by Ulick et al. (1964) indicated a defect in the oxidation of this compound. Little or no aldosterone or its metabolites are found. The excessive production of corticosterone and its metabolites is probably due to over-production of renin which has been found in increased amounts in the plasma of patients during sodium depletion. The defect is not necessarily permanent, since patients have been reported in whom treatment with salt and 11-deoxycorticosterone acetate could be withdrawn after a few years. It has been suggested (Visser, 1966) that this transient hypoaldosteronism is caused by delayed maturation of the zona glomerulosa, and that the permanent form of the disorder is due to deficiency of the enzyme system. Rösler et al. (1977) suggest that clinical variability with age, in the manifestiation of aldosterone deficiency, is not due entirely to changes in hormone secretion rate, but also to a changing biological requirement; thus aldosterone deficiency during the first year of life may have disastrous consequences, but may be well tolerated in adult life. Plasma aldosterone concentration is not a reliable index of the disorder since some patients achieve normal values through the high activity of plasma renin. The best diagnostic index is an enhanced ratio of the urinary metabolites of glomerulosa zone 18-hydroxycorticosterone and aldosterone.

18-Hydroxycorticosterone can originate from both the glomerulosa and fasciculata zones of the adrenal cortex. Abnormally high production from the fasciculata occurs in cases with a 17α-hydroxylase defect, where enhancement of the pathways of corticoster-

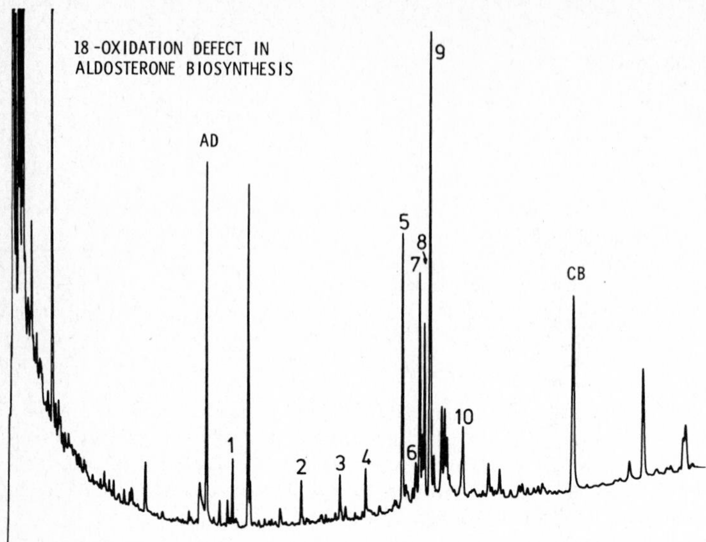

Figure 14.11. Capillary gas chromatographic analysis of urinary steroids (as methyloxime trimethylsilyl ethers) excreted by a 6-month-old infant with 18-oxygenation defect. The following steroids are indicated: AD and CB internal standards 5α-androstane-3α,17α-diol and cholesteryl butyrate; (1) androsterone; (2) 11β-hydroxyandrosterone; (3) 5-pregnene-3β,20α-diol; (4) 5-pregnene-3β,16α,20α-triol; (5) tetrahydrocortisone; (6) tetrahydrocorticosterone; (7) 5α-tetrahydrocorticosterone; (8) tetrahydrocortisol; (9) 5α-tetrahydrocortisol and (10) hexahydrocorticosterone. The peaks between (9) and (10) and α- and β-cortolone and a second peak of 5α-tetrahydrocorticosterone. The peak following androsterone (1) is an impurity present in the N-trimethylsilylimidazole. (Reproduced, by permission, from Shackleton et al., 1976)

one production leads to over-production of 18-hydroxycorticosterone. In this disorder, the high concentration of circulating 11-deoxycorticosterone leads to suppression of glomerulosa zona secretion. The two sources of production can be readily distinguished since the glomerulosa zone activity is easily suppressed by dexamethasone (Ulick, 1976).

The mechanism of biosynthesis of aldosterone from corticosterone has been proposed (Ulick, 1976) to be a two-stage reaction. A disorder involving the first step would lead to over-production of corticosterone only, but interference in the second step would give rise to an increase in both corticosterone and 18-hydroxycorticosterone. Ulick suggested that the nomenclature for the disorders should be: corticosterone methyl oxidase defects, type 1 and type 2.

14.7. INVESTIGATION OF ANDROGEN METABOLISM

Androgens are secreted directly by the adrenal cortex and by the gonads. The definition of an androgen is somewhat arbitrary and is usually taken to refer to certain naturally occurring C-19 steroids. These include testosterone and its metabolic product dihydrotestosterone; androst-5-ene-3β,17β-diol; 5α-androstane-3α,17β-diol; androstenedione;

androsterone; 11β-hydroxyandrostenedione, and dehydroepiandrosterone. It seems highly probable that testosterone and dihydrotestosterone are biologically the most important of these steroids, although both androstenediol and androstanediol are active androgens in some biological tests. General reviews of androgen metabolism are available in several monographs (James and Andre, 1974; Brooks, 1975; Clinics in Endocrinology and Metabolism, 1975). Androgen metabolism is complex; the inter-related metabolic pathways of the compounds involved have made it extremely difficult to use the estimation of urinary steroid metabolites as an index of the relevant steroid production rates. Most of the important recent progress in our understanding of androgen physiology and pathology has arisen from the use of radiolabelled tracers and from the development of methods, mostly radioimmunoassay, for measuring androgen concentrations in blood. In addition, it has become clear that the conversion of testosterone into dihydrotestosterone is an essential step in the expression of the androgenic activity of testosterone at the cellular level, and also that binding of testosterone to a specific plasma protein is an important factor in relation to the metabolism of this steroid.

Studies of radiolabelled androgens have shown that in addition to direct secretion, the production of androgens from precursor steroids can occur as an extra-glandular process; the conversion of androstenedione into testosterone is a particularly important example, and androstenedione is properly regarded as a "pre-hormone" in this context (Horton and Tait, 1966). Both the adrenal gland and the ovaries produce androstenedione, and in women the indirect production of testosterone is quantitatively much more important than is direct secretion.

The testes are the main source of androgens in adult men, about 19 μmol (7 mg) of testosterone being secreted daily. About 1.5 μmol (500 μg) of dihydrotestosterone is produced, largely from testosterone, although a little is secreted directly. Androstendione is derived mainly from the adrenal glands and conversion into testosterone is a relatively unimportant phenomenon in normal men, but may be significant in hypogonadism. In women, about 0.7 μmol/24 h (250 μg/24 h) of testosterone is produced, about 60% of which arises by conversion from androstenedione. Both the adrenals and the ovaries secrete similar amounts of androstenedione, and together they produce about 9 μmol/24 h (3 mg/24 h); the ovary may contribute more at mid-cycle.

In plasma, testosterone is largely bound to protein; only about 2% is unbound in men and 1% in women. Non-specific binding by albumin accounts for 40% of the bound fraction in men and 60% in women. The remainder is bound with high specificity and high affinity to a specific plasma protein, testosterone–oestradiol-binding protein (TEBG). As the name implies, this will also bind oestradiol. TEBG levels are decreased by androgens and increased by oestrogens, which explains why elevated levels of total testosterone occur in pregnancy and in patients receiving oestrogens, and why TEBG levels are lower in men than in women. Protein binding also influences metabolic clearance, since only the free and the albumin-bound fractions are easily cleared; hence metabolic clearances of testosterone are higher in men (1000 litre/day) than in women (600 litre/day). (For a review of TEBG activity see Anderson, 1974.)

The control of androgen secretion is not well understood. Androstenedione of adrenal origin is secreted in response to ACTH, and the plasma concentration follows that of cortisol. Leydig cells respond to stimulation by luteinizing hormone by increasing their output of testosterone; conversely, with deprivation, testosterone secretion diminishes. However, in contrast to the ACTH–cortisol mechanism, this process is sluggish, and responses require hours rather than minutes. Ovarian secretion of androstenedione is largely from the stroma, and it is not clear how this is influenced, if at all, by external factors.

The plasma testosterone concentration fluctuates throughout 24 hours, and secretion appears to be pulsatile. At any one time, swings of 30% on either side of the mean value may be found. The reason for this is entirely obscure. Studies in which luteinizing hormone and testosterone have been measured on repeated blood samples taken over an extended period have failed to show any correlation, suggesting that the hormone is not the mediator of these fluctuating steroid levels. The exception to this statement occurs in pubertal boys in whom sleep-associated bursts of hormone secretion do appear to relate to changes in plasma testosterone. Some authors have claimed that there is a diurnal rhythm in plasma testosterone concentrations; others have denied this, but it seems clear that any rhythm, if it exists, is not well marked and is certainly less pronounced than that seen for cortisol and androstenedione. Thus blood sampling for investigative purposes should be made with these points in mind, and there is nothing to be gained from taking specifically timed blood specimens.

In normal female subjects, using specific assay techniques for testosterone, plasma concentrations between 290 and 1700 pmol/litre (10 and 60 ng/dl) are found. The highest values are found at the time of mid-cycle. In men, concentrations range from 9000 to 13,000 pmol/litre (300 to 1100 ng/dl). Measurements have also been carried out in children (Ducharme et al., 1976). Plasma dehydroepiandrosterone was found to rise significantly between 6 and 8 years in girls and between 8 and 10 years in boys; in both sexes there was a further significant increase between 10 and 17 years. In neither sex was there a significant increase in plasma testosterone concentration until 12 years of age.

From the previous discussion, it will be clear that it may be necessary to make a fairly extensive investigation if androgen metabolism in a patient is to be properly evaluated. In practice, only measurements of plasma testosterone and 17-oxosteroid excretion are easily available; studies of protein binding, metabolic clearance and steroid interconversions require special facilities.

Requests are commonly made for androgen investigations in female patients with hirsutism, who sometimes demonstrate other clinical features of virilism. In the largest group, with "idiopathic" hirsutism, these features may include associated oligomenorrhoea, but manifestations of androgenicity other than hirsutism are usually lacking. It now seems likely that the cause is hypersecretion of testosterone and/or androstenedione by the ovary and/or the adrenal cortex. The increased secretion of androgen diminishes the concentration of TEBG, so that only minor increases in plasma testosterone concentration occur and many of these women have values which may be acceptable as normal. Some have polycystic ovaries, and in these women, androgen secretion is usually higher and plasma testosterone levels are increased, compared with women in whom no gross ovarian abnormality can be demonstrated.

There is a very large amount of literature describing various stimulation and suppression tests which attempt to define the pathology in patients with idiopathic hirsutism. However, so far it has not been convincingly demonstrated that any particular protocol will indicate accurately an adrenal or ovarian lesion; certainly, measurement of peripheral concentration of plasma testosterone does not appear to offer any useful information. On a few occasions, attempts have been made to catheterize and collect blood samples from ovarian and adrenal veins; by estimating the concentration of androgen it has been possible to demonstrate in this way that in particular patients one or both of the organs is secreting excess androgen (Kirschner and Jacobs, 1971). However, this is not a routine investigation, nor is it without risk. The information obtained is likely to contribute little to the treatment of the patient, so that the approach is rightly regarded as a research, rather than a diagnostic procedure.

Estimation of peripheral plasma testosterone concentration can be very helpful in the investigation of virilized patients, who may have an ovarian tumour. These are uncommon, but both arrhenoblastomas and hilar cell tumours can produce testosterone and may be too small to be discovered by other investigations. Indeed, they may only be detectable on ovarian section. The few reports in the literature record plasma testosterone values in or above the male range. Urinary 17-oxosteroid excretion is not necessarily increased and is often within normal limits. Administration of dexamethasone usually produces no change in plasma testosterone concentration. It is not possible to distinguish an adrenocortical tumour from an ovarian tumour on this basis, but adrenal tumours produce extremely large amounts of C_{19} steroids, with very high levels of urinary 17-oxosteroids; such findings should then direct attention to the adrenal glands. Radiography, venography or catheterization may be helpful in defining the site of the lesion.

REFERENCES

Abraham, G.E. (1974) Radioimmunoassay of steroid in biological materials. Acta Endocrinologica (Copenhagen), Suppl. 183, 1–42.

Aitchison, J., Brown, J.J., Ferris, J.B., Fraser, R., Kay, A.W., Lever, A.F., Neville, A.M., Symington, T. and Robertson, J.I.S. (1971) Quadric analysis in the preoperative distinction between patients with and without adrenocortical tumor in hypertension with aldosterone excess and low plasma renin. American Heart Journal, 82, 660–671.

Anderson, D.C. (1974) Sex-hormone-binding globulin. Clinical Endocrinology, 3, 69–96.

André, C.A. and James, V.H.T. (1972) A method for the assay of testosterone and androstenedione in human female plasma by competitive protein binding. Clinica Chimica Acta, 40, 325–333.

Appleby, J.I. and Norymberski, J.K. (1954) The indirect determination and identification of urinary 17-hydroxy-20-oxosteroids unsubstituted at $C_{(21)}$. Biochemical Journal, 58, xxix.

Appleby, J.I., Gibson, G., Norymberski, J.K. and Stubbs, R.D. (1955) Indirect analysis of corticosteroids. I. The determination of 17-hydroxycorticosteroids. Biochemical Journal, 60, 453–460.

Atherden, S.M., Edmunds, A.T. and Grant, D.B. (1974) Plasma 17-hydroxyprogesterone in newborn infants with congenital adrenal hyperplasia and in infants with normal adrenal function. Archives of Disease in Childhood, 49, 192–194.

Barberia, J.M. and Thorneycroft, I.H. (1974) Simultaneous radioimmunoassay of testosterone and dihydrostestosterone. Steroids, 23, 757–766.

Barnard, W.P. and Logan, R.W. (1971) An automated method for urinary "oestriol" determination in pregnant and non-pregnant subjects. Clinica Chimica Acta, 34, 377–386.

Barrett, S.A. and Brown, J.B. (1970) An evaluation of the method of Cox for the rapid analysis of pregnanediol in urine by gas-liquid chromatography. Journal of Endocrinology, 47, 471–480.

Baumann, G., Rappaport, G., Lemarchand-Béraud, T. and Felber, J.-P. (1975) Free cortisol index: a rapid and simple estimation of free cortisol in human plasma. Journal of Clinical Endocrinology and Metabolism, 40, 462–469.

Besser, G.M. (1973) ACTH and MSH assays and their clinical application. Clinical Endocrinology, 2, 175–186.

Biglieri, E.G., Stockigt, J.R. and Schambelan, M. (1972) Adrenal mineralocorticoids causing hypertension. American Journal of Medicine, 52, 623–632.

Binder, C. and Hall, P.E. (Eds.) (1972) Cushing's Syndrome. Heinemann, London.

Birchall, K. and Mitchell, F.L. (1965) Investigation of the Zimmermann reaction when used for the assay of groups of steroids in infants. Clinica Chimica Acta, 12, 125–136.

Bongiovanni, A.M., Eberlein, W.R., Goldman, A.S. and New, M. (1967) Disorders of adrenal steroid biogensis. Recent Progress in Hormone Research, 23, 375–449.

Borth, R., Linder, A. and Riondel, A. (1957) Urinary excretion of 17-hydroxycorticosteroids and 17-ketosteroids in healthy subjects, in relation to sex, age, body weight and height. Acta Endocrinologica, 25, 33–44.

Bowman, R.W. (1967) Ultramicro method for nonconjugated 17-hydroxycorticosteroids in one-half milliliter of monkey or human plasma. Analytical Biochemistry, 19, 166–176.

Brooks, R.V. (1975) Androgens: physiology and pathology. In Biochemistry of Steroid Hormones (Ed. H.L. Makin) Chap. 13, pp. 289–312, Blackwell Scientific Publications, Oxford.

Brown, J.B., MacLeod, S.C., MacNaughton, C., Smith, M.A. and Smythe, B. (1968) A rapid method for estimating oestrogens in urine using a semiautomatic extractor. Journal of Endocrinology, 42, 5–15.

Brown, J.J., Chinn, R.H., Davies, D.L., Düterdieck, G., Fraser, R., Lever, A.F., Robertson, J.I.S., Tree, M. and Wiseman, A. (1968) Plasma electrolytes, renin and aldosterone in the diagnosis of primary hyperaldosteronism. Lancet, ii, 55–59.

Brown, J.J., Ferriss, J.B., Fraser, R., Lever, A.F., Lever, D.R., Robertson, J.I.S. and Wilson, A. (1972) Apparently isolated excess deoxycorticosterone in hypertension. Lancet, ii, 243–247.

Burke, C.W. and Beardwell, C.G. (1973) Cushing's syndrome: an evaluation of the clinical usefulness of urinary free cortisol and other urinary steroid measurements in diagnosis. Quarterly Journal of Medicine, XLII, No. 165, 175–204.

Bush, I.E. (1961) The Chromatography of Steroids. Pergamon Press, Oxford.

Camacho, A.M., Kowarski, A., Migeon, C.J. and Brough, A.J. (1968) Congenital adrenal hyperplasia due to a deficiency of one of the enzymes involved in the biosynthesis of pregnenolone. Journal of Clinical Endocrinology and Metabolism, 28, 153–161.

Cameron, E.H.D. and Scarisbrick, J.J. (1973) Radioimmunoassay of plasma progesterone. Clinical Chemistry, 19, 1403–1408.

Cathro, D.M., Birchall, K., Mitchell, F.L. and Forsyth, C.C. (1963) The excretion of neutral steroids in the urine of newborn infants. Journal of Endocrinology, 27, 53–75.

Clinics in Endocrinology and Metabolism (1972) 1:2 (Ed. A.S. Mason) W.B. Saunders, London.

Clinics in Endocrinology and Metabolsim (1975) 4:3 (Eds. W.R. Butt and D.R. London) W.B. Saunders, London.

Cope, C.L. (1972) Adrenal Steroids and Disease. Pitman Medical, London.

Coyle, M.G. (1962) The urinary excretion of oestrogen in four cases of anencephaly and one case of foetal death from cirrhosis of the liver. Journal of Endocrinology, 25, viii-ix.

Dluhy, R.G., Greenfield, M. and Williams, G.H. (1977) Journal of Clinical Endocrinology and Metabolism, 45, 141–146.

Ducharme, J.-R., Forest, M.G., de Peretti, E., Sempé, M., Collu, R. and Bertrand, J. (1976) Plasma adrenal and gonadal sex steroids in human pubertal development. Journal of Clinical Endocrinology and Metabolism, 42, 468–476.

Einarsson, K., Gustafsson, J.-A., Ihre, T. and Ingelman-Sundberg, M. (1976) Specific metabolic pathways of steroid sulfates in human liver microsomes. Journal of Clinical Endocrinology and Metabolism, 43, 56–63.

Ernest, I., Håkansson, B., Lehmann, J. and Sjögren, B. (1964) Routine determinations of 17-ketosteroids and Porter–Silber chromogens compared with the chromatographic measurement of grouped and individual steroids. Acta Endocrinologica (Copenhagen), 46, 552–562.

Exley, D. and Norymberski, J.K. (1964) Urinary excretion of 17-deoxycorticosteroids by man. Journal of Endocrinology, 29, 293–302.

Farmer, R.W. and Pierce, C.E. (1974) Plasma cortisol determination: radioimmunoassay and competitive protein binding compared. Clinical Chemistry, 20, 411–414.

Forest, M.G. and Cathiard, A.M. (1975) Pattern of plasma testosterone and Δ^4-androstenedione in normal newborns: evidence for testicular activity at birth. Journal of Clinical Endocrinology and Metabolism, 41, 977–980.

Foster, L.B. and Dunn, R.T. (1974) Single-antibody technique for radioimmunoassay of cortisol in unextracted serum or plasma. Clinical Chemistry, 20, 365–368.

Fraser, R. and James, V.H.T. (1968) Double isotope assay of aldosterone, corticosterone and cortisol in human peripheral plasma. Journal of Endocrinology, 40, 59–72.

Fraser, R., James, V.H.T., Landon, J., Peart, W.S., Rawson, A., Giles, C.A. and McKay, A.M. (1968) Clinical and biochemical studies of a patient with a corticosterone secreting adrenocortical tumour. Lancet, ii, 1116–1120.

Furuyama, S., Mayes, D.M. and Nugent, C.A. (1970) A radioimmunoassay for plasma steroids. Steroids, 16, 415–428.

Ganguly, A., Chavarri, M., Luetscher, J.A. and Dowdy, A.J. (1977a) Transient fall and subsequent return of high aldosterone secretion by adrenal adenoma during continued dexamethasone administration. Journal of Clinical Endocrinology and Metabolism, 44, 775–779.

Ganguly, A., Meikle, A.W., Tyler, F.H. and West, C.D. (1977b) Assessment of 11β-hydroxylase activity with plasma corticosterone, deoxycorticosterone, cortisol and deoxycortisol: role of ACTH and angiotensin. Journal of Clinical Endocrinology and Metabolism, 44, 560–568.

Ganguly, A., Melada, G.A., Luetscher, J.A. and Dowdy, A.J. (1973) Control of plasma aldosterone in primary aldosteronism. Distinction between adenoma and hyperplasia. Journal of Clinical Endocrinology and Metabolism, 37, 765–775.

Glaz, E. and Vecsei, P. (1971) Aldosterone. Pergamon Press, Oxford.

Goldzieher, J.W. and Axelrod, L.R. (1962) A study of methods for the determination of total, grouped, and individual urinary 17-ketosteroids. Journal of Clinical Endocrinology and Metabolism, 22, 1234–1241.

Gray, C.H., Baron, D.N., Brooks, R.V. and James, V.H.T. (1969) A critical appraisal of a method of estimating urinary 17-oxosteroids and total 17-oxogenic steroids. Lancet, i, 124–127.

Himathongkam, T., Dluhy, R.G. and Williams, R.H. (1975) Potassium–aldosterone–renin interrelationships. Journal of Clinical Endocrinology and Metabolism, 41, 153–159.

Hoefnagels, W.H.L., Drayer, J.I.M., Hofman, J.A., Kloppenborg, P.W.C., Smals, A.G.H. and Benraad, Th.J. (1978) Dexamethasone-responsive hypertension in young women with suppressed renin and aldosterone. Lancet, i, 741–743.

Honda, M., Nowaczynski, W., Guthrie, Jr., G.P., Messerli, F.H., Tolis, G., Kuchel, O. and Genest, J. (1977) Response of several adrenal steroids to ACTH stimulation in essential hypertension. Journal of Clinical Endocrinology and Metabolism, 44, 264–272.

Honour, J.W. and Shackleton, C.H.L. (1977) Mass spectrometric analysis for tetrahydroaldosterone. Journal of Steroid Biochemistry, 8, 299–305.

Horton, R. and Tait, J.F. (1966) Androstenedione production and interconversion rates measured in peripheral blood and studies on the possible site of its conversion to testosterone. Journal of Clinical Investigation, 45, 301–313.

Ito, T., Woo, J., Haring, R. and Horton, R. (1971) A radioimmunoassay for aldosterone in human peripheral plasma including a comparison of alternate techniques. Journal of Clinical Endocrinology and Metabolism, 34, 106–112.

Ittrich, G. (1958) Eine neue Methode zur Chemischen Bestimmung der Östrogene Hormone im Harn. Hoppe-Seyler's Zeitschrift für Physiologische Chemie, 312, 1–14.

James, V.H.T. (1961) The excretion of individual 17-oxosteroids in Cushing's syndrome. Journal of Endocrinology, 23, 119–127.

James, V.H.T. and André, C.A. (1974) Androgen metabolism in the human female. In Biochemistry of Women: Clinical Concepts (Eds. A.S. Curry and J.V. Hewitt) pp. 23–40, CRC Press, Ohio.

James, V.H.T. and Jeffcoate, S.L. (1974) Steroids. British Medical Bulletin, 30, 50–54.

James, V.H.T., Tunbridge, R.D.G. and Wilson, G.A. (1976) Studies on the control of aldosterone secretion in man. Journal of Steroid Biochemistry, 7, 941–948.

Jiang, N.-S., Machacek, D. and Wadel, O.P. (1975) Comparison of clinical assays for serum corticosteroids. Clinical Chemistry, 21, 387–391.

Jurjens, H., Pratt, J.J. and Woldring, M.G. (1975) Radioimmunoassay of plasma estradiol without extraction and chromatography. Journal of Clinical Endocrinology and Metabolism, 40, 19–25.

Katz, F.H., Romfh, P. and Smith, J.A. (1975) Diurnal variation of plasma aldosterone, cortisol and renin activity in supine man. Journal of Clinical Endocrinology and Metabolism, 40, 125–134.

Kirschner, M.A. and Jacobs, J.B. (1971) Combined ovarian and adrenal vein catheterization to determine the site(s) of androgen overproduction in hirsute women. Journal of Clinical Endocrinology and Metabolism, 33, 199–209.

Klopper, A., Michie, E. and Brown, J.B. (1955) A method for the determination of urinary pregnanediol. Journal of Endocrinology, 12, 209–219.

Kober, S. (1931) Eine Kolorimetrische Bestimmung des Drunsthormons (Mensormon). Biochemische Zeitschrift, 239, 209–212.

Kowarski, A., de Lacerda, L. and Migeon, C.J. (1975) Integrated concentration of plasma aldosterone in normal subjects: correlation with cortisol. Journal of Clinical Endocrinology and Metabolism, 40, 205–210.

Krieger, D.T. and Gewirtz, G.P. (1974) The nature of the circadian periodicity and suppressibility of immunoactive ACTH levels in Addison's disease. Journal of Clinical Endocrinology and Metabolism, 39, 46–52.

Krieger, D.T., Allen, W., Rizzo, F. and Krieger, H.P. (1971) Characterization of the normal temporal pattern of plasma corticosteroid levels. Journal of Clinical Endocrinology and Metabolism, 32, 266–284.

Langan, J., Jackson, R., Adlin, E.V. and Chanwick, B.J. (1974) A simple radioimmunoassay for urinary aldosterone. Journal of Clinical Endocrinology and Metabolism, 38, 189–193.

Lee, P.A. and Gareis, F.J. (1975) Evidence for partial 21-hydroxylase deficiency among heterozygote carriers of congenital adrenal hyperplasia. Journal of Clinical Endocrinology and Metabolism, 41, 415–418.

Liddle, G.W. (1960) Tests of pituitary–adrenal suppressibility in the diagnosis of Cushing's syndrome. Journal of Clinical Endocrinology and Metabolism. 20, 1539–1560.

Mattingly, D. (1962) A simple fluometric method for the estimation of free 11-hydroxycorticosteroids in human plasma. Journal of Clinical Pathology, 15, 374–379.

McKenna, T.J., Miller, R.B. and Liddle, G.W. (1977) Plasma pregnenolone and 17-OH-pregnenolone in patients with adrenal tumours, ACTH excess, or idiopathic hirsutism. Journal of Clinical Endocrinology and Metabolism, 44, 231–241.

Mitchell, F.L. (1967) Steroid metabolism in the fetoplacental unit and in early childhood. Vitamins and Hormones, 25, 191–269.

Mitchell, F.L. and Shackleton, C.H.L. (1969) The investigation of steroid metabolism in early infancy. Advances in Clinical Chemistry, 12, 141–215.

Moscrop, K.H., Antcliff, A.C., Braunsberg, H., James, V.H.T., Goudie, J.H. and Burnett, D. (1974) An interlaboratory study of an automated technique for the assay of urinary oestrogens. Clinica Chimica Acta, 56, 265–280.

Murphy, B.E.P. (1967) Some studies of the protein-binding of steroids and their application to the routine micro and ultramicro measurement of various steroids in body fluids by competitive protein-binding radioassay. Journal of Clinical Endocrinology and Metabolism, 27, 973–990.

Nelson, D.H. and Samuels, L.T. (1952) A method for the determination of 17-hydroxycorticosteroids in blood: 17-hydroxycorticosterone in the peripheral circulation. Journal of Clinical Endocrinology and Metabolism, 12, 519–526.

New, M.I., Peterson, R.E., Saenger, P. and Levine, L.S. (1976) Evidence for an unidentified ACTH-induced steroid hormone causing hypertension. Journal of Clinical Endocrinology and Metabolism, 45, 1283–1293.

Nicholls, M.G., Espiner, E.A. and Donald, R.A. (1975) Plasma aldosterone response to low dose ACTH stimulation. Journal of Clinical Endocrinology and Metabolism, 41, 186–188.

Nieschlag, E. and Wickings, E.J. (1975) A review of radioimmunoassay for steroids. Zeitschrift für Klinische Chemie und Klinische Biochemie, 13, 261–271.

Norymberski, J.K. (1961) Methods of group corticosteroid estimation - II. In The Adrenal Cortex (Eds. G.K. McGowan and M. Sandler) pp. 88-109, Pitman, London.

Norymberski, J.K., Stubbs, R.D. and West, H.F. (1953) Assessment of adrenocortical activity by assay of 17-ketogenic steroids in urine. Lancet i, 1276–1281.

Porter, C.C. and Silber, R.H. (1950) A quantitative color reaction for cortisone and related 17,21-dihydroxy-20-ketosteroids. Journal of Biological Chemistry, 185, 201–207.

Reynolds, J.W. (1964) The isolation of 16-ketoandrostenediol (3β,17β-dihydroxyandrost-5-en-16-one) from the urine of a newborn infant. Steroids, 3, 77–83.

Rösler, A., Rabinowitz, D., Theodor, R., Ramirez, L.C. and Ulick, S. (1977) The nature of the defect in a salt-wasting disorder in Jews of Iran. Journal of Clinical Endocrinology and Metabolism, 44, 279–291.

Ross, E.J. (1975) Aldosterone and Aldosteronism. Lloyd-Luke Medical Books, London.

Roy, E.J. (1962) Application of the Ittrich extraction procedure to the fluorometric measurement of oestrogens in blood. Journal of Endocrinology, 25, 361–368.

Ruder, H.J., Guy, R.L. and Lipsett, M.B. (1972) A radioimmunoassay for cortisol in plasma and urine. Journal of Clinical Endocrinology and Metabolism, 35, 219–224.

Sann, L., Revol, A., Zachmann, M., Legrand, J.C. and Bethenod, M. (1976) Unusual low plasma renin hypertension in a child. Journal of Clinical Endocrinology and Metabolism, 43, 265–271.

Shackleton, C.H.L. (1976) Congenital adrenal hyperplasia caused by defect in steroid 21-hydroxylase. Establishment of definitive urinary excretion pattern during first weeks of life. Clinica Chimica Acta, 67, 287–298.

Shackleton, C.H.L., Biglieri, E.G. and Honour, J.W. (1978) Steroid excretion by eight patients with 17α-hydroxylase deficiency syndrome. Journal of Clinical Endocrinology and Metabolism (in press).

Shackleton, C.H.L., Gustafsson, J.-Å. and Mitchell, F.L. (1973) The changing pattern of urinary steroid excretion during infancy. Acta Endocrinologica, 74, 157–167.

Shackleton, C.H.L., Honour, J.W., Dillon, M. and Milla, P. (1976) Multicomponent gas chromatographic analysis of urinary steroids excreted by an infant with a defect in aldosterone biosynthesis. Acta Endocrinologica, 81, 762–773.

Shackleton, C.H.L., Mitchell, F.L. and Farquar, J.W. (1972) Difficulties in the diagnosis of the adrenogenital syndrome in infancy. Pediatrics, 49, 198–205.

Shackleton, C.H.L. and Snodgrass, G.H.A.I. (1974) Steroid excretion by an infant with an unusual salt-losing syndrome: a gas chromatographic-mass spectrometric study. Annals of Clinical Biochemistry, 11, 91–99.

Smeaton, T.C., Andersen, G.J. and Fulton, I.S. (1977) Study of aldosterone levels in plasma during pregnancy. Journal of Clinical Endocrinology and Metabolism, 44, 1–7.

Spark, R.F. (1971) Simplified assessment of pituitary–adrenal reserve: measurement of serum 11-deoxycortisol and cortisol after metyrapone. Annals of Internal Medicine, 75, 717–723.

Steinbeck, A.W. and Theile, H.M. (1974) The adrenal cortex (excluding aldosteronism). In Clinics in Endocrinology and Metabolism. Investigations of Endocrine Disorders Vol. 3:3 (Ed. R.I.S. Baylis) pp. 557–591, W.B. Saunders, London.

Stockigt, J.R. (1976) Mineralocorticoid Hormones. In Advances in Steroid Biochemistry and Pharmacology, Vol. 5, (Eds. M.H. Briggs and G.A. Christie) pp. 161–222, Academic Press, London.

Tait, J.F. and Burstein, S. (1964) In vivo studies of steroid dynamics in man. In The Hormones, Vol. 5 (Ed. G. Pincus, K.V. Thimann and E.B. Astwood) pp. 441–557, Academic Press, New York.

Taylor, N.F., Curnow, D.H. and Shackleton, C.H.L. (1978) Analysis of glucocorticoid metabolites in the neonatal period: catabolism of cortisone acetate by an infant with 21-hydroxylase deficiency. Clinica Chimica Acta, 85, 219–229.

Taylor, N.F. and Shackleton, C.H.L. (1977) 15α-Hydroxyoestriol and other polar oestrogens in pregnancy monitoring. Annals of Clinical Biochemistry, 15, 1–11.

Townsend, J. and James, V.H.T. (1968) A semi-automatic fluorimeteric procedure for the determination of plasma corticosteroids. Steroids, 11, 497–511.

Ulick, S. (1976) Diagnosis and nomenclature of the disorders of the terminal portion of the aldosterone biosynthetic pathway. Journal of Clinical Endocrinology and Metabolism, 43, 92–96.

Ulick, S., Gautier, E., Vetter, K.K., Markello, J.R., Jaffe, S. and Lowe, C.U. (1964) An aldosterone biosynthetic defect in a salt-losing disorder. Journal of Clinical Endocrinology and Metabolism, 24, 669–672.

Ulick, S., Ramirez, L.C. and New, M.I. (1977) An abnormality in steroid reductive metabolism in a hypertensive syndrome. Journal of Clinical Endocrinology and Metabolism, 44, 799–802.

Visser, H.K.A. (1966) The adrenal cortex in childhood. Part 2. Pathological aspects. Archives of Disease in Childhood, 41, 113–136.

Williams, R.H. (1974) Text-Book of Endocrinology, 5th edn. W.B. Saunders, London.

Zumoff, B., Fukushima, D.K. and Hellman, L. (1974) Intercomparison of four methods for measuring cortisol production. Journal of Clinical Endocrinology and Metabolism, 38, 169–175.

FURTHER READING

Burke, C.W. (1978) Disorders of cortisol production: diagnostic and therapeutic progress; London, D.R. and Shaw, R.W., Gynaecological endocrinology; O'Riordan, J.L.H., Hormonal control of mineral metabolism. All in Recent Advances in Endocrinology and Metabolism (Ed. J.L.H. O'Riordan) Churchill Livingstone, 1978.

Cope, C.L. (1972) Adrenal Steroids and Disease, 2nd edn. Pitman, London.

Glaz, E. and Vecsei, P. (1971) Aldosterone. Pergamon, Oxford.

Gray, C.H. and James, V.H.T. (Eds.) (1979) Hormones in Blood, Vol. 3, 3rd edn. Academic Press, London and New York.

James, V.H.T., Serio, M. and Martini, L. (Eds.) (1975) The Endocrine Function of the Human Testis. Academic Press, London and New York.

James, V.H.T., Serio, M. and Giusti, G. (Eds.) (1976) The Endocrine Function of the Human Ovary. Academic Press, London and New York.

James, V.H.T., Serio, M., Giusti, G. and Martini, L. (Eds.) (1978) The Endocrine Function of the Human Adrenal Cortex. Academic Press, London and New York.

Labhart, A. (Ed.) (1974) Clinical Endocrinology. Theory and Practice. Springer-Verlag, New York, Heidelberg and Berlin.

Loraine, J.A. and Bell, E.T. (Eds.) (1976) Hormone Assays and their Clinical Application, 4th edn. Churchill Livingstone, Edinburgh.

Makin, H.J.L. (Ed.) (1975) Biochemistry of Steroid Hormones. Blackwell Scientific Publications, Oxford, London, Edinburgh and Melbourne.

Mitchell, F.L. and Shackleton, C.H.L. (1969) The investigation of steroid metabolism in early infancy. In Advances in Clinical Chemistry. Academic Press, New York.

Ross, E.J. (Ed.) Aldosterone and Aldosteronism. Lloyd-Luke, London, 1975.

Vermeuler, A., Klopper, A., Sciarra, F., Jungblut, P. and Lerner, L. (Eds.) (1977) Research on Steroids. Transactions of the 7th Meeting of the International Study Group for Steroid Hormones, Vol. VII. North-Holland, Amsterdam.

Williams, R.H. (Ed.) (1974) Textbook of Endocrinology, 5th edn. W.B. Saunders, Philadelphia, London and Toronto.

ADDENDUM

14.5.3. Primary aldosteronism, hypermineralocorticism and hypertension

The implication of a deficiency of steroid reductive metabolism in the production of hypertension (Ulick et al., 1977) has been further investigated in the two patients demonstrating the syndrome, and shown to be due to a deficiency of 11β-hydroxydehydrogenase. In addition to hypertension, the syndrome is characterized by hypokalaemia and low levels of renin and ACTH, despite low secretions of aldosterone, cortisol and other adrenocorticosteroids. Free dihydrocortisol is increased in the urine. The main feature, however, is a considerable increase in the ratio of tetrahydrocortisol to tetrahydrocortisone, resting, during ACTH stimulation and cortisol treatment; presumably due to impairment of the metabolism of cortisol to cortisone prolonging the half-life of cortisol in plasma. It has been proposed that the hypertension is caused by the excess production of dihydrocortisol which has mineralocorticoid effect (New et al., 1978). Two further cases have since been investigated (N.F. Taylor and C.H.L. Shackleton, personal communication).

14.5.4. Secondary aldosteronism

High excretion of tetrahydroaldosterone with apparent renal unresponsiveness is demonstrated for an infant in Figure 14.5. Ten infants with this disorder (pseudohypoaldosteronism) have now been described and it may be more common than hitherto thought (Dillon et al., 1979). It can be confused with an aldosterone biosynthetic defect but differential diagnosis is established by demonstrating increased values of plasma renin activity and increased plasma aldosterone concentration, plus increased excretion of aldosterone and its metabolites in pseudohypoaldosteronism, compared with aldosterone normal or low and renin high, in the presence of the biosynthetic defect.

14.6.2. Pregnancy

Low levels of oestrogen excretion in pregnancy may have several causes including the presence of an anencephalic foetus which may now be diagnosed by the use of ultrasound. A specific defect in oestrogen biosynthesis may be due to failure of precursor production as in congenital adrenal hypoplasia in the foetus, suppression by exogenous corticosteroids, specific enzyme deficiencies in the foetus or an inability of the placenta to desulphurylate foetal oestrogen precursors. It is clinically important to differentiate these possibilities and diagnosis can be achieved by gas chromatographic analysis of maternal urine. With increasing awareness of the possibility of placental sulphatase deficiency, its incidence is proving to be relatively common (Taylor and Shackleton, 1979).

14.6.4.4. Corticosteroids

The 1β- and 6α-hydroxylated metabolites of cortisol in infants are distributed approximately equally between the free and glucuronide containing urinary fractions. Analysis of urine from a pregnant woman indicates that these polar metabolites can pass from the foetus to the mother where they undergo 11-reduction before excretion. It is possible that their measurement in maternal urine could give important information on the status of cortisol production in the foetus (Taylor and Shackleton, 1978).

14.6.6.1. Lipoid adrenal hyperplasia

Urine from a newborn infant with lipoid adrenal hyperplasia has been analyzed and found to contain no steroids which could be identified as of non-maternal origin; urinary cholesterol content was normal (N.F. Taylor, personal communication).

Dillon, M.J., Leonard, J.V., Buckler, J.M., Ogilvie, D., Lillystone, D., Honour, J.W. and Shackleton, C.H.L. (1979) Pseudohypoaldosteronism – Report of ten cases presenting in infancy. Archives of Disease in Childhood, submitted for publication.

New, M.I., Bradlow, L., Fishman, J., Gunczler, P., Zanconato, G., Rauh, W., Levine, L.S. and Ulick, S. (1978) Deficiency of cortisol 11-β-ketoreductase – a new metabolic defect. Pediatric Research, 12, 416.

Taylor, N.F. and Shackleton, C.H.L. (1978) Metabolism of cortisol by the foetus and neonate. Journal of Endocrinology, 79, 61P–62P.

Taylor, N.F. and Shackleton, C.H.L. (1979) Gas chromatographic steroid analysis for diagnosis of placental sulfatase deficiency: a study of 9 patients. Journal of Clinical Endocrinology and Metabolism, in press.

ADDITIONAL FURTHER READING

Gupta, D. (Ed.) (1975) Radioimmunoassay of Steroid Hormones. Verlag Chemie, Weinheim.

Pratt, J.J. (1978) Steroid immunoassay in clinical chemistry. Clinical Chemistry, 24, 1869–1890.

Chapter 15

Fertility, pregnancy and contraception

R. Angus Harkness

Division of Perinatal Medicine, Clinical Research Centre, Watford Road, Harrow, Middlesex HA1 3UJ, England

Nature to be commanded, must be obeyed (Francis Bacon 1561–1626)

CONTENTS

Chemical diagnosis of disease, edited by S.S. Brown, F.L. Mitchell and D.S. Young

15.1. INTRODUCTION

The final differentiation of male and female at puberty is the major extrauterine component of human development. It is a process which demands the successful working of the basic systems necessary for life, and it is therefore retarded by diseases of these systems, congenital or acquired. Perhaps it is a measure of the sensitivity of this final phase of growth and development to external influences that only within the last few years has the fall in age of menarche stopped in developed countries at about the age of 12 to 13 years. Nutrition is an important external influence; in "acute" undernutrition, reproductive functions are reduced before many other functions are affected.

Disease specific to the reproductive system is surprisingly common; even with apparently normal development in both partners, involuntary infertility is a feature of about 10% of marriages despite the overall success of human reproduction in the modern world with its consequent problem of overpopulation.

This Chapter seeks to outline the processes in human reproduction which are successfully studied by chemical methods with a view to determining diagnoses and for treatment. Emphasis has been given to areas of proven value in diagnosis rather than to the many studies of normal and abnormal human physiology and biochemistry which are detailed in the books and review articles listed in the bibliography. The general medical background to the subject is described in the relevant sections of some textbooks, for example, those of Passmore and Robson (1968, 1974); short and useful sections on many diseases are found in a reference book such as that of Beeson and McDermott (1975). The morbid anatomical aspects of obstetric and gynaecological pathology are described in the book edited by Novak and Woodruff (1974).

For assessment of the variables in biological systems it is useful to distinguish between measurements of overall function, such as linear or weight measurements of growth, and measures which are specific to one or a small number of biochemical steps. One measurement can sometimes be interpreted in two ways, e.g. oestriol excretion by a pregnant mother can be linked to overall rate of foetal growth in utero; such growth can be measured directly clinically, or more accurately by ultrasonic scanning. However, oestriol excretion is not an unfailing guide to failure of foetal growth. Specifically, oestriol excretion is a reliable guide to defects in central control of the foetal adrenal cortex, as in anencephaly, or to adrenocortical function itself in adrenocortical hypoplasia, or even closer, to oestrogen formation in "placental" sulphatase deficiency. The relative diagnostic success of endocrinology may be due to the inherent accessibility of hormones and their metabolites in body fluids, so allowing the detailed and virtually direct dissection of processes which in other areas of metabolism are partially or completely hidden within cells or "confounded" by conflicting changes. Such considerations certainly apply to pregnancy; direct sampling of the foetal compartment in the form at least of amniotic fluid, including its cells, has been needed to diagnose many defects. The overlap of α-foetoprotein concentrations in sera from mothers carrying children with open lesions of the CNS and from mothers carrying normal children, contrasts with the clear distinction generally possible from amniotic fluid concentrations. It seems that the further away a measurement is made from the site of the primary defect the greater the overlap of "normal" with "abnormal" until both become part of one continuous "normal" or "log normal" distribution. In such a distribution, abnormal values are those above or below some arbitrary point. A measured variable may be separated from the site of the primary defect by physiological and biochemical mechanisms, or by space or by time, separately or in combination. The importance of time has to be emphasized in the menstrual cycle of about 28 days. A single blood specimen or even a 24-hour urine collection must usually be precisely located in time in the cycle if the results are to be interpretable. For example, a single sample for plasma progesterone or urinary pregnanediol can provide useful information if it is timed to coincide with the possible presence of a corpus luteum producing its characteristic hormone progesterone. A more reliable diagnosis would be provided by follicular as well as luteal phase samples, say on days 7 and 21, thus eliminating the large differences between individuals. A knowledge of the pattern of events in the menstrual cycle is a basis for the investigation of ovarian function. The importance of serial sampling has been stressed by all who have tried to interpret endocrine data in the area of human reproduction.

The choice of test depends on the stage which the investigation has reached. At first it would appear that diagnosis should be relatively specific for a given defect, but this is only practical where a defect is fairly common; thus open developmental defects of the CNS can be diagnosed from high concentrations of amniotic fluid α-foetoprotein. In this case, it is possible that a number of rare basic causes combine to give one series of defects. Relatively specific tests have their place in initial investigation only to reveal common causes of disease. It is generally necessary to narrow the possibilities logically and progressively, guided by the basic physiology and biochemistry until a useful result is achieved.

15.2. METHODS OF DIAGNOSIS

The process starts with a clinical history and examination and continues with increasingly close liaison between clinical and laboratory staff. The patterns of clinical findings for common conditions are familiar; however for other diagnoses, reference books are often difficult to use because, understandably, conditions are described in the context of the final diagnosis rather than of the initial findings. An exception to this approach is Smith's (1976) book in which photographs of human malformations are linked with short texts which can sometimes be used to guide further investigation. The final diagnosis may rest completely on laboratory evidence. In the area of reproduction, the investigations generally start in an outpatient clinic and progress stepwise – with perhaps one inpatient admission – for an agreed series of tests at a late stage. Early discharge to an outpatient clinic appointment allows results from many areas to be gathered together and, when necessary, discussed in order to reach conclusions on diagnosis and on treatment.

A relevant example of a common problem might be hirsutism in a female, a condition in which it is rarely possible to reach a useful diagnosis. If this is linked with menstrual irregularity an ovarian source for the excess testosterone is probable. As a consequence of the long-term variations in ovarian function, a single sample of blood or urine for testosterone analysis affords a less valuable measure of excessive androgen production than the hirsutism itself, since this represents a cumulative record of raised androgen production. If hirsutism is severe, with other signs of masculinization and possibly amenorrhoea, a tumour may rarely be present. In this case, testosterone concentrations are markedly raised and relatively constant, sometimes staying raised despite suppression with oral oestrogens; however, three cases of adrenocortical adenomata which were controlled by gonadotrophins have now been described (see Larson et al., 1976). Localization of such a tumour is then the next problem prior to its surgical removal. It is perhaps a measure of the diagnostic ability of the whole team if such a tumour can be found without the exhaustive and impractical investigation of every case of such a common complaint as hirsutism.

15.3. PRINCIPLES OF DIAGNOSTIC METHODS

A knowledge of the nature and extent of masculinization or feminization is inherent. This can be refined by a staging or grading process – for further information see Brotherton (1976). The occurrence of menstrual bleeding indicates that the female reproductive tract, ovaries and their central controls are present. The time of such menstruation indicates the function of the various inter-relations in the control loop. When quantitative and specific estimates of the amount of stimulation by sex hormones is needed, measurement of the sex hormones themselves and their metabolites are available; these are the oestrogens oestradiol-17β and oestrone, with their metabolite oestriol; progesterone and its metabolite pregnanediol; and testosterone which, with its 5α-reduction product dihydrotestosterone, may be usefully regarded as the sole androgens. The measurement of the intermediates of steroid biosynthesis such as 17α-hydroxyprogesterone and its metabolite, pregnanetriol, and dehydroepiandrosterone are discussed in Chapter 14.

Overactivity of steroid secreting tissues and their control mechanisms is rather easier to diagnose than failures of secretion, so that emphasis is placed here on the failures. Using the principles described in this section, it should be possible to define and localize most causes of hyperfunction.

Testosterone and the oestrogens are tightly controlled by gonadotrophins, and the amount of gonadotrophin stimulation necessary to achieve a given rate of sex hormone production is a measure of gonadal responsiveness. The failing "menopausal" gonad may be detected by higher concentrations of gonadotrophins. In the male, luteinizing hormone controls testosterone secretion by the interstitial (Leydig) cells of the testis in a relatively simple negative feed-back system. The feedback is mediated, at least in part, by oestrogen produced by conversion of testosterone into oestrogen in peripheral tissues. Thus oestrogens are potent inhibitors of secretion of luteinizing hormone in males as well as females. The interaction of the metabolism of peripheral tissues with this control loop may account for the menstrual irregularities apparently sometimes produced by obesity and also for the gynaecomastia of hepatic cirrhosis in which C_{19} steroid conversion to oestrogens is increased. Steroid inactivation mechanisms in liver are generally slowed by hepatic cirrhosis. In general, slowing of steroid metabolism is associated with increased conversion into oestrogens (Baker et al., 1976b). It seems justifiable to accept that this conversion occurs in most tissues since the aromatization of androstenedione to oestrogens has been observed in cultured human fibroblasts (Schweikert et al., 1976).

Spermatogenesis in its early stages, for example the spermatogonia, seems to control follicle stimulating hormone secretion, although the nature of the postulated "inhibin" responsible for the negative feed-back is not understood (Figure 15.1). Thus complete failure of spermatogenesis, with or without Sertoli cells in the tubules, is associated with raised secretion of follicle stimulating hormone by the anterior pituitary. Isolated gonadotrophin deficiences, for example of luteinizing hormone in the "fertile eunuch", as with other pituitary hormones, are rare.

In the female, the hypothalamic control systems are more complex in that there is a marked positive feed-back effect of oestrogen, in the amounts normally secreted in the menstrual cycle, on secretion of luteinizing hormone. This stimulates a mature follicle to

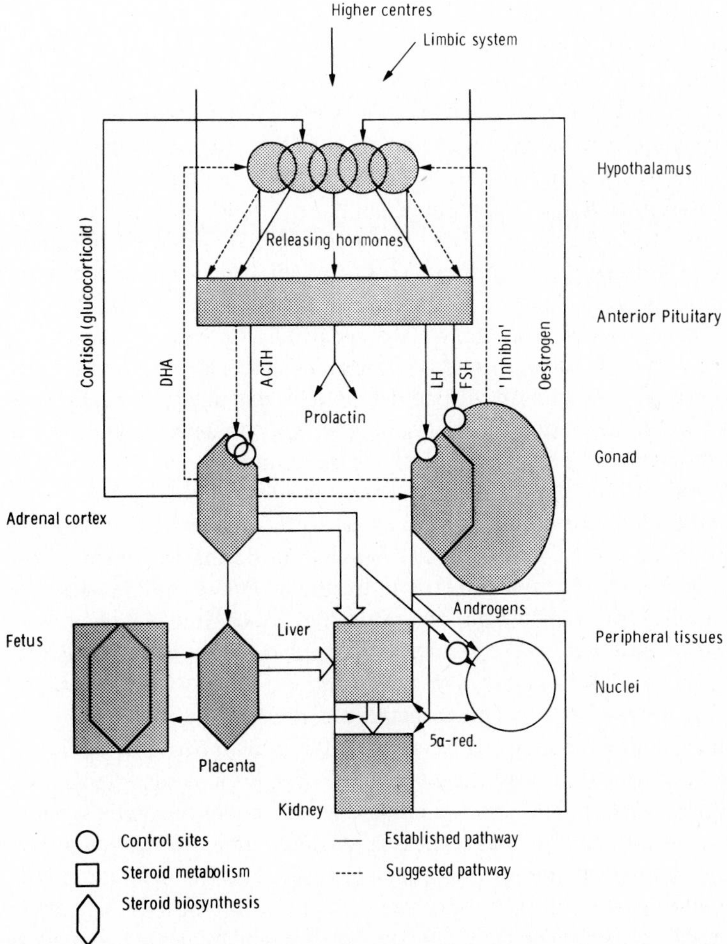

Figure 15.1. A scheme for steroid biosynthesis and metabolism as well as their inter-relationships and control in human reproduction. Inter-relationships between controls are indicated by overlap where possible.

ovulate and form a corpus luteum, which generally functions normally for the fixed span of about 14 days. Large amounts of oestrogen, associated with oral contraceptive therapy or pregnancy, inhibit secretion of luteinizing hormone as they do in the male. Sexual differentiation of the hypothalamus is retained by the female foetus despite her masculinization in the last trimester of pregnancy due to steroid 21-hydroxylation deficiency.

The link between the anterior pituitary and the hypothalamus appears to be a series of peptides passed from the hypothalamus to the pituitary. So far only one peptide has been characterized which, surprisingly, releases both luteinizing hormone and follicle stimulating hormone, despite the physiological independence of these two hormones. Despite many studies with this peptide, which is a decapeptide (LH/FSH-RH) which has also been called "gonadotrophin releasing hormone", and which is now available in pure form, diagnostic stimulation tests with the decapeptide (section 15.4.2.1.) have not yet proved useful (Hall and Gomez Pan, 1976).

The hypothalamus is probably the least satisfactory area to investigate. The negative feed-back effect of oestrogen and, to a lesser extent, of testosterone, and various analogues of both of these steroids, can be used to suppress gonadotrophin and thus gonadal activity. This manouevre can sometimes be used to detect steroid-secreting gonadal tumours, as in the widely used adrenocortical suppression tests, but there is little available experience. Suppression tests are most useful when there is raised steroid production, since suppression of gonadotrophin production to subnormal levels is difficult to demonstrate even by radioimmunoassay. In isosexual precocity, in which pubertal changes appear before the age of 10 years, there is a relative insensitivity of the hypothalamus to steroid suppression. This is normally determined therapeutically in that large doses of a powerful progesterone analogue, such as medroxyprogesterone acetate, must be used to control gonadal function. In view of the difficulties of achieving adequate suppression initially, it can be useful to monitor gonadal response in order to achieve an optimum dosage which can then be used largely without biochemical monitoring.

The most widely used test of hypothalamic function is subtle. Clomiphene, a weak oestrogen which can also block the action of strong oestrogens, can be used to stimulate gonadotrophin secretion; this results in testicular stimulation during treatment in the male, and ovulation at a highly variable time after treatment in the female. Doses of about 100 mg/day for 5 days are widely used. This positive effect of clomiphene does not appear until puberty. In interpreting the results of clomiphene stimulation, the small stimulation of adrenal steroid production during the dosage period should be remembered. Slight increases in progesterone and pregnanediol are otherwise puzzling.

Failure of gonadal endocrine function can be confirmed by gonadotrophin stimulation tests which have also been widely used. In the male, 3 to 5 days' stimulation of the testes is achieved with 1000 to 5000 units/day, intramuscularly, of human chorionic gonadotrophin. The testosterone production gives a measure of interstitial cell mass. The test is sensitive enough to detect small amounts of testicular tissue. Failure of response is an indication for replacement treatment with testosterone, if this is appropriate. The effective life of a testosterone implant, which is widely used in such replacement treatment, is relatively constant so that monitoring of its life by gonadotrophin or testosterone assays is rarely justifiable.

The ovaries are more variable than the testes in their response to gonadotrophins so that care is needed in searching for an optimum dose which avoids over-stimulation and the risk of multiple follicular rupture. The careful monitoring of oestrogen output from the follicles can be an adequate guide. Therapeutic stimulation of ovulation is the most frequently required procedure in which sequential "follicle-stimulating hormone-like" preparations are used, followed by a "luteinizing hormone-like" preparation, generally human chorionic gonadotrophin, to produce ovulation.

The precise test scheme and endpoints used should be those with which most experience is available, as long as the basic chemistry and biochemistry involved are satisfactory. Once a regime is chosen it should not be lightly altered because experience is difficult to acquire; it is only on the basis of this experience that normal can be distinguished from abnormal. It must be admitted that many procedures are arbitrary. The dose of human chorionic gonadotrophin for testicular stimulation has been raised by some workers from the earlier 1000 units/day to 5000 units/day without any correction for body weight, despite the widespread use of this test in small boys with failures of pubertal development. The answer would appear to be that all regimes are providing approximately maximal stimulation.

The role of prolactin in the initiation and maintenance of lactation is clear; thus galactorrhoea is a clear indication for measuring prolactin, but plasma concentrations are not markedly abnormal in gynaecomastia. High concentrations – 10 to 20 times normal values – are a clear indication of a pituitary tumour; in about 30% of cases of pituitary tumour there is a raised concentration. There are no marked differences in concentrations between men, women and children. The control of prolactin secretion is complex and appears to be inter-related with those for the gonadotrophins, thyrotrophin and growth hormone release. Stress causes marked elevations and there is a clear nocturnal maximum in secretion. Oestrogens, thyrotrophin, hypoglycaemia and psychotropic drugs, including phenothiazines and some tricyclic antidepressants, stimulate secretion; L-DOPA and bromocryptine inhibit secretion. From this it can be seen that the interpretation of a raised prolactin concentration demands close control and considerable knowledge and experience. This too is an area where, at present, reference ranges are especially dependent on the individual laboratory. The use of purer standards, possibly provided by the World Health Organization, may reduce the present inter-laboratory differences. An attempt to indicate some of the elements involved in the control of reproduction has been made in Figure 15.1.

In summary, biochemical tests of gonadal function are mainly tests of their endocrine function. The basic pattern of the tests of adrenocortical function is repeated in the tests of gonadal function. If steroid output is low, try to stimulate it and estimate trophic hormones. In cases where steroid output is high, trophic hormone measurements can often be at, or below the limits of sensitivity of the methods; in these cases suppression tests may have a place.

The basic components of a series of clinically useful tests have been defined above. After eliminating the common causes of a condition, it is necessary to narrow the alternative possibilities in a logical and stepwise series of investigations. Within limits, the details of these tests now depend on the existing experience of the investigating group and the available methods, since there may be a number of satisfactory routes to the solution of the problem.

After the common causes of abnormalities in the tests described have been given, it is not very helpful to list "all" the possible causes. The use of a single name from an encyclopaedic list can provide a false impression of homogeneity or relevance. In contrast, reading more limited review articles – and even the original papers – can provide good evidence for a useful diagnosis, and perhaps also an indication for treatment. References to more specialized review articles are therefore given as a key to the very large number of specific conditions.

15.4. PHYSIOLOGICAL AND PATHOLOGICAL STATES

This section is "problem oriented" in that chemical diagnosis is considered in two common states, pregnancy and failure of gonadal function.

15.4.1. Pregnancy

Changes in the concentrations of many compounds in blood and urine during pregnancy are defined in specialized monographs listed in Further Reading and References. One of the important series of patterns is the increase in human chorionic gonadotrophin in plasma and of oestriol and pregnanediol in urine already defined in Figure 1.9 in Chapter 1.

15.4.1.1. Diagnosis

Pregnancy is common enough to make it practicable to use a specific test for its presence. Less specific tests have been generally abandoned.

Reliable tests for pregnancy depend on the detection of human chorionic gonadotrophin in urine and serum, produced specifically by the trophoblast. Detailed and practical reviews of this topic are available (Hobson, 1966; 1974). Earlier biological methods for the measurement of human chorionic gonadotrophin, although reliable, have been replaced by a variety of simpler immunological methods, most of which are now available in kit form. The kits are by no means uniformly reliable. An evaluation of kits by Hobson (1966) showed that the Pregnosticon (Organon Laboratories Ltd.) and Prepuerin (Burroughs Wellcome and Co.) were about 98% accurate in normal pregnancy. Urine samples are taken 10 or more days after the first missed menstrual period. False negative results are mainly due to the small amounts of human chorionic gonadotrophin present being below the limit of sensitivity of the method. About 30% of tests using such kits are negative in ectopic pregnancy. If a highly sensitive system is used, false positives may occur due to cross-reactions with the similar α-subunit in luteinizing hormone (section 15.4.1.2.). Physiological elevations of luteinizing hormone near the menopause are a source of false positive reactions; such elevations may also occur after psychotropic drugs. The progress towards simplification of the methods used has been spectacular but it has also produced overconfidence in inexperienced workers, as well as a long list of factors associated with abnormal results; for example, non-specific agglutination or inhibition of agglutination of the erythrocytes commonly used. The literature on advances in pregnancy testing has been reviewed (Hobson, 1974).

15.4.1.2. Tumours of the trophoblast

Tumours of the trophoblast – hydatidiform mole and choriocarcinoma – also characteristically secrete human chorionic gonadotrophin, as do similar tumours from the gonads. Other secretions, such as human placental lactogen and progesterone, are often found but they are less reliable than human chorionic gonadotrophin as an indicator for the presence of a tumour, perhaps because it is secreted earlier in the development of the trophoblast. Although human chorionic gonadotrophin has many similarities to luteinizing hormone, sharing its α-subunit, the β-subunit is different and possesses an extra 30 aminoacid residues at its COOH end; this has formed the basis of a specific human chorionic gonadotrophin assay which can be automated. With this increase in specificity, it is possible to increase the sensitivity of the assay without cross-reactions to luteinizing hormone. Such sensitive assays can detect about 10^4 or 10^5 choriocarcinoma cells; a pregnancy test becomes positive when 10^8 or 10^9 cells are present (Bagshawe, 1976). It is thus possible to identify patients needing chemotherapy after surgical evacuation of hydatidiform mole, and also monitor the response to treatment and detect recurrences.

15.4.1.3. Assessment of gestational age

The estimation of the age of the foetus from the date of the last menstrual period is adequate in the majority of cases, but the history may be unreliable or menstruation may have been irregular or even absent before pregnancy started. Estimates of foetal length by ultrasound are related closely to age, but for estimates of foetal maturity, biochemical assessment is needed.

15.4.1.3.1. Estimation of gestational age in the first and second trimester. Biochemical methods at this time generally estimate the developmental maturity of the placenta which can be used to estimate the date of delivery. Between 10 and 20 weeks after conception, the rapid and opposite changes in concentration of maternal plasma human placental lactogen (which is rising) and of human chorionic gonadotrophin (which is falling) have been used to estimate maturation (Peeters et al., 1976). The rapid marked rise in serum diamine oxidase from 6 to 16 weeks of gestation, with no further increase thereafter, has been claimed to allow more accurate estimates of gestational age than the menstrual history (Elmfors and Tryding, 1976). Certainly, the requirement is for accurate dating to within about 1 week.

15.4.1.3.2. Foetal maturity in the last trimester. In the last 3 months of pregnancy, biochemical indices are a good guide to progress in the perinatal period. Perinatal morbidity has been improved by assessing pulmonary maturity from the amount of lecithin in the amniotic fluid, which is often expressed as a ratio to the relatively unchanging internal standard of sphingomyelin. A lecithin/sphingomyelin (L/S) ratio of 2 or more, as determined by thin-layer chromatography, is desirable before operative delivery.

Other major problems in the newborn are the maintenance of adequate plasma glucose and calcium concentrations and the susceptibility to infection. Such failures of adaptation to extrauterine existence and of homoeostatic mechanisms appear sometimes to be related to developmental immaturity; some may be related to "hypoxia" possibly during delivery. At present, there is no means of estimating foetal maturity in these areas and the biochemical events must be detected as they occur.

15.4.1.4. Foetal and/or placental function: foetal development in the first 3 months of pregnancy

The development of the embryo is mainly completed in the first 3 months of pregnancy. During this time, a series of well-defined and precisely timed changes occur. Thereafter, the growth of established systems occurs until, at about the time of delivery, there is a final phase of developmental changes in preparation for extrauterine existence, notably in lungs and in haemoglobin synthesis. In the last 3 months of pregnancy, most measured variables show increased scatters of results which make estimations of foetal age from such measurements inaccurate.

The detection of serious developmental anomalies, after the initial major developmental changes should have been completed and before the foetus becomes viable, is now an important part of preventive medicine. The major forms of serious congenital anatomical abnormality are those of the central nervous system and of the heart and great vessels. Only the former are at present accessible to antenatal diagnosis; even in the area of the central nervous system it must be admitted that many children with mental defects show no adequate cause of their developmental failure.

The successful use of assay of amniotic fluid α-foetoprotein for the detection of open defects of the central nervous system is now widespread, at least in the U.K. More detailed considerations of the amniotic fluid changes are given in Chapter 2 (section 2.4.3.). This section is mainly concerned with attempts to detect elevations of α-foetoprotein in maternal serum in cases of open lesions of the foetal central nervous system. Basically, this approach depends on abnormal leakage of foetal serum proteins into amniotic fluid without bleeding; bleeding itself can be detected from the presence of foetal haemoglobin. α-Foetoprotein appears in foetal serum in quantity at about the 6th week of pregnancy, the concentration rising rapidly to a peak of up to 3 to 4 mg/ml at about the 12th week of pregnancy when it is a major serum protein in the foetus, second only to albumin. Thereafter the concentration decreases. It is detectable in the sera of newborn infants at concentrations of 10 to 150 μg/ml. α-Foetoprotein is detectable in amniotic fluid at the μg/ml level but in maternal serum, ng/ml concentrations are found, necessitating radioimmunoassay.

An attempt to detect abnormal leakage of foetal proteins into amniotic fluid from changes in maternal serum is needed if any marked reduction is to be achieved in the overall incidence of open abnormalities of the foetal central nervous system; 90% of infants with anencephaly or spina bifida are born to mothers who have no history suggestive of an increased risk. At the most appropriate time, which is the 16th to 18th week of pregnancy (if the upper limit of normal concentration is taken at the 99th percentile), then 78% of the anencephalics and 63% of open spina bifida cases would be detected, according to preliminary data from the U.K. collaborative study on maternal serum α-foetoprotein (1977). The present state of the methods of diagnosis of neural tube defects has been reviewed in detail (Brock, 1976, 1977), and some other aspects of α-foetoprotein by Lau and Linkins (1976) and in Chapter 10. There are many problems remaining to be solved in this area, including appropriate standardization and quality control quite apart from the logistics and overall value of a screening programme. Since some of the answers to these questions are available from the report on the U.K. collaborative study (1977) it should be possible to reach a more rational decision on the allocation of resources to such a programme.

15.4.1.5. Placental function in early pregnancy

Chemical diagnosis in pregnancy rests largely on understanding the endocrinology of pregnancy which has been reviewed in the monograph edited by Fuchs and Klopper (1977).

The placenta "initially" produces large amounts of human chorionic gonadotrophin with later increases in the amounts of progesterone and human placental lactogen, a material initially detected from cross reactions with human growth hormone, but present in relatively high concentration (μg/ml) in plasma during pregnancy. The use of estimations of placental lactogen as a measure of foetoplacental function has been extensively evaluated (Chard, 1976): Niven and his colleagues (1972) used low or falling concentrations to differentiate between those pregnant women in danger of imminent abortion and those who were not. It must be admitted that apart from α-foetoprotein, other readily measurable variables in the first and second trimesters of pregnancy are of placental origin, including placental lactogen – like its predecessors in this area, progesterone and pregnanediol. Some other such variables have already been mentioned in considering the assessment of gestational age (section 15.4.1.3.1.).

The enzymes commonly studied appear to be placental in origin; for example placental alkaline phosphatase, which is normally measured as heat-stable enzyme activity in maternal plasma. The wide reference range has limited the clinical use of this and other enzyme assays (Wilde and Oakey, 1975). The main limitation of placental tests in clinical practice is that placental function can be apparently normal in the presence of a dead foetus. The search for clinically useful tests of foetal health, especially in the second trimester, therefore, appears likely to continue.

Concentrations of maternal intracellular proteins are also altered during pregnancy, but of these only haemoglobin is widely measured, generally to assess iron stores.

15.4.1.6. Foetoplacental function in late pregnancy

In the third trimester, the production of oestrogens is a useful index of the health of the foetoplacental unit. At present the assay of maternal urinary oestrogens is the most widely used and best validated test. If the long and complex process of synthesis of oestrogens by the foetoplacental unit is "normal", the general health of the foetus is usually "normal". One of the major benefits of oestrogen assay has been in reassuring obstetricians of the health of the foetus and thus avoiding the delivery of a premature infant. The importance of serial assays to reveal a trend, if any, is generally accepted; this allows the patient to act as her own control, thus eliminating the large differences between individuals, which are an important component of the range of reference values.

Dynamic tests of foetoplacental function have been little used, although the conversion of administered dehydroepiandrosterone sulphate into oestrogens, and indirect estimates of placental transfer have been studied.

The choice between the use of blood or urine for hormone estimations depends on many factors, apart from the information required (Klopper, 1977). In general, changes in blood are more rapid than those in urine; half-lives of most of the hormones in plasma are short, and thus a single blood sample gives information that is relevant to about 1 hour, compared to the effective integration over a whole day offered by a 24-hour urine. Plasma concentrations are more directly linked to secretion, whereas urinary outputs are complicated by the intervention of liver and kidney. The plasma concentration is a measure of the balance between production and further metabolism. In contrast, the urine specimen provides an estimate of mean production over a 24-hour period which is little affected by changes in the rate of metabolism. At present, despite recent methodological progress, especially in radioimmunoassay, the speed of hormone analyses seems to be too slow to take full advantage of the rapidity with which a trend might potentially be detected in plasma. The debate about blood versus urine arises in part because plasma is more convenient to handle and analyse; also it is obtained at one point in space and time by a medical worker. The answer would appear to be best provided by the established clinical benefit. In their critical review of biochemical tests of foetoplacental function, Wilde and Oakey (1975) included a reminder that much harm might be done if measurements of oestrogens in plasma were uncritically substituted for urinary assays. Thus, despite a strong positive correlation between the levels of oestrogens in blood and urine and no clear difference in their variability, it seems advisable to continue to use the proven procedures of urine analysis.

Consideration of the biochemical basis of the clinical use of oestrogen assays in the third trimester suggests that urinary procedures may persist. In the third trimester, total oestrogens in urine consist largely of the 16α-hydroxylation product of oestrogen metabolism, oestriol. This compound shows a disproportionately rapid increase with gestational age, so that a much greater proportion of oestrogen output is in the form of oestriol at the end of pregnancy. It is this measurement of oestriol in urine which is clinically valuable. The output of the 6α- and 6β-hydroxylation products of progesterone is also disproportionately increased at the end of pregnancy.

This increase in the output of hydroxylation products would appear to be related to an increase in the hydroxylation of steroids predominantly by the foetal and maternal livers. Such an increase is consistent with the widespread process of substrate induction of hydroxylation. Lesser increases in steroid 6-hydroxylation are detectable in the presence of the increased secretion of a corpus luteum (Harkness et al., 1974) as well as in states with increased cortisol production. It should also be noted that hydroxylation reaction products at C6 and C16, for example, are said to be largely foetal but this may only be true because the foetal liver is subjected to massive stimulation with "administered" steroids. The administration of 40 to 50 mg of steroid per day to adults allowed Fukushima and his colleagues (1962) to demonstrate "hepatic" 18-hydroxylation. From these considerations, it seems likely that the group measurement of many hydroxylation products – including, 16α-, 6α-, 6β-, 15- and even many 18-hydroxysteroids – may increase the discrimination of normal from abnormal levels; urine may be the fluid in which these changes are most obvious, since such water-soluble compounds are rapidly removed from the circulation and excreted in the urine.

There appears to be a need for a rapid and robust method of monitoring foetal well-being in the last trimester. Experience with oestrogen measurements has shown some successes as well as revealing the practical difficulties, especially in the speed of the analyses required. The value of maternal serum α-foetoprotein concentrations in the last trimester seems doubtful (Wilde and Oakey, 1975; Rodeck et al., 1976) despite it foetal origin. Direct monitoring of the foetal heart is widely used, but unequivocal proof of significant overall benefit is difficult to find and now to obtain, since the technique is now used widely. The problems of biochemical monitoring of foetal health include a precise understanding of normality and quality control. This latter problem also affects the direct measurement of foetal acid–base and blood gas variables during delivery; these measurements do provide information on the immediate status of the child at this critical stage in its life. Oestrogen measurements, foetal heart rate, and acid–base determinations – especially if used serially in this order – can provide useful information, but the cost is high and the reliability less than expected. Further details are provided in the book on "Perinatal Medicine" (Goodwin et al., 1976).

15.4.1.7. Toxaemia and renal disease in pregnancy

The occurrence of oedema, hypertension and proteinuria in pregnancy provides a working definition of toxaemia of pregnancy which is otherwise extremely ill understood. In general, varying types and degrees of renal failure, with widely different rates of development, are more liable to occur during or about the time of pregnancy; the conditions which are generally recognized are listed in "The Pathology of Pregnancy", edited by Hurley (1976). In monitoring the course of these disorders, measurement of the concentration of urate in serum or plasma is useful since it is better correlated with foetal prognosis than many other variables (Redman et al., 1976). Hyperuricaemia also occurs earlier than proteinuria and uraemia in pre-eclampsia. For monitoring renal function itself, serial estimations of creatinine in serum or plasma are a useful overall indication of renal clearance. Although the extent of the proteinuria is generally estimated, specific proteins are not usually identified or measured to characterize the renal damage.

15.4.2. Failures of gonadal function

15.4.2.1. Failures of sexual development. Physical

In any gross failure of the development of gonadal function it is advisable to check that the chromosomal constitution or karyotype corresponds to that of the body or phenotype. The usual simple preliminary test is to examine the cells in a buccal smear for the XX chromosone pair which is found as a triangular mass of chromatin generally at the periphery of 15 to 50% of cells. Females with the XO constitution, usually found in Turner's syndrome, and males with the XXY constitution of Klinefelter's syndrome should be detected. Other conditions are even less common and justify a more complete cytogenetic investigation and further biochemical investigation.

A useful guide to the next stages of such an investigation is the finding of a "female" lower genital tract. If this is present, then testosterone secretion or response has not been present. An androgenized female lower genital tract is suggestive of steroid 21-hydroxylation defect which shows itself after genital tract development is largely complete (see Chapter 7). The normal patterns of plasma concentrations of steroid sex hormones and gonadotrophins for both male and female throughout life are shown in Figure 15.2.

In order to check the functional capacity of a gonad, or even its presence in some problems of sexual differentiation, gonadotrophin stimulation tests are widely used, especially in the male. The human chorionic gonadotrophin stimulation test (section 15.3.) has been found by most groups (e.g. Grant et al., 1976) to be a sensitive method of detecting Leydig cells. Sometimes the basal values show gonadal activity which in 3 to 6 months will be apparent in pubertal development. If there is no response, a clear diagnosis

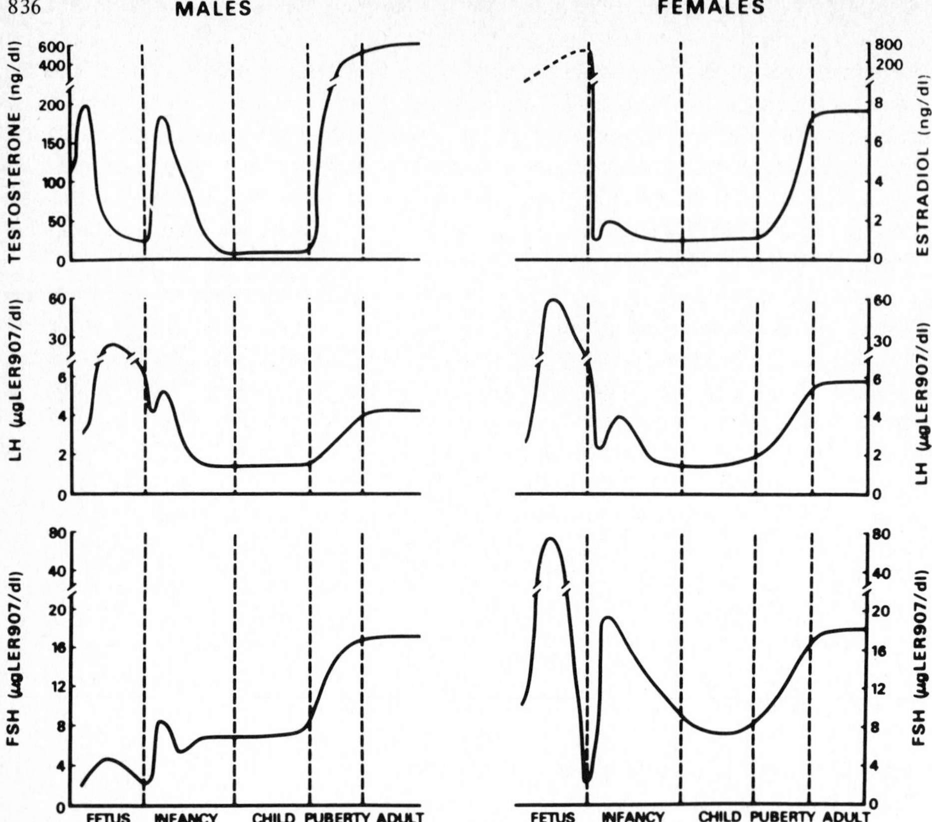

Figure 15.2. Developmental changes in plasma concentrations of gonadal steroids and gonadotrophins from foetal to adult life in males and females. (Reproduced, by permission, from Winter et al., 1976)

of interstitial cell failure or absence has been achieved and replacement therapy should be considered. If a clear testicular response is present, the defect may be higher up the controlling system. Measurement of the endogenous gonadotrophins before and after the decapeptide LH/FSH-RH administration (section 15.3.) has been tried and has usually not provided clinically useful information. The hypothalamus and higher controlling centres are especially difficult to test before puberty since clomiphene does not stimulate until after the onset of puberty. Neurological investigation of the central nervous system may reveal an associated, and sometimes possibly causal, defect although such disease is most often associated with sexual precocity.

The number of causes of failures of sexual development is large and each specific cause is rare. Diagnosis can be achieved by a stepwise logical narrowing of the possibilities. When some definite evidence has been obtained to guide the search, careful reading of the original articles which appear to be relevant is advisable before a conclusion is reached as to diagnosis or treatment.

Parallel investigations of other endocrine glands may also be helpful; there may be an associated insufficiency of thyroid or adrenal function.

15.4.2.2. Gynaecomastia

This occurs either at puberty or after about 50 years of age. In a case presenting at another time of life, it may be justifiable to suspect hepatic cirrhosis, an oestrogen-secreting tumour or even administered oestrogen as a cause. There is generally no obvious endocrine abnormality, so that diagnostic investigation is rarely justified. It does seem relevant that at puberty and especially after the age of 50, rather higher gonadotrophin concentrations are sometimes required to produce a given amount of testosterone. In the older age groups, in whom a wide variety of drug regimes may be associated with gynaecomastia, oestrogen production rises slightly with a fall in the mean concentrations of testosterone. The variations in plasma concentrations, especially of oestrogens, are large, and useful changes are only seen in mean values (Baker et al., 1976a, b). Prolactin assays also have not been valuable.

15.4.2.3. Behavioural

Problems of disordered sexual behaviour rarely have an obvious endocrine cause. Many published series do include some cases amongst males with hypo- or hyperfunction of their gonads as appropriate. These cases are probably distinguishable on purely clinical grounds as requiring endocrine investigation. There seem to be no grounds for the endocrine investigation of cases of homosexuality. When a normal plasma testosterone concentration could be predicted to have great therapeutic value in reassuring a man – for example in a case of impotence – the assay may be justified, but widespread measurements are not generally helpful.

The endocrine aspects of male gonadal dysfunction have been reviewed in Clinics in Endocrinology and Metabolism (Bayliss, 1974; Butt and London, 1975). The problems of puberty are also reviewed in this series (Bierich, 1975) especially the contribution from Sizonenko (1975). Female problems have been covered in the same series by Franchimont et al. (1974) and in similar detail in the "Biochemistry of Women" edited by Curry and Hewitt (1974).

15.4.2.4. Male infertility

Although spermatogenesis requires the stimulus of testosterone, failures of spermatogenesis are rarely due to inadequate androgen production. Male infertility is often associated with, and presumably due to, a low sperm count which can be caused by blockage of the duct system. This may be localized from the different secretions which are known to occur in the male reproductive tract. For example, the seminal vesicle secretes large amounts of fructose, and the prostate, acid phosphatase (Mann, 1964). In this way, a block distal to the seminal vesicles but proximal to the prostate would largely remove fructose from the seminal fluid which would still have a high acid phosphatase activity. Such studies are rarely performed, possibly due to the poor results of attempts to correct the obstruction. High concentrations of follicle stimulating hormone in plasma are associated with a marked lack of even the initial cells of the developmental series, the spermatogonia, on testicular biopsy. An arrest of the maturation of spermatogenic cells is not associated with such marked elevations of the hormone but both this assay and testicular biopsy still require further evaluation of their clinical benefit in the investigation of male infertility. Similarly cytogenetic studies have revealed abnormalities; for example, in 3.5% of 200 infertile males, such abnormalities frequently affect the Y chromosome (Hendry et al., 1976). Large doses of anabolic steroids as used by some athletes, depress the sperm count and androgen production; it is not yet known whether such changes can be irreversible in susceptible individuals.

It remains true that the majority of cases of male infertility have no detectable cause and that there is no effective treatment for nearly all cases.

15.4.2.5. Female infertility: oligomenorrhoea and secondary amenorrhoea

A pattern of investigation of these disorders is evolving with its first aim being treatment (Lunenfeld and Insler, 1974; Jacobs et al., 1976). Basically, oligomenorrhoea implies the presence of all the necessary apparatus and controls but with some imbalance in the controls. In view of the high incidence of oligomenorrhoea this is discussed under a separate heading. Primary amenorrhoea has already been considered as gonadal failure (section 15.4.2.1.) since the rare cases in which there is mechanical blockage to the outflow of menstrual blood should not provoke biochemical investigation.

An initial division of cases of secondary amenorrhoea can be made on the basis of the presence or absence of gonadal oestrogen production. This oestrogen can be measured directly in blood or urine, or indirectly by its effects in the presence or absence of bleeding following progestogen withdrawal, or by histological criteria. The results of simultaneous gonadotrophin estimations should be consistent with the level of oestrogen production. High levels of follicle stimulating hormone would suggest gonadal failure. Such estimations might justifiably be limited to follicle stimulating hormone but some laboratories are now able to interpret changes in the ratio of this hormone to luteinizing hormone which can sometimes be useful supplementary evidence. If the concentrations of gonadotrophins are normal or even low, and if the latter can be adequately distinguished by the methods used, failure in the pituitary could be detected by a subnormal response to the decapeptide LH/FSH-RH (section 15.3.). Hypothalamic failure might be detected by an absence of a response to clomiphene. Pregnancy or a trophoblastic tumour can be readily detected by estimation of human chorionic gonadotrophin. In general, a corpus luteum once formed functions normally, but some people – possibly with short cycles – have been found in whom progesterone production is deficient. Such defects have been found during the investigation of infertility. Since marked variation in progesterone production may be found in fertile women it may be dangerous to assume the relationship between low progesterone production and infertility is causal unless progesterone production is 10%, or less, of normal mean values. There seems to be approximately a 10-fold safety factor in many biological systems before function is affected, as shown in many studies of hereditary metabolic disease (Chapter 18).

In such a complex series of investigations a parallel series of anatomically based tests is often proceeding, e.g. on the genital tract to detect obstruction and on the pituitary and hypothalamus to find space-occupying lesions. The latter is often summarized by the listing of a skull X-ray. Interacting endocrine systems – such as thyroid and especially those related chemically in the pituitary and adrenal cortex – are also usually scanned clinically, and sometimes biochemical investigations are justified. The finding of definitely high levels of prolactin, associated in 30% of cases with radiologically definable pituitary tumours, has emphasized the value of this approach (Haesslein and Lamb, 1976; Jacobs et al., 1976). If there were no detectable pituitary tumour and normal thyroid function, as indicated by circulating thyroxine levels for example, then bromocryptine treatment could restore ovulation. As would be predicted from the above scheme of investigation, such patients with a prolactin-secreting tumour or tumours have a severe oestrogen deficiency and a failure to ovulate in response to clomiphene. Although galactorrhoea can be an abnormality which is associated with a high concentration of prolactin, this is not necessarily found. From this, it follows that prolactin determinations should certainly be performed on specimens from patients with galactorrhoea but its absence is not a reliable indication of normal prolactin concentrations. Considerable experience is necessary to interpret small apparent rises in the values since normality is difficult to define; stress, as from venepuncture, hypoglycaemia, oestrogenic stimulation at "pregnancy" levels, thyroid releasing hormone and many psychotropic drugs like chlorpromazine, increase prolactin concentrations. There is also a circadian variation, possibly due to predominantly nocturnal discharge; females are also more responsive than males to stimuli provoking prolactin release. A review of many basic endocrine studies of prolactin is provided by L'Hermite (1976) and in the monograph on the "Endocrinology of Pregnancy" (1977) listed in the Further Reading.

15.4.2.6. Polycystic ovary syndrome

The commonest cause of infertility and secondary amenorrhoea has been called a number of names, including the polycystic ovary or Stein–Leventhal syndrome. It is almost certainly not due to a single cause, and is generally suggested to be caused by an obscure defect or defects in control mechanisms. It is characterized by an oestrogen production equivalent to about 10 μg/24 h excretion of total oestrogen, and some gonadotrophic activity which overall shows more follicle stimulating than luteinizing hormone activity, but this is not definite enough for diagnostic use; luteinizing hormone apparently fails to be pushed to a high enough concentration to stimulate ovulation. There is either spontaneous bleeding or exogenous progesterone withdrawal bleeding. Clinically the two main problems are infertility and hirsutism. There may also be obesity. Ovulation can be produced in about 70% of patients a variable time after the administration of clomiphene, sometimes with added human chorionic gonadotrophin.

Marked hirsutism with other features of masculinization may rarely be due to a gonadal or adrenocortical tumour or to the late onset of the 21-hydroxylation defect. Such causes can generally be excluded by the absence of a raised urinary output of 17-hydroxycorticosteroids as measured by glycol cleaving methods (Chapter 7).

The problem of hirsutism is only partially resolved. Its presence is good cumulative evidence of raised androgen production and it therefore seems unnecessary to attempt the limited measurements of testosterone production which are possible, unless the constant higher levels found with tumours are suspected. The source of the increased testosterone production which is found in an increasingly large number of endocrine studies is obscure.

In view of the frequency of the condition and the continued and unresolved doubts as to the course of its investigation and treatment, some further discussion is justified although this must be largely speculative. Serial studies of ovarian function in the condition have shown slow variations in follicular activity and only intermittently raised testosterone production; this accounts for the occasional failure to demonstrate raised testosterone levels in association with hirsutism. Adrenal secretion of 17-oxosteroids, especially dehydroepiandrosterone, is frequently raised; these compounds are only androgenic after conversion into testosterone or 5α-dihydrotestosterone. Such a conversion will occur most efficiently in gonadal tissue. It therefore seems possible to reconcile the quantitative studies showing a predominantly adrenal source of androgen with the marked clinical effects of gonadal suppression, on hair growth for example, which could operate by selectively blocking the most efficient means of conversion of adrenal precursors into potent androgens.

Some suggestions as to the defects in at least some of these women can be made. Since the major accumulating enzyme substrates in this condition are 17-oxosteroids, it may be relevant that there are at least two enzymes catalyzing the final reduction of the 17-oxo to the active 17β-hydroxyl group, and these are under independent genetic control (Harkness et al., 1975). A defect in an ovarian enzyme responsible for the conversion of 17-oxo into 17β-hydroxyl groups could be partially compensated for by the parallel extragonadal pathways mediated by another enzyme or other enzymes. The transmission of biosynthetic intermediates from the adrenal cortex to a gonad to enable it to bypass, or otherwise overcome, other blocks in biosynthesis should be possible since the pathways of steroid biosynthesis "leak" to a surprisingly large extent: intermediates of steroid biosynthesis appear in the circulation in relatively large amounts. The existence of this exchange is suggested in Figure 15.1, in which the foetal adrenocortical placental exchange is also shown. A specifically ovarian series of defects in steroid biosynthesis could thus be masked.

The provision of intermediates by the adrenal cortex to the gonads is suggested from several items of evidence including the occurrence of "adrenarche". This is a series of changes in adrenocortical secretion leading to greater production of DHA and other 17-oxosteroids relative to that of cortisol and mineralocorticoids, and associated with the appearance of sexual hair. Adrenarche normally precedes puberty, as indicated in Figure 15.3, but can occur earlier, independently of puberty. This latter observation provides further evidence for the existence of an unknown trophic factor (Figure 15.1) which is potentially independent of ACTH or gonadotrophins. Related to the above evidence is the increasing recognition that the marked adrenocortical hypofunction found in familial congenital adrenocortical hypoplasia is associated with delayed puberty in children. More acute stimulation with clomiphene provides similar evidence in that the gonadal response to the drug is markedly reduced in "adrenalectomized" males (Harkness et al., 1968). The adrenal cortex thus seems to provide power to the final controlled process in the gonad, possibly as synthesized intermediates. It is therefore possible that a variety of endocrine defects in the gonads may be masked by adrenocortical secretion. The existence of parallel, partially self-compensatory pathways would thus account for the failure of endocrine studies in the whole woman, and even in gonadal and adrenocortical effluent, to reveal clear evidence of abnormality. These suggestions would also help to explain why the follicle rarely manages to produce an adequate rapid oestrogen surge to trigger luteinizing hormone release for ovulation since adrenocortical controls would be involved in any control loop. For many years it was hoped to be possible, by classical suppression tests, to guide treatment to adrenal or gonad, but more than a decade of intensive work has shown that this is not the case, although many patients continue to be subjected to such tests. The above explanations at least have the merit of being a reminder, explaining in part how such tests might have failed.

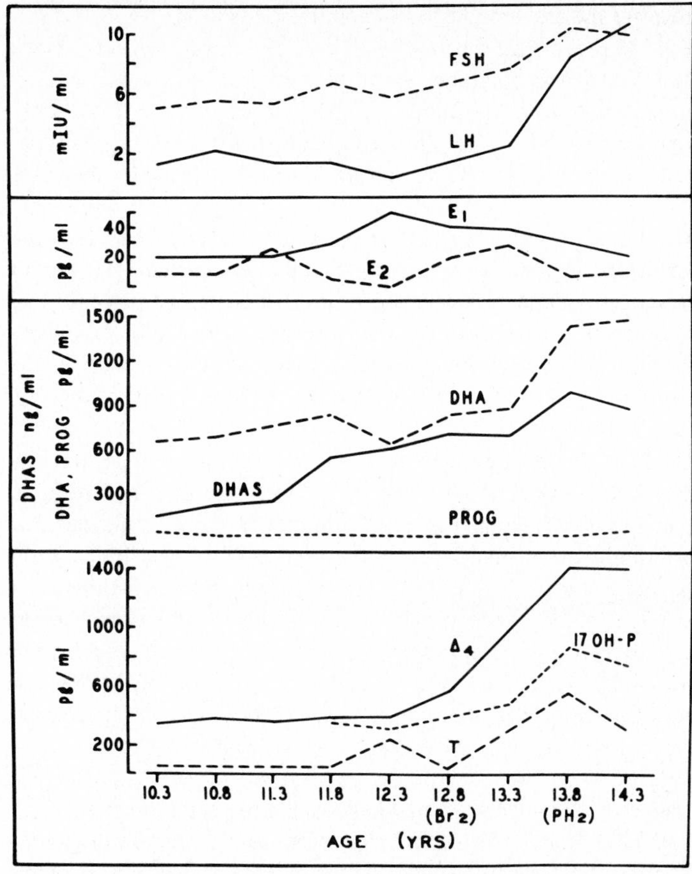

Figure 15.3. Developmental changes in one girl from the age of 10.3 to 14.3 years. Adrenal and gonadal steroids and gonadotrophin rises are shown sequentially with the earliest clearly demonstrable rise in plasma dehydroepiandrosterone sulphate. Breast development was noted at 12.8 years and pubic hair at 13.8 years. Bone age at the start of the study (10.3 years) was 8.5 years. (Reproduced, by permission, from Lee et al., 1976)

15.5. BIOCHEMICAL CHANGES AFTER ORAL CONTRACEPTIVES

The most biologically powerful compounds in the many oral contraceptive pills are the oestrogens, which are usually present as analogues such as ethinyloestradiol or its 3-methylether, mestranol. Varied doses are used, with a marked reduction in the dose in recent years. The metabolic effects of many pills are similar to those found in pregnancy, when it is clear that many of the widespread changes are produced by the oestrogen–progesterone combination, especially the oestrogenic component. The nature of the progestogen in the contraceptive has some clinical biochemical importance since 19-norprogestogens like 17α-alkylated androgens, can cause an intrahepatic cholestatic jaundice; in contrast, the analogues close to progesterone are rarely associated with jaundice.

The biochemical effects of oral contraceptives have been the subject of much work and the changes found are many and complex. Some indication of this complexity is shown in Table 15.1 from Briggs (1976). Further consideration of more commonly encountered changes is given in Chapter 1. It should be remembered that the relationships of these changes to disease, or even to undesirable changes in physiological mechanisms, are much more difficult to determine. Large retrospective and prospective series have shown a slightly increased incidence of thrombotic disease, but have been otherwise largely reassuring, suggesting that women are safer with the pill than pregnant. The use of oestrogens by women is common; about 50% of younger women and about 30 to 40% of women over 50 years of age took some preparation according to a survey of 10 diverse demographically defined North American populations (Wallace et al., 1977). Many of the present problems connected with contraception have been reviewed in a symposium proceedings (Short and Baird, 1976).

Similar metabolic changes after oral contraceptives are found in all women, but the diseases associated with blood clotting in very few. It may be possible, in future, to develop tests predicting an abnormal response to sex hormones and their analogues; for example, certain women respond to pregnancy and to exogenous oestrogens by developing jaundice. In the same way, menstrual irregularity before the pill is a reliable indicator of irregularity after the pill; similarly with psychiatric problems which may occur in women on the pill. If such idiosyncrasy has a simple genetic basis, then such defects need only be defined once in a family. There may also be ethnic or environmental differences; it was clear in early studies that some Scandinavians showed marked changes in classical liver function tests after oral contraceptives, whereas no such changes were seen in extensive British studies.

At first, the number and extent of changes in pregnancy and in a pseudopregnant state induced by oral contraceptives appear confusing, but they often seem to be useful modifications which preserve the health of mother and/or of the child. For example, it seems probable that evolution would select mothers who did not bleed easily through the highly vascular placental attachment; hence an increase in the activity of blood clotting mechanisms after oestrogens. In the same way, increases in binding proteins probably help overall function when another large series of "compartments", in the form of the foetoplacental unit, grows in the mother. The maintenance of a favourable glucose and oxygen gradient for the foetus would appear to be objectives of changes in carbohydrate metabolism and the regulation of respiration. The many such changes in pregnancy are reviewed in "The Physiology of Human Pregnancy" (Hytten and Leitch, 1971) and "Diagnostic Indices in Pregnancy" (Hytten and Lind, 1973).

Such hypotheses may point to useful biochemical investigations in failures of normal foetoplacental and maternal function. For example, detailed consideration of the available records of the labours of patients with placental sulphatase deficiency and very low oestrogens, less than 10% of normal, suggests that some may have prolonged labour possibly due to poor dilatation of the cervix, a tissue on which oestrogen effects have been recognized for many years. Since this condition may be diagnosed antenatally, some warning of the possibility to the obstetrician may save a child and a great deal of trouble for all concerned. However, the rarity of placental sulphatase deficiency is a warning against generalizations.

TABLE 15.1.

BIOCHEMICAL EFFECTS OF ORAL CONTRACEPTIVES IN WOMEN

(Reproduced, by permission, from Briggs, 1976)

Parameter	Type of product	Reported effect
1. Serum calcium	Combined o.c.	Small increase
2. Serum phosphate	Combined o.c.	Small decrease
3. Platelet calcium	Combined o.c.	Increase
4. Erythrocyte magnesium	Combined o.c.	Transient decrease
5. Platelet magnesium	Combined o.c.	Increase
6. Milk sodium	Combined o.c.	Decrease
	Mini-pill	No change
7. Milk potassium	Combined o.c.	Increase
	Mini-pill	Increase
8. Milk calcium	Combined o.c.	Variable
	Mini-pill	No change
9. Milk magnesium	Combined o.c.	Increase
	Mini-pill	Increase
10. Milk phosphate	Combined o.c.	Decrease
	Mini-pill	Decrease
11. Serum magnesium	Combined o.c.	Variable (mainly decrease)
12. Serum iron	Combined o.c.	Increase
	Mini-pill	Variable
13. Serum copper	Combined o.c.	Increase
	Mini-pill	Small increase or no change
14. Hair copper	Combined o.c.	Increase
15. Plasma or serum zinc	Combined o.c.	Decrease
	Mini-pill	No change
16. Plasma retinol	Combined o.c.	Increase
17. Plasma carotene	Combined o.c.	No change
18. Leucocyte ascorbate	Combined o.c.	Decrease
	Sequential o.c.	Decrease
	Mini-pill	No change
19. Platelet ascorbate	Combined o.c.	Decrease
20. Plasma ascorbate	Combined o.c.	Decrease
21. Urinary ascorbate	Combined o.c.	Decrease
22. Serum folate	Combined o.c.	Variable
23. Erythrocyte folate	Combined o.c.	Decrease
24. Urinary forminoglutamate	Combined o.c.	Increase
25. Serum pyridoxal phosphate	Combined o.c.	No change
26. Urinary pyridoxic acid	Combined o.c.	No change
27. Serum vitamin B_{12}	Combined o.c.	Decrease
28. Erythrocyte vitamin B_{12}	Combined o.c.	Variable
29. Plasma tocopherol	Combined o.c.	Increase
30. Plasma LH	Combined o.c.	Mid-cycle peak absent
	Sequential o.c.	Mid-cycle peak absent
	Mini-pill	Variable
31. Plasma FSH	Combined o.c.	Mid-cycle peak absent
	Sequential o.c.	Mid-cycle peak absent
	Mini-pill	Variable
32. Plasma progesterone	Sequential o.c.	Luteal phase decrease

TABLE 15.1. (continued)

Parameter	Type of product	Reported effect
33. Plasma estradiol	Combined o.c.	Basal unchanged, peaks decreased
34. Urinary estrogens	Mini-pill	Decrease
35. Plasma testosterone	Combined o.c.	Increase
36. Plasma dehydroepiandrosterone sulfate	Combined o.c.	Decrease
37. Plasma androsterone sulfate	Combined o.c.	Decrease
38. Plasma total corticosteroids	Combined o.c.	Decrease
	Mini-pill	Variable
39. Plasma free corticosteroids	Combined o.c.	Increase
40. Urinary corticosteroids	Combined o.c.	Increase
41. Plasma aldosterone	Combined o.c.	Increase
42. Urinary tetrahydroaldosterone	Combined o.c.	Increase
43. Plasma angiotensin-II	Combined o.c.	Increase
44. Plasma renin substrate	Combined o.c.	Increase
45. Plasma renin activity	Combined o.c.	Increase
46. Plasma renin concentration	Combined o.c.	Decrease
47. Plasma angiotensin-I	Combined o.c.	Increase
48. Plasma angiotensinase	Combined o.c.	Increase
49. Fasting plasma insulin	Combined o.c.	Increase
	Sequential o.c.	Increase
	Mini-pill	Variable
50. Plasma growth hormone	Combined o.c.	Increase
	Sequential o.c.	Increase
51. Serum protein-bound iodine	Combined o.c.	Increase
52. T^3-resin uptake	Combined o.c.	Decrease
53. Electrophoretic index	Combined o.c.	Increase
54. Free thyroxine index	Combined o.c.	Increase
55. Urinary noradrenaline	Combined o.c.	Increase
	Sequential o.c.	Increase
56. Urinary adrenaline	Combined o.c.	Increase
	Sequential o.c.	Decrease
57. Plasma α-amino N	Combined o.c.	Decrease (luteal phase)
58. Plasma tyrosine	Combined o.c.	Decrease
59. Serum amino acids	Combined o.c.	Altered pattern
60. Urinary 3-hydroxyanthranilate	Combined o.c.	Increase
61. Urinary kynurenine	Combined o.c.	Increase
62. Urinary 3-β-hydroxykynurenine	Combined o.c.	Increase
63. Urinary xanthurenate	Combined o.c.	Increase
64. Urinary quinolinate	Combined o.c.	Increase
65. Red cell hemoglobin	Combined o.c.	No change
66. Serum haptoglobin	Combined o.c.	Decrease
	Mini-pill	No change
67. Serum transferrin	Combined o.c.	Increase
	Sequential o.c.	Increase
	Mini-pill	No change
68. Serum TIBC	Combined o.c.	Increase
	Sequential o.c.	Increase
	Mini-pill	Variable

TABLE 15.1. (continued)

Parameter	Type of product	Reported effect
69. Serum ceruloplasmin	Combined o.c.	Increase
	Sequential o.c.	Increase
	Mini-pills	Variable
70. Serum transcortin	Combined o.c.	Increase
71. Serum α_2-macroglobulin	Combined o.c.	Increase
72. Serum albumin	Combined o.c.	Decrease
	Mini-pill	No effect
73. Serum orosomucoid	Combined o.c.	Decrease
	Mini-pill	Variable
74. Serum α_1-glycoprotein	Combined o.c.	Decrease
75. Serum α_1-lipoprotein	Combined o.c.	Increase
76. Serum α_1-antitrypsin	Combined o.c.	Increase
77. Serum α_2-SH- glycoprotein	Combined o.c.	Increase
78. Serum β_1-lipoprotein	Combined o.c.	Increase
79. Serum antinuclear antibody	Combined o.c.	Increase
80. Serum rheumatoid factor	Combined o.c.	Increase
81. Serum C-reactive protein	Combined o.c.	Increase
82. Plasma fibrinogen	Combined o.c.	Variable
83. Factor V	Combined o.c.	No change
84. Factor IX	Combined o.c.	Increase
85. Factor VIII (1st stage)	Combined o.c.	Increase
86. Factor VIII (2nd stage)	Combined o.c.	No change
87. Plasma plasminogen	Combined o.c.	Increase
88. Serum or plasma antithrombin-III	Combined o.c.	Decrease
	Mini-pill	No change
89. Fasting blood glucose	Combined o.c.	No change
	Sequential o.c.	No change
	Mini-pill	No change
90. Serum total lipids	Combined o.c.	Increase
	Sequential o.c.	Increase
91. Serum triglycerides	Combined o.c.	Increase
	Sequential o.c.	Increase
	Mini-pill	No change
92. Glucose-tolerance test	Combined o.c.	Increased % abnormal
	Sequential o.c.	Increased % abnormal
93. Blood pyruvate	Combined o.c.	Increase
94. Serum fucose	Combined o.c.	No change
95. Milk total protein	Combined o.c.	Decrease
	Mini-pill	Decrease
96. Milk fat	Combined o.c.	Small decrease
97. Milk lactose	Combined o.c.	Variable
98. Serum phospholipids	Combined o.c.	Increase
	Mini-pill	No change
99. Cervical mucus lipids fatty acids	Combined o.c.	Altered pattern
100. Serum NEFA	Combined o.c.	Decrease
	Mini-pill	No change
101. Serum cholesterol	Combined o.c.	Variable (mainly increased)
	Sequential o.c.	Increase
102. Menstrual blood cholesterol	Combined o.c.	Decrease
103. Plasma glycerol	Combined o.c.	Decrease

TABLE 15.1. (continued)

Parameter	Type of product	Reported effect
104. Serum β-hydroxybutyrate	Combined o.c.	Increase
105. Erythrocyte aminotransferases	Combined o.c.	Small increase
106. Serum aminotransferases	All types	Variable
107. Serum alkaline phosphatase	All types	Variable
108. Serum γ-glutamyltransferase	All types	Increase
109. Serum amylase	Combined o.c.	Variable
110. Erythrocyte-catechol-*O*-methyl transferase	Combined o.c. Mini-pill	Variable Decrease
111. Erythrocyte-carbonic anhydrase-B	Combined o.c.	Increase
112. Lipolytic activity	Combined o.c.	Variable
113. Cervical mucus glucose-6-phosphate isomerase	Combined o.c.	Increase
114. Serum monoamine oxidase	Combined o.c.	Decrease
115. Blood fibrinolytic activity	Combined o.c.	Variable
116. Urinary fibrinolytic activity	Combined o.c.	Increase

15.6. CONCLUSION

In human reproduction there are many examples of the successful use of biochemistry and of chemical methods of diagnosis. Recent advances have included the identification of open defects of the central nervous system in the foetus before it becomes viable. To an increasing extent, it is to be hoped that the biochemist will help to prevent many more diseases rather than struggling, along with his clinical colleagues, from one crisis to the next.

ACKNOWLEDGEMENTS

I should like to thank past and present colleagues for our many discussions.

REFERENCES

Bagshawe, K.D. (1976) Endocrinology and treatment of trophoblastic tumours. Journal of Clinical Pathology, 29, suppl. (Royal College of Pathologists) 10, 140–144.

Baker, H.W.G. and Hudson, B. (1974) Male gonadal dysfunction. In Investigation of Endocrine Disorders (Ed. R.I.S. Bayliss) Clinics in Endocrinology and Metabolism, 3 (3) pp. 507–531.

Baker, H.W.G., Burger, H.G., de Kretser, D.M., Hudson, B., O'Connor, S.O., Wang, C., Mirovics, A., Court, J., Dunlop, M. and Rennie, G.C. (1976a) Changes in the pituitary–testicular system with age. Clinical Endocrinology, 5, 349–372.

Baker, H.W.G., Burger, H.G., de Kretser, D.M., Dulmanis, A., Hudson, B., O'Connor, S., Paulsen, C.A., Purcell, N., Rennie, G.C., Seah, C.S., Taft, H.P. and Wang, C. (1976b) A study of the endocrine manifestations of hepatic cirrhosis. Quarterly Journal of Medicine, 45 (N.S.), 145–178.

Bayliss, R.I.S. (Ed.) (1974) Investigation of Endocrine Disorders. Clinics in Endocrinology and Metabolism 3 (3).

Beeson, P.B. and McDermott, W. (Ed.) (1975) Textbook of Medicine. W.B. Saunders Co., Philadelphia.

Bierich, J.R. (Ed.) (1975) Disorders of Puberty. Clinics in Endocrinology and Metabolism, 4 (1).

Briggs, M.H. (1976) Biochemical effects of oral contraceptives. Advances in Steroid Biochemistry and Pharmacology, 5, 66–160.

Brock, D.J.H. (1976) Alphafetoprotein and neural tube defects. Journal of Clinical Pathology, 29, suppl. (Royal College of Pathologists) 10, 157–164.

Brock, D.J.H. (1977) Biochemical and cytological methods in the diagnosis of neural tube defects. Progress in Medical Genetics (new series) II, 1–38.

Brotherton, J. (Ed.) (1976) Sex Hormone Pharmacology. Academic Press, London and New York.

Butt, W.R. and London, D.R. (Ed.) (1975) The Testis. Clinics in Endocrinology and Metabolism, 4 (3).

Chard, T. (1976) Assessment of fetoplacental function by biochemical determinations. Journal of Clinical Pathology, 29, suppl. (Royal College of Pathologists) 10, 18–26.

Curry, A.S. and Hewitt, J.V. (Eds.) (1974) Biochemistry of Women: Clinical Concepts and Methods for Clinical Investigation. CRC Press, Cleveland.

Dewhurst, C.J. (1974) Abnormal sex differentiation. In A companion to Medical Studies, Vol. 3 (Eds. R. Passmore and J.S. Robson) Chap. 29, Blackwell Scientific Publications, Oxford and Edinburgh.

Elmfors, B. and Tryding, N. (1976) Date of confinement prediction from serum diamine oxidase determination in early pregnancy. British Journal of Obstetrics and Gynaecology, 83, 6–10.

Franchimont, P., Valcke, J.C. and Lambotte, R. (1974) Female gonadal dysfunction. In Investigation of Endocrine Disorders (Ed. R.I.S. Bayliss) Clinics in Endocrinology and Metabolism, 3 (3) pp. 533–556.

Fuchs, F. and Klopper, A. (Eds.) (1977) Endocrinology of Pregnancy. Harper Row, New York and London.

Fukushima, D.K., Bradlow, H.L., Hellman, L. and Gallagher, T.F. (1962) Isolation and characterization of 18-hydroxy-17-ketosteroids. Journal of Biological Chemistry, 237, 3359–3363.

Glenister, T.W., Hytten, F.E. and Kerr, M.G. (1968) Human reproduction. In A Companion to Medical Studies, Vol 1 (Eds. R. Passmore and J.S. Robson) Chap. 37, Blackwell, Oxford and Edinburgh.

Goodwin, J.W., Godden, J.O. and Chance, G.W. (Eds.) (1976) Perinatal Medicine – The Basic Science Underlying Clinical Practice. Williams and Wilkins, Baltimore.

Grant, D.B., Laurance, B.M., Atherden, S.M. and Tyness, J. (1976) HCG stimulation test in children with abnormal sexual development. Archives of Diseases in Childhood, 51, 596–601.

Haesslein, H.C. and Lamb, E.J. (1976) Pituitary tumours with secondary amenorrhoea. American Journal of Obstetrics and Gynecology, 123, 759–767.

Hall, R. and Gomez-Pan, A. (1976) Hypothalamic regulatory hormones and their clinical application. Advances in Clinical Chemistry, 18, 174–212.

Harkness, R.A., Bell, E.T., Loraine, J.A., Ismail, A.A.A. and Morse, W.I. (1968) The effects of clomiphene on endocrine function in male patients with adrenocortical insufficiency and following castration. Acta Endocrinologica (Kbh.), 58, 38–48.

Harkness, R.A., Scott, R.D.M. and Strong, J.A. (1974) Physiological and pharmacological factors affecting the 6β-hydroxylation and 17-epimerization of methandrostenedione. Biochemical Society Transactions, 2, 119–121.

Harkness, R.A., Thistlethwaite, D., Darling, J.A.B., Skakkebaek, N.E. and Corker, C.S. (1975) 17β-Hydroxysteroid oxidoreductase deficiency causing male pseudohermaphroditism in a child. Journal of Endocrinology, 67, 16–17P.

Hendry, W.F., Polani, P.E., Pugh, R.C.B., Sommerville, I.F. and Wallace, D.M. (1976) 200 Infertile males: correlation of chromosome, histological, endocrine and clinical studies. British Journal of Urology, 47, 899–908.

Hobson, B.M. (1966) A review: pregnancy diagnosis. Journal of Reproduction and Fertility, 12, 33–48.

Hobson, B.M. (1974) Advances in human pregnancy testing. Bibliography of Reproduction, 24, 110–112.

Hurley, R. (Ed.) (1976) The Pathology of Pregnancy. Journal of Clinical Pathology, suppl. 10 (Royal College of Pathologists).

Hytten, F.E. and Leitch, I. (1971) The Physiology of Human Pregnancy. Blackwell, Oxford.

Hytten, F.E. and Lind, T. (1973) Diagnostic Indices in Pregnancy. pp. 77–83, Ciba-Geigy, Basle.

Jacobs, H.S., Franks, S., Murray, M.A.F., Hull, M.G.R., Steele, S.J. and Nabarro, J.D.N. (1976) Clinical and endocrine features of hyperprolactinaemic amenorrhoea. Clinical Endocrinology, 5, 439–454.

Kerr, M.G. and Parboosingh, I.J.T. (1974) Disorders of the female reproductive tract. In A Comparison to Medical Studies, Vol. 3 (Eds. R. Passmore and J.S. Robson) Chap. 28, Blackwell Scientific publications, Oxford and Edinburgh.

Klopper, A. (1977) Choice of hormone in the assessment of fetoplacental function. In Endocrinology of Pregnancy (Eds. F. Fuchs and A. Klopper) pp. 350–364, Harper and Row, New York and London.

Larson, B.A., Vanderlaan, W.P., Judd, H.L. and McCullough, D.L. (1976) Testosterone producing adrenalcortical adenoma in an elderly woman. Journal of Clinical Endocrinology, 42, 882–887.

Lau, H.L. and Linkins, S.E. (1976) Alphafetoprotein. American Journal of Obstetrics and Gynecology, 124, 533–554.

Lee, P.A., Xenakis, T., Winer, J. and Matsenbaugh, S. (1976) Puberty in girls: correlation of serum levels of gonadotrophins, prolactin, androgens, estrogens and progestins with physical changes. Journal of Clinical Endocrinology, 43, 775–784.

L'Hermite, M. (1976) Prolactin. In Hormone Assays and Their Clinical Application (Eds. J.A. Loraine and E.T. Bell) pp. 350–364, Churchill-Livingstone, Edinburgh.

Loraine, J.A. and Bell, E.T. (Eds.) (1976) Hormone Assays and their Clinical Application. Churchill-Livingstone, Edinburgh.

Lunenfeld, B. and Insler, V. (1974) Classification of amenorrhoeic states and their treatment by ovulation induction. Clinical Endocrinology, 3, 223–237.

Mann, T. (1964) Biochemistry of Semen and of the Male Reproductive Tract, Methuen, London.

Niven, P.A.R., Landon, J. and Chard, T. (1972) Placental lactogen levels as a guide to the outcome of threatened abortion. British Medical Journal, 3, 799–801.

Novak, E.R. and Woodruff, J.D. (Eds.) (1974) Gynècologic and Obstetric Pathology, W.B. Saunders, Philadelphia.

Peeters, L.L., Lemons, J.A., Niswender, G.D. and Battaglia, F.C. (1976) Serum levels of human placental lactogen and human chorionic gonadotrophin in early pregnancy: a maturation index of the placenta. American Journal of Obstetrics and Gynecology, 126, 707–715.

Redman, C.W.G., Beilin, L.J., Bonnar, J. and Wilkinson, J.H. (1976) Plasma urate measurements in predicting fetal death in hypertensive pregnancy. Lancet, i, 1370.

Rodeck, C.H., Campbell, S. and Biswas, S. (1976) Maternal plasma alphafetoprotein in normal and complicated pregnancies. British Journal of Obstetrics and Gynaecology, 83, 24–32.

Schweikert, H.U., Milewich, L. and Wilson, J.D. (1976) Aromatization of androstenedione by cultured human fibroblasts. Journal of Clinical Endocrinology, 43, 785–795.

Short, R.V. and Baird, D.T. (1976) Contraceptives of the future. Proceedings of the Royal Society (London) Series B, 195, 1–224.

Smith, D.W. (1976) Recognizable Patterns of Human Malformation, 2nd edn. W.B. Saunders, Philadelphia.

Sizonenko, P.C. (1975) Endocrine laboratory findings in pubertal disturbances. In Disorders of Puberty (Ed. J.R. Bierich) Clinics in Endocrinology and Metabolism, 4 (1), pp. 173–206.

U.K. Collaborative Study (1977) Maternal serum alphafetoprotein measurement in antenatal screening for anencephaly and spina bifida in early pregnancy. Lancet, i, 1323–1332.

Wallace, R.B., Hoover, J., Sandler, D., Rifkind, B.M. and Tyroler, H.A. (1977) Altered plasma lipids associated with oral contraceptive or oestrogen consumption. Lancet, ii, 11–14.

Wilde, C.E. and Oakey, R.E. (1975) Biochemical tests for the assessment of feto-placental function. Annals of Clinical Biochemistry, 12, 83–118.

Winter, J.S.D., Hughes, I.A., Reyes, F.E. and Faiman, C. (1976) Pituitary–gonadal relations in infancy: 2. Patterns of serum gonadal steroid concentrations in man from birth to two years of age. Journal of Clinical Endocrinology, 42, 679–686.

FURTHER READING

Brotherton, J. (Ed.) (1976) Sex Hormone Pharmacology. Academic Press, London and New York.

Curry, A.S. and Hewitt, J.V. (Eds.) (1974) Biochemistry of Women: Clinical Concepts and Methods for Clinical Investigation. CRC Press, Cleveland.

Fuchs, F. and Klopper, A. (Eds.) (1977) Endocrinology of Pregnancy, Harper Row, New York and London.

Goodwin, J.W., Godden, J.O. and Chance, G.W. (Eds.) (1976) Perinatal Medicine – The Basic Science Underlying Clinical Practice. William and Wilkins, Baltimore.

Hytten, F.E. and Leitch, I. (1971) The Physiology of Human Pregnancy. Blackwell, Oxford.

Loraine, J.A. and Bell, E.T. (Eds.) (1976) Hormone Assays and their Clinical Application. Churchill-Livingstone, Edinburgh.

Passmore, R. and Robson, J.S. (Eds.) (1968) A Companion to Medical Studies, Vol. 1. Chap. 37. Blackwell, Oxford and Edinburgh.

Passmore, R. and Robson, J.S. (Eds.) (1974) A Companion to Medical Studies, Vol. 3. Chaps. 28 and 29, Blackwell, Oxford and Edinburgh.

Recent Progress in Hormone Research. Yearly. Academic Press, London and New York.

Chapter 16

Haematological biochemistry

Israel Chanarin

Department of Haematology, Northwick Park Hospital, Harrow, Middlesex HA1 3UJ, England

CONTENTS

Chemical diagnosis of disease, edited by S.S. Brown, F.L. Mitchell and D.S. Young

This chapter is concerned with the interpretation of data that may be generated in the haematology laboratory but which is relevant to the chemical diagnosis of disease. Blood corpuscular enzymes are dealt with in Chapter 7.

16.1. INTERPRETATION OF BLOOD COUNT VALUES

Routine blood cell counts and other haematological measurements are now generally carried out on automatic instruments which generate data on the haemoglobin concentration, haematocrit, mean corpuscular volume (MCV), mean corpuscular haemoglobin (MCH), mean corpuscular haemoglobin concentration (MCHC), red cell count, total white cell count, and sometimes also the platelet count. The results are highly reproducible in the same patient from day to day, and the mean values for large numbers of samples may be used for quality control purposes.

16.1.1. The haemoglobin concentration (Hb)

Measurement of haemoglobin concentration remains the most commonly used means of assessing anaemia. Estimation by the cyanmethaemoglobin technique is preferred to older methods since it measures haemoglobin, methaemoglobin and carboxyhaemoglobin but not, however, sulphaemoglobin. An additional advantage of the cyanmethaemoglobin technique is that stable cyanmethaemoglobin standard solutions are available or may be prepared with relative ease.

Reference values for total haemoglobin concentration are 15.0 ± 0.8 (S.D.) g/dl in males at sea level and 12.7 ± 0.6 (S.D.) g/dl in women; the sex difference only emerges at puberty. Any group of normal individuals, particularly women of child-bearing age, will include a significant number of persons whose haemoglobin values will increase if they are given iron medication (Garby, 1970). In Western societies, some 15% of apparently normal females respond in this way.

16.1.2. The venous haematocrit

The normal true haematocrit values on venous blood for adult males at sea level are $44.5 \pm 2.2\%$ (S.D.) and for adult females $39.5 \pm 2.0\%$ (S.D.) (Garby, 1970). When estimated by a centrifugation method, the packed cell volume (PCV) includes an average of 2.7% trapped plasma. Thus the true haematocrit is on the average about 1.4% less than that recorded on centrifugation. In addition, the haematocrit varies with blood samples collected from various sites in the body. In organs, blood moves in an axial stream with a sleeve of plasma around the walls of the vessel. Thus the haematocrit of blood from tissue is lower than in that taken directly from veins; the ratio, tissue haematocrit/venous haematocrit, is generally taken to be 0.91.

The haematocrit estimation in some automatic instruments is computed by summation of measurement of red cell size and numbers. In these circumstances, the result can be adjusted to exclude trapped plasma and so give a true haematocrit value. When this is done there are significant effects on the calculated values of the MCV and the MCHC.

16.1.3. Mean corpuscular volume (MCV)

This measurement refers to the average volume of the red blood cells. Normal values using a true haematocrit are 80 to 92 fl. The MCV and the MCH have emerged as exceptionally valuable measurements in the interpretation of blood count data.

A low MCV (and MCH) is found in iron-deficiency anaemia, anaemia of chronic disorders and the thalassaemia syndromes. In addition, some microcytosis may occur in hyperthyroidism and in other haemoglobinopathies, when it often indicates associated α-thalassaemia trait. Iron deficiency or anaemia of chronic disorders is suggested when the red cell count is less than 5.0 million/μl and thalassaemia when it is more than 5.5 million/μl. An MCV below 60 fl suggests combined iron deficiency and thalassaemia trait. The blood picture in a patient with iron deficiency and polycythaemia can mimic the blood picture more usually found in thalassaemia trait.

A modest increase in the MCV (up to 94 fl) is common among patients in hospital, but persistent elevations above this level require investigation. Macrocytosis with a megaloblastic marrow is due to folate or vitamin B_{12} deficiency as well as to drugs that interfere with pyrimidine or purine metabolism (cytosine arabinoside, pyrimethamine, mercaptopurine, thioguanine and methotrexate) or to rare inborn errors of metabolism (orotic aciduria, Lesch–Nyhan syndrome).

Macrocytosis associated with a normoblastic marrow and normal vitamin B_{12} and folate stores may be due to chronic alcoholism, liver disease, disseminated neoplasms, aplastic and hypoplastic anaemia, pure red cell aplasia, sideroblastic anaemia, chronic haemolytic states, hypothyroidism and drug therapy, e.g. with melphalan. In some cases no explanation for a patient's macrocytosis is found. About 50% of patients with untreated myxoedema have large red cells and virtually all patients with hypothyroidism show a decline in MCV on treatment with thyroxine, including those patients whose initial MCV was within the normal range. Macrocytosis is present in 80% of chronic alcoholics.

16.1.4. Mean corpuscular haemoglobin (MCH)

The normal haemoglobin content of the red blood cell is 27 to 32 pg. A small red cell contains less, and a large red cell more, haemoglobin than normal. The values, therefore, match the changes in red cell size and the parallellism of these two measurements is a useful addition to quality control. In effect, (Hb/PCV) = (MCH/MCV) = MCHC. Only in severe iron-deficiency anaemia is haemoglobinization more severely impaired than the decline in red cell size: then the MCHC declines.

16.1.5. Mean corpuscular haemoglobin concentration (MCHC)

The mean corpuscular haemoglobin concentration has lost much of its diagnostic value with the development of automatic blood counters. With manual counting methods and a PCV derived by centrifugation, the MCHC is low in iron deficiency and other conditions associated with small red cells. This "early" fall in the MCHC is not seen when estimation is made with automatic counters. The probable explanation is that the abnormal red cells in iron deficiency trap more plasma in the haematocrit than do normal cells; hence a falsely high PCV is obtained. This causes an apparent fall in MCHC which is obtained from the ratio of Hb/PCV. Whatever the setting in the automatic cell counter (including or excluding trapped plasma), it does not reflect the *variation* in amounts of trapped plasma present in the centrifugation haematocrit. With automatic counters, the MCHC falls only in severe iron deficiency and in other defects of haemoglobin synthesis of comparable severity. The MCHC remains within the normal range in early iron deficiency. Thus, in iron deficiency, the red cell decreases in size first and only later does haemoglobinization fail.

16.1.6. The red cell count

The normal red cell count is 5.0 ± 0.6 (2 S.D.) million/μl in males and 4.6 ± 0.5 (2 S.D.) million/μl in females.

16.1.7. The white cell count

The normal range in adults is 4,000 to 11,000/μl. Children have higher lymphocyte levels and hence higher total white cell counts until the age of about seven years, and some increase may be encountered up to puberty.

16.1.8. Platelet counts

These are normally in the range 150,000 to 450,000/μl. While there are many causes of low platelet levels, an increase in platelets is due to myeloproliferative disorders (polycythaemia, chronic myeloid leukaemia, myelofibrosis), loss of the spleen (operative or atrophic) or to chronic blood loss.

16.2. ASSESSMENT OF IRON STATUS

16.2.1. The blood picture

The characteristic blood picture in iron-deficiency anaemia is that of a variable fall in haemoglobin, haematocrit and red cell count, associated with a fall in the MCV and MCH and subsequently a fall in MCHC. The blood film shows hypochromic red cells, with occasional elongated red cells sometimes called pencil cells. Platelets tend to be increased in numbers. The blood may be similar to that seen in the anaemia of chronic disorders and in thalassaemia, although in the latter the red cell count is often significantly higher.

16.2.2. The bone marrow

The bone marrow in iron deficiency is of normal cellularity. Late erythroblasts tend to have an irregular nuclear pattern rather than a round nucleus, and the cytoplasm is ragged. This cell has been called the micronormoblast. Normal marrow which is stained for iron by the Prussian blue method shows iron in reticuloendothelial cells, most readily seen in marrow fragments. This storage iron is absent in iron deficiency. In addition, at least 10% of erythroblasts normally show one or more iron granules in the cytoplasm – these cells are called sideroblasts. Such cells become relatively scanty in iron deficiency. On the other hand, in the anaemia of chronic disorders and in thalassaemia, adequate iron stores are present unless there is additional iron deficiency. Excessive iron is present in these cells in iron overload. Liver biopsy material has also been used to assess iron stores.

16.2.3. Serum ferritin

Ferritin is the iron-storage protein, present in large amounts in liver, spleen and marrow, whereas transferrin is the iron-transport protein. Ferritin has a molecular mass of 450,000 and consists of a spherical protein shell made up of 24 subunits. Iron in the form of ferric-oxide-phosphate accumulates in the centre of the protein core and each molecule may hold up to about 4000 iron atoms. The last iron stored is the first released on demand. Synthesis of ferritin is induced by the presence of iron in the cell; it occurs intracellularly as well as in serum where it may be measured by a radioimmunoassay (Addison et al., 1972). Serum ferritin appears to be closely related to reticuloendothelial ferritin since there is a close correlation between the amount of iron and the ferritin level at the two sites. The protein itself is termed apoferritin. The range of normal serum concentrations is wide, from 12 to 250 μg/l, with a distribution skewed to the right. The mean concentration is 123 μg/l in males and 56 μg/l in females (Jacobs et al., 1972). In iron deficiency the concentration is below 12 μg/l, and in iron overload it is increased considerably. In the anaemia of chronic disorders the serum ferritin is either normal or raised.

The serum ferritin is abnormally high in liver disease including hepatitis, obstructive jaundice and carcinoma of the liver. It is high in leukaemia, Hodgkin's disease and, particularly, haemochromatosis. The serum ferritin level declines to normal with successful phlebotomy treatment of haemochromatosis although the serum iron concentrations remain elevated.

16.2.4. Serum iron and iron-binding capacity

There is sufficient transferrin in plasma to bind 40 to 70 μmol iron per litre. Normally about one-third of the transferrin carries iron, the normal serum iron concentration being

12 to 27 μmol/l. There is a significant sex difference in serum iron values which appears at puberty. The serum iron in males is 10 to 20% higher than in females. This difference is unrelated to the higher incidence of iron deficiency in women and to menstruation; it is not influenced by iron treatment (Verloop et al., 1959).

Low serum iron concentrations are frequently found in the first two years of life, but normal adult values are achieved after two years of age. There is a marked diurnal variation, with a fall in concentration in the late afternoon and evening to near 21.00 h, followed by an increase to a maximum value between 07.00 and 10.00 h (Bowie et al., 1963).

Measurement of serum iron should always be combined with measurement of the iron-binding capacity. In iron deficiency, a low serum iron concentration is present with an increase in the total iron-binding capacity. By contrast, in anaemia of chronic disorders a low serum iron concentration indicates impaired delivery of iron from the reticuloendothelial system and is accompanied by a low iron-binding capacity. The measurements are normal in uncomplicated thalassaemia. Results may be expressed as the percentage of transferrin which carries, or is saturated with iron. This is normally 30%; the saturation is low in iron deficiency and increased in iron overload.

16.2.5. Red cell protoporphyrin

Protoporphyrin accumulates in iron deficiency because of lack of iron at the stage of insertion of iron into the tetrapyrrole ring. Red cell protoporphyrin in iron deficiency is greater than 40 μg/dl. It is also raised in anaemia of infection.

16.2.6. Iron chelating methods

Attempts have been made to assess iron stores by measuring the urinary excretion of iron following an injection of an iron-chelating agent such as desferrioxamine. Following an injection of 500 mg, there is an increased iron excretion over the next six hours and this amount is increased in patients with iron overload (Wöhler, 1964). Diethylenetriamine penta-acetic acid (DTPA) has also been used in assessment of iron stores (Barry and Sherlock, 1971). These tests have been applied in managing patients with haemochromatosis undergoing phlebotomy where the desferrioxamine-induced iron excretion correlated well with iron stores assessed by phlebotomy (Olsson, 1972). The test has only limited value in clinical work.

16.2.7. Iron overload (haemochromatosis)

Excessive iron stores may arise from excessive absorption of normal dietary iron, as in idiopathic haemochromatosis; from an abnormally high dietary iron intake, as in the South African Bantu; or from repeated blood transfusions. Over many years as much as 50 g of iron may accumulate, producing skin pigmentation, liver disease, diabetes and cardiac failure. The plasma iron concentration is high and transferrin saturation is between 80 and 100%. The plasma ferritin concentration is increased and iron chelation tests give an abnormally high urinary excretion. Liver biopsy confirms excessive amounts of iron as well as providing evidence of cirrhosis. Liver function tests, evidence of diabetes and an abnormal electrocardiogram may be found. When idiopathic haemochromatosis has been diagnosed, other family members should be screened by determining the serum iron concentration and measuring the percentage saturation of transferrin.

16.2.8. Iron kinetics

Isotopically labelled iron (usually ^{59}Fe) can be used to obtain information about haemopoiesis and, in a more limited way, about iron storage and metabolism. The labelled iron (10 μCi of ^{59}Fe) is added to 5 ml defibrinated plasma and after five minutes equilibration at room temperature, any iron not complexed to transferrin is removed by passing the plasma through a cation exchange resin (Cavill, 1971).

16.2.8.1. Plasma iron clearance

The rate of disappearance of ^{59}Fe from plasma following i.v. injection is measured and the half-clearance time plotted; this is normally about 90 minutes, with a range of 45 to 175 minutes. An abnormally fast clearance is found in iron deficiency, in anaemia of chronic disorders, and in all disorders with increased erythropoiesis including haemolytic anaemia and megaloblastic anaemia. An abnormally slow clearance is found in underactive marrows as in hypoplastic and aplastic anaemia.

16.2.8.2. Plasma iron turnover

With a knowledge of the plasma iron concentration, plasma volume, and plasma iron clearance, the amount of iron passing through the plasma in 24 hours can be calculated. This is normally 30 to 40 mg per day. Data can also be expressed in relation to plasma iron turnover per dl of whole blood, normal values being 0.65 mg/dl per day. In both iron deficiency and haemochromatosis the plasma iron turnover is normal, despite wide variation in the serum iron concentration. The turnover is reduced in marrow hypoplasia and increased in overactive marrow states, as in haemolytic anaemia.

16.2.8.3. Incorporation of ^{59}Fe into red cells

Following a dose of labelled iron, there is a rapid increase in ^{59}Fe in red cells for the first seven days and thereafter a slower rise up to 14 days. Normally 80 to 90% of iron is incorporated into red cells, and in iron deficiency almost all is taken up. In ineffective haemopoiesis, as in megaloblastic anaemia, iron incorporation is decreased despite increased plasma iron turnover, and may be as low as 10 to 30%. It is low in hypoplastic and aplastic anaemia. Using the plasma iron turnover and percentage incorporation of iron into red cells, the red cell iron turnover can be calculated: this value is 0.56 mg/dl blood per day (Finch et al., 1970).

16.2.8.4. Surface counting

Following injection of ^{59}Fe, radioactivity is usually monitored over the sacrum (marrow) and, to a lesser extent, the spleen and liver. With the rise in red cell radioactivity, ^{59}Fe disappears from these sites. In myelofibrosis, haemopoiesis may be largely extramedullary in the spleen and liver; ^{59}Fe counts will be high in those sites initially, with little activity in the sacrum (marrow), where it is barely above that over the heart (blood).

16.2.8.5. Response to iron

Sometimes the response to iron is used in the diagnosis of iron deficiency anaemia if diagnosis still remains in doubt. In general, treatment should provide 150 to 200 mg of elemental iron daily by mouth, as ferrous sulphate or another suitable preparation. Haemoglobin concentration rises at the rate of 0.1 to 0.25 g/dl per day. The reticulocyte response is much less dramatic than in megaloblastic anaemia, rising to 10 or 15% in about ten days.

16.2.8.6. Iron absorption

A test of iron absorption may be carried out by whole body counting following an appropriate dose of labelled iron. The test is of greater value in assessing the availability of food iron rather than as a means of testing intestinal absorption. When 0.1 mg of iron, as ferric chloride with ^{59}Fe, is added to food, the mean absorption of the inorganic iron is the same as the absorption of the food iron. This applies to a wide range of food items as well as to whole meals (Martinez-Torres and Layrisse, 1973). Iron from the ferric salt enters into a pool of iron from the food, and absorption of such added iron reflects the absorption of non-haem iron in that pool. This test has shown that iron is much better absorbed from some foods (veal, liver, fish, soybean, wheat) than from others (spinach, maize, black beans, eggs, rice). Normally only about 1 to 2 mg is absorbed from a normal average daily iron intake of about 14 mg. Iron absorption is enhanced in iron deficiency and in pregnancy; it is also enhanced when erythropoiesis is increased.

Iron absorption can also be assessed by giving an oral dose of ^{59}Fe and following its incorporation into red cells over the next two weeks. About 40% of a 1 mg dose of iron is absorbed in iron deficiency, and most of this will appear in red cells. Normally only 5 to 10% of such a dose is absorbed. A good response indicates that the iron has been absorbed, but a low response has little value since it may merely indicate that iron has not been utilised.

16.2.9. Tests for blood loss

Detection of blood loss in the gastrointestinal tract is one of the most important investigations carried out in the laboratory. It is the pointer to the clinician to a bleeding lesion in the gut that may need radical surgery, or may be amenable to cure by simple methods: otherwise it may have to be tolerated. Unfortunately chemical tests for blood in faeces remain unsatisfactory. When over 20 ml of blood is lost into the gut daily, just over half the tests for occult blood are likely to be positive. Intermittent blood loss indicates that it is necessary to test many samples of faeces (Holt et al., 1968).

Labelling the patient's red cells with ^{51}Cr and collecting faeces provides a more reliable and quantitative method of measuring intestinal blood loss. A blood sample is required to serve as standard with each batch of faeces. Normally about 1 ml of blood is lost each day; daily blood loss greater than 6 ml cannot be compensated for by increased iron absorption from the normal diet and anaemia will follow.

Iron loss from the gastrointestinal tract may be increased when there is rapid turnover of epithelial cells lining the stomach or gut as in atrophic gastritis and coeliac disease. This may contribute to iron deficiency.

16.3. ASSESSMENT OF MEGALOBLASTIC ANAEMIA

16.3.1. Recognition of a megaloblastic process

Diagnosis of megaloblastic anaemia depends on recognition of the appropriate changes in the blood measurements, blood film and bone marrow. Low concentrations of vitamin B_{12} and folate in plasma and tissues are commonplace in the absence of any blood changes, and hence such measurements are not relevant when a decision is required whether haemopoiesis is normoblastic or megaloblastic.

The earliest change in the peripheral blood is a rise in the MCV. This is followed by a fall in the red cell count and the presence in the stained blood film of variation in cell size (anisocytosis), pear-shaped cells (poikilocytes) and oval macrocytes. The total white cell count falls when megaloblastosis is well established. The neutrophil polymorphs tend to have an increase in the number of nuclear lobes. This is not seen in early cases which show only an increased MCV. In severe cases the platelet count falls.

The marrow shows megaloblastic erythropoiesis replacing a normoblastic form. In early cases this change in appearance is recognizable by erythoblasts showing evidence of haemoglobinization, but later all stages are abnormal. Giant metamyelocytes are usually present in well developed cases. Minor marrow changes are of no importance and must not be termed megaloblastic.

16.3.2. Deoxyuridine suppression test

If dividing marrow cells are incubated with deoxyuridine, they take up this compound and convert it into thymidine which is incorporated into DNA; [^{3}H]thymidine added to a second aliquot of marrow suspension is taken up in a similar way and incorporated into DNA. If, however, the marrow cells are first exposed to deoxyuridine and then later to thymidine, the requirement for thymidylate by the salvage pathway is satisfied by the initial uptake of deoxyuridine (which is methylated by the cells to thymidine); thus very little of the added thymidine is used. In fact, less than 10% of the added thymidine appears in DNA using normal marrow cells. With marrow cells from megaloblastic patients, however, there is a failure to convert uridine into thymidine because of lack of normal folate coenzyme, and hence the requirements of the cells for thymidine are not met by supplying uridine. Under these circumstances, a significantly larger proportion of [^{3}H]thymidine (added after the uridine) is taken up and incorporated into DNA. This amount is greater than 10%. This test is abnormal in the majority of patients with megaloblastic anaemia and it has been suggested that it can be used as a test for megaloblastosis (Herbert et al., 1973). Experience with this test in clinical practice confirms that this is the case.

16.3.3. Diagnosis of vitamin B_{12} deficiency

Vitamin B_{12} deficiency is diagnosed either by measuring the B_{12} concentration in serum, by measuring the excretion of methylmalonic acid in the urine, or by noting the response of the blood to B_{12} treatment.

16.3.3.1. Serum vitamin B_{12}

The concentration of vitamin B_{12} in serum may be measured by either microbiological assay or saturation analysis methods. The assay organisms used most frequently are *Lactobacillus Leichmannii* and *Euglena gracilis.* The reference range with microbiological and some saturation analysis methods is 170 to 1000 ng/l. With other methods using saturation analysis it is significantly higher, for example 300 to 1600 ng/l (Raven and Robson. 1974). The various methods may give significantly different results with certain sera, e.g. from patients who have undergone a partial gastrectomy. Patients giving low results with microbiological assay may show normal values when saturation analysis is used (Raven et al., 1972). Rarely the presence of antiobiotic or antimitotic drugs in serum may inhibit microbiological assay but have no effect on assay by saturation analysis.

All patients suffering from vitamin B_{12} deficiency have low serum vitamin B_{12} concentrations. However, a reduced value may also be associated with other conditions. Thus in normal pregnancy the serum vitamin B_{12} concentration falls because of preferential transfer of absorbed B_{12} to the placenta and foetus, at the expense of maintaining the plasma compartment. In 5% of pregnant women, the serum concentration falls below 170 ng/l although tissue stores of B_{12} remain adequate. The value rises to normal within two weeks of birth of the child.

In iron deficiency complicating partial gastrectomy, low serum B_{12} concentrations may be found which rise to normal on treatment with iron alone. About one-third of patients with megaloblastic anaemia due to folate deficiency have low serum B_{12} values. In these patients, treatment with folic acid alone restores the serum B_{12} concentration to normal within about ten days. All these patients are able to absorb vitamin B_{12} normally. In contrast, patients with low serum B_{12} values due to B_{12} deficiency have malabsorption of vitamin B_{12}.

Low serum vitamin B_{12} concentrations are commonplace among vegetarians (usually Hindus) who take no meat, eggs or milk in their diets. Patients with severe atrophic gastritis without pernicious anaemia commonly have low B_{12} values. These patients usually have normal blood and marrow haematology.

16.3.3.2. Vitamin B_{12} in other tissues

Sometimes vitamin B_{12} concentrations are assayed in red cells and liver. The reference range for red cell B_{12} is 100 to 500 ng/l of packed cells, with a mean of 150 ng/l. Liver B_{12} is normally about 1 μg/g wet liver; in pernicious anaemia the value is of the order of 0.1 μg/g.

16.3.3.3. Urinary excretion of methylmalonic acid

Methylmalonic acid arises through the metabolism of propionate, leucine, isoleucine and valine. It is normally converted into succinic acid by the enzyme methylmalonyl-CoA mutase. Each mole of the mutase carries two molecules of cobamide (B_{12}) coenzyme, so that shortage of B_{12} results in shortage of coenzyme. In clinical practice, the urinary excretion of methylmalonate is measured in a 24-hour urine specimen after an oral dose of 10 g L-valine, or of an equimolar amount of isoleucine. Colorimetric methods do not readily differentiate other weak organic acids in urine from methylmalonic acid, and hence are unreliable when the excretion is low. Gas chromatography after ether extraction is the analytical method of choice. The excretion is related to the degree of vitamin B_{12} deficiency as assessed by the serum B_{12} concentration. After ingestion of valine, healthy subjects may excrete as much as 23 mg methylmalonate in 24 hours, but the mean is about 1.8 mg. There is a significantly greater excretion of methylmalonic acid in the urine in B_{12} deficiency, but patients with early deficiency, relatively higher serum B_{12} concentrations and little anaemia, give normal results. There are no false positive results. Children with congenital methylmalonylaciduria will excrete very large amounts in the urine. Most of these children are not anaemic and their marrows are haematologically normal.

16.3.3.4. Response to vitamin B_{12}

A favourable haematological response following injections of 2 μg of vitamin B_{12} daily is evidence of B_{12} deficiency. This is only possible in relatively anaemic patients with red cell counts of less than 2.5 million/μl. An optimal response after the first injection, on day zero, requires a rise in the reticulocyte count on day five, six or seven, and a rise in the red cell count in the third week. The height of the reticulocyte peak depends on the severity of anaemia, and is about 30% when the red cell count is less than 1.5 million/μl and only 10% when the red cell count is greater than 2.5 million/μl. The red cell count should always reach 3 million/μl in the third week, but higher values are required to establish positive response in less anaemic patients. In nutritional B_{12} deficiency, the test should be carried out by giving 2 to 5 μg of vitamin B_{12} daily by mouth.

Failure to obtain an optimal response may indicate a wrong diagnosis or the presence of factors preventing a response, such as renal failure, intercurrent infection or a neoplasm.

16.3.4. Diagnosis of folate deficiency

In patients with megaloblastic anaemia, folate deficiency is diagnosed by excluding deficiency of vitamin B_{12}, by finding a low serum folate level, a low red cell folate level and a raised urinary formiminoglutamic acid (figlu) excretion. A favourable haematological response to 200 μg of folate per day is also evidence of folate deficiency.

16.3.4.1. Exclusion of vitamin B_{12} deficiency

Vitamin B_{12} deficiency can be excluded by finding a normal serum B_{12} concentration and by demonstrating B_{12} absorption in a patient taking a mixed diet. In these circumstances megaloblastic anaemia must be due to folate deficiency. Failure to response haematologically to vitamin B_{12} with persistence of a megaloblastic marrow also suggests folate deficiency.

16.3.4.2. Serum folate

The reference range is 3 to 15 μg/l, but will vary from laboratory to laboratory. A low value is found in about one-third of patients in hospital, and a very low concentration (less than 1.5 μg/l) in most patients with megaloblastic anaemia due to folate deficiency. A low serum folate concentration indicates a negative folate balance, but not necessarily folate deficiency. However, the majority of patients with B_{12} deficiency have normal serum folate concentrations because of a defect in uptake of methyltetrahydrofolate by cells.

16.3.4.3. Red cell folate

The folate content of normal red cells varies from 160 to 600 ng/ml packed cells. The folate content of the cell is determined during erythropoiesis, reticulocytes having a higher folate content than mature red cells. Thereafter the folate is locked in the red cell and released at the end of its life span. Changes in red cell folate, therefore, are due to production of new red cells with a different folate content. A low red cell folate value is unequivocal evidence of folate deficiency and is found in about 8% of old people and in about one-quarter of pregnant women near term who have not received folate supplements. Low values are found in megaloblastic anaemia due to folate deficiency, but if megaloblastic anaemia is of recent onset – as in pregnancy – sufficient time may not have elapsed to allow replacement of old red cells with a new population of low folate content. Hence only half the patients with megaloblastic anaemia in pregnancy have low values. Megaloblastic anaemia complicating haemolytic anaemia may also be associated with somewhat higher red cell folate values because of the high proportion of young red cells.

16.3.4.4. Formiminoglutamic acid excretion

The degradation of histidine to glutamic acid is by way of urocanic acid and formiminoglutamic acid. The formimino group of the latter is transferred to tetrahydrofolate by formiminotransferase. In folate deficiency, formiminoglutamic acid accumulates and is excreted into the urine.

In clinical practice, the test is carried out by collecting urine into acid for eight hours after an oral dose of 15 g of L-histidine. Formiminoglutamic acid is best estimated by an enzymatic method (Chanarin and Bennett, 1962). The normal excretion is 1 to 17 mg over the 8-hour period.

Frequently the enzyme urocanase, which converts urocanic acid into formiminoglutamic acid, has very low activity, particularly in protein malnutrition and as a result of a feed-back inhibition from high levels of tissue formiminoglutamic acid. Thus urocanic acid may appear in large amounts and very little formiminoglutamic acid is present following oral histidine.

In the uncomplicated case, a high excretion of formiminoglutamic acid, which can exceed 1000 mg, occurs in folate deficiency and disappears four to six days after treatment with folate. Because of changes in intestinal absorption of amino acids, including histidine during pregnancy, and changes in renal threshold leading to marked loss of histidine in the urine, the test is of little value during pregnancy. Patients with primary vitamin B_{12} deficiency may also have a raised excretion of formiminoglutamic acid as well as a reduced red cell folate.

16.3.4.5. Response to folate

Treatment with 200 μg of pteroylglutamic acid per day, either by mouth or injection, should produce a favourable haematological response in megaloblastic anaemia due to folate deficiency but not to vitamin B_{12} deficiency. In some patients megaloblastic anaemia is due to an abnormally increased requirement for folate (e.g. in pregnancy or haemolytic anaemia) and a larger dose (500 μg/day) may be needed in these patients.

16.3.5. The absorption of vitamin B_{12}

Two γ-emitting isotopes are commonly used in absorption tests – ^{57}Co and ^{58}Co. ^{57}Co provides the least radiation exposure with the highest counting efficiency. It is relatively easy to count each isotope in the presence of the other, since ^{57}Co emits γ-radiation over a relatively restricted energy range. The usual dose of vitamin B_{12} given in absorption tests is 1 μg, with a specific activity of 0.5 to 1.0 μCi.

16.3.5.1. The urinary excretion test

This test is carried out by giving an oral dose of labelled vitamin B_{12} accompanied by an intramuscular injection of 1000 μg of unlabelled cyanocobalamin. After the plasma vitamin B_{12}-binding proteins (transcobalamin I and II) have been saturated, the remaining unbound B_{12} is handled like inulin, i.e. it is excreted quantitatively by the glomeruli and not reabsorbed by the renal tubules. Labelled B_{12} which is absorbed joins the plasma pool of unlabelled cyanocobalamin and is carried into the urine with it. One-third of the labelled dose that is absorbed appears in the urine. Results are expressed as a percentage of the oral labelled dose which is excreted in urine. Normal subjects excrete more than 10% of the oral dose and patients with malabsorption less than 10%.

Collection of the urine should be accompanied by measurement of labelled B_{12} in plasma between 8 and 12 hours after the oral dose. Normally more than 0.65% of the oral dose is present per litre plasma at this time.

An alternative method of measuring absorption of vitamin B_{12} is by whole body counting in a specially constructed room containing a sensitive crystal detector.

16.3.5.2. Vitamin B_{12} malabsorption

Malabsorption of B_{12} which is corrected by the addition of intrinsic factor (either dried hog pyloric mucosa or pooled neutralized normal human gastric juice) indicates lack of intrinsic factor, as in pernicious anaemia, post-gastrectomy and severe atrophic gastritis (Whiteside et al., 1964). Failure to correct impaired B_{12} absorption with added intrinsic factor indicates an intestinal lesion, but it also occurs in pernicious anaemia with potent intrinsic factor antibodies in the gastric secretion (Rose and Chanarin, 1971). In the case of an intestinal lesion, temporary improvement in B_{12} absorption may be obtained with a wide spectrum antibiotic, such as tetracycline, in cases where there is an abnormal gut flora with the ileum remaining intact and not by-passed, for example, by surgery.

Malabsorption of vitamin B_{12} occurs in gluten-sensitive enteropathy; tropical sprue; anatomical abnormalities of the small gut; in pancreatic disease with either chronic pancreatitis or cystic fibrosis (Deren et al., 1973); and after drug therapy, including metformin and phenformin (Tomkin, 1973), colchicine (Race et al., 1970), para-aminosalicylic acid (Heinivaara and Palva, 1964) and cholestyramine (Coronato and Glass, 1973). Absorption can also be impaired in giardiasis (Ament and Rubin, 1972). Radiotherapy to the lower abdomen may damage the ileum and lead to impaired B_{12} absorption (McBrien, 1973).

Long-standing vitamin B_{12} deficiency per se impairs ileal function; hence after treatment with B_{12} there is an improvement in response to added intrinsic factor in pernicious anaemia over the course of six months or more.

The absorption of free vitamin B_{12} and intrinsic factor-bound B_{12} can be tested simultaneously by using both ^{57}Co and ^{58}Co. In normal subjects both isotopes are absorbed equally, since intrinsic factor is available from gastric juice. In pernicious anaemia, only the intrinsic factor-bound isotope is well absorbed whereas in intestinal disease both are poorly absorbed. Only an aliquot of urine is required to determine the ratio of absorption of the two isotopes.

16.3.6. The absorption of folic acid

Tests of folate absorption should be carried out after the patient has received substantial amounts of folate to overcome lack of tissue saturation of the vitamin. Two methods are available. In one, 40 μg of folate per kg body weight is given orally and the plasma concentration measured hourly for three hours; samples should be assayed microbiologically with *Streptococcus faecalis,* and a rise in plasma folate concentration above 40 μg/l is normal.

Tritium-labelled folate may be given orally accompanied by an intramuscular injection of 15 mg of unlabelled folate. Urine is collected for 24 hours and its tritium activity measured. Freedman et al. (1973), using an oral dose of 300 μg folate, found a urinary excretion of 45 ± 7 (S.D.) % in normal subjects. The excretion in eight coeliac patients ranged from 7 to 21%.

16.3.7. Biochemical changes in megaloblastic anaemia

16.3.7.1. Lactate dehydrogenase and hydroxybutyrate dehydrogenase

Although the serum activities of a variety of enzymes, including aldolase, phosphohexoisomerase and malate dehydrogenase, are raised in untreated megaloblastic anaemia, lactate dehydrogenase (LD_1 and LD_2) and hydroxybutyrate dehydrogenase activities may be particularly high. The increase in lactate dehydrogenase is due to the death of a considerable number of immature erythroblasts in the marrow. Enzyme activities are normal in mildly anaemic patients. On treatment of megaloblastic anaemia, there are marked falls in serum enzyme activities within the first week of treatment, with normal values obtained at the end of the second week.

16.3.7.2. Serum iron

The serum iron concentration is elevated in untreated megaloblastic anaemia, the highest values being found in the most anaemic patients. The concentration falls abruptly within 24 hours of treatment and may remain abnormally low for several weeks.

16.3.7.3. Plasma potassium

Following treatment of megaloblastic anaemia there is a fall in plasma potassium concentration, and in some cases a fall in red cell potassium (Lawson et al., 1972). The fall is rarely of sufficient importance to warrant supplementation (Hesp et al., 1975). There is an increase in whole body potassium on treatment due to an increase in red cell mass and body weight.

16.3.7.4. Bilirubin

The plasma bilirubin concentration (both conjugated and total) is increased in untreated megaloblastic anaemia with moderate to severe degrees of anaemia, and there is an increase in urinary urobilinogen. These effects are due to the premature destruction of the patient's red cells. Haptoglobins are generally absent but normal concentrations are found two to three weeks after commencing treatment.

16.3.8. Antibodies in megaloblastic anaemia

Parietal-cell antibodies are found in serum in 85% of patients with pernicious anaemia, as well as in 5 to 15% of control subjects. Intrinsic factor antibodies are present in serum in 57% of patients with pernicious anaemia, but are found only rarely in patients with Graves' disease and atrophic gastritis. An equally high proportion of patients with pernicious anaemia have intrinsic factor antibodies in gastric secretion. The serum antibodies are usually IgG immunoglobulins and the antibodies in gastric juice are IgA. In addition, over 80% of patients with pernicious anaemia have evidence of cell-mediated immunity against intrinsic factor.

16.4. ASSESSMENT OF TOTAL HAEMOPOIESIS

16.4.1. Marrow failure

Marrow failure may occur following drug exposure, particularly to chloramphenicol and phenylbutazone (Butazolidine); many other drugs, on rare occasions, can also produce this effect. In some patients no cause can be found. The patient presents either with symptoms of anaemia or with bruising and purpura due to a low platelet count; the white cell count is also low.

The blood count demonstrates a pancytopaenia, and the marrow shows fatty hypocellular fragments, cells being mainly plasma cells and iron-storage reticulum cells. Occasionally surviving foci of marrow remain; should aspiration be made from such a site, there will be a paradoxical finding of blood pancytopaenia with apparently normal marrow. In this circumstance, marrow trephine and aspiration from other sites are required. Help in diagnosis may be obtained from the serum iron concentration, which is abnormally high, and plasma transferrin may be fully saturated.

Ferrokinetics show a very slow clearance of radioactive iron from plasma and a very poor incorporation of iron into new red cells.

A very short-lived isotope of iron (^{52}Fe), if given intravenously, can provide a picture of active sites of haemopoiesis using a gamma camera.

16.4.2. Polycythaemia

Over-production of blood occurs in primary or secondary polycythaemia. The disorder must be distinguished from polycythaemia of stress wherein there is a fall in plasma volume with haemoconcentration, increased red cell count, a high haemoglobin concentration, but a normal red cell mass.

16.4.2.1. Estimation of red cell and plasma volume

Red cell volume is measured by labelling an aliquot of red cells with ^{51}Cr and returning a measured amount to the circulation. Mixing is normally complete after three minutes except in a patient with a large spleen when 30 minutes should be allowed. Plasma volume is measured using ^{125}I-labelled albumin. Reference values for red cell volume are: men, 26 to 33 ml per kg body weight; women, 22 to 29 ml per kg; plasma volume, 35 to 45 ml per kg (men and women); and total blood volume, 55 to 75 ml per kg (men and women).

The difference in apparent blood volume between the result of calculation from a sample collected three minutes after re-injecting the labelled red cells and that from one collected after 30 minutes is a measure of the volume of blood in the spleen.

16.4.2.2. Arterial oxygen saturation

Measurement of arterial oxygen saturation is essential to recognize secondary polycythaemia due to failure of normal oxygenation of blood. It is normal in primary polycythaemia.

16.4.2.3. Oxygen dissociation curve

Characterization of the oxygen dissociation curve is required to recognise polycythaemia due to a high-affinity haemoglobin. In this condition there is inadequate release of oxygen from haemoglobin so that the oxygen dissociation curve is shifted to the left. Measurement is conveniently expressed as the oxygen tension (P_{50}) when the blood is 50% saturated. The normal P_{50} is 25 to 27 mm Hg. It is low in the case of a high-affinity haemoglobin.

16.2.2.4. Erythropoietin estimation

Erythropoietin is probably a hormone arising from the kidney which is concerned with stimulating development of erythroblasts from stem cells. It appears to be responsible for maintaining the normal concentration of circulating haemoglobin. Its plasma concentration is high in anaemia, including anaemia in marrow failure; in patients undergoing venesection, as in blood donation; and in individuals subject to hypoxia, for example at high altitude. Descent from high altitude to sea level is accompanied by disappearance of erythropoietin.

The concentration of erythropoietin in plasma is immeasurably low in polycythaemia rubra vera and normal or raised in other polycythaemias. This also applies to those rare forms of polycythaemia associated with erythropoietin-producing tumours such as myomata, cerebellar tumours, hepatoma or renal tumours.

16.5. ASSESSMENT OF WHITE BLOOD CELL FUNCTION

16.5.1. Granulopoiesis

Assessment of neutrophil function is made by measuring the total number of these cells in the blood; the count is normally in the range 2000 to 7500 per μl. When the number is reduced below 500 per μl there may be recurrent infection or painful mouth ulcers. A history of repeated infection with normal neutrophil count but without immunoglobulin deficiency, may suggest impairment of neutrophil function. Three types of disorder may be found (Douglas, 1970). (a) A defect of neutrophil chemotaxis; there may be a defect in the mechanism whereby normal neutrophils are attracted to bacteria by a process called chemotaxis. (b) A defect in phagocytosis of bacteria by neutrophils. (c) Failure of intracellular killing of bacteria which have been ingested (granulomatous disease of childhood).

16.5.2. Nitroblue tetrazolium test

Nitroblue tetrazolium (NBT) acts as a hydrogen ion receptor for both NADH and NADPH. In the presence of infection in the patient, neutrophils rapidly reduce this dye. Patients with defective neutrophils fail to reduce the dye.

16.5.3. Bactericidal activity of neutrophils

Leucocytes are incubated with organisms such as *Staphylococcus aureus* and *S. marcescens.* Opsonin (complement provided by fresh normal serum) is added. After a standard period of incubation the remaining viable bacteria are assessed by plating out the suspension.

16.5.4. B-lymphocytes

These are the lymphocytes which are transformed into plasma cells and produce humoral antibody. Their activity is indicated by the immunoglobulin (IgG, IgA and IgM) concentrations in sera, and assessed by measuring antibodies against common antigens, such as *Escherichia coli*, and by the response to challenge with antigens such as pneumococcal polysaccharide.

16.5.5. T-lymphocytes

T-lymphocytes are responsible for cell-mediated immunity and their activity is assessed in vivo by response to dinitrochlorobenzene. Following a sensitizing dose placed on the skin, a second test dose applied a week later should produce an appropriate skin reaction if a normal T-lymphocyte response has occurred. A positive tuberculin skin test is evidence of cell-mediated immunity against the tubercle bacillus. The patient's lymphocytes may be tested in vitro for the release of products of a cell-mediated reaction, as in migration inhibition tests using appropriate antigens (Bendixen and Søborg, 1969).

16.6. ASSESSMENT IN HAEMOLYTIC STATES

16.6.1. Is there haemolysis?

If there is excessive breakdown of red blood cells, the plasma bilirubin concentration is generally increased to between 20 and 50 μmol/l (1 and 3 mg/dl). Higher concentrations can be due to an exacerbation of haemolysis or to liver disease. The bilirubin is unconjugated (indirect) and not excreted by the kidney.

There is increased urobilinogen and stercobilinogen in urine and stools respectively. Haptoglobin concentrations are absent, or in the mildest cases decreased. The finding of free haemoglobin in plasma and urine is rare except in acute haemolysis, e.g. that following drug ingestion in glucose-6-phosphate dehydrogenase deficiency. Altered haemoglobin may be excreted in the presence of an unstable haemoglobin such as Hb Koln, Zurich or Hammersmith. Excess iron in the urine is present in chronic haemolysis.

Methaemoglobin may also occur in long-standing haemolysis. The characteristic haemochromogen absorbing at 558 nm is detected in Schumm's test.

The extent of red cell breakdown may be indicated by measuring red cell survival after labelling the cells with ^{51}Cr. Normal mean red cell life is 110 days. In moderate haemolysis, survival is reduced to 15 to 20 days, and in severe cases to less than ten days. With more severe degrees of red cell breakdown, marrow compensation fails and anaemia results. Often evidence of abnormal red cells may be detected on inspection of the blood film; this might include the presence of spherocytes, red cell fragments, agglutinates, etc.

Destruction of red cells is accompanied by evidence of increased red cell regeneration. In the blood film this is shown by increased polychromasia and by a reticulocytosis which varies from 3% to over 50%. The marrow shows marked erythroid hyperplasia, and in lifelong hereditary disorders there are radiological changes in bones indicative of marrow expansion such as "hair-on-end" appearance of the cranium.

16.6.2. Classification of haemolytic disorders

Haemolytic disorders may be classified as follows, under the headings of intrinsic or extrinsic defects.

Intrinsic red cell defects

Congenital
- membrane defects – spherocytosis, elliptocytosis
- enzymic defects – particularly glucose-6-phosphate dehydrogenase deficiency and phenylketonuria; rarely other defects in glycolytic or reducing pathways
- haemoglobinopathies

Acquired
- paroxysmal nocturnal haemoglobinuria

Extrinsic defects

Autoimmune
- warm autobodies
- cold agglutinins
- haemolytic diseases of newborn
- drug-dependent

Drugs
- such as dapsone

Mechanical	– artificial heart valves
	– march haemoglobinuria
	– damage by fibrin strands (haemolytic uraemic syndrome)
Infections	– malaria, *Clostridium welchii.*

16.6.3. Investigations

16.6.3.1. Blood picture

The blood haemoglobin concentration may be normal or reduced, depending on whether the marrow has been able to compensate for the reduced red cell life span or not. The MCV is generally raised because reticulocytes are larger than mature red cells. The reticulocyte count is raised.

Spherocytes in the blood film occur in both hereditary spherocytosis and in autoimmune haemolytic anaemia. In the latter, the direct antiglobulin test on the red cell is positive, indicating an antibody on the red cell surface.

The red cells may be agglutinated in a haemolytic anaemia due to cold antibodies. They are essentially normal in appearance in enzyme deficiencies, paroxysmal nocturnal haemoglobinuria and many haemoglobinopathies. Sickle cells or target cells may appear in HbS disease and other haemoglobinopathies.

Occasionally severe haemolytic anaemia may be associated with marked red cell fragmentation, although this is more characteristic of a haemolytic–uraemic-type situation.

16.6.3.2. Red cell fragility tests

Fragility tests are used to confirm the presence of spherocytes suspected in the blood film. More spherical red cells are haemolyzed relatively soon, as the saline concentration is reduced. Abnormally flat cells (target cells) are more resistant than normal to saline haemolysis.

16.6.3.3. Autohaemolysis

Incubation of blood at 37°C for 24 hours produces a small degree of haemolysis. In spherocytosis haemolysis is more marked, but if glucose is added, haemolysis is reduced significantly in hereditary spherocytosis; however, this also obtains in some other diseases like glucose-6-phosphate dehydrogenase deficiency.

A patient with spherocytosis and a negative antiglobulin test probably has hereditary spherocytosis. A relevant family history is often discovered.

16.6.3.4. Enzyme tests

The commonest enzyme deficiency giving rise to non-spherocytic haemolytic anaemia is glucose-6-phosphate dehydrogenase deficiency. Of the rest, the least uncommon is pyruvate kinase deficiency; thereafter some cases with deficiency of hexokinase, triosephosphate isomerase, diphosphoglycerate mutase, phosphoglycerate kinase and ATPase deficiency have been described.

A screening test for glucose-6-phosphate dehydrogenase deficiency should be done, and if there is an abnormal finding, an assay of the enzyme activity is carried out. The deficiency can also present as neonatal jaundice, or as acute attacks of haemolysis following ingestion of a wide variety of oxidizing drugs or because of sensitivity to beans (*Vicia faba*).

The next enzyme to be assayed is pyruvate kinase. Other enzymic deficiencies should not be sought until the less common disorders have been excluded.

16.6.3.5. Acid serum (Ham's) test

In the very rare disorder paroxysmal nocturnal haemoglobinuria (PNH), a small amount of haemolysis occurs when the pH of plasma is reduced to about 6. Complement is required, so that the test is done by incubating the patient's cells with ABO compatible fresh serum which has been acidified. A positive result may sometimes occur in aplastic anaemia and in some rare dyserythropoietic anaemias.

Clinically, patients with PNH have haemoglobinuria often occurring at night, and may indeed become iron-deficient as a result of loss of iron in the urine.

16.6.3.6. Sucrose-lysis test

Here red cells are suspended in isotonic sucrose, of low ionic strength, with normal serum. PNH cells become susceptible to complement lysis under these circumstances.

16.6.4. Haemolysis due to drugs

A few drugs like the sulphones, e.g. dapsone, produce destruction of normal red cells. This drug is used in treatment of dermatitis herpetiformis, and related drugs are used in the treatment of leprosy. The blood film shows the presence of occasional irregularly crenated red blood cells; some elevation of reticulocytes; low or absent haptoglobins; and sometimes Heinz bodies.

16.6.4.1. Heinz bodies

Heinz bodies are precipitated globin derived from haemoglobin within the red cell. They are detected by examining a blood film after the blood has been incubated with methyl violet. Heinz bodies appear when an unstable haemoglobin is present or after an oxidizing drug has been ingested by a patient with a defective reducing enzyme system such as glucose-6-phosphate dehydrogenase deficiency or lack of glutathione. Small numbers of Heinz bodies are removed by the spleen. They accumulate under oxidative stress and after splenectomy.

Reducing conditions within the red cell are required to maintain iron in the ferrous state and to prevent oxidation of the thiol bonds of globin. Normally some methaemoglobin is formed as a result of oxidation of ferrous iron to ferric iron, and this action is reversed by NADH-methaemoglobin reductase. The second important reducing system is glutathione, which is maintained in the reduced state by NADPH produced by the aerobic glycolysis of glucose (pentose phosphate shunt) in which glucose-6-phosphate dehydrogenase is concerned. Glutathione may be concerned with preventing oxidation of disulphide links in globin. Substances which affect these systems are drugs like sulphonamides, phenacetin, antimalarials such as primaquine, quinine and quinidine, acetylsalicylic acid, nitrofurantoin and many others.

These drugs are particularly effective in glucose-6-phosphate dehydrogenase deficiency which affects millions of subjects throughout the world; it is inherited as a sex-linked characteristic and affected males are hemizygous. The haemolytic episode starts acutely three days after taking the drug, with jaundice and haemoglobinuria, followed by anaemia and a reticulocytosis. Young red cells are more resistant to drugs, so that the episode is self-limiting. Sensitivity to broad beans (favism) has a similar presentation. Other patients, however, present with chronic non-spherocytic haemolytic anaemia and some with neonatal jaundice.

A third way in which drugs produce haemolysis is by an autoimmune mechanism. Some, like methyldopa, produce an autoimmune haemolytic anaemia indistinguishable from the idiopathic type. Penicillin and cephalosporin combine with the red cell and an antibody is formed against this complex (hapten–cell mechanism).

Phenacetin, sulphonamides, chlorpromazine and other drugs bind to serum proteins and an antibody is formed. The antigen (drug–protein) and antibody complex absorb to the red cells causing haemolysis (immune–complex mechanism). In these patients, a positive direct antiglobulin test in the presence of the drug is obtained.

16.6.5. The direct antiglobulin test

This test detects antibody on the red cell surface. The antiglobulin serum will bridge immunoglobulin molecules across red cells and produce agglutination which is visible to the naked eye. The antiglobulin reagent should not only detect IgG immunoglobulins, but also complement on the red cell surface which may have attached to IgM molecules.

A positive result is obtained in autoimmune haemolytic anaemia. Such cells are usually spherocytic. In haemolytic disease of the newborn due to antirhesus antibody, the test is also positive; however, weak or even negative reactions are obtained in haemolytic disease of the newborn due to anti-A or anti-B.

Autoimmune haemolytic anaemia with a positive direct antiglobulin test may be associated with DLE, lymphomas, chronic lymphocytic leukaemia or methyldopa treatment. Sometimes no apparent cause is found (idiopathic).

16.6.6. Cold agglutinins

The "cold-type" haemolytic anaemia is due to IgM antobodies. These antibodies may be of very high titre and may be active at relatively high temperatures, for example 25 to 30 °C. Anaemia can be severe with Raynaud's phenomenon, often with a relatively poor reticulocyte response suggesting marrow depression by the antibody. Such antibodies may be associated with a lymphoma but may be transient, following *Mycoplasma pneumoniae* infection.

16.7. ASSESSMENT IN BLEEDING DISORDERS

Arrest of bleeding is brought about by contraction of the blood vessel, followed by plugging the break in the vessel with a haemostatic plug which consists of an admixture of platelets and a fibrin meshwork.

16.7.1. Role of platelets

When platelets come into contact either with collagen – present in the wall of a damaged blood vessel – or with ADP, thrombin, immune complexes, etc., they start to adhere to one another and to other tissues; they lose their normal discoid shape and form aggregates. Within each platelet, a layer containing a contractile protein – thrombasthenin – undergoes contraction, and various structures within the platelet are forced into the centre and thereafter are discharged through a system of fine canals into the surrounding plasma. This phase of contraction is an energy-dependent process. The substances secreted in this way are ADP, ATP, Ca^{2+}, platelet factor 4, and others whose function in coagulation is less well understood. Platelet factor 3 is a phospholipid which is present on the platelet surface and reacts in the coagulation sequence. Platelet factor 4 neutralizes heparin.

16.7.1.1. Assessment of platelet function
Platelet function may be assessed by several means.

(a) *The platelet count.* The reference range is 150,000 to 450,000 per μl. Purpura is unlikely until the count is below 50,000 per μl.

(b) *Platelet aggregation.* When substances such as ADP, adrenaline, collagen or ristocetin are added to plasma, containing platelets in suspension, aggregation of the platelets ensues, which may be monitored by optical means. There are normally two waves of aggregation. Aspirin and many other anti-inflammatory drugs interfere with the secondary wave of platelet aggregation. Diseases associated with impaired platelet function (thrombasthaenia, Bernard Soulier syndrome and platelet storage pool disease) show an abnormal pattern to particular aggregating agents. Aggregation is absent following ristocetin in Von Willebrand's disease.

(c) *Retention of platelets on glass beads.* Platelet "stickiness" can be measured by carrying out a platelet count before and after passing the blood through a column of glass beads. Stickiness is increased after surgery, and sometimes in diseases of blood vessels; it is decreased in uraemia and thrombasthaenia.

(d) *Platelet factor 3 availability.* The availability of a phospholipid on the platelet surface is measured by carrying out the kaolin–cephalin test with platelet-rich and platelet-poor plasmas. The factor is poorly available in uraemia, thrombasthaenia and myeloma.

16.7.2. Blood coagulation

Coagulation involves the interaction of a series of proteins present in plasma. These factors are activated by conversion of inactive precursors; most function as enzymes, and two (factor V and VIII) are co-factors in this activation.

Vessel injury activates factor XII (Hageman factor) which in turn activates factor XI, which again activates factor IX (Christmas factor).

Factor IX (with platelets, factor VIII or antihaemophilic factor and Ca^{2+}) activates factor X (Stuart–Prower factor).

Tissue injury, via release of a tissue factor, activates factor VII which acts on factor X directly. Active factor X (termed factor Xa) with factor V, platelets and Ca^{2+} then convert prothrombin into thrombin. Thrombin then converts fibrinogen into fibrin which forms the meshwork of the blood clot.

The stages up to the formation of thrombin take 5 to 10 minutes. The subsequent stages only take 10 to 20 seconds.

Intravascular coagulation is prevented by a variety of plasma inhibitors to the various stages of coagulation. One of the better known is antithrombin III which inactivates factor Xa, thrombin, and activated factors IX and XI; its action is greatly potentiated by heparin.

The fibrin clot is finally removed by a proteolytic enzyme called plasmin which exists as inactive plasminogen. Inhibitors to this system are also present in plasma.

16.7.2.1. Tests of blood coagulation

(a) *Clinical history.* A history of prolonged bleeding after a relatively minor procedure such as tooth extraction, or of spontaneous bleeding in joints and tissues, favours the diagnosis of a bleeding disorder. On the other hand, a patient who has undergone such stress without undue blood loss is not likely to have a congenital bleeding disorder, although he or she may be suffering from an acquired disorder of coagulation.

(b) *Bleeding time.* This is the time taken for bleeding to stop from a small puncture into the skin; it is usually less than seven minutes, and is abnormal if the platelet count is low or if the platelets are functionally abnormal.

(c) *Hess's test.* This consists of applying a tight cuff around the arm, so as to impede venous return, and noting the number of purpuric spots produced. It is abnormal if platelets are low or are malfunctioning.

Capillaries can be inspected directly in the nail bed and may be seen to be abnormal in hereditary telangiectasia.

(d) *Whole blood clotting time.* The time taken for blood to clot in a glass tube is normally five to ten minutes. This is a crude test that is abnormal in severe haemophilia but not necessarily abnormal in mild cases.

(e) *Kaolin–cephalin time.* This is carried out by noting the time plasma takes to clot when it is mixed with kaolin, brain extract and Ca^{2+}. The normal time is 30 to 60 seconds. An abnormal result is obtained if there are reduced levels of factors V, VIII, IX, XI, XII as well as reduced prothrombin or fibrinogen. It is a good screening test for many of the factors concerned in coagulation, particularly those that precede the generation of thrombin.

(f) *Prothrombin time.* This is carried out by noting the time plasma takes to clot when mixed with brain extract and calcium. It is normally 11 to 20 seconds. It measures the later stages of coagulation, viz. factors V, VII, X, prothrombin and fibrinogen.

(g) *Fibrinogen estimation.* Fibrinogen estimation is particularly useful in disseminated intravascular coagulation.

(h) *Thrombin time.* This measures the time plasma takes to clot after addition of thrombin and Ca^{2+}. It is prolonged when fibrinogen levels are low or when fibrin degradation products are present, as in disseminated intravascular coagulation.

16.7.3. Haemophilia A

The gene for deficiency of factor VIII is transmitted on the X-chromosome, carried by females, and the disease is present in males. Patients with haemophilia A have very low levels of factor VIII, and female carriers intermediate levels. However, factor VIII identified immunologically (factor VIII antigen) is present, implying the presence of an abnormal factor VIII molecule rather than its absence. Laboratory tests show normal bleeding time and normal prothrombin time, but whole blood clotting and kaolin–cephalin times are prolonged and assay of factor VIII is low.

16.7.4. Haemophilia B (Christmas disease)

Haemophilia B is due to deficiency of factor IX. Clinically it is indistinguishable from haemophilia A and the results of laboratory tests are the same. Factor VIII assay is normal but factor IX is low. Mixing tests show that haemophiliac A plasma can correct the clotting deficit in Christmas disease plasma, and vice versa.

16.7.5. Von Willebrand's disease

Unlike haemophilia, severe cases of this disease have a prolonged bleeding time due to defective platelets as well as a low level of factor VIII on assay. However, unlike haemophilia A, factor VIII antigen is also low. The platelets do not adhere normally to glass beads and fail to aggregate on exposure to ristocetin.

16.7.6. Disseminated intravascular coagulation

A host of clinical disorders, including shock, accidents, septicaemia, pulmonary embolism and neoplasia, may initiate coagulation in the circulation. Thus coagulation factors are consumed with deposition of fibrin which in turn may stimulate fibrinolysis. The patient may or may not have active bleeding. A large variety of abnormal coagulation tests may appear depending on the acuteness of the process, the extent of fibrinolysis and the removal of products of fibrin breakdown by the phagocytic system.

In general, the thrombin time is prolonged, platelets and fibrinogen levels are reduced, and fibrin-split products are present. In addition, prothrombin time and kaolin–cephalin time may be prolonged.

16.7.7. Liver disease

Liver disease is associated with a failure of production of vitamin K-dependent factors (prothrombin, factors VII, IX and X), particularly in obstructive jaundice. The prothrombin time is prolonged and it may be corrected by administration of vitamin K.

In more severe liver failure, the levels of other liver-produced coagulation factors may decline, including factor V and fibrinogen.

16.7.8. Local fibrinolysis

This may be responsible for local bleeding after operations on the prostate or uterus. It is doubtful if generalized fibrinolysis occurs, apart from its involvement in disseminated intravascular coagulation.

16.8. ANTICOAGULANT THERAPY

Oral anticoagulants interfere with the synthesis of vitamin K-dependent factors by the liver. These coumarin or indanedione compounds result in falls in the levels of prothrombin, and factors VII, IX and X in plasma. After a dose of warfarin their disappearance rates depend on their half-lives, which are shortest with factor VII and longest with prothrombin. The anticoagulant drugs bind strongly to albumin and only a small unbound portion is active. Drugs which displace warfarin from albumin enhance its anticoagulant action, and other drugs which stimulate hepatic enzymes enhance degradation of warfarin, and hence reduce its anticoagulant effect. Illness, too, alters the responsiveness of patients to warfarin.

The test employed to control anticoagulant therapy is the prothrombin time. Results are expressed as a ratio of the prothrombin time of a control plasma to that of the test plasma. A patient is adequately anticoagulated when the ratio is between 1.8 and 3.0.

16.9. THE ANAEMIA OF CHRONIC DISORDERS OR SECONDARY ANAEMIA

Anaemia commonly accompanies many disease processes and is commonplace in patients with rheumatoid arthritis, renal and hepatic disease and malignancy. The anaemia may be complicated by any of the anaemias previously discussed, including true iron deficiency.

When the anaemia is not complicated by other factors it may still resemble the anaemia of iron deficiency in some detail. Differentiation from iron deficiency is of considerable importance.

The degree of anaemia is variable, being moderate but sometimes quite severe, particularly in severe renal failure. The red cells may be either normal in size or microcytic, as in iron deficiency.

The serum iron concentration is low but, unlike iron deficiency, the iron-binding capacity is also reduced in the anaemia of chronic disorders. This is an important point in the differentiation from true iron deficiency. The serum ferritin concentration is low in iron deficiency but normal or even raised in the anaemia of chronic disorders.

Marrow aspirates stained for iron by the Prussian blue method show adequate, or even increased, iron in the anaemia of chronic disorders but an absence of stainable iron in true iron deficiency.

The anaemia of chronic disorders is due to a failure of iron release from iron stores in reticulum storage cells. In addition, the mean red cell life span is reduced, sometimes to as low as 30 days. The marrow remains normocellular despite anaemia, indicating a failure of the usual response.

REFERENCES

Addison, G.M., Beamish, M.R., Hales, C.N., Hodgkins, M., Jacobs, A. and Llewellin, P. (1972) An immunoradiometric assay for ferritin in the serum of normal subjects and patients with iron deficiency and iron overload. Journal of Clinical Pathology, 25: 326–329.

Ament, M.E. and Rubin, C.E. (1972) Relation of giardiasis to abnormal intestinal structure and function in gastrointestinal immunodeficiency syndromes. Gastroenterology, 62: 216–226.

Barry, M. and Sherlock, S. (1971) Measurement of liver iron concentration in needle-biopsy specimens. Lancet, 1: 100–103.

Bendixen, G. and Søborg, M. (1969) A leucocyte migration technique for in vitro detection of cellular (delayed type) hypersensitivity in man. Danish Medical Bulletin, 16: 1–6.

Bowie, E.J.W., Tauxe, W.N., Sjoberg, W.E., Jr. and Yamaguchi, M.Y. (1963) Daily variation in the concentration of iron in serum. American Journal of Clinical Pathology, 40: 491–494.

Cavill, I. (1971) The preparation of Fe-labelled transferrin for ferrokinetic studies. Journal of Clinical Pathology, 24: 472–474.

Chanarin, I. and Bennett, M.C. (1972) A spectrophotometric method for estimating formiminoglutamic acid and urocanic acid. British Medical Journal, 1: 27–29.

Coronato, A. and Glass, G.B.J. (1973) Depression of the intestinal uptake of radio-vitamin B_{12} by cholestyramine. Proceedings of Society for Experimental Biology and Medicine, 142: 1341–1344.

Croft, D.N. (1970) Body iron loss and cell loss from epithelia. Proceedings of Royal Society of Medicine, 63: 1221–1224.

Deren, J.J., Arora, B., Toskes, P.P., Hansell, J. and Sibinga, M.S. (1973) Malabsorption of crystalline vitamin B_{12} in cystic fibrosis. New England Journal of Medicine, 288: 949–950.

Douglas, S.D. (1970) Analytic review: disorders of phagocyte function. Blood, 35: 851–866.

Finch, C.A., Denbelbeiss, K., Cook, J.D., Eschbach, J.W. Harker, L.A., Funk, D.D., Marsaglia, G., Hillman, R.S., Slichter, S., Adamson, T.W., Ganzoni, A. and Giblett, E.R. (1970) Ferrokinetics in man. Medicine, 49: 17–53.

Freedman, D.S., Brown, J.P., Weir, D.G. and Scott, J.M. (1973) The "reproducibility" and use of the tritiated folic acid urinary excretion as a measure of folate absorption in clinical practice: effect of methotrexate on absorption of folic acid. Journal of Clinical Pathology, 26: 261–267.

Garby, L. (1970) The normal haemoglobin level. British Journal of Haematology, 19: 429–434.

Heinivaara, O. and Palva, I.P. (1964) Malabsorption of vitamin B_{12} during treatment with para-aminosalicylic acid. A preliminary report. Acta Medica Scandinavica, 175: 469–471.

Herbert, V., Tisman, G., Go, L.T. and Brenner, L. (1973) The dU suppression test using ^{125}I-UdR to define biochemical megaloblastosis. British Journal of Haematology, 24: 713–723.

Hesp, R., Chanarin, I. and Tait, C.E. (1975) Potassium changes in megaloblastic anaemia. Clinical Science and Molecular Medicine, 49: 77–79.

Holt, J.M., Mayet, F.G.H., Warner, G.T., Callender, S.T. and Gunning, A.J. (1968) Iron absorption and blood loss in patients with hiatus hernia. British Medical Journal, iii: 22–25.

Jacobs, A., Miller, F., Worwood, M., Beamish, M.R. and Wardrop, C.A. (1972) Ferritin in the serum of normal subjects and patients with iron deficiency and iron overload. British Medical Journal, 4: 206–208.

Lawson, D.H., Murray, R.M. and Parker, J.L.W. (1972) Early mortality in the megaloblastic anaemias. Quarterly Journal of Medicine, New Series, 41: 1–14.

Martinez-Torres, C. and Layrisse, M. (1973) Nutritional factors in iron-deficiency: food iron absorption. Clinics in Haematology, 2: 339–352.

McBrien, M.P. (1973) Vitamin B_{12} malabsorption after cobalt teletherapy for carcinoma of the bladder. British Medical Journal, 1: 648–650.

Olsson, K.S. (1972) Iron stores in normal man and male blood donors as measured by desferrioxamine and quantitative phlebotomy. Acta Medica Scandinavica, 192: 401–407.

Race, T.F., Paes, I.C. and Faloon, W.W. (1970) Intestinal malabsorption induced by oral colchicine. American Journal of Medical Science, 259: 32–41.

Raven, J.L. and Robson, M.B. (1974) Experience with a commercial kit for the radioisotopic assay of vitamin B_{12} in serum: the Phadebas B_{12} test. Journal of Clinical Pathology, 27: 59–65.

Raven, J.L., Robson, M.B., Morgan, J.O. and Hoffbrand, A.V. (1972) Comparison of three methods for measuring vitamin B_{12} in serum: radioisotopic, *Euglena gracilis* and *Lactobacillus leichmannii.* British Journal of Haematology, 22: 21–31.

Rose, M.S. and Chanarin, I. (1971) Intrinsic-factor antibody and the absorption of vitamin B_{12} in pernicious anaemia. British Medical Journal, 1: 25–26.

Tomkin, G.H. (1973) Malabsorption of vitamin B_{12} in diabetic patients treated with phenformin: a comparison with metformin. British Medical Journal, 3: 673–675.

Verloop, M.C., Blokhuis, E.W. and Bos, C.C. (1959) Causes of the differences in haemoglobin and serum-iron between men and women. Acta Haematologica, 21: 199–205.

Whiteside, M.G., Mollin, D.L., Coghill, N.F., Williams, A.N. and Anderson, B. (1964) The absorption of radioactive vitamin B_{12} and the secretion of hydrochloric acid in patients with atrophic gastritis. Gut, 5: 385–399.

Wöhler, F. (1964) Diagnosis of iron storage disease with desferrioxamine (Desferal test). Acta Haematologica, 31: 321–337.

FURTHER READING

Williams, W.J., Beutler, E., Erslev, A.J. and Rundles, R.W. (1972) Hematology, McGraw-Hill, New York.

Wintrobe, M.M., Lee, G.R., Boggs, D., Bethell, T.C., Athens, J.W. and Foerster, J. (1974) Clinical Hematology, Lea and Febiger, Philadelphia.

Chapter 17

Abnormal haemoglobins

Robin W. Carrell and Hermann Lehmann

MRC Abnormal Haemoglobin Unit, Addenbrooke's Hospital, Hills Road, Cambridge CB2 2QR, England

CONTENTS

Chemical diagnosis of disease, edited by
S.S. Brown, F.L. Mitchell and D.S. Young

17.1. THE HAEM GROUP

17.1.1. Porphyrin and haem molecular structure and spectra

The protoporphyrin ring owes its central role in biochemistry to its ability to undergo changes in electron distribution. This property results from its structure which, as shown in Figure 17.1, is a linked series of conjugated bonds.

The doughnut-shaped cloud of shared electrons of the porphyrin ring is readily excited into a higher energy state by light in the near ultraviolet range (Corwin, 1973). This gives the characteristic high intensity absorption of both the porphyrins and haem proteins, the Soret band, with a maximum near 400 nm. Excitation of the free porphyrins by light of this wavelength is followed by emission, explaining their ready fluorescence.

This fluorescence is lost in iron–porphyrin complexes and consequently neither haem nor haemoglobin is fluorescent. However, when there is some porphyrin present without iron, as in iron deficiency anaemia or lead poisoning, then an apparent fluorescence of haemoglobin is detectable. This is due to the formation of a zinc haemoglobin in which zince replaces iron in the haem groups (Lamola and Yaman, 1974). The characteristic fluorescence of this zinc "haemoglobin" provides a simple screening test for lead poisoning and iron deficiency anaemia.

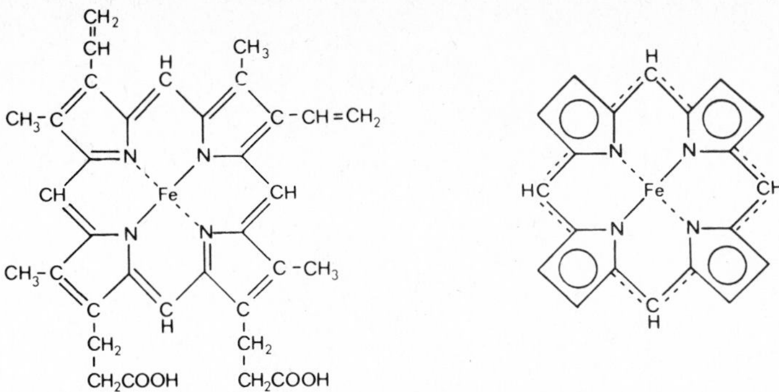

Figure 17.1. The haem group. An essential feature is the complete system of unsaturated carbon bridges (–C=) between the four pyrrole rings. The simplified depiction of the haem group on the right emphasizes the extended electron orbitals which are responsible for its characteristic properties.

The electron cloud of the porphyrin ring can readily allow a charge transfer to a co-ordinated metal (e.g. the iron atom in haem). The controlled use of this ability of the haem group to transfer charge is essential to its biological function, but the ability to undergo reversible charge transfers also means that the porphyrins can function as general electron transfer, or redox, intermediates. This immediately makes them potentially dangerous, since in the presence of metal ions (e.g. Cu^{2+}), or oxygen, or light of Soret band wavelength, they can catalyze the formation of toxic free radicals and other high energy products. It is therefore essential for its physiological role that the haem group should be compartmented in such a way that access to it is carefully controlled. Thus a prime function of the globin molecule is to protect the haem group. Any abnormality of the globin structure may not only disturb its function as an oxygen carrier but may also place the red cell at risk due to the formation of various free radicals (Carrell et al., 1975).

Similar safeguards exist in both the synthesis and catabolism of haem. The porphyrin synthetic pathway occurs via the porphyrinogens, in which saturated bonds between the pyrrole rings break the series of double bonds and prevent the formation of extended delocalised orbitals. Not until the last step, the conversion of protoporphyrinogen into protoporphyrin, does the ring gain its "electron cloud". Multiple safeguards also exist against the release of free haem in the form of the haptoglobin, haemopexin and albumin systems.

The redox properties of the haem group allow it to act as a pseudoperoxidase, catalyzing the oxidation, by hydrogen peroxide, of amines such as benzidine, *o*-tolidine, and diphenylamine. This provides a sensitive test for the presence of any of the haem derivatives, including haematin and myoglobin, as well as the various forms of haemoglobin. The dyes involved are potentially carcinogenic although a tetramethyl derivative of benzidine has now been produced that is claimed to be non-carcinogenic (Holland et al., 1974).

The iron of the haem group forms four bonds with the protoporhyrin and can readily

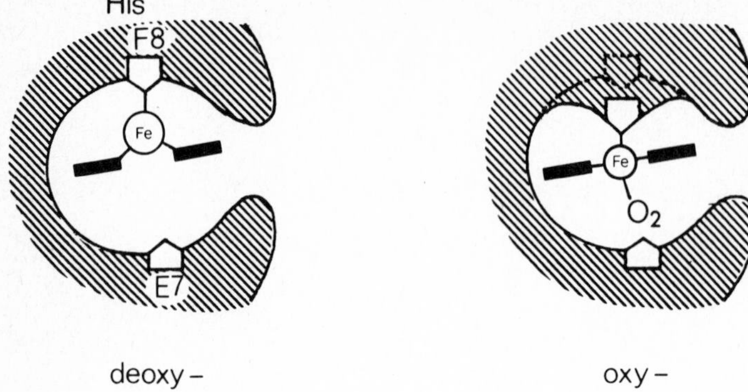

Figure 17.2. Schematic representation of the haem pockets of deoxy- and oxyhaemoglobins. The porphyrin ring with its four bonds is shown in planar section. The proximal histidine (F8) forms the fifth co-ordinate, the sixth co-ordinate being formed by the ligand, oxygen in this case, which lies between the iron and the distal histidine (E7). Note the linked movement of the globin and the iron as change in the radius of the iron causes it to move into and out of the haem plane.

take up one or two additional ligands to form altogether a five or six co-ordinate structure. In haemoglobin, the fifth co-ordinate is the proximal histidine (F8) of the globin molecule. The sixth co-ordinate is free to bond with other ligands, the physiologically important one being oxygen (Figure 17.2).

17.2. GLOBIN

The function of globin is to combine with the haem to render it soluble and provide it with a non-polar environment. This depends on structural features at two levels; the overall conformation of the globin to form the haem pocket, and the precise specification of the aminoacid side chains that line this pocket.

17.2.1. Overall conformation of globin

The globin molecule is formed of eight helices (A–H), linked by short interhelical segments (AB, CD etc.) as indicated in Figure 17.3.

The length and primary structure of the different globins varies considerably, with the haemoglobin α-chain having 141 aminoacid residues, the β, γ and δ-chains 146, and myoglobin 153. At first sight, the aminoacid sequence of the various globins has little in common, but when they are aligned according to helical positions their homologous structure is immediately apparent. For example, in all globins the eighth position of the F helix is occupied by a histidine which links with the haem iron (the proximal histidine). Similarly, in almost all globins there is a histidine in position E7 which forms a hydrogen bond with the haem ligand (the distal histidine).

The concept of homologous residues enables the important structural features of the globin molecule to be deduced by comparing all known globins and looking for residues which have been protected during evolutionary change. Four residues are present in almost all the 90 globin chains of animals and plants so far examined – phenylalanine, CD1; leucine, F4; histidine, F8; and tyrosine HC2. Not surprisingly, three of these are in the haem pocket (Phe, CD1; Leu, F4; and His, F8). All globins contain Phe, CD1 and His, F8 but even these have been found substituted in some human pathological variants. Many residues are not totally invariant but show relatively little variation. In particular, there are a number of positions which are consistently occupied by non-polar residues. It is this regular pattern of hydrophobic side chains which determines the overall structure of the globin, as the molecule will fold on itself to bring these side chains together in the centre of the molecule. The molecule therefore consists of a central hydrophobic core and a largely polar surface which renders it soluble. It is important to realize that the globin also folds itself about the haem group, thereby burying more hydrophobic residues. This removal of hydrophobic side chains from the surrounding water makes haemoglobin more soluble. Thus factors which increase the ordered structure of the globin increase its solubility; conversely solubility is decreased by factors which lessen ordered structure. Thus loss of the haem group, extremes of pH and increased temperature will lead to exposure of hydrophobic residues, loss of solubility and precipitation. These changes, together with the random aggregation that occurs during precipitation, constitute the process of denaturation. Clearly, any aminoacid substitution that affects ordered structure will also hasten denaturation. This loss of stability is a characteristic feature of pathological protein variants and occurs with other proteins such as glucose-6-phosphate dehydrogenase and α-1-antitrypsin, as well as with haemoglobin (Sutton and Wagner, 1975). The use of stability tests, usually at increased temperature, is consequently an important diagnostic test in identifying and characterizing many mutant proteins.

17.2.2. The haem pocket

The haem group is embedded in a pocket in the globin with just the two propionic acids emerging from the surface of the molecule. Although it is useful to depict the structure of globin in terms of the open backbone structure which is shown in Figure 17.3, a truer picture is seen in the space filling model illustrated in Figure 17.4 (between pp. 884 and 885). This shows that the molecule is actually tightly packed, with the side chains of aminoacids forming van der Waals bonds with each other and with the haem group. The stability of the molecule depends on the sum of these van der Waals bonds along with the associative forces that bring the non-polar groups together; the overall process is referred to as hydrophobic bonding.

The hydrophobic bonding of the haem group is particularly important for the stability of the molecule, involving bonding to some 20 aminoacids (Perutz et al., 1968). Obviously the steric relationships in this area are critical and it is not surprising that the aminoacids lining the haem pocket of haemoglobin and myoglobin have remained relatively constant throughout evolution. The replacement of any of these aminoacids may disrupt the whole molecule and result in an unstable haemoglobin haemolytic anaemia (section 17.6.3).

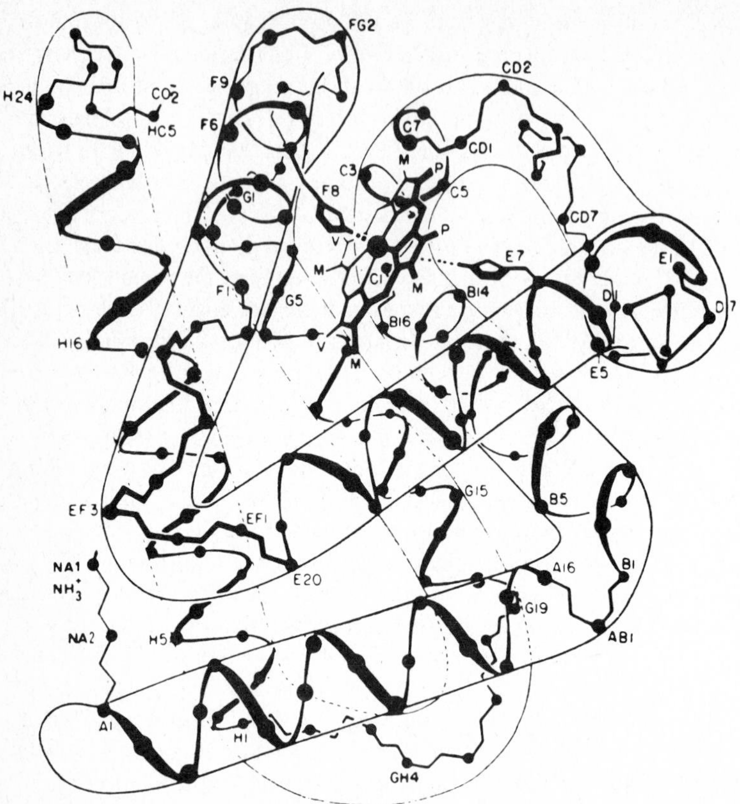

Figure 17.3. Structure of myoglobin, which exemplifies those of all the globins: 80% of the molecule is in the helical form, each helix being designated by a letter and number, and non-helical portions by two letters and a number according to their position (thus A1–A16, helical; CD1–CD7, non-helical).

17.2.3. Haem–globin derivatives

17.2.3.1. Myoglobin

This is a monomer of molecular mass 17,200, found in striated muscle where it is thought to assist diffusion of oxygen and to act as an oxygen reservoir to meet requirements during muscle contraction. Mutant, i.e. abnormal, myoglobins have been identified, but as yet none have been found to be associated with disease or dysfunction (Lehmann and Huntsman, 1974). Medical interest in myoglobin largely centres on its abnormal release into the plasma. This occurs in various myopathies, following violent exercise, and in idiopathic paroxysmal myoglobinuria. Its presence in urine is tested for by first screening for the presence of haem pigments (section 17.1.1.). The method of choice for confirmation that the pigment is myoglobin, and for subsequent quantitation, is by radial immunodiffusion aginst specific antisera. Spectrophotometric identification of oxymyoglobin (absorption maxima 418, 542 and 582 nm) is possible, but this is not a convenient method due to the tendency of myoglobin to oxidize to metmyoglobin.

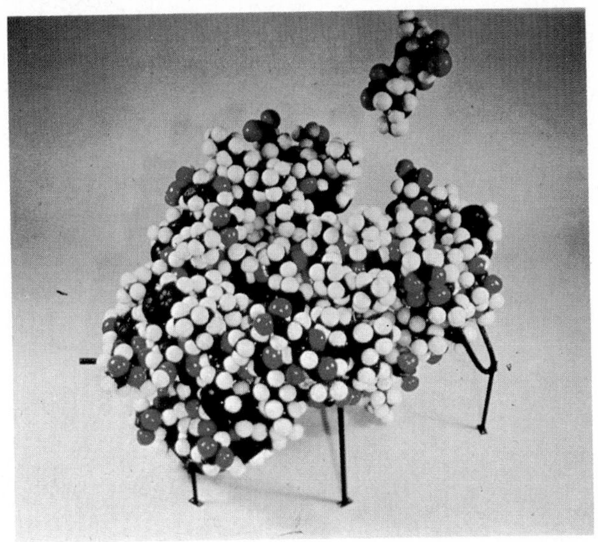

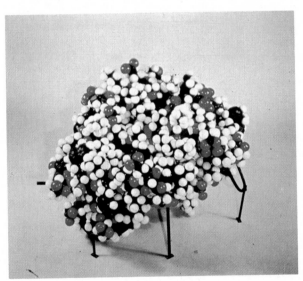

Figure 17.4. Space filling model: myoglobin. The usual skeletal representations of globin (as in Figure 17.3) give a false sense of space within the molecule. If the effective space occupied by each atom is represented as in this Figure, the molecule is seen to be tightly packed. This is particularly true about the haem group, as shown by removal of the haem (top model) and its replacement (below). The oxygen atoms are shown in red in the model, so demonstrating the exterior placement of the haem propionic acid side chains. (Photograph by courtesy of Prof. H.C. Watson).

17.2.3.2. Haemoglobin

This has molecular mass 67,000 and is a tetramer formed by two pairs of unlike globin chains, designated $\alpha_2\beta_2$. Its prime role is that of an oxygen carrier, with the two physiological components being deoxyhaemoglobin (dull purple) and oxyhaemoglobin (red).

The absorption spectra of the haemoglobin derivatives are shown in Figure 17.5. There

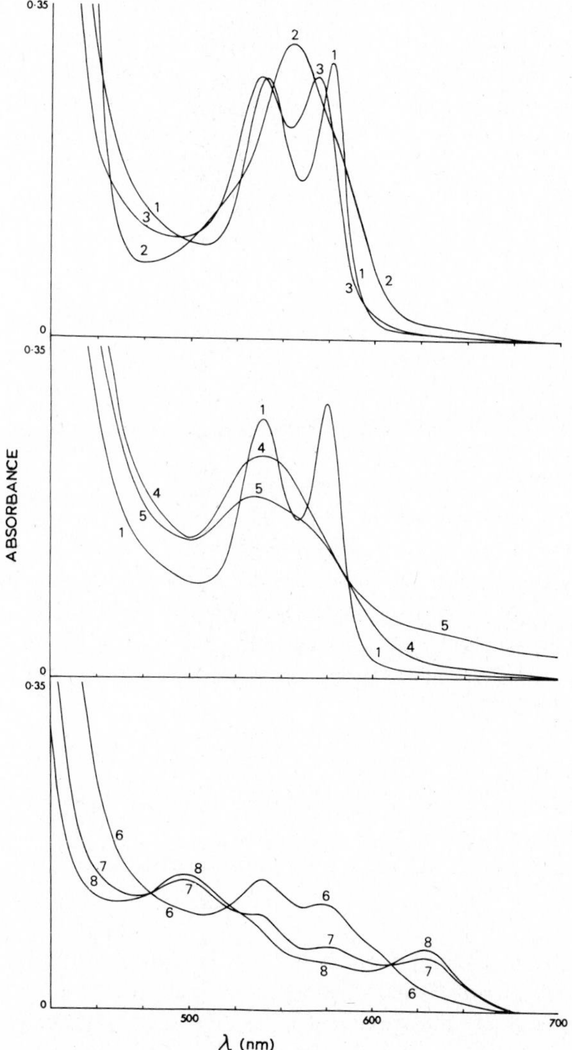

Figure 17.5. Absorption spectra of haemoglobin derivatives measured in phosphate buffer, pH 7.4 except as indicated below. (Beckman model 25 spectrophotometer, Miss. B.M. McGrath). 1. oxyhaemoglobin, 2. deoxyhaemoglobin, 3. carboxyhaemoglobin, 4. cyanmethaemoglobin, 5. haemichrome, 6. methaemoglobin, in pH 6.0 phosphate buffer; 7. methaemoglobin, 8. methaemoglobin, in pH 11.0 glycine buffer.

are two major contributions to the spectrum of haemoglobin: the Soret band absorption of the electron cloud of the protoporphyrin, and the charge transitions of the iron and its ligand. The last depends on the oxidation state of the iron (Fe^{2+} or Fe^{3+}), its spin state, and the electronegativity of the ligand.

Both ferrous and ferric iron can exist in high- or low-spin states according to the pairing of their outer orbital electrons. Fe^{2+} has six outer electrons and Fe^{3+} five. These can be arranged to give either a maximum or minimum number of unpaired electrons, the minimum being known as the low-spin state and the maximum as the high-spin state. The radius of the iron atom increases in the high-spin state and it is this that produces the lengthening of Fe–porphyrin bonds. As a consequence, there is a movement of iron out of the plane of the haem when, for example, the low-spin oxyhaemoglobin is converted to high-spin deoxyhaemoglobin (Figure 17.2). This lengthening of the Fe–porphyrin bonds will affect the charge transfer between the iron and porphyrin and hence the absorption spectrum.

17.2.3.3. Oxyhaemoglobin

Oxygen binds in an angular situation to the haem, with the partial negative charge of the oxygen balanced by hydrogen bonding to the distal histidine. The iron is low-spin and is in the plane of the haem. It is in the ferrous state, although there is additional partial positive charge due to polarization of an electron to the oxygen.

17.2.3.4. Deoxyhaemoglobin

With the loss of oxygen, the iron becomes five co-ordinated and takes up the high-spin state with movement out of the plane of the haem. In deoxymyoglobin, the movement is of the order of 0.5 Å, but in deoxyhaemoglobin this is increased to 0.75 Å, presumably due to the change in tertiary conformation that occurs in the deoxygenated haemoglobin tetramer. This change in conformation of the globin gives an additional pull on the iron, amplifying its movement out of the haem and hence speeding the loss of oxygen (section 17.2.4.1 and Figure 17.12).

17.2.3.5. Carboxyhaemoglobin

Carbon monoxide reacts with haemoglobin more avidly than oxygen and will displace it to give carboxyhaemoglobin. Though similar in structure to oxyhaemoglobin, there is a slight shift in the absorption spectrum to a brighter red, almost pink, appearance.

17.2.3.6. Methaemoglobin

This chocolate brown derivative of haemoglobin is formed by the oxidation of ferrous to ferric iron. This can be brought about directly by oxidizing agents such as ferricyanide or nitrite. Methaemoglobin is also formed by the spontaneous oxidation of oxyhaemoglobin which occurs in ageing blood samples, and can be formed in vivo with oxidative stress. About 3% of the circulating haemoglobin is normally oxidized to methaemoglobin each day. Several mechanisms exist for its reduction, the most important of which is the NADH-linked diaphorase (methaemoglobin reductase I). The reductase is thought to act indirectly by first reducing cytochrome b_5 which then directly reduces the methaemoglobin (Hultquist et al., 1975). It is therefore probably more correct to name the enzyme

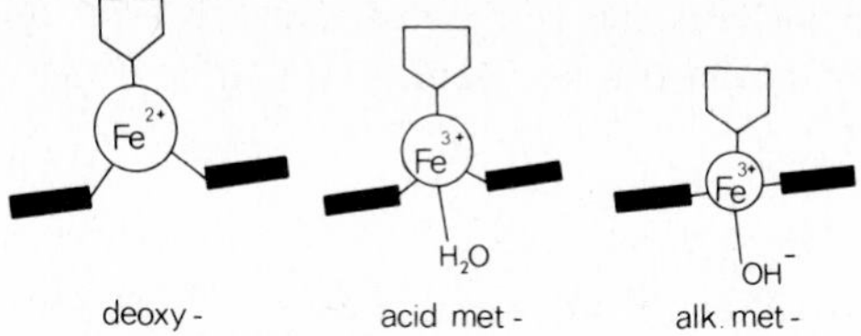

Figure 17.6. Deoxyhaemoglobin and acid and alkaline methaemoglobins, showing the changes in charge and relationship of iron to the haem plane that produce changes in absorption spectra. Note how the iron shrinks and moves into the plane of the haem with linked movement of the proximal histidine (cf. Figure 17.2).

cytochrome b_5 reductase. Deficiency of this enzyme is a cause of hereditary methaemoglobinaemia (section 17.6.4.2). The absorption spectrum of methaemoglobin varies with pH, since it exists in both an acid form with water as the sixth ligand, and an alkaline form with hydroxyl as the ligand (Figure 17.6). The pK of transition is near 8. The iron in methaemoglobin is a mixture of high- and low-spin states, mainly high-spin in the acid form (pH 6.5) and an equal mixture of high- and low-spin at pH 10.0.

17.2.3.7. Cyanmethaemoglobin

One of the problems of handling haemoglobin solutions is that oxyhaemoglobin readily oxidizes to methaemoglobin, which in turn is readily denatured to form haemichromes (section 17.2.3.8). It is therefore useful to stabilize a solution by oxidation and concurrent addition of cyanide which displaces the water from methaemoglobin to form the stable cyanmethaemoglobin. Conversion into cyanmethaemoglobin is now the reference method of measurement of haemoglobin concentration (Makarem, 1974). This overcomes the problem of assaying solutions of haemoglobin containing several derivatives, e.g. oxyhaemoglobin, carboxyhaemoglobin and methaemoglobin, since all the haemoglobin is converted into methaemoglobin and then stabilized as cyanmethaemoglobin.

17.2.3.8. Haemichromes

These are denaturation products of methaemoglobin involving the formation of an internal sixth ligand by the side chains of the globin. The distal, usually non-liganded, histidine is of particular importance since, if the structure of the globin is distorted it can bend to the iron, forming the reversible globin haemichrome I (Figure 17.7). If further

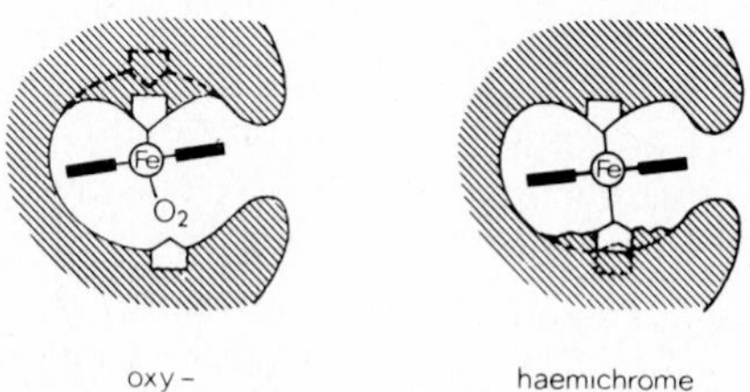

Figure 17.7. Comparison of oxyhaemoglobin and haemichrome I. A first stage in the denaturation of methaemoglobin is the formation of a bond between the distal histidine and the iron, with consequent distortion of the globin to give haemichrome.

distortion occurs, other side chains in the globin may displace the histidine to form an irreversible globin haemichrome II, with resultant denaturation and precipitation (Rachmilewitz, 1974).

17.2.3.9. Sulphaemoglobin

This appears in some individuals after ingestion of drugs such as phenacetin and sulphonamides. It is probable that it is formed by complexing of a sulphur to the haem in a manner which still allows the haem iron to react with other ligands (Berzofsky et al., 1971). It is likely that circulating haemichromes have been included in the past under the general heading of sulphaemoglobinaemia.

17.2.4. Oxygen carriage and co-operative effects

Adult haemoglobin (Hb A) is a tetramer formed of two pairs of unlike chains, $\alpha_2\beta_2$. The tetrameric structure modifies the oxygen binding properties of the monomer to make it more suitable for oxygen transport by the blood. As shown in Figure 17.8, in comparison with haemoglobin, myoglobin has a hyperbolic oxygen dissociation curve that only gives appreciable release of oxygen at very low partial pressures. Blood has to release oxygen at the much higher tensions of working tissues, and haemoglobin is able to meet this requirement because of co-operation between its subunits. Deoxygenation of one subunit decreases the oxygen affinity of the others, resulting in much earlier oxygen release. This allosteric interaction gives haemoglobin a sigmoid oxygen dissociation curve with efficient uptake of oxygen at alveolar pressures and release as the partial pressure moves below the mean venous level of 40 mm Hg (5 kPa).

The allosteric interaction of haemoglobin can be treated quantitatively. The oxygenation of myoglobin or of a single haemoglobin subunit follows first order kinetics –

$$\begin{array}{lll} \mathrm{Mb} & + \mathrm{O_2} \rightleftharpoons & \mathrm{MbO_2} \\ (1-Y) & (P) & (Y) \end{array}$$

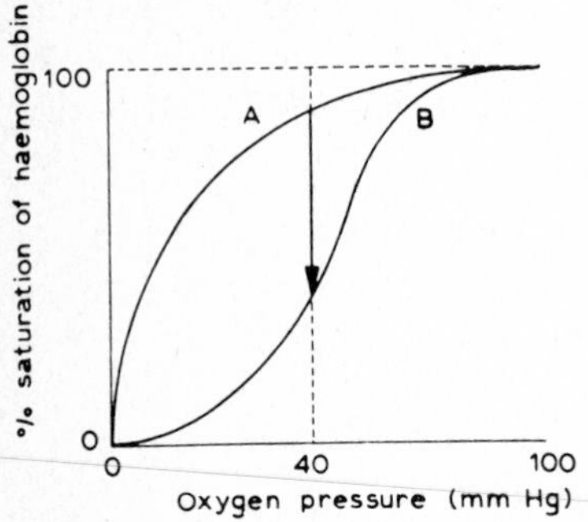

Figure 17.8. Comparison of the hyperbolic oxygen dissociation curve of myoglobin (A) with the sigmoid curve of haemoglobin (B). Note the increased efficiency of release of oxygen of the sigmoid curve at the mean venous tension of 40 mm Hg. (Reproduced, with permission, from Lehmann and Huntsman, 1974)

where Y is the fractional saturation and P the partial pressure. If K is the equilibrium constant, then the fractional (percentage) saturation is the hyperbolic function

$$Y = \frac{KP}{1 + KP}$$

Hill showed that in the case of the haemoglobin tetramer, the oxygen dissociation could be represented by the sigmoid function –

$$Y = \frac{KP^n}{1 + KP^n}$$

where n indicates the degree of subunit interaction. Normally its value is 2.8, but it will be lower in mutant haemoglobins with decreased co-operativity. Myoglobin, with no co-operative interaction and very high oxygen affinity, has an n value of 1.

It can be seen that the co-operative interaction of the haemoglobin subunits results in changes that lower their oxygen affinity. The high-affinity of myoglobin can be regarded as the primitive state to which haemoglobin will revert if its chains are separated, or if it is subject to major molecular modifications. In allosteric terminology, this natural high-affinity state is referred to as the relaxed, R, state. The low-affinity, high-energy, deoxygenated, conformation of the haemoglobin tetramer is referred to as the tense, T, state. This use of the term "tense" is quite descriptive, as it is now known that as deoxygenation occurs, a number of inter-chain bonds are formed that tense the whole molecule and so favour loss of oxygen. A simple analogy would be to that of a sponge which in its relaxed form will readily take up water, but if constrained, it will readily lose, and less readily take up, water.

This change in the haemoglobin molecule affects the whole tetramer, which at some stage during deoxygenation will switch over from the R to the T form with a consequent decrease in affinity of all subunits. Statistically, the changing proportions of the R and T forms are represented by the sigmoid shape of the dissociation curve.

A summary of the molecular changes that occur on deoxygenation follows, but for fuller accounts the reader is referred to Perutz and TenEyck (1971), Perutz (1972), Lehmann and Huntsman (1974), and Charache (1974).

17.2.4.1. Molecular changes on deoxygenation

The haemoglobin molecule, as already stated, can be considered as being formed of two dimers with the major bonding being between two unlike chains to form the $\alpha\beta$ dimer. Figure 17.9 illustrates the terminology which is applied to their interfaces. There are two types of bonding contacts; $\alpha_1\beta_1$ (synonymous with $\alpha_2\beta_2$) and $\alpha_1\beta_2$ (synonymous with $\alpha_2\beta_1$). The $\alpha_1\beta_1$ contact that holds the dimer together is particularly strong, involving 34 aminoacid side chains in mainly hydrophobic bonding (section 17.2.2). It glues the dimer together and is important structurally, but does not play an active part in the changes occurring during deoxygenation. The active movement in the change from the R to the T state occurs at the $\alpha_1\beta_2$ contact due to a sliding rotation of the $\alpha_1\beta_1$ dimer with respect to the $\alpha_2\beta_2$ dimer (Figure 17.10). The $\alpha_1\beta_2$ contact is therefore critical to the transport

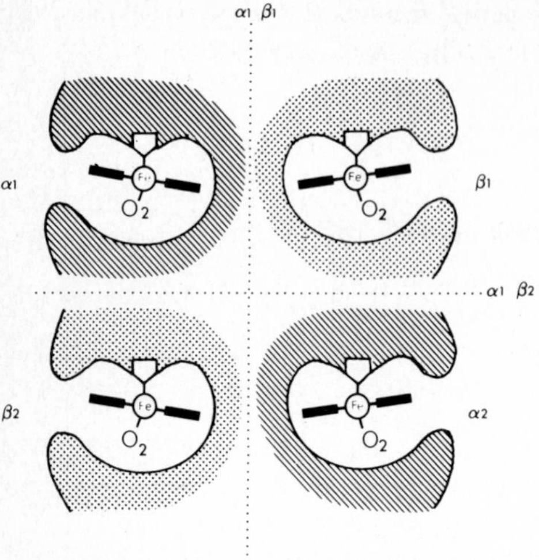

Figure 17.9. Quaternary structure of the R-form (oxyhaemoglobin) showing the nomenclature of the four subunits and their junctions.

function of haemoglobin and it is not surprising that it shows virtually no variation in composition from the haemoglobin of one species to another. It also follows that mutations involving the $\alpha_1\beta_2$ contact are liable to produce major changes in oxygen affinity (section 17.6.5).

The rotation that occurs at the $\alpha_1\beta_2$ junction on deoxygenation produces a widening

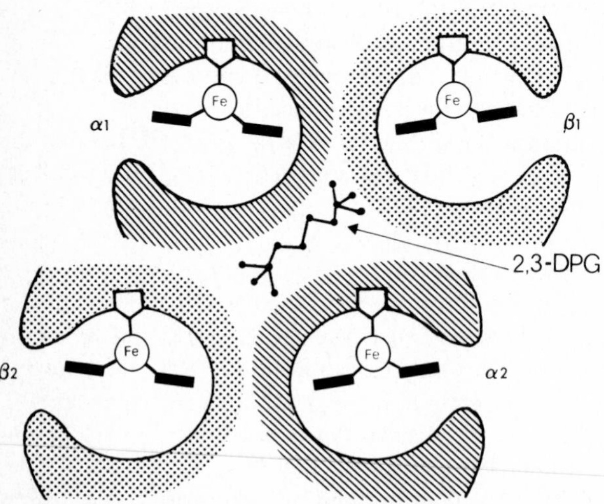

Figure 17.10. Quaternary structure of the T-form (deoxyhaemoglobin) after sliding movement at the $\alpha_1\beta_2$ junction. The α-chains have moved closer to each other, and the gap between the β-chains has widened, allowing the entry of 2,3-diphosphoglycerate (2,3-DPG).

of the gap between the two β chains in the central axis of the molecule. The opening of this gap allows the entry of a molecule of 2,3-diphosphoglycerate (section 17.2.5), which strengthens the deoxy-configuration. On oxygenation, the $\alpha\beta$ dimers rotate back again, the β chains move closer together and expel the 2,3-diphosphoglycerate from the central cavity.

Although these shifts in overall or quaternary structure are the most obvious changes, the most significant changes are occurring at the subunit or tertiary level. This can be seen by examining the sequence of events that takes place on deoxygenation.

The triggering factor is the loss of oxygen from the first subunit, assumed here to be an α-chain. With the loss of oxygen, the iron changes from low- to high-spin and moves out of the plane of the haem. In doing so, it pushes on the F helix opening a gap between the F and H helices. In deoxyhaemoglobin this gap is of the right dimensions to accept the aromatic side chain of tyrosine HC2, the penultimate aminoacid of both the α- and β-chains. The non-helical terminal portion of the globin which had been free to take up random positions in oxyhaemoglobin is thus fixed in the deoxygenated subunit by the binding of this penultimate tyrosine. This fixes the position of the terminal arginine of the α-subunit (Figure 17.11). This arginine has both a negatively charged carboxyl and a positively charged guanidine group, both of which can form salt bridges with oppositely charged side-chains on the other α-subunit. Other salt bridges are formed, but these bondings between subunits can only occur if they are correctly spaced one to another, i.e. if the molecule has undergone the quaternary shift to the T state. Hence from the time of loss of the first oxygen, changes accrue which favour the switching of the molecule to the T conformation. Deoxygenation of the next subunit will similarly result in fixation of its penultimate tyrosine and the potential formation of further salt bridges. At a critical stage, which may vary from molecule to molecule, there will be a "clicking" over of the whole haemoglobin molecule to the T formation. As stated earlier, this clicking over involves a sliding rotation about the $\alpha_1\beta_2$ interface with a widening of the space

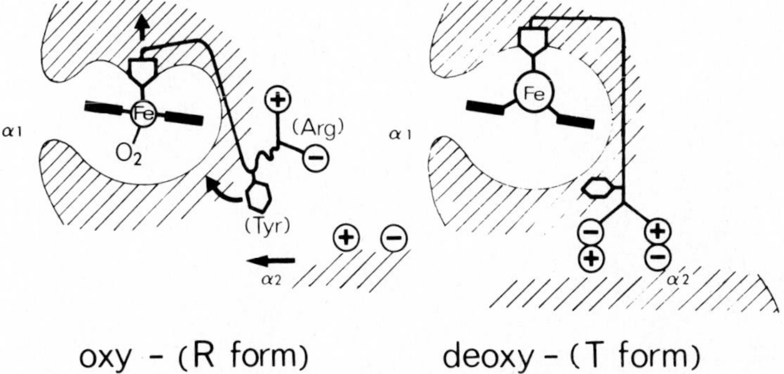

Figure 17.11. Representation of the change in tertiary structure from the R- to the T-form, involving a movement of the iron from the plane of the haem, shifting and holding the position of the penultimate tyrosine and terminal arginine. The other α-chain moves across, as in Figure 17.10, to form an ionic bond (salt bridge). Similar changes occur with the β-chains, but additionally there is a closure of the haem pocket hindering reoxygenation.

between the β-chains. 2,3-Diphosphoglycerate enters this space and its phosphates form three ionic bonds with positively charged side chains on each of the two β-chains. Thus, 2,3-diphosphoglycerate acts as a stabilizer to the deoxygenated T state, hindering it from spontaneously reverting to the R state.

In the example given, the haemoglobin now has two oxygenated and two deoxygenated subunits but the overall conformation has switched to that of the deoxy (T) state, The two remaining oxygenated subunits of the tetramer are thus forced into the tertiary deoxy state (Figure 17.12). In the β-subunits, this means a narrowing of the haem pocket, and in all subunits a tension at the haem tending to pull the iron into the high-spin deoxy state. All these forces will facilitate the release of the remaining oxygen to give complete deoxygenation. Thus the globin can be compared to a pump, moving into and out of the T state and forcing the iron out of and into the plane of the haem with consequent loss and gain of oxygen.

17.2.4.2. The Bohr effect

Within the physiological pH range, the oxygen affinity of haemoglobin decreases with increasing acidity. This is the alkaline Bohr effect, an important physiological mechanism which ensures the increased release of oxygen to active acid-forming tissues such as exercising muscles. The decrease in affinity continues until the pH drops below 6 (Figure 17.13) at which stage the affinity begins to rise again. This is the non-physiological "acid" Bohr effect.

As the alkaline Bohr effect is associated with uptake of hydrogen ion, it has the added advantage of buffering the acid released by working tissues. The change from oxy- to deoxy-conformation brings some negative charges into closer proximity to amine and histidine residues. This increases their positive charge with a consequent uptake of hydrogen ions and stabilizing of the deoxy state.

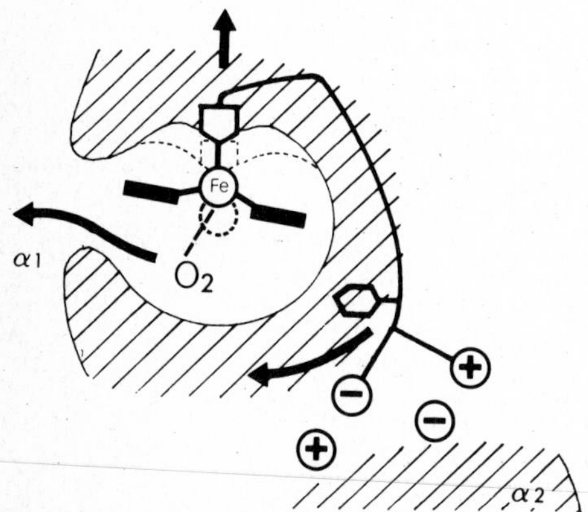

Figure 17.12. Representation of decreased oxygen affinity of subunit α_1 which occurs when the whole molecule switches to the quaternary T-state. The terminal arginine of the subunit endeavours to form a salt bridge with the α_2 subunit and this tends to pull the iron out of the plane of the haem with consequent loss of the oxygen.

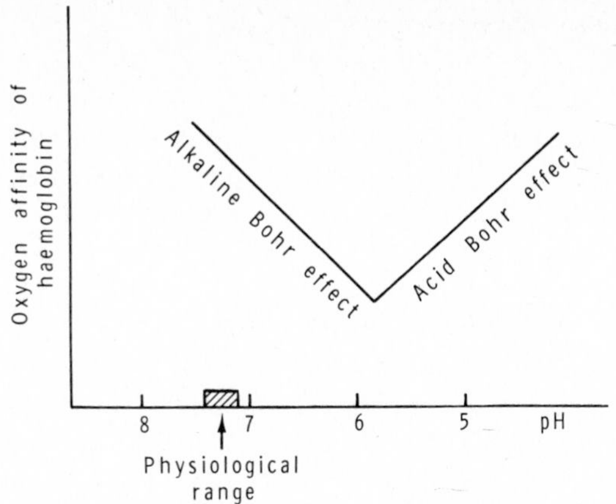

Figure 17.13. The Bohr effect, showing the minimal oxygen affinity of haemoglobin at pH 6. The acid Bohr effect lies well outside the physiological range. The alkaline Bohr effect assists the release of further oxygen when the pH is reduced in the venous capillaries. (Reproduced, with permission, from Lehmann and Huntsman, 1974)

The overall result is that haemoglobin acts as a carrier of hydrogen ion from the peripheral tissues to the lungs, where it is neutralized by combination with bicarbonate ion.

17.2.4.3. Carbon dioxide transport

Carbon dioxide can combine with the N-terminal amino groups of proteins to form carbamino groups, which can form stabilizing salt bridges in deoxy- but not oxyhaemoglobins. Hence, increased carbon dioxide concentration will encourage the haemoglobin to release oxygen by lowering its oxygen affinity (Kilmartin, 1976).

17.2.5. 2,3-Diphosphoglycerate and oxygen transport

One concept that must be guarded against in clinical chemistry is the tendency to think in terms of concentration of a substance rather than of its function. The blood's ability to transport oxygen is an excellent illustration of this problem, as it is still assessed solely by measurement of the haemoglobin concentration or the packed cell volume. Instead, there should also be some emphasis on the haemoglobin's oxygen affinity which, with the haemoglobin concentration, determines oxygen delivery.

The shape of the oxygen dissociation curve of haemoglobin is such that small shifts will produce large changes in the amount of oxygen released. As shown in Figure 17.14, 100 ml of blood normally carry 20 ml of oxygen, but only some 25% of this amount is released at the mean venous tension of 40 mm Hg (5 kPa), the remaining 75% returning to the lungs in the oxygenated form. There is therefore a considerable potential for improving oxygen delivery by decreasing the oxygen affinity of the haemoglobin. This "shift to the right" of the oxygen dissociation curve will release a larger proportion of oxygen without the need to lower the tissue oxygen tension. Such a shift occurs in exer-

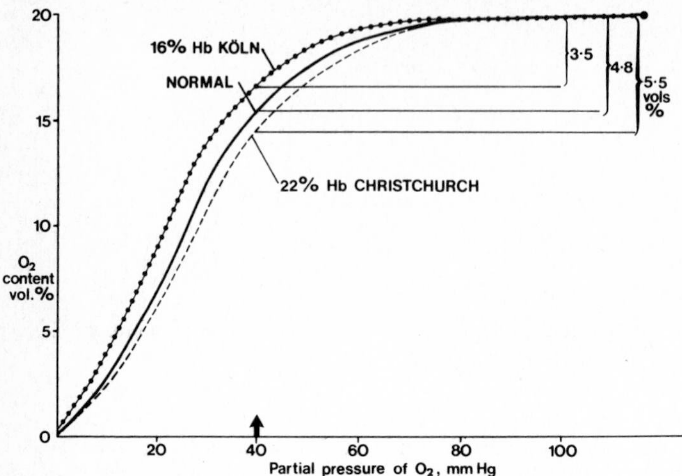

Figure 17.14. Oxygen dissociation curves. Only a small proportion of the total oxygen which is carried is released at the mixed venous pO_2 of 40 mm Hg. A very slight shift in the curve causes an appreciable change in oxygen release, as illustrated by whole cells from patients with Haemoglobins Köln and Christchurch.

cise and stress owing to the resultant increases in temperature, pCO_2 and hydrogen ion concentration.

However, the most critical adjustments to oxygen supply result from changes in 2,3-diphosphoglycerate concentration which provide a subtle and long-term means of controlling the efficiency of oxygen transport. This mechanism is of considerable clinical importance, and detailed accounts of its role are given by Torrance et al. (1970), Bellingham (1974), Duhm and Gerlach (1974) and Huehns (1975).

2,3-Diphosphoglycerate is a glycolytic pathway side product, formed in the Rapoport–Luebering cycle which by-passes the phosphoglycerate kinase step of the main pathway (Scheme 17.1). This cycle occurs in a number of tissues, but is obviously of special importance in the red cell where the concentration of 2,3-diphosphoglycerate is 100 times greater than that of other glycolytic intermediates, and nearly equimolar with that of haemoglobin. The explanation for this high concentration was provided by Chanutin and Curnish (1967) and Benesch and Benesch (1967) who showed that 2,3-diphosphoglycerate functioned as an allosteric modifier of oxygen dissociation, stabilizing the deoxy state.

The synthesis of 2,3-diphosphoglycerate is controlled by a number of factors which compensate for any changes in oxygen delivery. For example, the shift in the oxygen dissociation curve to the right which occurs when the pH drops (section 17.2.4.2) will be compensated by an equal shift to the left, due to inhibition of 2,3-diphosphoglycerate synthesis by the lowered pH. Thus there is an automatic correction of the oxygen dissociation in acid–base disturbances. However, whereas the Bohr effect acts immediately on the oxygen dissociation, the alteration of 2,3-diphosphoglycerate concentration takes place over some 8 hours. For this reason correction of acid–base disturbances should be

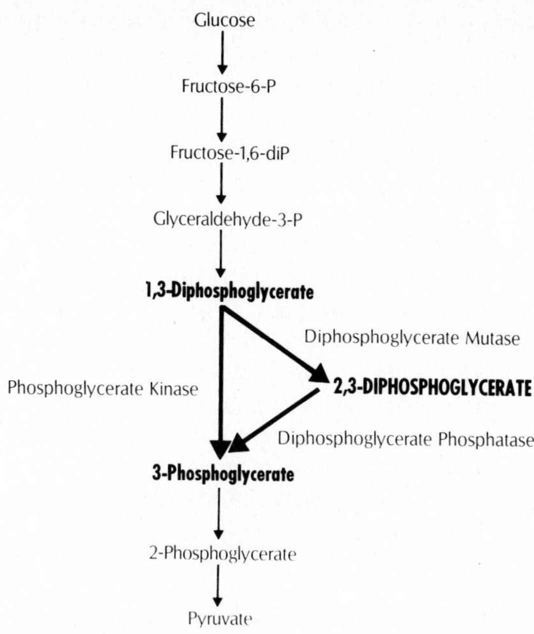

Scheme 17.1. The Rapoport–Luebering cycle for the production of 2,3-diphosphoglycerate.

carried out cautiously. In a long term acidosis, 2,3-diphosphoglycerate concentration will be low, and sudden correction of the blood pH will result in a marked swing to the left (Bellingham et al., 1971). The only way the body can then meet the oxygen demand is by increasing cardiac output. Thus the end result of a sudden correction of acidosis in an elderly diabetic may be cardiac failure.

Differences in haemoglobin levels in response to changes in 2,3-diphosphoglycerate may give a lead in the diagnosis of enzyme defects of the glycolytic pathway. A deficiency of an enzyme beyond the Rapoport–Luebering cycle, e.g. of pyruvate kinase, will cause a build up in 2,3-diphosphoglycerate, a decreased oxygen affinity, and hence a low haemoglobin concentration. Alternatively, an enzyme defect above the cycle, e.g. hexokinase deficiency, will give rise to decreased 2,3-diphosphoglycerate and a compensatory erythropoietic response leading to a relatively high haemoglobin concentration.

The syntheses of both haemoglobin and 2,3-diphosphoglycerate are stimulated by anoxia. Thus the high altitude climber will undergo two compensatory changes – the first, occurring over some 8 to 12 hours, will be an increase in 2,3-diphosphoglycerate; the second, occurring over several weeks, will be an increase in haemoglobin concentration stimulated by erythropoietin.

In the long term, there is a balance in a number of conditions between haemoglobin and 2,3-diphosphoglycerate concentrations. In anaemia, increases in 2,3-diphosphoglycerate produce a detectable shift in oxygen dissociation at a level of 10 g/dl with an overall increase of 25% in oxygen released at a haemoglobin concentration of 7.5 g/dl. Below this value, or in anaemia due to sudden blood loss, compensation occurs by increase in cardiac output or fall in tissue oxygen tension.

The importance of the reciprocal relationship between haemoglobin and 2,3-diphosphoglycerate concentrations cannot be too strongly stressed. It contributes to a number of real and apparent anaemias. Increased phosphate and sulphate concentrations stimulate 2,3-diphosphoglycerate synthesis and hence contribute to the anaemia of renal failure and the apparent anaemia of childhood. The last of these is a good example, as it is a "physiological" anaemia with perfectly normal oxygen delivery and arises from the normal increase in phosphate concentration that occurs before puberty (Card and Brain, 1973). As with most other biochemical constituents, there are probably considerable individual variations of this type in which an apparently low haemoglobin is matched by a high 2,3-diphosphoglycerate. This provides an explanation for earlier observations of individual variations in carriage of oxygen by haemoglobin. This is well illustrated by the comment of J.S. Haldane many years ago that people had as different haemoglobins as they had noses. Until the diagnostic services recognize this individuality and provide a measurement of oxygen carrying ability, rather than of haemoglobin alone, some patients are liable to receive unnecessary transfusion and therapy.

17.2.6. Physiological haemoglobins

Haemoglobin A, $\alpha_2\beta_2$, is the most important of the human haemoglobins, forming 96% of the adult pigment. The other 4% consists of Haemoglobin A_2, $\alpha_2\delta_2$, a minor constituent whose concentration may be raised or lowered in thalassaemia, and Haemoglobin F. Haemoglobin F, $\alpha_2\gamma_2$, forms more than half of the haemoglobin of the newborn, but disappears almost completely during infancy, contributing less than 0.8% to the haemoglobin of the adult (Figure 17.15). Early in foetal development, other haemoglobins appear formed from the embryonic ζ and ϵ chains. Of diagnostic significance are the haemoglobins that are found when α chain synthesis is suppressed in α-thalassaemia. These are the tetramers Haemoglobins H (β_4) and Barts (γ_4).

Measurement of Haemoglobin F is diagnostically important as raised concentrations may occur in a number of the haemoglobinopathies, particularly in the thalassaemias.

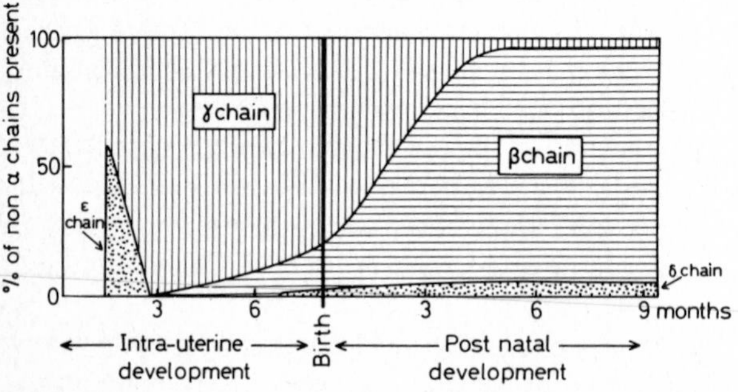

Figure 17.15. The changing pattern of production of non-α-chains in man during the months preceding and following birth. (Reproduced, with permission, from Lehmann and Huntsman, 1974)

A raised concentration may also occur with any lifelong anaemia, and occasionally with disordered erythropoiesis, as in some leukaemias. The concentration of Haemoglobin F can be readily measured because of its relative resistance to alkaline denaturation. This results from the absence of alkali-ionizable cysteine and tyrosine residues in the γ-chain that are internally situated in the β- and δ-chain. (Perutz, 1974).

Similarly the γ-chain lacks some of the β-chain residues which are involved in binding 2,3-diphosphoglycerate. Haemoglobin F consequently has an increased affinity for oxygen. This must be of advantage in the transport of oxygen from the maternal to the foetal circulation.

17.2.7. Multiple genes

The haemoglobins have emphasized the significance of gene duplication as an evolutionary mechanism and also as a complicating factor in the interpretation of hereditary disease. The evolution of the different globin chains has occurred by the process of duplication, with subsequent mutation and divergence. This chain duplication is a continuing process and it is known that both the γ and α chains are represented by multiple genetic loci. In the case of the γ-chain, there are at least two loci which differ at position 136; one gene ($^{A}\gamma$) having alanine, the other ($^{G}\gamma$) having glycine. At position 75 of the γ-chain, the substitution isoleucine to threonine (Haemoglobin F Sardinia) is unusually frequent, and it has been suggested that it represents evidence for a third γ-chain locus.

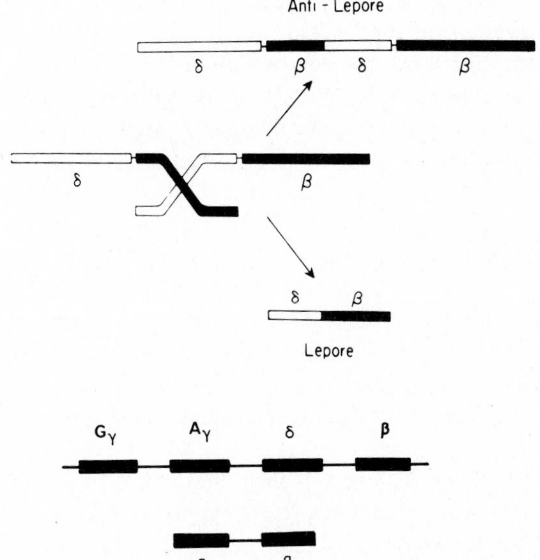

Fig. 17.16. Top: unequal crossing over of chromosomes carrying the δ- and β-polypeptide chains. One new product is a $\delta-\beta$ gene which would be responsible for a Haemoglobin Lepore. The other chromosome has one δ gene, one $\beta-\delta$ gene and one β gene. The $\beta-\delta$ fusion gene would produce a Haemoglobin Miyada or Nilotic. Bottom: the two chromosomes responsible for the globin chains showing the sequence of the genes.

However, it is most likely to represent a straight-forward polymorphism of the $^{G}\gamma$ chain.

It is now also agreed that there is duplication of the α-chain gene, but in this case the duplicated loci are identical in sequence. This doubling of the number of genes lessens the effect of a harmful mutation. For example an α-chain mutant will generally affect only one out of four genes (two pairs of alleles). However, having duplicated genes also increases the risk of unequal crossing over of genetic material, as is later illustrated (Figure 17.16) with the Haemoglobins Lepore. In the case of the duplicated α-chain, this could lead to some individuals having one or three genes. This would explain the apparently contradictory findings both on the proportions of α-chain variants and the genetics of α-thalassaemia (Lehmann and Lang, 1974).

17.3. BIOSYNTHESIS AND MUTATION

This account concentrates on the way in which the study of abnormal haemoglobins has provided insights into the complex process of protein biosynthesis. A fuller account of haemoglobin synthesis is given by Clegg (1974).

The synthesis of haemoglobin occurs in the red cell precursors of the bone marrow, the ability to synthesize messenger-RNA ceasing with loss of the cell nucleus. However, some synthetic ability is retained by the immature red cell, the reticulocyte. Though this lacks a nucleus, it still has some residual messenger-RNA, which explains both its partial synthetic ability and its characteristic basophilic staining.

Protein synthesis involves a number of sequential steps. These include the steps from chromatin to a committed DNA; *transcription* of the DNA of the gene into messenger-RNA; the *initiation* of peptide synthesis by the ribosomes; the *translation* of the RNA message into the polypeptide sequence; and the *termination* of the polypeptide chain and its release from the polyribosomes. Errors can occur anywhere along this pathway. In this respect, the haemoglobinopathies illustrate the familiar laboratory maxim, that whatever can go wrong will go wrong.

17.3.1. The fusion haemoglobins

The ultimate template from which haemoglobin is formed is contained in the chromosomal DNA of the nucleus. Each of the haemoglobin chains is coded by a separate locus (gene) most of which are closely linked on the one chromosome. However, the α-chain genes segregate independently from those of the other globin chains and hence are on a separate chromosome.

The best evidence for the close linkage of the γ-, δ- and β-chain loci comes from the fusion haemoglobins. These are abnormal haemoglobins formed by non-equal homologous cross-overs. They can most readily be described by reference to the best known examples, the Haemoglobins Lepore. These result from a fusion of the δ- and β-chains as illustrated in Figure 17.16. The δ- and β-chains are very similar in sequence, differing only in 10 residues distributed along their length. In the crossing over of genetic material that occurs during germ cell division, it is possible for misalignment of similar sequences of DNA to occur. In the case of the Haemoglobin Lepore, the N-terminal part of the fusion product is derived from the δ-chain gene and the C-terminal portion from the β-chain gene. The point of fusion differs with the different variants, the commonest, Lepore Boston, having the linkage between residues 88 and 115. As shown in Figure 17.16, the corollary of a Lepore haemoglobin is the other product of the cross-over, the anti-Lepore haemoglobins with a $\beta\delta$ structure. In these instances, there is normal synthesis of the β- and δ-chains as well as production of the anti-Lepore haemoglobin. One other fusion haemoglobin has been of value in deciding the sequence of haemoglobin genes. This is Haemoglobin Kenya which is a Lepore-type haemoglobin, but formed by a fusion of the $^{A}\gamma$- and β-chains. Overall, the fusion haemoglobins provide evidence that the non-α-chain genes lie on the one chromosome in the sequence $^{G}\gamma^{A}\gamma\delta\beta$ (Figure 17.16).

17.3.2. Thalassaemia: imbalanced chain synthesis

Equal formation of α- and non-α-chains is an essential requirement for normal red cell function. Isolated haemoglobin chains are unstable, and an excess of one chain will result in its intracellular precipitation, inclusion bodies and resultant haemolysis. This is the process that underlies the thalassaemias, a heterogeneous group of diseases in which there is imbalanced chain synthesis. The severity of the disease depends on the degree of imbalance. In its most severe form, with gross excess of one chain, a large proportion of the red cell precursors are disrupted before they leave the bone marrow, giving a presentation similar to the diseases of red cell production, the dyserythropoieses. On the other hand, if there is only mild imbalance, there may merely be a slight shortening of red cell survival.

The heterozygous Haemoglobins Lepore are an example of mild imbalance. There is a reduced synthesis of $\delta\beta$-chain, its proportion (near 10%) being a compromise between the proportion of the normal allelic β-chain (50%) and δ-chain (1.5%). Thus the Haemoglobin Lepore heterozygote has a very mild β-thalassaemia, due to inadequate β-chain synthesis.

There are two main types of β-thalassaemia: β^0 thalassaemia, due to a failure in transcription or translation, has no β-chain production; β^+ thalassaemia arises from decreased production of messenger-RNA and gives small but inadequate synthesis of β-chain. The findings to date emphasize the heterogeneous nature of even these separate classes of β-thalassaemia, some β^0 thalassaemias being due to gene deletion and others to production of an abnormal messenger (Orkin and Nathan, 1976). Since there are a pair of allelic genes coding for the β-chain, β-thalassaemia can occur as either a mild heterozygous form, β-thalassaemia minor; or as the severe homozygous form, β-thalassaemia major.

The inheritance of α-thalassaemia is complex. As described in section 17.2.7, there is now general agreement that most humans have two pairs of genes coding for the α-chain. Thus four levels of suppression are proposed (Table 17.1). Suppression of one gene would give the undetectable carrier state; suppression of two genes would give a clinically mild α-thalassaemia minor; suppression of three genes would give Haemoglobin H disease with moderately severe haemolytic anaemia; and suppression of four genes would give the fatal hydrops foetalis state. The four states can be additionally described (Table 17.1) by the amount of Haemoglobin Bart's at birth. Positive confirmation of these proposals has come from measurements of the number of α-chain genes in thalassaemic states, using annealing techniques with labelled complementary-DNA (Ottolenghi et al., 1974; Taylor

TABLE 17.1.

α-THALASSAEMIA: NOMENCLATURE AND INHERITANCE

One gene deleted	1-α-thalassaemia; no red cell abnormalities	1–2% Hb Bart's at birth	Previously α-thalassaemia trait type 2 "α-thal$_2$"
Two genes deleted	2-α-thalassaemia; mild red cell abnormalities	5% Hb Bart's at birth	Previously α-thalassaemia trait type 1 "α-thal$_1$"
Three genes deleted	3-α-thalassaemia; major red cell abnormalities and splenomegaly	15% Hb Bart's at birth	Hb H disease heterozygote state for 1- and for 2-α-thalassaemia
Four genes deleted	4-α-thalassaemia; Hb Bart's hydrops foetalis, lethal	90% Hb Bart's at birth (the rest Hb Portland, $\zeta_2\gamma_2$)	Homozygote for 2-α-thalassaemia

et al., 1974; Kan et al., 1975). To do this, the messenger-RNA for the chain is first isolated and the labelled DNA complement is produced with use of a viral enzyme, reverse transcriptase. The DNA complement can be annealed by heat to the native DNA, the number of loci being indicated by the radioactivity of the product. These studies showed that no α-chain genes were present in hydrops foetalis, and they provided strong evidence of the presence of four genes in the normal individual, but only one gene in a patient with Haemoglobin H disease. This also provides clear evidence that the underlying defect is a deletion, rather than suppression, of the α-chain genes in at least some types of α-thalassaemia. It is emphasized that there are likely to be multiple causes of both α- and β-thalassaemia. One other quite different cause of α-thalassaemia has been identified in the structural variants arising from chain-termination mutations as discussed in the next section.

17.3.3. Mutation and haemoglobin variants

The sequence of aminoacids in a polypeptide is determined by the genetic code, which is an arrangement in triplets of the four bases cytosine (C), guanine (G), adenine (A) and thymine (T) (uracil in DNA). The code was determined from work with bacteria but its universal nature and application to higher organisms has been confirmed by studies of the abnormal haemoglobins. The coding for each aminoacid in the messenger-RNA is given in Table 17.2. This shows, for example, that glutamic acid is coded by the triplets GAG and GAA and valine is coded by GUU, GUC, GUA and GUG.

The great majority of abnormal haemoglobins arise from point mutations with the substitution of one base by another. An example is Haemoglobin S where there is a replacement of glutamic acid by valine. This must be due to a point mutation in the DNA resulting in a replacement in the RNA of adenine by uracil, i.e.

G*A*A GU*A*

G*A*G G*U*G

(glutamic acid) (valine)

TABLE 17.2.

THE MESSENGER-RNA TRIPLET CODE FOR AMINOACIDS

		Second base									
		U		C		A		G			
First base	U	UUU	Phe	UCU	Ser	UAU	Tyr	UGU	Cys	U	Third base
		UUC	Phe	UCC	Ser	UAC	Tyr	UGC	Cys	C	
		UUA	Leu	UCA	Ser	UAA	Stop	UGA	Stop	A	
		UUG	Leu	UCG	Ser	UAG	Stop	UGG	Trp	G	
	C	CUU	Leu	CUU	Pro	CAU	His	CGU	Arg	U	
		CUC	Leu	CCC	Pro	CAC	His	CGC	Arg	C	
		CUA	Leu	CCA	Pro	CAA	Gln	CGA	Arg	A	
		CUG	Leu	CCG	Pro	CAG	Gln	CGG	Arg	G	
	A	AUU	Ile	ACU	Thr	AAU	Asn	AGU	Ser	U	
		AUC	Ile	ACC	Thr	AAC	Asn	AGC	Ser	C	
		AUA	Ile	ACA	Thr	AAA	Lys	AGA	Arg	A	
		AUG	Met	ACG	Thr	AAG	Lys	AGG	Arg	G	
	G	GUU	Val	GCU	Ala	GAU	Asp	GGU	Gly	U	
		GUC	Val	GCC	Ala	GAC	Asp	GGC	Gly	C	
		GUA	Val	GCA	Ala	GAA	Glu	GGA	Gly	A	
		GUG	Val	GCG	Ala	GAG	Glu	GGG	Gly	G	

Most of the 200 haemoglobin variants now known (Lehmann and Kynoch, 1976) are of this type, with their abnormality being due to the replacement of one aminoacid by another. The majority of these are apparently functionally normal, though they may be

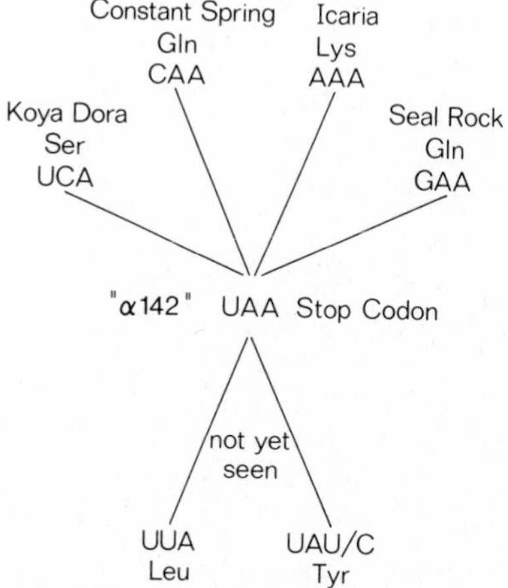

Figure 17.17. Mutation of Stop codon: six point mutations of the α142 Stop codon are theoretically possible. Four of these have already been observed, as indicated above, to give the elongated Haemoglobins: Koya Dora, Constant Spring, Icaria and Seal Rock. Two point mutations as in the lower part of the diagram, have yet to be observed.

slightly disadvantageous as their altered charge could affect the carefully adjusted water and ion distribution within the red cell.

Interesting examples of point mutations have been provided by variants, present as minor components. These have provided evidence for the chain termination mechanism and have also shown that thalassaemia can arise from mutations at the structural level. These variants arise from a translation of the non-structural part of the messenger-RNA. They can be due to a mutation of the stop codon (Figure 17.17) which allows a continued reading of the messenger-RNA beyond the part which is normally translated. Alternatively, an intra-codon crossing over, due to misalignment of the DNA, can alter the stop codon with the same result (Scheme 17.2). Haemoglobins Constant Spring and Icaria have elongated α-chains with 172 rather than the normal 141 residues; presumably each has a mutation of the terminating codon in position 142 as shown in Figure 17.17.

Haemoglobin abnormalities may also occur due to deletions of portions of the amino-acid sequence. These usually result from unequal cross-overs, as has been seen in a gross form with the mixed $\delta\beta$ and $\gamma\beta$ haemoglobins, Lepore and Kenya. But more examples exist on a smaller scale that result in deletions of sequence within a chain. Usually this occurs in an area which is preceded and succeeded by the same minor sequence allowing mismatching to occur on crossing over. An example is Haemoglobin Gun Hill where there is a deletion of the sequence between two leucine–histidine sequences in the β-chain –

Leu–His–Cys–Asp–Lys *Leu–His*
91 92 93 94 95 96 97

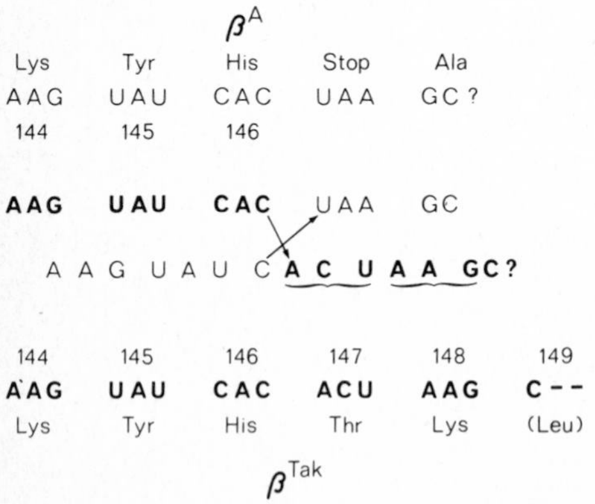

β^A

Lys	Tyr	His	Stop	Ala
AAG	UAU	CAC	UAA	GC ?
144	145	146		

AAG UAU CAC UAA GC

A A G U A U C **A C U A A GC?**

144	145	146	147	148	149
AAG	**UAU**	**CAC**	**ACU**	**AAG**	**C - -**
Lys	Tyr	His	Thr	Lys	(Leu)

β^{Tak}

A possible mechanism for the Tak sequence formed by unequal crossing over

Scheme 17.2. Chain elongation due to unequal cross-over. The elongated β-chain variant, Haemoglobin Tak, is explicable by a misalignment of DNA at the time of cross-over. This gives a frame shift alteration of each codon subsequent to the point of crossing over, the first codon to be affected being the Stop codon UAA which becomes ACU, the codon for threonine.

17.4. DIAGNOSTIC TECHNIQUES

17.4.1. Initial investigations

The suggestion of a haemoglobinopathy usually originates from a haematological problem, and it is important that there should be co-operation between the haematologist and biochemist in its further investigation. As in most diagnostic work, it is useful to have a preliminary screen established that can be routinely followed by laboratory staff. It is tempting to haemolyse all the sample and to proceed directly to the identification of an abnormal component, but the significance of the findings often depends on other measurements such as the level of Haemoglobin A_2, or the presence of red cell inclusion bodies. These measurements may not be subsequently available due to deterioration of the specimen and lack of further material.

The scope of the initial screen may have to be modified by the amount of blood available, but with an adequate specimen (5 ml or more) the following should be included – initial haematological investigations including a film for red cell morphology, red cell indices, prolonged incubation for inclusion bodies, and plasma iron. A 10% (10 g/dl) haemolysate should be prepared, with subsequent measurement of Haemoglobin A_2 and F, performance of haemoglobin stability tests, and electrophoresis at alkaline pH. This provides a good general screen for haemoglobinopathies, though other tests may be added such as sickling tests, spectrophotometric scanning of the haemolysate, screening for glucose-6-phosphate dehydrogenase deficiency and the use of more than one electrophoretic system. The procedures involved in the initial screen are discussed in general terms in the next few sections, but for more detailed accounts, reference should be made to Efremov and Huisman (1974), Lehmann and Huntsman (1974) and Schmidt et al. (1974).

17.4.1.1. Specimen collection and transportation

A preferred specimen for haemoglobin studies would be 10 to 15 ml of anticoagulated whole blood, but 2 to 3 ml suffices for standard investigations. Haemoglobin deteriorates in haemolysates, and it is far preferable to transport the sample as whole blood, utilizing the red cell enzyme systems to keep it in a condition suitable for oxygen dissociation studies as well as for standard diagnostic procedures. Any anticoagulant is suitable, though a heparinized specimen should also be accompanied by a small specimen containing EDTA, as heparinized blood is not satisfactory for assessment of red cell morphology. The addition of a few mg of a 99:1 mixture of glucose and chloramphenicol should suffice to keep a sample in good condition at room temperature for as long as a week or more. Thus airmail transport is quite adequate for most purposes.

17.4.1.2. Haematological investigations

The use of automated equipment enables accurate determination of the red cell indices. These assist in the differentiation of two common conditions, β-thalassaemia minor and iron deficiency anaemia. Both are microcytic anaemias, but in β-thalassaemia minor the red cell count is higher, and the mean cell haemoglobin concentration is usually lower in iron deficiency anaemia. This could arise from a disproportion of haem to globin in these conditions. One would expect free globin in iron deficiency anaemia, but only haemoglobin in thalassaemia. Hence for their small size and volume, the cell haemoglobin content would be lower in iron deficiency anaemia.

The finding of red cell inclusion bodies is an important help in the diagnosis of thalassaemia and the unstable haemoglobins. The inclusions are formed by precipitated haemoglobin and stain with methyl violet. However, they are removed by the spleen, so that in the non-splenectomized patient they are best demonstrated by prolonged incubation of the red cells with a redox dye; brilliant cresyl blue is usually used (Papayannopoulou and Stamatoyannopoulos, 1974). The inclusions can vary in form from the multiple punctate, gold-ball-like inclusions of Haemoglobin H disease, to the large amorphous inclusions of the very unstable haemoglobins.

17.4.1.3. Specific tests for sickle cell haemoglobin

The microscopic sickling test provides a simple means of demonstrating the presence of Haemoglobin S by the cellular distortion that appears in deoxygenated blood. Although the procedure is straightforward, the interpretation of results may be difficult for the biochemical laboratory. For this reason, the solubility screening test for Haemoglobin S provides a more robust test. The principle is the comparitive insolubility of reduced Haemoglobin S in concentrated phosphate buffer. The reagents are available commercially but can also be easily prepared. The test is influenced by major changes in the plasma proteins and increased γ-globulins can give false positive results. Reduced red cell to plasma ratios, as in severe anaemia, may give false negative results. For this reason, Efremov and Huisman (1974) recommend the use of haemolysates or washed red cells. Details of both the microscopic sickling test and the solubility screening test are given by Lehmann and Huntsman (1974).

An efficient screening test for Haemoglobin S is provided by electrophoresis, and this should always be carried out to confirm a positive, or unexpected negative, result from a sickling or solubility test.

17.4.1.4. Preparation of a haemolysate

The starting point of most haemoglobin studies is the preparation of a haemolysate. The plasma proteins are removed from the red cells by thorough washing with isotonic saline and the cells are then lysed with water. The cell debris is removed by vigorous shaking with a small volume of carbon tetrachloride and centrifuging. It is useful to adjust the concentration of the supernatant haemolysate to 10% (10 g/dl) as this simplifies subsequent quantitation of the various haemoglobin fractions and allows valid visual comparisons to be made on electrophoretic strips.

Haemolysates can be stored indefinitely in liquid nitrogen, but at –20 °C gradual deterioration takes place. This can be minimized by converting the oxyhaemoglobin to the carbon monoxide form, and/or by the addition of cyanide. EDTA should also be added to remove copper which is the major accelerant of methaemoglobin formation. Addition of cyanide and conversion to the carbon monoxide form should wait until stability tests have been completed, as both can mask haemoglobin instability.

17.4.1.5. Measurement of Haemoglobin A_2

The concentration of Haemoglobin A_2 serves a useful diagnostic purpose as an indicator of imbalanced chain synthesis. The value is raised in β-thalassaemia and with β-chain abnormal unstable haemoglobins. Lower values are associated with some forms of α-thalassaemia and with Haemoglobin Lepore. An extra A_2 band on electrophoresis is a useful index of an α-chain abnormality.

Measurement of Haemoglobin A_2 can be carried out using cellulose acetate electrophoresis at pH 8.9 (Marengo-Rowe, 1965). The strip is heavily loaded, with the test and a control sample both being assayed at the same time. The A_2 and A bands separate after about 90 minutes and can be eluted from the strips. the percentage of Haemoglobin A_2 may be calculated from the relative absorbances of the eluates at 413 nm. Efremov and Huisman (1974) described a simple microchromatographic technique which is particularly suitable for laboratories carrying out many Haemoglobin A_2 estimations. Whichever method is used, careful attention to detail is required to get reliable results. The reference range, spanning 2.6 to 3.5%, leaves little room for experimental error. There are, as yet, few efficient quality control techniques and each laboratory should carefully determine its own reference range and run frequent normal controls to check its technique. Reliable standards are now being prepared, mainly by using EDTA to remove copper.

17.4.1.6. Measurement of Haemoglobin F

A raised concentration of foetal haemoglobin may be a secondary accompaniment of a lifelong anaemia such as sickle cell disease. It may also occur in the adult as an inherited defect of the mechanisms that control the switch from foetal to adult haemoglobin. In this condition – hereditary persistence of foetal haemoglobin – there is usually, though not always, an even distribution of foetal haemoglobin through all cells which distinguishes it from secondary causes of raised foetal haemoglobin.

Measurement of the total foetal haemoglobin is based on its increased resistance to alkaline denaturation (section 17.2.6). An alkaline ammonium sulphate solution is added to a haemolysate of known concentration and after a fixed period, to allow the precipitation of adult haemoglobin, a filtrate is prepared whose concentration gives a measure of Haemoglobin F. The various modified techniques for this procedure are discussed in the references given in section 17.4.1 but as with Haemoglobin A_2 the main requirement is for a careful and practised technique. After infancy, foetal haemoglobin forms no more than 0.8% of the total haemoglobin, a value above 2% indicating haematological disease.

The determination of the distribution of foetal haemoglobin through all cells can be carried out by the technique of Kleihauer (1974). An acid buffer adjusted to the pK of Haemoglobin F is used to wash out the non-foetal haemoglobins from an alcohol-fixed blood film, followed by staining for haemoglobin.

An immunofluorescent anti-Haemoglobin F serum detects very small traces of that haemoglobin and reveals a considerable difference between the percentage of Haemoglobin F measured chemically, and the percentage of Haemoglobin F-containing-cells, say in a case of sickle cell anaemia.

There is often a need to determine whether an unidentified component on electrophoresis or chromatography is a foetal or adult haemoglobin. Use can be made of the increased absorption, at 290 nm, of the foetal haemoglobin due to the presence of an extra tryptophan in the γ-chain. The sensitivity of detection is increased by differential scanning (Owen, 1975).

17.4.1.7. Detection of unstable haemoglobins

The simplest means of detecting haemoglobin variants is by screening for changed electrophoretic mobility. However, it is now realized that a better index of abnormality for the pathological haemoglobin variants is their changed molecular stability. Some 50 haemoglobins with markedly reduced stability are now known, many of them resulting in an inclusion body haemolytic anaemia in the heterozygote (section 17.6.3). As a group, they form an appreciable proportion of the known haemoglobin variants and the major portion of the known pathological haemoglobins. All have changed molecular stability but only some show appreciable electrophoretic abnormalities. For this reason, any screen for haemoglobinopathies in a medical laboratory should include stability testing as well as the more standard electrophoretic techniques.

The haemoglobin molecule can be stressed by increasing the temperature in the heat test or by changing the polarity of the solvent in the isopropanol test. Conditions are chosen under which Haemoglobin A is just stable whereas haemoglobins of decreased stability undergo denaturation to give a flocculent precipitate. The isopropanol test of Carrell and Kay (1972) provides a simple screening test with addition of 0.2 ml of a 10% (10 g/dl) haemolysate to 2 ml of a 17% isopropanol buffer in pH 7.4 Tris buffer at 37 °C. A normal adult haemolysate gives precipitation after 30 minutes, the presence of an unstable haemoglobin being indicated by flocculent precipitation before 20 minutes and usually by 5 minutes. The test is sensitive, but false positives may occur due to raised concentration of methaemoglobin or foetal haemoglobin, both of these having a decreased stability as compared to Oxyhaemoglobin A. It is important for specimens to be fresh and to contain no methaemoglobin.

The heat instability of these haemoglobins (Grimes and Meisler, 1962) provides a useful diagnostic test at 50 °C (Dacie and Lewis, 1975) and should be used to check positive results obtained from the isopropanol test. A dilute haemolysate in pH 7.4 Tris (rather than phosphate!) buffer is incubated for 2 hours at 50 °C. A major unstable haemoglobin will give an obvious precipitate, usually before the end of the first hour's incubation. This test is less sensitive than the isopropanol test and has the advantage of giving fewer false positive results. However, it is also more likely to miss abnormalities which cause minor degrees of instability. Some workers recommend raising the temperature of the test to 55 or 60 °C. This increases its sensitivity but again increases the possibility of false positives, which are a time consuming problem in the laboratory. Overall, the procedure recommended is to use the isopropanol technique as the screening test with careful checking of positives by the standard heat test.

Huehns (1975) has also described the use of the sulphydryl reagent *p*-chloromercuribenzoate as a precipitant. Examples of its use, both preparatively and as a diagnostic test, are given by Efremov and Huisman (1974).

17.4.1.8. Glucose-6-phosphate dehydrogenase and the glutathione enzymes

A general consideration of red cell enzymes is beyond the scope of this chapter, but it is important to take into account the reductive mechanisms of the red cell in the investigation for haemoglobinopathies. Deficiencies in the mechanisms which are responsible for the maintenance of reduced glutathione can result in an anaemia with similar haematological findings to those seen in thalassaemia and in the unstable haemoglobin diseases.

The enzymes involved include those of the pentose phosphate shunt, particularly glucose-6-phosphate dehydrogenase, as well as the reductase, peroxidase and synthetase of glutathione. The ascorbate cyanide test of Jacob and Jandl (1966) provides a broad screening procedure that covers all these enzymes and at least some unstable haemoglobins. The test depends on the catalyzed production of peroxide and superoxide, by ascorbate, from oxyhaemoglobin. Cyanide inhibits the protective role of catalase, and the consequent accumulation of peroxide stresses the glutathione system. If this fails to cope, then there is oxidation of haemoglobin to methaemoglobin and the formation of further denaturation products to give brown discolouration.

A specific screening test for glucose-6-phosphate dehydrogenase deficiency such as the fluorescent spot test of Beutler and Mitchell (1968) may be more useful as a routine procedure due to its simplicity and the relative predominance of this deficiency over the other abnormalities.

17.5. DETECTION AND IDENTIFICATION OF VARIANTS

Genetic disease always has as its underlying basis a variation in the production and/or structure of a protein. This is obviously so in the case of the haemoglobinopathies, and well established techniques have been developed for identification of variations in haemoglobin structure. However, the same is true of the inborn errors of metabolism and there is now greater incentive for biochemists to pursue the investigation of these diseases to the level of the structural abnormality of the aberrant enzyme. The principles described in this section for the haemoglobinopathies are equally applicable to protein variants in general.

The detection of variants is required at two levels. The first is the relatively straightforward task of screening populations to detect obvious electrophoretic variants, as in anthropological surveys or in population testing for sickle cell disease. The second task, which is much more difficult, is investigation of individuals in whom an abnormality is suspected which may not necessarily be obvious on electrophoresis. This requires careful performance of functional tests such as stability measurements and determination of oxygen dissociation curves. Alternatively, a variant may have a change in charge that is suppressed at the usual alkaline pH. This occurs with several of the haemoglobins which are best detected by electrophoresis at acid pH.

Thus there are two levels of investigation in the laboratory. Simple electrophoresis at pH 8 to 9 on paper, cellulose acetate, or starch gel, suffices as a screening process for general purposes. However, a defined investigative protocol is required for individual cases where a new or obscure haemoglobinopathy is suspected. In the present authors' laboratories, this consists of most of the initial investigations outlined in section 17.4.1, with standardized performance of stability tests, starch gel electrophoresis in two or three buffers, fractionation on DEAE–Sephadex and often the measurement of oxygen dissociation curves. The details of the protocol will depend on the facilities available: many laboratories will be content to limit their investigations to the identification of the common haemoglobinopathies. A basic approach using well established techniques is detailed in a broadsheet prepared for the Association of Clinical Pathologists by Lehmann and Huntsman (1975).

17.5.1. Electrophoresis – principles and available media

The choice of paper, cellulose acetate and starch gel as electrophoretic media may seem unadventurous at a time when much more discriminating media are available, such as gradient pore acrylamide gels and isoelectric focussing gels. However, there are problems in using too selective a medium, as difficulties occur in differentiating true genetic variation of the protein from storage-induced changes such as polymerization or deamidation.

Almost all electrophoresis is now carried out with zone rather than open boundary separation. A sample is applied to the origin on a supporting medium whose ends are immersed in a buffer with a potential difference being applied between the two ends. The migration of haemoglobin on electrophoresis is dependent on its net charge, its molecular size (mass), its interaction with the supporting medium, and the buffer flow from one electrode to the other. The conditions of electrophoresis can be varied to affect each of these factors and hence obtain maximal separation.

The net charge of a protein depends on the pH of the medium; the net charge of normal adult haemoglobin is zero at its isoelectric point near pH 7. Most haemoglobin electrophoresis is carried out at alkaline pH, and consequently the haemoglobin is negatively charged and moves to the anode. This approach is so standard that variants are often classified as "fast" or "slow"; a fast variant has increased negative charge and hence moves more rapidly than Haemoglobin A to the anode on alkaline electrophoresis, and a slow variant has an increased positive charge. The isoelectric point of haemoglobin changes when there is a replacement involving aminoacid residues with charged side chains, such as positively charged lysine, arginine and histidine, and negatively charged aspartic and glutamic acids. However, this is not invariably true. A change in isoelectric point may also occur in association with a neutral (uncharged) substitution, or another change that affects the overall conformation of the molecule and/or the loss of haem with its negatively charged propionic acid such as occurs with Haemoglobin Köln (β98 valine → methionine). Alternatively, there may be a substitution involving a change in charge in the interior of the molecule that does not appreciably affect the net molecular charge. In Haemoglobin Volga, replacement of an alanine by an aspartic acid at position 27 of the β-chain is masked by its being internally situated. Standard electrophoresis at alkaline pH will not separate this variant from Haemoglobin A, but it becomes immediately apparent on electrophoresis in buffers containing high concentrations of urea. This causes the molecule to unfold and its net charge then becomes a true summation of all the charged side chains (Figures 17.18 and 17.19).

The net charge will also vary with the pH of the buffer since various aminoacid side chains will have their ionization suppressed as the pH varies. Histidine is the most important of these, as the imidazole ring has a pK of near 6.5. Thus at pH 7.5 and above there will be almost total suppression of the protonation of the histidine side chain. Therefore electrophoresis at pH 7, or below, is desirable in order to detect substitutions involving a histidine. The technique of isoelectric focussing has the advantage of separating out each protein according to its isoelectric point, and thus avoids the need to use separate

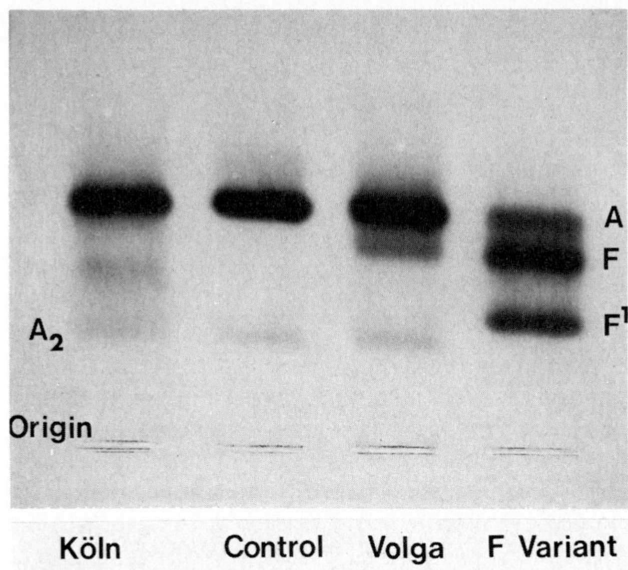

Figure 17.18. Starch gel electrophoresis at pH 8.6 of the unstable haemoglobins Köln and Volga. Hb A (control) and a cord blood haemolysate (with a variant Hb F) are included as markers. Hb Köln shows a slow band between Hb A and Hb A_2; Hb Volga is electrophoretically normal except for a raised Hb F.

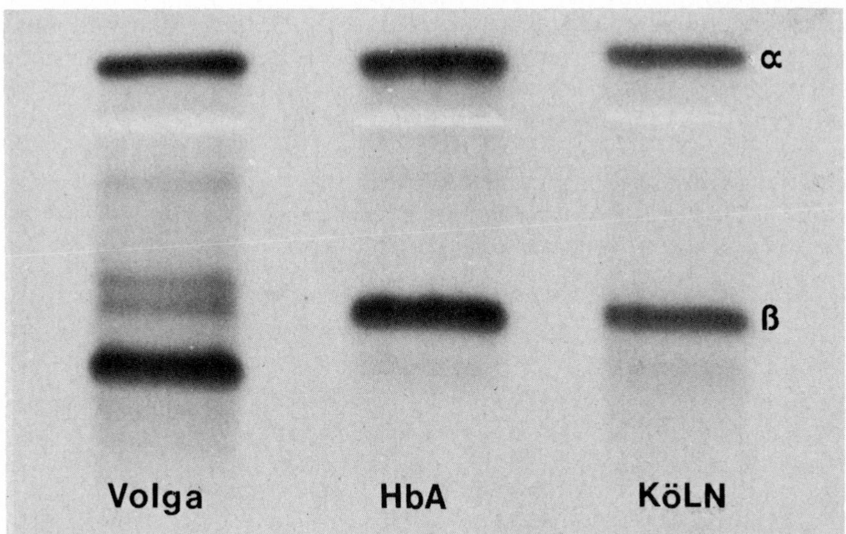

Figure 17.19. Electrophoresis in 6 M urea with chain separation of two unstable haemoglobins (cf. Figure 17.18). A charge change is revealed in the β-chain of Hb Volga but not Hb Köln. The Hb Volga has been purified by precipitation and traces of co-precipitated normal β- and γ-chain are also present.

procedures at various pH. This also separates out minor, often artefactual, components of haemoglobin (section 17.6.6). These are not of genetic consequence and hence interpretation can be difficult.

The electrophoretic mobility is dependent on molecular size and varies according to the supporting medium. Wide pore media, such as paper and cellulose acetate, provide little hindrance to the movement of proteins, but the tighter pore structures in starch or acrylamide gels do give separations which are influenced by molecular size. In particular, polyacrylamide gels can be cross-linked to give a wide range of pore sizes and have a pronounced molecular sieving effect. This is only of limited value in haemoglobin electrophoresis as it is exceptional for variants to have a significant change in molecular size. With haemoglobins, use of selective pore gels may be something of a disadvantage as changes in molecular size usually arise due to polymerization on ageing of the sample. However, molecular size determination is useful in some haemoglobin studies and is of particular use as a general clinical laboratory technique in the investigation of aberrant plasma proteins. For this reason a more detailed account of the determination of molecular size is given in section 17.5.4. This uses polyacrylamide gel electrophoresis in the presence of a detergent, sodium dodecyl sulphate, that denatures the protein and dissociates its subunits.

The other factors that affect electrophoresis are interaction with the supporting medium and buffer flow. Various media interact with protein side chains to a different extent. Cellulose acetate and polyacrylamide gels are relatively inert and there is little interaction with proteins. Paper shows some interaction, as does starch gel, but a more important interaction is that between agar gel and haemoglobin. Agar gel electrophoresis at pH 6 separates foetal from adult haemoglobin, as well as Haemoglobins C and E, and Haemoglobins D and S, respectively. These haemoglobins are difficult to separate by any other simple electrophoretic procedure.

Although the cause of electrophoretic separation is the electric field, an important contributor is the flow of buffer. Charged groups, such as the carboxylate anion of the paper or starch, induce a positive charge in the surrounding buffer and consequently there is a steady flow of water to the cathode. This electro-osmotic flow carries the protein with it and explains the dependence of separation efficiency on factors such as the positioning of sample application and the height of the buffer compartments. As a consequence there is a need for a trial and error approach to obtain the best conditions for electrophoretic separations in individual laboratories.

17.5.2. Column chromatography

Although electrophoresis on paper or starch block can be used as a preparative procedure, the method of choice for isolation of an abnormal component is column chromatography. As with electrophoresis there is a wide choice of media and either cation exchange resins (e.g. carboxymethylcellulose) or anion exchange resins (e.g. DEAE–cellulose) may be used. The choice of resin and conditions of elution can be varied to meet different requirements, as outlined by Huisman (1974).

DEAE–Sephadex A-50 provides a simple and reproducible means of separating most abnormal haemoglobins and its use illustrates the principles of column chromatography.

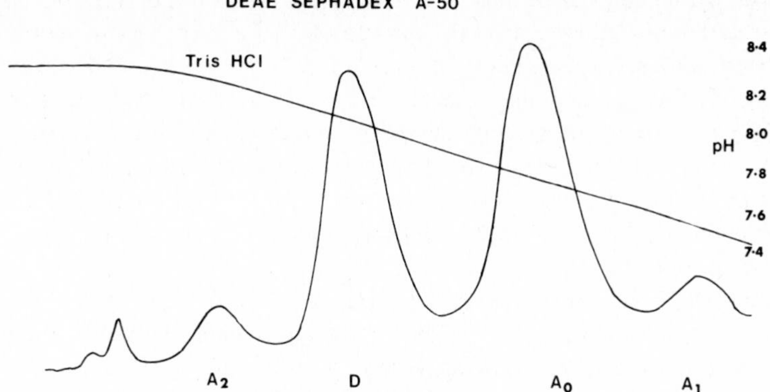

Figure 17.20. The separation of Haemoglobins A and D on DEAE–Sephadex. A Tris–HCl pH gradient has been used and absorbance monitored at 280 nm. For quantitation it is important that allowance is made for the artefact A_1, a modified product of A_0, and also D_1, a similar product of D, which is present in the same proportions but obscured by the much larger A_0 peak.

The DEAE matrix is positively charged and therefore binds negatively charged molecules, such as haemoglobin, in alkaline buffer. The column is equilibrated and the haemoglobin applied in a buffer more alkaline than its isoelectric point. As the buffer pH is slowly decreased, the more positively charged haemoglobins such as A_2, C and E are eluted. These are followed by less positively charged variants such as S and D, then Haemoglobin A, and finally the negatively charged haemoglobins such as J and H. The separation is therefore in accord with that of alkaline electrophoresis but with the important exception that foetal haemoglobin is eluted between haemoglobins A and J. whereas in electrophoresis it moves between haemoglobins A and S. Instead of changing the pH the salt concentration can be raised, the Cl^- replacing the Hb^- on the column and the Na^+ forming the soluble Hb^-Na^+. Column effluent can be monitored spectrophotometically (Figure 17.20) and the fractions collected. It is a useful practice to routinely pool each peak and calculate the relative proportions from their Soret band absorbance (420 nm). Some of the most significant information to be obtained from studying the abnormal haemoglobins comes from their relative proportions. Unfortunately in the past these have seldom been recorded.

17.5.3. Chain separation

Chain separation, either diagnostically or preparatively, greatly simplifies the identification of an abnormal haemoglobin. As in most proteins, the bonds between the haemoglobin subunits are non-covalent and are readily disrupted by denaturing agents or detergents such as urea and sodium dodecyl sulphate respectively. These also cause an unfolding of the polypeptide chains allowing access to cysteine residues with risk of oxidation and hence polymerization. For this reason, procedures for chain separation are usually accompanied throughout by use of a reducing agent such as mercaptoethanol or dithiothreitol.

Diagnostically, chain separation can be carried out using starch gel electrophoresis of globin in an alkaline buffer containing urea and mercaptoethanol (Chernoff and Pettit, 1964). A more recent modification uses electrophoresis on cellulose acetate of haemolysates in a solution of urea containing a high concentration of mercaptoethanol (Schneider, 1974). In both systems the α- and β-chains are well separated, the presence of an abnormal chain with altered charge being clearly apparent, along with an index of the magnitude of the change. These procedures have the added advantage of measuring the strict algebraic summation of charges in each polypeptide and of being unaffected by conformational changes (Figure 17.19).

Preparatively, this principle has been applied by Clegg et al. (1965) to separate the chains on CM-cellulose columns. The column buffers contain urea and dithiothreitol and the chains are eluted with an ionic gradient. Because the pH used, 6.4 to 7.0, is near the pK of imidazole groups, the system has the added advantage that it can separate chains differing in only a histidine residue. Since the chains are obtained from the column in unfolded form they can be conveniently modified by aminoethylation of the cysteine residues (section 17.5.5.3). The whole procedure now forms a standard part of the process of characterizing haemoglobin variants and determining α/β globin ratios.

17.5.4. Molecular size determination

The determination of molecular size (mass) is a valuable help in the investigation of aberrant proteins, though only occasionally is it required for the haemoglobinopathies. The techniques involved have been greatly simplified by the use of polyacrylamide gel electrophoresis. Sodium dodecyl sulphate unfolds proteins and binds to them in an amount that is dependent on their molecular size. The negative charge of the bound detergent overwhelms the inherent charge of the protein. Consequently, the electrophoretic mobility of the complex reflects the size of the protein, the relative mobility being proportional to the logarithm of the molecular mass of the protein. Weber et al. (1972) applied this principle by measuring the mobilities of several proteins of known size relative to bromophenol blue: the molecular mass of the unknown was determined from a plotted calibration curve.

Relative mobilities are independent of buffer pH provided that it is above 6.5. Mobility will depend on the pore size of the acrylamide gel. For large proteins 5% gels should be used; for smaller ones, 10% or 15% gels.

17.5.5. Peptide mapping

The identification of an aminoacid abnormality in a polypeptide is greatly simplified if an enzymic digestion is carried out to give numbers of small peptides. The peptides can then be separated by electrophoresis in one direction followed by chromatography at right angles to give a peptide map that represents a unique "fingerprint" for each polypeptide.

An alteration in the position of a peptide from that of a normal control indicates the presence of an aminoacid substitution. This procedure is firmly established for the investigation of haemoglobin abnormalities, as described in the following sections, but it is applicable to all protein variants, including those whose primary aminoacid sequence is undetermined.

17.5.5.1. Preparation of enzyme digest

Trypsin is still the enzyme of choice because of its almost complete specificity for cleavage of peptide bonds C-terminal to lysine or arginine residues. The haemoglobin is first irreversibly denatured, usually by addition to acid/acetone, to give precipitation of the globin. The globin is redissolved in an ammonium bicarbonate buffer near pH 8, and trypsin added. Digestion is complete after 1 hour at 37 °C, the process being stopped by the addition of acetic acid to take the pH to between 4.5 and 6.5. A brief period of heating precipitates the insoluble "core", and aliquots of the supernatant are lyophilized to remove the volatile buffers. About 1.5 mg of globin is required for the usual peptide map.

17.5.5.2. Preparation of peptide maps

Paper is still the most suitable medium for separation of peptides, having the advantages of cheapness, reproducibility and, most importantly, being suitable for high yield preparative procedures. The digested material is redissolved in the electrophoretic buffer and applied to the origin with gentle drying. Electrophoresis is usually carried out at pH 6.5, which gives partial ionization of histidine side chains and maximum discrimination between peptides. In order to obtain good peptide separation, high voltages (above 1000 V) and relatively high currents are used. This incurs heat dissipation problems that are only satisfactorily solved by immersing the paper in an organic solvent with good heat conductivity, such as toluene. Electrophoresis is stopped after about an hour and the paper is dried and prepared for chromatography.

Chromatography is either ascending or descending, at right angles to the direction of electrophoresis. The separation depends on a partition of the peptides between the bound water of the paper and the relatively non-polar chromatography solvent. Hence, peptides that contain largely non-polar residues (such as phenylalanine, valine, leucine) will tend to move with the non-polar solvent, whereas there will be little movement of peptides containing largely polar residues (such as aspartic acid, serine, lysine) which preferentially dissolve in water. The combination of changes in charge (indicated from the first dimension) and changes in polarity (indicated from the second) provide deductive evidence of the likely aminoacid change in a peptide. The peptides can be visualized, as in Figure 17.21, by staining with fluorescamine or ninhydrin; extra information can be obtained by specific colour stains for histidine, tyrosine, arginine, methionine and tryptophan residues. Besides the use of observational deduction, estimates can also be made of the molecular size of peptides if markers are included in the electrophoretic separation. By all these means a good deal of evidence is provided than often allows the specific aminoacid abnormality to be deduced, particularly if it is assumed that there has been a point mutation compatible with the genetic code (Table 17.2).

17.5.5.3. The insoluble "core"

In most proteins there is a proportion of insoluble material left after incubation with trypsin. In haemoglobin this insoluble "core" consists of nearly one-third of the mole-

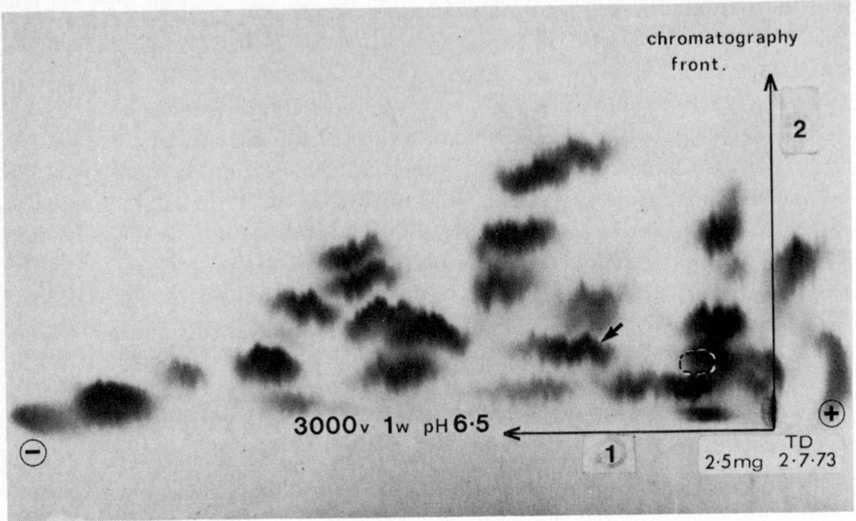

Figure 17.21. Peptide map of Haemoglobin D Punjab. Electrophoresis in the horizontal dimension (1) followed by chromatography in the vertical dimension (2). The new peptide βXIII (arrowed) has shifted towards the cathode and moved further in chromatography than does the same peptide in Haemoglobin A (dotted outline). This shift results from the substitution of an uncharged glutamine for the negatively charged glutamic acid of Haemoglobin A.

cule. It primarily consists of large peptides with mainly hydrophobic residues, and is complicated by random disulphide bonds between cysteine residues. The problem is largely overcome by blocking the sulphydryl groups by aminoethylation which converts cysteine residues to the lysine analogue, aminoethylcysteine. This provides an additional point for tryptic cleavage as well as preventing polymerization. Subsequent to aminoethylation, all the β-chain is represented on the tryptic peptide map, but a quarter of the α-chain still remains insoluble. It can be further digested with other enzymes. A different approach to analysis of the α-chain may be taken by the initial cleavage of methionine residues using cyanogen bromide.

17.5.6. Aminoacid analysis and sequence determination

Peptides that have been stained with fluorescamine can be eluted directly from a heavily loaded peptide map. Elution with hydrochloric acid into a capillary tube is often used. The tube is sealed, heated at 105 °C for 18 hours, and then diluted with buffer and directly applied to the column of an automatic aminoacid analyzer.

Confirmation of the aminoacid substitution and its position, can be obtained by Edman "degradation" which sequentially removes N-terminal aminoacids by reaction with phenylisothiocyanate. This can be carried out on a micro scale in conjuction with fluorescent labelling by the combined Edman–dansyl procedure (Hartley, 1970). This will readily allow sequences of five to eight aminoacids to be determined on peptides eluted from paper maps. Larger peptides may need a second enzyme treatment, e.g. with chymotrypsin or thermolysin, to break them into smaller peptides before being sequenced.

17.5.7. Assessment of oxygen affinity

The full characterization of an abnormal haemoglobin requires the measurement of the oxygen dissociation curve. The P_{50}, the partial pressure at half saturation, should be determined, the Hill coefficient calculated and the influence of 2,3-diphosphoglycerate assessed.

Various approaches to oxygen dissociation curve measurement are available as discussed by Rosa et al. (1975). These authors give a full account of the overall approach to the assessment of oxygen affinity. The simplest technique for the clinical laboratory is the discontinuous spectrophotometric method (Dacie and Lewis, 1975) adapted from Benesch et al. (1965). This uses a tonometer with a cuvette at one end and at the other a stop-cock that allows the measured inflow of atmospheric oxygen. The diluted sample is placed in the tonometer which is then evacuated to effect complete deoxygenation. Sequential measurements are made of changes in absorbance at 578 and 560 nm, as known increments of air are added. Equilibration is carried out at a fixed temperature, usually 37 °C. The oxygen dissociation curve is calculated from the measurements as described by Benesch et al. (1965) taking into account the oxygen content of the air. The Hill coefficient is the slope of the straight line obtained when the data are plotted on log/log paper.

Washed red cells are usually used for the initial assessment. The 2,3-diphosphoglycerate concentration is determined on an aliquot of packed red cells by the method of Rose and Leibowitz (1970). The P_{50} obtained from the oxygen dissociation curve can be adjusted for varying 2,3-diphosphoglycerate concentrations using tables for normal red blood cells (Bellingham et al., 1971).

A thorough study of oxygen affinity also involves measurements of haemolysates stripped of 2,3-diphosphoglycerate. This is conveniently carried out by standard DEAE–Sephadex column chromatography which additionally isolates each haemoglobin fraction. To study the intrinsic oxygen affinity of the haemoglobin all phosphates should be excluded and measurements carried out in a buffer of the Tris type. The addition of a molar excess of 2,3-diphosphoglycerate then gives an index of its effectiveness in interacting with the haemoglobin under study.

The determination of the oxygen dissociation by measurement of a small number of points does not allow accurate definition at the two ends where the curve becomes almost horizontal. This can be overcome by the use of an oxygen electrode for continuous determination of the whole of the curve. The oxygen electrode is in contact with the haemoglobin which is at first fully oxygenated, and then progressively deoxygenated by the passage of nitrogen. An XY recorder simultaneously plots the oxygen tension and concentration of oxyhaemoglobin. By this means it is possible to demonstrate that the upper part of the curve has a slightly different shape at different pH values, reflecting the dependence of deoxygenation on salt bridges. The original apparatus (Imai et al., 1970) was relatively complex, but now simplified, semi-automatic machines are commercially available.

17.6. SPECIFIC HAEMOGLOBINOPATHIES – INVESTIGATION AND INTERPRETATION

17.6.1. Sickle cell disease

The identification of Haemoglobin S is relatively straightforward by electrophoresis, with confirmation from solubility or sickling tests (section 17.4.1.3). However, assessment of accompanying disability may be complicated by the association of Haemoglobin S with other haemoglobinopathies.

Sickle cell disease is due to the enhanced tendency of Haemoglobin S to form unidirectional crystals in deoxygenated solutions. The crystallization process involves the formation of strands by end-to-end association of haemoglobin molecules, six or more of these strands winding about a central core to form tubular fibrils. In the process, water is lost from the cell and there is a general distortion of shape to give the characteristic sickled appearance. It is important to note that while Haemoglobin S enhances this process of crystallization, other haemoglobins also take part with varying readiness. Haemoglobins C and O Arab will more readily co-polymerize with S than will Haemoglobin F which does not appear to take part in filament formation. Hence, even in homozygous Haemoglobin S disease, foetal haemoglobin values above 10% usually ensure a milder clinical course, and a value near or above 20% protects against most symptoms. The process of crystallization is also concentration dependent, and reduction of the haemoglobin concentration within the cell may protect against sickling. The low mean cell haemoglobin concentration of β-thalassaemia affords some protection, and sickle cell β-thalassaemia is clinically less severe than the homozygous disorder, even if almost all the haemoglobin is type S; α-thalassaemia also modifies sickle cell disease.

The investigation of Haemoglobin S, therefore, requires the definition of whether it is homozygous, heterozygous with Haemoglobin A, or heterozygous with some other abnormality including α- and β-thalassaemia or another haemoglobin variant. There should also routinely be a quantitative estimation of foetal haemoglobin.

Further details on the interaction of Haemoglobin S with other abnormal haemoglobins and its clinical significance are given by Milner (1974).

17.6.2. Thalassaemia – diagnostic summary

The pathology of thalassaemia is due to the relative excess of one chain, rather than to an overall deficiency in haemoglobin synthesis. Thus in β-thalassaemia the damage to the red cell is caused by the breakdown and precipitation of the excess α-chains. This fundamental observation by Fessas laid the foundation for the recognition of the disease process – not only of thalassaemias but of most haemoglobinopathies. Much of the damage occurs within the bone marrow which becomes hyperplastic; in severe forms of the disease the overgrowth can lead to major bone distortion. The precipitation of the excess chains gives inclusion body formation (section 17.4.1.2) and the decreased synthesis of haemoglobin gives a low mean cell volume and mean cell haemoglobin.

The complex genetics of α-thalassaemia has been referred to in section 17.3.2 and the clinical presentation is summarized in Table 17.1. The severe forms are not difficult to diagnose, the complete homozygous form leading to death in utero, i.e. hydrops foetalis. The intermediate form of α-thalassaemia is also known as Hb H disease because of the presence of large amounts (5 to 30%) of Haemoglobin H (β_4) in the mature individual and Haemoglobin Barts (γ_4) in the infant. There may also be small amounts of Haemoglobin Constant Spring, especially in patients of South-East Asian origin.

Whereas the diagnosis of the major forms is usually straightforward, the diagnosis of the minor forms is difficult. In the immediate newborn period there may be the presence of small amounts of Haemoglobin Barts – usually less than 5% of the total haemoglobin. In the adult, the only finding will be a mild anaemia of similar morphology to that of iron deficiency. The diagnosis otherwise rests on differential labelling rates. Reticulocyte-rich preparations are incubated with ^{14}C-labelled aminoacids and the chains subsequently separated. Whereas the relative rates of synthesis of α- and β-chains in the normal are close to 1.00, in α-thalassaemia trait there may be a decrease of this ratio; however, in the mildest forms this will fall within the range of technical error.

The diagnosis of β-thalassaemia minor is very dependent on accurate measurement of Haemoglobin A_2 (section 17.4.1.5). A value above 3.5% of the total haemoglobin strongly supports the diagnosis. The presence of β-thalassaemia major is usually obvious, with the Haemoglobin F value being greater than that of the Haemoglobin A. However, the diagnosis of all the thalassaemias can be complicated by the presence of other haemoglobinopathies. A full description of the differential diagnosis and pathophysiology of α-thalassaemia is given by Wasi et al. (1974) and of the β-thalassaemias by Fessas and Loukopoulos (1974).

17.6.3. The unstable haemoglobin haemolytic anaemias

The unstable variants now form the largest single group of abnormal haemoglobins. They are associated with a characteristic haemolytic anaemia and all share the common feature of a decreased stability when stressed by heat or other means (section 17.4.1.7). The instability is due to mutations that affect critical structural features of the molecule, particularly the haem pocket and the $\alpha_1\beta_1$ interface (sections 17.2.1 and 17.2.2). The consequent molecular distortion results in: increased rates of methaemoglobin production; the formation of haemichromes (section 17.2.3.8); and intracellular precipitation of haemoglobin to give inclusion body formation (section 17.4.1.2). The loss of haem groups from the globin can lead to a dipyrroluria with the passage of dark urine.

The diagnosis ultimately rests on the demonstration of the unstable haemoglobin (section 17.4.1.7) but presumptive evidence is provided by the clinical findings. There should be a history of a familial or congenital haemolytic anaemia. In the usual case of a β-chain variant, the anaemia has an onset a few months after birth and may be related to an oxidative crisis. These crises can occur following administration of drugs, such as sulphonamides, but more usually are associated with a childhood infection. Circulating inclusion bodies are usually only apparent after splenectomy.

The change in structure of the unstable haemoglobins is frequently associated with an altered oxygen dissociation curve. This should be measured before the severity of the disease can be fully assessed (Huehns, 1975).

17.6.4. Methaemoglobinaemia

The production and nature of methaemoglobin has been discussed in section 17.2.3.6. The major causes of methaemoglobin accumulation are given below, but diagnostically one of the most important points is the clinical recognition of the possibility of methaemoglobinaemia. It should always be considered in the differential diagnosis of cyanosis, particularly in children, but unfortunately it is frequently not thought of until after extensive cardiac investigations, including catheterization, have proved negative.

Methaemoglobin is readily detected by the technique of West, detailed by Huehns (1975). This relies on a difference spectrum between the patient's fresh haemolysate with and without added dithionite. The dithionite reduces any Methaemoglobin A present and this acts as a baseline for the unmodified aliquot. The appearance of a peak at 632 nm confirms the presence of methaemoglobin and allows its quantitation.

17.6.4.1. Acquired methaemoglobinaemia

Some patients seem to be susceptible to methaemoglobin formation, based on a decreased activity of their reductive mechanisms or of the detoxifying systems for some drugs. Newborn infants, in particular, have poorly developed red cell reductive mechanisms and are susceptible to oxidant drugs and dyes such as aromatic amines. Another significant cause is the presence of nitrate in foodstuffs or water, which can be converted in the bowel into nitrite which is then absorbed, with resultant methaemoglobin formation.

The diagnosis can usually be made from the history of exposure and a normal methaemoglobin reduction test, as described in the following section.

17.6.4.2. Congenital methaemoglobinaemia

This arises from a deficiency of the NADH-linked methaemoglobin (cytochrome b_5) reductase (section 17.2.3.6). As with other enzymopathies, there appear to be many underlying causes, indicating both a deficiency of enzyme production and various structural abnormalities. All of them result, in the homozygote, in an accumulation of some 10 to 20% methaemoglobin in the blood. The defect may be limited to the red cell enzyme or there can be a generalized deficiency of cytochrome b_5 reductase, in which case the methaemoglobinaemia is associated with mental retardation (Leroux et al., 1975).

The diagnosis is confirmed by demonstrating a decreased reductase activity. A simple screening method is that of Tönz (1968). Red cells are oxidized with nitrite, any excess being removed by further washing. The cells are then incubated in the presence of lactate along with similarly treated cells from two normal controls. Normally about 10% of the methaemoglobin is reduced each hour. The method is robust and simple to interpret. A more definitive method for measurement of NADH reductase is that of Hegesh et al. (1968) which utilised the specificity of the NADH-linked enzyme for the reduction of a ferrocyanide–methaemoglobin complex.

Patients with a congenital methaemoglobinaemia of this type respond to treatment with methylene blue or ascorbic acid, and this can be a useful diagnostic test. These and other means of differentiating the enzymic defects from the abnormal Haemoglobins M are discussed in the following section.

17.6.4.3. The Haemoglobins M

Cyanosis may be due to the presence of an abnormal haemoglobin in which the iron is maintained permanantly in the ferric form. This will occur if there is a substitution which brings an electronegative group close to the haem iron. Replacement of the distal histidine E7 by the larger tyrosine allows the hydroxyl of the tyrosine to bond to the haem iron converting it into the ferric form. This occurs in the β-chain in Haemoglobin M Saskatoon (β63 His → Tyr) and in the α-chain in Haemoglobin M Boston (α58 His → Tyr). The substitution of the proximal histidine by tyrosine will also cause a displacement of the iron such that it can bond directly with the distal histidine as fifth co-ordinate, and form a sixth co-ordinate with the hydroxyl of the tyrosine. This is the case with Haemoglobin M Hyde Park (β92 His → Tyr) and Haemoglobin M Iwate (α87 His → Tyr). Another important example is Haemoglobin M Milwaukee in which a glutamic acid is substituted for valine β67 (E11) close to the distal aspect of the haem. As a consequence, the carboxylic group of the glutamic acid can readily bond to the iron, again converting it into the ferric form.

Cyanosis will be apparent from birth in the case of an α-chain abnormal Haemoglobin M and be seen a few months after birth in the case of the β-chain haemoglobinopathies. The condition is dominant, in that all known cases have been heterozygotes. This may help in its differentiation from a methaemoglobin reductase deficiency which only gives rise to cyanosis in the homozygote. However, the usefulness of this as a guide is limited, as numbers of recorded cases of Haemoglobins M have arisen from new mutations.

A useful clinical test for identifying the cause of a methaemoglobinaemia is the administration of methylene blue to the patient (1 to 3 mg/kg body weight). This will decrease methaemoglobin levels to near normal in individuals with the reductase deficiency, as methylene blue by-passes this pathway to give direct reduction utilizing NADPH. There will be no appreciable improvement in patients whose methaemoglobinaemia is due to a haemoglobin abnormality.

In examining a case of methaemoglobinaemia, a portion of whole cells should be fully converted into methaemoglobin and used to check the rate of methaemoglobin reduction as outlined in section 17.6.4.2. This rate of reduction should be near normal with the Haemoglobins M, but markedly decreased with an enzymic methaemoglobinaemia. Haemolysate can be prepared from the methaemoglobin sample and used for electrophoretic studies, particularly near pH 7.0. The Haemoglobins M, with His → Tyr mutations, have a different mobility from Haemoglobin A at this pH because it is low enough to ionize the imidazole side chain of histidine. An aliquot may also be used to check the spectrum of the haemolysate, the Haemoglobins M all having characteristic changes in their visible spectrum (Lehmann and Huntsman, 1974). However, the spectral changes are of most value if a preliminary purification of the abnormal component can be carried out.

17.6.5. Haemoglobins with disordered oxygen affinity

The possibility of an abnormal haemoglobin should always be considered in the investigation of either a polycythaemia or an unexplained cyanosis. Suspicion is increased if the condition has been present from an early age, particularly in the case of polycythaemia occurring before the age of 30 years. Although it was thought that a normal white cell count with erythraemia indicated the likelihood of a high-affinity haemoglobin, experience has shown that the white count may well be raised and that such a finding should not contraindicate a measurement of the oxygen affinity. The likelihood of an abnormal haemoglobin is also increased if there is a family history of the complaint though, as with the unstable haemoglobins, new mutations are relatively common. Again, as with the unstable haemoglobins, the absence of an electrophoretic abnormality does not exclude a haemoglobin variant, since many of the haemoglobins with altered oxygen affinity have no change in electrophoretic mobility.

The investigations involved in the assessment of oxygen affinity have been described in section 17.5.7. There should be measurement of 2,3-diphosphoglycerate concentration in a fresh haemolysate and the P_{50} of the whole cells should be determined, along with normal controls. A deviation of the P_{50} by more than 3 mm Hg from that of the control is of significance and should be checked. This requires measurement of the dissociation curve of haemolysates, both in the presence of excess phosphate or 2,3-diphosphoglycerate and when stripped of phosphates. The demonstration of a consistent change in oxygen affinity confirms the presence of a haemoglobin abnormality.

An appreciable decrease in the P_{50}, i.e. a rise in oxygen affinity, will result in an increase in the packed cell volume. There will be a normal arterial pO_2 but a decreased mixed venous pO_2. In severe cases, an increase in cardiac output may occur in order to meet tissue oxygen requirements. In the converse situation where there is an increase in the P_{50}, i.e. a low oxygen affinity, it might be expected that there would be a compensatory anaemia due to the increased oxygen carrying capacity of the blood under resting conditions. However this is not a consistent feature and most cases with decreased oxygen affinity have come to medical attention because of their cyanotic appearance resulting from the increased levels of circulating deoxyhaemoglobin.

The first point to be made concerning the molecular abnormalities resulting in changed oxygen affinity is that the high-affinity form is the natural or relaxed (R) state of the haemoglobin molecule Evolution has resulted in a number of modifications that have resuled in the co-operative effects between the four subunits of haemoglobin to give a low affinity (T) state as outlined in section 17.2.4. It is not surprising, therefore, that most mutations affecting oxygen affinity result in a regression to the relaxed, high-affinity state whereas low-affinity variants are rare.

The abnormalities that result in changed affinity have been discussed in detail by Morimoto et al. (1971). Not surprisingly, they arise from alterations in the structural features involved in oxygenation and deoxygenation as described in section 17.2.4.

The most frequent cause is a mutation at the $\alpha_1\beta_2$ interface about which the sliding rotation takes place in the change from the oxygenated to the deoxygenated form. There may either be a steric hindrance to this movement or a disruption of one of the salt bridges that stabilizes the deoxy-form. Examples are the substitutions that occur in the aspartic acid position 99 (G1) in the β-chain. This residue is part of the $\alpha_1\beta_2$ junction and forms an important stabilizing hydrogen bond in the deoxy-conformation. All the substitutions affecting this position are associated with a polycythaemia, i.e. Haemoglobin Yakima (β99 His), Kempsey (β99 Asn), Radcliffe (β99 Ala), and Ypsilanti (β99 Tyr). An increased affinity will also occur if there is a replacement of the penultimate tyrosine that locks the tertiary structure in the deoxy form, as occurs with Haemoglobins Bethesda (β145 Tyr → His) and Rainier (β415 Tyr → Cys). A similar effect occurs if there is an alteration in the pocket in the globin into which the penultimate tyrosine fits, as in Haemoglobin Hirose (β37 Tyr → Ser). An increased oxygen affinity will also occur if a mutation affects the binding site of 2,3-diphosphoglycerate as in Haemoglobin Rahere (β82 Lys → Thr) or Helsinki (β82 Lys → Met).

An interesting group of variants is that in which there is alteration in the oxygen affinity by allowing movement of the haem plate. Normally the haem plate is fixed, with the proximal histidine above and the distal histidine below. Movement of the proximal histidine down towards the haem plate will occur on change from the deoxy- to oxy-form. This shift will tend to push the iron back into the plane of the haem, increasing the oxygen affinity. If, however, a spacer group from beneath the haem is replaced by a smaller group, the haem plate can move without the iron being forced back into the plane of the haem. Thus the iron remains out of the plane of the haem and in the deoxy-form. This occurs with Haemoglobin Hammersmith and Haemoglobin Christchurch, both of which have the replacement below the haem of the large phenylalanine, by the smaller serine. As a result both have a decreased oxygen affinity. The converse can occur with the same type of substitution above the plane of the haem, as occurs with Haemoglobin Heathrow, a high-affinity variant, in which phenylalanine above the haem is replaced by a smaller leucine. Because these substitutions affect the haem pocket, they are all unstable haemoglobins and illustrate the way in which a change in oxygen affinity may be a useful additional means of confirming the presence of a haemoglobin abnormality in an atypical Heinz body anaemia.

17.6.6. Isoelectric focussing and minor components

When haemoglobin is electrophoresed in acrylamide, containing ampholytes, in the range pH 6 to 8, a series of minor components can be seen (Figure 17.22). Some of these are

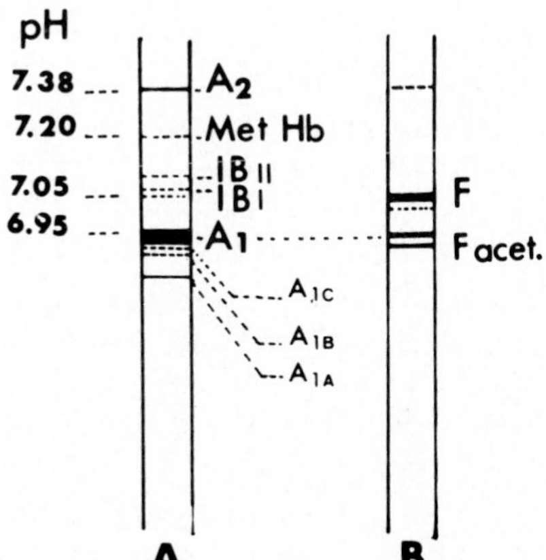

Figure 17.22. Isoelectric focussing of: A, adult haemolysate; B, neonatal haemolysate. IBI is now known to be the β-oxidized hybrid (αIIβIII) and IBII is the α-oxidized hybrid (αIIIβII). (Reproduced, with permission, from Krishnamoorthy et al. 1976)

due to modifications of amino-terminal groups, acetylation of the γ-chain giving a modified Haemoglobin F and glycosylation of the β-chain giving Haemoglobin A_{1c}. A more diffuse fraction, Haemoglobin A_{1a} is due to a combination of the β-chain terminus with mono- and diphosphates of various hexoses. A further component, A_{1b}, appears to be due to loss of an amide group from the β-chain. Also, oxidation of haemoglobin produces not only methaemoglobin, with all iron atoms in the ferric form, but also the intermediate hybrids $(\alpha II\beta III)_2$ and $(\alpha III\beta II)_2$ with only one of the two pairs of chains oxidized.

Interest in these modified haemoglobins has been stimulated by the use of isoelectric focussing. This has been standardized in gel column form (e.g. Krishnamoorthy et al., 1976) but the simpler thin-layer techniques are probably more suitable for general laboratory use.

17.6.7. Glycosylated haemoglobin and diabetes

Glucose combines with the N-terminal of haemoglobin β-chains to give the glycosylated haemoglobin A_{1c}. The proportion of this can be estimated by column chromatography (Kynoch and Lehmann, 1977) or more approximately by electrophoretic techniques. A simple chemical technique has also been introduced (Flückiger and Winterhalter, 1976) which depends on the conversion of the bound glucose to a furfural with subsequent hydrolysis and colorimetric measurement.

Koenig et al. (1976) found that the normal adult has 3 to 6% of haemoglobin in the form of A_{1c} but that this proportion rises above 6% in diabetics, the degree of the rise indicating the mean blood sugar level over the previous weeks. Thus it seems likely that the measurement of haemoglobin A_{1c} levels will provide a useful index of the long-term control of hyperglycaemia in the diabetic.

REFERENCES

Bellingham, A.J. (1974) The red cell in adaptation to anaemic hypoxia. Clinics in Hematology, 3, 577–594.

Bellingham, A.J., Detter, J.C. and Lenfant, C. (1971) Regulatory mechanisms of hemoglobin oxygen affinity in acidosis and alkalosis. Journal of Clinical Investigation, 50, 700–706.

Benesch, R. and Benesch, R.E. (1967) The effect of organic phosphates from the human erythrocyte on the allosteric properties of haemoglobin. Biochemical and Biophysical Research Communications, 26, 162–167.

Benesch, R., MacDuff, G. and Benesch, R.E. (1965) Determination of oxygen equilibria with a versatile new tonometer. Analytical Biochemistry, 11, 81–87.

Berzofsky, J.A., Peisach, J. and Blumberg, W.E. (1971) Sulfheme proteins. I Optical and magnetic properties of sulfmyoglobin and its derivatives. Journal of Biological Chemistry, 246, 3367–3377.

Beutler, E. and Mitchell, M. (1968) Special modifications of the fluorescent screening method for glucose-6-phosphate dehydrogenase deficiency. Blood, 32, 816–818.

Brosious, E.M., Morrison, B.Y. and Schmidt, R.M. (1976) Effects of hemoglobin F levels, KCN, and storage on the isopropanol precipitation test for unstable hemoglobins. American Journal of Clinical Pathology, 66, 878–882.

Card, R.T. and Brain, M.C. (1973) The anemia of childhood: evidence for a physiologic response to hyperphosphatemia. New England Journal of Medicine, 288, 388–392.

Carrell, R.W. and Kay, R. (1972) A simple method for the detection of unstable haemoglobins. British Journal of Haematology, 23, 615–619.

Carrell, R.W., Winterbourn, C.C. and Rachmilewitz, E.A. (1975) Activated oxygen and haemolysis (Annotation). British Journal of Haematology, 30, 259–264.

Chanutin, A. and Curnish, R.R. (1967) Effect of organic and inorganic phosphates on the oxygen equilibrium of human erythrocytes. Archives of Biochemistry and Biophysics, 121, 96–102.

Charache, S. (1974) Hemoglobins with altered oxygen affinity. Clinics in Haematology, 3, 357–381.

Chernoff and Pettit (1964) A qualitative method for identifying abnormalities of the polypeptide chains of haemoglobin. Blood, 24, 750–756.

Clegg, J.B. (1974) Haemoglobin synthesis. Clinics in Haematology, 3, 225–250.

Clegg, J.B., Naughton, M.A. and Weatherall, D.J. (1965) An improved method for the characterisation of human haemoglobin mutants. Nature (London) 207, 945–947.

Corwin, A.H. (1973) Interpretations of porphyrin spectra. Annals of The New York Academy of Sciences, 206, 201–209.

Dacie, J.V. and Lewis, S.M. (1975) In Practical Hematology, 5th edn. pp. 227–233, Churchill Livingstone, Edinburgh.

Duhm, J. and Gerlach, E. (1974) Metabolism and function of 2-3 diphosphoglycerate in red blood cells. In The Human Red Cell in Vitro (Eds. T.J. Greenwalt and G.A. Jamieson) pp. 111–148, Grune and Stratton, New York.

Efremov, G.D. and Huisman, T.H.J. (1974) The laboratory diagnosis of the haemoglobinopathies. Clinics in Haematology, 3, 527–570.

Fessas, P. and Loukopoulos, D. (1974) The β-thalassaemias. Clinics in Haematology, 3, 411–435.

Flückiger, R. and Winterhalter, K.H. (1976) In vitro synthesis of hemoglobin AIc. FEBS Letters, 71, 356–360.

Grimes, A.J. and Meisler, A. (1962) Possible cause of Heinz bodies in congenital Heinz body anaemia. Nature (London), 194, 190–191.

Hartley, B.S. (1970). Strategy and tactics in protein chemistry. Biochemical Journal, 119, 805–822.

Hegesh, E., Calmanovici, N. and Avron, M. (1968) New method for determining ferrihemoglobin reductase (NADH methemoglobin reductase) in erythrocytes. Journal of Laboratory and Clinical Medicine, 72, 339–344.

Holland, V.R., Saunders, B.C., Rose, F.L. and Walpole, A.L. (1974) A safer substitute for benzidine in the detection of blood. Tetrahedron, 30, 3299–3302.

Huehns, E.R. (1975) The structure and function of haemoglobin: clinical disorders due to abnormal haemoglobin structure. In Blood and its Disorders (Eds. R.M. Hardisty and D.J. Weatherall) pp. 526–629, Blackwell Scientific Publications, Oxford.

Huisman T.H.J. (1974) Chromatography of hemoglobin variants. In The Detection of Hemoglobinopathies (Eds. R. Schmidt, T.H.J. Huisman and H. Lehmann) pp. 43–48, CRC Press, Cleveland.

Hultquist, D.E., Douglas, R.H. and Dean, R.T. (1975) The methemoglobin reduction system of erythrocytes. In Erythrocyte structure and function (Ed. G.J. Brewer) pp. 297–300, Liss, New York.

Imai, K., Morimoto, H., Kotani, M., Watari, H., Hirata, W. and Kuroda, M. (1970) Studies on the function of abnormal hemoglobins I. An improved method for automatic measurement of the oxygen equilibrium curve of hemoglobin. Biochimica et Biophysica Acta, 200, 189–196.

Jacob, H.S. and Jandl, J.H. (1966) A simple visual screening test for glucose-6-phosphate dehydrogenase deficiency employing ascorbate and cyanide. New England Journal of Medicine, 274, 1162–1167.

Kan, Y.W., Dozy, A.M., Varmus, H.E., Taylor, J.M., Holland, J.P., Lei-Injo, L.E., Ganesan, J. and Todd, D. (1975) Delection of α-globin genes in Haemoglobin-H disease demonstrates multiple α-globin structural loci. Nature (London), 255, 255–256.

Kilmartin, J.V. (1976) Interaction of haemoglobin with protons, CO_2, and 2,3-diphosphoglycerate. British Medical Bulletin, 32, 209–212.

Kleihauer, E. (1974) Determination of fetal hemoglobin: elution technique. In The Detection of Hemoglobinopathies (Eds. R. Schmidt, T.H.J. Huisman and H. Lehmann) pp. 20–22, CRC Press, Cleveland.

Koenig, R.J., Peterson, C.M., Jones, R.L., Saudek, C., Lehrman, M. and Cerami, A. (1976) Correlation of glucose regulation and Hemoglobin A_{Ic} in Diabetes Mellitus. New England Journal of Medicine, 295, 417–420.

Krishnamoorthy, R., Wajcman, H. and Labie, D. (1976) Isoelectric focusing: a method of multiple application for hemoglobin studies. Clinica Chimica Acta, 69, 203–209.

Kynoch, P.A.M. and Lehmann, H. (1977) Rapid estimation (2½ hours) of glycosylated haemoglobin for routine purposes. Lancet, ii, 16.

Lamola, A.A. and Yamane, T. (1974) Zinc protoporphyrin in the erythrocytes of patients with lead intoxication and iron deficiency anaemia. Science, 186, 936–938.

Lehmann, H. and Huntsman, R.G. (1974) Man's Haemoglobins, 2nd edn. North-Holland, Amsterdam.

Lehmann, H. and Huntsman, R.G. (1975) Laboratory detection of haemoglobinopathies. Broadsheet 33 (revised 1975) Published by Journl of Clinical Pathology, BMA House, London.

Lehmann, H. and Lang, A. (1974) Various aspects of α-thalassaemia. Annals of New York Academy of Sciences, 232, 152–158.

Leroux, A., Junien, C., Kaplan, J. and Bamberger, J. (1975) Generalised deficiency of cytochrome b_5 reductase in congenital methaemoglobinaemia with mental retardation. Nature (London), 258, 619–620.

Makarem, A. (1974) Hemoglobins, hemoglobin binding proteins. In Clinical Chemistry: Principles and Technics (Eds. R.J. Henry, D.C. Cannon, J.W. Winkelman) pp. 1111–1215, Harper and Row, New York.

Marengo-Rowe, A.J. (1965) Rapid electrophoresis and quantitation of haemoglobins on cellulose acetate. Journal of Clinical Pathology, 18, 790–792.

Milner, P.F. (1974) The sickling disorders. Clinics in Hematology, 3, 289–331.

Morimoto, H., Lehmann, H. and Perutz, M.F. (1971) Molecular pathology of human haemoglobin. Stereochemical interpretation of abnormal oxygen affinities. Nature (London), 232, 408–413.

Orkin, S.H. and Nathan, O.G. (1976) The thalassaemias (Medical Intelligence). New England Journal of Medicine, 295, 710–714.

Ottolenghi, S., Lanyon, W.G., Paul, J., Williamson, R. et al. (1974) Gene deletion as the cause of α-thalassaemia. Nature (London), 251, 389–392.

Owen, M.C. (1975) A sensitive technique by differential scanning for detecting haemoglobins of fetal origin. Journal of Clinical Pathology, 28, 16–17.

Papayannopoulou, T. and Stamatoyannopoulos, G. (1974) Stains for inclusion bodies, In The Detection of Hemoglobinopathies (Eds. R. Schmidt, T.H.J. Huisman and H. Lehmann) pp. 32–38, CRC Press, Cleveland.

Perutz, M.F. (1972) Nature of haem–haem interaction. Nature (London), 237, 495–499.

Perutz, M.F. (1974) Mechanism of denaturation of hemoglobin by alkali. Nature (London), 247, 341–344.

Perutz, M.F. and TenEyck, L.F. (1971) Stereochemistry of co-operative effects in hemoglobin. Cold Spring Harbor Symposia on Quantitative Biology, 36, 295–310.

Perutz, M.F., Muirhead, H., Cox, J.M. and Goaman, L.C.G. (1968) Three dimensional Fourier synthesis of horse oxyhaemoglobin at 2.8 Å resolution. The atomic model. Nature (London), 219, 131–139.

Rachmilewitz, E.A. (1974) Denaturation of the normal and abnormal haemoglobin molecule. Seminars in Hematology, 11, 441–462.

Rosa, J., Beuzard, Y., Thillet, J., Gerel, M.C. and Caburi, J. (1975) Testing for hemoglobins with abnormal oxygen affinity curves. In Abnormal Haemoglobins and Thalassaemia Diagnostic Aspects. (Ed. R.M. Schmidt) pp. 79–116, Academic Press, New York.

Rose, Z.B. and Leibowitz, J. (1970) Direct determination of 2,3-diphosphoglycerate. Analytical Biochemistry, 35, 177–180.

Schmidt, R.M., Huisman, T.H.J. and Lehmann, H. (Eds.) (1974) The Detection of Haemoglobinopathies. C.R.C. Press, Cleveland.

Schneider, R.G. (1974) Identification of hemoglobins by electrophoresis. In The Detection of Hemoglobinopathies (Eds. R. Schmidt, T.H.J. Huisman and H. Lehmann) pp. 11–15, C.R.C. Press, Cleveland.

Sutton, H.E. and Wagner, R.P. (1975) Mutation and enzyme function in humans. Annual Review of Genetics, 9, 187–212.

Taylor, J.M., Dozy, A., Kan, Y.W., Varmus, H.E. and Lie-Injo, L.E. (1974) Genetic lesion in homozygous α thalassaemia (hydrops fetalis). Nature (London), 251, 392–393.

Tönz, O. (1968) The Congenital Methaemoglobinaemias. S. Karger, Basel.

Torrance, J., Jacobs, P., Rostrepo, A., Esbach, J., Lenfant, C. and Finch, C. (1970) Intraerythrocytic adaptation to anaemia. New England Journal of Medicine, 283, 165–169.

Wasi, P., Na-Nakorn, S. and Pootrakul, S.N. (1974) The α thalassaemias. Clinics in Haematology, 4, 383–410.

Weber, K., Pringle, J.R. and Osborn, M. (1972) Measurement of molecular weights by electrophoresis on SDS-acrylamide gel. In Methods in Enzymology. Enzyme Structure, Part C, Vol. 26 (Eds. C.H.W. Hirs and S.N. Timasheff) pp. 3–27, Academic, New York.

FURTHER READING

Antonini, E. and Brunori, M. (1971) Hemoglobin and Myoglobin in their Reactions with Ligands. North-Holland, Amsterdam.

Brewer, G.J. (Ed.) (1975) Erythrocyte Structure and Function. Proceedings of the Third International Conference on Red Cell Metabolism and Function. Alan Liss Inc., New York.

Bunn, H.F., Forget, B.G. and Ranney, H.M. (1977) Human Hemoglobins. W.B. Saunders, Philadelphia.

Lehmann, H. and Huntsman, R.G. (1974) Man's Haemoglobins, 2nd edn. North-Holland, Amsterdam.

Lehmann, H. and Huntsman, R.G. (1975) Laboratory detection of haemoglobinopathies. Broadsheet 33 (revised 1975). Published by Journal of Clinical Pathology, BMA House, London.

Lehmann, H. and Kynoch, P.A.M. (1976) Human Haemoglobin Variants and their Characteristics. North-Holland, Amsterdam.

Makarem, A. (1974) Hemoglobins, hemoglobin derivatives and hemoglobin binding proteins. In Clinical Chemistry: Principles and Techniques (Eds. R.J. Henry, D.C. Cannon and J.W. Winkelman) pp. 1111–1215, Harper and Row, New York.

Schmidt, R.M. (1975) Abnormal Haemoglobins and Thalassaemia – Diagnostic Aspects. Academic Press, New York.

Schmidt, R.M., Huisman, T.H.J. and Lehmann, H. (1974) The Detection of Haemoglobinopathies. C.R.C. Press, Cleveland.

Schroeder, W.A. (1968) The Primary Structure of Proteins – Principles and Practices for the Determination of Amino Acid Sequence. Harper and Row, New York.

Special recommendation

Haemoglobin: structure, function and synthesis (1976) British Medical Bulletin, 32 (3), 193–287.

ADDENDUM

Mapping of the globin gene

It is now possible to obtain relatively detailed maps of the globin gene using restriction endonucleases which cleave DNA at precisely specified points. In the first place, the DNA responsible for a particular globin is synthesized from the relevant messenger RNA by reverse transcriptase. The materials used for this synthesis are isotopically labelled, so that the "complementary" DNA (cDNA) is radioactive. The DNA to be investigated is broken down by restriction enzymes and the fragments are separated by agarose gel electrophoresis. Those which contain the globin gene can be identified by hybridization with labelled cDNA. The autoradiograph of the gel gives a restriction map of the globin gene fragments which will vary with each specific endonuclease.

The technique has exciting prospects as a tool for the diagnosis of thalassaemia. There is the advantage that a wide range of tissues can be used as source material. Amniotic fluid fibroblasts allow the technique to be used for prenatal diagnosis. As yet the application is largely limited to the diagnosis of gene deletion. Readily identifiable changes have been demonstrated in restriction maps from individuals with α, β and δ/β thalassaemias due to gene deletions. As the range of endonucleases increases it should be possible to detect even the minor changes in the DNA that produce non-deletional thalassaemia or aminoacid substitutions which prevent production of a viable globin chain.

Some of the abnormal haemoglobins are already identifiable from restriction maps. For example, the cleavage point of the restriction enzyme Eco RI is the DNA sequence GAATTC which occurs at codons β121–122 and is altered in Haemoglobin O Arab (β121 Glu–Lys) to AAATTC. Thus fragments of the O Arab gene have a readily identifiable change in their Eco RI restriction map.

The use of restriction enzymes has led to knowledge of the intervening sequences of DNA that separate, and are inserted into, the globin genes. Even closely related genes such as those responsible for the δ and β globin respectively are separated by approximately 7000 base-pairs of DNA. Both genes also have their sequence interrupted by intervening sequences, "Introns", some 1000 base-pairs in length. These are transcribed into the nuclear RNA but are excised before the release of the messenger RNA. Hence they are not represented in the cDNA prepared from messenger RNA.

These intervening sequences show much more variability between species than is seen in the genes themselves and there is a suggestion of variation (? polymorphism) within our own species. Current findings indicate that the β-chain gene of Haemoglobin S in American Blacks has arisen from an individual bearing a clonal variation of this type. As a consequence Haemoglobin S disease may be diagnosable in them from restriction differences due not to the structural gene mutation (β6 Glu–Val) but to coincidental variation in the DNA sequences not within the globin gene.

Nienhuis, A.W. (1978) Mapping the human genome: Editorial. New England Journal of Medicine, 299, 195–196.

Tolstoshev, P. (1978) Of mice and men: Annotation. Nature, 276, 13–15.

Chapter 18

Inborn errors of metabolism

D. Noel Raine

Department of Clinical Chemistry, The Children's Hospital, Ladywood Middleway, Birmingham B16 8ET, England

CONTENTS

Chemical diagnosis of disease, edited by
S.S. Brown, F.L. Mitchell and D.S. Young

18.1. INTRODUCTION

The concept of disease characterized by chemical abnormality from birth in children born to closely related parents was propounded in its most complete and recognizable form by Archibald Garrod in the Croonian lectures of 1908: he gave as examples of such "Inborn Errors of Metabolism" albinism, alkaptonuria, cystinuria and pentosuria. Cystinuria derives its name from a bladder (cystic) calculus which was analyzed by W.H. Wollaston in 1810. Cases of alkaptonuria, characterized by the excretion of urine which is black or darkens on standing, were undoubtedly known to mediaeval uroscopists, and accounts exist from the sixteenth century. In 1902, Garrod discovered that the parents of his patient with alkaptonuria were first cousins; further enquiry revealed that, of the 40 known cases, 18 derived from 10 marriages, two-thirds of which were first-cousin unions. Meanwhile, William Bateson was reviewing the evidence from plant studies that lead to the rediscovery of Mendel's laws of inheritance, and he remarked in a footnote to a report to the Royal Society that these laws would explain Dr. Garrod's findings in alkaptonuria (see Raine, 1966).

Phenylketonuria was recognized in 1934 and galactosaemia in 1935. Thereafter the number of new examples increased logarithmically, stimulated by the development of paper and gas chromatography, by the discovery of lysosomes and co-ordinated by the whole concept of molecular genetics.

18.2. GENETIC CONSIDERATIONS

In this chapter, the term "inherited" implies that the metabolic disease is caused by a defect in a single gene responsible for the production of an enzyme. This is not to imply that other metabolic diseases, such as diabetes mellitus, are not genetically determined or that diseases with inherited tendencies, such as schizophrenia, may not have a metabolic cause. This use of a stricter definition allows certain useful rules to be derived that would not otherwise apply. Thus no dominantly inherited disease has, as its primary cause, an inherited enzyme deficiency, and all examples of the latter lead to recessive or X-linked disorders. Moreover, it can be predicted that both the parents of a patient with an autosomal recessive disorder must be heterozygous carriers, each with one normal and one abnormal gene controlling the synthesis of the appropriate enzyme. (In X-linked recessive disorders only the mother is a carrier.)

For autosomal recessive genes, a sibship containing an affected individual will statistically comprise, for each genotypically and phenotypically abnormal patient, one genotypically normal subject and two heterozygotes, although these last three will all be phenotypically normal. The risk that further siblings will be affected is always 1 in 4, and consequently – but rarely emphasized – the chance that another sibling will be completely healthy is 3 in 4. In X-linked disorders only boys are affected by the disease, and usually only the mother carries the abnormal gene. Again, 1 in 4 of a total sibship will be affected, but this means that half of the boys are at risk and, while all the girls will be healthy, half will be heterozygotes and carry the abnormal gene. The occasional departures from these rules are due to the rare instances where one of the parents is a homozygote, and if this is established, here too the chances of further children being affected can be calculated.

It is desirable that all close relatives of a propositus with an inherited metabolic disease, including cousins and their parents and offspring, should be examined for evidence of the disorder; where this may lead to treatment or to prophylactic advice, such a search is obligatory. In practice, the clinical chemist is as likely as the clinician to be moved to make the effort to do this.

With increasing familiarity with genetic disease, the distinction between the terms "dominant" and "recessive" becomes blurred. If the disease can only be recognized on clinical grounds the issue is usually clear – when homozygotes are affected and heterozygotes not, the inheritance is recessive; when, however, as with Haemoglobin S, the abnormality can easily be demonstrated by laboratory tests in the carrier as well as the homozygote, this defect may be, and is by some, regarded as dominantly inherited. What then of angiokeratoma, diffuse (Fabry's disease), an X-linked enzyme deficiency in which female carriers can be recognized by careful examination of their eyes? Nevertheless, the distinction between dominant and recessive inheritance continues to be useful although it is of doubtful fundamental significance.

None of these single gene defects is recognizable from microscopic examination of the chromosomes: the known disorders of the latter such as trisomy, short arms, and ring formations, result in abnormalities which are quite different from the inherited metabolic diseases and are usually characterized by malformations of the face or limbs.

All of the inherited metabolic diseases are rare. Table 18.1 shows phenylketonuria to be one of the commonest while others such as maple syrup urine disease are exceedingly

TABLE 18.1.

INCIDENCE AND GENE FREQUENCY OF SOME INHERITED METABOLIC DISEASES

(Reproduced, with permission, from Raine, 1974a)

Disease	Incidence	Gene frequency	Heterozygote incidence
Phenylketonuria	0.000 1 (1 in 10,000)	0.0100	0.020 (1 in 50)
Histidinaemia	0.000 07 (1 in 14,000)	0.0084	0.017 (1 in 60)
Cystinuria	0.000 07 (1 in 14,000)	0.0084	0.017 (1 in 60)
Homocystinuria	0.000 06 (1 in 17,000)	0.0077	0.015 (1 in 65)
Argininosuccinic aciduria	0.000 05 (1 in 20,000)	0.0071	0.014 (1 in 71)
Galactosaemia	0.000 03 (1 in 33, 000)	0.0055	0.011 (1 in 92)
Tyrosinaemia	0.000 004 (1 in 250,000)	0.002	0.004 (1 in 250)
Maple syrup urine disease	0.000 0003 (1 in 333,000)	0.0017	0.003 (1 in 289)

rare. Where a disease appears to be more common than 1 in 10,000, e.g. the adrenogenital syndrome (1 in 7000), it is probable that no distinction has been made between several (three in this case) different enzyme deficiencies resulting in similar clinical disorders. The only exceptions to this occur in geographically isolated areas where the chances of inbreeding are greatly increased, as in part of Quebec, where the incidence of tyrosinosis is 1 in 2000, and in the Celts of Norway, Western Scotland and Ireland, where the incidence of phenylketonuria is 1 in 5000, twice that in England.

For some considerations, it is necessary to differentiate between the frequency of a recessive disease and that of the abnormal gene. The latter is much greater than the former since it includes the two abnormal genes in all homozygotes and the one each in all heterozygotes. For an autosomal recessive disease, the abnormal gene frequency (q) is usually calculated from the square root of the incidence of the disease. Thus for phenylketonuria, with an incidence of 1 in 10,000 (0.0001), the square root is 1 in 100 (0.01). For diseases as rare as phenylketonuria, the incidence of heterozygotes is obtained by multiplying the abnormal gene frequency by 2 (a factor which has a mathematical derivation), i.e. 1 in 50 (0.02).

These calculations make the reasonable assumption that the population has reached equilibrium through random mating. However, new mutations do occur and their frequency probably varies considerably with different diseases. Thus, two unrelated children with Haemoglobinopathy M studied by the present Author were the only subjects affected and more than 35 close relatives in each family had only normal haemoglobin (Farmer et al., 1964). Both children must therefore have been new – and were in fact different (Pick and Raine, 1964) – mutations. Almost nothing is known about mutation rates in the enzyme deficiency diseases.

Female cells are recognized cytogenetically by the presence of a Barr body, a dense clump of chromatin in the nucleus. This is believed to be a degenerate X chromosome. This observation, and experimental evidence from the colouring of some animals, led Mary Lyon to postulate that, in the female, one of the X chromosomes is always suppressed and that selection of the survivor is a random process. A consequence of this random suppression – known as lyonization – in the field of inherited metabolic disease is that in the female carriers of an X-linked disorder, half the chromosomes bearing the abnormal gene will be suppressed and these cells will be dominated by the normal gene: in the remainder, the reverse will hold and the cell will be dominated by the defective gene. Thus, while the activity of the enzyme determined by the gene overall will be half the normal activity, that in individual cells will be either normal or completely deficient. This contrasts with the situation in autosomal recessive carriers, all of whose cells contain half the normal enzyme activity. This fact is utilized, for instance, in examining females for glucose-6-phosphate dehydrogenase deficiency by histochemical means, where the carriers show two populations of red blood cells and the normal homozygote only one.

Mosaicism – the situation where only some of the cells of a particular tissue have an abnormal genetic constitution – is clearly established for the trisomy syndromes where the karyotype can be seen in individual cells. Such patients have less severe clinical manifestations than those in whom all cells of the tissue are affected. (Not all enzyme deficiency diseases show the defect in all tissues of the body.) There is no reason to suppose that mosaicism does not also occur in the enzyme deficiency diseases (although it would be much more difficult to detect) and a case, known to the present Author, of albinism in a Negro child in whom there are only patches of depigmentation, is probably analogous to the chromosomal mosaic patients.

18.3. PATHOGENETIC MECHANISMS

18.3.1. Genetic abnormalities

Most defects in enzyme biosynthesis seem likely to be the result of defective structural genes. Although there is evidence, in some organisms, of the activities of structural genes being regulated by control genes, and it is possible that defects in these could account for some diseases, there is little evidence, as yet, for this type of abnormality in man. The structural gene is a strand of DNA consisting of a series of nucleotide triplets – the genetic code – which determines the sequence of aminoacids in the polypeptide chain, whose biosynthesis it controls. In the haemoglobinopathies at least, there is evidence that the protein abnormality is due to a single mistake in this code. Thus the sixth aminoacid in the β-chain of haemoglobin is glutamic acid, the code for which is GAA. In haemoglobins S and C, this is replaced by valine and lysine respectively, and the codes for these aminoacids are GUA and AAA, each differing from GAA by one nucleotide only. Because the aminoacid sequences in enzymes are not yet known, similar mistakes have not yet been demonstrated, but there is good reason to suppose that they will be in time.

Using one of the pair of DNA strands of the gene as a template, the enzyme RNA polymerase synthesizes a single strand of messenger RNA. Separate units of RNA – transfer-RNA – are attached by specific enzymes to individual aminoacids after these have been activated by phosphorylation under the influence of a specific kinase. Each transfer-RNA bears a triplet of nucleotides – an anticodon – which is complementary to the triplet in the messenger-RNA – the codon. Thus the aminoacids are assembled in the correct order at the site of, and under the influence of, the constituents of a ribosome. There is every possibility that some genetic diseases will be shown to be due to defects in any one of this series of biosynthetic steps. Most, however, are expected to be due to a mistake in the nucleotide sequence in the DNA, leading to the formation of a faulty codon in the messenger RNA. This in turn results in the wrong aminoacid becoming incorporated at a particular site in the polypeptide, brought about by normally functioning ribosomes and transfer RNA.

18.3.2. Enzymic abnormalities

Enzymes may be malformed in this way, and have different physical properties – such as electrophoretic mobility – without this affecting the active site and hence the enzyme activity. Thus there are almost 100 different forms of glucose-6-phosphate dehydrogenase known in man, but in only about five is the activity diminished sufficiently to have pathological consequences. Abnormal enzyme structure in the region of the binding site can affect activity by a change in the affinity of the site for either substrate or co-enzyme, and there are examples of closely similar diseases resulting from different degrees and types of interference with the same enzyme. Thus in methylmalonic aciduria due to inactivity of methylmalonyl CoA isomerase, the activity of this enzyme is unaffected by increasing the concentration of cobalamin in certain cases (defects of the substrate binding site) whereas in others (defects of the co-enzyme binding site) the activity can be increased in this way. In still other cases, inactivity of this enzyme may be due to failure of biosynthesis of the co-enzyme, but this is a matter distinct from the present discussion. Such variation in the affinity of the substrate for the enzyme may have an effect in vivo and yet be difficult to detect in vitro where the enzyme is assayed under "optimal" conditions. It is therefore necessary sometimes to assay the enzyme whose diminished activity is suspected to be the cause of the disease under varying substrate or co-enzyme concentrations. Such K_m variants are known for pyruvate kinase-deficient haemolytic anaemia, the thiamine-responsive form of pyruvate decarboxylase deficiency, and the thiamine-responsive form of branched-chain ketoacid decarboxylase-deficient form of maple syrup urine disease.

Where such an affinity involves a co-enzyme, the diminished enzyme activity may be enhanced by administering larger amounts of the vitamin precursor: since, in practice, even a small increase in the activity of an enzyme can have a large biological effect, this may be of considerable therapeutic value. Thus those cases of homocystinuria in whom

TABLE 18.2.

SOME VITAMIN-RESPONSIVE DISORDERS

Vitamin	Disorder
Thiamine (B_1)	Pyruvate carboxylase deficiency
	Maple syrup urine disease
	Megaloblastic anaemia, thiamine responsive
Pyridoxine (B_6)	Pyridoxine-dependency with seizures
	Anaemia, hypochromic
	Cystathioninuria
	Xanthurenic aciduria
	Homocystinuria, type 1
	Oxalosis, type 1 (glycolic aciduria)
Cobalamin (B_{12})	Methylmalonic aciduria, type 2
	Vitamin B_{12} metabolic defect
	Transcobalamin deficiency
Folic acid	Homocystinuria, type 2
	Formiminotransferase deficiency
	Megaloblastic anaemia due to dihydrofolate reductase deficiency
	Folic acid, transport defect involving
Biotin	Glycinaemia – propionic acidaemia
	β-Hydroxyisovaleric aciduria and β-methylcrotonylglycinuria
Cholecalciferol (D)	Pseudovitamin D deficiency rickets
	Hypophosphataemia (X-linked)

hepatic cystathionine synthetase is reduced to 2 to 4% of normal are improved by large doses of pyridoxine, after which the enzyme activity may double. Other cases in whom there is no measurable activity, and hence no basis for even a slight increase, do not respond to the vitamin and must be treated by restriction of dietary methionine. Several other vitamin-dependent inherited metabolic diseases are already known, and since these may be eminently treatable, they are listed in Table 18.2; however in some (e.g. the methylmalonic acidurias) it is most important to take those specimens that will enable the correct diagnosis to be established *before* administering the vitamin. Otherwise subsequent investigations can be obscured, with delay in establishing the most appropriate therapy.

18.3.3. Effects of enzyme deficiency

Given that the activity of a particular enzyme is deficient, the pathological consequences may arise in several different ways. The most familiar one is the accumulation of the normal substrate of the defective enzyme, as in phenylketonuria (phenylalanine) and galactosaemia (galactose-1-phosphate). Such accumulation may interfere with various vital functions, causing disease, and with other metabolic paths, producing secondary metabolic abnormalities. In other cases, deficiency of the immediate or more remote product is of more serious consequence, as in adrenal hyperplasia type 1 (lipoid hyperplasia) (cortisol) and the several forms of thyroid dyshormonogenesis (thyroxine). Sometimes accumulation of the substrate causes unusual side reactions with the formation of unusual products, and it is these that have the adverse effect. Thus in galactosaemia the formation of galactitol is the probable cause of the cataracts; certain forms of adrenal hyperplasia show both a deficiency of the product (cortisol) and the consequences (virilization and pseudohermaphroditism) of abnormal products (androgens) formed in this way. Another mechanism is illustrated by hypoxanthine–guanine phosphoribosyl transferase deficiency (Lesch–Nyhan syndrome) where there is a deficiency of the products guanylic and inosinic acids. These products normally inhibit the first – rate-limiting – step in purine biosynthesis and their absence allows this to proceed excessively, resulting in a greatly increased urinary excretion of uric acid, the normal waste product of purines. Thus this is a failure of feed-back control.

18.3.4. Tissue specificity of enzymes

Not all enzymes occur in all tissues. This sometimes has a bearing on the manifestation of an inherited abnormality and is of obvious importance in the approaches to be made in the diagnosis of the consequent disorder. For example, phosphofructokinase in erythrocytes and muscle are closely similar when examined by immunochemical methods but the two enzymes are different; whereas in glycogen storage disease type 7 the activity of the enzyme in muscle is almost totally absent, about half of the normal activity remains in the erythrocyte, so that if the latter were used for diagnosis a quite misleading conclusion might be drawn. In galactosaemia, galactose-1-phosphate uridyltransferase is deficient in both liver and erythrocytes and it is quite safe to use the latter for diagnostic purposes; however, there is another form of galactosaemia known as the "Negro variant" in which the leucocyte enzyme deficiency is less marked in heterozygotes than in carriers of the more usual form of the disorder.

In other instances, the distribution of an enzyme abnormality can explain differences between one disease and another to which it is apparently related. Thus of all the enzymopenic haemolytic anaemias, triosephosphate isomerase and phosphoglycerate kinase deficiencies are exceptional in that they are associated with neurological manifestations. In these instances, the enzyme deficiency is not only present in erythrocytes but also in leucocytes and presumably in other tissues not so far examined. Similarly, cytochrome b_5 reductase deficiency, a form of methaemoglobinaemia, is associated with neurological damage and here too the enzyme deficiency can be demonstrated in both erythrocytes and leucocytes; however the two abnormal forms of methaemoglobin reductase, associated with uncomplicated methaemoglobinaemia, can only be demonstrated as an enzyme deficiency in erythrocytes.

18.4 CLASSIFICATION OF INHERITED METABOLIC DISEASE

On first meeting this group of diseases, hardly any of which will have been encountered – even as single cases – by a clinical chemist or clinician, their large number can be forbidding. There are already 947 recessively inherited and 171 X-linked human diseases catalogued by McKusick (1975) and in 141 of these the precise enzyme deficiency is known. In these circumstances, the broad classifications used later in this chapter are helpful but, for those who seek to be more than superficially involved, these conventional groupings have disadvantages. For example, glycogen storage diseases types 2 and 5, which present with muscle weakness and pain respectively, have no clinical resemblance with types 1, 3, 4 and 6, in which enlargement of the liver and some other organs predominates. Similarly, angiokeratoma, diffuse (Fabry's disease) with renal and respiratory failure in young adults, although chemically related to other sphingolipidoses, is quite unlike the various types of GM_1- and GM_2-gangliosidoses, neurodegenerations likely to have proved fatal at an age well before that at which Fabry's disease will be diagnosed. At an early stage in the education of the clinical chemist the diseases should be regarded individually and care should be taken to define them precisely by using a standard nomenclature (perhaps with the McKusick number); earlier terms such as Tay Sachs disease, glycinuria, gargoylism and von Gierke's disease should be strictly avoided. At any time, an apparent disease entity may have to be split in the light of more recent knowledge, as, for example, the mucopolysaccharidosis type 3 – the Sanfilippo syndrome – into types A and B. More rarely, two or more separately described conditions may be recognized as having the same underlying cause (e.g. multiple sulphatase deficiency which was formerly listed as three distinct disorders) or represent different defects of the same enzyme (e.g. mucopolysaccharidoses types 1 and 5 now designated types 1H and 1S).

18.5. INHERITED BIOCHEMICAL ABNORMALITIES NOT ASSOCIATED WITH DISEASE

Because the first subjects with the particular disorder of phenylalanine metabolism happened to be inmates of mental subnormality hospitals, such hospitals became the hunting ground for those searching for new inherited diseases, all of which were associated with mental subnormality. An increasing number of the biochemical abnormalities discovered there and elsewhere is now proving to have been coincidentally associated with the disease in which they were first observed. There is no doubt that cystathioninuria, iminoglycinuria, prolinaemia type 1 and histidinaemia are biochemically unusual and that they are inherited, but in the first three there is no link with disease and in the fourth the link is, at most, very tenuous. (It should be noted that non-inherited cystathioninuria can be a dramatic and important association of hepatoblastoma and neuroblastoma, and prolinaemia type 2 may not be as benign as type 1.) Designation of another syndrome, comprising mental subnormality, hiatus hernia and sucrosuria, resulted from the failure to recognize that all babies readily excrete any ingested sugar in the first months of life (Haworth and McCredie, 1956; Haworth and MacDonald, 1957). Such mistakes may be avoided by seeking the biochemical abnormality in all close relatives of an apparently affected subject; in this way inherited variants will be found among healthy relatives, and if these are older than the propositus, this is a strong indication that the biochemical defect is benign.

18.6. SCREENING HEALTHY POPULATIONS FOR EARLY DETECTION OF INHERITED METABOLIC DISEASE

Following the discovery by Bickel et al. (1953) that rearing phenylketonuric infants on a phenylalanine-restricted diet prevented, but did not correct, the severe mental subnormality associated with this disease, it was clearly important that the disorder should be detected at the earliest possible age. Thus a dip-stick version of the ferric chloride test for phenylpyruvic acid in urine, "Phenistix", was introduced as a screening method, and by 1960 all babies born in Britain were being tested at 3 weeks of age. This test, however, failed to detect all cases of phenylketonuria and alternatives were developed. Woolf (1967) used one-dimensional chromatography of urine for detecting *o*-hydroxyphenylacetic acid, in combination with some simple tests for sugars, protein and sulphur compounds, and this was used for several years in parts of England and Wales (Bradley, 1975). In the U.S.A., Guthrie and Susi (1963) looked for an abnormal rise in blood phenylalanine concentration using a phenylalanine-requiring mutant coliform bacterium whose growth was suppressed by chemical inhibition. The presence of phenylalanine allowed a circle of growth, the size of which was proportional to the phenylalanine concentration, to occur round a disc of blood-soaked paper applied to an agar plate containing the bacteria. Because of its convenience and its established reliability – provided it is not performed before the sixth day of life (Medical Research Council Working Party, 1968) – this test has now replaced the ferric chloride test.

Except for Woolf's scheme, which can detect several diseases, the early tests only recognized phenylketonuria. Techniques that will discover several aminoacid disorders, based on one-dimensional paper or thin-layer chromatography applied to plasma, urine or to blood from the same spot used for the Guthrie test, have proved valuable (Efron et al., 1964; Scriver et al., 1964; Ireland and Read, 1972). Their application in several centres has shown that the incidence of both prolinaemia type 1 and histidinaemia is comparable with that of phenylketonuria. Other diseases such as tyrosinosis, tyrosine transaminase deficiency, maple syrup urine disease, homocystinuria and lysinaemia have also been recognized using these methods. When plasma is used, its creamy appearance has revealed several cases of hyperlipidaemia as early as the second week of life (Levy et al., 1968; Raine et al., 1972).

Screening methods for some other diseases – galactosaemia, tyrosinosis and glucose-6-phosphate dehydrogenase deficiency – have been devised and are suitable for application to healthy populations, but none of these has found significant application. Screening the Ashkenazi Jewish population for GM_2-gangliosidosis (Tay Sach's disease) has been applied more widely, with rather more interest in North America and Israel than elsewhere. The techniques are not simple, but a high proportion of this population are at risk and the effort is therefore rewarding. The technology of screening methods is always much simpler than their application in the community and no total population screening for any disease should be initiated without careful consideration of the criteria laid down by the McKeown Committee (Nuffield Provincial Hospitals Trust, 1968) and summarized by Raine (1969; see also Raine, 1974b, 1977).

18.7. SCREENING A PATIENT FOR EVIDENCE OF METABOLIC DISEASE

The first suggestion that a patient may be suffering from a metabolic disease will normally come from a physician who will have been alerted by some clinical feature. However, the analyses he requests will usually be limited or even inappropriate: the clinical chemist should ascertain the nature of the condition, for only then will he be able to institute the appropriate diagnostic procedures, either in his own laboratory or elsewhere. No single laboratory can expect to offer more than a selection of the necessary tests. In this way, as many as possible of the inherited metabolic diseases associated with a particular symptom or sign can be considered: there are at least 90 such causes of mental subnormality, 16 of haemolytic anaemia, 3 of ectopia lentis and 20 of hepatomegaly.

Where the clinical features are specially indicative, for example an unexplained metabolic acidosis in the organic acidurias, brittle hair in argininosuccinic aciduria, red macular spot in some sphingolipidoses, or Kayser–Fleischer rings in Wilson's disease, the definitive diagnostic tests may be performed immediately. However, in many instances there is little more than a family history of death or disorder in childhood, or a symptom or sign that could have causes other than an inherited metabolic disease, such as mental subnormality, a degenerative neurological disease, corneal or lens opacities or skeletal deformity. These circumstances call for a series of tests designed to indicate whether or not the condition has a metabolic cause and, if so, which group of substances is likely to be involved. Such tests can all be simple and there is no reason why they should not be offered by all laboratories. Indeed, several can be performed by the clinician (Perry et al., 1966; Buist and Jhaveri, 1973; see also Thomas and Howell, 1973; Shih, 1975). The selection of investigations in Table 18.3 is within the scope of most clinical chemistry departments; it affords considerable discrimination, and those disorders it will detect are indicated in the listing of Table 18.7.

TABLE 18.3.

SEVEN LABORATORY INVESTIGATIONS SUITABLE FOR SCREENING A PATIENT WITH AN UNKNOWN METABOLIC DISORDER

Abbreviation used in Table 18.7	Technique	Interpretation
A	Assessment of the colour and odour of urine freshly passed and after standing.	(Cone, 1968a, b)
B	Two-dimensional chromatography or high-voltage electrophoresis of urinary aminoacids	(Smith, 1969)
C	One- or two-dimensional chromatography of plasma aminoacids	(Smith, 1969; Scriver et al., 1964; Ireland and Read, 1972)
D	Cyanide nitroprusside test applied to urine	Some sulphur compounds (Brand et al., 1930; Roesel and Coryell, 1974)
E	Tablet copper-reducing test or Benedict's test *and* a glucose oxidase stick test applied to urine followed when positive by chromatography for sugars.	Reducing sugars (Smith, 1969)
F	Test for sulphite in fresh urine. (Test papers available from Machery, Nagel and Co., D-516 Duren, G.F.R.)	(Kutter and Humbel, 1969)
G	Alcian Blue spot test applied to urine followed by other related tests, including electrophoresis.	Mucopolysaccharides (Lewis et al., 1974)

These tests may be followed by a scheme of investigation involving chromatographic and other techniques such as that suggested by Berry et al. (1968). Here it is not the technique itself but the interpretation that discourages those without experience. This should not deter a clinical chemist from trying. If the result or its meaning is in doubt, reference should then be made to a specialized centre which expects to assist in this way. There is no other way of gaining experience with rare conditions.

18.8. RECOGNITION OF HETEROZYGOTES

There is ample evidence that the amount of protein produced by a cell is proportional to the number of structural genes controlling its synthesis. Thus in patients with trisomy, some enzyme activities are increased by 50%; generally, there is a reduction by 50% in subjects heterozygous for an abnormal gene whose product is almost without enzyme activity. If the genetic abnormality has a less severe effect on enzyme activity, then the reduction in the heterozygote will be masked, and may even be within, albeit at the lower limit of, the normal range.

Heterozygotes may be recognized by two methods: first, by determining the enzyme activity in a suitable body fluid, cell or tissue; second, by stressing the defective enzyme step with a load of its normal substrate, and demonstrating decreased tolerance, as revealed either by an increased and prolonged blood concentration, or by the excretion of unusual metabolites not produced by normal homozygotes. Neither method in any instance provides the basis for a complete and certain separation of heterozygotes from normal homozygotes.

The direct approach to enzyme activity is best but if it is applied to tissue, the parameter to which activity is referred must be considered. Thus enzyme activity has been referred by most authors to the protein concentration of the homogenate used for assay, but this gives less discrimination than when activity is referred to that of another enzyme believed to be unaffected in the disease under investigation. When cultured cells (leucocytes or fibroblasts) are used, further discrimination is claimed if they are brought to a more uniform stage of development under the influence of phytohaemagglutinin. Needless to say, the most precise enzyme assay available should be employed, even if this is less convenient than an alternative suitable for the recognition of an abnormal homozygote.

The loading tests are an indirect measure of the enzyme block, but they may provide the only reasonable approach as, for example, in phenylketonuria where useful direct enzyme assay cannot be performed without liver biopsy. The existence of tests for the heterozygous state and their basis – whether direct enzyme assay or a more indirect test – is indicated in the listing of Table 18.7.

Because of the inevitable difficulty of interpretation, it cannot be expected that the use of any one technique will determine the heterozygous status of any subject with absolute certainty. It is better to state a probability, using the methods described by Westwood and Raine (1973, 1975).

18.9. PRENATAL DETECTION OF AN AFFECTED FOETUS

In some countries, changes in the laws relating to abortion have encouraged the development of new attitudes towards the management of a foetus affected by genetically determined disease. However, these ideas are still new and there will undoubtedly be further changes in social attitudes, in laws governing these forms of technical intervention, and in the availability and form of medical genetic counselling services. It is most important that those concerned with genetic disease should remain sensitive to these changes and adapt to them. A useful summary of such medicosocial problems is given by Jones and Bodmer (1974) and Raine (1977).

Already there is a small demand, by those who risk carrying an affected foetus, for examination of amniotic fluid, in order that the births of infants with untreatable diseases may be prevented, and to allow the earliest introduction of treatment in those for whom it is available. The technology of these investigations is very new and it is unlikely that all the considerations necessary to ensure their reliability have yet been elucidated. Examination may be made of the amniotic fluid, of the cells suspended in it – some of which are dead – and of living cells obtained after a period of their growth in vitro. The composition of amniotic fluid at different stages of gestation is not yet well documented, so that attempts at the confident recognition of deviations from normality due to metabolic disease can be hazardous. Examination of uncultured cells can reveal the sex of the foetus, which is very relevant when the disease causing concern is X-linked: if female, health is assured; if male, the risk is 1 in 2. Microscopic examination of the cells may reveal a convincing number with inclusions, vacuoles or other unusual features from which affection of the foetus can be predicted. Enzyme assays on uncultured cells are without value because of the unknown proportion of dead cells in the sample, and it has been shown that even slight contamination with blood during amniocentesis can mask an enzyme deficiency (Sutcliffe and Brock, 1971). The safest procedure but one which conflicts most with the simpler methods of abortion, because of the time involved, is to examine living cells cultured from those obtained at amniocentesis. Here there are small risks that contaminating maternal cells may be cultured with, or in preference to, foetal cells, and that unrecognized multiple pregnancies may also confuse the diagnosis. Measurement of enzyme activity referred to that of an enzyme believed to be unaffected may be more discriminating than when referred to protein (section 18.8).

It should be remembered that a foetal heterozygote will have diminished enzyme activity and yet be clinically unaffected. At least one unnecessary abortion is recorded because a moderate lowering of activity was misinterpreted as indicating a homozygously abnormal foetus. The availability of tests suitable for prenatal examination is indicated in the listing of Table 18.7. Whenever possible, material should be sent to more than one laboratory because if cells fail to grow in one, there is rarely time to repeat the amniocentesis; agreement in results from two laboratories will increase the confidence of all concerned. In all cases, adequate explanation of the uncertainties should be given to the parents requiring prenatal examination, and the abortus should always be examined to discover whether or not the prediction was correct.

18.10 MONITORING TREATMENT

The details of therapeutic management vary greatly with the disease, and at any given time may not be fully worked out. Hence there is often the opportunity to combine something safe, according to established practice, with new developments conducted in a sufficiently controlled manner to allow unequivocal conclusions to be drawn. There are still many disorders for which no useful proposals for treatment have been made, and only symptomatic management can be offered. Indications of the status of some 200 disorders are given by Raine (1975).

The most usual approach to treatment of the aminoacid and carbohydrate disorders is to remove from the diet the constitutent whose metabolism is inhibited. Diseases for which treatment of established value is based on this principle include phenylketonuria, maple syrup urine disease, homocystinuria, galactosaemia and fructose intolerance. Because natural foods are replaced by artificial or synthetic mixtures, based on casein hydrolysates or, more recently, mixtures of synthetic L-aminoacids, it is important to remember that these may be inadequate with respect to some constituents such as vitamins, calcium and trace metals. Much useful information is contained in the pocket-book by Wood (1977) and in Raine (1975). The latter lists the locations of agents throughout the world from whom these special preparations can be obtained. Some lessons of general importance have been learned empirically from the experience gained in treating phenylketonuria. Phenylalanine restriction which is sufficient to reduce the plasma phenylalanine concentration to normal, often results in growth retardation, skin excoriation and other adverse signs. If too severe a restriction is imposed, and the phenylalanine concentration falls to a dangerously low value, catabolism of body tissue occurs with the release of phenylalanine; the plasma concentration then rises, which may lead the inexperienced physician to restrict dietary phenylalanine further. It is safer to reduce the plasma concentration to only 350 μmol/litre, and to monitor this value weekly at first, and thereafter montly. One-dimensional paper chromatography of plasma with appropriate standards can be a valuable guide if automated aminoacid analysis is not available. During any intercurrent illness, however minor, weekly checks should be made since dramatic changes in stabilization can occur. Nevertheless, the diet should not be altered if these disturbances are likely to be of short duration.

An important part of the management of homocystinuria is to avoid conditions predisposing to thrombosis; if anaesthesia or surgery, however minor, is contemplated the patient should be given pyridoxine (600 mg/day) until homocystine, methionine and the mixed disulphide in plasma each falls to a nearly normal concentration and that of plasma cystine shows a rise. (If there is no response in 3 days, a low-methionine diet with cystine supplements should bring about the same results.) This treatment should be maintained until 2 weeks after the operation, when pyridoxine should be gradually reduced to the minimum dose required to maintain normal concentrations of the sulphur aminoacids. When pyridoxine is used, plasma folate concentration should be checked and supplements given when this falls below normal.

Other diseases are monitored in other ways and details should be sought from those with experience of particular disorders. For example, methylmalonic aciduria may be treated with vitamin B_{12} until the urinary concentration of the metabolite falls.

There are several possible approaches to developing new treatments (Raine, 1972, 1975) and since opportunities come rarely, these should be explored within an ethical framework (Franklin et al., 1973), especially where no satisfactory treatment is yet available. However, it is essential that such experiments should be conducted with the full knowledge of all concerned and in a manner that allows reliable conclusions to be drawn from which others can benefit. Only in this way can progress be made with the treatment of these difficult and rare conditions.

18.10.1. Practical precautions and pitfalls

Some diets based on protein hydrolysates are supplemented with DL-aminoacids. The D-isomers are not metabolized but excreted promptly and usually in large amounts, thus interfering with any chromatographic studies made on urine. Even L-methionine may provide a special problem in monitoring the treatment of maple syrup urine disease. In these patients an important isomer, alloisoleucine, is obscured by methionine in analyses of plasma by ion-exchange chromatography, and it is necessary to treat the specimen with hydrogen peroxide to convert methionine into its sulphoxide which does not obscure alloisoleucine (Figure 18.1).

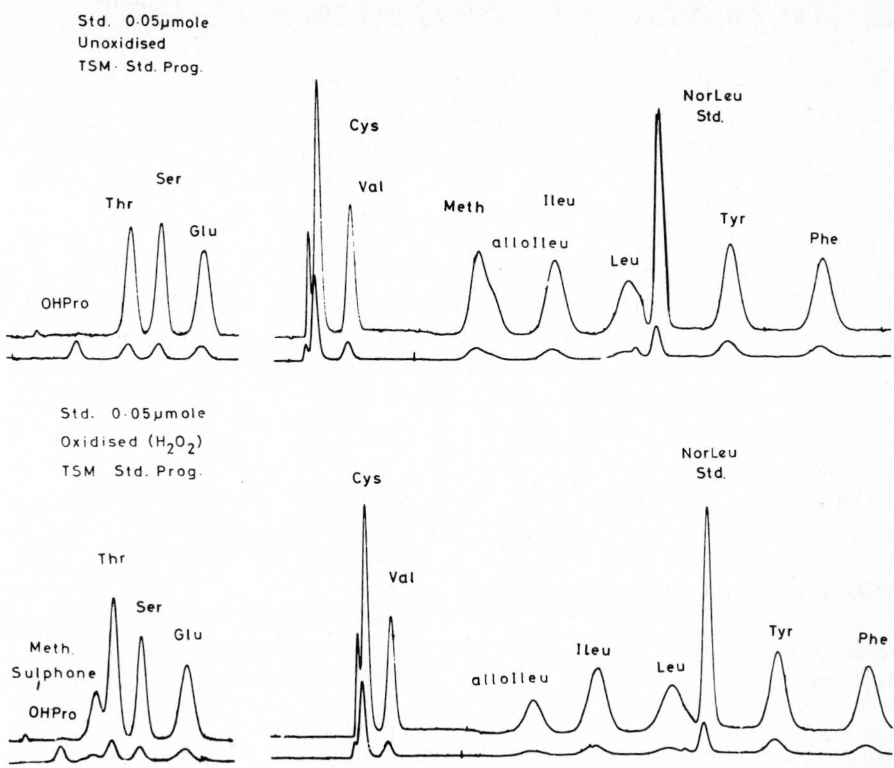

Figure 18.1. Chromatogram of mixture of aminoacids simulating maple syrup urine disease. (Technicon TSM analyzer with standard program.) The upper part, before oxidation, shows alloisoleucine as a shoulder on the right side of the methionine peak. The lower part, after oxidation of the sample with hydrogen peroxide, shows only alloisoleucine in this position so that this can be quantitated; methionine (as sulphone) now appears to the left of the figure. The two parts of each chart are not continuous.

Another dietary artefact is the urinary excretion of homocitrulline by infants fed on a formulation containing condensed milk. This aminoacid is formed during manufacture of the milk and stains pink with Ehrlich's reagent when this is used in the screening method of Scriver et al. (1964). In monitoring the treatment of homocystinuria, or investigating any other disorder of sulphur aminoacids, it is important to separate the plasma promptly and to deproteinize within 30 minutes of taking the blood, otherwise the sulphur aminoacids become bound to protein, leading to falsely low values on analysis.

Perry and Hansen (1969) give much valuable advice on avoiding contamination of plasma by leucocytes (which contain high concentrations of aminoacids), the avoidance and effects of haemolysis, the effects of storage of specimens and the extent to which different anticoagulants can interfere with analysis. The warning of Hamilton (1965) of the aminoacid content of a single finger-print should also be heeded by all staff concerned with any aspect of aminoacid analysis.

18.11. SOME GROUPS OF INHERITED METABOLIC DISEASES

The following sections of this chapter are headed by lists of relevant diseases (and the corresponding McKusick catalogue numbers) that may be encountered. Thus, all in the first section will present with an aminoacid or organic acid manifestation and may be detectable on a simple aminoacid chromatogram – even though, as explained in section 18.11.1), there are reasons why the former may not all be regarded as disorders of aminoacid metabolism. Where disorders come under more than one heading they are repeated in the appropriate lists. Further details for all these diseases are given in the listing of Table 18.7, the length of which emphasizes the futility of trying to commit this subject to memory. Instead the student should locate the appropriate reference works and only study certain diseases because they are clinically important or represent some general aspect of inherited metabolic disease. These diseases are marked with an asterisk in each sectional list. Thus, if the principles enumerated in sections 18.2 to 18.10 are understood and some 20 disorders are studied in greater depth, the student will have, in return for minimal effort, a knowledge of inherited metabolic disease which is distinctly above average.

18.11.1. Aminoacid and organic acid disorders

*Alkaptonuria (20350)
Argininaemia (20780)
Argininosuccinic aciduria (29790)
Aspartylglycosaminuria (20840)
Ataxia, intermittent (20880)
Blue diaper syndrome (21100)
Carnosinaemia (21220)
Citrullinaemia (21570)
Cystathioninuria (21950)
Cystinuria (22010)
*hyper*Cystinuria, isolated (23820)
Dibasic aminoaciduria, type 1 (12600)
Dibasic aminoaciduria, type 2, (22260)
*hyper*Glycinaemia, non-ketotic form (23830)
Hartnup disease (23450)
Histidinaemia (23580)
*Homocystinuria, type 1 (23620)
Homocystinuria, type 2 (23625)
β-Hydroxyisovaleric aciduria and β-methylcrotonylglycinuria (21020)
Hydroxyprolinaemia (23700)
Iminoglycinuria (24260)
Isovaleric acidaemia (24350)
Ketoacidosis, infantile (24505)
Leighs necrotizing encephalomyelopathy (25600)
*hyper*Lysinaemia (23870)
Lysine intolerance (24790)
Maple syrup urine disease (24860)
Methionine malabsorption (25090)
*Methylmalonic aciduria, type 1 (25100)
Methylmalonic aciduria, type 2 (25110)
Methylmalonic aciduria, type 3 (25112)
Ornithinaemia (25887)
Orotic aciduria, type 1 (25890)
Orotic aciduria, type 2 (25892)
*Oxalosis, type 1 (25990)
Oxalosis, type 2 (26000)
*Phenylketonuria (26160)
Prolinaemia, type 1 (23950)
Prolinaemia, type 2 (23951)
Propionic acidaemia (23200)
Pyruvate carboxylase deficiency (20880)
Richner–Hanhart syndrome (24480)
Sarcosinaemia (26890)
Sulphite oxidase deficiency (27230)
Tyrosinaemia, type 1 (27670)
Tyrosinaemia, type 2 (27660)
Valinaemia (27710)

---

* See introductory comments to section 18.11.

Although alkaptonuria is the archetype of the inborn errors of metabolism, a more familiar and typical example is phenylketonuria. Here, because of the low activity of liver phenylalanine hydroxylase, phenylalanine is converted into tyrosine at a very slow rate. There is no shortage of tyrosine in these patients, since they absorb more than is needed from dietary sources, but the plasma concentration of phenylalanine increases 30-fold. Values of 1500 μmol/litre are usual in untreated older children, and infants may have 5000 μmol/litre when first detected. As a result, the normal development of the brain is impaired and there appears to be a slight deficiency of myelination. However, the impairment of mental function is much more severe than would be accounted for by this alone and clearly damage of a different sort is also sustained. Why such concentrations of this aminoacid should be harmful is still not clear but there is evidence that several metabolic processes are interfered with. For example, the various indole derivatives excreted in the urine of phenylketonurics are due to secondary interference with tryptophan metabolism and the dilution of hair colour (fair in light-skinned races; red in the normally black-haired Japanese) is due to interference with melanin formation, a process requiring Cu^{2+} which is strongly chelated by aminoacids. The most favoured view of the effect of phenylalanine on the brain is that it inhibits protein synthesis; this effect can be demonstrated in rats at phenylalanine concentrations as low as 500 μmol/litre. The concentration at which treatment should be instituted has been set as high as 1000 μmol/litre, but many feel that concentrations sustained above 600 μmol/litre should be treated, and it has been cogently argued by Bickel (1970) that values higher than 400 μmol/litre may be harmful.

In infants, there are a number of causes of hyperphenylalaninaemia, some of which are transient, but in others concentrations of plasma phenylalanine of about 400 μmol/litre are sustained. These subjects do not show such severe, or indeed may not show any, clinical features. However they, and the occasional true phenylketonuric subject who escapes detection, may reach much higher phenylalanine concentrations during pregnancy; it is well established that this can cause microcephaly in the infant, even though the foetus is genetically normal. There is, therefore, every reason to test all women in early pregnancy for abnormal plasma phenylalanine concentration (by Guthrie or similar test) or for phenylpyruvic acid in urine (with ferric chloride). Pregnancy continues quite satisfactorily when those who need a low phenylalanine diet are maintained in this way.

Alkaptonuria is associated with the dramatic feature of black urine, but homogentisic acid – the precursor of the pigment – also reacts with cartilage; where this lies just beneath the skin, as in the external ear and bridge of the nose and in the sclera of the eye, the discolouration can be detected clinically. The associated degeneration of the cartilage may lead to narrowing of the intervertebral discs and consequently sciatic pain, but it is now recognized that arterial degeneration also occurs, and many patients die prematurely with coronary thrombosis. Diets low in phenylalanine and tyrosine are being tested but their value in the treatment of this disease is not yet established. Homogentisic acid is a reducing substance and alkaptonuric urine will therefore give a positive test with Benedict's reagent.

Reference to homocystinuria has been made already. It is important that the disease be managed well, either by pyridoxine or methionine restriction and, because of the tendency to thrombosis, hypotensive and dehydrating situations should be avoided. Where-ever possible, for example prior to surgery, more frequent monitoring should be performed and, if the patient is not being treated, the consequences of delaying surgery until this can be initiated should be weighed against those of thrombosis of which there is a substantial risk.

Maple syrup urine disease is well known, but because of its extreme rarity can hardly be regarded as an important disorder. It does, however, explain why this section combines a discussion of both aminoacid and organic acid disorders. Although usually recognized by an excessive excretion of branched-chain aminoacids – leucine, isoleucine and valine – maple syrup urine disease is a metabolic defect of the corresponding ketoacids. Scheme 18.1 shows this and also illustrates three further disorders – isovaleric acidaemia, β-methylcrotonyl CoA carboxylase deficiency and α-methylacetoacetic and α-methyl-β-hydroxybutyric aciduria.

Methylmalonic aciduria appears to be more common than other organic acidaemias, perhaps because it has several underlying causes. Scheme 18.2 shows that increased methylmalonic acid excretion can result from a deficiency of the enzyme proteins of methylmalonyl CoA racemase and mutase as well as from a deficiency of adenosyl-B_{12} reductase and of the enzyme that links the reduced hydroxy-B_{12} with adenosine. There is, in addition, a known inherited deficiency of transcobalamin II – the protein which is concerned with transport of vitamin B_{12} across the cell membrane. A further complication of this area of metabolism derives from the role of reduced hydroxy-B_{12} in the biosynthesis of methyl-B_{12} which is a co-enzyme for homocysteine – methyltetrahydrofolate transmethylase, the enzyme involved with remethylation of homocysteine to methionine. Thus in the deficiency of hydroxy-B_{12} reductase, there is interference with both methylmalonic acid and homocysteine metabolism and these patients present with both methylmalonic aciduria and homocystinuria.

All of the organic acid disorders may present either as acute (and often fatal) conditions in infancy or in a more chronic, even intermittent, form in older children. The symptoms are failure to thrive, vomiting, lethargy and hypotonia; these disorders should be suspected in any patient with an unexplained metabolic acidosis, with a base deficit which may be of the order of only 6 mmol/litre. Several cases have been discovered in children admitted to hospital for other reasons on no more biochemical evidence than this. Urine specimens should be analyzed by gas chromatography, preferably in an experienced centre, as the availability of mass spectrometry may be crucial in reaching a precise diagnosis speedily. Although thin-layer chromatographic techniques are available for methylmalonic acid, these will not detect all the organic acid disorders and hence they may be misleading if the patient has something other than methylmalonic aciduria. Once a specimen has been submitted for analysis it is a wise precaution to restrict protein until the results are available. Some disorders respond to vitamins (section 18.3.2 and Table 18.2) but it is most important that a specific diagnosis should be established before such treatment is initiated.

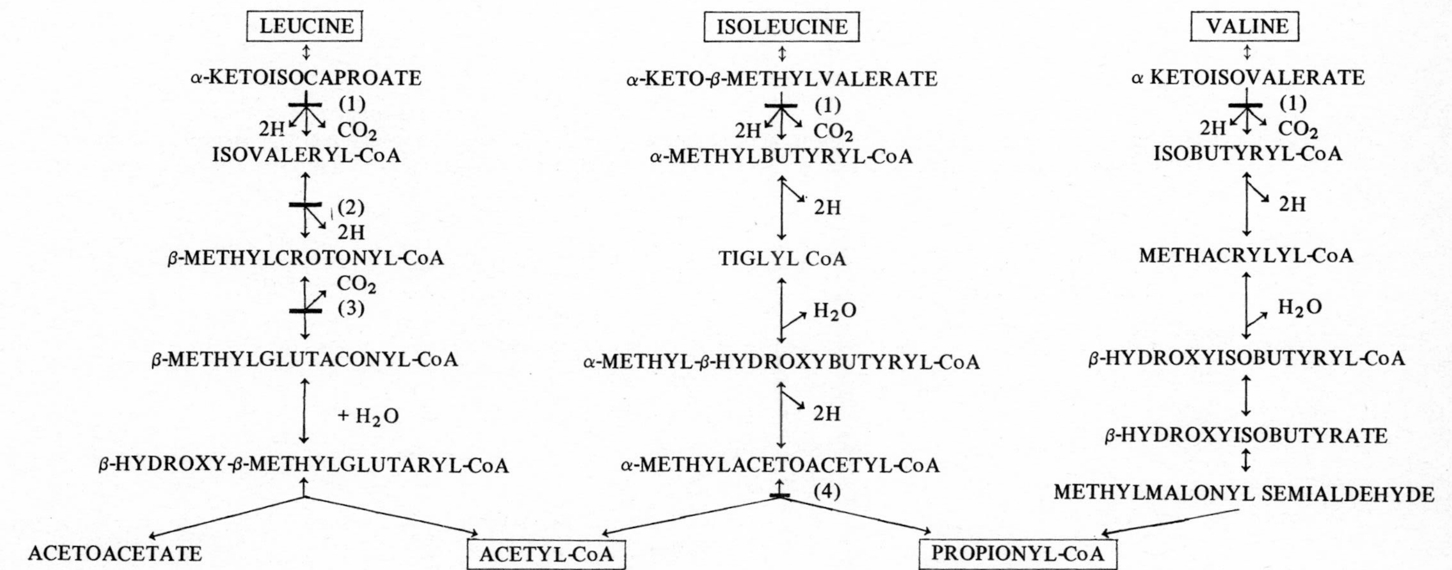

Scheme 18.1. Metabolism of the three branched chain aminoacids showing metabolic blocks in (1) maple syrup disease, (2) isovaleric acidaemia, (3) β-methylcrotonyl-CoA carboxylase deficiency and (4) α-methylacetoacetic and α-methyl-β-hydroxybutyric aciduria. (Reproduced, with permission, from Raine, 1975)

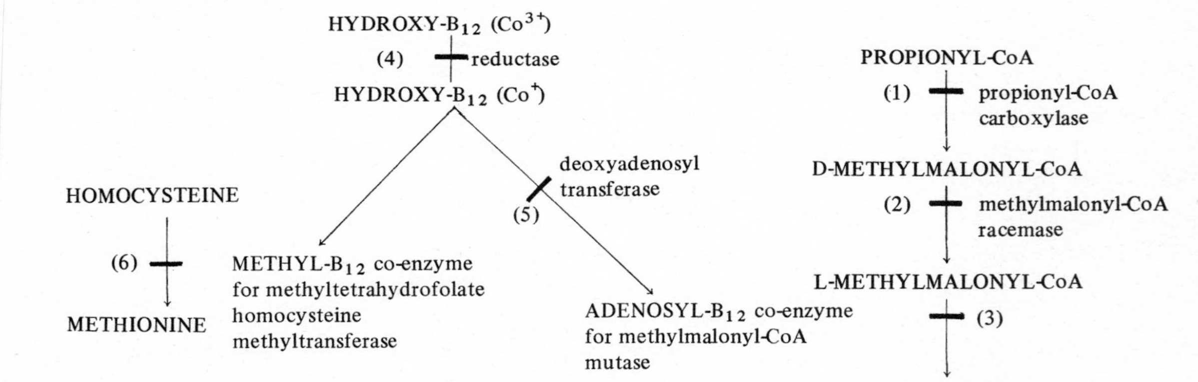

Scheme 18.2. Further metabolism of propionyl-CoA (see Scheme 18.1) with the several causes of methylmalonic aciduria and showing metabolic blocks: (1) propionic acidaemia, (2) methylmalonic aciduria type 3, (3) methylmalonic aciduria type 1, (4) vitamin B_{12} metabolic defect, (5) methylmalonic aciduria type 2, and (6) homocystinuria type 2.

18.11.2. Carbohydrate disorders

*Fructose intolerance (22960)
Fructosuria (22980)
Galactokinase deficiency (23020)
*Galactosaemia (23040)
Galactose epimerase deficiency (23035)
Glycogen storage disease, type 1 (23220)
Glycogen storage disease, type 2 (23230)
*Glycogen storage disease, type 3 (23240)
Glycogen storage disease, type 4 (23250)
*Glycogen storage disease, type 5 (23260)
*Glycogen storage disease, type 6 (23270)
Glycogen storage disease, type 7 (23280)
Glycogen storage disease, type 8
Glycogen storage disease, type 9 (McKusick type 8 (30600)
Glycogen storage disease, type 10
Glycosuria, renal (23310)
Hypoglycaemia due to glycogen synthetase deficiency (24060)
Pentosuria (26080)
Phosphoglucomutase deficiency

18.11.2.1. Glycogen storage diseases

The several disorders of glycogen metabolism are detailed in the listing of Table 18.7 but it is convenient to regard types 1, 3 and 6 (and the variants of type 6, types 8, 9 and 10) together, as they all present with the syndrome of hypoglycaemia, ketosis, enlargement of the liver and to a less extent of the kidney, all of which features diminish in severity after puberty. Type 2 is a distinct disorder due to lysosomal maltase deficiency which may present either with enlargement of the heart or with the clinical picture of muscular dystrophy. Type 5 is also a muscle disorder presenting in teenagers and adults, and it is not associated with organ enlargement. Type 4 is very rare and it is associated with enlargement and other abnormal changes in the liver.

The conditions can be distinguished using the following tests (Steinitz, 1967); measurement of plasma glucose concentration half-hourly for 3 hours after glucagon (which is more specific than adrenaline), both in the fasting state and 2 hours after a carbohydrate meal, and after an infusion of galactose; measurement of red cell glycogen; measurement of lactate after ischaemic exercise (type 5 only) and measurement of leucocyte acid maltase (type 2 only). The scheme of Fernandes et al. (1969, 1974) may be followed. Liver biopsy is usually only required to confirm a diagnosis reached by clinical chemical investigation. When biopsy is performed, the specimen should be submitted to an experienced centre both for enzyme assay – which may be less than straightforward – and for an examination of glycogen structure in terms of the relative lengths of inner and outer chains. In type 3 disease, in the fasting state, the outer chains will be very short and glucagon stimulation will not cause the plasma glucose concentration to rise. After a carbohydrate meal, the outer chains are reformed and glucagon can then stimulate a normal glucose response by hydrolysis of the glucose residues until the branch points in the glycogen structure are reached.

Treatment of glycogen storage diseases requires as much attention to the lipidaemia that accompanies some forms as to the hypoglycaemia, and the advice of Fernandes (1975) should be studied carefully.

---

* See introductory comments to section 18.11.

18.11.2.2. *Galactose disorders*

Galactose is normally converted into galactose-1-phosphate under the influence of galactokinase, and this then reacts with UDP-glucose to form UDP-galactose and glucose-1-phosphate under the influence of galactose-1-phosphate uridyltransferase. Deficiency of the latter enzyme occurs in galactosaemia, and deficiency of the kinase is associated with cataract formation in adults. Galactosuria in childhood, which may be due to either deficiency, is strongly suggested if on testing urine with both a copper-reducing test and a glucose oxidase test, the first shows reduction but there is no reaction with the second. If both are either positive or negative, the galactose disorders cannot be excluded since many infants excrete dietary sugars, which may include glucose, but dietary galactose will only be found in urine if it has been ingested in the previous 12 hours. Since in galactosaemia vomiting is a common symptom, this may have caused milk to be withdrawn and the infant to be fed on glucose–saline.

Galactosaemia may present in infancy with jaundice prolonged beyond the "physiological" period (10 days), enlargement of the liver and reluctance to feed with vomiting, but it is not uncommon for this to be mild or transient. Thus the diagnosis may only be made at 2 or 3 years of age when mental subnormality and cataracts are well established and irreversible. Whenever these disorders are suspected, the appropriate enzyme should be assayed in erythrocytes, and all infants born into families at risk should be tested using cord blood.

18.11.2.3. *Fructose disorders*

Fructose is converted into fructose-1-phosphate under the influence of fructokinase and thence into a mixture of trioses by the action of fructose-1-phosphate aldolase. Inherited defects of both enzymes are known in man; the first is entirely benign and recognized by the excretion of fructose in the urine; the second is a more serious disorder leading to vomiting, jaundice and hepatomegaly in infancy – very like the infantile symptoms of galactosaemia. However, many subjects learn to avoid sweet foods in later life and only reveal themselves by this unusual dietary habit, by their tendency to vomit when inadvertently exposed to fructose and by their total absence of dental caries consequent upon their life-long avoidance of glucose, the taste of which they are unable to distinguish from the affecting sugar.

18.11.2.4. *Glucose–triose defects in erythrocytes*

Glucose-triose defects, which are confined to the erythrocyte, all lead to haemolytic anaemia because of interference with the main source of ATP necessary to maintain the integrity of the red cell. The same clinical features occur in a group of defects in glutathione biosynthesis and metabolism which maintain the redox balance in the red cell necessary for its preservation. The stability of redox balance is also affected in a deficiency of the first step in the hexosemonophosphate pathway – glucose-6-phosphate dehydrogenase. The conditions are discussed in Chapter 7 but are also included in the listing of Table 18.7.

18.11.3. Mucopolysaccharidoses and related disorders

Mucopolysaccharidoses		Disorders clinically related to the mucopolysaccharidoses
Mucopolysaccharidosis	* type 1H (25280)	Aspartylglycosaminuria (20840)
	type 1S (25310)	Farber's lipogranulomatosis (22800)
	type 2 (30990)	Fucosidosis (23000)
	* type 3A (25290)	* GM_1-gangliosidosis (23050)
	type 3B (25292)	Mannosidosis (24850)
	type 4 (25300)	
	type 6 (25320)	
	type 7 (25322)	

This group of storage diseases derives from the early observations of Hunter, Hurler and others, who described children with skeletal deformity and a grotesque appearance, placing them under the collective name "gargoyle". It is now recognized that this description encompasses several distinct entities characterized by the urinary excretion of acid mucopolysaccharides (glycosaminoglycans). There are three such substances present in normal urine – chondroitin 4 and 6 sulphates and hyaluronic acid. An excessive excretion of one or both of the first two appears to characterize some patients, but most representatives of the group are associated with one or more of the abnormal glycosaminoglycans dermatan sulphate, heparan sulphate and keratan sulphate. These are polysaccharides with a characteristic repeating disaccharide linked by a series of monosaccharide units to protein. A knowledge of their structures, as indicated in Scheme 18.3 (which is in parts tentative and simplified), helps in the understanding of their clinical chemistry. The groups known to be present in the different glycosaminoglycans are shown in Table 18.4, which also records the precise enzyme deficiencies characterizing the several mucopolysaccharidoses; hence the particular glycosaminoglycans excreted in each disorder can be inferred (Table 18.5). Note how dermatan sulphate correlates with skeletal deformity and heparan sulphate with mental subnormality, particularly in the Sanfilippo syndrome where only heparan sulphate is excreted and mental subnormality is extreme.

The laboratory diagnosis of the mucopolysaccharidoses should proceed in stages: rarely should reliance be placed on one test, and never if this is performed on a urine collection of less than 24 hours duration. (The clinical chemist should retain a collection of results of the Alcian Blue test performed on random specimens of urine from a known case of the Hurler syndrome, type 1H, to convince the paediatrician of the need for this, as he will always be reluctant to make 24 hour collections of urine from these difficult patients.) Two qualitative tests, the Alcian Blue spot test and the albumin turbidity test are reliable and may be performed on urine collections of 18 hours or longer. The two quantitative tests – cetylpyridinium chloride-precipitable total uronic acid and the quantitative Alcian Blue test – require complete 24 hour collections of urine. The urine

* See introductory comments to section 18.11.

TABLE 18.4.

GLYCOSIDIC AND SULPHAMIDE LINKAGES IN MUCOPOLYSACCHARIDES (after Dorfman et al., 1975)

	Glycosides						
	β-Xylose	β-Galactose	β-N-Acetyl-glucosamine	α-N-Acetyl-glucosamine	α-Glucosamine-N-sulphate	β-N-Acetyl-galactosamine	β-Aspartyl-N-acetyl-glucosamine
Chondroitin-4-(and-6-) sulphate	+	+				+	
Dermatan sulphate	+	+				+	
Heparan sulphate	+	+		+	+		
Keratan sulphate 1 (cornea)		+	+				+
Keratan sulphate 2 (bone)		+	+			+	
Hyaluronic acid			+				
				↑ MPS IIIB α-N-Acetyl glucosaminidase			

The linkages enclosed in boxes are those which connect the repeating disaccharide chain with the protein chain (see Scheme 18.3). Below the table the different mucopolysaccharidoses with their associated enzyme deficiencies are indicated opposite to the linkage whose hydrolysis is impaired. Thus the mucopolysaccharides affected, and hence excreted, in each disorder can be inferred.

should be kept cold during collection and frozen thereafter since bacteria degrade the mucopolysaccharides giving false negative results. A positive result with any of these tests, which are all described by Lewis et al. (1974), should be followed by cellulose acetate electrophoresis of the urinary glycosaminoglycans. This will allow the almost certain diagnosis of mucopolysaccharidoses types 1S, 3A, 3B and 4, and the recognition of a group comprising types 1H and 2. Follow-up should be done, where possible, by the assay of the appropriate enzyme in cultured skin fibroblasts, and the diagnosis finally confirmed by cross-culture of these fibroblasts with those from a known case of the condition suspected. These last investigations will usually need to be done in a reference laboratory.

		Sulphatides					
β-Glucuronic acid	α-Iduronic acid	N-Acetylglucosamine-6-sulphate	N-Acetylgalactosamine-6-sulphate	N-Acetylgalactosamine-4-sulphate	Galactose-6-sulphate	Iduronic acid-2-sulphate	Glucosamine-N-sulphate
+			+(6)	+(4)			
+	+		+	+		+	
+	+	+				+	+
	+				+		
	+				+		
+							
↑ MPS VII β-glucoronidase	↑ MPS IH + S α-iduronidase	↑ MPS IV glucosamine-6-suphate sulphatase		↑ MPS VI galactosamine-4-sulphate sulphatase		↑ MPS II Sulphoiduronate-2-sulphatase	↑ MPS IIIA Glucosamine-N-sulphate sulphamidase

TABLE 18.5.
URINARY GLYCOSAMINOGLYCANS AND THE PREDOMINANT CLINICAL FEATURES IN THE SEVERAL MUCOPOLYSACCHARIDOSES

Mucopolysaccharidosis type	Urinary glycosaminoglycans	Predominant clinical features		
		Mental subnormality	Skeletal deformity	Eye defect
1H (Hurler)		+	+	+
1S (Scheie)	Dermatan and heparan sulphates	–	+	+
2 (Hunter)		+	+	–
3A 3B (Sanfilippo)	Heparan sulphate	+	–	–
4 (Morquio)	(Keratan sulphate)	–	+	+
6 (Maroteaux Lamy)	(Dermatan sulphate)	–	+	+
7 (β-Glucuronidase deficiency)	Dermatan and heparan sulphates and chondroitin-4- and -6-sulphates	+	+	–

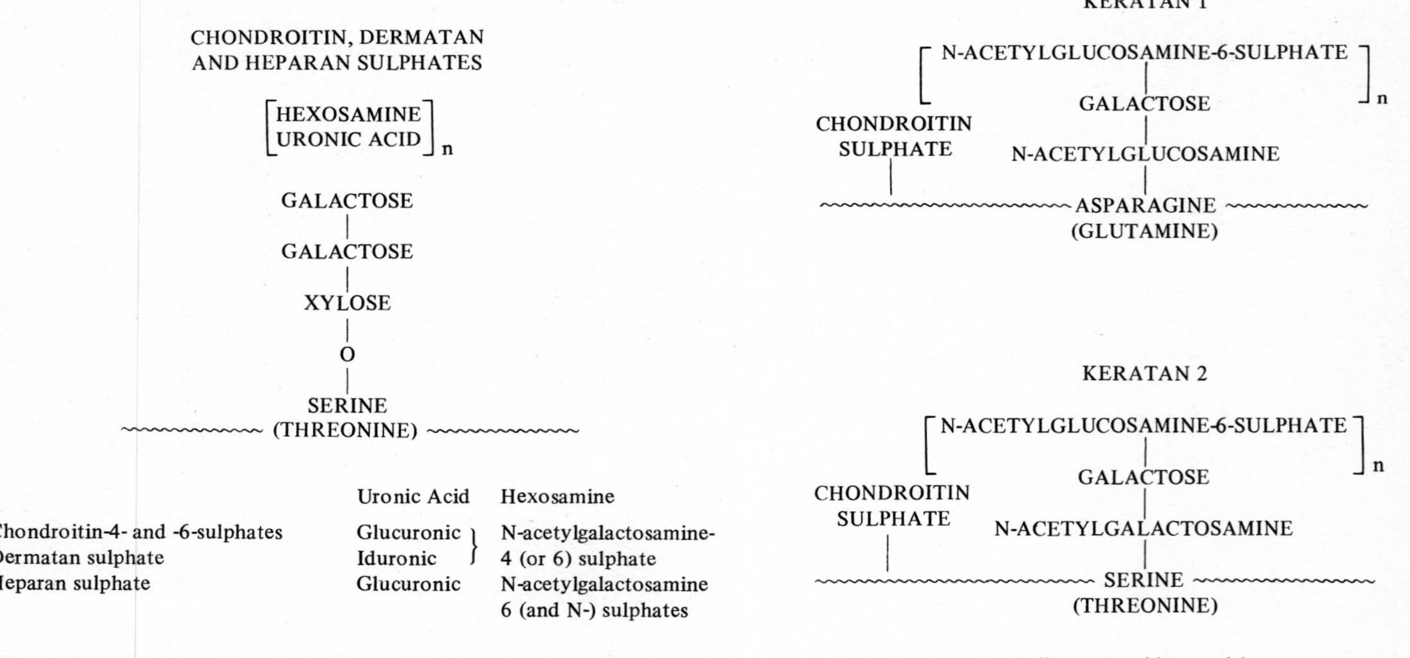

	Uronic Acid	Hexosamine
Chondroitin-4- and -6-sulphates	Glucuronic }	N-acetylgalactosamine-
Dermatan sulphate	Iduronic }	4 (or 6) sulphate
Heparan sulphate	Glucuronic	N-acetylgalactosamine 6 (and N-) sulphates

Scheme 18.3. The structures of some mucopolysaccharides

A valuable feature of the electrophoretic separation of urinary glycosaminoglycans is that when (together with negative findings of the other tests) a normal pattern is obtained in a patient with some clinical features of a mucopolysaccharidosis, this result can definitely exclude the latter diagnosis and allow a number of related syndromes, listed at the head of this section, to be considered. The full extent of this list of alternative diagnoses has yet to be determined, but meanwhile a number of differentiating investigations are already available and should be instituted.

18.11.4. Lysine intolerance, hyperammonaemia and urea cycle disorders

α-Aminoadipic aciduria
*hyper*Ammonaemia, type 1 (23720)
*hyper*Ammonaemia, type 2 (23730)
Argininaemia (20780)
Argininosuccinic aciduria (20790)
Citrullinaemia (21570)
Cystinuria (22010)
Dibasic aminoaciduria, type 1 (12600)
Dibasic aminoaciduria, type 2 (22260)
*hyper*Lysinaemia (23870)
Lysine intolerance (24790)
*hyper*Lysinuria with hyperammonaemia (23875)
Ornithinaemia (25887)
Orotic aciduria, type 1 (25890)
Orotic aciduria, type 2 (25892)
*hyper*Pipecolataemia (23940)
Saccharopinuria (26870)

A group of inherited disorders that well illustrate the disadvantages of a rigid chemical classification are those whose manifestations range from lysinuria and lysinaemia alone, through a subgroup with these biochemical abnormalities accompanied by vomiting and intermittent or more sustained hyperammonaemia, into the subgroup of metabolic defects of the urea cycle, some of which have similar, but others quite different, clinical features. It is still not possible to give a completely satisfactory account of these disorders, but the causes of confusion are becoming more apparent and the directions for further study clearer. The group is associated with more than its share of unusual observations and explanations, and a number of earlier studies have been, and perhaps still are being, misinterpreted because of failure to appreciate and control factors such as the following.

(1) Not all of the urea cycle enzymes are stable, and the efficiency of their extraction from tissues varies considerably with the buffers used (Maier et al., 1974). A report that in hyperammonaemia type 2 the liver carbamyl phosphate synthetase activity is only reduced to 20% of normal, provides unconvincing evidence that this enzyme deficiency is the primary cause of the disorder: on the other hand, see point (4) below.

(2) Some urea cycle and related enzymes are inhibited by ammonia, and arginase is inhibited by lysine; thus an apparent reduction in enzyme activity or the excretion of metabolites characteristic of certain disorders may be secondary phenomena.

(3) Ammonia production in some diseases depends very much on protein intake, and the results of metabolic studies in a basal state may be very different from those obtained after feeding.

(4) Hyperammonaemia type 1, due to ornithine transcarbamylase deficiency, is apparently inherited as an X-linked dominant. This is out of character with other enzyme

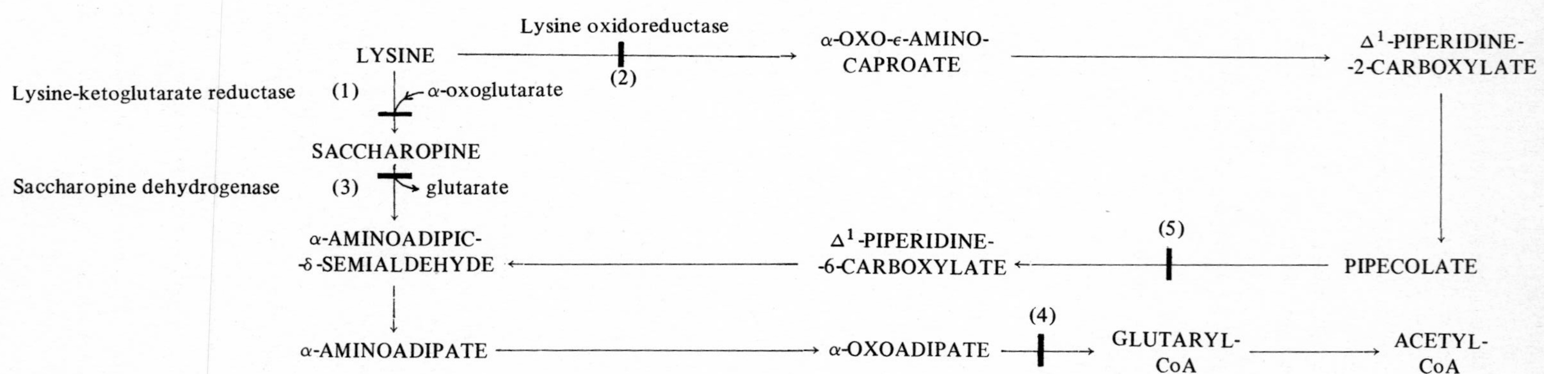

Scheme 18.4. Some metabolic defects of lysine metabolism. See Table 18.6 for summary explanations of metabolic blocks (1) to (5).

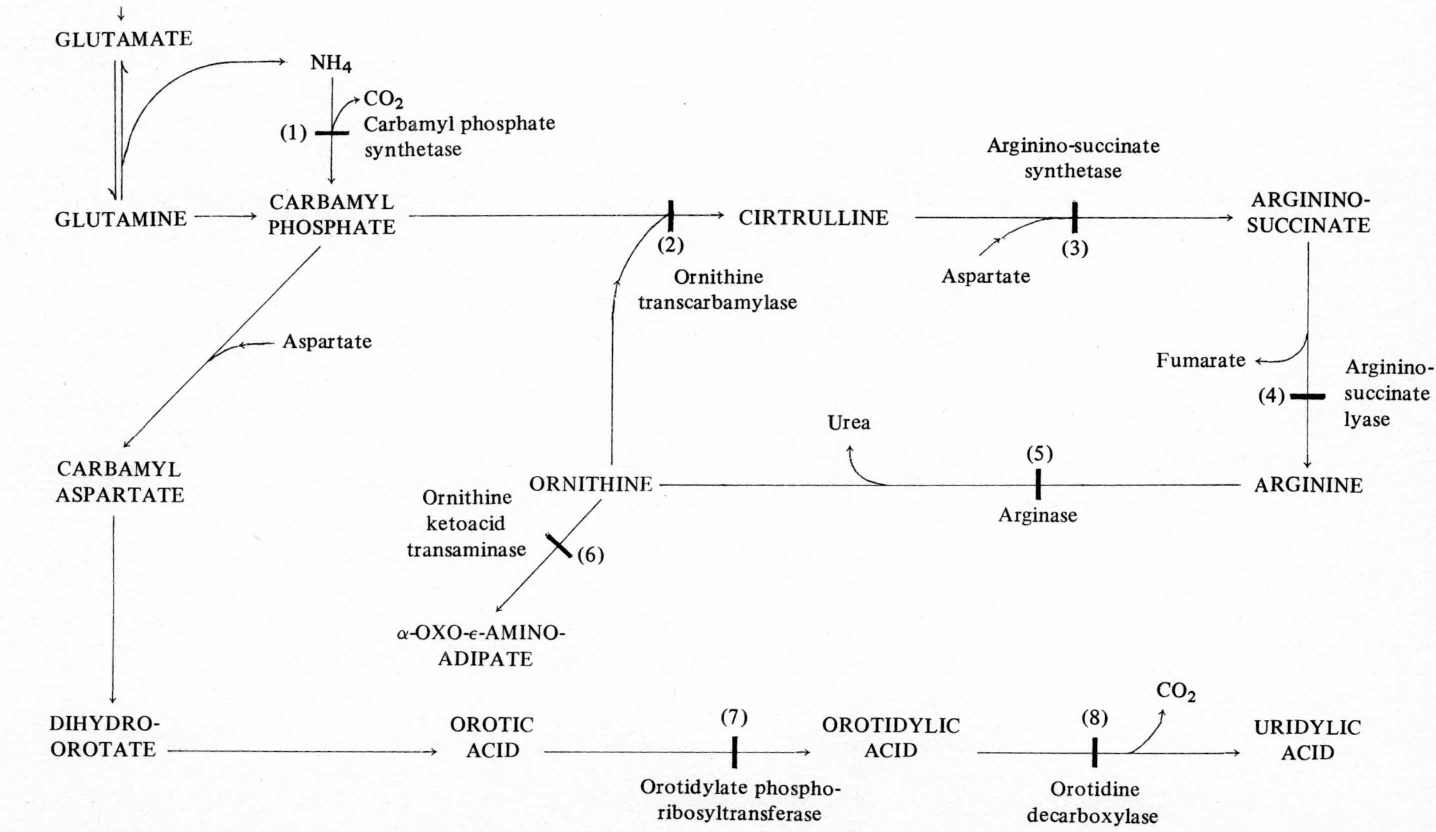

Scheme 18.5. Some metabolic defects of urea cycle substrates. See Table 18.6 for summary explanations of metabolic blocks (1) to (8).

TABLE 18.6.

DIAGNOSTIC CRITERIA OF METABOLIC DISORDERS OF LYSINE, AMMONIA, THE UREA CYCLE AND RELATED PATHWAYS

Disorder and enzyme deficiency	Plasma metabolites	Plasma ammonia	Urinary metabolites	Protein intolerance	Remarks
*hyper*Ammonaemia type 2 (23730) *Carbamylphosphate synthetase* see Scheme 18.5 (1)	Increased glycine and glutamine	Increased after protein	Increased glycine	Present	Liver enzyme must be assayed fresh. Reduction to 20% of normal in one case at autopsy. Association of hyperammonaemia with some organic acid disorders had led the existence of this defect to be questioned.
*hyper*Ammonaemia type 1 (23720) *Ornithine transcarbamylase* see Scheme 18.5 (2)	Increased glutamine	Increased	Increased glutamine and orotic acid (but less than in orotic aciduria)	Present	Sex-linked dominant inheritance. Liver enzyme 10% of normal in females. Complete deficiency in males.
Citrullinuria (21570) *Arginino-succinic acid synthetase* see Scheme 18.5 (3)	Increased citrulline	Increased after protein	Increased citrulline	Present	Liver enzyme less then 5% of normal; that in cultered cells may need low substrate concencentration in assay to demonstrate defect.
Arginino-succinic aciduria (20970) *Arginino-succinic acid lyase* see Scheme 18.5 (4)	Increased arginino-succinic acid, citrulline and glutamine	Normal fasting, increased after protein	Increased arginino-succinic acid and its anhydrides	Present	Enzyme deficiency demonstrable in most tissues including erythrocytes.
Argininaemia (20780) *Arginase* see Scheme 18.5 (5)	Increased arginine	Increased	Increased dibasic amino acids and cystine (due to competitive inhibition of tubular reabsorption)	Present	Enzyme deficiency demonstrable in erythrocytes.

Ornithinaemia (25887) (Shih et al., 1969; Fell et al., 1974; Shih and Mandell, 1974)	Increased ornithine	Increased	Increased ornithine and homocitrulline	Present	Presumed ornithine decarboxylase deficiency. Some evidence for this in fibroblasts, but may be mitochondrial transport defect for ornithine.
Ornithinaemia (25887) *Ornithine ketoacid aminotransferase* see Scheme 18.5 (6)	Increased ornithine ×3	Normal	Increased ornithine	Absent	Enzyme deficiency in liver; jaundice in infancy.
Ornithinaemia and gyrate optic atrophy (25887) (Simell and Takki, 1973)	Increased ornithine ×10	Normal	Increased ornithine	Absent	Gyrate optic atrophy.
Orotic aciduria (25890, 25892) see Scheme 18.5 (7 and 8)	–	–	Increased orotic acid	Absent	Two types, one with deficiencies of orotidylate phosphoribosyltransferase and orotidine decarboxylase (25890), the other with the latter only 25892).
*hyper*Lysinaemia (23870) *Lysine-ketoglutarate reductase* see Scheme 18.4 (1)	Increased lysine × 4	Normal	Increased lysine, homocitrulline, homoarginine and pipecolate	Absent	Mental subnormality not constant. Disorder may be benign.
Lysine intolerance (24790) *L-Lysine NAD oxidoreductase* see Scheme 18.4 (2)	Increased lysine (×2 to 5) and arginine (×2 to 7) on normal protein intake	Slight and moderate increases on low and normal protein intakes	–	Present	Liver enzyme reduced to 25% of normal. Hyperammonaemia may be due to inhibition of arginase by lysine.
*hyper*Lysinuria with hyperammonaemia (23875)	Decreased lysine and arginine	Increased following protein	Increased lysine, arginine and glutamate	Present	Resembles dibasic aminoaciduria type 2 but intestinal absorption of arginine and lysine defective.
Lysinuria (Oyanagi et al., 1970)	Decreased lysine, arginine and ornithine.	–	Increased lysine, arginine and ornithine	Absent	Resembles dibasic aminoaciduria type 1, but recessive inheritance and some clinical differences.

TABLE 18.6. (continued)

Disorder and enzyme deficiency	Plasma metabolites	Plasma ammonia	Urinary metabolites	Protein intolerance	Remarks
Saccharopinuria (26870) see Scheme 18.4 (3)	Increased lysine (×5) saccharopine and sometimes citrulline.	Normal	Increased lysine, saccharopine, homocitrulline, α-aminoadipic acid and sometimes citrulline.	Absent	Presumed deficiency of aminoadipic semialdehyde glutamate reductase.
α-Aminoadipic aciduria. (Lormans and Lowenthal, 1974; Przyrembel et al., 1975) see Scheme 18.4 (4)	Increased α-aminoadipic acid. Lysine normal.	Normal	Increased α-aminoadipic acid.	Absent	Two patients with mental subnormality. Fibroblast studies indicate a probable defect in oxidative decarboxylation of α-oxoadipate.
*hyper*Pipecolataemia (23940) see Scheme 18.4 (5)	Increased pipecolic acid (×10 to 40 depending on protein intake). Lysine normal.	Normal	Mild generalized aminoaciduria.	Absent	Enzyme deficiency inferred.
Dibasic aminoaciduria type 1 (12600)	Normal	–	Increased lysine, arginine and ornithine. (cystine normal)	Absent	Benign dominant renal and intestinal transport defect.
Dibasic aminoaciduria type 2 (22270)	Decreased lysine and arginine	Increased following protein intake.	Increased lysine, arginine and ornithine; sometimes cystine.	Present	Defective renal transport of dibasic aminoacids. Normal intestinal absorption of arginine and lysine.
Cystinuria types 1, 2 and 3 (22010)	Normal	Normal	Increased cystine, lysine, arginine and ornithine.	Absent	Renal tubular and intestinal transport defects. For differentiation, see Scriver and Rosenberg (1973).

deficiency diseases which seem to be invariably recessively inherited. This must mean that a reduction to about 50% in enzyme activity – the value usually found in heterozygotes – is sufficient to produce symptoms. In other diseases, a reduction by more than 90% is usual before the subject is clinically affected.

Those with the opportunity to study these disorders further should try to correlate simultaneously as many measurements as possible in blood and urine (lysine, ammonia, orotic acid, citrulline, homocitrulline, pipecolate and other metabolites); to investigate the patient both in the fasting state and on a low and high protein (or specific amino-acid) intake; and to perform enzyme studies whenever possible.

(5) Inhibition by substrate is also used to explain the fact that there appear to be two forms of orotic aciduria, one due to deficiency of two enzymes, orotidylate phosphoribosyltransferase and orotidine decarboxylase, and the other due to deficiency of the latter only. It has been suggested that the double enzyme deficiency, which was postulated because concentrating procedures and other forms of experimental interference affect the two enzymes equally, may be a defect in a structure linking them. Before such novel theories are espoused it is reasonable to consider whether a simpler and yet unknown factor is affecting the primary observations on which they are based.

Some of the disorders which are believed to reflect specific enzyme deficiencies are indicated in Schemes 18.4 and 18.5: because they are particularly difficult to distinguish from the medical and scientific literature and even from some text books, they are further detailed in Table 18.6.

18.11.5. Complex lipidoses

Fabry's disease (30150)
Farber's lipogranulomatosis (22800)
*Gaucher's disease (23100)
*GM_1-gangliosidosis (23050)
*GM_2-gangliosidosis, type 1 (27280)
GM_2-gangliosidosis, type 2 (26880)
GM_2-gangliosidosis, type 3 (23070)
Krabbe's disease (24520)
Lactosyl ceramidosis (24550)
*Metachromatic leucodystrophy (25010)
Niemann–Pick disease (25720)

The complex lipids – substances composed of a base (often sphingosine or glycerol), fatty acids, neutral monosaccharides, amino-sugars and neuraminic acid derivatives – are involved in cell membrane structure throughout the body and with myelin. There are several known inherited myelin disorders but in only two or three is the biochemical cause known: more progress has been made with the metabolic disorders of gangliosides, lipids which are quantitatively much less important in the brain than myelin, but of vital importance for normal neuronal function.

Several disorders are included on the metabolic chart in Scheme 18.6. Most are progressive degenerations of the nervous system, beginning after a few months of normal development and lasting about 2 years. GM_1-gangliosidosis is distinguished by hepatomegaly and spinal changes, the latter identical with those seen in mucopolysaccharidosis type 1H, but without the accompanying mucopolysacchariduria. GM_2-gangliosidosis types 1 and 2 are distinguished respectively by the absence of hexosaminidase A in the

* See introductory comments to section 18.11.

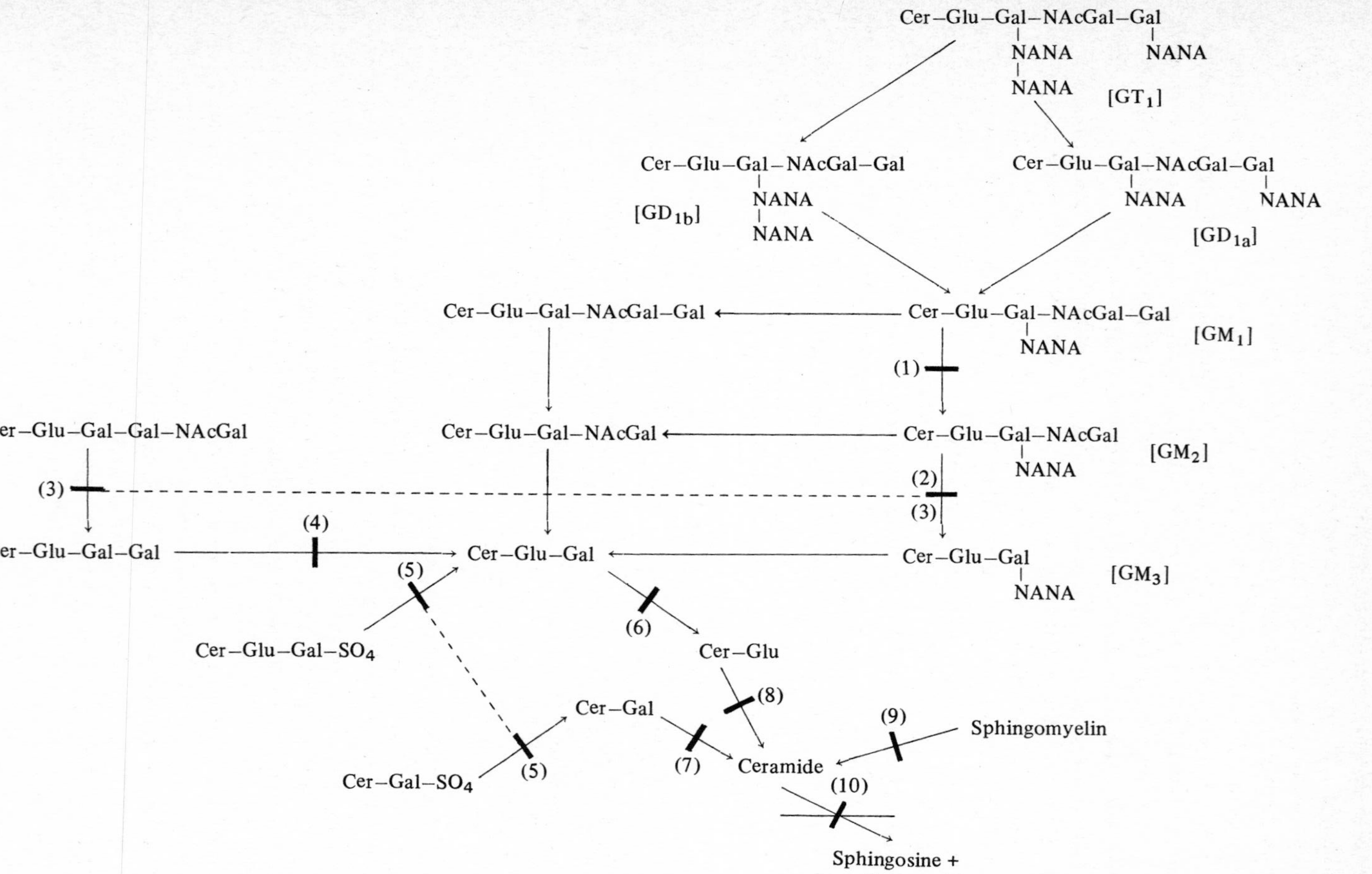

Scheme 18.6. Ganglioside metabolism. The chemical structures are represented by Cer = ceramide; Gal = galactose; Glu = glucose; NAcGal = N-acetylgalactosamine; NANA = N-acetylneuraminic acid. The metabolic blocks correspond to (1) GM$_1$-gangliosidosis; (2) GM$_2$-gangliosidosis, type 1 (Tay–Sachs disease); (3) GM$_2$-gangiosidosis, type 2 (Sandhoff's disease); (4) angiokeratoma, diffuse (Fabry's disease); (5) metachromatic leucodystrophy; (6) lactosyl ceramidosis; (7) Krabbe leucodystrophy; (8) Gaucher disease; (9) Niemann Pick disease; (10) Farber lipogranulomatosis.

first and both hexosaminidases A and B in the second. Total leucocyte hexosaminidase activity is absent in type 2 but normal in type 1, and the latter requires electrophoretic separation to demonstrate the absence of the A isoenzyme which establishes the diagnosis. Fabry's disease (angiokeratoma, diffuse) is unlike the other sphingolipidoses, presenting in young adults with skin nodules and progressive respiratory and renal failure, all caused by infiltration of the tissues with ceramide trihexoside whose further metabolism is prevented by deficiency of α-galactosidase.

Gaucher's disease, which is usually characterized by gross splenomegaly in adults, may present in infancy as a neurodegeneration. Here the enzyme is difficult to assay in a clinical situation; demonstration of the accumulated ceramide glucoside in biopsy material, in bone marrow, or in large amounts of urine sediment may be preferred for diagnosis.

The only disorders of myelin which at present can easily be investigated chemically are metachromatic leucodystrophy, the diagnosis of which is confirmed by the near absence of leucocyte arylsulphatase A (an artificial substrate is used instead of cerebroside sulphate which is not readily available), and Krabbe's leucodystrophy by assay of β-galactosidase using radioactively labelled galactocerebroside.

18.11.6. Transport disorders

Blue diaper syndrome (21100)
Chloride diarrhoea, familial (21470)
*Cystinuria (22010)
*hyper*Cystinuria, isolated (23820)
Diabetes insipidus, nephrogenic (30480)
Dibasic aminoaciduria, type 1 (12600)
Dibasic aminoaciduria, type 2 (22260)
Glucose–galactose malabsorption (23160)
Glycosuria, renal (23310)
Hartnup disease (23450)
Iminoglycinuria (24260)
Methionine malabsorption syndrome (25090)
Pernicious anaemia, juvenile (26110)
**hypo*Phosphataemia (30780)
Pseudohypoparathyroidism (26440)
Renal tubular acidosis, type 1 (17980)
Renal tubular acidosis, type 2 (31240)
Renal tubular acidosis with deafness (26730)

The transport of small molecules across membranes and across cellular boundaries such as the intestinal mucosa and the renal tubule, is an active process mediated by a molecular mechanism almost certainly involving carrier molecules which, like enzymes, have a catalytic function. It may be for this reason that, when a carrier mechanism fails, the disease, or a less serious biochemical consequence, shows recessive inheritance. Several studies have shown that in a number of conditions first recognized as transport defects of the kidney, these are accompanied by a similar defect in the intestine (Morikawa et al., 1966; Goodman et al., 1967), although this is not always the case (Rosenberg et al., 1966). This raises the possibility that the transport process may be defective at other sites less accessible to study, such as the blood–brain barrier or the liver.

There are five main transport mechanisms concerned with reabsorption of amino-acids in the renal tubule, and superimposed on these are some specific mechanisms,

* See introductory comments to section 18.11.

notably one for cystine. The five transport systems are concerned with the following aminoacids:

(1) Neutral aminoacids

leucine	*asparagine*	*serine*	*phenylalanine*	*glycine*	*cysteine*
isoleucine	*glutamine*	*threonine*	*tyrosine*	*alanine*	*methionine*
valine			*tryptophan*		*histidine*

(2) Basic amino acids and cystine

cystine *lysine* *arginine* *ornithine*

(3) Acidic aminoacids

aspartic acid *glutamic acid*

(4) Iminoacids and glycine

proline *hydroxyproline* *glycine*

(5) β-Aminoacids

β-alanine *β-aminoisobutyric acid* *taurine*

An almost complete failure of the first transport system occurs in Hartnup disease in which, but for the absence of proline and hydroxyproline, there is a generalized aminoaciduria. The symptoms of Hartnup disease are a pellagra-like rash and ataxia, and both could result from the wastage of tryptophan, the precursor of nicotinic acid.

Cystinuria results from a failure of the second transport system. Here the only symptoms arise from the presence of renal calculi; this is to be contrasted with cystinosis, which is a much more serious disorder. Symptoms of cystinuria may occur in childhood but some homozygotes remain trouble-free throughout life. Patients should avoid dehydration, and in some penicillamine is given because the mixed disulphide of this and cysteine is more soluble than is cystine. Most patients, however, are managed by regulating the fluid intake.

A patient who excretes proline with glutamic and aspartic acids may represent a defect of the third transport system (Teijema et al., 1974). Iminoglycinuria is due to an inherited abnormality of the fourth system; this is completely benign although it was once thought to be associated with disease (Joseph's syndrome). A defect of the β-aminoacid transport system has not yet been described.

A transport defect of the monosaccharides glucose and galactose associated with severe fluid diarrhoea is known, and glycosuria may also occur as a result of a less severe defect in the renal tubules. The condition is distinguished from the disaccharidase lactase deficiency by noting the clinical effect on the gastrointestinal tract and the rise in the concentration of reducing substances in the blood after oral loads of glucose, galactose and lactose. In lactase deficiency, the monosaccharides are well absorbed and do not cause diarrhoea, whereas in glucose–galactose malabsorption all these sugars are poorly absorbed (Meeuwisse and Melin, 1969). A number of renal tubular defects are referred to in Chapter 9.

18.11.7. Pharmacogenetics

Acetophenetidin sensitivity (20030)
Glucose-6-phosphate dehydrogenase deficiency (30590)
Isoniazid inactivation (24340)
Suxamethonium sensitivity (27240)

The term "pharmacogenetics" includes a number of phenomena which arise from genetically determined differences in a subject's response to the administration of a drug. These differences may be in the rate of excretion or metabolic inactivation of the drug, or in the production of adverse side effects in some subjects and not in others. For example, when the urinary concentration of *p*-aminosalicylic acid is determined after its administration to a normal population, the frequency with which different concentrations occur has a bimodal distribution. Similarly, the rate of acetylation of isonicotinic acid hydrazide, by which mechanism the drug is inactivated in the liver, is more rapid in some subjects than in others due to an underlying inherited enzymic difference. The proportions of "fast" and "slow" inactivators of isonicotinic acid hydrazide varies with different populations, fast excretors being more common in Japanese than in Caucasians. Clearly, the dose schedule required to maintain effective plasma concentrations of these two antitubercular drugs will depend on the genotype of the subject: it is probable that the failure of antituberculosis programmes in some countries where minimal doses were administered on economic grounds can be partly explained in this way.

There are other more serious examples of pharmacogenetics in which drugs produce side effects in some subjects. The haemolytic anaemia which was seen in some American soldiers of African origin when given prophylactic doses of antimalarial drugs during the Korean war led to the recognition of glucose-6-phosphate dehydrogenase deficiency – a completely benign trait as long as the subject does not receive one of a now long list of drugs which interfere with redox balance within the erythrocyte. Suxamethonium sensitivity is another inherited deficiency which remains unrecognized until the subject is given this muscle relaxant. The near absence of plasma cholinesterase prolongs the paralysis induced by the drug from a few minutes to a few hours. This defect is of special interest since it provides a good example of multiple allelic defects, and determination of the extent to which the enzyme activity (however low) can be inhibited by various chemicals (notably dibucaine and fluoride) allows the different genotypes to be identified. Thus apart from the normal gene in the homozygous state (UU), there are homozygous variants of the dibucaine type (DD), fluoride type (FF), a type in which activity is absent – the silent type (SS) – and every possible combination of normal and mixed heterozygote (UD, UF, US, DF, DS and FS); human examples are now known for all of these classes. The precipitation of symptoms by barbiturates and other drugs in patients with porphyria may depend on similar, but as yet unidentified, factors concerned with the metabolism of these drugs.

Evidence for a genetic basis for the difference in the rates of metabolism of drugs has been obtained from a study of the response in pairs of twins when given the same dose. Dependence on a genetic factor is strongly suggested if homozygous twins, who have the same genetic constitution, show the same degree of response while dizygous twins, who are as likely to be as genetically different as any other pair of siblings, show a mixture of

(continued on p. 1002)

TABLE 18.7

CLINICAL FEATURES AND INVESTIGATIONAL POSSIBILITIES OF SOME INHERITED METABOLIC DISEASES

Such a table can be neither complete nor wholly accurate. It may be scanned either for the disease or for symptoms. The "Clinical Features" column does not contain sufficient information for diagnosis and is only intended to lead to further sources of information.

Disorder. The alphabetical system adopted is that of McKusick (1975), modified to accord with British spelling. Prefixes indicating quantity – for example *hyper-*, *hypo-*, *a-* and Greek letters – are ignored for listing purposes. The number in brackets is that of McKusick; those starting with 2 and 3 are recessive and X-linked respectively.

Clinical features. The severity of the condition is graded 1 to 4. Benign disorders are designated 1; 2 includes those benign conditions which underlie drug-induced diseases; 3 = mild to moderate; 4 = severe to lethal. The main presentation is indicated by M = mental subnormality, N = neurological degeneration, E = eye abnormalities, and O = other features. The last two are subdivided.

Biochemical diagnosis. This column has up to three entries.

(S) denotes a screening test of the type discussed in section 18.6 and the most suitable tests are designated A to G as detailed in Table 18.3.

(I) denotes further chemical investigations that will help to establish the diagnosis but which alone may not be definitive.

(D) indicates the definitive investigation which generally will involve the assay of a specific enzyme. + The assay of those so marked is discussed by Raine and Westwood in Wilkinson (1976).

Treatability. This is designated Est = established, Prom = promising results with initial trials, Exp = still experimental, Symp = there is no specific therapy and treatment should be directed to relieve unpleasant symptoms.

** Those disorders for which specific advice on treatment is given in Raine (1975) are marked with a double asterisk.

* Those for which only references relating to attempts at treatment are given in an appendix in Raine (1975) are marked with a single asterisk.

Heterozygote test. Enz = based on enzyme assay, Indir = indirect – i.e. loading tests and other studies, Lyon = staining for two populations of cells as predicted by the Lyon hypothesis.

Prenatal diagnosis. The criteria for this are not yet established with certainty in any instance. "Cells" denotes diagnosis reached by morphological examination of amniotic cells. "Fluid" denotes diagnosis by examination of a soluble constituent. "Enz" denotes that the enzyme is present in amniotic cells almost always after culture or cultures of skin fibroblasts and therefore an affected foetus might be expected to be associated with cells deficient in the enzyme.

Enzyme. The number in brackets is that of The Enzyme Commission (Commission on Biochemical Nomenclature, 1972 and Biochimica et Biophysica Acta (1976), Supplement).

Disorder (McKusick No.)	Clinical features	Biochemical diagnosis	Treat-ability	Hetero-zygote detec-tion	Prena-tal diag-nosis	Enzyme deficiency (E.C. number)
Acetophenetidin sensitivity (20030)	2O – anaemia, cyanosis	S A I blood methaemoglobin; urine ferric chloride test D –	Est.	Indir.	–	–

Acid phosphatase deficiency (20095)	4O – vomiting, anaemia, hepatomegaly	S I D	– – fibroblast enz.	Symp. *	–	Enz.	Acid phosphatase (3.1.3.2)
Acrodermatitis enteropathica (20110)	4O – alopecia, dermatitis, diarrhoea	S I D	– plasma zinc –	Est. *	–	–	–
Addison disease and cerebral sclerosis (30010)	**4MNO** – skin pigmentation	S I D	– plasma cortisol, glucose and electrolytes; glucose tolerance test; ACTH stimulation test –	Symp.	–	–	–
Addison disease and spastic paraplegia (20150)	4NO – skin pigmentation, hypoglycaemia	S I D	– plasma cortisol, glucose and electrolytes; glucose tolerance test; ACTH stimulation test –	Symp. *	–	–	–
Adenosine triphosphatase deficiency, anaemia due to (10280)	3O – anaemia	S I D	– – erythrocyte enz.	Symp.	Enz.	–	Adenosine triphosphatase (3.6.1.3)
Adenylate kinase deficiency, anaemia due to (20160)	4O – anaemia	S I D	– erythrocyte starch gel electrophoresis of enz. erythrocyte enz.	Symp. *	Enz.	–	Adenylate kinase (2.7.4.3)
Adrenal hyperplasia type 1 (20171)	4O – genital abnormalities	S I D	– serum cortisol, aldosterone –	Est. *	–	–	20,22-Cholesterol desmolase
Adrenal hyperplasia type 2 (20181)	4O – genital abnormalities	S I D	– urine dehydroepiandrosterone, plasma cortisol (dec.), urine 5-pregnene-3α,17α,20β-triol –	Est.	–	–	3β-Hydroxy-Δ^5-steroid dehydrogenase (1.1.1.145)
Adrenal hyperplasia type 3 (with defect in 21-hydroxylase) (20191)	4O – genital abnormalities	S I D	– serum 17α-hydroxyprogesterone; urine pregnanetriol –	Est.	Indir.	–	Steroid 21-monooxygenase (1.14.99.10)

Table 18.7 (continued)

Disorder (McKusick No.)	Clinical features	Biochemical diagnosis	Treat-ability	Hetero-zygote detec-tion	Prena-tal diag-nosis	Enzyme deficiency (E.C. number)
Adrenal hyperplasia type 4 (20201)	**4O** – genital abnormalities, hypertension	S – I serum 11-deoxycortisol; urine tetrahydro-11-deoxycortisol D –	Est.	–	–	Steroid 11β-monooxygenase (1.14.15.4)
Adrenal hyperplasia type 5 (20211)	**3O** – genital abnormalities, hypertension	S – I serum cortisol, deoxycorticosterone, luteinising hormone and follicle stimulating hormone D –	Est.	–	–	Steroid 17-α-monooxygenase (1.14.9.99)
Adrenal unresponsiveness to ACTH (20220)	**4O** – pigmentation, hypoglycaemia	S – I serum ACTH and cortisol; urine aldosterone D –	Est.	–	–	–
hyper-β-Alaninaemia (23740)	**4N**	S B I quant. urine and plasma aminoacids D –	Symp. *	–	–	–
Alaninuria with microcephaly, dwarfism, enamel hypoplasia, diabetes mellitus (20290)	**3MNO** – microcephaly, dwarfism, teeth	S B, C, E I quant. urine and plasma aminoacids; blood alanine, pyruvate and lactate following oral glucose D –	Symp. *	–	–	
Albinism, type 1 (20310)	**3E** – depigmentation **O** – skin and hair depigmentation	S – I hair bulb enz. D –	Symp.	–	–	Monophenol monooxygenase (1.14.18.1)

Aldolase A deficiency (20335)	**3MO** – hepatomegaly, anaemia	S – I – D erythrocyte enz.	Symp.	–	–	Fructose bisphosphate aldolase (4.1.2.13)
Aldosterone deficiency (20340)	**4O** – dehydration, growth retardation	S – I serum or urine aldosterone, cortisol and corticosterone; urine tetrahydrocorticosterone D 18-hydroxytetrahydrocorticosterone	Est. *	Indir.	–	18-Hydroxysteroid oxidoreductase
Alkaptonuria (20350)	**3NE** – ochronosis **O** – arthritis, black urine	S A I urinary homogentisic acid chromatog. D liver enz. +	Prom. *	–	–	Homogentisate 1,2-dioxygenase (1.13.11.5)
β-Aminoisobutyric acid (BAIB), urinary excretion of (21010)	1	S B I blood and urine quant. amino-acid analysis D –	None req'd	Indir.	–	–
*hyper*Ammonaemia type 1 (23720)	**4MNO** – vomiting	S B C I quant. plasma and urine amino-acids ($GluNH_2$); blood ammonia D liver enz. + (note sex difference)	Exp. *	–	–	Ornithine carbamoyltransferase (2.1.3.3.)
*hyper*Ammonaemia type 2 (23730)	**4MNO** – vomiting	S B C I quant. plasma and urine amino-acids, (Gly, $GluNH_2$); blood ammonia D liver enz. +	Exp. *	–	–	Carbamoylphosphate synthase (ammonia) (1.7.2.5)
Anaemia, hypochromic (30130)	**4O** – anaemia	S – I – D bone marrow enz.	Est. *	Lyon	–	δ-Aminolaevulinate synthetase (2.3.1.37)
Angiokeratoma, diffuse (Fabry disease) (30150)	**3E** – cataracts, retinal pigmentation **O** – skin, renal and pulmonary failure	S – I urine sediment lipids D leucocyte or urine enz. +	Exp. *	Enz.	Enz.	α-Galactosidase (3.2.1.22)

Table 18.7 (continued)

Disorder (McKusick No.)	Clinical features	Biochemical diagnosis	Treat-ability	Hetero-zygote detec-tion	Prena-tal diag-nosis	Enzyme deficiency (E.C. number)
Angioneurotic oedema (10610)	**3O** – oedema	S – I – D serum C_1 esterase inhibitor	Symp.	Quant. C_1 esterase inhibitor	–	C_1 esterase inhibitor
Antitrypsin deficiency of plasma (20740)	**3O**-respiratory, liver	S – I – D serum α_1-antitrypsin including genotype	Symp. *	Quant. anti-trypsin	–	α_1-Antitrypsin
Argininaemia (20780)	**3MN**	S B C I quantitative plasma and urine aminoacids; blood ammonia D erythrocyte enz. +	Symp. *	–	–	Arginase (3.5.3.1)
Argininosuccinic aciduria (20790)	**3MNO** – hepatomegaly, hair	S B C I quant. plasma, C.S.F. and urine aminoacids (before and after hydrolysis) D erythrocyte and fibroblast enz. +	Exp. *	Enz.	Enz.	Argininosuccinate lyase (4.3.2.1)
spartylglycosaminuria (20840)	**3MNO** – skin, bone	S B I – D leucocyte enz. +	Symp.	Enz.	Enz.	Aspartylglucosyl-aminase (3.5.1.26)
taxia, intermittent with pyruvate dehydrogenase (decarboxylase) deficiency (20880)	**3NE** – nystagmus	S B C I urine and plasma lactate and pyruvate D leucocyte enz.	Symp.	Enz.	Enz.	Pyruvate decarb-oxylase (4.1.1.1.)

Ataxia-telangiectasia (20890)	**3NO** – telangiectasia, infection	S – I serum immunoglobulin; α-foetoprotein; lymphocyte and fibroblast chromosome and enz. studies D –	Symp.	–	–	DNA excision (γ-radiation damage) repair enzyme
*hyper*Bilirubinaemia, Arias type (14380)	3O – jaundice	S – I serum unconjugated bilirubin; menthol conjugation test D liver enz.	Symp.	–	–	UDP-glucuronosyl-transferase (2.4.1.17)
*hyper*Bilirubinaemia, shunt (23780)	3O – jaundice	S – I serum unconjugated bilirubin; urine and faecal urobilinogen D –	Symp. *	–	–	–
*hyper*Bilirubinaemia, transient familial neonatal (23790)	3O – jaundice	S – I serum conjugated and unconjugated bilirubin; maternal serum inhibition of conjugation of bilirubin by rat liver slices D –	Symp. *	–	–	–
*hyper*Bilirubinaemia type 1 (Gilbert) (14350)	2O – jaundice	S – I serum conjugated and unconjugated bilirubin before and after 24 hours on 400 calorie diet, or the same measurements before and after 50 mg nicotinic acid i.v. D liver enz.	Symp.	–	–	UDP-glucuronosyl-transferase (2.4.1.17)
*hyper*Bilirubinaemia type 2 (Dubin–Johnson) (23750)	2O – jaundice	S – I serum unconjugated and conjugated bilirubin; bromosulphthalein retention test; ratio of isomers I and III of coproporphyrin in urine D –	Symp.	–	–	Defect in excretion of bilirubin from liver to biliary tract

Table 18.7 (continued)

Disorder (McKusick No.)	Clinical features	Biochemical diagnosis	Treat-ability	Hetero-zygote detec-tion	Prena-tal diag-nosis	Enzyme deficiency (E.C. number)
*hyper*Bilirubinaemia type 3 (Rotor) (14370)	3O – jaundice	S – I serum conjugated and unconjugated bilirubin; bromosuphthalein retention; absence of black pigment in liver biopsy D –	Symp.	–	–	–
Bloom syndrome (21090)	4O – skin, dwarf	S – I spontaneous chromosome breakage in peripheral lymphocytes and chromatid interchange between homologous chromosomes D –	Symp.	–	–	DNA polymerase
Blue diaper syndrome (21100)	**4MO** – constipation	S – I hypercalcaemia; indole chromatog. urine and faeces before and after Try load D –	Symp.	Indir.	–	Intestinal tryptophan absorption defect
Byler disease (21160)	4O – jaundice, hepatosplenomegaly, malabsorption	S – I serum bilirubin, transaminase, alkaline phosphatase, cholesterol, bile salts; bromosulphthalein retention D –	Exp.	–	–	–
*hyper*Calcaemia, idiopathic (23800)	**3MO** – aortic stenosis	S – I serum calcium (total and ionized), phosphate; calcium infusion test D –	Symp.	–	–	–

*hyper*Calciuria (23810)	3O – skeletal	S – I urine calcium; calcium balance D –	Exp.	–	–	–
Carnosinaemia (21220)	**4MN**	S B C I quant. plasma and urine amino-acids (carnosine); serum enz. (low values not definitive) D –	Symp.	–	–	Aminoacylhistidine dipeptidase (3.4.13.3)
*a*Catalasaemia (20020)	3O – gum hypertrophy	S – I decol. acid $KMnO_4$ by haemolysate added to H_2O_2 D erythrocyte enz.	Symp.	Enz.	–	Catalase (1.11.1.6)
Cerebral cholesterinosis (cerebrotendinous xanthomatosis) (21370)	**4MN** **E** – cataracts **O** – tendon xanthomata	S – I serum and duodenal fluid cholestanol D –	Exp. *	–	–	–
Chloride diarrhoea, familial (21470)	4O – diarrhoea	S – I faecal chloride D –	Est. *	–	–	Colonic chloride transport defect
Cholesterol ester storage disease of liver (21500)	3O – hepatomegaly	S – I serum cholesterol and bile acids; liver cholesterol ester D liver enz.	Symp.	Enz.	–	Acid lipase
Citrullinuria (21570)	**4MNO** – vomiting	S B C I quant. plasma and urine aminoacids D fibroblast or liver enz. +	Exp. *	Enz.	Enz.	Argininosuccinate synthetase (6.3.4.5)
Cockayne syndrome (21640)	**4MNO**-skeletal	S – I clinical observations only D –	Symp.	–	–	Slow DNA synthesis
Complement component C1r, deficiency of (21695)	3O – recurrent infections, skin, joints	S – I serum C1r D	Symp.	–	–	Complement C1r

Table 18.7 (continued)

Disorder (McKusick No.)	Clinical features	Biochemical diagnosis	Treat-ability	Hetero-zygote detec-tion	Prena-tal diag-nosis	Enzyme deficiency (E.C. number)
Complement component C_2, deficiency of (21700)	1	S – I serum C_2 D –	None req'd.	Quant. C_2	–	Complement C_2
Complement component C_3 (12070)	3O – recurrent infections	S – I serum C_3 assay and electro-phoresis D –	Est.	–	–	Complement C_3
Complement component C_4 (12080)	1	S – I serum C_4 assay and electro-phoresis D –	None req'd.	–	–	Complement C_4
Complement component C_5, deficiency of (12090)	3O – recurrent infections	S – I leucocyte phagocytosis of yeast suspension; serum C_5 D –	Exp.	–	–	Complement C_5
Complement component C_6, deficiency of (21708)	1	S – I serum C_6 D –	None req'd.	Quant. C_6	–	Complement C_6
Crigler–Najjar syndrome (21880)	4O – jaundice	S – I serum conjugated and uncon-jugated bilirubin D liver enz.	Symp. *	–	–	UDP-glucuronosyl-transferase (2.4.1.17)
Cystathioninuria (21950)	1	S B C I quant. plasma and urine amino-acids D liver or fibroblast enz.	None req'd.	Indir.	–	Cystathionase (4.4.1.1)

Cystinosis type 1 (21980)	**4E** – photophobia **O** – bone	S B C D I leucocyte and fibroblast cystine D –	Exp. *	Indir.	Cells	–
Cystinosis type 2 (21990)	**3E** – photophobia, retinal pigmentation	S B C D I leucocyte, fibroblast cystine D –	Exp.	Indir.	–	–
Cystinosis type 3 (22000)	**1E** – corneal crystals	S – I leucocyte and fibroblast cystine D –	None req'd.	Indir.	–	–
Cystinuria (22010)	**2O** – calculi	S B D I – D urine aminoacid clearance and intestinal uptake of Cys	Est. *	Indir.	–	Renal and intestinal transport defect of Cys, Orn and Lys (3 subtypes)
*hyper*Cystinuria, isolated, (23820)	1	S B D I quant. urine and plasma aminoacids D –	None req'd	–	–	Renal tubular cystine transport defect
Diabetes insipidus, nephrogenic (30480)	**3O** – dehydration	S – I urine and plasma osmolality; absent response to vasopressin D –	Est.	–	–	Renal tubular water transport defect
Dibasic aminoaciduria type 1 (12600)	1	S B I quant. urine aminoacids; aminoacid loading tests D –	None req'd	–	–	Renal tubular and intestinal transport defect of lysine, arginine and ornithine.
Dibasic aminoaciduria type 2 (22270)	**3MNO** – diarrhoea, vomiting, hepatomegaly	S B C I quant. plasma and urine aminoacid loading tests D –	Exp. *	–	–	Defect in renal tubular transport of lysine, arginine and ornithine
Diphosphoglycerate mutase deficiency (22280)	**3O** – splenomegaly, haemolytic anaemia	S – I – D erythrocyte enz.	Exp. *	Enz.	–	Bisphosphoglyceromutase (2.7.5.4.)

Table 18.7 (continued)

Disorder (McKusick No.)	Clinical features	Biochemical diagnosis	Treat-ability	Hetero-zygote detec-tion	Prena-tal diag-nosis	Enzyme deficiency (E.C. number)
Disaccharide intolerance type 1 (22290)	3O – diarrhoea	S – I blood sugar after glucose + fructose and sucrose load D intestinal mucosal enz.	Est. *	–	–	Invertase (3.2.1.26)
Disaccharide intolerance type 2 (22300)	4O – diarrhoea	S – I blood sugar after glucose + galactose and lactose load D intestinal mucosal enz.	Est. *	–	–	Lactase (3.2.1.23)
Disaccharide intolerance type 3 (22310)	4O – diarrhoea	S – I blood sugar after glucose + galactose and lactose load D intestinal mucosal enz.	Est. *	–	–	Lactase (3.2.1.23)
Ehlers Danlos syndrome type 5 (30520)	3O – lax skin and digital joints	S – I – D tissue enz.	Symp.	–	–	Lysyl oxidase
Ehlers Danlos syndrome type 6 (22540)	3E – retinal detachment O – lax skin and joints, scoliosis	S – I skin hydroxylysine–hydroxyproline ratio D fibroblast enz.	Exp.	Enz.	–	Collagen lysyl hydroxylase
Ehlers Danlos syndrome type 7 (22541)	3O – dwarf, lax skin and joints	S – I skin collagen fractions D fibroblast enz.	Symp.	–	–	Procollagen peptidase
Enterokinase deficiency (22620)	3O – diarrhoea, steatorrhoea, vomiting, oedema	S – I duodenal juice trypsin with and without enterokinase added to assay D intestinal mucosal enz.	Prom. *	–	–	Enteropeptidase (3.4.21.9)

Enteropathy, protein losing (22630)	3O – anaemia, oedema	S – I serum protein; [^{131}I] PVP excretion test D –	Symp.	–	–	–
Fanconi pancytopaenia (22765)	4O – anaemia	S – I spontaneous chromosome breakage in peripheral lymphocytes D –	Exp.	–	–	DNA excision (cross-linkage) repair enzyme
Fanconi syndrome type 2 (22780)	3O – bone, muscle weakness	S B E I blood acid–base; serum and urine phosphorus D –	Symp.	–	–	Renal tubular transport defects
Farber lipogranulomatosis (22800)	4MNO – skin	S – I urine sediment sphingolipid chromatog. D kidney or brain enz.	Symp.	–	–	Acylsphingosine deacylase (3.5.1.23)
Folic acid reductase, deficiency of (22903)	3O – anaemia	S – I urine formiminoglutamic acid following histidine load D liver enz.	Exp.	–	–	Folic acid reductase
Formiminotransferase deficiency (22910)	3M	S B I blood folate; FIGLU before and after His load D liver enz.	Symp. *	Indir.	–	Formiminotransferase (2.1.2.5)
Fructose and galactose intolerance (22950)	3O – fits	S – I fructose and galactose tolerance test D –	Est. *	–	–	–
Fructose-1,6-diphosphatase deficiency (22970)	3NO – acidosis, hepatomegaly	S B C E I glycerol tolerance test D leucocyte or liver enz.	Exp. *	Enz.	–	Hexose diphosphatase (3.1.3.11)

Table 18.7 (continued)

Disorder (McKusick No.)	Clinical features	Biochemical diagnosis	Treat-ability	Hetero-zygote detec-tion	Prena-tal diag-nosis	Enzyme deficiency (E.C. number)
Fructose intolerance, hereditary (22960)	3O – vomiting	S E I intravenous fructose load, (fructosuria, hypoglycaemia) and hypophosphataemia D liver or intestinal mucosal enz. +	Est. **	–	–	Hepatic fructose-1-phosphate aldolase, fructose bisphosphate aldolase (4.1.2.13) secondarily inhibited.
Fructosuria (22980)	1	S E I uptake of labelled fructose by liver biopsy + D –	None req'd.	–	–	Ketohexokinase (2.7.1.3)
Fucosidosis (23000)	**4MNO** – skeletal	S – I – D liver enz. +	Symp.	Enz.	Enz.	α-L-fucosidase (3.2.1.51)
Galactokinase deficiency (23020)	**3E** – cataract	S E I – D erythrocyte enz. +	Est. **	Enz.	Enz.	Galactokinase (2.7.1.6)
Galactosaemia (23040)	**4ME** – cataract **O** – jaundice, hepatomegaly	S B E I – D erythrocyte enz. +	Est. **	Enz.	Enz.	Hexose-1-phosphate uridylyltransferase (2.7.7.12)
Galactose epimerase deficiency (23035)	1	S E I blood galactose D erythrocyte enz.	None req'd	Enz.	–	UDP-glucose-4-epimerase (5.1.3.2)
Gangliosidosis, generalized, GM_1 type 1 (23050)	**4MNE** – macular spot **O** – hepatomegaly, skeletal	S – I – D leucocyte enz.	Symp.	Enz.	Enz.	β-Galactosidase (3.2.1.23)

Gangliosidosis, generalized GM_1 type 2 (late infantile) (23060)	**4MN** **O** – bone, hepatosplenomegaly	S – I fibroblast and leucocyte enz. + including electrophoresis D –	Symp.	Enz.	Enz.	β-D-Galactoside galactohydrolase (3.2.1.23)
Gangliosidosis GM_2 type 1 (Tay–Sachs disease) (27280)	**4NE** – macular spot	S – I – D leucocyte enz. and electrophoresis of isoenz. (A defic.) +	Symp.	Enz.	Enz.	β-N-Acetylhexosaminidase (3.2.1.52)
Gangliosidosis GM_2 type 2 (Sandhoff) (26880)	**4NE** – macular spot	S – I – D leucocyte or fibroblast enz. + and isoenzyme electrophoresis	Symp.	Enz.	Enz.	β-N-Acetylhexosaminidase isoenzymes A + B (3.2.1.52)
Gangliosidosis GM_2 type 3 (juvenile) (23070)	**4MNE** – macular spot	S – I – D leucocyte or fibroblast enz. + and electrophoresis	Symp.	–	–	β-N-Acetylhexosaminidase isoenzyme A (3.2.1.52)
Gangliosidosis GM_3 (23075)	**4MNO** – hepatosplenomegaly	S – I liver and brain lipid (TLC) D brain enz.	Symp.	–	–	GM_3-UDP-N-acetylgalactosaminyltransferase
Gaucher disease type 1 (non-cerebral, juvenile) (23080)	**3O** – hepatosplenomegaly, anaemia	S – I bone marrow microscopy; urine lipid chromatog; serum acid phosphatase D leucocyte, fibroblast or spleen enz. +	Symp.	–	–	β-Glucosidase (3.2.1.21)
Gaucher disease type 2 (infantile, cerebral) (23090)	**4MNO** – hepatosplenomegaly	S – I bone marrow microscopy; urine lipid chromatog; serum acid phosphatase D leucocyte or fibroblast enz. +	Symp.	–	Enz.	β-Glucosidase (3.2.1.21)
Gaucher disease type 3 (23100)	**3O** – splenomegaly, anaemia	S – I bone marrow and tissue lipid chromatog; serum acid phosphatase D fibroblast enz. +	Exp.	Enz.	–	β-Glucosidase (3.2.1.21)

Table 18.7 (continued)

Disorder (McKusick No.)	Clinical features	Biochemical diagnosis	Treat-ability	Hetero-zygote detec-tion	Prena-tal diag-nosis	Enzyme deficiency (E.C. number)
*agamma*Globulinaemia, Swiss or alymphocytotic type (20250)	4O – recurrent infections	S – I serum immunoglobulins D –	Exp.	–	–	–
Glucose–galactose malabsorption (23160)	4O – diarrhoea	S – I faecal sugar chromatog. after glucose and galactose load D uptake of labelled sugars by intestinal mucosa	Est. *	Indir.	–	Intestinal and renal glucose and galactose transport defect
Glucose-6-phosphate dehydrogenase deficiency (30590)	2O – anaemia, jaundice	S – I Beutler fluorescence screening of erythrocytes; D erythrocyte enz. assay and electrophoresis	Exp. *	Lyon	–	Glucose-6-phosphate dehydrogenase (1.1.1.49)
Glutamate–aspartate transport defect (23165)	3O-hypoglycaemia	S B C I quant. plasma and urine aminoacids D –	Symp.	–	–	Renal dicarboxylic acid transport defect
γ-Glutamyl-cysteine synthetase deficiency, haemolytic anaemia due to (23045)	3O – anaemia, cholelithiasis	S – I erythrocyte reduced glutathione D erythrocyte enz.	Symp.	Enz.	–	γ-Glutamyl-cysteine synthetase (6.3.2.2)
Glutaric acidaemia (23167)	**4MNO** – athetosis, acidosis	S – I serum and urine amino- and organic acids D leucocyte enz.	Symp.	–	–	Glutaryl CoA dehydrogenase (1.3.99.7)
Glutathione peroxidase deficiency, haemolytic anaemia due to, (23170)	2O – haemolytic anaemia	S – I Heinz bodies in erythrocytes D erythrocyte enz.	Symp. *	Enz.	–	Glutathione peroxidase (1.11.1.9)

Glutathione reductase, haemolytic anaemia due to deficiency in red cells (23180)	**3O** – anaemia	S – I Heinz bodies in blood film D erythrocyte enz.	Exp. *	Enz.	–	Glutathione reductase (1.6.4.2)
Glutathione synthetase deficiency of erythrocytes, haemolytic anaemia due to (23190)	**3O** – anaemia, jaundice	S – I methaemoglobin reduction test; cyanide-ascorbate test D erythrocyte enz.	Symp. *	Enz.	–	Glutathione synthetase (6.3.2.3.)
*hypo*Glycaemia, ketotic, of childhood (24065)	**3N**	S C I blood, glucose, β-hydroxybutyrate and alanine D –	Symp.	–	–	–
*hypo*Glycaemia, leucine induced (24080)	**3N**	S – I blood glucose and insulin following oral leucine D –	Symp.	–	–	–
*hypo*Glycaemia, neonatal, simulating fetopathica diabetica (24090)	**4N**	S – I blood glucose D –	Symp.	–	–	–
*hypo*Glycaemia with absent pancreatic alpha cells (24055)	**4O** – hypoglycaemia	S – I blood glucose and insulin D –	Symp.	–	–	–
*hypo*Glycaemia with deficiency of glycogen synthetase in the liver (24060)	**3M**	S – I blood glucose and lactate after galactose load D liver enz.	Symp.	–	–	Glycogen synthase (2.4.1.11)
*hyper*Glycinaemia, isolated (23830)	**4MNO** – fits	S B C I quant. plasma, C.S.F. and urine aminoacids D liver enz.	Exp.	–	–	Glycine synthase (2.1.2.10) ? others in some cases
Glycogen storage disease type 1 (23220)	**3O** – hepatomegaly	S – I glucagon test; galactose infusion test D thrombocyte, intestinal mucosal or liver enz.	Prom. **	Enz.	–	Glucose-6-phosphatase (3.1.3.9)

Table 18.7 (continued)

Disorder (McKusick No.)	Clinical features	Biochemical diagnosis	Treat-ability	Hetero-zygote detec-tion	Prena-tal diag-nosis	Enzyme deficiency (E.C. number)
Glycogen storage disease type 2 (23230)	4O – cardiomegaly, myopathy	S – I muscle glycogen D leucocyte, fibroblast or liver enz.	Exp. **	Enz.	Cells, Enz.	Exo-1,4-α-glucosidase (3.2.1.3)
Glycogen storage disease type 3 (23240)	3O – hepatomegaly	S – I glucagon test before and after carbohydrate; erythrocyte glycogen; liver glycogen – quantity and structure D erythrocyte, muscle or liver enz.	Exp. **	Enz.	–	Amylo-1,6-glucosidase (3.2.1.33)
Glycogen storage disease type 4 (23250)	4O – hepatomegaly	S – I spectrophotometry of erythrocyte glycogen–iodine complex. D leucocyte, fibroblast or liver enz.	Exp. **	Enz.	Enz.	1,4-α-Glucan (glycogen) branching enzyme (2.4.1.18)
Glycogen storage disease type 5 (23260)	3O – muscle weakness	S – I blood lactate after ischaemic exercise; muscle glycogen D muscle enz.	Exp. *	–	–	Phosphorylase (muscle) (2.4.1.1.)
Glycogen storage disease type 6 (23270)	3O – hepatomegaly	S – I glucagon test before and after carbohydrate meal; blood glucose and lactate after galactose infusion; liver glycogen D leucocyte or liver enz.	Prom. **	Enz.	–	Phosphorylase (liver) (2.4.1.1.)

Glycogen storage disease type 7 (23280)	3O – muscle weakness	S – I blood lactate after ischaemic exercise; muscle glycogen D erythrocyte or muscle enz.	Symp. *	Enz.	–	6-Phosphofructokinase (2.7.1.11)
Glycogen storage disease type 8 (designated type 9 by others) (30600)	3O – hepatomegaly	S – I liver glycogen I leucocyte or liver enz.	Exp. **	Enz.	–	Phosphorylase kinase (liver) (2.7.1.38)
Glycogen storage disease limited to heart (23210)	4O – cardiomegaly	S – I heart and skeletal muscle glycogen D –	Symp.	–	–	–
Glycosuria, renal (23310)	1	S E I renal tubular T_{max} glucose D –	None req'd.	–	–	Renal glucose transport defect
Glyoxylase type 2 (23320)	1	S – I – D erythrocyte enz.	None req'd.	enz.	–	Hydroxyacylglutathione hydrolase (3.1.2.6)
*hypo*Gonadism male, and ataxia (30740)	3NO – delayed puberty	S – I serum LH, FSH, testosterone D –	Exp.	Quant. LH and FSH after LHRH	–	–
Granulomatous disease due to leucocyte malfunction (23370)	3O – hepatosplenomegaly, skin, lymphadenitis	S – I NBT test; bactericidal test; leucocyte glutathione peroxidase D –	Exp.	–	–	–
Granulomatous disease due to leucocyte malfunction (30640)	4O – hepatosplenomegaly, skin, lymphadenitis	S – I NBT test; bactericidal test; NADPH oxidase D –	Exp.	–	–	–
Hartnup disease (23450)	3MNO – skin	S B I faecal aminoacid chromatog. before and after Try load D –	Exp. *	Indir.	–	Renal and intestinal monoaminomonocarboxylic acid transport defect

Table 18.7 (continued)

Disorder (McKusick No.)	Clinical features	Biochemical diagnosis	Treat-ability	Hetero-zygote detec-tion	Prena-tal diag-nosis	Enzyme deficiency (E.C. number)
Hexokinase deficiency, haemolytic anaemia (23570)	**3O** – anaemia, jaundice	S – I osmotic fragility of erythrocytes; erythrocyte glucose-6-phosphate D erythrocyte enz.	Symp. *	Enz.	–	Hexokinase (2.7.1.1.)
Histidinaemia (23580)	(**3M**) Possibly 1	S B C I sweat urocanic acid D skin enz.	Est. or none req'd. *	–	–	Histidine ammonia-lyase (4.3.1.3)
Homocystinuria (23620)	**3ME** – ectopia lentis **O** – marfanoid stature	S B C I quant. urine and plasma aminoacids D fibroblast or liver enz. +	Est. **	Enz. Indir.	Enz.	Cystathionine β-synthase (4.2.1.22)
Homocystinuria due to deficiency of N-(5,10)-methylenetetrahydrofolate reductase activity (23625)	**4M**	S B C I quant. urine and plasma aminoacids D fibroblast enz.	Symp.	–	–	Methylenetetrahydrofolate reductase (1.5.1.5)
β-Hydroxyisovaleric aciduria and β-methylcrotonylglycinuria (21020)	**3NO** – odour	S A I urine fatty and organic acids by G.L.C. D leucocyte enz.	Exp. **	Indir.	–	Methylcrotonyl-CoA carboxylase (6.4.1.4)
Hydroxykynureninuria (23680)	**4MO** – anaemia, short stature	S A I urine tryptophan metabolites D –	Symp. *	Indir.	–	Kynureninase (3.7.1.3)
Hydroxylysinuria (23690)	**3MN**	S B I quant. serum and urine amino-acids before and after acid hydrolysis of urine D –	Symp.	–	–	–

Hydroxyprolinaemia (23700)	(**3MO** – haematuria, hyperactive) Probably 1	S B C I quant. plasma and urine aminoacids D liver enz. +	Exp. ** Probably none req'd.	–	–	Hydroxyproline oxidase
Hypoxanthine, guanine phosphoribosyltransferase (Lesch–Nyhan syndrome) (30800)	**4MNO** – self-mutilation	S – I urine uric acid/creatinine ratio D erythrocyte enz. +	Symp. *	Enz.	Enz.	Hypoxanthine phosphoribosyltransferase (2.4.2.8)
Iminoglycinuria (24260)	1	S B I – D renal clearance of glycine, and infused proline and hydroxyproline	None req'd.	Indir.	–	Renal and small intestinal transport defect of GlyPro and Hypro
Immune defect with deficiency of adenosine deaminase (24275)	**4O** – recurrent infection	S – I – D erythrocyte enz.	Exp.	Enz.	Enz.	Adenosine deaminase (3.5.4.4.)
Isoniazid (INH) inactivation (24340)	1	S – I plasma INH and urine INH metabolites D –	None req'd	Indir.	–	–
Isovaleric acidaemia (24350)	**4NO** – vomiting, acidosis, odour	S A I urine isovalerylglycine; plasma isovaleric acid following leucine load D leucocyte enz. +	Est. **	Enz.	Enz.	Isovaleric acid dehydrogenase
Jaundice, familial obstructive, of infancy (30860)	**2O** – jaundice	S – I serum conjugated and unconjugated bilirubin D –	Symp.	–	–	–
*hypo*Kalaemic alkalosis (Bartter syndrome) (24120)	**3NO** – muscle weakness	S – I serum potassium, renin and aldosterone; renal biopsy – juxtaglomerular hyperplasia; pressor effect of angiotensin D –	Exp.	–	–	–

Table 18.7 (continued)

Disorder (McKusick No.)	Clinical features	Biochemical diagnosis	Treat-ability	Hetero-zygote detec-tion	Prena-tal diag-nosis	Enzyme deficiency (E.C. number)
Keratosis palmo-plantaris with corneal dystrophy (Richner–Hanhart syndrome) (24480)	**4M** **E** – corneal dystrophy **O** – skin	S C I urine phenolic acids D may be identical with tyrosine transaminase deficiency (27660)	Exp.	–	–	Tyrosine amino-transferase (cytosol) (2.6.1.5)
Ketoacidosis of infancy (24505)	**4O** – acidosis	S – I blood pH, bicarbonate and ketones D fibroblast enz.	Symp.	–	–	3-Ketoacid CoA transferase (2.8.3.5)
Krabbe disease (globoid cell sclerosis) (24520)	**4N** **E** – optic atrophy **O** – deafness	S – I – D leucocyte enz. +	Symp.	–	Enz.	β-Galactosidase (3.2.1.23)
Lactic acidosis, chronic adult form (15017)	**3O** – intermittent breathlessness and muscle weakness	S – I blood lactate and pyruvate and arterial pH before and after exercise D –	Symp.	–	–	–
Lactic acidosis, familial infantile (24540)	**4NO** – respiratory	S B I blood lactate and pyruvate D –	Exp. **	–	–	–
Lactosylceramidosis (24550) May be identical with Gangliosidosis GM_3 (23075)	–	– –	–	–	–	–
Lecithin cholesterol acyltransferase deficiency (24590)	**3E** – corneal deposits **O** – anaemia, proteinuria	S – I plasma lipoprotein electrophoresis; plasma lipid chromatog. D plasma enz. +	Symp. *	–	–	Lecithin acyltransferase (2.3.1.43)

Lipase, congenital absence of pancreatic (24660)	**3O** – steatorrhoea	S – I faecal fat D duodenal juice enz.	Exp. *	–	–	Triacylglycerol lipase (3.1.1.3)
an α-Lipoproteinaemia (20540)	**3NO** – enlarged tonsils, hepatosplenomegaly	S – I serum cholesterol; lipoprotein electrophoresis D lipoprotein immunoelectrophoresis	Exp.	Quant. lipoprotein	–	Absence of α-lipoprotein
a,β-Lipoproteinaemia (20010)	**3MNE** – retinitis pigmentosa **O** – steatorrhoea, anaemia	S – I acanthocytes on wet blood film; serum cholesterol (dec.) D immunoelectrophoresis of lipoproteins	Exp. *	–	–	Absence of β-lipoprotein
*hyper*Lipoproteinaemia type 1 (23860)	**3O** – splenomegaly	S – I serum cholesterol, triglycerides, lipoprotein electrophoresis D plasma enz.	Prom.	Enz.	–	Diacylglycerol lipase (3.1.1.34)
Lowe oculocerebrorenal syndrome (30900)	**4MNE** – cataracts **O** – acidosis, hypotonia, rickets, retarded growth	S B E I quant. urinary aminoacids before and after ornithine load D –	Exp. *	Indir.	–	–
*hyper*Lysinaemia (23870)	**3MO** – ectopia lentis	S B C I quant. plasma and urine aminoacids D fibroblast enz.	Symp.	–	Enz.	Lysine ketoglutarate reductase
Lysine intolerance (24790)	**4NO** – vomiting	S B C I quant. plasma and urine aminoacids; blood ammonia D liver enz.	Prom. *	–	–	L-Lysine NAD oxidoreductase
*hyper*Lysinuria with hyperammonaemia (23875)	**4MN**	S B C I quant. plasma and urine aminoacids; blood ammonia after feed D –	Symp.	–	–	–

Table 18.7 (continued)

Disorder (McKusick No.)	Clinical features	Biochemical diagnosis	Treat-ability	Hetero-zygote detec-tion	Prena-tal diag-nosis	Enzyme deficiency (E.C. number)
*hypo*Magnesaemia, primary (24130) see *hypo*Magnesaemic tetany (30760)	–	– –	–	–	–	–
*hypo*Magnesaemic tetany (30760) may be identical with hypo-magnesaemia, primary (24130)	**4O** – fits	S – I serum calcium, magnesium, and acid phosphatase D –	Est.	–	–	–
Male pseudohermaphroditism (30915)	**3O** – genital abnor-malities	S – I urine or serum testosterone; urine pregnanetriol and pregnanetriolone D –	Symp.	–	–	Testicular 17,20-steroid desmolase
Mannosidosis (24850)	**4MNE** – cataract **O** – hepatospleno-megaly, skeletal	S – I – D leucocyte, fibroblast or liver enz. +	Symp.	–	Enz.	α-Mannosidase (3.2.1.24)
Maple syrup urine disease (24860)	**4MO** – odour	S A B C I quant. aminoacids; urine keto-acids D leucocyte enz. +	Prom. **	Enz.	Enz.	Branched-chain ketoacid oxi-dative decar-boxylase
Menkes syndrome (30940)	**4MNO** – hair	S – I plasma copper and caerulo-plasmin D –	Exp. *	Quant. copper and caerulo-plasmin	–	–

Mercaptolactate–cysteine disulphiduria (24965)	(3M) probably 1	S B D I quant. urine aminoacids, before and after cysteine load D –	(Symp.) probably none req'd.	–	–	–
Metachromatic leukodystrophy, late infantile (25010)	4MN	S – I urine lipid chromatog. (sulphatide) D leucocyte enz. +	Exp. *	Enz.	Enz.	Arylsulphatase (isoenzyme A) (3.1.6.1.)
Methaemoglobin reductase (NADPH) deficiency (25070)	2O – anaemia	S – I blood methaemoglobin D erythrocyte enz.	None req'd.	Enz.	–	NADPH-linked methaemoglobin reductase
Methaemoglobinaemia due to deficiency of methaemoglobin reductase (diaphorase) (25080)	3MO – cyanosis	S – I blood methaemoglobin D erythrocyte and leucocyte enz.	Exp. *	Enz.	–	NADH-linked methaemoglobin reductase
*hyper*Methioninaemia (23890)	4O – liver, bleeding tendency	S A B C I quant. plasma and urine aminoacids; urine ketoacids D –	Symp.	–	–	–
Methionine adenosyltransferase deficiency (25085)	3O – liver	S B C I quant. plasma aminoacids D liver enz.	Symp.	–	–	Methionine adenosyltransferase (2.5.1.6)
Methionine malabsorption syndrome (25090)	4MO – odour, diarrhoea	S A I faecal aminoacid chromatog. (Meth); urine organic acid chromatog. (α-hydroxybutyric) D –	Exp. *	Indir.	–	Small intestinal methionine transport defect
α-Methyl-acetoacetic aciduria (20375)	4O – acidosis, coma, vomiting	S – I urine ketone bodies and organic acids before and after isoleucine load D fibroblast enz.	Symp. **	Indir.	–	–
Methylmalonic aciduria type 1 (vitamin B_{12} unresponsive) (25100)	4MO – acidosis, vomiting	S – I urine organic acids (G.L.C) D leucocyte enz. +	Exp. **	–	Fluid, Enz.	Methylmalonyl-CoA mutase (5.4.99.2)

Table 18.7 (continued)

Disorder (McKusick No.)	Clinical features	Biochemical diagnosis	Treat-ability	Hetero-zygote detec-tion	Prena-tal diag-nosis	Enzyme deficiency (E.C. number)
Methylmalonic aciduria type 2 (vitamin B_{12} responsive) (25110)	**4MO** – vomiting, acidosis, retarded growth	S – I urine organic acids (G.L.C.) D leucocyte enz. +	Prom. **	–	Enz.	5′-Deoxyadenosylcobalamin transferase
Methylmalonic aciduria type 3 (25112)	**4O** – acidosis	S – I urine organic acids (G.L.C.) D fibroblast enz. +	–	–	–	Methylmalonyl-CoA racemase (5.1.99.1)
Mitochondrial myopathy with lactic acidosis (25195)	**3O** – muscle	S B I blood lactate and pyruvate; larger and more numerous mitochondria on E.M. of muscle biopsy D –	Symp.	–	–	–
Mucolipidosis type 2 (I-cell disease) (25250)	**4MN** **O** – bone	S – I microscopic inclusions in fibroblasts; increased plasma and fibroblast acid hydrolases D –	Symp.	–	Enz.	–
Mucolipidosis type 3 (25260)	**3E** – corneal clouding **O** – bone	S – I serum and fibroblast acid hydrolases D –	Symp.	–	–	–
Mucopolysaccharidosis type 1H (Hurler) (25280)	**4ME** – cataract **O** – bone, hepatosplenomegaly	S G I – D leucocyte or fibroblast enz. +	Exp. *	Enz.	Enz., fluid	L-Iduronidase (3.2.1.76)
Mucopolysaccharidosis type 1S (Scheie) (25310)	**3E** – cataract **O** – skeletal	S G I – D leucocyte or fibroblast enz. +	Symp.	Enz.	Enz.	L-Iduronidase (3.2.1.76)

Mucopolysaccharidosis type 2 (Hunter syndrome) (30990)	**4MO** – skeletal, hepatomegaly	S G I – D fibroblast enz. +	Exp. *	Enz.	Cells, Enz.	Sulphoiduronate sulphatase
Mucopolysaccharidosis type 3A (Sanfilippo A) (25290)	**4MO** – bone, hepatosplenomegaly	S G I – D leucocyte or fibroblast enz. +	Exp. *	Enz.	Cells	Heparan sulphate sulphamidase
Mucopolysaccharidosis type 3B (Sanfilippo B) (25292)	**4MO** – bone, hepatosplenomegaly, deafness	S G I – D serum or fibroblast enz. +	Exp. *	Enz.	Cells	α-N-Acetylglucosaminidase (3.2.1.50)
Mucopolysaccharidosis type 4 (Morquio) (25300)	**3E** – corneal opacities **O** – bone, deafness	S G I – D fibroblast enz.	Symp. *	–	–	N-Acetyl-hexosamine-6-sulphate sulphatase
Mucopolysaccharidosis type 6 (Maroteaux–Lamy) (25320)	**3E** – corneal clouding **O** – bone, heart, hepatosplenomegaly	S G I – D fibroblast enz. +	Symp.	Enz.	Enz.	Arylsulphatase isoenzyme B (3.1.6.1)
Mucopolysaccharidosis type 7 (β-glucuronidase deficiency) (25322)	**4MO** – bone, hepatosplenomegaly	S G I leucocyte granular inclusions D fibroblast or leucocyte enz. +	Symp.	Enz.	Cells	β-Glucuronidase (3.2.1.31)
Myeloperoxidase deficiency (25460)	**3O** – recurrent infection	S – I – D leucocyte enz.	Exp.	–	–	Myeloperoxidase
Myopathy with abnormal lipid metabolism (25510)	**3O** – myopathy	S – I serum creatine kinase (fasting); muscle carnitine palmityltransferase and lipid. D –	Exp.	–	–	–
Myopathy with carnitine deficiency (25513)	**3O** – myopathy	S – I muscle carnitine and lipid D –	Exp.	–	–	–
Myopathy with lactic acidosis (25514)	**3O** – intermittant breathlessness and muscle weakness	S – I blood lactate and pyruvate and arterial pH before and after exercise; abnormal mitochondria on EM of muscle biopsy D –	Symp.	–	–	–

Table 18.7 (continued)

Disorder (McKusick No.)	Clinical features	Biochemical diagnosis	Treat-ability	Hetero-zygote detec-tion	Prena-tal diag-nosis	Enzyme deficiency (E.C. number)
Necrotizing encephalopathy, infantile subacute, of Leigh (25600)	**4N**	S B I blood lactate, pyruvate, erythrocyte transketolase with and without thiamine pyrophosphate added to assay; urine inhibition of thiamine phosphorylation D –	Exp.	–	–	–
Nieman–Pick disease (sphingomyelin lipidosis) (25720)	**4MNE** – macular spot **O** – hepatosplenomegaly	S – I leucocyte, liver or urine sediment lipid chromatog. D fibroblast or liver enz. +	Symp. *	–	Enz.	Phosphatidylcholine cholinephosphohydrolase (3.1.4.3)
Ornithinaemia (25887)	**3ME** – retinal atrophy	S B C I quant. plasma, urine and C.S.F. aminoacids D liver enz.	Symp.	–	–	Ornithine oxoacid aminotransferase (2.6.1.13)
Ornithine transcarbamylase deficiency (31125)	**4M**	S B I quant. urine aminoacids; blood ammonia D liver enz.	Symp.	–	–	Ornithine carbamoyltransferase (2.1.3.3)
Oroticaciduria type 1 (25890)	**3O** – anaemia	S – I urinary orotic acid D erythrocyte or fibroblast enz.	Exp. *	Enz.; urinary orotic acid	–	Orotate phosphoribosyltransferase (2.4.2.10) and and orotidine-5′phosphate decarboxylase (4.1.1.23)

Orotic aciduria type 2 (25892)	3O – anaemia	S – I urine orotic acid D erythrocyte enz.	Exp. *	–	–	Orotidine 5′-phosphate decarboxylase (4.1.1.23)
Oxalosis type 1 (25990)	3O – calculi	S – I urine oxalate D liver enz.	Symp.	–	–	2-Oxoglutamate-glyoxylate carboligase
Oxalosis type 2 (26000)	2O – calculi	S – I urine oxalate; urine chromatog. for L-glyceric acid D leucocyte enz.	Symp.	–	–	Glycerate dehydrogenase (1.1.1.29)
Pendred syndrome (26070)	3O – deafness, goitre	S – I radioactive I uptake and perchlorate discharge D –	Prom.	–	–	–
Pentosuria (L-xylulosuria) (26080)	1	S E I – D erythrocyte enz. +	None req'd	–	–	L-Xylulose reductase (1.1.1.10)
Periodic paralysis type 1 (hypokalaemic type) (17040)	3O – muscle	S – I serum and urine potassium D –	Est.	–	–	–
Periodic paralysis type 2 (hyperkalaemic type) (17050)	3O – muscle	S – I serum potassium D –	Est.	–	–	–
Pernicious anaemia, juvenile due to selective intestinal malabsorption of vitamin B_{12} (26110)	3O – anaemia	S B I serum vitamin B_{12}; Schilling test. D –	Prom.	–	–	Small intestinal vitamin B_{12} transport defect
Phenylketonuria (26160)	4M	S B C I quant. plasma aminoacids D liver enz. +	Est. **	Indir.	–	L-Phenylalanine tetrahydropteridine:oxygen oxidoreductase (1.14.16.1)

Table 18.7 (continued)

Disorder (McKusick No.)	Clinical features	Biochemical diagnosis	Treat-ability	Hetero-zygote detec-tion	Prena-tal diag-nosis	Enzyme deficiency (E.C. number)
*hypo*Phosphataemia (vitamin D resistant rickets) (30780)	3O – bone	S – I serum and urine phosphate D –	Prom.	–	–	renal tubular calcium and phosphate transport defect
*hypo*Phosphatasia (phosphoethanolaminuria) (24150)	4O – bone	S – I urine and plasma phosphoethanolamine D serum enz. and isoenz. (bone diminished)	Symp. *	Enz.	Enz., Fluid phosphoethanolamine	Alkaline phosphatase (3.1.3.1)
Phosphoglycerate kinase (31180)	3O – anaemia	S – I – D erythrocyte enz. in both young and old cells (young def.)	Symp. *	Enz.	–	Phosphoglycerate kinase (2.7.2.3)
Phosphoglycerate kinase deficiency of erythrocyte (26170)	2O – anaemia	S – I – D erythrocyte enz. in both young and old cells (old def.)	Symp. *	–	–	Phosphoglycerate kinase (2.7.2.3)
Phosphohexoseisomerase (17240)	3O – anaemia	S – I erythrocyte survival, starch gel electrophoresis of erythrocyte enz. D erythrocyte enz.	Symp.	Enz.	–	Glucose phosphate isomerase (5.3.1.9)
*hyper*Pipecolataemia (23940)	4N O – hepatomegaly	S C I serum pipecolate D –	Symp. *	–	–	–
Polysaccharide, storage of unusual (26360)	4O – hepatosplenomegaly, anaemia	S – I liver polysaccharide D –	Symp.	–	–	–

Porphyria, acute intermittent (17600)	**4NO** – abdominal pain, vomiting, fits in children	S A I urine porphobilinogen, aminolaevulinic acid and porphyrins before and after ALA load; erythrocyte enz. D –	Exp.	Enz.	–	Uroporphyrinogen I synthase (4.3.1.8)
Porphyria, congenital erythropoietic (26370)	**4O** – photosensitivity, anaemia, splenomegaly	S A I erythrocyte, urine and faecal porphyrins and isomer distribution D erythrocyte enz.	Exp.	Enz.	–	Uroporphyrinogen III cosynthetase
Prader–Willi syndrome (26400)	**3NO** – hypogonadism, obesity	S – I glucose tolerance; serum LH, testosterone (males) or oestradiol (females) – all low D –	Symp.	Testosterone after HCG; LH after LH-RH	–	–
*hyper*Prolinaemia type 1 (23950)	(**3MO** – haematuria, deafness) Probably 1	S B C I plasma and urine quant. aminoacids D liver enz. +	Exp. ** Probably none req'd.	–	–	Pyrroline-5-carboxylate reductase (1.5.1.2)
*hyper*Prolinaemia type 2 (23951)	**3MO** – fits	S B C I quant. plasma and urine aminoacids; urine pyrroline carboxylate D fibroblast or liver enz. +	Exp. **	–	–	1-Pyrroline dehydrogenase (1.5.1.12)
Propionic acidaemia (23200)	**4O** – acidosis	S B C I quant. plasma and urine aminoacids and organic acids D leucocyte enz. +	Exp. **	Enz.	Enz.	Propionyl-CoA carboxylase (6.4.1.3)
Pseudohermaphroditism, incomplete male type 1 (31210)	**3O** – genital abnormalities	S – I serum testosterone, oestradiol and luteinising hormone D –	Symp.	Testosterone and L.H. after pituitary–gonadal stimulation	–	Steroid binding protein deficiency

Table 18.7 (continued)

Disorder (McKusick No.)	Clinical features	Biochemical diagnosis	Treat-ability	Hetero-zygote detec-tion	Prena-tal diag-nosis	Enzyme deficiency (E.C. number)
Pseudohermaphroditism, male with gynaecomastia (26430)	3O – virilisation, gynaeco-mastia	S – I serum Δ^4-androstenedione D –	Symp.	–	–	β-Hydroxysteroid dehydrogenase (1.1.1.51)
Pseudohypoparathyroidism type 2 (26440)	**4MNO** – skeletal	S – I serum Ca, ionized Ca; urinary cyclic AMP D –	Exp.	–	–	Renal tubular cal-cium and phos-phate transport defect
Pseudouridinuria and mental defect (26450)	**3M**	S – I urine pseudouridine D –	Symp.	–	–	
Pseudovaginal perineoscrotal hypo-spadias (incomplete male type 2) (26460)	3O – male pseudoherma-phrodite, no breasts at puberty	S – I serum testosterone, LH and 5α-dihydrotestosterone D –	Prom.	5α-Di-hydro-testoster-one after HCG	–	Steroid 5α-reduc-tase
Pyridoxine dependency with seizures (26610)	**4N**	S – I xanthurenic acid excretion after Try D kidney enz.	Est.	–	–	Glutamate decar-boxylase (4.1.1.15)
Pyrimidine 5′-nucleotidase deficiency, haemolytic anaemia from (26612)	4O – anaemia	S – I spectrophotometry of erythro-cyte (deproteinized) pyrimidine nucleotides D erythrocyte enz.	Enz.	–	–	Pyrimidine 5′nucleotidase

Pyroglutamic aciduria (26613)	**3MNO** – vomiting, acidosis	S B C I quant. plasma and urine aminoacids D urine pyroglutamic acid	Symp.	–	–	
Pyruvate carboxylase deficiency (26615)	**4MN**	S C I blood lactate and pyruvate D liver enz.	Symp.	–	–	Pyruvate carboxylase (6.4.1.1.)
Pyruvate kinase deficiency of erythrocyte (26620)	**4O** – splenomegaly, anaemia, jaundice	S – I erythrocyte autohaemolysis with and without added glucose D erythrocyte enz.	Symp. *	Enz.	–	Pyruvate kinase (2.7.1.40)
Refsum syndrome (26650)	**3NE** – retinal pigmentation **O** – skin	S – I plasma lipid chromatog. D́ fibroblast enz. +	Exp. *	Enz.	Enz.	Phytanic acid α-oxidase
Renal tubular acidosis type 1 (distal type) (17980)	**3O** – acidosis, nephrocalcinosis, osteomalacia, weakness	S – I blood acid–base; urine pH NH_4Cl load D –	Est.	–	–	Renal tubular H^+ transport defect
Renal tubular acidosis type 2 (proximal bicarbonate wasting type) (31240)	**3O** – acidosis	S – I blood acid–base; urine pH following NH_4Cl load D –	Est.	–	–	Renal tubular bicarbonate–H^+ transport defect
Renal tubular acidosis type 3 (bicarbonate wasting) (26720)	**3O** – nephrocalcinosis, osteomalacia, periodic paralysis	S – I serum potassium and immunoglobulins; blood acid–base; urine pH D –	Est.	–	–	Renal tubular bicarbonate transport defect
Renal tubular acidosis with progressive nerve deafness (26730)	**3O** – deafness, nephrocalcinosis, vomiting	S – I blood acid–base; urine pH D erythrocyte enz.	Symp.	–	–	Carbonate dehydratase isoenzyme B (4.2.1.1)
Rhabdomyolysis, acute recurrent (26820)	**4O** – fits, muscle pain	S A I urine myoglobin D –	Symp.	–	–	–

Table 18.7 (continued)

Disorder (McKusick No.)	Clinical features	Biochemical diagnosis	Treat-ability	Hetero-zygote detec-tion	Prena-tal diag-nosis	Enzyme deficiency (E.C. number)
Saccharopinuria (26870)	**3M**	S B C I quant. urine and plasma aminoacids D fibroblast or muscle enz.	Symp.	–	–	Saccharopine dehydrogenase (1.5.1.9)
Sarcosinaemia (26890)	1	S B C I sarcosine loading test D –	None req'd.	Indir.	–	Sarcosine dehydrogenase (1.5.99.1)
*hyper*Serotonaemia (23960)	**3NO** – flushing	S – I serum serotonin; urine 5-hydroxyindole D –	Symp.	–	–	–
Sialuria (26990)	**3O** – acidosis, hepato-megaly, retarded growth	S – I urine sialic acid D –	Symp.	–	–	–
β-Sitosterolaemia (21025)	**3O** – tendon xantho-mata	S – I plasma or erythrocyte sterol G.L.C. D absorption of labelled β-sitos-terol	Symp.	–	–	
Sulphatidosis, juvenile, Austin type (27220)	**4MNO** – hepatomegaly	S G I urine sulphatide chromatog. D leucocyte or fibroblast enz.	Symp.	–	–	Arylsulphatase iso-enzymes A, B and C
Sulphocysteinuria (sulphite oxidase deficiency) (27230)	**4MNE** – dislocated lens	S B F I urine thiosulphate D liver enz.	Symp.	–	–	Sulphite oxidase (1.8.3.1)

Suxamethonium sensitivity (27240)	**2O** – apnoea	S – I – D plasma enz. and inhibition by dibucaine and fluoride	Symp. *	Enz.	–	Acylcholine acyl-hydrolase (3.1.1.8)
Testicular feminization (incomplete male) type 1 (31370)	**4O** – male pseudohermaphroditism (breasts at puberty), cryptorchidism	S – I serum testosterone, LH and 5α-dihydrotestosterone D –	Symp.	Quant. serum 5α-dihydrotestosterone and LH	–	End-organ receptor deficiency
Thyroid hormone unresponsiveness (27430)	**3O** – deafness, goitre	S – I serum T_4, TSH D –	Symp.	T_4, TSH	–	–
Thyroid hormonogenesis, genetic defect in, type 1 (trapping defect) (27440)	**4MO** – goitre	S – I serum T_4; radio-iodine uptake D –	Est. *	–	–	–
Thyroid hormonogenesis, genetic defect in, type 2A (organification defect, type 1) (27450)	**4MO** – goitre	S – I radio-iodine uptake and perchlorate discharge; all other thyroid tests normal D –	Est. *	–	–	–
Thyroid hormonogenesis, genetic defect in, type 2B (organification defect type 2) (27460)	**4MO** – goitre	S – I serum T_4; TSH; radioiodine uptake and thiocyanate discharge D –	Est. *	Quant. T_4 and iodine uptake	–	– –
Thyroid hormonogenesis, genetic defect in, type 3 (coupling defect) (27470)	**4MO** – goitre	S – I serum T_4; TSH; butanol extractable iodine D –	Prom.	T_4 and butanol extractable iodine	–	–
Thyroid hormonogenesis, genetic defect in, type 4 (27480)	**4MO** – goitre	S – I serum inorganic iodine, T_4; radio-iodine uptake D –	Prom. *	Radio-iodine uptake	–	Iodotyrosine-dehalogenase

Table 18.7 (continued)

Disorder (McKusick No.)	Clinical features	Biochemical diagnosis	Treat-ability	Hetero-zygote detec-tion	Prena-tal diag-nosis	Enzyme deficiency (E.C. number)
Thyroid hormonogenesis, genetic defect in, type 5 (iodoprotein defect) (27490)	**4MO** – goitre	S – I serum T_3; thyroid tissue thyroglobulin; serum iodo-tyrosine–albumin complex D –	Est.	T_3 and tissue thyro-globulin	–	–
Thyroxine binding globulin of serum, variants of (31420)	**2N**	S – I serum T_4, TBG D –	Symp.	T_4 and TBG	–	–
*a*Transferrinaemia (20930)	**3O** – anaemia	S – I serum total iron binding capacity D serum transferrin	Prom.	Indir.	–	Transferrin
Tricarboxylic acid cycle, defect of (27537)	**3MN**	S – I blood lactate D fibroblast enz.	Symp.	–	–	Pyruvate dehydro-genase complex
Trichorrhexis nodosa syndrome (27555)	**4MNO** – hair	S – I hair cystine D –	Symp.	–	–	–
Trimethylaminuria (fish-odour syndrome) (27570)	**3O** – smell, spleno-megaly, infection	S A I urine trimethylamine (G.L.C.) before and after oral tri-methylamine D –	Symp.	–	–	–
Triosephosphate isomerase deficiency (27580)	**3NO** – haemolytic anaemia	S – I – D erythrocyte enz.	Symp.	Enz.	–	Triosephosphate isomerase (5.3.1.1.)

Trypsinogen deficiency (27600)	3O – diarrhoea, anaemia	S – I show enterokinase active D duodenal juice enz.	Exp. *	–	–	Trypsinogen
T-substance anomaly (27620)	3M	S B I – D –	Symp.	Indir.	–	–
Tuftsin deficiency (19115)	3O – recurrent infections	S – I tuftsin effect on phagocytosis D –	Exp.	–	–	–
Tyrosinaemia (27670)	4O – liver, bone	S B C I urinary phenolic acids; quant. tyrosine D liver enz.	Exp. *	–	–	4-Hydroxyphenyl pyruvate dioxygenase (1.13.11.27)
Tyrosine transaminase deficiency (27660)	3M	S B C I quant. urine and plasma amino-acids; urine phenolic acids D liver enz.	Exp. *	–	–	Tyrosine amino-transferase (2.6.1.5)
Uridine monophosphate kinase (19173)	1	S – I – D erythrocyte enz.	None req'd.	Enz.	–	Uridine monophos-phate kinase
Valinaemia (27710)	3MO – vomiting	S B C I – D leucocyte enz.	Exp. *	–	Enz.	Valine aminotrans-ferase (2.6.1.32)
Vitamin B_{12} metabolic defect (27740)	4MO – anaemia	S B C I urine homocystine and methyl-malonic acid; plasma cobal-amine coenzymes D –	Symp.	–	–	–
Wilson disease (27790)	3NE – Kayser–Fleischer rings O – liver	S B I serum and urine copper, serum enz. (caeruloplasmin) D –	Est. **	Indir.	–	Ferroxidase (1.16.3.1)

Table 18.7 (continued)

Disorder (McKusick No.)	Clinical features	Biochemical diagnosis	Treatability	Heterozygote detection	Prenatal diagnosis	Enzyme deficiency (E.C. number)
Wolman disease (27800)	4O – hepatosplenomegaly vomiting, diarrhoea	S – I – D leucocyte enz. +	Symp.	Enz.	Enz.	Triacylglycerol lipase (3.1.1.3)
Wolman disease with hypolipoproteinaemia and acanthocytosis (27810)	4O – vomiting hepatosplenomegaly, steatorrhoea	S – I wet blood film for acanthocytes; plasma lipoprotein electrophoresis; plasma total lipid and cholesterol D –	Symp.	–	–	–
Xanthinuria (27830)	2O – calculi	S – I low serum urate, urinary purine chromatog. D intestinal or liver enz.	Symp. *	–	–	Xanthine oxidase (1.2.3.2)
Xanthurenicaciduria (27860)	3M	S – I urine indole chromatog. before and after Try load D liver enz.	Exp. *	–	–	Kynureninase (3.7.1.3)
Xeroderma pigmentosum (27870)	4O – skin	S – I – D fibroblast enz.	Symp.	–	Enz.	DNA excision (UV damage) repair enzyme (5 types)
Xerodermic idiocy of de Sanctis and Cacchione (27880)	4MNO – skin	S – I fibroblast enz. D –	Symp.	Indir.	–	DNA excision repair enzyme
Xylosidase deficiency (27890)	3NO – vomiting	S – I – D cultured lymphocyte enz.	Symp.	–	–	Exo-1,4-β-xylosidase (3.2.1.37)

TABLE 18.8.

SOME INHERITED METABOLIC DISEASES DISCUSSED IN OTHER CHAPTERS OR WHOSE ESSENTIAL BACKGROUND IS COVERED IN OTHER CHAPTERS

Haematological (Chapter 16)

Adenosine triphosphatase deficiency (10280)
Adenylate kinase deficiency (20160)
Aldolase A deficiency (20335)
Anaemia, hypochromic (30130)
Diphosphoglycerate mutase deficiency (22280)
Glucose-6-phosphate dehydrogenase deficiency (30590)
Glutathione peroxidase deficiency (23170)
Glutathione reductase deficiency (23180)
Glutathione synthetase deficiency (23190)
γ-Glutamylcysteine synthetase deficiency (23045)
Hexokinase deficiency (23570)
Hexose phosphate isomerase deficiency (23575)
Methaemoglobin reductase deficiency, NADPH (25070)
Methaemoglobin reductase deficiency, NADH (25080)
Phosphoglycerate kinase deficiency (31180)
Pyrimidine 5′-nucleotidase deficiency (26612)
Pyruvate kinase deficiency (26620)
Triose phosphate isomerase deficiency (27580)

Plasma lipids (Chapter 5)

Lecithin-cholesterol acyltransferase deficiency (24590)
*hyper*Lipoproteinaemia, type 1 (23860)

Purines and pyrimidines (Chapter 21)

Hypoxanthine-guanine phosphoribosyltransferase deficiency (30800)
Xanthinuria (27830)

Disorders of the immune systems

Granulomatous disease (30640)
Immunodeficiency disease (24275)
Immunodeficiency disease (19173)
Myeloperoxidase deficiency (25460)

Intestinal (Chapter 12)

Congenital absence of pancreatic lipase (24660)
Disaccharide intolerance, type 1 (22290)
Disaccharide intolerance, type 2 (22300)
Disaccharide intolerance, type 3 (22310)
Trypsinogen deficiency (27600)

Renal (Chapter 9)

Glycosuria, renal (23310)
*hypo*Phosphataemia (30780)
Pseudohypoparathyroidism (26440)
Renal tubular acidosis, type 1 (17980)
Renal tubular acidosis, type 2 (31240)
Renal tubular acidosis, type 3 (26730)

TABLE 18.8. (continued)

Hepatic (Chapter 10)
Crigler–Najjar syndrome (21880)
Porphyrins (Chapter 20)
Porphyria, acute intermittent (17600)
Porphyria, congenital (26370)
Steroid hormones (Chapter 14)
Adrenal hyperplasia, type 1 (20170)
Adrenal hyperplasia, type 2 (20180)
Adrenal hyperplasia, type 3 (20190)
Adrenal hyperplasia, type 4 (20200)
Adrenal hyperplasia, type 5 (20210)
Aldosterone deficiency (20340)
Male pseudohermaphroditism (30915)
Male pseudohermaphroditism (26430)
Thyroid hormones (Chapter 13)
Thyroid dyshormonogenesis, type 1 (27440)
Thyroid dyshormonogenesis, type 2A (27450)
Thyroid dyshormonogenesis, type 2B (27460)
Thyroid dyshormonogenesis, type 3 (27470)
Thyroid dyshormonogenesis, type 4 (27480)
Thyroid dyshormonogenesis, type 5 (27490)

responses with some pairs falling into one or other part of a bimodal response and other pairs separating, with one member giving each of the two possible responses.

18.11.8. Inherited metabolic diseases in other chapters

Table 18.7 details features of clinical chemical interest for all inherited metabolic diseases for which the information could be assembled. It is important that the common concepts for genetic disease should be broadened and he who investigates unknown genetic and metabolic situations by "doing the urine aminoacids" only should examine his motives carefully. Many inherited metabolic diseases are quite appropriately discussed in chapters on haematological and intestinal biochemistry, on liver and kidney disorders and elsewhere. These are listed in Table 18.8, so that the relevant chapters may be referred to, but further details are included in Table 18.7 to emphasize that the same underlying principles will apply to their understanding and investigation.

REFERENCES

* Useful for background reading.
** Useful reference works.

Berry, H.K., Leonard, C., Peters, H., Granger, M. and Chunekamrai, N. (1968) Detection of metabolic disorders: chromatographic procedures and interpretation of results. Clinical Chemistry, 14, 1033–1065.

Bickel, H. (1970) Phenylalaninaemia or classical phenylketonuria (PKU) ? Neuropädiatrie, 1, 379–382.

Bickel, H., Gerrard, J. and Hickmans, E.M. (1953) Influence of phenylalanine intake on phenylketonuria. Lancet, ii, 812–813.

Bradley, D.M. (1975) Screening for inherited metabolic disease in Wales using urine-impregnated filter paper. Archives of Disease in Childhood, 50, 264–268.

Brand, E., Harris, M.M. and Biloon, S. (1930) Cystinuria: excretion of cystine complex which decomposes in urine with liberation of free cystine. Journal of Biological Chemistry, 86, 315–331.

Buist, N.R.M. and Jhaveri, B.M. (1973) A guide to screening newborn infants for inborn errors of metabolism. Journal of Pediatrics, 82, 511–522.

Commission on Biochemical Nomenclature (1972) Enzyme Nomenclature, Elsevier, Amsterdam and Biochimica Biophysica Acta (1976) Suppl., 429, 1–45.

Cone, T.E. (1968a) Diagnosis and treatment: some syndromes, diseases and conditions associated with abnormal coloration of the urine or diaper – a clinician's viewpoint. Pediatrics, 41, 654–658.

Cone, T.E. (1968b) Diagnosis and treatment: some diseases, syndromes and conditions associated with an unusual odour. Pediatrics, 41, 993–995.

Dorfman, A., Matalon, R., Thompson, J.N., Cifonelli, J.A., Dawson, G., Stoolmiller, A.C. and Lamberg, S.J. (1975) Genetic defects of the degradation of glycosaminoglycans: the mucopolysaccharidoses. In Inborn Errors of Skin, Hair and Connective Tissue (Eds. J.B. Holton and J.T. Ireland) pp. 163–178, Medical and Technical Publishing Co. Ltd., Lancaster.

Efron, M.L., Young, D., Moser, H.W. and MacCready, R.A. (1964) A simple chromatographic test for the detection of disorders of amino acid metabolism. New England Journal of Medicine, 270, 1378–1383.

Farmer, M.D., Lehmann, H. and Raine, D.N. (1964) Two unrelated patients with congenital cyanosis due to Haemoglobinopathy M. Lancet, ii, 786–789.

Fell, V., Pollitt, R.J., Sampson, G.A. and Wright, T. (1974) Ornithinaemia, hyperammonaemia and homocitrullinuria: a disease associated with mental retardation and possibly caused by defective mitochondrial transport. American Journal of Diseases of Children, 127, 752–756.

Fernandes, J. (1975) Hepatic glycogen storage diseases. In The Treatment of Inherited Metabolic Disease (Ed. D.N. Raine) pp. 115–149, Medical and Technical Publishing Co. Ltd., Lancaster.

Fernandes, J., Huijing, F. and Van de Kamer, J.H. (1969) A screening method for liver glycogen diseases. Archives of Disease in Childhood, 44, 311–317.

Fernandes, J., Koster, J.F., Grose, W.F.A. and Sorgedrager, N. (1974) Hepatic phosphorylase deficiency: its differentiation from other hepatic glycogenoses. Archives of Disease in Childhood, 49, 186–191.

Franklin, A.W., Porter, A.M.W. and Raine, D.N. (1973) Research investigations in children. British Medical Journal, 2, 402–407.

* Garrod, A.E. (1902) The incidence of alkaptonuria: a study in chemical individuality. Lancet, ii, 1616–1620.

Garrod, A.E. (1908) Inborn errors of metabolism. Lancet, ii, 1, 73, 142 and 214.

Goodman, S.I., McIntyre, C.A. and O'Brien, D. (1967) Impaired intestinal transport of proline in a patient with familial iminoaciduria. Journal of Pediatrics, 71, 246–249.

Guthrie, R. and Susi, A. (1963) A simple phenylalanine method for detecting phenylketonuria in large populations of newborn infants. Pediatrics, 32, 338–343.

Hamilton, P.B. (1965) Amino acids on hands. Nature (London), 205, 284–285.

Haworth, J.C. and McCredie, D. (1956) Chromatographic separation of reducing sugars in the urines of newborn babies. Archives of Disease in Childhood, 31, 189–190.

Haworth, J.C. and MacDonald, M.S. (1957) Reducing sugars in the urine and blood of premature babies. Archives of Disease in Childhood, 32, 417–421.

Ireland, J.T. and Read, R.A. (1972) A thin-layer chromatographic method for use in neonatal screening to detect excess amino acidaemia. Annals of Clinical Biochemistry, 9, 129–132.

* Jones, A. and Bodmer, W.F. (1974) Our Future Inheritance: Choice or Chance. Oxford University Press, London.

Kutter, D. and Humbel. R. (1969) Screening for sulfite oxidase deficiency. Clinica Chimica Acta, 24, 211–214.

Levy, H.L., Shih, V.E., Madigan, P.M., Karolkewicz, V. and MacCready, R.A. (1968) Results of a screening method for free amino acids. 1. Whole blood. 2. Urine. Clinical Biochemistry, 1, 200–207 and 208–215.

Lewis, P.W., Raine, D.N. and Kennedy, J.F. (1974) Recognition of the mucopolysaccharidoses by four screening tests, including a refinement of the albumin turbidity test, and their differentiation by electrophoretic separation of urinary glycosaminoglycans. Annals of Clinical Biochemistry, 11, 67–71.

Lormans, S. and Lowenthal, A. (1974) α-Amino adipic aciduria in an oligophrenic child. Clinica Chimica Acta, 57, 97–101.

Maier, K.P., Helbig, C.L., Hoppe-Seyler, G., Talke, H., Fröhlich, J., Schollmeyer, P. and Gerok, W. (1974). Extractability and intracellular localisation of urea cycle enzymes from rat liver. Zeitschrift für Klinische Chemie und Klinische Biochemie, 12, 524–529.

** McKusick, V.A. (1975) Mendelian Inheritance in Man, 4th edn. The Johns Hopkins University Press, Baltimore.

Medical Research Council Working Party on Phenylketonuria (1968) British Medical Journal, 4, 7–13.

Meeuwisse, G.W. and Melin, K. (1969) Glucose–galactose malabsorption: a clinical study of 6 cases. Acta Paediatrica Scandinavica, Suppl., 188, 3–18.

Morikawa, T., Tada., K., Ando, T., Yoshida, T., Tokoyama, Y. and Arakawa, T. (1966) Prolinuria: defect in intestinal absorption of imino acids and glycine. Tohoku Journal of Experimental Medicine, 90, 105–116.

* Nuffield Provincial Hospitals Trust (1968) Screening in Medical Care. Oxford University Press, London.

Oyanagi, K., Miura, R. and Yamanouchi, T. (1970) Congenital lysinuria: a new inherited transport disorder of dibasic amino acids. Journal of Pediatrics, 77, 259–266.

Perry, T.L., Hansen, S. and MacDougall, L. (1966) Urinary screening tests in the prevention of mental deficiency. Canadian Medical Association Journal, 95, 89–95.

Perry, T.L. and Hansen, S. (1969) Technical pitfalls leading to errors in the quantitation of plasma amino acids. Clinica Chimica Acta, 25, 53–58.

Pik, C. and Raine, D.N. (1964) The chemical identification of two cases of HbM (HbM Boston and HbM Saskatoon) occurring in England. Clinica Chimica Acta, 10, 90–92.

Przyrembel, H., Bachmann, D., Lombeck, I., Becker, K., Wendel, U., Wadham, S.K. and Bremer, H.J. (1975) Alpha-ketoadipic aciduria, a new inborn error of lysine metabolism: biochemical studies. Clinica Chimica Acta, 58, 257–269.

Raine, D.N. (1966) Inborn errors of metabolism – the development of an idea. In Basic Concepts of Inborn Errors and Defects of Steroid Biosynthesis (Eds. K. Holt and D.N. Raine) pp. 2–8, E. and S. Livingstone, Edinburgh.

Raine, D.N. (1969) Screening for inherited metabolic disease. Annals of Clinical Biochemistry, 6, 29–33.

Raine, D.N. (1972) Management of inherited metabolic disease. British Medical Journal, 2, 329–336.

Raine, D.N. (1974a) The need for a national policy for the management of inherited metabolic disease. In Molecular Variants in Disease (Ed. D.N. Raine), Journal of Clinical Pathology, 27, Suppl. (Royal College of Pathologists), 8, 156–163 (reprinted with corrections in Raine, 1977).

Raine, D.N. (1974b) Screening for disease: inherited metabolic disease. Lancet, ii, 996–998.

** Raine, D.N. (1975) The Treatment of Inherited Metabolic Disease. Medical and Technical Publishing Co. Ltd., Lancaster.

Raine, D.N. (1977) Medicosocial Management of Inherited Metabolic Disease. Medical and Technical Press Ltd., Lancaster.

Raine, D.N., Cooke, J.R., Andrews, W.A. and Mahon, D.F. (1972) Screening for inherited metabolic disease by plasma chromatography (Scriver) in a large city. British Medical Journal, 3, 7–13.

Roesel, R.A. and Coryell, M.E. (1974) Determination of cystine excretion by the nitroprusside method during drug therapy of cystinuria. Clinica Chimica Acta, 52, 343–346.

Rosenberg, L.E., Downing, S.J., Durant, J.L. and Segal, S. (1966) Cystinuria: biochemical evidence for three genetically distinct diseases. Journal of Clinical Investigation, 45, 365–371.

Scriver, C.R., Davies, E. and Cullen, A.M. (1964) Application of a simple micromethod to the screening of plasma for a variety of aminoacidopathies. Lancet, ii, 230–232.

** Scriver, C.R. and Rosenberg, L.E. (1973) Amino Acid Metabolism and its Disorders. W.B. Saunders, Philadelphia.

** Shih, V.E. (1975) Laboratory Techniques for the Detection of Hereditary Metabolic Disorders. C.R.C. Press, Cleveland.

Shih, V.E., Efron, M.L. and Moser, H.W. (1969) Hyperornithinemia, hyperammonemia and homocitrullinuria. American Journal of Diseases of Children, 117, 83–92.

Shih, V.E. and Mandell, R. (1974) Metabolic defect in hyperornithinaemia. Lancet, ii, 1522–1523.

Simell, O. and Takki, K. (1973) Raised plasma ornithine and gyrate atrophy of the choroid and retina. Lancet, i, 1031–1033.

Smith, I. (1969) Chromatographic and Electrophoretic Techniques, Vol. 1, Chromatography. Heineman Medical Ltd., London.

Steinitz, K. (1967) Laboratory diagnosis of glycogen diseases. Advances in Clinical Chemistry, 9, 227–354.

Sutcliffe, R.G. and Brock, D.J.H. (1971) Enzymes in uncultured amniotic fluid cells. Clinica Chimica Acta, 31, 363–365.

Teijema, H.L., van Gelderen, H.H., Giesberts, M.A.H. and Laurent de Angulo, M.S.L. (1974) Dicarboxylic amino aciduria: an inborn error of glutamate and aspartate transport with metabolic implications in combination with hyperprolinemia. Metabolism, 23, 115–123.

** Thomas, G.H. and Howell, R.R. (1973) Selected Screening Tests for Genetic Metabolic Diseases. Year Book Medical Publishers Inc., Chicago.

Westwood, A. and Raine, D.N. (1973) Some problems of heterozygote recognition in inherited metabolic disease with special reference to phenylketonuria. In Treatment of Inborn Errors of Metabolism (Eds. J.W.T. Seakins, R.A. Saunders and C. Toothill) pp. 63–77, Churchill-Livingstone, Edinburgh.

Westwood, A. and Raine, D.N. (1975) Heterozygote detection in phenylketonuria: measurement of discriminatory ability and interpretation of the phenylalanine loading test by determination of the heterozygote likelihood ratio (HLR). Journal of Medical Genetics, 12, 327–333.

** Wilkinson, J.H. (1976) The Principles and Practice of Diagnostic Enzymology. Edward Arnold, London.

Wood, B. (1977) Paediatric Vade-Mecum, 9th edn. Lloyd-Luke, London.

Woolf, L.I. (1967) Large-scale screening for metabolic disease in the newborn in Great Britain. In Phenylketonuria and Allied Metabolic Diseases. (Eds. J.A. Anderson and K.F. Swaiman) pp. 50–61, U.S. Department of Health, Education and Welfare, Washington.

FURTHER READING

Background (In addition to those marked * above)

Carter, C.O. (1962) Human Heredity. Penguin Books, Harmondsworth.

Cavalli-Sforza, L.L. and Bodmer, W.F. (1971) The Genetics of Human Populations. W.H. Freeman, San Francisco.

Griffiths, M.I. (Ed.) (1973) The Young Retarded Child – Medical Aspects of Care. Churchill Livingstone, Edinburgh and London.

Knox, W.E. (1958) Sir Archibald Garrod's Inborn Errors of Metabolism. 1. Cystinuria. 2. Alkaptonuria. 3. Albinism. 4. Pentosuria. American Journal of Human Genetics, 10, 3–32, 95–124, 249–267, 385–397.

Motulsky, A.G. (1974) Brave New World. Science, 185, 653–663.

Raine, D.N. (Ed.) (1974) Molecular Variants in Disease. Journal of Clinical Pathology (Royal College of Pathologists) 27, Suppl.

Works of reference (In addition to those marked ** above)

Bondy, P.K. and Rosenberg, L.E. (1974) Duncan's Diseases of Metabolism, 7th edn. (2 vols). W.B. Saunders, Philadelphia.

Carter, C.O. and Fairbank, T.J. (1974) The Genetics of Locomotor Disorders. Oxford University Press, London.

Emery, A.E.H. (1973) Antenatal Diagnosis of Genetic Disease, Churchill-Livingstone, Edinburgh.

Geeraets, W.J. (1969) Ocular Syndromes, 2nd edn. Lea and Febiger, Philadelphia.

McKusick, V.A. (1972) Heritable Disorders of Connective Tissue, 4th edn. C.V. Mosby and Co., Saint Louis.

Milunsky, A. (1973) The Prenatal Diagnosis of Hereditary Disorders. Charles C. Thomas, Springfield.

Pratt, R.T.C. (1967) The Genetics of Neurological Disorders. Oxford University Press, London.

Slater, E. and Cowie, V. (1971) The Genetics of Mental Disorders. Oxford University Press, London.

Stanbury, J.B., Wyngaarden, J.B. and Fredrickson, D.S. (1978) The Metabolic Basis of Inherited Disease, 4th edn. McGraw-Hill Book Co., New York.

Wynne-Davies, R. (1973) Heritable Disorders in Orthopaedic Practice. Blackwell Scientific Publications, Oxford.

Publications of the Society for the Study of Inborn Errors of Metabolism

1. Holt, K.S. and Milner, J. (Eds.) (1964) Neurometabolic Disorders in Childhood. E. and S. Livingstone, Ltd., Edinburgh.
2. Allan, J.D. and Holt, K.S. (Eds.) (1965) Biochemical Approaches to Mental Handicap in Childhood. E. and S. Livingstone, Ltd., Edinburgh.
3. Holt, K.S. and Raine, D.N. (Eds.) (1966) Basic Concepts of Inborn Errors and Defects of Steroid Biosynthesis. E. and S. Livingstone, Ltd., Edinburgh.
4. Holt, K.S. and Coffey, V.P. (Eds.) (1968) Some Recent Advances in Inborn Errors of Metabolism. E. and S. Livingstone, Ltd., Edinburgh.
5. Allan, J.D. and Raine, D.N. (Eds.) (1969) Some Inherited Disorders of Brain and Muscle. E. and S. Livingstone, Ltd., Edinburgh.
6. Allan, J.D., Holt, K.S., Ireland, J.T. and Pollitt, R.J. (Eds.) (1969) Enzymopenic Anaemias, Lysosomes and other Papers. E. and S. Livingstone, Ltd., Edinburgh.
7. Hamilton, W. and Hudson, F.P. (Eds.) (1970) Errors of Phenylalanine, Thyroxine and Testosterone Metabolism. E. and S. Livingstone, Ltd., Edinburgh.
8. Carson, N.A.J. and Raine, D.N. (Eds.) (1971) Inherited Disorders of Sulphur Metabolism. Churchill-Livingstone, Edinburgh.
9. Stern, J. and Toothill, C. (Eds.) (1972) Organic Acidurias. Churchill-Livingstone, Edinburgh.
10. Seakins, J.W.T., Saunders, R.A. and Toothill, C. (Eds.) (1973) Treatment of Inborn Errors of Metabolism. Churchill-Livingstone, Edinburgh.
11. Ireland, J.T. and Holton, J. (Eds.) (1975) Inborn Errors of Skin, Hair and Connective Tissue. Medical and Technical Publishing Co. Ltd., Lancaster.
12. Bickel, H. and Stern, J. (Eds.) (1975) Inborn Errors of Calcium and Bone Metabolism. Medical and Technical Publishing Co. Ltd., Lancaster.
13. Raine, D.N. (Ed.) (1976) Medicosocial Management of Inherited Metabolic Disease. Medical and Technical Publishing Co. Ltd., Lancaster.
14. Harkness, R.A. and Cockburn, F. (1977) The Cultured Cell and Inherited Metabolic Disease. Medical and Technical Press Publishing Co. Ltd., Lancaster.
15. Güttler, F., Seakins, J. and Harkness, R.A. (1978) Inborn Errors of Immunity of Phagocytosis. Medical and Technical Publishing Co. Ltd., Lancaster (in press).
16. Burman, D., Holton, J.B. and Pennock, C.A. (1979) Inherited Disorders of Carbohydrate Metabolism. Medical and Technical Publishing Co. Ltd., Lancaster.

ADDENDUM

18.9. PRENATAL DETECTION OF AN AFFECTED FOETUS

This subject is developing rapidly. Experience of 3000 amniocenteses (Golbus et al., 1979) has shown, amongst other things, that the procedure fails to yield fluid in 0.7% of taps (in three cases from one centre maternal urine was obtained and routine determination of urea is recommended): the foetus may be damaged (limbs have been amputated) but abortions following amniocentesis when compared with the spontaneous abortion rate show only a very slight excess. Culture of amniotic cells failed in 1.7% requiring the test to be repeated; in three certain and three more probable cases maternal rather than foetal cells were grown; 12 chromosomal mosaics were recognized and there is no reason to suppose that unrecognized biochemical mosaics are less common. This study provides a valuable perspective and confirms the need for caution expressed earlier under this heading.

Most of the ethical guidelines recently recommended (Powledge and Fletcher, 1979) to those involved in prenatal diagnosis will find ready acceptance in most countries.

Legal aspects of genetic diagnosis

A genetic diagnosis has not only a life-long effect on the presenting patient, but has implications for all his close relatives and for the generations as yet unborn. It is therefore imperative that any information given should be as accurate and detailed as it is possible to make it at the time it is given, and the possibility should be recognized that the diagnosis may require review in the light of new knowledge. A system or reviewing and, where necessary, re-investigating patients with genetic disease should exist wherever these diagnoses are made. There is already considerable case law and much more pending in both the United Kingdom and North America, and developments should be followed while standards of practice in this very new field are being established (Milunsky and Annas, 1976; Ratner, 1977). Patients grateful for the help given by their physician have often submitted silently to all but the most flagrant mistakes; healthy relatives given wrong, misleading or even inadequate advice are likely to be much less tolerant.

18.11.1. Phenylketonuria

The enzyme phenylalanine hydroxylase requires, as an essential co-factor, tetrahydrobiopterin (BH_4) which, as phenylalanine is converted to tyrosine, is changed to a quinonoid form of dihydrobiopterin (qBH_2). Normally this is re-converted to BH_4 by the action of dihydrobiopterin reductase. Two inherited enzyme deficiencies which reduce the supply of this essential co-factor, and hence the activity of the otherwise normal phenylalanine hydroxylase, are now recognized; one is concerned with the biosynthesis of biopterin and the other with the regeneration of BH_4. The form of phenylketonuria that results is particularly severe since BH_4 is the co-factor for a number of enzymes other than phenylalanine hydroxylase. Treatment by provision of the products of these enzymes in addition to the usual dietary restriction of phenylalanine is giving promising results but it is essential that these varieties of phenylketonuria are recognized at the time of diagnosis and not after the more usual treatment of this condition has been shown to fail (Danks et al., 1978; Editorial, 1979).

18.11.2.1. Glycogen storage disease type 5

The ischaemic exercise test used to recognize this disorder will also serve to recognize a new disease of muscle with a similar presentation – myoadenylate deaminase deficiency – if ammonia as well as lactate is determined in the blood (Fishbein et al., 1978).

Danks, D.M. et al. (1978) Pteridines and phenylketonuria: report of a workshop. Journal of Inherited Metabolic Disease, 1, 47–65.

Editorial (1979) New varieties of P.K.U. Lancet, 1, 304–305.

Fishbein, W.N., Armbrustmacher, V.W. and Griffin, J.L. (1978) Myoadenylate deaminase deficiency: a new disease of muscle. Science, 200, 545–548.

Goldbus, M.S., Loughman, W.D., Epstein, C.J., Halbasch, G., Stephens, J.D. and Hall, B.D. (1979) Prenatal genetic diagnosis in 3000 amniocenteses. New England Journal of Medicine, 300, 157–163.

Milunsky, A. and Annas, G.J. (Eds.) (1976) Genetics and the Law. Plenum Press, New York. (The proceedings of a second conference on this subject, under the same editorship, will be published in 1980.)

Powledge, T.M. and Fletcher, J. (1979) Guidelines for the ethical, social and legal issues in prenatal diagnosis. New England Journal of Medicine, 300, 168–172.

Ratner, G.A. (1977) The coming of the second genetic code: eugenic abortion in the United Kingdom. In Medico-Social Management of Inherited Metabolic Disease (Ed. D.N. Raine) pp. 119–139, Medical and Technical Publishers Ltd., Lancaster.

Chapter 19

Trace elements

F. William Sunderman, Jr.

Department of Laboratory Medicine, University of Connecticut School of Medicine, Farmington, CONN 06032, U.S.A.

CONTENTS

Chemical diagnosis of disease, edited by S.S. Brown, F.L. Mitchell and D.S. Young

19.1. INTRODUCTION

Clinical interest in trace metal analyses for the diagnosis and prognosis of diseases has recently been stimulated by (a) increasing awareness of the prevalence of poisonings from occupational and environmental exposures to toxic metals; (b) recognition that measurements of serum copper furnish a prognostic index in patients with lymphomas and leukaemias; and (c) discoveries that deficiencies of specific trace metals (e.g. copper and zinc) may be involved in the pathogenesis of certain hitherto idiopathic conditions, such as Menkes' disease (trichopoliodystrophy) and Danbolt's disease (acrodermatitis enteropathica). The practicality of assessing trace metal concentrations in body fluids and tissues of patients with various disorders has been enhanced by the addition of atomic absorption spectrometers to the instrumentation of many clinical laboratories. These various developments have led the editors of this textbook on chemical diagnosis of disease to the innovation of including a separate chapter on trace metals.

The scope of this chapter is limited to applications of trace metal analyses which have achieved practical importance in clinical diagnosis. This chapter does not include any consideration of iron metabolism, since this topic is discussed in the context of Haematological Biochemistry (Chapter 16). This chapter is intended to supplement recent treatises on (a) clinical and nutritional aspects of trace metals (Underwood, 1971; Davies, 1972; Burch et al., 1975; Mertz, 1975; Reinhold, 1975); (b) metabolism of trace metals in animals (Mills, 1970; O'Dell and Campbell, 1971; Hoekstra et al., 1974); (c) biochemistry of trace metals (Williams, 1971; Dhar, 1972; Friedman, 1973); (d) atomic absorption spectrometry of trace metals (Berman, 1969; Christian and Feldman, 1970; Sunderman, 1973, 1975a); and (e) comprehensive reviews of the metabolism and toxicology of chromium, copper, lead, manganese, nickel, vanadium and zinc (National Research Council, 1972–75), cadmium (Friberg et al., 1971) and mercury (Friberg and Vostal, 1972). These articles and monographs are listed under "Further Reading" at the end of this Chapter.

19.2. ZINC

19.2.1. Zinc metabolism

Adult persons ingest approximately 200 to 300 μmol (13 to 20 mg) of zinc per day. Absorption of zinc occurs primarily in the small intestine, and probably involves mucosal transport by a zinc-binding protein (Kowarski et al., 1974). Most of the ingested zinc remains unabsorbed within the intestinal tract and is excreted in the faeces. In addition, a major portion of the zinc that is absorbed from the intestines is subsequently excreted in saliva, bile, and pancreatic and intestinal fluids, and is eliminated in the faeces. Excretion of zinc in urine normally averages 5 μmol (325 μg)/day, and excretion of zinc in sweat averages only 1.5 μmol (100 μg)/day. Under conditions of profuse perspiration, the excretion of zinc in sweat can increase to 10 to 20 μmol (650 to 1300 μg)/day. Additional routes of zinc elimination include hair and dermal detritus, menses, semen, prostatic fluid and milk. For comprehensive discussions of ^{65}Zn-kinetics and tissue distributions of zinc, the reader is referred to a review by Mikac-Devic (1970).

Giroux (1975) has shown that zinc is present in human plasma in two distinct pools: (a) loosely bound or exchangeable zinc, and (b) firmly bound or non-exchangeable zinc. The exchangeable zinc pool includes zinc that is bound to plasma albumin and to aminoacids, such as histidine and cysteine. These ligands form complexes with zinc in vivo and in vitro. The non-exchangeable zinc pool includes zinc that is bound to an α_2-macroglobulin and the traces of zinc that occur in zinc metalloenzymes, such as alkaline phosphatase and lactate dehydrogenase. These metalloproteins do not form complexes with zinc in vitro. In erythrocytes, hepatocytes and other cells, zinc is bound to numerous metalloproteins and metalloenzymes (Parisi and Vallee, 1969). In particular, a major fraction of intracellular zinc is bound to metallothioneins (cysteine-rich proteins with molecular mass of approximately 6600) which also form complexes with cadmium, mercury and copper (Bühler and Kägi, 1974).

19.2.2. Acrodermatitis enteropathica

In 1974, Moynahan reported that acrodermatitis enteropathica (Danbolt's disease) may be a genetically determined disorder of zinc metabolism. As summarized by Sunderman (1975a), acrodermatitis enteropathica is a lethal, autosomal trait, which usually occurs in infants of Italian, Armenian or Iranian lineage. The disease is not present at birth, but typically develops in the early months of life, soon after weaning from breast feeding. Dermatological manifestations include progressive bullous-pustular dermatitis of the extremities and the oral, anal and genital areas, combined with paronychia and generalized alopecia. Infection with *Candida albicans* is a frequent complication. Ophthalmic signs may include blepharitis, conjunctivitis, photophobia and corneal opacities. Gastrointestinal disturbances are usually severe, including chronic diarrhoea, malabsorption, steatorrhoea and lactose intolerance. Neuropsychiatric signs include irritability, emotional disorders, tremor and occasional cerebellar ataxia. The patients generally have retarded growth and hypogonadism. Prior to the serendipitous discovery of diiodohydroxyquinolone therapy, patients with acrodermatitis enteropathica invariably died from cachexia, usually with terminal respiratory infection. Although diiodohydroxyquinolone has been used successfully for the therapy of this condition for more than 20 years, the mechanism of drug action has never been elucidated. It now seems possible that its efficacy might be related to the formation of an absorbable zinc-chelate, inasmuch as diiodohydroxyquinolone is a derivative of 8-hydroxyquinoline, a chelating agent.

Moynahan and Barnes (1973) studied a 2-year-old girl with acrodermatitis enteropathica who was being treated with diiodohydroxyquinolone and a lactose-deficient synthetic diet. The clinical response to this therapy was not satisfactory, and the physicians sought to identify contributory factors. They found that the concentration of zinc in the patient's serum was markedly reduced, and they decided to administer oral zinc sulphate. The patient's skin lesions and gastrointestinal symptoms cleared completely, and the patient was discharged from the hospital. When zinc sulphate was inadvertently omitted from the regimen, the patient suffered a relapse which promptly responded when oral zinc sulphate was reinstituted. Moynahan (1974) recognized that the dermatitis and alopecia in acrodermatitis enteropathica were similar to the dermal lesions which occur in zinc-deficient rats, and he suspected that a genetic abnormality of zinc metabolism might be fundamental to the pathogenesis of acrodermatitis enteropathica. Moynahan (1974) tested this hypothesis by administration of zinc sulphate to nine additional children with acrodermatitis enteropathica, while completely withdrawing diiodohydroxyquinolone from their therapeutic regimens. The children became free of symptoms, and the prepubertal children experienced rapid increase in rate of growth. The therapeutic efficacy of zinc sulphate in acrodermatitis enteropathica has been independently confirmed (Michaelsson, 1974; Portnoy and Molokhia, 1974).

Studies of the metabolism of ^{65}Zn in patients with acrodermatitis enteropathica (Lombeck et al., 1975) have demonstrated reduced intestinal absorption of zinc and normal elimination of zinc into faeces, urine and sweat. Amador et al. (1975) have shown that concentrations of zinc in hair samples from patients with acrodermatitis enteropathica were significantly lower than in hair samples from healthy infants and children, and from patients with other diseases. It may be speculated that patients with acrodermatitis enteropathica are genetically deficient in the soluble zinc-binding protein which has been isolated from intestinal mucosa by Kowarski et al. (1974) and which may be involved in active transport of zinc. Endre et al. (1975) have suggested that zinc deprivation in patients with acrodermatitis enteropathica produces a lymphocyte malfunction, which leads to impairment of cellular immunity, and thus predisposes to bacterial and fungal infections. Although the molecular pathogenesis of acrodermatitis remains to be elucidated (Henkin and Aamodt, 1975), it seems clear that measurements of zinc concentrations in plasma and other body fluids are valuable for diagnosis and monitoring the therapy of patients with this disorder (Strain et al., 1975).

19.2.3. Hypogonadal dwarfism

The syndrome of zinc-deficient hypogonadal dwarfism was first reported by Prasad et al. (1963). According to Prasad (1972), most of the zinc-deficient subjects whom he and his colleagues have studied have been adolescent males with dwarfism, retardation of sexual maturation, iron-deficiency anaemia and hepatosplenomegaly, who live in rural Iran and Egypt. The laboratory and clinical evidence of zinc-deficiency in these subjects has included: low concentrations of zinc in plasma, erythrocytes and hair; low excretions of zinc in urine and sweat; increased turnover of ^{65}Zn in plasma; low cumulative excretions of ^{65}Zn in urine and faeces; and increased rate of skeletal growth and gonadal development after dietary zinc supplementation. Zinc deficiency in these subjects apparently is the result of interference with zinc absorption from the gastrointestinal tract owing to the large amount of phytate which is present in the native diet. Ronaghy et al. (1974) have reported a 2-year study of zinc supplementation in malnourished Iranian schoolboys. Administration of oral zinc sulphate to these subjects provided an unequivocal stimulus to skeletal growth.

Cases of hypogonadal dwarfism with zinc deficiency have also been found in the United States. Caggiano et al. (1969) reported a 21-year-old man with dwarfism, hypogonadism and zinc deficiency. Within 3 months after zinc supplementation was instituted, this man's height increased by 7 cm; his genitalia became significantly larger; and he developed secondary sexual characteristics. Sandstead (1973) described a 20-year-old man with regional enteritis, growth failure and hypogonadism who responded to oral zinc supplementation. Prasad et al. (1975) reported the occurrence of zinc deficiency and hypogonadal dwarfism in several male patients with sickle cell disease. Administration of oral zinc sulphate resulted in increase in body height and growth of genitalia in some of these young men. On the basis of these several reports, zinc deficiency can be regarded a pathogenetic factor in certain cases of human hypogonadal dwarfism.

19.2.4. Impaired wound healing

In 1966, Pories and Strain reported that oral administration of zinc sulphate to patients with pilonidal sinuses was attended by a 2-fold increase in the rate of re-epithelialization. The authors' conclusion that zinc sulphate can promote the healing of cutaneous sores and wounds has been a subject of continuing controversy. Carruthers (1973), Henkin (1974) and Sunderman (1975b) have reviewed the conflicting clinical evidence, and have concluded that administration of zinc sulphate to patients who are zinc-deficient is one of the factors which accelerates the healing of cutaneous wounds. This conclusion is supported by studies in experimental animals which have demonstrated that: healing of incised wounds is impaired in rats with dietary zinc deficiency; synthesis of desoxyribonucleic acid (DNA), ribonucleic acid (RNA), collagen and non-collagen proteins is reduced in skin and connective tissues from rats with dietary zinc deficiency; zinc supplementation does *not* augment wound healing in normal rats; and zinc supplementation *does* augment wound healing in chronically ill rats. If a clinician accepts the conclusion that zinc supplementation may promote wound healing in zinc-deficient patients, the clinician is then confronted with the difficult question of how to diagnose zinc deficiency. As Henkin (1974) and Prasad et al. (1975) have emphasized, there is no ready answer to this question, owing to the complex interactions of pathophysiological mechanisms which influence zinc metabolism and which produce hypozincaemia.

19.2.5. Pathophysiological mechanisms of hypozincaemia

According to Sunderman (1975b), the pathophysiological mechanisms which have been implicated in the production of hypozincaemia include: nutritional deficiency and/or intestinal malabsorption of zinc; increased urinary excretion of zinc, secondary to aminoaciduria (e.g. histidine and cysteine), frequently associated with tissue catabolism; zinc losses in sweat during profuse perspiration; diminution of serum zinc secondary to hypoalbuminaemia; alteration of body zinc pools and increased urinary excretion of zinc secondary to adrenal release of cortisol and pituitary release of growth hormone (e.g. following stress); alteration of body zinc pools produced by endogenous estrogens (e.g. pregnancy) or exogenous estrogens (e.g. oral contraceptives); and alteration of body zinc pools produced by "leucocytic endogenous mediator". Leucocytic endogenous mediator is a heat-labile protein released from sensitized polymorphonuclear leucocytes, which produces prompt hypozincaemia with concommitant increase in hepatic zinc (Pekarek et al., 1972). Leucocytic endogenous mediator is involved in many facets of the "acute phase reaction", and there is evidence that leucocytic endogenous mediator may be responsible for the hypozincaemia which occurs during acute infections and inflammatory conditions (Powanda et al., 1973; Beisel et al., 1974). The hypozincaemia which is produced by leucocytic endogenous mediator is the result of redistribution of zinc within body pools, without zinc deficiency necessarily being present. Therefore, reliance cannot be placed solely upon measurements of plasma zinc for the diagnosis of zinc deficiency.

The many clinical conditions which are associated with hypozincaemia include: myocardial infarction; acute infections; viral hepatitis; hepatic cirrhosis; hypogeusia (diminished perception of taste); hyposomia (decreased sense of smell); nyctalopia (night blindness); carcinomatosis; leukaemias and lymphomas; pernicious anemia and sickle cell anaemia; chronic uraemia; malabsorption states and kwashiorkor; alcoholism; mongolism; psoriasis; surgical stress; acromegaly; pregnancy; chronic debilitation (e.g. paraplegia, cystic fibrosis); and the effects of various drugs (e.g. oestrogens, oral contraceptives and corticosteroids) (Sunderman, 1975b). The pathophysiological mechanisms which have been cited may function to varying degrees in these several disorders. In order to assess zinc nutriture in patients, it is frequently desirable to measure zinc in diverse biological samples, including urine, blood cells, hair, sweat, saliva, and amniotic fluid. Studies of ^{65}Zn are invaluable for clinical research, but should be approached with caution for diagnostic purposes, owing to the long residence time of ^{65}Zn in the human body and the presence of zinc in DNA polymerase and reverse transcriptase. As additional approaches to assessment of zinc nutriture, measurements of zinc in plasma ultrafiltrates and spinal fluid may be attempted. Consideration may also be given to measurements of urinary excretion of zinc before and after infusion of chelating agents such as calcium-EDTA (ethylenediaminetetraacetate) or calcium-DTPA (diethylenetriaminepentaacetate). Finally, in many cases it is desirable to perform a therapeutic trial of oral supplementation with zinc sulphate. For an excellent example of the difficulties of establishing the presence of zinc deficiency, readers may consult the study by Prasad et al. (1975) of zinc metabolism in sickle cell disease.

19.2.6. Hyperzincaemia

A high serum zinc concentration may occur as a result of industrial exposure or in patients undergoing haemodialysis against a dialysate containing a large amount of zinc, as has occurred in one dialysis centre in which a galvanized iron water softener was used. The serum zinc concentration in the haemodialysis patients may be sufficiently high to cause anaemia (Petrie and Row, 1977).

TABLE 19.1.

REFERENCE INTERVALS FOR ZINC IN BODY FLUIDS OF HEALTHY ADULTS [a]

Body fluid	No. of subjects	Zn concentration or excretion		Authors
		Mean ± S.D.	Units	
Serum	37 ♂	14.5 ± 0.5	μmol/litre	Meret and Henkin (1971)
	45 ♀	13.9 ± 0.5	μmol/litre	
Erythrocytes	14 ♂	0.18 ± 0.02	μmol/10^{10} cells	Rosner and Gorfien (1968)
	9 ♀	0.19 ± 0.04	μmol/10^{10} cells	
Urine	37 ♂	5.5 ± 0.3	μmol/24 hours	Meret and Henkin (1971)
	45 ♀	5.4 ± 0.7	μmol/24 hours	
Sweat	33 ♂	7.7 ± 7.3	μmol/litre	Hohnadel et al. (1973)
	15 ♀	19.1 ± 11.8	μmol/litre	
Saliva	11 ♂	0.81 ± 0.17	μmol/litre	Henkin et al. (1975)
	23 ♀	0.76 ± 0.24	μmol/litre	

[a] SI unit conversion for zinc, μmol × 65 = μg

19.2.7. Measurements of zinc in biological materials

Methods for the analysis of zinc in biological materials have been reviewed by Mikac-Devic (1970) and Sunderman (1973). Most clinical laboratories currently employ atomic absorption spectrometry for zinc analyses. It should be emphasized that inadequacies in specimen collection and errors from contamination during analysis frequently contribute to the difficulties of clinical evaluation of zinc metabolism. Blood for zinc analysis should be collected in the morning while the patient remains in bed after an overnight fast, in order to minimize the effects of circadian variations. All glassware which is used for specimen collection, processing and analysis must be acid-washed in order to avoid zinc contamination. Since the zinc content of erythrocytes is 14-fold that of plasma, scrupulous precautions should be observed in order to minimize haemolysis. It is preferable to analyze plasma rather than serum, since the concentration of zinc in serum averages 16% higher than in plasma, owing in part to platelet release of zinc during clotting.

Reference intervals for zinc concentrations in biological fluids from healthy adults are summarized in Table 19.1, based upon a critical evaluation of published values. Measurements of the concentrations of zinc in plasma from healthy infants and children have been reported by Henkin et al. (1973).

19.3. COPPER

19.3.1. Copper metabolism

Adult persons ingest approximately 50 to 80 μmol (3.2 to 5.1 mg) of copper per day in their diet. Strickland et al. (1972) found that healthy subjects absorb an average of 56%

(range, 40 to 70%) of orally administered copper. Most of the absorbed copper is subsequently excreted in the bile and eliminated in the faeces. Copper is absorbed by the mucosa of the small intestine and released into the plasma by active transport processes, which may be impaired in patients with diffuse gastrointestinal diseases in patients with Menkes' disease, as discussed in section 19.3.2.

Copper is transported from the intestine to the liver by binding to plasma albumin and to aminoacids. Copper which is transported by these ligands in plasma is avidly taken up into hepatocytes. Within the hepatocytes, copper becomes reversibly bound to two cytosol proteins: hepatocuprein and metallothionein. Minor fractions of hepatic copper also become reversibly bound to an acidic chromatin protein in the nucleus which is involved in regulation of DNA transcription, and to an intramitochondrial polypeptide. In hepatic microsomes and endoplasmic reticulum, copper becomes irreversibly incorporated into metalloenzymes for intracellular functions within hepatocytes (e.g. cytochrome c oxidase), and into caeruloplasmin which is released into the serum. Detoxification and biliary excretion of copper is accomplished by the hepatic lysosomes.

The lysosomes excrete approximately 8 to 15 μmol of copper per day into bile in the form of a copper–taurochenodesoxycholate–lecithin micellar complex, which impairs the intestinal reabsorption of copper (Lewis, 1973). Intestinal loss of caeruloplasmin amounts to only 1.5 μmol (95 μg) of copper per day. Salivary, gastric and pancreatic-jejunal secretions account for the remainder of the gastrointestinal excretion of copper. Normally, the urinary excretion of copper is very low (≃0.3 μmol (19 μg) per day). Minor routes for copper elimination also include sweat, hair, dermal detritis, menses and milk.

Copper which is firmly bound to caeruloplasmin comprises approximately 95% of the total plasma copper. Caeruloplasmin is a blue glycoprotein (molecular mass 130,000 to 160,000) which posseses oxidase activity. The physiological role of this enzyme remains obscure, although it has been suggested that it functions both as a ferroxidase and as a histaminase. Caeruloplasmin does not serve as a transport protein for copper en route from the intestine to the liver, but it may possibly play a role in transport of copper from the liver to other tissues (Owen, 1975). For enzymatic analyses of caeruloplasmin in clinical laboratories, *p*-phenylenediamine is usually employed as the substrate (Sunderman and Nomoto, 1970; Hohnadel et al., 1975). Copper is a constituent of important metalloenzymes and metalloproteins in various organs and tissues, e.g. dopamine-β-hydroxylase (EC 1.14.17.1) in adrenal and brain; lysyloxidase in cartilage; tyrosinase (EC 1.14.18.1) in skin and eye; tryptophan dioxygenase (EC 1.13.11.11) in liver; superoxide dysmutase (EC 1.15.1.1) in erythrocytes, liver and brain; albocupreins I and II in brain; and cytochrome c oxidase (EC 1.9.3.1) in most tissues. For comprehensive reviews of the biochemistry and physiology of copper in mammals, the reader may consult articles by Sass-Kortsak (1965); Malkin and Malmstrom (1970); and Evans (1973).

There are five principal clinical situations in which hospital laboratories are required to measure copper concentrations in serum, urine, liver or other biological materials: Menkes' disease; acquired copper deficiency; Wilson's disease; copper toxicity; and malignant diseases (especially lymphomas and leukaemias). Each of these topics will be considered in the following sections.

19.3.2. Menkes' disease (trichopoliodystrophy)

Menkes' disease is a progressive inherited brain disease of male infants which usually causes death before 3 years of age, and which is characterized by severely retarded growth and development, "kinky" or "steely" hair (pili torti), hypothermia, arterial tortuosity, scorbutic bone changes, and cerebral gliosis with cystic degeneration. Danks et al. (1972, 1973) discovered that Menkes' disease is associated with profound hypocupraemia, hypocaeruloplasminaemia, hypocupruria, and diminished concentrations of copper in hair and other tissues (excepting duodenal mucosa, which contains abnormally large amounts of copper). The malabsorption of copper in Menkes' disease apparently results from defective transport of copper within the intestinal epithelial cells or across the serosal membrane, since copper uptake into the epithelial cells from the gut lumen is normal. It may be speculated that an X-linked absence or abnormality of a copper transport protein causes impaired release of copper from mucosal cells, thus leading to post-natal copper deprivation. The pathogenesis of the disease can hypothetically be explained on the basis of copper deficiency, assuming that diminished activity of lysyloxidase (a copper metalloenzyme) may cause impaired elastin and collagen biosynthesis, and thereby produce arterial tortuosity and scorbutic bone changes, and that diminished activities of cytochrome c oxidase, dopamine-β-hydroxylase, and superoxide dysmutase (copper metalloenzymes) may cause neuronal degeneration and demyelination of brain tissue. Copper deficiency is presumed to induce alterations in free sulphydryl groups of the hair, resulting in its tendency to twist. The defect of trace metal metabolism may involve nickel as well as copper, based upon a finding by the present author of profound reduction of nickel concentrations in serum and hair from a patient with Menkes' disease.

Several investigators (Bucknall et al., 1973; Walker-Smith et al., 1973; Dekaban and Steusing, 1974; Wehinger et al., 1975) have administered copper salts by parenteral injections to patients with Menkes' disease who were more than 3 months of age. Copper administration consistently resulted in increased concentrations of serum copper and caeruloplasmin. According to Bucknall et al. (1973), caeruloplasmin synthesis and decay are normal in these patients when copper is available. Regrettably, parenteral copper therapy has not been attended by improvement of neurological status in any patient who was more than 3 months of age. On the other hand, Grover and Scrutton (1975) treated an infant with Menkes' disease who was diagnosed at the age of 3 days. Parenteral copper therapy was started at the age of 28 days, and the preliminary response was encouraging, with no convulsions and some developmental progress. At 6 months of age, this infant had reached a functional level of 4 months. These observations suggest that the neurological and biochemical dysfunctions of Menkes' disease may be ameliorated by infusion of a copper salt within the first weeks of life. In response to this finding, clinical laboratories are being requested to perform analyses of copper in serum from newborn infants as a possible screening test for Menkes' syndrome.

19.3.3. Acquired copper deficiency

Nutritional copper deficiency has been recognized in infants and in adults. In both groups of patients, the syndrome is characterized by severe anaemia and neutropenia. In addition, copper deficient infants develop scurvy-like bone changes. Infantile copper deficiency was first described in marasmic infants in Peru who were admitted to a hospital because of malnutrition and chronic diarrhoea, and who were rehabilitated on a calorie-rich milk diet that was deficient in copper (Cordano et al., 1966; Graham, 1971). In these infants, the concentrations of serum copper became profoundly reduced and bone marrow examinations revealed granulocytic maturation arrest and erythroid hypoplasia. Al Rashid and Spangler (1971), Seely et al. (1972) and Ashkenazi et al. (1973) have reported that premature infants in the United States developed neutropenia, anaemia, scorbutic bone changes and impaired growth while receiving copper-deficient milk diets. In these infants, there was profound hypocupraemia and hypocaeruloplasminaemia. Oral copper supplementation in these infants resulted in prompt clinical improvement and increases of serum copper and caeruloplasmin concentrations to normal ranges. Ashkenazi et al. (1973) have recommended that 1.5 to 8 μmol of copper be added to the daily diet of premature infants until they are receiving other foods beside milk. Karpel and Peden (1972) and Ashkenazi et al. (1973) have also observed profound hypocupraemia associated with anaemia and neutropenia in infants who were receiving prolonged intravenous alimentation as supportive therapy for impaired gastrointestinal function. These infants improved dramatically following copper supplementation.

Copper deficiency in adults was reported by Sternlieb and Janowitz (1964) as a result of defective absorption of copper, usually as a manifestation of severe disease of the small intestine. Case reports of adult copper deficiency have been published by Dunlap et al. (1974) and Vilter et al. (1974). The patient described by Vilter et al. (1974) suffered from severe systemic sclerosis of the intestine with malabsorption, and copper deficiency developed after 10 weeks of intravenous hyperalimentation. This patient had anaemia, leukopenia and marked neutropenia which disappeared when copper was administered. Dunlap et al. (1974) described two adult patients with copper deficiency who had had extensive bowel surgery and had received long-term parenteral hyperalimentation. One of these patients was neutropenic and anaemic. Marrow examination showed a predominance of early granulocytes and cytoplasmic vacuolization of erythroid and myeloid elements. Erythroid development was megaloblastoid with increased sideroblasts. These abnormalities disappeared after oral copper therapy; reappeared when therapy was withdrawn, and again disappeared after intravenous copper therapy. The other patient was neutropenic but not anaemic, and bone marrow revealed normoblastic erythropoiesis with cytoplasmic vacuolization or erythroid and myeloid precursors and a predominance of early granulocytes. The neutropenia was corrected after oral copper therapy. On the basis of these reports, the syndrome of adult copper deficiency is well established. Measurement of serum copper concentration appears to be a reliable index of copper deprivation in such patients.

19.3.4. Wilson's disease

Wilson's disease (hepatolenticular degeneration) is a familial disease of copper metabolism which is inherited as an autosomal recessive trait. The basic metabolic defect appears to be impairment of hepatic lysosomal excretion of copper into bile, usually (but *not* always) associated with diminution of hepatic caeruloplasmin synthesis (Sternlieb, 1972;

Sternlieb et al., 1973). Copper progressively accumulates within hepatocytes until parenchymal degeneration and necrosis result in release of copper into the plasma. Increase in the plasma non-caeruloplasmin copper concentration, which develops rapidly, may precipitate acute haemolysis. More commonly, gradual increase of plasma non-caeruloplasmin copper results in progressive accumulation of copper in brain, kidney and cornea, leading to psychiatric, neurological and renal functional disturbances, and to the development of characteristic Kayser-Fleischer corneal rings. In children and adolescents, hepatic manifestations usually dominate the symptomatology of Wilson's disease, whereas in adults, neuropsychiatric manifestations (e.g. tremors, incoordination, dysarthria, athetosis, salivation and emotional lability) are very common symptoms (Bearn, 1972).

The laboratory diagnosis of Wilson's disease has been authoritatively summarized by Sternlieb (1968). The following laboratory abnormalities are present in almost all patients with Wilson's disease, and therefore they possess major diagnostic value:

(a) Deficiency or virtual absence of serum caeruloplasmin. The caeruloplasmin concentrations in sera of healthy persons range from 200 to 350 mg/litre; the majority of patients with Wilson's disease have concentrations below 100 mg/litre.

(b) Increased concentration of copper in liver biopsy. The concentration of copper in normal liver tissue is less than 1.6 mmol (100 mg) per kg dry weight. Livers of untreated patients with Wilson's disease usually contain more than 3.9 mmol (250 mg) of copper per kg dry weight.

(c) Diminished incorporation of ^{64}Cu into caeruloplasmin. Following oral or intravenous administration of $^{64}CuCl_2$, there is a characteristic lack of incorporation of ^{64}Cu into caeruloplasmin, even in those patients with Wilson's disease who have measurable concentrations of serum caeruloplasmin.

The following additional laboratory abnormalities are commonly observed in patients with Wilson's disease who have developed hepatic, neurological and renal impairment:

(a) Increase in non-caeruloplasmin fraction of total serum copper. Normally, serum non-caeruloplasmin copper (copper bound to serum albumin and aminoacids) is present in concentrations less than 1.6 μmol (102 μg) per litre. Increase in serum non-caeruloplasmin copper is found in patients with Wilson's disease, especially in the presence of hemolytic anaemia.

(b) Increase in urinary copper excretion. Excretion of copper in urine of patients with Wilson's disease usually exceeds 0.8 μmol/day.

(c) Renal functional disturbances. Generalized aminoaciduria, proteinuria, phosphaturia, uricosuria, calciuria and glucosuria are frequently noted in patients with Wilson's disease.

(d) Hepatic functional disturbances. Hyperbilirubinaemia, increased activities of serum alkaline phosphatase and 5′-nucleotidase, hypoalbuminaemia, and hypoprothrombinaemia are frequently noted in patients with Wilson's disease.

Sternlieb (1968) has emphasized that laboratory tests (especially assays of caeruloplasmin and analyses of liver copper) are indispensible in establishing the diagnosis of Wilson's disease in early, asymptomatic subjects. Laboratory testing of siblings of known patients with Wilson's disease may lead to a definite diagnosis of Wilson's disease long before the appearance of clinical abnormalities. Similarly, laboratory testing for Wilson's disease is indispensible for differential diagnosis of patients with juvenile cirrhosis. On the other hand, laboratory tests are often unnecessary for diagnosis of patients with advanced, symptomatic Wilson's disease. Patients with neurological manifestations of Wilson's disease almost invariably exhibit Kayser-Fleischer corneal rings. In the presence of bilateral Kayser-Fleischer rings, seen on slit-lamp examination by an experienced ophthalmologist, an unequivocal diagnosis of Wilson's disease can be made clinically. In such cases, laboratory tests serve only to confirm the diagnosis and to provide base-line data for monitoring therapy. During chelation therapy with D-penicillamine, the oral intake of copper is restricted with a low-copper diet and the dosage of the chelating agent is regulated in order to keep the patient in negative copper balance. Urinary excretion of about 16 μmol (1.0 mg) of copper per day is considered by Sternlieb (1968) to be satisfactory evidence of negative copper balance. Periodic measurements of urinary copper excretion should be performed in patients with Wilson's disease at approximately three month intervals, in order to adjust the dosage of D-penicillamine. In some patients, however, the urinary excretion of 16 μmol (1.0 mg) of copper per day cannot be attained, and the elimination of lesser amounts of copper in the urine has to be accepted.

19.3.5. Copper toxicity

Acute copper intoxication has been described as a complication of renal haemodialysis (Bloomfield et al., 1971) and neonatal exchange transfusion (Bloomfield, 1969), as well as in subjects who have ingested copper salts (Fairbanks, 1967; Holtzman et al., 1966). Measurements of copper in serum, erythrocytes and urine are desirable for the diagnosis of acute copper poisoning, and are useful in the management of the haemolytic anaemia and hepatic insufficiency which are the usual systemic manifestations.

19.3.6. Serum copper in malignant diseases

Hypercupraemia owing to hypercaeruloplasminaemia develops in many patients with malignant neoplasms, and resembles the response that occurs in the "acute phase reaction" following trauma and infections, during pregnancy, and during administration of certain drugs (e.g. oestrogens and phenytoin). Little is known regarding the pathophysiologic mechanisms of hyperceruloplasminaemia in malignant diseases. There is no evidence that tumours per se synthesize and release caeruloplasmin into the serum. Rather, it appears possible that certain neoplasms produce a metabolite which stimulates hepatocytes to synthesize and release caeruloplasmin. Because of the non-specificity of hypercupraemia, measurements of serum copper are not useful as a diagnostic or screening test for neoplastic diseases. However, measurements of serum copper are definitely valuable as a prognostic index in patients with leukaemias and lymphomas. Hrgovcic et al. (1968, 1973), Delves et al. (1973), Tessmer et al. (1972) and Ray et al. (1973) have demonstrated that serum copper concentrations are almost invariably increased in patients with lymphomas and acute leukaemias; that diminution of the concentration of serum copper is often the earliest sign of a favourable response to chemotherapy or radiation therapy, preceding the usual signs such as normalization of the sedimentation rate, fever and leucocytosis; and that renewed increase of serum copper is often the first sign of relapse. Tessmer et al. (1972) reported correlation between the concentrations of serum copper and the proportions of blast cells in bone marrow of patients with acute leukaemia; they suggested that measurements of serum copper may serve as a supplement or as a partial substitute for frequent bone marrow examinations to monitor treatment in patients with acute leukaemia.

19.3.7. Pathophysiology of copper metabolism

In addition to the various abnormalities of copper metabolism that have been discussed, it may be noted that hypocupraemia occurs in patients with kwashiorkor, sprue, and nephrotic syndrome. Increased concentration of serum copper is observed in most patients with hepatic diseases (excepting Wilson's disease); acute myocardial infarction; collagen diseases; infections; after trauma and stress; and in various haematological disorders such as thalassaemia, aplastic anaemia, pernicious anaemia and sickle cell anaemia (Sass-Kortsak, 1965; Sinha and Gabrieli, 1970; Olatunbosun et al., 1975). Hormonal effects upon copper metabolism have been reviewed by Evans (1973) and Burch et al. (1975).

19.3.8. Measurements of copper in biological materials

Spectrophotometric methods for measurement of copper in body fluids and tissues have been reviewed by Sass-Kortsak (1965) and atomic absorption spectrometry of copper has been summarized by Sunderman (1973, 1975a). Reference intervals for copper concentrations in biological fluids from healthy adults are summarized in Table 19.2. Measurements of concentration of serum copper in healthy infants and children have been reported by Henkin et al. (1973), Sass-Kortsak and Sarkar (1973) and Tessmer et al. (1973).

TABLE 19.2.

REFERENCE INTERVALS FOR COPPER IN BODY FLUIDS OF HEALTHY ADULTS [a]

Body fluid	No. of subjects	Cu concentration or excretion		Authors
		Mean ± S.D.	Units	
Serum	25 ♂	16.2 ± 2.8	μmol/litre	Versieck et al. (1974a)
	21 ♀	17.8 ± 4.6	μmol/litre	
Erythrocytes	25 ♂	10.4 ± 0.9	μmol/kg	Versieck et al. (1974a)
	21 ♀	10.4 ± 1.6	μmol/kg	
Urine	21 ♂	0.28 ± 0.13	μmol/24 hours	Sunderman and Roszel (1967)
Sweat	33 ♂	8.7 ± 5.5	μmol/litre	Hohnadel et al. (1973)
	15 ♀	23.3 ± 9.6	μmol/litre	

[a] SI unit conversion for copper, μmol × 63.5 = μg.

19.4. CHROMIUM

19.4.1. Chromium metabolism

Although chromium has been established as an essential element for mammalian nutrition (Mertz et al., 1974), reliable data are not available for the dietary intake of chromium by healthy adults. Transport of absorbed $^{51}Cr^{3+}$ is accomplished primarily by binding to plasma albumin and to plasma transferrin. Excretion of chromium occurs primarily in the urine, and to a minor degree in faeces (Doisy et al., 1971).

19.4.2. Relationship of chromium to carbohydrate metabolism

Clinical interest in chromium metabolism was stimulated by the report of Mertz and Schwarz (1961) that trivalent chromium is an active ingredient of the "glucose tolerance factor", a dietary agent that is required for maintenance of normal intravenous glucose tolerance in rats. Evidence of possible clinical relevance of chromium to human diabetes has included: the report by Glinssmann et al. (1966) that oral glucose administration causes a prompt increase in plasma chromium concentrations in normal men, but not in diabetic patients unless trace amounts of trivalent chromium are given as a dietary supplement; the finding of Levine et al. (1968) that oral chromium supplementation has a beneficial effect on glucose tolerance in elderly human subjects; and the observation by Hambidge et al. (1968) that concentrations of chromium in hair of diabetic children were significantly lower than in the hair of normal children. Studies in four countries (Jordan, Nigeria, Egypt and Turkey) have indicated that chromium deficiency is one facet of protein-calorie malnutrition of marasmic infants, and that improvement of glucose tolerance occurs in such infants following administration of chromium (Hambidge, 1974). Davidson et al. (1974) reported that the ingestion by normal adults of a standard oral glucose load resulted in a significant decrease of the rate of urinary excretion of chromium. Hambidge and Rodgerson (1968) and Hambidge and Droegemueller (1974) found that concentrations of chromium in hair and serum of pregnant women were significantly lower than in non-pregnant women, and they speculated that depletion of tissue chromium stores might occur during pregnancy. Burt and Davidson (1973) also found that chromium concentrations in hair and plasma were significantly lower in pregnant women at term than in non-pregnant, nulliparous women. They concluded that altered chromium metabolism may be related to the diabetogenic features of pregnancy. In contrast to the findings of Glinssman et al. (1966) and Hambidge and Droegemueller (1974), Burt and Davidson (1973) observed a fall rather than an increase in plasma concentrations of chromium after administration of glucose or insulin to healthy non-pregnant subjects, and they observed that this response to glucose or insulin was abolished during late pregnancy. On the basis of these several clinical studies, there is apparently a poorly defined relationship between chromium nutrition and carbohydrate metabolism in man. Present knowledge of the metabolic role of chromium has been reviewed by Mertz et al. (1974).

19.4.3. Measurements of chromium in biological materials

Analyses of chromium in biological materials by gas chromatography have been summarized by Savory et al. (1970), and analyses of chromium by atomic absorption spectrometry have been reviewed by Sunderman (1973). In order to measure the minute traces that are normally present in human serum and urine, electrothermal atomic absorption spectrometry is currently the method of choice (Pekarek et al., 1974). Reference intervals for chromium concentration in body fluids from healthy adults have not as yet been established with sufficient validity to merit citation in this text (Mertz, 1975).

19.5. MANGANESE

19.5.1. Manganese metabolism

The daily consumption of manganese in the human diet ranges from 50 to 125 μmol (2.8 to 6.9 mg). A small fraction of the ingested manganese is absorbed from the intestine. In human and rabbit serum, trivalent manganese is bound to two β_1-globulins. One of these proteins has a molecular mass of approximately 70,000 and is indistinguishable from transferrin. The second protein has a molecular mass of 200,000 to 250,000 and has been named "plasmanganin" (Hancock et al., 1973). Studies of human and rabbit serum have demonstrated that divalent manganese is bound to albumin (Chapman et al., 1973; Nandekar et al., 1973). Biliary excretion is the principal route for elimination of manganese, although traces of manganese are present in other intestinal secretions (Bertinchamps et al., 1966). Manganese is considered to be an essential element for mammalian nutrition, and it is a constituent of a metalloenzyme, pyruvate carboxylase (Scrutton et al., 1966). Manganese also plays metabolic roles in the synthesis of chondroitin sulphate (Leach et al., 1969) and in the regulation of nucleic acid synthesis (Kehoe et al., 1969; Luck and Zimmer, 1972; Brynes et al., 1974). Manganese deficiency has been reported in a human volunteer who was being subjected to vitamin K deficiency under metabolic ward conditions (Doisy, 1973). This patient developed hypocholesterolaemia, loss of body mass, dermatitis, changes in hair and beard, and gastrointestinal symptoms, which were attributed to omission of manganese from the diet mixture. The clinical biochemistry of manganese has been thoroughly reviewed by Burch et al. (1975).

19.5.2. Manganese poisoning

Chronic manganese poisoning is an industrial problem among manganese miners, refinery and battery workers (Emara et ai., 1971; Chandra et al., 1974; Cook et al., 1974; Mena, 1974). The initial symptom of manganism is usually an acute psychosis which may last from 1 to 3 months before the onset of neurological manifestations. The progressive neurological disease is characterized by extrapyramidal signs (facial rigidity, bradykinesia, "cock-walk", scanning speech, tremor, and occasionally athetosis and ataxia). Central nervous system degeneration occurs primarily in the basal ganglia, associated with disturbances of dopamine, homovanillic acid and serotonin metabolism which may be the result of inhibition of tyrosine hydroxylase activity. Therapy with levodopa (L-DOPA) has been beneficial in some clinical trials (Rosenstock et al., 1971; Mena, 1974) and edetic acid (EDTA) therapy has also resulted in an apparently favourable response (Cook et al., 1974).

Chronic manganese poisoning is difficult to substantiate by laboratory tests, since individuals with increased urinary concentrations of manganese do not necessarily have symptoms, and symptomatic patients do not necessarily have a high urinary excretion of manganese (Tanaka and Lieben, 1969). Measurements of increased manganese excretion following edetic acid infusion have been used as a diagnostic test (Rosenstock et al., 1971), but Cook et al. (1974) questioned the validity of this test because control patients without any history of exposure to manganese also showed an increase in urinary manganese excretion following administration of edetic acid. Rosenstock et al. (1971) found increased concentration of manganese in hair of a patient with chronic manganism. Chandra et al. (1974) noted that hypercalcaemia may be a useful laboratory indication of chronic manganese poisoning in its early stages. The pathophysiologic mechanism of hypercalcaemia in patients with manganism has not been elucidated.

19.5.3. Measurements of manganese in biological materials

Neutron activation analysis has been employed for analyses of manganese concentrations in serum and erythrocytes by Versieck et al. (1973, 1974a, b, 1975). Atomic absorption spectrometry of manganese in various biological materials has been reported by Ajemian and Whitman (1969), Mahoney et al. (1969), Bek et al. (1972), Van Ormer and Purdy (1973) and Suzuki and Wacker (1974). Reference intervals for manganese concentrations in body fluids from healthy adults are listed in Table 19.3. Versieck et al. (1975) have measured the concentration of manganese in sera of patients with acute myocardial infarction. Contrary to earlier reports, they did not find any significant increase in serum manganese concentrations following acute myocardial infarction. Hambidge and Droegemueller (1974) reported that mean concentrations of manganese in plasma samples from pregnant women did not differ from corresponding values in non-pregnant women. Versieck et al. (1974a) observed that serum manganese concentrations are invariably increased during the active phase of acute hepatitis, the mean concentration being approximately four times that observed in sera from healthy control subjects.

TABLE 19.3.

REFERENCE INTERVALS FOR MANGANESE IN BODY FLUIDS OF HEALTHY ADULTS [a]

Body fluid	No. of subjects	Mn concentration or excretion		Authors
		Mean ± S.D.	Units	
Serum	25 ♂	10.7 ± 2.2	nmol/litre	Versieck et al. (1974b)
	25 ♀	10.0 ± 2.6	nmol/litre	
Erythrocytes	25 ♂	250 ± 60	nmol/kg	Versieck et al. (1974a)
	21 ♀	310 ± 110	nmol/kg	

[a] SI unit conversion for manganese, nmol × 55 = ng.

19.6. NICKEL

19.6.1. Nickel metabolism

The usual oral intake of nickel is 3 to 10 μmol (180 to 590 μg) per day. Most of the nickel that is ingested orally is excreted in the faeces. Horak and Sunderman (1973) reported that faecal nickel excretion in healthy adults averaged 4.4 ± 2.1 (S.D.) μmol (260 ± 120 μg) per day (range = 1.4 to 9.2 μmol (83 to 540 μg) per day). In healthy individuals, the excretion of nickel in the faeces is approximately 100 times greater than in the urine, which averages 41 ± 18 nmol (2.4 ± 1.0 mg) per day (Nomoto and Sunderman, 1970). Nickel is present in normal human serum in three forms: ultrafilterable nickel, albumin-bound nickel, and a nickel metalloprotein that has been named "nickeloplasmin" (Hendel and Sunderman, 1972; Sunderman et al., 1972; Asato et al., 1975). Nickel is excreted in urine as low-molecular mass complexes with ninhydrin-positive substances, which are believed to include histidine and aspartic acid (Asato et al., 1975). The concentration of nickel in sweat from healthy men averages 0.9 ± 0.6 μmol (53 ± 35 μg) per litre (Hohnadel et al., 1973) which is approximately 20 times greater than the mean concentration of nickel in urine. Under conditions of profuse sweating, appreciable amounts of nickel are excreted in sweat, which may be responsible for the diminished concentrations of serum nickel which have been reported by Szadkowski et al. (1969) in workmen who were chronically exposed to extreme heat. Based upon the studies of Sunderman et al. (1972) and Nielsen and Ollerich (1974) it seems likely that nickel is an essential element for nutrition. However, its metabolic role remains to be elucidated.

19.6.2. Abnormalities of nickel metabolism in man

Sunderman et al. (1970) and McNeely et al. (1971) found increased concentrations of serum nickel in patients with acute myocardial infarction, acute stroke and extensive thermal burns. Based upon unpublished studies in the present author's laboratory, it seems probable that the hypernickelaemia in these conditions is a secondary manifestation of leukocytosis and leukocytolysis. McNeely et al. (1971) observed hyponickelaemia in patients with hepatic and renal diseases, presumably as a consequence of hypoalbuminaemia. The principal clinical applications of measurements of nickel in body fluids are in the diagnosis of cases of acute nickel poisoning, and in monitoring the chelation therapy of patients with nickel poisoning who are being treated with diethyldithiocarbamate. Poisoning from inhalation of nickel carbonyl is a serious industrial problem (Von Ludewigs and Thiess, 1970; Vuopala et al., 1970; Sunderman, 1971) and measurements of nickel in urine have been shown to be correlated with the clinical severity of nickel carbonyl intoxication (Nomoto and Sunderman, 1970; Sunderman, 1971). Analyses of nickel in urine and serum also serve as laboratory indices of chronic environmental exposures to nickel (McNeely et al., 1972).

19.6.3. Measurements of nickel in biological fluids

Atomic absorption spectrometry is the only practical technique that has sufficient sensitivity for measurement of nickel in normal human serum and other body fluids, as

TABLE 19.4.

REFERENCE INTERVALS FOR NICKEL IN BODY FLUIDS AND EXCRETA OF HEALTHY ADULTS [a]

Body fluid	No. of subjects	Ni concentration or excretion		Authors
		Mean ± S.D.	Units	
Serum	23 ♂	44 ± 14	nmol/litre	Nomoto and Sunderman (1970)
	17 ♀	46 ± 12	nmol/litre	
Whole blood	10 ♂	77 ± 24	nmol/litre	Nomoto and Sunderman (1970)
	7 ♀	89 ± 19	nmol/litre	
Urine	14 ♂	44 ± 22	nmol/24 hours	Nomoto and Sunderman (1970)
	12 ♀	37 ± 14	nmol/24 hours	
Sweat	33 ♂	0.9 ± 0.6	μmol/litre	Hohnadel et al. (1973)
	15 ♀	2.2 ± 1.1	μmol/litre	
Faeces	10 ♂ + ♀	4.4 ± 2.1	μmol/24 hours	Horak and Sunderman (1973)
Hair	13 ♂	4.1 ± 1.5	μmol/kg	Nechay and Sunderman (1973)
	7 ♀	3.2 ± 0.7	μmol/kg	

[a] SI unit conversion for nickel, nmol × 59 = ng.

described by Nomoto and Sunderman (1970), Sunderman and Nechay (1974) and Zachariasen et al. (1975). Reference intervals for concentrations of nickel in body fluids from healthy subjects are given in Table 19.4.

19.7. LEAD

19.7.1. Lead metabolism

Thompson (1971) carefully investigated lead balance in a small group of healthy subjects. He found that the dietary intake of lead averaged 1.32 μmol (270 μg) per day, and that the daily excretion of lead in the faeces averaged 1.16 μmol (240 μg) per day. The urinary excretion of lead in these subjects averaged 0.12 μmol (25 μg) per day. These data are consistent with the results of investigations in other studies, which have been summarized by Barry (1973). Significant excretion of lead has been found in sweat of healthy adults who have no occupational exposure to lead (Hohnadel et al., 1973).

Barry (1973) estimated the body burden of lead in adult men (age >50 years) based upon analyses of post-mortem tissues. In 15 men who had not had occupational exposures to lead, the body burden of lead averaged 1.07 mmol, range 0.53 to 1.69 mmol (222 mg, range 110 to 350 mg) of which 1.03 mmol, range 0.48 to 1.64 mmol (213 mg, range 99 to 340 mg) was deposited in bone, and 0.04 mmol, range 0.02 to 0.06 mmol (8.3 mg, range 4.1 to 12.4 mg) was present in soft tissues, including especially aorta, liver and kidney. Lead in whole blood is predominantly in the erythrocytes, and less than 5% of total lead in blood is in the plasma. Barltrop and Smith (1971) showed that erythrocyte lead is not bound to the stromal fraction but is present within the soluble corpuscular contents. Fractionations of corpuscular contents by gel-filtration and by density-gradient ultracentrifugation showed that a minor fraction of erythrocyte lead is present in a low molecular mass fraction. However, the major component of erythrocyte lead is bound to haemoglobin (Barltrop and Smith, 1971). In vitro binding of lead to haemoglobin is not prevented by chemical blockage of the free sulphydryl groups of haemoglobin (Barltrop and Smith, 1972), which indicates that free sulphydryl groups are not essential for formation of the lead–haemoglobin complex. Barltrop and Smith (1972) found that there were no significant differences in the binding of lead to adult and foetal haemoglobins, and they concluded that the binding sites for lead are independent of the β-chain components of the haemoglobins.

Rosen and Trinidad (1974) measured the concentrations of lead in plasma samples from healthy children and from children with lead poisoning. No significant differences were observed in the mean concentrations of plasma lead in the healthy and lead-intoxicated children, despite the finding of marked differences in the concentrations of lead in whole blood. Rosen and Trinidad (1974) noted that a small fraction of plasma lead is ultrafilterable, and that the remainder is bound to plasma proteins.

Barry (1973) emphasized that the concentration of lead in whole blood furnishes an index of lead concentrations in the soft tissues of the body. However, the concentration of lead in whole blood does not bear any direct relationship to the concentration of lead in bone. Hence, analyses of blood lead do not reflect the body burden of lead. Measurements of lead excretion in urine after administration of calcium ethylenediaminetetraacetate may provide a guide to the body burden of lead (Pterovska and Teisinger, 1970; Emmerson, 1963). Measurements of lead concentrations in dentine of decidous teeth from school children have also been suggested as an index of the body burden of lead (Needleman and Shapiro, 1974).

19.7.2. Lead poisoning

For discussions of the clinical manifestations and pathogenesis of lead poisoning in children and adults, the reader may consult reviews by Goyer and Chisholm (1972) and Hamilton and Hardy (1974). Current knowledge of the toxicity of low levels of environmental lead has been summarized by Pfitzer (1974) and Waldron (1975). The toxic effects of lead upon haem synthesis are attributable primarily to inhibition of the activities of: erythrocyte δ-aminolaevulic dehydratase, an enzyme that catalyzes the coupling of two molecules of δ-aminolaevulic acid to form porphobilinogen; and haem synthetase, an enzyme that catalyzes the coupling of iron with protoporphyrin-IX to form the haem molecule. The combination of these effects upon haem synthesis leads to the biochemical abnormalities that are commonly monitored for the diagnosis of lead intoxication: increased concentration of erythrocyte zinc-protoporphyrin; increased urinary excretion of coproporphyrin; increased urinary excretion of δ-aminolaevulic acid; and diminished activity of erythrocyte δ-aminolaevulic dehydratase. Lead inhibition of δ-aminolaevulic acid dehydratase activity may be related to the toxic effects of lead upon the central nervous system, since Millar et al. (1970) found that administration of lead to rats resulted in diminished δ-aminolaevulic acid dehydratase activity in the brain as well as in erythrocytes. Secchi et al. (1973) reported inhibition of sodium–potassium-activated adenosine triphosphatase activity in erythrocyte membranes of urban inhabitants who had had no occupational exposure to lead.

Waldron (1975) has emphasized that lead inhibition of Na^+–K^+-ATPase should be viewed with concern, especially since this enzyme may possibly be inhibited at other membrane sites, such as in the brain. Subclinical lead poisoning has been demonstrated to produce varied manifestations in experimental animals, including enhanced susceptibility to infection, impairment of reproductive ability, teratogenicity, and behavioural effects and learning disabilities. In Waldron's view, the most serious effects of subclinical lead poisoning in man may be the production of hyperactivity in children (and possibly in some adult delinquents). Hyperactivity may be observed when the concentration of blood lead is within the range that has hitherto been regarded as safe.

No single laboratory test can be employed reliably for the detection of lead poisoning in the varied populations that are subjected to occupational or environmental exposures to lead. Measurements of lead in blood and urine are widely used for the monitoring of industrial workers. Barltrop and Killala (1967) have shown that determination of faecal lead is a sensitive index of ingested lead, and these workers have emphasized the importance of analyses of faecal lead in population screening programs. Thorough laboratory evaluation of lead exposure requires measurements of lead in blood, urine, faeces and possibly sweat, as well as measurements of the key enzymes and metabolites in the haem synthetic pathway, as indicated above. In persons who have not had recent exposures to lead, but who are suspected of suffering from delayed manifestations of lead poisoning (e.g. lead nephropathy), lead-mobilization tests after the administration of calcium-EDTA, or analyses of lead in bone biopsy specimens may be necessary.

19.7.3. Measurements of lead in biological materials

A few laboratories rely upon spectrophotometric measurements of lead by the dithizone reaction, and some other laboratories use anodic-stripping voltametry for estimations of blood lead. However, the overwhelming majority of clinical laboratories currently employ atomic absorption techniques for analyses of lead in biological materials. Atomic absorption spectrometry of lead has been reviewed by Berman (1969) and Sunderman (1973, 1975a), and critical evaluations of atomic absorption systems for determinations of lead in whole blood have been published by Hicks et al. (1973) and Anderson et al. (1974). Sources of errors and interlaboratory variations in analyses of blood lead by atomic absorption spectrometry have been discussed by Keppler et al. (1970), Browne et al. (1974), Kopito et al. (1974) and Lathe (1974). Davies and Rainsford (1967) noted that most of the lead in blood is present in erythrocytes, and that one of the toxic effects of lead is to cause erythrocytopenia. Therefore, they emphasized that measurements of lead in whole blood may be misleading unless the results are corrected for the anaemia that may be present. It is now common practice to adjust the observed concentration of blood lead against the normal mean value for erythrocyte mass by multiplying by 44% – assuming a normal packed cell volume (haematocrit) of 44% – divided by the observed haematocrit of the patient's blood. Reference intervals for lead concentrations or excretion in body fluids from healthy adults are summarized in Table 19.5. Reference intervals for

TABLE 19.5.

REFERENCE INTERVALS FOR LEAD IN BODY FLUIDS OF HEALTHY ADULTS [a]

Body fluid	No. of subjects	Pb concentration or excretion		Authors
		Mean ± S.D.	Units	
Blood	19 ♂	0.77 ± 0.24	μmol/litre	Hohnadel et al. (1973)
	26 ♀	0.51 ± 0.14	μmol/litre	
Urine	40 ♂ + ♀	54 ± 38	nmol/24 hours	Piper and Higgins (1967)
Sweat	33 ♂	0.25 ± 0.20	μmol/litre	Hohnadel et al. (1973)
	26 ♀	0.53 ± 0.29	μmol/litre	

[a] SI unit conversion for lead, μmol × 207 = μg.

lead in blood and excreta from infants and children may be found in reports by Barltrop and Killala (1967), Murphy et al. (1971) and Haas (1972a, b).

19.8. GOLD

19.8.1. Chrysotherapy of rheumatoid arthritis

Gold compounds have been used for the treatment of rheumatoid arthritis for approximately 40 years. Although the manner in which gold compounds produce their beneficial effects is not known, and although other agents have been found which help to suppress rheumatoid disease, gold continues to have a favoured place in the therapeutic program for rheumatoid arthritis. There is controversy whether or not measurements of gold in plasma or urine are helpful in monitoring chrysotherapy of rheumatoid arthritis. Lorber et al. (1973) found significantly improved clinical response in patients who received dosages of gold thiomalate that were adjusted on the basis of serum gold analyses, when compared to patients who received the drug on a fixed dosage schedule. According to DeBosset and Bitter (1973), patients noted to have high concentrations of plasma gold (>25 μmol (4.9 mg) per litre) during therapy were more likely to obtain an early improvement (i.e. before 20 weeks), and patients who were considered to be non-responders to gold therapy often did not achieve adequate (25 μmol (4.9 mg) per litre) plasma concentrations of gold. Toxic manifestations generally developed when plasma gold concentrations exceeded 38 μmol (7.5 mg) per litre. On the other hand, Gottlieb et al. (1974) reported that serum concentrations of gold failed to correlate with clinical course or toxicity in patients with rheumatoid arthritis. Measurements of urinary and faecal excretion of gold during chrysotherapy of rheumatoid arthritis have been reported by Harth (1974), but the results of such measurements did not appear to be correlated with clinical response or toxicity. On the basis of these conflicting reports, no firm conclusions can currently be reached regarding the clinical value of gold analyses for monitoring of chrysotherapy. To date, there have not been any reported measurements of the concentrations of serum ultrafilterable gold in patients during chrysotherapy. Since serum ultrafilterable gold represents the intravascular gold compartment which is directly exchangeable with extravascular and intracellular gold compartments, it would seem desirable to attempt to measure the ultrafilterable fraction and to assess its prognostic value. Atomic absorption methods for analysis of gold have been tabulated by Sunderman (1973).

19.9. OTHER TRACE METALS

Measurements of essential trace elements such as cobalt and molybdenum in body fluids are currently of great interest for research purposes, but these determinations have not yet achieved clinical importance or practicability. Measurements of cadmium, mercury, arsenic, bismuth, thallium and antimony are of increasing importance in industrial and environmental toxicology. For references to measurements of these metals in body fluids by atomic absorption spectrometry, the readers are referred to articles by Berman (1969), Christian and Feldman (1970) and Sunderman (1973), cited under Further Reading.

REFERENCES

Zinc

Amador, M., Pena, M., Garcia-Miranda, A., Gonzalez, A. and Hermelo, M. (1975) Low hair-zinc concentrations in acrodermatitis enteropathica. Lancet, 1, 1379.

Beisel, W.R., Pekarek, R.S. and Wannemacher, W.R., Jr. (1974) The impact of infectious disease on trace-element metabolism of the host. In Trace Element Metabolism in Animals, Vol. 2 (Eds. W.G. Hoekstra, J.W. Suttie, H.E. Ganther and W. Mertz) pp. 217–240, Park Press, Baltimore, Maryland.

Bühler, R.H.O. and Kägi, J.H.R. (1974) Human hepatic metallothioneins. Federation of European Biochemical Societies Letters, 39, 229–234.

Caggiano, V., Schnitzler, R., Strauss, W., Baker, R.K., Carter, A.C., Josephson, A.S. and Wallach, S. (1969) Zinc deficiency in a patient with retarded growth, hypogonadism, hypogammaglobulinemia and chronic infection. American Journal of Medical Sciences, 257, 305–319.

Carruthers, R. (1973) Oral zinc in cutaneous healing. Drugs, 6, 161–164.

Endre, L., Katona, Z. and Gyurkovits, K. (1975) Zinc deficiency and cellular immune deficiency in acrodermatitis enteropathica. Lancet, 1, 1196.

Giroux, E.L. (1975) Determination of zinc distribution between albumin and α_2-macroglobulin in human serum. Biochemical Medicine, 12, 258–266.

Henkin, R.I., Schulman, J.D., Schulman, C.B. and Bronzert, D.A. (1973) Changes in total, nondiffusible and diffusible plasma zinc and copper during infancy. Journal of Pediatrics, 82, 831–837.

Henkin, R.I. (1974) Zinc in wound healing. New England Journal of Medicine, 291, 675–676.

Henkin, R.I. and Aamodt, R.L. (1975) Zinc absorption in acrodermatitis enteropathica and in hypogeusia and hyposmia. Lancet, 1, 1379–1380.

Henkin, R.I., Mueller, C.W. and Wolf, R.O. (1975) Estimation of zinc concentration of parotid saliva by flameless atomic absorption spectrophotometry in normal subjects and in patients with idiopathic hypogeusia. Journal of Laboratory and Clinical Medicine, 86, 175–180.

Hohnadel, D.C., Sunderman, F.W., Jr., Nechay, M.W. and McNeely, M.D. (1973) Atomic absorption spectrometry of nickel, copper, zinc and lead in sweat collected from healthy subjects during sauna bathing. Clinical Chemistry, 19, 1288–1292.

Kowarski, S., Blair-Stanek, C.S. and Schachter, D. (1974) Active transport of zinc and identification of zinc-binding protein in rat jejunal mucosa. American Journal of Physiology, 226, 401–407.

Lombeck, I., Schnippering, H.G., Ritzl, F., Feinendegen, L.E. and Bremer, H.J. (1975) Absorption of zinc in acrodermatitis enteropathica. Lancet, 1, 855.

Meret, S. and Henkin, R.I. (1971) Simultaneous direct estimation by atomic absorption spectrophotometry of copper and zinc in serum, urine and cerebrospinal fluid. Clinical Chemistry, 17, 369–373.

Michaelsson, G. (1974) Acrodermatitis enterophathica – successful new therapy. Lakartidningen, 71, 1959–1961.

Mikac-Devic, D. (1970) Methodology of zinc determinations and the role of zinc in biochemical processes. Advances in Clinical Chemistry, 13, 271–333.

Moynahan, E.J. (1974) Acrodermatitis enteropathica. A lethal inherited human zinc deficiency disorder. Lancet, 2, 399–400.

Moynahan, E.J. and Barnes, P.M. (1973) Zinc deficiency and a synthetic diet for lactose intolerance. Lancet, 1, 676–677.

Parisi, A.F. and Vallee, B.L. (1969) Zinc metalloenzymes – characteristics and significance in biology and medicine. American Journal of Clinical Nutrition, 22, 1222–1239.

Pekarek, R.S., Wannemacher, R.W., Jr. and Beisel, W.R. (1972) The effect of leukocytic endogenous mediator (LEM) on the tissue distribution of zinc and iron. Proceedings of the Society for Experimental Biology and Medicine, 140, 685–688.

Petrie, J.J.B. and Row, P.G. (1977) Dialysis anaemia caused by subacute zinc toxicity. Lancet, 1, 1178–1180.

Pories, W.J. and Strain, W.H. (1966) Zinc and wound healing. In Zinc Metabolism (Ed. A.S. Prasad) pp. 378–394, C.C. Thomas Company, Springfield, Illinois.

Portnoy, B. and Molokhia, M. (1974) Zinc in acrodermatitis enteropathica. Lancet, 2, 663–664.

Powanda, M.C., Cockerell, G.L. and Pekarek, R.S. (1973) Amino acid and zinc movement in relation to protein synthesis early in inflammation. American Journal of Physiology, 225, 399–401.

Prasad, A.S. (1972) Zinc deficiency syndrome in man: a historical review. International Review of Neurobiology, Supplement 1, 1–6.

Prasad, A.S., Miale, A., Jr., Farid, Z., Sandstead, H.H. and Schulert, A.R. (1963) Zinc metabolism in patients with the syndrome of iron deficiency anemia, hepatosplenomegaly, dwarfism and hypogonadism. Journal of Laboratory and Clinical Medicine, 61, 537–549.

Prasad, A.S., Schoomaker, E.B., Ortega, J., Brewer, G.J., Oberleas, D. and Oelshlegel, F.J., Jr. (1975) Zinc deficiency in sickle cell disease. Clinical Chemistry, 21, 582–587.

Ronaghy, H.A., Reinhold, J.G., Mahloudji, M., Ghavami, P., Fox, M.R.S. and Halsted, J.A. (1974) Zinc supplementation of malnourished schoolboys in Iran: increased growth and other effects. American Journal of Clinical Nutrition, 27, 112–121.

Rosner, R. and Gorfien, P.C. (1968) Erythrocyte and plasma zinc and magnesium levels in health and disease. Journal of Laboratory and Clinical Medicine, 72, 213–219.

Sandstead, H.H. (1973) Zinc nutrition in the United States. American Journal of Clinical Nutrition, 26, 1251–1260.

Strain, W.H., Hirsh, F.S. and Michel, B. (1975) Increased copper/zinc ratios in acrodermatitis enteropathica. Lancet, 1, 1196–1197.

Sunderman, F.W., Jr. (1973) Atomic absorption spectrometry of trace metals in clinical pathology, Human Pathology, 4, 549–582.

Sunderman, F.W., Jr. (1975a) see Further Reading.

Sunderman, F.W., Jr. (1975b) Current status of zinc deficiency in the pathogenesis of neurological, dermatological and musculoskeletal disorders. Annals of Clinical and Laboratory Science, 5, 132–145.

Copper

Al-Rashid, R.A. and Spangler, J. (1971) Neonatal copper deficiency. New England Journal of Medicine, 285, 841–843.

Ashkenazi, A., Levin, S., Djaldetti, M., Fishel, E. and Benvenisti, D. (1973) The syndrome of neonatal copper deficiency. Pediatrics, 52, 525–533.

Bearn, A.G. (1972) Wilson's disease. In Metabolic Basis of Inherited Disease, 3rd edn. (Eds. J.B. Stanbury, J.G. Wyngaarden and D.S. Fredrickson) pp. 1033–1050, McGraw Hill Company, New York.

Blomfield, J. (1969) Copper contamination in exchange transfusions. Lancet, 1, 731–732.

Blomfield, J., Dixon, S.R. and McCredie, D.A. (1971) Potential hepatotoxicity of copper in recurrent hemodialysis. Archives of Internal Medicine, 128, 555–560.

Bucknall, W.E., Haslan, R.H.A. and Holtzman, N.A. (1973) Kinky hair syndrome: response to copper therapy. Pediatrics, 52, 653–657.

Burch, R.E., Hahn, H.K.J. and Sullivan, J.F. (1975) Newer aspects of the roles of zinc, manganese and copper in human nutrition. Clinical Chemistry, 21, 501–520.

Cordana, A., Placko, R.P. and Graham, G.G. (1966) Hypocupremia and neutropenia in copper deficiency. Blood, 28, 280–283.

Danks, D.M., Campbell, P.E., Walker-Smith, J., Stevens, B.J., Gillespie, J.M., Blomfield, J. and Turner, B. (1972) Menkes' kinky-hair syndrome. Lancet, 1, 1100–1103.

Danks, D.M., Cartwright, E., Stevens, B.J. and Townley, R.R.W. (1973) Menkes' kinky-hair disease: further definition of the defect in copper transport. Science, 179, 1140–1141.

Dekaban, A.S. and Steusing, J.K. (1974) Menkes' kinky-hair disease treated with subcutaneous copper sulfate. Lancet, 2, 1523.

Delves, H.T., Alexander, F.W. and Lay, H. (1973) Copper and zinc concentration in the plasma of leukaemic children. British Journal of Haematology, 24, 525–531.

Dunlap, W.M., James, G.W. and Hume, D.M. (1974) Anemia and neutropenia caused by copper deficiency. Annals of Internal Medicine, 80, 470–476.

Evans, G.W. (1973) Copper homeostasis in the mammalian system. Physiological Reviews, 53, 535–570.

Fairbanks, V.F. (1967) Copper sulfate-induced hemolytic anemia. Archives of Internal Medicine, 120, 428–432.

Graham, G.G. (1971) Human copper deficiency. New England Journal of Medicine, 285, 857–858.

Grover, W.D. and Scrutton, M.D. (1975) Copper infusion therapy in trichopoliodystrophy. Journal of Pediatrics, 86, 216–220.

Henkin, R.I. et al. (1973) See reference under **Zinc**.

Hohnadel, D.C. et al. (1973) See reference under **Zinc**.

Hohnadel, D.C., McNeely, M.D. and Sunderman, F.W., Jr. (1975) Automated bichromatic analysis of serum ceruloplasmin. Annals of Clinical and Laboratory Science, 5, 65–70.

Holtzman, N.A., Elliott, D.A. and Heller, R.N. (1966) Copper intoxication. New England Journal of Medicine, 275, 347–352.

Hrgovcic, M., Tessmer, C.F., Minckler, T.M., Mosier, B. and Taylor, G.H. (1968) Serum copper levels in lymphoma and leukemia. Cancer Research, 21, 743–755.

Hrgovcic, M., Tessmer, C.F., Thomas, F.B., Ong, P.S., Gamble, J.F. and Shullenberger, C.C. (1973) Serum copper observations in patients with malignant lymphoma. Cancer, 32, 1512–1524.

Karpel, J.T. and Peden, V.H. (1972) Copper deficiency in long-term parenteral nutrition. Journal of Pediatrics, 80, 32–36.

Lewis, K.O. (1973) The nature of the copper complexes in bile and their relationship to the absorption and excretion of copper in normal subjects and in Wilson's disease. Gut, 14, 221–232.

Malkin, R. and Malmstrom, B.G. (1970) The state and function of copper in biological systems. Advances in Enzymology, 33, 177–194.

Olatunbosun, D.A., Isaacs-Sodeye, W.A., Adeniyi, F.A. and Adadevoh, B.K. (1975) Serum copper in sickle-cell anemia. Lancet, 1, 285–286.

Owen, C.A., Jr. (1975) Uptake of ^{67}Cu by ceruloplasmin in vitro. Proceedings of the Society for Experimental Biology and Medicine, 149, 681–682.

Ray, G.R., Wolf, P.H. and Kaplan, H.S. (1973) Value of laboratory indicators in Hodgkin's disease: preliminary results. National Cancer Institute Monograph, 36, 315–323.

Sass-Kortsak, A. (1965) Copper metabolism. Advances in Clinical Chemistry, 8, 1–67.

Sass-Kortsak, A. and Sarkar, B. (1973) Age-related changes in copper and the biological transport of copper: a commentary. Journal of Pediatrics, 82, 905–907.

Seely, J.R., Humphrey, G.B. and Matter, B.J. (1972) Copper deficiency in a premature infant fed an iron-fortified diet. New England Journal of Medicine, 286, 109–110.

Sinha, S.N. and Gabrieli, E.R. (1970) Serum copper and zinc levels in various pathologic conditions. American Journal of Clinical Pathology, 54, 570–577.

Sternlieb, I. (1968) Laboratory diagnosis of hepatolenticular degeneration. In Laboratory Diagnosis of Liver Diseases (Eds. F.W. Sunderman and F.W. Sunderman, Jr.) pp. 189–192, Warren H. Green Company, St. Louis, Missouri.

Sternlieb, I. (1972) Evolution of the hepatic lesion in Wilson's disease (hepatolenticular degeneration). In Progress in Liver Diseases, Vol. IV (Eds. H. Popper and F. Schaffner) pp. 511–525, Heinemann.

Sternlieb, I. and Janowitz, H.D. (1964) Absorption of copper in malabsorption syndromes. Journal of Clinical Investigation, 43, 1049–1055.

Sternlieb, I., Van Den Hamer, C.J.A., Morell, A.J., Alpert, S., Gregoriadis, G. and Scheinberg, I.H. (1973) Lysosomal defect of hepatic copper excretion in Wilson's disease (hepatolenticular degeneration). Gastroenterology, 64, 99–103.

Strickland, G.T., Bechner, W.M. and Leu, M.L. (1972) Absorption of copper in homozygotes and heterozygotes for Wilson's disease and controls: isotope tracer studies with ^{67}Cu and ^{64}Cu. Clinical Science, 43, 617–625.

Sunderman, F.W., Jr. (1973) Atomic absorption spectrometry of trace metals in clinical pathology. Human Pathology, 4, 549–582.

Sunderman, F.W., Jr. (1975a) Electrothermal atomic absorption spectrometry of trace metals in biological fluids. Annals of Clinical and Laboratory Science, 5, 421–434.

Sunderman, F.W., Jr. and Nomoto, S. (1970) Measurement of serum ceruloplasmin by the p-phenylenediamine oxidase reaction. Clinical Chemistry, 16, 903–910.

Sunderman, F.W., Jr. and Roszel, N.O. (1967) Measurements of copper in biological materials by atomic absorption spectrometry. American Journal of Clinical Pathology, 48, 286–300.

Tessmer, C.F., Hrgovcic, M., Brown, B.W., Wilbur, J. and Thomas, F.B. (1972) Serum copper correlations with bone marrow. Cancer, 29, 173–179.

Tessmer, C.F., Krohn, W., Johnston, D., Thomas, F.B., Hrgovcic, M. and Brown, B. (1973) Serum copper in children (6–12 years old). American Journal of Clinical Pathology, 60, 870–878.

Versieck, J., Barbier, F., Speecke, A. and Hoste, J. (1974a) Manganese, copper and zinc concentrations in serum and packed blood cells during acute hepatitis, chronic hepatitis and post hepatic cirrhosis. Clinical Chemistry, 20, 1141–1145.

Vilter, R.W., Bozian, R.C., Hess, E.V., Zellner, D.C. and Petering, H.G. (1974) Manifestations of copper deficiency in a patient with systemic sclerosis on intravenous hyperalimentation. New England Journal of Medicine, 291, 188–191.

Walker-Smith, J.A., Turner, B., Blomfield, J. and Wise, G. (1973) Therapeutic implications of copper deficiency in Menkes' steely-hair syndrome. Archives of Disease in Childhood, 18, 958–962.

Wehinger, H., Witt, I., Losel, I., Denz-Seibert, G. and Sander, C. (1975). Intravenous copper in Menkes' kinky-hair syndrome. Lancet, 1, 1143–1144.

Chromium

Burt, R.L. and Davidson, I.W.F. (1973) Carbohydrate metabolism in pregnancy: a possible role of chromium. Acta Diabetologica Latina, 10, 770–778.

Davidson, I.W.F., Burt, R.L. and Parker, J.C. (1974) Renal excretion of trace elements: chromium and copper. Proceedings of the Society for Experimental Biology and Medicine, 147, 720–725.

Doisy, R.J., Streeter, D.H.P., Souma, M.L., Kalafe, M.E., Rekant, S.I. and Dalakos, T.G. (1971) Metabolism of ^{51}chromium in human subjects, normal, elderly and diabetic subjects. In Newer Trace Elements in Nutrition (Eds. W. Mertz and W.E. Cornatzer) pp. 155–168, Marcel Dekker, Inc., New York.

Glinssmann, W.H., Feldman, F.J. and Mertz, W. (1966) Plasma chromium after glucose administration. Science, 152, 1243–1245.

Hambidge, K.M. (1974) Chromium nutrition in man. American Journal of Clinical Nutrition, 27, 505–514.

Hambidge, K.M. and Droegemueller, W. (1974) Changes in plasma and hair concentrations of zinc, copper, chromium and manganese during pregnancy. Obstetrics and Gynecology, 44, 666–672.

Hambidge, K.M. and Rodgerson, D.O. (1969) Comparison of hair chromium levels of nulliparous and parous women. American Journal of Obstetrics and Gynecology, 103, 320–321.

Hambidge, K.M., Rodgerson, D.O. and O'Brien, D. (1968) Concentration of chromium in the hair of normal children and children with juvenile diabetes mellitus. Diabetes, 17, 517–519.

Levine, R.A., Streeten, D.H.P. and Doisey, R.J. (1968) Effects of oral chromium supplementation on glucose tolerance of elderly human subjects. Metabolism, 17, 114–125.

Mertz, W. (1975) Trace element nutrition in health and disease: contributions and problems of analysis. Clinical Chemistry, 21, 468–475.

Mertz, W. and Schwarz, K. (1961) Chromium (III) and the glucose tolerance factor. In Measurements of Exocrine and Endocrine Functions of the Pancreas (Eds. F.W. Sunderman and F.W. Sunderman, Jr.) pp. 123–127, J.B. Lippincott Company, Philadelphia, Pennsylvania.

Mertz, W., Toepffer, E.W., Roginski, E.E. and Polansky, M.M. (1974) Present knowledge of the role of chromium. Federation Proceedings, 33, 2275–2280.

Pekarek, R.S., Hauer, E.C., Wannemacher, R.W., Jr. and Beisel, W.R. (1974) The direct determination of serum chromium by an atomic absorption spectrometer with a heated graphite atomizer. Analytical Biochemistry, 59, 283–292.

Savory, J., Mushak, P., Sunderman, F.W., Jr., Estes, R.H. and Roszel, N.O. (1970) Microdetermination of chromium in biological materials by gas chromatography. Analytical Chemistry, 42, 294–300.

Sunderman, F.W., Jr. (1973) Atomic absorption spectrometry of trace metals in clinical pathology. Human Pathology, 4, 549–582.

Manganese

Ajemian, R.S. and Whitman, N.E. (1969) Determination of manganese in urine by atomic absorption spectrometry. American Industrial Hygiene Association Journal, 30, 52–56.

Bek, F., Janouskova, J. and Moldan, B. (1972) Direct determination of manganese and strontium in human blood serum by means of the graphite furnace Perkin-Elmer HGA-70. Chemické Listy, 66, 867–875.

Bertinchamps, A.J., Miller, S.T. and Cotzias, G.C. (1966) Interdependence of routes for excreting manganese. American Journal of Physiology, 211, 217–224.

Brynes, J.J., Doroney, K.M. and So, A.G. (1974) Metabolic regulation of cytoplasmic DNA synthesis. Proceedings of the National Academy of Sciences, U.S.A., 71, 205–208.

Burch, R.E., Hahn, H.K.J. and Sullivan, J.F. (1975) Newer aspects of the roles of zinc, manganese and copper in human nutrition. Clinical Chemistry, 21, 501–520.

Chandra, S.V., Seth, P.K. and Mankeshwar, J.K. (1974) Manganese poisoning: clinical and biochemical observations. Environmental Research, 7, 374–380.

Chapman, B.E., MacDermott, T.E. and O'Sullivan, W.J. (1973) Studies on manganese complexes of human serum albumin. Bioinorganic Chemistry, 3, 27–38.

Cook, D.G., Fahn, S. and Brait, K.A. (1974) Chronic manganese intoxication. Archives of Neurology, 30, 59–64.

Doisy, E.A., Jr. (1973) Micronutrient control of biosynthesis of clotting proteins and cholesterol. In Proceedings of the Conference on Trace Substances in Environmental Health, Vol. 6 (Ed. D.D. Hemphill) pp. 193–197, University of Missouri Press, Columbia, Missouri.

Emara, A.M., El-Ghawabi, S.H., Madkour, O.I. and El-Samra, A.G. (1971) Chronic manganese poisoning in the dry battery industry. British Journal of Industrial Medicine, 28, 78–82.

Hambidge, K.M. and Droegemueller, W. (1974) See Reference under **Chromium.**

Hancock, R.G.V., Evans, D.J.R. and Fritze, K. (1973) Manganese proteins in blood plasma. Biochimica et Biophysica Acta, 320, 486–493.

Kehoe, J.M., Lust, G. and Beisel, W.R. (1969) Lymphoid tissue–corticosteroid interaction: an early effect on both Mg^{2+} and Mn^{2+}-activated RNA polymerase activities. Biochimica et Biophysica Acta, 174, 761–763.

Leach, R.M., Muenster, A. and Wien, E.M. (1969) Studies on the role of manganese in bond formation. II. Effect upon chondroitin sulfate synthesis in chick epiphyseal cartilage. Archives of Biochemistry and Biophysics, 133, 22–28.

Luck, G. and Zimmer, C. (1972) Conformational aspects and reactivity of DNA: effects of manganese and magnesium ions on interaction with DNA. European Journal of Biochemistry, 29, 528–536.

Mahoney, J.P., Sargent, K., Greland, M. and Small, W. (1969) Studies on manganese. I. Determination in serum by atomic absorption spectrophotometry. Clinical Chemistry, 15, 312–322.

Mena, I. (1974) The role of manganese in human disease. Annals of Clinical and Laboratory Science, 4, 487–491.

Nandekar, A.K.N., Nurse, C.E. and Friedberg, F. (1973) Mn(II)-binding by plasma proteins. International Journal of Peptide Research, 5, 279–281.

Rosenstock, H.A., Simons, D.G. and Meyers, J.S. (1971) Chronic manganism. Journal of the American Medical Association, 217, 1354–1358.

Scrutton, M.C., Utter, M.F. and Mildvan, A.S. (1966) Pyruvate carboxylase. VI. The presence of tightly bound manganese. Journal of Biological Chemistry, 231, 3480–3487.

Suzuki, M. and Wacker, W.E.C. (1974) Determination of manganese in biological materials by atomic absorption spectroscopy. Analytical Biochemistry, 57, 605–613.

Tanaka, S. and Lieben, J. (1969) Manganese poisoning and exposure in Pennsylvania. Archives of Environmental Health, 19, 674–684.

Van Ormer, D.G. and Purdy, W.C. (1973) The determination of manganese in urine by atomic absorption spectrometry. Analytica Chimica Acta, 64, 93–105.

Versieck, J. et al. (1974a) See reference under **Copper**.

Versieck, J., Barbier, F., Speecke, A. and Hoste, J. (1974b) Normal manganese concentrations in human serum. Acta Endocrinologica, 76, 783–788.

Versieck, J., Barbier, F., Speecke, A. and Hoste, J. (1975) Influence of myocardial infarction on serum manganese, copper and zinc concentrations. Clinical Chemistry, 21, 578–581.

Versieck, J., Speecke, A., Hoste, J. and Barbier, F. (1973) Determination of manganese, copper, and zinc in serum and packed blood cells by neutron activation analysis. Zeitschrift für Klinische Chemie und Klinische Biochemie, 11, 193–196.

Nickel

Asato, N., van Soestbergen, M. and Sunderman, F.W., Jr. (1975) Binding of ^{63}Ni(II) to ultrafiltrable constituents of rabbit serum in vivo and in vitro. Clinical Chemistry, 21, 521–527, 1975.

Hendel, R.C. and Sunderman, F.W., Jr. (1972) Species variations in the proportions of ultrafiltrable and protein-bound serum nickel. Research Communications in Chemical Pathology and Pharmacology, 4, 141–146.

Hohnadel et al. (1973) See reference under **Zinc**.

Horak, E. and Sunderman, F.W., Jr. (1973) Measurements of nickel excretion in feces of healthy adults. Clinical Chemistry, 19, 429–430.

McNeely, M.D., Nechay, M.W. and Sunderman, F.W., Jr. (1972) Measurements of nickel in serum and urine as indices of environmental exposure to nickel. Clinical Chemistry, 18, 992–995.

McNeely, M.D., Sunderman, F.W., Jr., Nechay, M.W. and Levine, H. (1971) Abnormal concentrations of serum nickel in myocardial infarction, stroke, burns, hepatic cirrhosis and uremia. Clinical Chemistry, 17, 1123–1128.

Nechay, M.W. and Sunderman, F.W., Jr. (1973) Measurements of nickel in hair by atomic absorption spectrometry. Annals of Clinical and Laboratory Science, 3, 30–35.

Nielsen, F.H. and Ollerich, D.A. (1974) Nickel: a new essential trace element. Federation Proceedings, 33, 1767–1772.

Nomoto, S. and Sunderman, F.W., Jr. (1970) Measurements of nickel in serum and other biological materials by atomic absorption spectrometry. Clinical Chemistry, 16, 477–485.

Sunderman, F.W. (1971) The treatment of acute nickel carbonyl poisoning with sodium diethyldithiocarbamate. Annals of Clinical Research, 3, 182–185.

Sunderman, F.W., Jr., Decsy, M.I. and McNeely, M.D. (1972) Nickel metabolism in health and disease. Annals of the New York Academy of Science, 199, 300–312.

Sunderman, F.W., Jr. and Nechay, M.W. (1974) Measurements of serum nickel by flameless atomic absorption spectrometry. Zeitschrift für Klinische Chemie und Klinische Biochemie, 12, 220.

Sunderman, F.W., Jr., Nomoto, S., Pradhan, A.M., Levine, H., Bernstein, S.H. and Hirsch, R. (1970) Increased concentrations of serum nickel following acute myocardial infarction. New England Journal of Medicine, 283, 896–899.

Szadkowski, D., Kohler, G. and Lehnert, G. (1970) Serumelektrolyte und elektrischmechanische Herzaction unter chronischer industrieller Hitzebelastung. Arztliche Forschung, 23, 271–284.

Von Ludewigs, H.J. and Thiess, A.M. (1970) Occupational medical importance of nickel carbonyl poisoning. Zentralblat Arbeitsmedicine, 20, 329–339.

Vuopala, V.E., Hahti, E., Takkunen, J. and Huikko, M. (1970) Nickel carbonyl poisoning: report of 25 cases. Annals of Clinical Research, 2, 214–222.

Zachariasen, H., Andersen, I. and Barton, R. (1975) Technique for determining nickel in blood by flameless atomic absorption spectrophotometry. Clinical Chemistry, 21, 562–567.

Lead

Anderson, W.N., Broughton, P.M.G., Dawson, J.B. and Fisher, G.W. (1974) An evaluation of some atomic absorption systems for the determination of lead in blood. Clinica Chimica Acta, 50, 129–136.

Barltrop, D. and Killala, N.J.P. (1967) Faecal excretion of lead by children. Lancet, 2, 1017–1019.

Barltrop, D. and Smith, A. (1971) Interaction of lead with erythrocytes. Experientia, 27, 92–93.

Barltrop, D. and Smith, A. (1972) Lead binding to human haemoglobin. Experientia, 28, 76–77.

Barry, P.S.I. (1973) Lead in man – a review. In Medical Aspects of Lead Absorption in Industrial Processes (Ed. P.J. Lawther) pp. 5–13, Lead Development Association, London.

Berman, E. (1969) Applications of atomic absorption spectrometry to trace metal analyses of toxicological materials. In Progress in Chemical Toxicology, Vol. 4 (Ed. A. Stolman) pp. 155–178, Academic Press, New York.

Browne, R.C., Ellis, R.W. and Weightman, D. (1974) Inter-laboratory variation in measurement of blood-lead levels. Lancet, 2, 1112–1113.

Davies, T.A.L. and Rainsford, S.G. (1967) Reporting blood-lead values. Lancet, 2, 834–835.

Emmerson, B.T. (1963) Chronic lead nephropathy: the diagnostic use of calcium EDTA and the association with gout. Australasian Annals of Medicine, 12, 310–324.

Goyer, R.A. and Chisholm, J.J. (1972) Lead. In Metallic Contaminants and Human Health (Ed. D.H.K. Lee) pp. 57–95, Academic Press, New York.

Haas, T., Mache, K., Schaller, K.H., Mache, W. and Valentin, H. (1972a) Investigations into ecological lead levels in children. Zentralblatt für Bakteriologie und Hygeine, 156, 353–360.

Haas, T., Wieck, A.G., Schaller, K.H. Mache, K. and Valentin, H. (1972b) The usual lead load in newborn infants and their mothers, Zeitschrift für Bakteriologie und Hygeine, 155, 341–349.

Hamilton, A. and Hardy, H.L. (1974) Industrial Toxicology, Publishing Sciences Group, Inc., Acton, Massachusetts, pp. 85–121.

Hicks, J.M., Gutierrez, A.N. and Worthy, B.E. (1973) Evaluation of the Delves microsystem for blood lead analysis. Clinical Chemistry, 19, 322–326.

Hohnadel et al. (1973) See reference under **Zinc**.

Keppler, J.F., Maxfield, M.E., Moss, W.D., Tietjen, G. and Linch, A.L. (1970) Interlaboratory evaluation of the reliability of blood lead analyses. American Industrial Hygiene Association Journal, 31, 412–429.

Kopito, L.E., Davis, M.A. and Shwachman, H. (1974) Sources of error in determining lead in blood by atomic absorption spectrophotometry. Clinical Chemistry, 20, 205–211.

Lathe, G.H. (1974) Errors of lead analyses: dependability of laboratories and clinicians. Lancet, 2, 1568–1569.

Millar, J.A., Cumming, R.L.C., Battistini, V., Carswell, F. and Goldberg, A. (1970), Lead and δ-aminolaevulinic acid dehydratase in mentally retarded children and in lead-poisoned suckling rats. Lancet, 2, 695–698.

Murphy, T.F., Nomoto, S. and Sunderman, F.W., Jr. (1971) Measurements of blood lead by atomic absorption spectrometry. Annals of Clinical and Laboratory Science, 1, 57–63.

Needleman, H.L. and Shapiro, I.M. (1974) Dentine lead levels in asymptomatic Philadelphia school children: subclinical exposure in high and low risk groups. Environmental Health Perspectives, 7, 27–31.

Pfitzer, E.A. (1974) An overview of the conference on low level lead toxicity. Environmental Health Perspectives, 7, 247–252.

Piper, K.G. and Higgins, G. (1967) Estimation of trace metals in biological material by atomic absorption spectrophotometry. Proceedings of the Association of Clinical Biochemists, 4, 191–197.

Pterovska, I. and Teisinger, J. (1970) Excretion of lead and its biological activity several years after termination of exposure. British Journal of Industrial Medicine, 27, 352–355.

Rosen, J.F. and Trinidad, E.E. (1974) Significance of plasma lead levels in normal and lead-intoxicated children. Environmental Health Perspectives, 7, 139–214.

Secchi, G.C., Alessio, L. and Cambiagni, G. (1973) Na^{+}/K^{+}-ATPase activity of erythrocyte membranes in urban populations not occupationally exposed to lead. Archives of Environmental Health, 27, 399–400.

Sunderman, F.W., Jr. (1973) Atomic absorption spectrometry of trace metals in clinical pathology. Human Pathology, 4, 549–582.

Sunderman, F.W., Jr. (1975a) Electrothermal atomic absorption spectrometry of trace metals in biological fluids. Annals of Clinical and Laboratory Science, 5, 421–434.

Thompson, J.A. (1971) Balance between intake and output of lead in normal individuals. British Journal of Industrial Medicine, 28, 189–194.

Waldron, H.A. (1975) Subclinical lead poisoning: a preventable disease. Preventive Medicine, 4, 135–153.

Gold

DeBosset, P.L. and Bitter, T. (1973) Near cytotoxic gold salt therapy in long-standing drug-refractory rheumatoid arthritis. Schweitzer Medizinische Wochenschrift, 103, 1153–1158.

Gottlieb, N.L., Smith, P.M. and Smith, E.M. (1974) Pharmacodynamics of ^{197}Au and ^{195}Au-labelled aurothiomalate in blood. Archives of Rheumatology, 17, 171–183.

Harth, M. (1974) Serum gold levels during chrysotherapy with relation to urinary and fecal excretion. Clinical Pharmacology and Therapeutics, 15, 354–360.

Lorber, A., Atkins, C.J., Chang, C.C., Lee, Y.B., Starrs, J. and Bovy, R.A. (1973) Monitoring serum gold values to improve chrysotherapy in rheumatoid arthritis. Annals of Rheumatic Diseases, 32, 133–138.

Sunderman, F.W., Jr. (1973) Atomic absorption spectrometry of trace metals in clinical pathology. Human Pathology, 4, 549–582.

FURTHER READING

Berman, E. (1969) Applications of atomic absorption spectrometry to trace metal analyses of toxicological materials. In Progress in Chemical Toxicology, Vol. 4 (Ed. A. Stolman) pp. 155–178, Academic Press, New York.

Brown, S.S. (Ed.) (1977) Clinical Chemistry and Chemical Toxicology of Metals, 398 pp. Elsevier, Amsterdam.

Burch, R.E., Hahn, H.K.J. and Sullivan, J.F. (1975) Newer aspects of the roles of zinc, manganese and copper in human nutrition. Clinical Chemistry, 21, 501–520.

Christian, C.D. and Feldman, F.J. (1970) Atomic Absorption Spectroscopy: Applications in Agriculture, Biology and Medicine, 490 pp. Wiley-Interscience Publishing Company, New York.

Davies, I.J.T. (1972) The Clinical Significance of the Essential Biological Metals, 126 pp. C.C. Thomas, Springfield, Illinois.

Dhar, S.K. (1972) Metal Ions in Biological Systems, 306 pp. Plenum Press, New York.

Friberg, L., Piscator, M. and Nordberg, G. (1971) Cadmium in the Environment, 165 pp. Chemical Rubber Company, Cleveland, Ohio.

Friberg, L. and Vostal, J. (1972) Mercury in the Environment. An Epidemiological and Toxicological Appraisal, 215 pp. Chemical Rubber Company, Cleveland, Ohio.

Friedman, M. (1973) Protein–Metal Interactions, 692 pp. Plenum Press, New York.

Hoekstra, W.G., Suttie, J.W., Ganther, H.E. and Mertz, W. (1974) Trace Element Metabolism in Animals – 2, 775 pp. University Park Press, Baltimore, Maryland.

Mertz, W. (1975) Trace element nutrition in health and disease: contributions and problems of analysis. Clinical Chemistry, 21, 468–475.

Mills, C.F. (1970) Trace Element Metabolism in Animals, 550 pp. Livingstone Ltd., Edinburgh.

National Research Council, Committee on Medical and Biologic Effects of Environmental Pollutants (1972–75) Monograph Series: Chromium, Copper, Lead, Manganese, Nickel, Vanadium and Zinc. National Academy of Sciences, Washington, D.C.

O'Dell, B.L. and Campbell, B.J. (1971) Trace elements: metabolism and metabolic function. In Comprehensive Biochemistry, Vol. 21 (Eds. M. Florkin and E.H. Stotz) pp. 179–266, Elsevier, New York.

Reinhold, J.G. (1975) Trace elements – a selective survey. Clinical Chemistry, 21, 476–500.

Sunderman, F.W., Jr. (1973) Atomic absorption spectrometry of trace metals in clinical pathology. Human Pathology, 4, 549–582.

Sunderman, F.W., Jr. (1975a) Electrothermal atomic absorption spectrometry of trace metals in biological fluids. Annals of Clinical and Laboratory Science, 5, 421–434.

Underwood, E.J. (1971) Trace Elements in Human and Animal Nutrition, 543 pp, Academic Press, 3rd edn.

Williams, D.R. (1971) The Metals of Life, 172 pp. Van Nostrand/Reinhold Company, London.

Chapter 20

Porphyrins

Donald P. Tschudy

Molecular Disease Branch, National Cancer Institute, National Institutes of Health, Bethesda, MD 20014, U.S.A.

CONTENTS

20.1 PORPHYRIN AND HAEM CHEMISTRY AND BIOCHEMISTRY

In order to understand the chemical basis for the diagnosis of each type of porphyria it is necessary to have a knowledge of the fundamentals of porphyrin nomenclature and the steps of the haem biosynthetic pathway.

20.1.1. Porphyrin structure and nomenclature

The basic ring structure common to all porphyrins is the compound, porphin (Figure 20.1). This structure, originally proposed in 1912 by Küster, was thought at the time by

Chemical diagnosis of disease, edited by S.S. Brown, F.L. Mitchell and D.S. Young

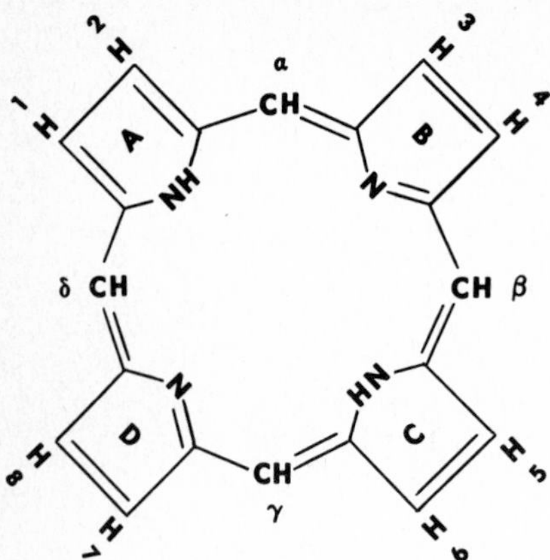

Figure 20.1. The structure of porphin, showing the eight numbered positions in which substitutions occur in the various porphyrins.

many to be unlikely as the correct structure, since such a large complicated molecule was presumed to be chemically less stable than porphin was known to be. It is now known that the chemical stability of porphin results from the conjugated double bond system which imparts a resonance stability to the ring, which possesses aromatic properties in that treatment with electrophilic reagents such as nitric and sulphuric acid results in substitution reactions, rather than ring cleavage.

On examination of the porphin ring, it is seen that, aside from the four hydrogens of the methene bridges, there are only eight positions (the eight β-positions of the pyrrole rings) in which substitutions can occur. These positions are numbered in Figure 20.1. Porphyrins differ primarily in the nature of the substituents which occur in these eight positions. The sequence in which particular substituents occur around the ring can vary, thus permitting the existence of isomeric sequences. There are two systems of isomeric nomenclature of porphyrins, the first based on the aetioporphyrins and the second on the mesoporphyrins. These two sets of reference compounds are used because many naturally occurring porphyrins can be converted into the corresponding aetio- or mesoporphyrin by the proper chemical manoeuvres, thus permitting conclusions regarding the sequence of substituents in the naturally occurring porphyrin.

If each pyrrole ring bears a methyl and ethyl substituent, there are four possible isomeric sequences which can exist. These are aetioporphyrins I–IV (Figure 20.2). This system of nomenclature is widely used because naturally occurring porphyrins have been shown to be isomer types I and III, a phenomenon which Fischer termed the "dualism" of the porphyrins. It appears, however, that porphyrins only function in living systems as metal chelates of type III isomers, and that type I isomers are "dead end" side products. The isomer type has some relevance to the chemical abnormalities of certain porphyrias and other disorders.

When each of two adjacent pyrrole rings bears a methyl and an ethyl substituent and the remaining two pyrrole rings each bear methyl and propionic acid substituents, one ob-

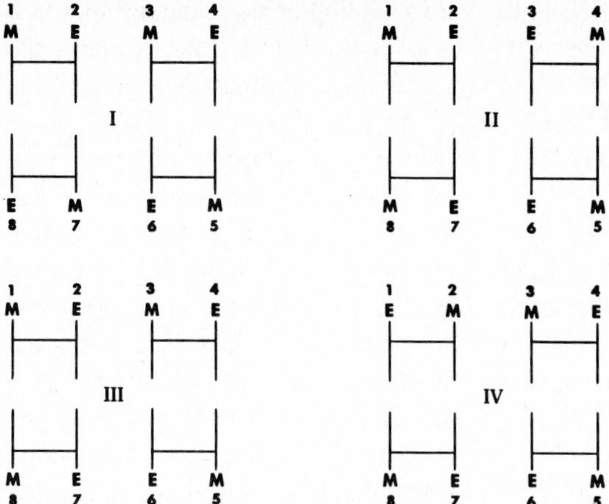

Figure 20.2. The sequence of methyl (M) and ethyl (E) substituents in the four isomeric aetioporphyrins.

tains a mesoporphyrin, of which there are 15 isomeric forms. Naturally occurring protoporphyrin corresponds to type 9 mesoporphyrin, since it is converted into this compound by reduction of its two vinyl groups.

20.1.2. Chemical and physical properties of porphyrins

In acid solution porphyrins have a red-violet colour and in alkaline solution or organic solvents a red-brown colour. Porphyrins have an absorption spectrum which is characterized by strong absorption in the neighbourhood of 400 nm – the Soret band – in addition to much weaker absorption bands in the visible region. The Soret band is significant from both a clinical and analytical chemical standpoint. Since the action spectrum, i.e. the spectrum producing photosensitivity reactions, corresponds to the absorption spectrum, it is radiation in the neighbourhood of wavelength 400 nm which is most active in producing skin lesions in the porphyrias. This wavelength is much longer than the sunburn wavelength and passes through window glass. Of importance to the analytical chemist is the active red fluorescence of porphyrins when irradiated by radiation of Soret band wavelength. This is the basis of screening methods which involve an extraction of porphyrins followed by visual estimation of fluorescence when the extract is irradiated with near ultraviolet (Wood's) light. It is also the basis for quantitative determination of minute quantities of porphyrins by fluorometric or spectrophotofluorometric methods.

The physical and chemical properties of porphyrins have been discussed in detail by Schwartz et al. (1960) and Falk (1964).

20.1.3. Haem biosynthesis

The haem biosynthetic pathway is thought to be present in all mammalian tissues, and indeed in all organisms, with a few exceptions, such as viruses and also probably obligatory anaerobes.

For the purposes of understanding the patterns of metabolites excreted in the various porphyrias, the haem biosynthetic pathway can be considered to consist of essentially eight steps, as shown in Figure 20.3. Details beyond the present discussion can be found in the writings of Burnham (1969), Shemin (1970), Granick and Sassa (1971), Marver and Schmid (1972) and Tschudy (1974). Step 1 involves the "activation" of glycine by reaction with pyridoxal phosphate, followed by condensation of the activated glycine with succinyl CoA. The immediate product, α-amino-β-oxoadipic acid, undergoes rapid spontaneous decarboxylation to form δ-aminolaevulic acid (δ-aminolaevulinic acid), the aliphatic precursor of porphyrins. This reaction occurs in mitochondria and is catalyzed by δ-aminolaevulate synthase (E.C. 2.3.1.37; ALA synthase; δ-aminolaevulic acid synthetase), the rate controlling enzyme of the pathway. In liver, the rate of synthesis of δ-aminolaevulinate synthase is controlled by a closed negative feedback loop in which haem acts to repress the synthesis of the enzyme and probably affects its uptake into mitochondria as well as directly inhibiting it (Tschudy, 1974). Present evidence indicates that in those hepatic porphyrias which can cause neurological disease, acute intermittent porphyria, variegate porphyria and hereditary coproporphyria, the activity of hepatic δ-aminolaevulinate synthase can vary from normal to greatly increased levels. These diseases are thought to result from mutations which lower the levels of specific enzymes of the path-

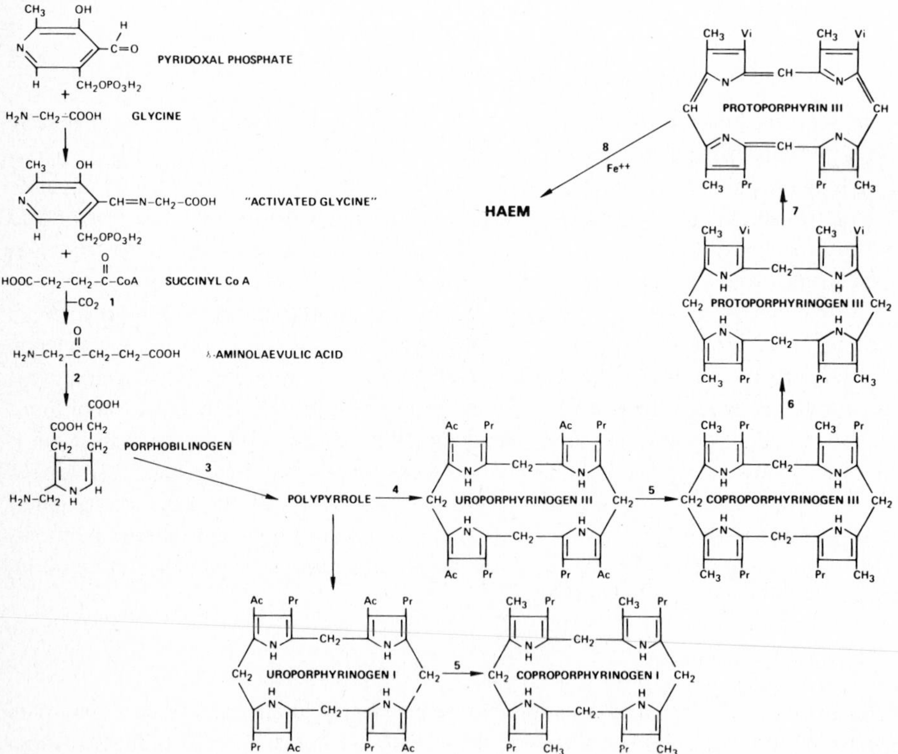

Figure 20.3. The haem biosynthetic pathway.

way and hence diminish haem synthesis. This results in diminished repression of hepatic δ-aminolaevulinate synthase. These diseases, therefore, are characterized chemically by both decreased utilization of metabolites at the level of the partial block in the pathway and increased production of precursors by the liver when hepatic δ-aminolaevulinate synthase levels are high.

Step 2 involves the self condensation of two molecules of δ-aminolaevulic acid to form porphobilinogen, the monopyrrole precursor of porphyrins. Since the Knorr-type condensation results in the removal of two molecules of water, the enzyme catalyzing this reaction has been named porphobilinogen synthase (E.C. 4.2.1.24; ALA dehydratase). This reaction occurs in the soluble portion of the cell, after δ-aminolaevulic acid has moved out of mitochondria. Porphobilinogen reacts with the Ehrlich aldehyde reagent (*p*-dimethylaminobenzaldehyde) to form a pink pigment. As discussed later, this is the basis of the Watson–Schwartz test, which is of great value in diagnosing acute intermittent, variegate and hereditary coproporphyria during attacks of neurologic dysfunction which may occur in these diseases.

Steps 3 and 4 convert porphobilinogen into uroporphyrinogen III. It is important to note that the intermediates between porphobilinogen and protoporphyrin are not the porphyrins, but their reduced forms, the hexahydroporphyrins, known as porphyrinogens. These compounds differ from the porphyrins in that they lack the conjugated double bond system of porphyrins and are colourless and non-fluorescent. In the presence of light and of oxygen or weak oxidizing agents, they are readily oxidized to the corresponding porphyrins. A significant portion of urinary coproporphyrin is excreted as coproporphyrinogen. It is at this stage of the pathway where isomeric forms are involved. Enzyme 3, uroporphyrinogen I synthase, catalyzes the polymerization of porphobilinogen to a linear polypyrrole, which is normally acted on by enzyme 4, uroporphyrinogen III cosynthase, to cyclize the linear polypyrrole to the asymmetric type III isomer, uroporphyrinogen III. Enzyme 4 is heat labile, in contrast to enzyme 3, and when this system is heated, allowing enzyme 3 to act alone on porphobilinogen, type I uroporphyrinogen is formed. This is significant in relation to the chemical findings in congenital erythropoietic porphyria (Günther's disease), since there are preliminary findings which indicate that the mutation in this disease markedly impairs the catalytic activity of uroporphyrinogen III cosynthase, resulting in conversion of much porphobilinogen into uroporphyrinogen I (Romeo and Levin, 1969). Evidence suggests that there is also an induction of δ-aminolaevulinate synthase in the normoblasts in this disease, resulting in both overproduction and diminished utilization of the linear polypyrrole produced by uroporphyrinogen I synthase. The type I isomer is not utilized physiologically and is excreted in the urine in large quantities.

Step 5 can be considered to be the decarboxylation of the four acetic acid side chains of uroporphyrinogen to form coproporphyrinogen. The four decarboxylations probably occur in stepwise fashion, leading to the production of hepta-, hexa-, and pentacarboxylic porphyrinogens which have been found in urine as the corresponding porphyrins, particularly in the disorder porphyria cutanea tarda. When porphyrins are separated by extraction methods, these intermediates partition between the uro- (8-carboxyl) and copro- (4-carboxyl) fractions. This enzyme, uroporphyrinogen decarboxylase (E.C. 4.1.1.37), acts on uroporphyrinogen I and III. It is for this reason that relatively large amounts of coproporphyrin I are excreted in congenital erythropoietic porphyria as well as uroporphyrin I.

Step 6 is the conversion of coproporphyrinogen into protoporphyrinogen. The two propionic acid side chains of the two adjacent A and B pyrrole rings of the tetrapyrrole structure are decarboxylated and oxidized to vinyl groups. This reaction occurs in mitochondria and is followed by the oxidation of protoporphyrinogen to protoporphyrin by removal of six hydrogen atoms (step 7). It is thought that this reaction involves an enzyme which is separate from that which converts coproporphyrinogen into protoporphyrinogen.

The final step is the chelation of Fe^{2+} by protoporphyrin to form haem. This is catalyzed by the mitochondrial enzyme ferrochelatase (haem synthase).

Those steps which involve oxidations or the use of oxidatively generated substrates (succinyl CoA) occur in mitochondria; those which involve primarily polymerization and decarboxylation occur in the soluble portion of the cell. Thus the enzymes of the pathway are compartmentalized within the cell, those at the beginning and end of the pathway being located in mitochondria and the intermediate steps in the soluble portion of the cell.

20.2. CLASSIFICATION OF THE PORPHYRIAS

The porphyrias can be divided into two general categories – erythropoietic and hepatic – depending on the main site of origin of the excess metabolites which are excreted. Each of the two groups is subdivided into specific clinical entities as shown in Table 20.1.

TABLE 20.1

CLASSIFICATION OF THE PORPHYRIAS

Erythropoietic
Congenital erythropoietic porphyria (Günther's disease) – recessive
Erythropoietic protoporphyria (erythrohepatic porphyria) – dominant
Erythropoietic coproporphyria (erythrohepatic coproporphyria)
Hepatic
Acute intermittent porphyria (pyrroloporphyria, Swedish porphyria) – dominant
Variegate porphyria (mixed porphyria, South African genetic porphyria) – dominant
Hereditary coproporphyria
Porphyria cutanea tarda

20.3. CLINICAL ASPECTS OF THE PORPHYRIAS

A porphyria can be defined as a primary disorder of porphyrin metabolism which is an inborn error, with the exception of certain cases of acquired porphyria cutanea tarda. The Turkish epidemic of hexachlorobenzene porphyria proved that this can sometimes be a toxic phenomenon (Ockner and Schmid, 1961). The porphyrias must be distinguished from those numerous disorders which produce secondary porphyrinuria, usually an increase of urinary coproporphyrin.

The clinical manifestations of these diseases (Marver and Schmid, 1972; Tschudy, 1974) can be mentioned briefly before their chemical diagnosis is discussed. The erythropoietic porphyrias and porphyria cutanea tarda produce variable types of cutaneous manifestations without neurologic disease. Congenital erythropoietic porphyria also produces haemolytic anaemia which can be severe. Erythropoietic protoporphyria is probably better named erythrohepatic porphyria, since excess protoporphyrin can probably originate in both liver and marrow cells in this condition. It may not be as innocuous as previously thought, since some patients are now dying of hepatic failure, probably related to excess deposition of protoporphyrin in the liver.

Acute intermittent, variegate and hereditary coproporphyria are all diseases which can exist indefinitely in latent form, but which can produce attacks of neurologic dysfunction, involving any portion of the nervous system. Although attacks may occur spontaneously, they are often precipitated by any of four groups of factors: certain drugs (of which barbiturates are the most notorious), certain hormones (oestrogen and possibly certain progestational type compounds), infections and starvation or dieting. The mechanism by which precipitating factors cause the attacks of neurological dysfunction is not yet known. Acute intermittent porphyria does not produce cutaneous lesions, but these may occur in the other types. Cutanea tarda porphyria, often precipitated by alcohol, oestrogen or iron, is a cutaneous disease which may be associated with clinically significant liver disease, but not neurological complications.

20.4. CHEMICAL FINDINGS IN THE PORPHYRIAS

It should be emphasized that the definitive diagnosis of each of the porphyrias is a chemical diagnosis. The correct diagnosis today is even more important than in years past, since specific modes of therapy have been developed for these diseases. The ideal method of diagnosis of the individual porphyrias would be a specific measurement of the defective enzyme in tissue or blood from the suspected patient – an enzyme test for each porphyria. At the present time a practical enzyme test has been achieved only for acute intermittent porphyria, as discussed later. For the others it is necessary to rely on demonstration of the pattern of metabolites in blood, urine and faeces which is characteristic of each disorder. One of the fundamental biochemical problems of these diseases is to relate in quantitative terms the specific enzyme defect to the observed pattern of metabolites for each disease. This problem underlies the basic understanding of the chemical findings in these diseases and is much more complex than it appears on cursory examination. An introduction to this problem with mathematical analysis of a steady state model of the pathway has been published (Tschudy, 1973; Tschudy and Bonkowsky, 1973). It is important to realize that there are certain patients who present patterns of chemical abnormalities which do not fit neatly into those categories described below. A summary of the abnormal chemical patterns in the porphyrias is presented in Table 20.2. Before

TABLE 20.2

THE PATTERNS OF METABOLITE EXCRETION IN THE VARIOUS PORPHYRIAS

The Table is only a general guide which attempts to be inclusive – exceptions to the patterns do occur. Abbreviations: N, normal: +–+++, slight to marked increase; X, porphyrin X; P_1, isocoproporphyrin series; ALA, δ-aminolaevulic acid; PBG, porphobilinogen; URO, uroporphyrins; COPRO, coproporphyrin; PROTO, protoporphyrin.

	Urine				Faeces					Erythrocytes		
	ALA	PBG	URO	COPRO	URO	COPRO	PROTO	X	P_1	URO	COPRO	PROTO
Congenital-erythropoietic porphyria	N	N	+++	++–+++	++	+++	N	N	?	+++	++	N–+
Erythropoietic protoporphyria	N	N	N	N	N	N–+	N–+++			N	N–+	+–+++
Latent	+–+++	+–+++	N–++	+	N–+	±	±	±	N	N	N	N
Acute intermittent porphyria												
Manifest	++–+++	++–+++	+–++	+	+–++	+	+	?	?	N	N	N
Latent	N–+	N–+	N–+	+–++	N	+++	+++	++–+++	N	N	N	N
Variegate porphyria												
Manifest	++–+++	++–+++	++	+–++	++	+++	+++	?	?	N	N	N
Latent	N–+	N–+	N–+	N–++	?	++–+++	N–+	N–+	N	N	N	N
Hereditary coproporphyria												
Manifest	++–+++	++–+++	++–+++	++–+++	?	+++	N–+			N	N	N
Cutanea tarda porphyria	N–+	N	+++	++–+++	++	+–++	N–+	N–+	++–+++	N	N	N
Normal values	<3 mg/day *	<2.5 mg/day	<50 μg/day	<300 μg/day	10–60 μg/day	<40 μg/ g dry wt	<100 μg/ g dry wt	<20 μg/ g dry wt **		0	0–2 μg/ 100 ml cells	15–75 μg/ 100 ml cells

* Excludes urinary aminoacetone, ** (Elder et al., 1974).

discussing the findings in the individual porphyrias, the routes of excretion of porphyrins and porphyrin precursors will be presented as an aid to understanding the patterns observed in the specific diseases.

20.4.1. Routes of excretion of porphyrins

The route of excretion of porphyrins and porphyrinogens is partly determined by their number of carboxyl groups, which, in turn, plays a major role in determining their water solubility. Protoporphyrin, with only two carboxyl groups, is excreted by the liver, but not by the kidney. Normal liver appears to clear blood coproporphyrin readily from the blood, but clears coproporphyrinogen less rapidly. A sufficiently high blood concentration of coproporphyrinogen can occur under normal circumstances to allow for some glomerular filtration of this substance, which explains the fact that most urinary coproporphyrin is excreted as coproporphyrinogen. Thus coproporphyrin, with four carboxyl groups, is excreted by both liver and kidney. Uroporphyrin and uroporphyrinogen, with eight carboxyl groups, are excreted almost exclusively in the urine. Uroporphyrin can be found in the faeces under certain conditions, but this often results from excess porphobilinogen which can be converted into uroporphyrinogen and uroporphyrin in the gut.

20.4.2. Congenital erythropoietic porphyria (Günther's disease)

This disease is characterized by the production of large quantities of uroporphyrinogen I and also increased amounts of coproporphyrinogen I. Because these are readily converted into the corresponding porphyrins, large quantities of uroporphyrin I and coproporphyrin I are found in the urine. The amount of uroporphyrin is greater than the amount of coproporphyrin. Uroporphyrin excretion may be up to 50 mg/day, as much as 1000 times the upper limit of total uroporphyrin in healthy individuals. Occasionally, even greater amounts than this have been reported. These quantities of porphyrin impart the classical "port wine" colour to the urine. Evidence of the disease may appear from the time of birth to a few years thereafter. The diagnosis is relatively simple. The onset of bullous skin disease and the appearance of red urine within the first few years of life are characteristic. The teeth may be discoloured (brown or pink) by porphyrin deposition (erythrodontia), since uroporphyrin has a high affinity for calcium phosphate. When erythrodontia is not obvious, fluorescence of the teeth is demonstrable. Haemolytic anaemia is common and fluorescence of a significant proportion of circulating red cells and marrow normoblasts can be demonstrated by fluorescence microscopy.

Quantitative measurements of urinary excretion and red cell uroporphyrin provide the conclusive evidence for the diagnosis of the disease. Because the combination of findings presented above is unique to congenital erythropoietic porphyria, it is difficult to confuse this disease with any other. There is no increased excretion of the porphyrin precursor porphobilinogen, and hence the Watson–Schwartz test is negative.

Evidence has been presented which suggests that there are decreased amounts of uroporphyrinogen III cosynthase in the red cells of these patients (Romeo and Levin, 1969) as well as in cattle with this disease. Because of the complexity of the method of measuring this enzyme, it must be considered at present only as a research procedure. Since the disease is relatively easy to diagnose, the need for an enzyme diagnostic test is not great. However, this is not the case for the heterozygous "carriers" who are asymptomatic. At present, the rarity of the defect and complexity of the enzyme test make screening for these carriers impractical.

20.4.3. Erythropoietic protoporphyria (erythrohepatic porphyria)

Although this disease has a much higher incidence than congenital erythropoietic porphyria, it was not defined as a specific clinical entity until 1961. The reason for this is undoubtedly because this is the only type of the well defined porphyrias in which there are no abnormal chemical findings in the urine. This statement, however, excludes the very rare erythropoietic coproporphyria and those patients with hereditary coproporphyria who have no increase of urinary coproporphyrin.

The enzyme defect in this disease appears to be a deficiency of ferrochelatase (Bonkowsky et al., 1975; Bottomley et al., 1975) which can result in accumulation of protoporphyrin. Since protoporphyrin is not excreted in urine, it is clear why no abnormalities are found in urine. There is evidence that indicates that excess protoporphyrin can originate from liver as well as erythrocytic cells in this disease. Hence, the separate variation in alternate sources of excess protoporphyrin may explain why different patterns of chemical findings can be seen in patients and in clinically unaffected ("carrier") parents. The three chemical patterns which may occur are: (1), increased free erythrocyte, plasma and faecal protoporphyrin; (2), increased free erythrocyte protoporphyrin with no increase of plasma or faecal protoporphyrin; and (3), increased faecal protoporphyrin with no increase of plasma or erythrocyte protoporphyrin. The third pattern is less frequent than the other two and has usually been seen in asymptomatic relatives of patients. There is also some increase of red cell and faecal coproporphyrin, but not to the extent seen with protoporphyrin. Symptomatic patients usually have an increase of red cell, plasma and faecal protoporphyrin. There can be great variation of the protoporphyrin concentrations in this disease, sometimes down to normal values. But red cell protoporphyrin levels can also approach values as high as 30 times the normal.

The diagnosis of this disease cannot be made without demonstration of an increased erythrocyte protoporphyrin concentration in individuals with the characteristic symptomatology. A high erythrocyte protoporphyrin concentration alone is not sufficient, since this may occur in other conditions such as lead intoxication or iron deficiency. In the latter conditions, however, photosensitivity does not occur. Likewise, an increased faecal protoporphyrin excretion is not pathognomonic, since this also occurs in other conditions, such as variegate porphyria.

Red cell and normoblast fluorescence can be demonstrated by fluorescence microscopy, which again is not pathognomonic, since this also occurs in congenital erythropoietic porphyria.

20.4.4. Erythropoietic coproporphyria

This extremely rare disease resembles erythropoietic protoporphyria clinically, but is accompanied by an increase of erythrocyte coproporphyrin with little or no increase of erythrocyte protoporphyrin (Heilmeyer and Clotten, 1964).

The diagnosis of the first three types of hepatic porphyria in the above classification is particularly important, even in individuals with the latent disease, because the simple expedient of warning these individuals of the known precipitating factors of the acute attacks of neurological disease may be a life-saving procedure. It is, therefore, important to examine the genetic relatives of afflicted individuals, so that those who bear the defect can be forewarned.

20.4.5. Acute intermittent porphyria

The most common misunderstanding concerning the chemical diagnosis of this disease is the failure to realize that it is the porphyrin precursors, δ-aminolaevulic acid and porphobilinogen, which are important and not the porphyrins. Since the partial block in the pathway is in the conversion of porphobilinogen into porphyrinogens (Figure 20.3, step 3) (Heilmeyer and Clotten, 1969; Strand et al., 1970; Miyagi et al., 1971), one might actually expect lower than normal porphyrin production. The fact is that urinary uroporphyrin excretion may be normal or increased in this disease. Increased uroporphyrin can be explained by two possible mechanisms. Porphobilinogen can undergo polymerization, particularly in acid solution, to various pigments. These include uroporphyrinogen and porphobilin, a brown pigment of unknown structure. The increased urinary uroporphyrin excretion sometimes observed in the presence of high concentrations of porphobilinogen may, therefore, merely result from in vitro polymerization of porphobilinogen. A second theoretical possibility is that under certain conditions excessive induction of hepatic δ-aminolaevulic synthase may expand the size of the porphobilinogen pool sufficiently to increase uroporphyrinogen production above normal. At any rate, urinary porphyrin measurements alone are not adequate for the diagnosis of this disease.

20.4.5.1. Enzyme diagnostic method

The two definite methods for the diagnosis of this disease involve the measurement of erythrocyte uroporphyrinogen I synthase or urinary porphyrin precursors. There are certain qualifications to this statement, in that both approaches have certain limitations. Four methods for the measurement of erythrocyte uroporphyrinogen I synthase have been developed (Granick et al., 1972; Strand et al., 1972; Meyer, 1973; Magnussen et al., 1974). There is a small overlap in the ranges of normal and porphyric values, thus creating a zone of values which is indeterminate when compared to the range observed in the normal population.

It was thought, on the basis of previous studies of excretion of porphyrin precursors in siblings of known patients, that practically all afflicted individuals could be shown to have an increased urinary porphobilinogen excretion after puberty (Haeger-Aronsen, 1963; Wetterberg, 1967), when porphobilinogen was measured quantitatively by chromatographic methods. The great utility of the enzyme determination is the fact that it can detect those afflicted individuals who have no increase of urinary porphobilinogen, a situation which undoubtedly is more frequent than previously suspected, particularly among teenage individuals (Strand et al., 1972). The enzyme method should have considerable application to prepubertal children in whom the increased urinary porphobilinogen is usually not demonstrable. The definitive method of diagnosis, therefore, of acute intermittent porphyria is the demonstration of an erythrocyte uroporphyrinogen I synthase activity which is approximately half that of normals. The techniques for measurement of the enzyme involve both micro- and macro-methods, which can be adapted for use in well-equipped clinical laboratories.

20.4.5.2. Urine methods

Patients with acute intermittent porphyria can be divided into two groups in terms of methods of diagnosis – latent and active. The enzyme method discussed above is applicable at all times, whereas there are certain limitations to the urine methods. The two substances, δ-aminolaevulic acid and porphobilinogen differ in relative diagnostic importance. Porphobilinogen is usually present in greater amount (when expressed as mg/day) than δ-aminolaevulic acid, and the proportion of patients with acute intermittent porphyria who excrete increased amounts of porphobilinogen is greater than that in whom an increased amount of δ-aminolaevulic acid is excreted. An increase of porphobilinogen with little or no increase of δ-aminolaevulic acid is seen in some patients with acute intermittent porphyria, but the opposite finding, i.e. increased δ-aminolaevulic acid without an increase of porphobilinogen, is not seen in acute intermittent porphyria (at least to the author's present knowledge) and indeed is characteristic of lead intoxication. This is particularly important to emphasize, since the clinical manifestations of lead intoxication can closely resemble those of acute intermittent porphyria. Thus, in the presence of clinical manifestations suggesting acute intermittent porphyria, a finding of increased urinary δ-aminolaevulic acid and coproporphyrin with normal porphobilinogen, is virtually diagnostic of lead intoxication. While increases of urinary δ-aminolaevulic acid are a sensitive indicator of lead exposure, some increase of δ-aminolaevulic acid and coproporphyrin may also occur in cutanea tarda porphyria. Neurological manifestations are not a part of the latter disease, however.

During both the latent and acute periods of acute intermittent porphyria, the diagnosis by examination of the urine requires demonstration of increased amounts of porphobilinogen. This can be done in two ways – quantitative measurement using chromatographic methods or by the qualitative Watson–Schwartz test (Watson et al., 1961; Watson et al., 1964).

The quantitative measurement of porphyrin precursors in urine involves passage of urine over an ion exchange column at a pH which causes retention of porphobilinogen but allows δ-aminolaevulic acid to pass through. Porphobilinogen is then eluted and measured spectrophotometrically after formation of the red pigment by reaction with Ehrlich's aldehyde reagent, *p*-dimethylaminobenzaldehyde. This reaction is subject to a number of modifiers as well as to false positives and negatives which will be discussed in relation to the Watson–Schwartz test. While most of these problems are circumvented by use of the column method, patients receiving large doses of phenothiazines may excrete a substance which can cause errors in the quantitative chromatographic determination of porphobilinogen (Wetterberg, 1967). The Ehrlich-positive material derived from phenothiazines has a spectral curve which differs from that derived from porphobilinogen, thus allowing differentiation of these substances from porphobilinogen. When the quantitative method is used in individuals with the *active* disease, it will closely approach 100% accuracy as a diagnostic method. Even in the latent disease it is of great value, but an exact figure for its diagnostic accuracy in the latent disease cannot be given. Wetterberg (1967) and Haeger-Aronsen (1963) found 55% and 46%, respectively, of positive urine tests by the quantitative method among siblings of known patients. Since these values are near the expected figure of 50%, it appears that this method will detect a high percentage of latent cases. The fact that asymptomatic individuals with normal urine values, but a low level of erythrocyte uroporphyrinogen I synthase, later experienced an acute attack associated with increased urinary porphobilinogen excretion proves conclusively that the quantitative urine method does not detect all latent cases (Strand et al., 1972).

There is little published information on urine values of prepubertal children of a porphyric parent, but the impression is that they usually do not excrete increased amounts of urinary porphobilinogen. The enzyme method will detect afflicted individuals before puberty.

The urinary excretion of porphobilinogen and δ-aminolaevulic acid can fluctuate greatly within a particular patient, and also can vary greatly from one patient to another. Therefore, in general, absolute values cannot be used as criteria for determining whether certain symptoms may be caused by the disease. Some asymptomatic patients excrete much more porphobilinogen than others who are experiencing activity of the disease. However, it is generally true that values for a particular patient increase when there is activity of the disease and decline when the patient recovers. Urinary excretion of porphobilinogen may reach 150 to 200 mg/day, or even higher, and that of δ-aminolaevulic acid can reach 180 mg/day. Thus the difference in porphyrin precursor excretion between the active and latent disease here is usually one of the magnitude of increase – not an all-or-none phenomenon as is often seen in variegate and hereditary coproporphyria. In these disorders, porphyrin precursor excretion may be abnormal during attacks of neurologic dysfunction, but often declines to normal during latent periods.

The Watson–Schwartz test is a qualitative test which is very useful as a quick method for diagnosing the acute attack of acute intermittent, variegate and hereditary coproporphyria. When properly performed and interpreted, it will detect these disorders in practically all cases during the acute attack. Since the acute attack is similar in all three of these disorders, the chemical differentiation of the three (discussed later) is actually academic. The test will be discussed in detail because it is so frequently misinterpreted. Step 1 involves addition of urine (2 ml) to an equal volume of Ehrlich's aldehyde reagent. This reagent is capable of reacting with pyrroles with an unsubstituted α position (such as porphobilinogen), urobilinogen, resorcinol, certain furans and various indoles. The conditions such as temperature, pH, etc. at which the rates of these various reactions are optimal vary considerably, as well as the colour of the product of the reaction. When there is an immediate production of a red pigment at room temperature after addition of the Ehrlich reagent to urine, it is usually indicative of either increased quantities of porphobilinogen or of the presence of a dye which is red at low pH. Substances such as pyridium (or its metabolites), beet pigment and melanogen (5,6-dihydroxyindole) can produce various colours when treated with strong acid. These colours usually differ from the characteristic colour formed when porphobilinogen reacts with the Ehrlich reagent. To rule out false positives of this type, it is necessary to determine whether addition of a strong acid (such as 22% hydrochloric acid) alone will produce the colour.

Urobilinogen does not react sufficiently rapidly at the low pH of the Ehrlich aldehyde reagent to produce an immediate colour. After addition of saturated sodium acetate, however, urobilinogen reacts rapidly to produce a purple-pink pigment. The original test was completed by chloroform extraction, which left the porphobilinogen pigment in the aqueous phase and extracted the urobilinogen pigment into the chloroform. The problem with the original test was that there was sometimes a residual weak pink, orange or violet colour, not caused by the porphobilinogen pigment, which remained in the aqueous phase. It is undoubtedly because of the misinterpretation of these atypical reactions that surveys of various types of populations by means of the Watson–Schwartz test have reported such a highly variable incidence of positives. These atypical pigments are extracted with butanol and the original test has, therefore, been modified so that the aqueous phase is extracted with butanol after chloroform extraction.

Some indoles, such as melanogen and indoleacetic acid, react with Ehrlich's reagent to form chloroform-insoluble pigments (Ludwig, 1958), suggesting that certain indoles may be responsible for the atypical pigments which have confused some observers in the past. Specific examples of certain diseases which have produced "atypical reactions" include malignant melanoma and pellagra. There are also several indoles which produce pigments of various colours with the Ehrlich reagent which are chloroform soluble (Watson et al., 1964).

There also are rare instances of false negative Watson–Schwartz tests. Certain indoles such as indole, indican or 5-hydroxyindoleacetic acid, when present in appropriate concentration, can form a colourless compound with porphobilinogen and the Ehrlich aldehyde reagent (Taddeini et al., 1967); however, excesses of these indoles produce a red or orange chloroform-soluble pigment. There are compounds which can be present in certain circumstances which apparently can inhibit the Ehrlich reaction, but they have not been identified. The colour of the reaction develops at a rate which depends on the nature of the reactant, temperature, pH, etc., and also fades at variable rate. High concentrations of certain compounds such as sulphydryl derivatives and urea, may augment the rate of colour fading.

Despite these limitations, the Watson–Schwartz test is the easiest and quickest method for diagnosing patients with acute intermittent, variegate or hereditary coproporphyria during the acute attacks of neurological dysfunction. It will also detect some patients with acute intermittent porphyria during latent periods. The concentration of porphobilinogen in the urine at which the test becomes positive varies, undoubtedly because of the factors discussed above as well as the visual interpretation involved.

Another qualitative screening procedure utilizing the Ehrlich aldehyde reagent is the Hoesch test (Lamon et al., 1974). The reaction of urobilinogen with the Ehrlich aldehyde reagent is inhibited completely by the use of a much higher concentration of acid than is used in the Watson–Schwartz test.

20.4.6. Variegate porphyria

The chemical pattern of this disease is different during the acute attack of neurological dysfunction than at other times. The faecal protoporphyrin excretion is increased at all times in patients with this disease as well as there being some increase of faecal coproporphyrin. Eales (1974) found a mean faecal protoporphyrin excretion in 45 patients of 632 μg/g dry faeces (range 129 to 1805) and 95% exceeded 200 μg/g. Mean faecal coproporphyrin was 325 μg/g (range 39 to 986) and 95% exceeded 100 μg/g. Porphobilinogen (and often δ-aminolaevulic acid) excretion is increased during acute attacks of neurologic dysfunction, but tends to return to normal afterward. This is in contrast to acute intermittent porphyria where excretion rates are often increased at all times, moving even higher during acute attacks. There is an increased urinary excretion of coproporphyrin and uroporphyrin. When the patient is not experiencing an acute attack of neurologic dysfunction, urinary coproporphyrin usually exceeds urinary uroporphyrin. In Eales's (1974) series, urinary coproporphyrin ranged from 17 to 5100 μg/litre whereas uroporphyrin ranged from 0 to 1410 μg/litre. These urine porphyrin values differ from the typical finding in cutanea tarda porphyria, where urinary uroporphyrin usually exceeds urinary coproporphyrin.

During remission, urine porphyrin excretion is low relative to faecal porphyrin. The large amounts of faecal copro- and protoporphyrin excreted (during both the acute attack and remission phases) are not accompanied by great increases of porphyrins with more than four carboxyl groups during the remission phase. However, in the acute attack there is a pronounced increase of both faecal and urinary uroporphyrin, so that urinary uroporphyrin frequently exceeds urinary coproporphyrin, thus reversing the pattern seen during the remission phase. Undoubtedly much of the urine and faecal uroporphyrin found during the acute attack is formed non-enzymatically from the excess porphobilinogen.

Patients with variegate porphyria have been shown to excrete ether-insoluble hydrophilic porphyrin peptide conjugates which have collectively been called porphyrin X (Rimington et al., 1968; Eales et al., 1971; Moore et al., 1972; Elder et al., 1974). Early work on porphyrin X indicated the presence of a porphyrin–peptide complex containing a thioether linkage, as seen in cytochrome c. It has generally been measured by the original method of Rimington et al. (1968), i.e. extraction by concentrated urea solution containing non-ionic detergent, of the faecal residue that remained after ether–acetic acid-soluble porphyrins had been extracted. Porphyrin X is not unique to variegate porphyria, although the highest values are commonly encountered in this disease. Small amounts are found in normal faeces using urea–Triton extraction – <12 μg/day reported by Eales (1974) and <20 μg/g dry faeces (mean = 3) reported by Elder et al. (1974).

Increases have been observed in porphyria cutanea tarda (Eales, 1974: mean = 31 μg/g dry faeces, range 0 to 98; Elder et al., 1974: untreated patients, mean = 133 μg/g dry faeces, range 0 to 358; treated patients, mean = 56). The increases in variegate porphyria are greater (Eales, 1974: mean = 156 μg/g dry faeces, range 13 to 805; Elder et al., 1974: mean = 368 μg/g dry faeces). Slight increases of faecal porphyrin X also occur in acute intermittent porphyria (Elder, 1974). Since there is some overlap in the ranges of the values for porphyrin X observed in variegate and cutanea tarda porphyria, measurement of this porphyrin alone cannot be relied on to make the distinction between the two diseases in individual patients. More important is the nature of the composition of the X porphyrin fraction in the two diseases. In variegate porphyria, it appears to be mainly the porphyrin--peptide conjugates, whereas in porphyria cutanea tarda it is largely a hepta-carboxylic porphyrin (Elder et al., 1974). These differences can be shown by electrophoretic methods.

20.4.7. Hereditary coproporphyria

Clinically this disease is similar to variegate porphyria. It can exist in latent form, or it can produce acute attacks of neurologic dysfunction or photosensitivity. During acute attacks, as in variegate porphyria, there is an increase of porphyrin precursor excretion which is associated with an increased level of hepatic δ-aminolaevulate synthase. During other periods there may or may not be an increase of urinary coproporphyrin. Faecal coproporphyrin III is increased (sometimes to several mg/g dry faeces) and is the most consistent finding in all phases of the disease. During acute attacks, the increased excretion of porphobilinogen is definitive in defining an acute attack of hepatic porphyria. Differentiation from acute intermittent and variegate porphyria is academic, but can be achieved by combined clinical and chemical analysis. If the porphyrin precursor excretion returns to normal after the attack and there is a high faecal coproporphyrin (with or without high urine coproporphyrin) excretion, acute intermittent porphyria is much less likely than hereditary coproporphyria. Skin lesions similar to those of variegate porphyria, further rule out the former. Variegate porphyria is distinguished by the high faecal protoporphyrin excretion seen in this disease. However, values of faecal protoporphyrin above the normal amount have been reported in hereditary coproporphyria.

In the patients who have not experienced an acute attack and who have no abnormalities in the urine, a high faecal porphyrin may be the only finding. Furthermore, in those who have an increase of urinary coproporphyrin during remission periods, the problem becomes one of distinguishing this disease from secondary porphyrinuria.

20.4.8. Cutanea tarda porphyria

The diagnosis of this disease involves the problem mainly of accurately differentiating it from variegate porphyria and hereditary coproporphyria. The skin lesions of these two conditions are similar to those of cutanea tarda porphyria, and in those patients with variegate porphyria or hereditary coproporphyria who have experienced no neurological problems, clinical differentiation may be difficult. There are two main reasons for accurately making the distinction between cutanea tarda porphyria and the other hepatic porphyrias. First is the fact that patients with cutanea tarda porphyria do not experience the acute attacks of neurologic dysfunction seen in the other hepatic porphyrias and hence need not fear the precipitating factors for these attacks. This is particularly relevant with regard to the use of the drugs which are dangerous in the other hepatic porphyrias. It should be pointed out, however, that there are three chemical agents which can play a role in precipitating clinical activity of cutanea tarda porphyria. These are alcohol, iron and oestrogen. In addition, chloroquine can precipitate a severe acute illness in these patients accompanied by the excretion of huge amounts of urinary porphyrin.

The second reason for accurate differentiation from the other hepatic porphyrias is that the treatment is different. Phlebotomy is highly successful in the treatment of cutanea tarda porphyria, whereas the other hepatic porphyrias are treated by a more complicated combination of pharmacological and dietary methods. Intravenous haemin, now under study, appears to be promising in the treatment of the other hepatic porphyrias.

The chemical pattern is a considerable increase of urinary uroporphyrin and coproporphyrin, with the former usually exceeding the latter. In Eales' (1974) series of 66 cases, mean urinary uroporphyrin concentration was 2819 μg/litre (range 80 to 9204) with 70% exceeding 1000 μg/litre. Mean coproporphyrin concentration was 560 μg/litre (range 55 to 3480). There are often significant amounts of porphyrins with seven, six or five carboxyl groups, as well as the octa- and tetra-carboxyl porphyrins. There is sometimes an increase of faecal porphyrin which is mainly coproporphyrin with significant amounts of heptacarboxylic porphyrin and smaller amounts of uro-, hexa- and pentacarboxylic porphyrins in addition to protoporphyrin. When increases of faecal copro- or protoporphyrin are found, they do not usually reach the amounts found in variegate porphyria. Thus in Eales' (1974) series, faecal protoporphyrin was below 100 μg/g dry faeces in 95% of patients, and exceeded 200 μg/g in only 2% (mean = 49). Porphyrin X levels in this disease have been discussed in the section on variegate porphyria. A more recent finding, which appears to be highly significant in this disease, is the isolation of a group of porphyrins of the isocoproporphyrin series (Elder, 1972; Elder, 1974). These porphyrins are excreted in the faeces of patients with porphyria cutanea tarda and also of rats treated with hexachlorobenzene, a compound which produces porphyria cutanea tarda in man. They may have a specific relationship to this disease. Porphyrins of the isocoproporphyrin series contain three propionate (in substituent positions 4, 6 and 7 of the porphin ring), one acetate (position 3) and three methyl substituents (positions 1, 5 and 8) in the β positions, but differ in the nature of the remaining β substituent (position 2). This is an ethyl group in isocoproporphyrin, a vinyl in dehydroisocoproporphyrin, and an hydroxyethyl group in hydroxyisocoproporphyrin; there is no substituent in this position in desethylisocoproporphyrin.

The main components of this series in the faeces of patients with cutanea tarda porphyria are isocopro- and desethylisocoproporphyrin. Data suggest that dehydroisocoproporphyrin is the main component of this series in bile, and that microorganisms in the gut may, by reduction and de-ethylation, convert it into the above compounds, in the same manner that protoporphyrin is converted into meso- and deuteroporphyrin. In clinically active porphyria cutanea tarda, Elder (1974) has found that porphyrins of the isocoproporphyrin series are a major component of the porphyrins excreted. In five patients, the isocoproporphyrin series accounted for 15 to 35% (mean 24%) of faecal porphyrin and 9 to 21% (mean 15%) of total urine and faecal porphyrin. Although they are excreted mainly in the faeces, they have been detected in smaller amounts in the urine also. They have been found in the faeces of one patient with congenital erythropoietic porphyria, and in small amounts in normal individuals and in patients with variegate porphyria. The measurement of these porphyrins in the faeces may ultimately prove to be a specific method for the chemical diagnosis of cutanea tarda porphyria.

Patients with cutanea tarda porphyria do not excrete increased amounts of porphobilinogen and do not have a positive Watson–Schwartz test. However, there may be small increases of urinary δ-aminolaevulic acid – on rare occasions as high as 8 to 10 mg/day.

20.4.9. Porphyrin metabolism in other diseases

Secondary porphyrinuria (almost always coproporphyrinuria) occurs in chemical and heavy metal toxicity: this includes alcohol, benzene, carbon tetrachloride, lead, gold and arsenic. It also may be seen in a variety of diseases, including leukaemia, Hodgkin's disease, aplastic anaemia, pernicious anaemia, haemolytic anaemia and liver disease.

The amount of erythrocyte protoporphyrin can be increased by factors which diminish iron incorporation into haem – iron deficiency, infection and lead intoxication. Some increase may also occur in Hodgkin's disease, leukaemia, azotaemia and haemolytic anaemia.

Considerable increases of urinary δ-aminolaevulic acid are seen in lead intoxication, as discussed previously, but lesser increases have been reported in hereditary tyrosinaemia, diabetic acidosis and the third trimester of pregnancy.

REFERENCES

Bonkowsky, H.L., Bloomer, J.R., Ebert, P.S. and Mahoney, M.J. (1975) Heme synthetase deficiency in human protoporphyria. Demonstration of the defect in liver and cultured skin fibroblasts. Journal of Clinical Investigation, 56: 1139–1148.

Bottomley, S.S., Tanaka, M. and Everett, M.A. (1975) Diminished erythroid ferrochelatase activity in protoporphyria. Journal of Laboratory and Clinical Medicine, 86: 126–131.

Burnham, B.F. (1969) Metabolism of porphyrins and corrinoids. In Metabolic Pathways, Vol. 3 (Ed. D.M. Greenberg) Chapter 18, pp. 403–537, Academic Press, New York.

Eales, L. (1974) The porphyrias, In Current Diagnosis, 4th ed. (Eds. H.F. Conn and R.B. Conn Jr.) W.B. Saunders Co., London.

Eales, L., Grosser, Y. and Sano, S. (1971) The porphyrin peptides: practical implications. South African Journal of Laboratory and Clinical Medicine, 17: 160–163.

Elder, G.H. (1972) Identification of a group of tetracarboxylate porphyrins, containing one acetate and three propionate β-substituents, in faeces from patients with symptomatic cutaneous hepatic porphyria and from rats with porphyria due to hexachlorobenzene. Biochemical Journal, 126: 877–891.

Elder, G.H. (1974) The metabolism of porphyrins of the isocoproporphyrin series. Enzyme, 17: 61–68.

Elder, G.H., Magnus, I.A., Handa, F. and Doyle, M. (1974) Faecal "X porphyrin" in the hepatic porphyrias. Enzyme, 17: 29–38.

Falk, J.E. (1964) Porphyrins and Metallo-Porphyrins. Elsevier, Amsterdam.

Granick, S. and Sassa, S. (1971) δ-Aminolevulinic acid synthetase and the control of heme and chlorophyll synthesis. In Metabolic Pathways, Vol. 5 (Ed. H.J. Vogel) pp. 77–141, Academic Press, New York.

Granick, S., Sassa, S., Granick, J.L., Levere, R.D. and Kappas, A. (1972) Assays for porphyrins, δ-aminolevulinic acid dehydratase and porphyrinogen synthetase in microliter samples of whole blood; applications to metabolic defects involving the heme pathway. Proceedings of the United States National Academy of Sciences, 69: 2381–2385.

Haeger-Aronsen, B. (1963) Various types of porphyria in Sweden. South African Journal of Laboratory and Clinical Medicine, 9: 288–295.

Heilmeyer, L. and Clotten, R. (1964) Congenital erythropoietic coproporphyria. German Medical Monthly, 9: 353–357.

Heilmeyer, L. and Clotten, R. (1969) Zur biochemischen Pathogenese der Porphyria acuta intermittens. Klinische Wochenschrift, 47: 71–74.

Lamon, J., With, T.K. and Redeker, A.G. (1974) The Hoesch test: bedside screening for urinary porphobilinogen in patients with suspected porphyria. Clinical Chemistry, 20: 1438–1440.

Ludwig, G.D. (1958) Urinary excretion of indoles causing false positive Watson–Schwartz tests for porphobilinogen. Journal of Clinical Investigation, 37: 914–915.

Magnussen, C.R., Levine, J.B., Doherty, J.M., Cheesman, J.O. and Tschudy, D.P. (1974) Blood, 44: 857–868.

Marver, H.S. and Schmid, R. (1972) The porphyrias. In The Metabolic Basis of Inherited Disease, 3rd ed. (Eds. J.B. Stanbury, J.B. Wyngaarden and D.S. Fredrickson) Chap. 45, pp. 1087–1140, McGraw-Hill, New York.

Meyer, U.A. (1973) Intermittent acute porphyria. Clinical and biochemical studies of disordered heme biosynthesis. Enzyme, 16: 334–342.

Miyagi, K., Cardinal, R., Bossenmaier, I. and Watson, C.J. (1971) The serum porphobilinogen and hepatic porphobilinogen deaminase in normal and porphyric individuals. Journal of Laboratory and Clinical Medicine, 78: 683–695.

Moore, M.R., Thompson, G.G. and Goldberg, A. (1972) Amount of faecal porphyrin–peptide conjugates in the porphyrias. Clinical Science, 43: 299–302.

Ockner, R.K. and Schmid, R. (1961) Acquired porphyria in man and rat due to hexachlorobenzene intoxication. Nature, 189: 499.

Rimington, C., Lockwood, W.H. and Belcher, R.V. (1968) The excretion of porphyrin peptide conjugates in porphyria variegata. Clinical Science, 35: 211–247.

Romeo, G. and Levin, E.Y. (1969) Uroporphyrinogen III cosynthetase in human congenital erythropoietic porphyria. Proceedings of the United States National Academy of Sciences, 63: 856–863.

Schwartz, S., Berg, M.H., Bossenmaier, I. and Dinsmore, H. (1960) Determination of porphyrins in biological materials. In: Methods of Biochemical Analysis, Vol. 8 (Ed. D. Glick) pp. 221–293, Interscience Publishers, New York.

Shemin, D. (1970) On the synthesis of heme. Naturwissenschaften, 57, 185–190.

Strand, L.J., Felsher, B.F., Redeker, A.G. and Marver, H.S. (1970) Heme biosynthesis in intermittent acute porphyria. Decreased hepatic conversion of porphobilinogen to porphyrins and increased delta-aminolevulinic acid synthetase activity. Proceedings of the United States National Academy of Science, 67: 1315–1320.

Strand, L.J., Meyer, U.A., Felsher, B.F., Redeker, A.G. and Marver, H.S. (1972) Decreased red cell uroporphyrinogen I synthetase activity in intermittent acute porphyria. Journal of Clinical Investigation, 51: 2530–2536.

Taddeini, L., Kay, I.T. and Watson, C.J. (1967) Inhibition of Ehrlich's reaction of porphobilinogen by indican and related compounds. Clinica Chimica Acta, 7: 890–891.

Tschudy, D.P. (1973) Enzyme aspects of acute intermittent porphyria. Molecular and Cellular Biochemistry, 2: 63–70.

Tschudy, D.P. (1974) Porphyrin metabolism and the porphyrias. In Duncan's Diseases of Metabolism, 7th ed. (Eds. P.K. Bondy and L. Rosenberg) Chap. 12, Saunders, Philadelphia.

Tschudy, D.P. and Bonkowsky, H.L. (1973) A steady state model of sequential irreversible enzyme reactions. Molecular and Cellular Biochemistry, 2: 55–62.

Watson, C.J., Bossenmaier, I. and Cardinal, R. (1961) Acute intermittent porphyria–urinary porphobilinogen and other Ehrlich reactors in the diagnosis. Journal of The American Medical Association, 175: 1087–1091.

Watson, C.J., Taddeini, L. and Bossenmaier, I. (1964) Present status of the Ehrlich aldehyde reaction for urinary porphobilinogen. Journal of the American Medical Association, 190: 501–504.

Wetterberg, L. (1967) A Neuropsychiatric and Genetical Investigation of Acute Intermittent Porphyria. Svenska Bokförlaget, Stockholm.

FURTHER READING

Fuhrhop, J.-H. and Smith, K.M. (1975) Laboratory Methods in Porphyrin and Metalloporphyrin Research. Elsevier, Amsterdam.

Smith, K.M. (Ed.) (1975) Porphyrins and Metalloporphyrins. Elsevier, Amsterdam.

Tschudy, D.P. (1973) Enzyme aspects of acute intermittent porphyria. Molecular and Cellular Biochemistry, 2: 63–70.

Tschudy, D.P. (1974) Porphyrin metabolism and the porphyrias. In Duncan's Diseases of Metabolism, 7th ed. (Eds. P.K. Bondy and L. Rosenberg) pp. 775–824, Saunders, Philadelphia.

Tschudy, D.P. and Bonkowsky, H.L. (1973) A steady state model of sequential irreversible enzyme reactions. Molecular and Cellular Biochemistry, 2: 55–62.

Chapter 21

Purines and nucleotides

Richard W.E. Watts

Division of Inherited Metabolic Diseases, Clinical Research Centre, Harrow, Middlesex HA1 3UJ, England

CONTENTS

Chemical diagnosis of disease, edited by
S.S. Brown, F.L. Mitchell and D.S. Young

21.1. BIOCHEMISTRY, PHYSIOLOGY AND PHARMACOLOGY

Abnormal concentrations of uric acid in the blood and urine are chemical indicators of a disorder of purine metabolism. The need for uric acid measurements arises mainly from rheumatological and urological practice and more rarely in relation to some aspects of paediatric neurology.

21.1.1. Some aspects of purine chemistry

Much of the present detailed knowledge of purine metabolism in all classes of living organisms, including man, has been derived by the use of purines labelled with radioactive or stable isotopes in specific positions in the purine ring.

Scheme 21.1 shows the chemical structures of the pathophysiologically important purine bases and of the pharmacologically active pyrazolo(3,4-d)pyrimidines, allopurinol and oxipurinol, which are structural analogues of hypoxanthine and xanthine respectively. The ribonucleotides adenylic acid (AMP) and guanylic acid (GMP), which together provide half of the bases for the triplet code of deoxyribonucleic acid (DNA) and ribonucleic acid (RNA), are shown together with their 3′,5′-cyclic derivatives (cAMP and cGMP) in Scheme 21.2. The cyclic ribonucleotides are of profound physiological importance as regulators of enzyme activity and mediators of hormonal function.

Uric acid is the most highly oxidized of these purines, being formed in vivo by the xanthine oxidase (EC 1.2.3.2) catalyzed oxidation of hypoxanthine and xanthine (Scheme 21.3). Further catalytic oxidation by uricase (EC 1.7.3.3) opens the pyrimidine ring to

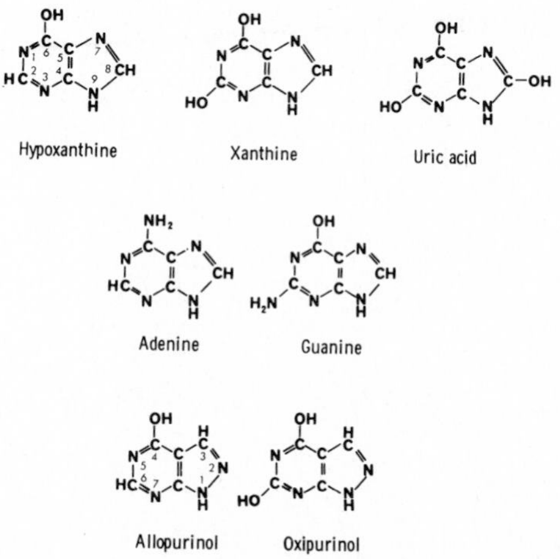

Hypoxanthine Xanthine Uric acid

Adenine Guanine

Allopurinol Oxipurinol

Scheme 21.1. The structural formulae of hypoxanthine, xanthine, uric acid, adenine, guanine, allopurinol (4-hydroxypyrazolo(3,4-d)pyrimidine) and oxipurinol (4,6-dihydroxypyrazolo(3,4-d)pyrimidine). The structures are all shown in the fully lactim (enol) form, although the relative proportions of the lactam (oxo) and lactim forms depend upon the conditions under which the compounds are studied. Allopurinol and oxipurinol are structural isomers of hypoxanthine and xanthine respectively. The numbering of the individual atoms of the heterocyclic ring systems is shown.

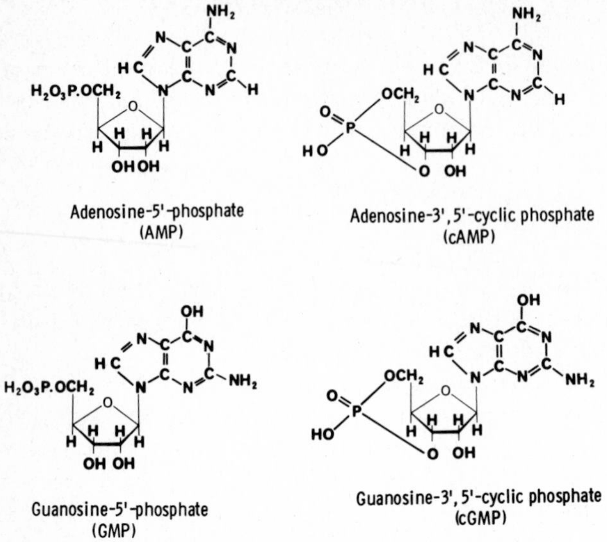

Adenosine-5'-phosphate (AMP)

Adenosine-3',5'-cyclic phosphate (cAMP)

Guanosine-5'-phosphate (GMP)

Guanosine-3',5'-cyclic phosphate (cGMP)

Scheme 21.2. The structural formulae of adenylic acid (adenosine-5′-phosphate, AMP), guanylic acid (guanosine-5′-phosphate, GMP), adenosine-3′,5′-cyclic phosphate (3′,5′-cyclic AMP, cAMP) and guanosine-3′,5′-cyclic phosphate (3′,5′-cyclic GMP, cGMP).

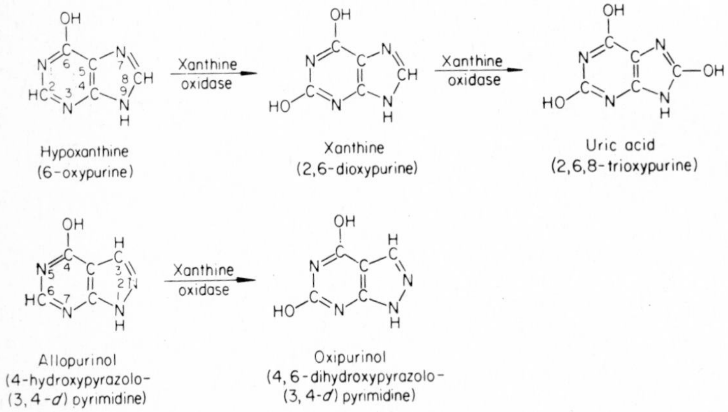

Hypoxanthine (6-oxypurine) → Xanthine oxidase → Xanthine (2,6-dioxypurine) → Xanthine oxidase → Uric acid (2,6,8-trioxypurine)

Allopurinol (4-hydroxypyrazolo-(3,4-*d*) pyrimidine) → Xanthine oxidase → Oxipurinol (4,6-dihydroxypyrazolo-(3,4-*d*) pyrimidine)

Scheme 21.3. The oxidation of purines and pyrazolo(3,4-d)pyrimidines catalyzed by xanthine oxidase (EC 1.2.3.2).

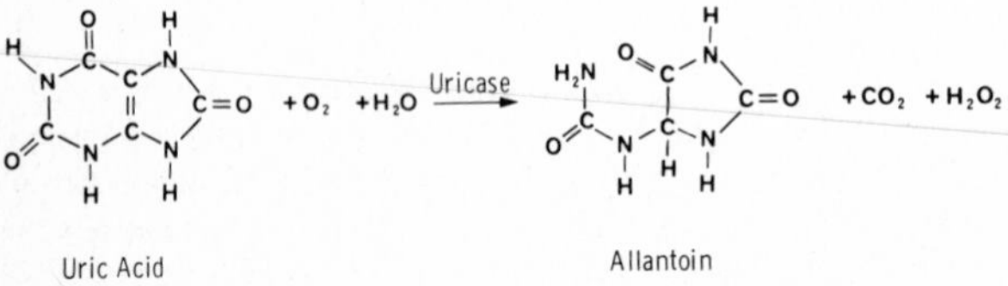

Uric Acid $+ O_2 + H_2O$ → Uricase → Allantoin $+ CO_2 + H_2O_2$

Scheme 21.4. The oxidation of uric acid catalyzed by uricase (EC 1.7.3.3).

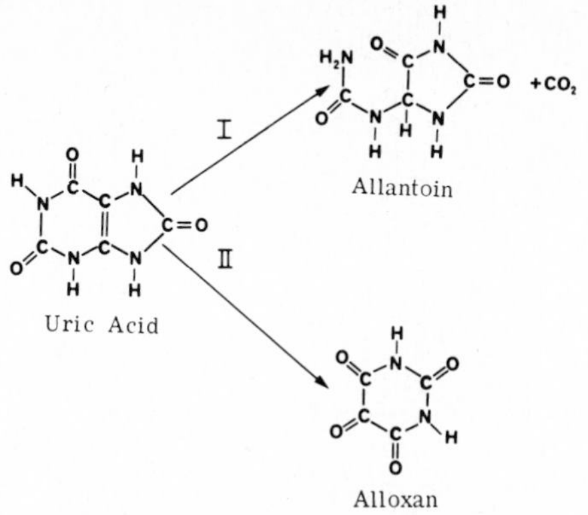

Scheme 21.5. The chemical oxidation of uric acid under neutral or alkaline conditions (I) and acidic conditions (II).

give allantoin, liberating carbon atom 6 as carbon dioxide and generating hydrogen peroxide (Scheme 21.4). The chemical oxidation of uric acid yields allantoin under alkaline or neutral conditions, and alloxan at acid pH values (Scheme 21.5). The qualitative murexide test for uric acid, which is also given by some other purines, depends upon oxidation with nitric acid to alloxantin (Scheme 21.6).

The limited solubilities of uric acid and monosodium urate underlie their pathophysiological significance. The hydrogen atoms at positions 3 and 9 are weakly ionized, with pK_a values of 10.3 and 5.75 respectively; the hydrogen atoms at positions 1 and 7 do not ionize significantly, so that the molecule largely exists as the monovalent urate ion at pH 7.4. It has been calculated that the solubility of sodium urate in serum should be about 0.39 mmol/litre (6.49 mg/dl); direct measurements have found it to be about 0.42 mmol/litre (7.0 mg/dl), and this agrees with the observation that deposits of sodium urate monohydrate in the tissues (tophi) only disappear if the serum uric acid concentration is kept below this level. Plasma or serum readily form stable supersaturated solutions of sodium urate, and this presumably explains the very high serum uric acid concentrations (up to 6 mmol/litre (100 mg/dl)), which are sometimes observed during cytotoxic drug therapy. Although tophi occur in the renal parenchyma, urinary stones are composed mainly of uric acid because they are formed in the urine, which is predominantly acidic. The solubilities of uric acid, xanthine and hypoxanthine in serum and in urine are compared in Table 21.1.

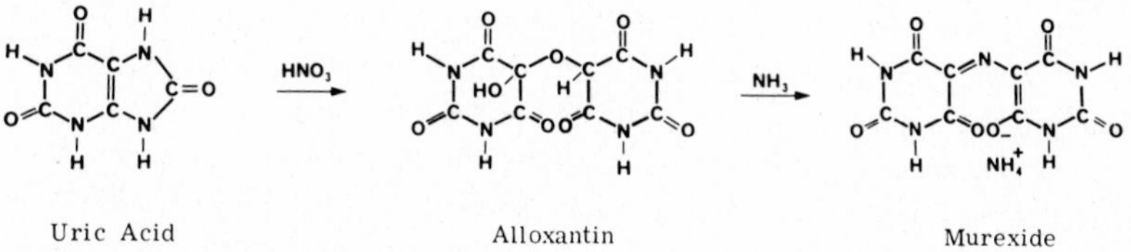

Scheme 21.6. The murexide reaction.

TABLE 21.1.
THE SOLUBILITIES OF URIC ACID, XANTHINE AND HYPOXANTHINE
(Data from Klinenberg et al., 1965)

Fluid	pH	Solubility (mg/dl)		
		Uric acid	Xanthine	Hypoxanthine
Serum	7.4	7	10	115
Urine	5	15	5	140
Urine	7	200	13	150

21.1.2. Purine biosynthesis de novo

Purines are derived either from the diet, or synthesized de novo, mainly in the liver, as shown in Scheme 21.7 and as discussed below. The biosynthetic sources of the individual atoms of the purine ring are shown in Scheme 21.8.

The intracellular concentration of α-5-phospho-D-ribosyl-1-pyrophosphate ("phosphoribosylpyrophosphate", PRPP) is important in regulating the rate of purine synthesis de novo. The synthesis of PRPP is catalyzed by ribosephosphate pyrophosphokinase (PRPP synthetase, EC 2.7.6.1). Kinetic studies have shown that the ribose-5-phosphate binds first to the enzyme, followed by binding of Mg^{2+}-ATP and release of AMP, and finally release of PRPP. Ribose-5-phosphate is formed by the oxidation of glucose via the 6-phosphogluconate shunt pathway. Human PRPP synthetase shows reversible association and dissociation. The molecular mass of the smallest native form of the enzyme is 60,000, and this is composed of two equal subunits. The enzyme associates into two heavy forms, molecular masses about 1.2×10^6 and 7.2×10^6, in the presence of ATP and Mg^{2+}. Ribose-5-phosphate does not alter the aggregation of the enzyme. The aggregated form appears to be the active and most stable form of the enzyme, the activity of which is regulated by: ADP, which inhibits competitively with respect to ATP; inhibition by 2,3-diphosphoglycerate (2,3-DPG) and PRPP; non-competitive inhibition by other nucleotides (Fox and Kelley, 1974; Kelley and Wyngaarden, 1974).

Evidence that the intracellular concentration of PRPP modulates the rate of purine synthesis de novo is provided by the results of in vitro studies of cultured human fibroblasts. Thus, orotic and nicotinic acids combine with PRPP under the influence of specific phosphoribosyltransferases. This lowers the intracellular concentration of PRPP and is associated with reduced purine biosynthesis de novo. Conversely, increasing the concentration of PRPP in cultured fibroblasts by adding methylene blue increases the rate of purine synthesis de novo. Methylene blue oxidizes NADPH to $NADP^+$, thereby increasing glucose oxidation and the supply of ribose-5-phosphate. Glucose, fructose and mannose increase the de novo synthesis of purines, and the acute administration of these sugars or of xylitol produces hyperuricaemia and hyperuric aciduria in man. Several different mechanisms may be involved, including rapid degradation of adenine nucleotides.

The formation of β-phosphoribosylamine from PRPP and glutamine is the first reac-

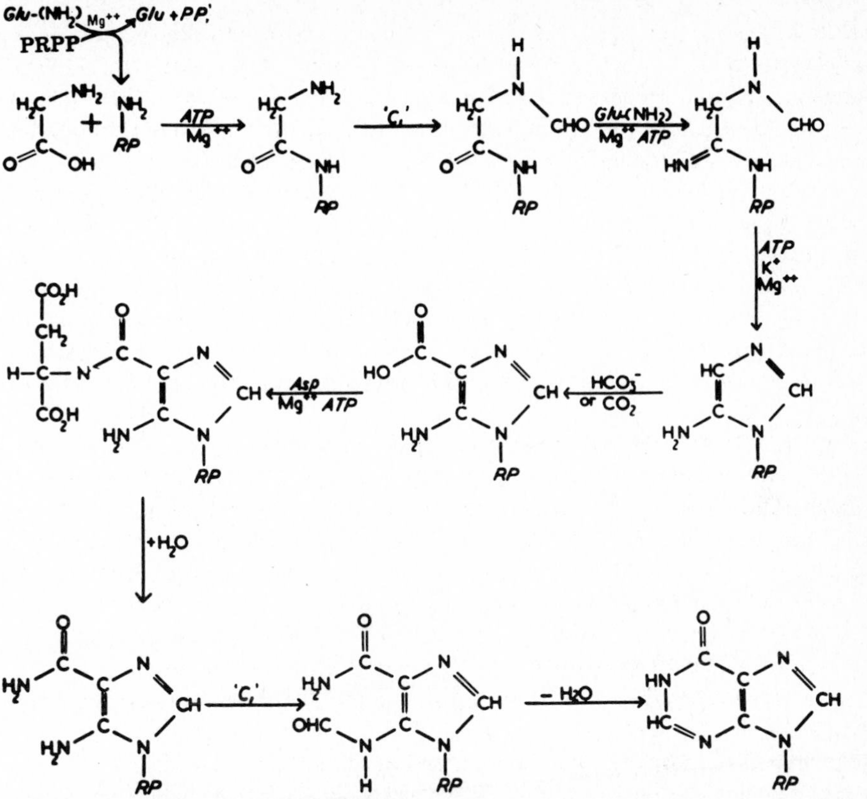

Scheme 21.7. The biosynthesis of inosinic acid. The reaction catalyzed by amidophosphoribosyltransferase (PRPP-amidotransferase, EC 2.4.2.14), which is the first specific reaction of the biosynthetic pathway, is shown in the top left of the diagram. Glu(NH_2) = glutamine; $NH_2 \cdot RP$ = β-phosphoribosylamine (PRA); Glu = glutamate; PPi = inorganic pyrophosphate; Asp = aspartate; "C_1" = the active one carbon fragment designated formyl (Reproduced, by permission, from Watts, 1966 and 1972, with minor modifications).

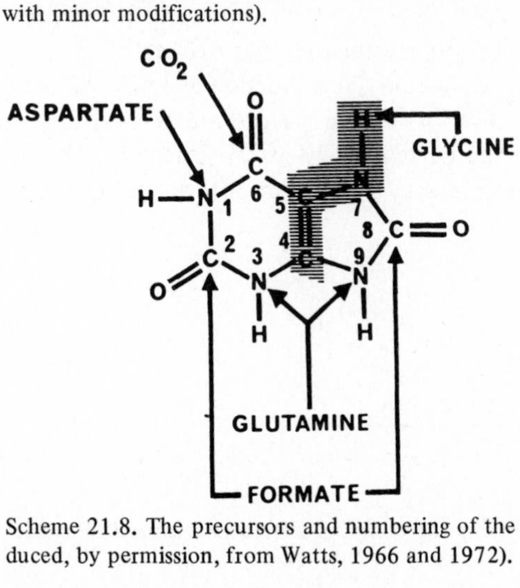

Scheme 21.8. The precursors and numbering of the individual atoms of the uric acid molecule (Reproduced, by permission, from Watts, 1966 and 1972).

tion which is specific for purine biosynthesis. This reaction is the rate-limiting step on the metabolic pathway and is catalyzed by amidophosphoribosyltransferase (EC 2.4.2.14, PRPP-amidotransferase). Holmes et al. (1973c) gathered evidence which indicates that the catalytic activity of this enzyme is modulated by PRPP and by the purine-5′-ribonucleotides which are the end products of the biosynthetic sequence: these factors alter the subunit structure of PRPP-amidotransferase (Figure 21.1). Purine ribonucleotides promote aggregation of the enzyme into a dimeric form (molecular mass 270,000) which is catalytically inactive, with PRPP converting it into the catalytically active monomeric form (molecular mass 133,000). Wood and Seegmiller (1973) studied the PRPP-amidotransferase activity of human lymphoblasts and reported that PRPP and purine ribonucleotides compete with one another for binding to the enzyme. Kelley and Wyngaarden (1974) have reviewed the properties of PRPP-synthetase preparations from different sources.

Reem (1972, 1974) studied the early steps of purine synthesis in some human tissues and reported that ammonia can replace glutamine in the PRPP-amidotransferase reaction and that phosphoribosylamine can be synthesized directly from ribose-5-phosphate and ammonia. The latter reaction is catalyzed by an enzyme which can be separated from PRPP-amidotransferase. These results suggest that the regulation of purine synthesis may be more complex than was formerly thought, depending upon two alternative pathways which can share a common substrate, ammonia, rather than on the single rate-limiting reaction of glutamine with PRPP. It is also noteworthy that ribose-5-phosphate is one of the substrates for PRPP synthetase, so increasing the possibility for the interplay of control mechanisms.

In the synthesis of inosine-5′-phosphate (inosinic acid, IMP), as shown in Scheme 21.7, the linking of β-phosphoribosylamine to glycine yields ribosylglycineamide-5′-phosphate, the glycineamide portion of which becomes carbon atoms 4, 5, 7 and 9 of the purine ring, with the sugar phosphate moeity already in its final position. This reaction is catalysed by phosphoribosylglycineamide synthetase (EC 6.3.4.13) and requires ATP and Mg^{2+}. Transformylation from N^5,N^{10}-anhydroformyltetrahydrofolate yields 5′-phosphoribosylformylglycinamide (FGAR). Addition of a nitrogen atom from L-glutamine, at the carbonyl group under the influence of phosphoribosylformylglycinamide synthetase (EC 6.3.5.3) and ATP yields 5′-phosphoribosylformylglycinamidine. This reaction is 100-fold more sensitive to inhibition by azaserine than is the PRPP-amidotransferase reaction. Thus, purine synthesis in intact cells can be interrupted selectively at this stage by azaserine treatment, and the incorporation of $[^{14}C]$glycine or $[^{14}C]$formate into the accumulated

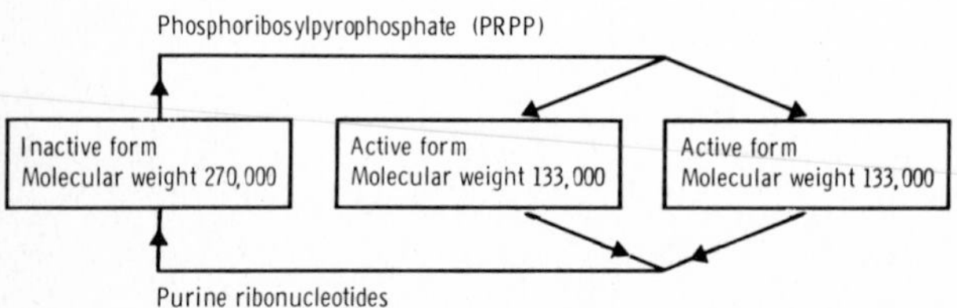

Figure 21.1. Mechanism proposed for the regulation of amidophosphoribosyltransferase (PRPP-amidotransferase, EC 2.4.2.14) (Holmes et al., 1973c).

FGAR may be used as an index of the overall activity of the earliest steps of purine synthesis de novo (Henderson, 1962; Seegmiller et al., 1967). This technique has been used because specific assays for PRPP-amidotransferase, which catalyzes the rate-limiting step of the metabolic pathway, have only recently been developed.

Ring closure of FGAR in the presence of ATP yields 5′-phosphoribosyl-5-aminoimidazole (AIR). The carboxyl group at position 4 is added by a biotin-dependent carbon dioxide fixation reaction, and condensation with aspartate provides the N_1 of the purine ring. Hydrolytic cleavage yields 5′-phosphoribosyl-5-amino-4-imidazole carboxamide (AICAR). Transformylation from N^{10}-formyltetrahydrofolate and cyclodehydration completes the biosynthesis of inosinic acid (Scheme 21.7).

4-Amino-5-imidazole carboxamide (AIC) has been isolated from sulphonamide-inhibited cultures of *Escherichia coli*. This compound is converted directly into its ribonucleotide (AICAR) by hypoxanthine guanine phosphoribosyltransferase (EC 2.4.2.8, HGPRT) and it can therefore enter the purine biosynthetic sequence directly at a late stage. It has been used extensively in studies of purine synthesis in man (Seegmiller et al., 1955).

21.1.3. Purine salvage pathways

The free purine bases, adenine, guanine and hypoxanthine, from either dietary or endogenous origin, are converted into the corresponding purine-5′-ribosemonophosphate by purine phosphoribosyltransferase (pyrophosphorylase) enzymes; these are the so-called purine salvage pathways. Adenine phosphoribosyltransferase (EC 2.4.2.7, APRT) catalyzes the formation of adenosine-5′-phosphate (AMP) from adenine and PRPP. Hypoxanthine phosphoribosyltransferase (EC 2.4.2.8, HGPRT) catalyzes the formation of guanosine-5′-phosphate (GMP) and inosine-5′-phosphate (IMP) from guanine and hypoxanthine respectively. HGPRT also converts xanthine into xanthosine-5′-phosphate (XMP), although this reaction occurs more slowly than the corresponding reactions with guanine or hypoxanthine. The substrate specificity of HGPRT includes AIC and the drugs 6-mercaptopurine, azathioprine, 8-azaguanine, 6-thioguanine and allopurinol. Other phosphoribosyltransferases catalyze the reaction of PRPP with orotic acid, uracil, nicotinamide and nicotinic acid.

HGPRT as a homogenous purified enzyme has a molecular mass of 68,000 with two subunits (34,000); its enzymology was reviewed by Kelley and Wyngaarden (1974).

The purine salvage pathways are particularly important in tissues which have a large requirement for purines but low activity with respect to purine biosynthesis de novo. Bone marrow and brain are in this category, whereas liver has high activity for both purine synthesis de novo and purine salvage. The quantitative significance of muscle as a source of purines during exercise is unknown. AMP-deaminase (EC 3.5.4.6) catalyzes the deamination of AMP to IMP during anaerobic muscle contraction, and although reamination occurs via adenylosuccinate, some of the IMP is converted into inosine and hypoxanthine. Muscular work is associated with increased hypoxanthine and xanthine excretion, and although uric acid excretion decreases during severe exertion, there is a net increase in uric acid excretion during the 48 to 72 hour period after the beginning of a bout of vigorous exercise.

Erythrocytes have high purine phosphoribosyltransferase activities, and this may be related to their function in the transport of purines in the blood; this subject is discussed in section 21.1.5. The overall biological significance of the purine salvage pathways has been well reviewed by Murray (1971).

21.1.4. Purine ribonucleotide interconversion reactions and the production of uric acid

IMP is converted into GMP and AMP by the reactions which are shown in Scheme 21.9 together with the purine salvage pathways and the steps which lead to uric acid.

The formation of AMP involves condensation of IMP with aspartate to form adenylosuccinate, which is then cleaved to AMP and fumarate. GMP is formed from IMP via xanthosine-5′-phosphate (XMP), and amination of XMP to GMP requires ATP and glutamine as a source of amino groups.

The activity of IMP dehydrogenase (EC 1.2.1.14) is regulated by the end products of purine biosynthesis, and it may be another point on the purine biosynthetic pathway at which some drugs (e.g. allopurinol and 6-mercaptopurine) and their metabolic products exert their pharmacological effects.

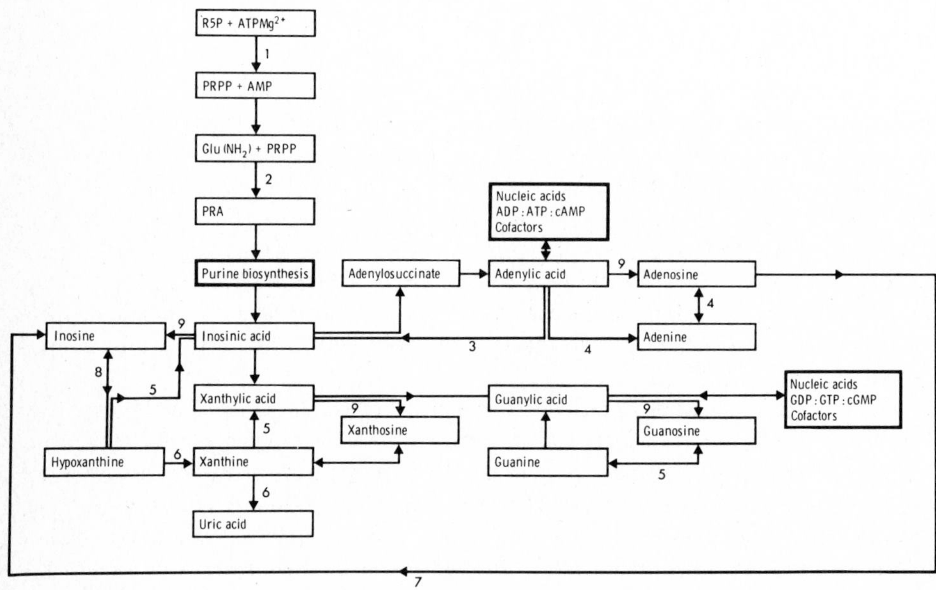

Scheme 21.9. The purine ribonucleotide interconversion reactions. R5P = ribose-5-phosphate; PRPP = phosphoribosylpyrophosphate; PRA = β-phosphoribosylamine; 1 = ribosephosphate pyrophosphokinase (PRPP synthetase, EC 2.7.6.1); 2 = amidophosphoribosyltransferase (PRPP amidotransferase, EC 2.4.2.14); 3 = adenylic acid deaminase (EC 3.5.4.6); 4 = adenine phosphoribosyltransferase (APRT, EC 2.4.2.7); 5 = hypoxanthine phosphoribosyltransferase (HGPRT, EC 2.4.2.8); 6 = xanthine oxidase (EC 1.2.3.2); 7 = adenosine deaminase (EC, 3.5.4.4); 8 = purine nucleoside phosphorylase (EC 2.4.2.1); 9 = 5′-nucleotidase (EC 3.1.3.5).

The free purines which are formed by the actions of 5′-nucleotidase (EC 3.1.3.5) and purine nucleoside phosphorylase (EC 2.4.2.1) are either salvaged as described above or converted into uric acid. Guanine deaminase (EC 3.5.4.3) catalyzes the conversion of guanine into xanthine, but human tissues lack adenine deaminase (EC 3.5.4.2) which converts adenine into hypoxanthine.

Xanthine oxidase (EC 1.2.3.2) occurs mainly in human milk, liver and small intestinal mucosa, and its activity in other tissues is very low. It catalyzes the oxidation of hypoxanthine to xanthine, and xanthine to uric acid; this two-step reaction involves the release of xanthine and re-binding of this, as a second substrate, to a possibly different active site. The enzyme has a wide substrate specificity which includes aldehydes, pteridines, other purines such as adenine (which is oxidized to 2,8-dioxyadenine) and purine analogues such as 6-mercaptopurine. It is usually regarded as an oxygenase using molecular oxygen as the terminal electron acceptor; this reflects a conformational change from a dehydrogenase using NAD^+ as the terminal electron acceptor. The relative activity of the enzyme as a dehydrogenase or oxygenase varies between species, and storage at –20°C or treatment with thiol binding reagents causes the liver enzyme to change from one form to the other. The mechanism of action of the enzyme has been extensively studied by Bray and his colleagues (Bray, 1975).

21.1.5. Purine transport

Biosynthesis de novo can meet all the body's purine needs, so that salvage of dietary purine is not necessary to achieve overall purine balance. Conversely, purine salvage is of vital significance in individual tissues, which have a high purine requirement and little or no capacity for purine synthesis de novo, as is shown by the brain damage and bone marrow dysfunction associated with gross HGPRT deficiency of the Lesch–Nyhan syndrome (section 21.6). Since purine synthesis de novo occurs mainly in the liver, purines have to be transported to their sites of utilization. Plasma contains only low concentrations of hypoxanthine and xanthine (less than about 10 mmol/litre) with no guanine and no nucleotides or nucleosides, but it has been shown experimentally that purines are continually leaving the liver, entering the nucleotide pools of erythrocytes and passing from there to extrahepatic tissues.

Purines are synthesized as their 5′-nucleotides which do not normally cross cell boundaries, but have powerful pharmacological effects if they do gain access to the extracellular fluid compartments. The liver cell nucleotides which are destined for other organs are converted into nucleosides by the 5′-nucleotidase on the plasma membrane of the liver cell. Human erythrocytes contain transport systems for both purine nucleosides and free purine bases, and it is uncertain if the conversion of nucleoside into purine base by the purine nucleoside phosphorylase occurs before or after the purine enters the erythrocyte, where its reconversion into a 5′-nucleotide is catalyzed by the appropriate phosphoribosyltransferase. The same overall reaction occurs in reverse in the tissues to which the purines are transported. Human blood has guanase but no xanthine oxidase activity, and guanine is thought to be the main physiological substrate for HGPRT. This suggestion, which is based on the results of in vitro enzyme assays performed with saturating substrate concentrations, ignores the possible effects on the overall pattern of purine metabolism in erythrocytes, of physiological activators and inhibitors, of substrate concentration, and the relative affinities of guanine deaminase and of HGPRT for guanine.

Human tissues lack adenase, so that the direct conversion of adenine into AMP, which is catalyzed by APRT, may be more important in man from the viewpoint of purine salvage than in some other species.

The turnover of nucleotides by erythrocytes is wholly due to the uptake and release of purine bases or purine nucleosides, because these cells do not contain the enzymes which are needed for purine synthesis de novo. The turnover times of the individual nucleotides are appreciably different from one another, being 9 days for the adenine nucleotides, 1 hour for IMP and 7 hours for GMP. The pool sizes are 1.3, 0.05 and 0.03 μmol/ml of erythrocytes for the adenine nucleotides, inosinic acid and guanylic acid respectively. Assuming a total erythrocyte volume of 2350 ml (based on a total body weight of 70 kg, haematocrit of 45%, and total blood volume of 75 ml/kg) the total nucleotide turnover has been calculated to be 3300 μmol/24 hours; this is equivalent to 1.28 grams of nucleotide or 450 mg of purine base per 24 hours and corresponds to 6 mg of purine base per 24 hours per kg body weight (Murray, 1971). The ATP content of erythrocytes decreases as the cells age; it has been shown that this phenomenon, and the replacement of labelled cells by new cells containing unlabelled ATP, does not account for the apparent turnover of adenine nucleotides.

21.1.6. Uricolysis

The birds, higher apes and man lack uricase. However in man, about 25% of the uric acid which is synthesized de novo is disposed of by mechanisms other than renal excretion. These are collectively termed uricolysis and are mainly due to bacterial degradation of uric acid in the intestinal tract. This increases in hyperuricaemia. A small proportion of in vivo uricolysis in man is attributed to the actions of peroxidase (EC 1.11.1.7) and cytochrome oxidase (EC 1.9.3.1). Polymorphonuclear leucocytes ingest and destroy urate crystals, by virtue of their peroxidase activity. The infusion of highly purified uricase reduces the plasma uric acid concentration in man, but antibody formation rapidly diminishes the effect, so that it is of no therapeutic benefit.

21.1.7. Renal handling of uric acid

The renal handling of urate in man was reviewed by Milne (1966) and by Steele (1971), and in non-human primates by Fanelli and Beyer (1974). The overall renal clearance of urate varies between about 5 and 10% of the simultaneously measured glomerular filtration rate, ignoring any possible effect of plasma binding. This value is attained by the age of 6 months, the urate clearance being 35% of the glomerular filtration rate during the first week of life. Although this difference between the neonate and older infant is clear cut, its magnitude should be viewed with reservation because the overall clearance of creatinine was used to measure the glomerular filtration rate; the renal handling of creatinine may change, at least quantitatively, during the period of rapid postnatal renal maturation.

The finite, but low, renal clearance of urate was initially ascribed to incomplete renal tubule reabsorption of uric acid. Increasing the filtered load of urate appeared to increase urate re-absorption until a maximum value (re-absorption T_m) was reached. The classical studies of Gutman et al. (1959), in which a net secretion of urate was produced experimentally in patients with mild chronic renal disease by a combination of urate infusion, osmotic diuresis and uricosuric drug administration, showed that the flux across the renal tubule epithelium was bidirectional. Consideration of a hypouricaemic patient whose uric acid excretion rate was more than 40% greater than the filtered load of uric acid, indicated that the renal tubules could excrete uric acid in man (Praetorius and Kirk, 1950). The more recently developed micropuncture and microdissection techniques have yielded data which are compatible with the operation of a carrier-mediated mechanism for urate reabsorption, which is probably located at the luminal border of the proximal tubule epithelium in the rat. No definitive evidence for urate secretion was obtained by these techniques. This negative finding is less significant than the positive one because small influxes into the medullary portion of the nephron may be masked by slow medullary circulation and by concomitant diffusion (Kramp et al., 1971).

Pyrazinamide and pyrazinoic acid inhibit urate excretion markedly, and stop-flow studies in the dog have shown that the former drug abolished uric acid excretion in part of the nephron. The decrement in uric acid excretion after pyrazinamide administration has been regarded as a measure of the secretion of urate (TS_{Ur}) by the renal tubules in man, but the relationship (Steele, 1971) between plasma urate concentration and TS_{Ur} was non-linear, as shown in Figure 21.2. Investigations with pyrazinamide have shown that secretion accounts for at least 80% of the urinary uric acid, whereas 98% of the filtered urate load is reabsorbed.

Studies with pyrazinamide have been very helpful in relation to human renal physiology, but the results must be interpreted cautiously in the light of more critical evaluations in experimental animals. Thus, because of the bidirectional flux of uric acid across the renal tubule epithelium, it is difficult to prove conclusively that pyrazinamide com-

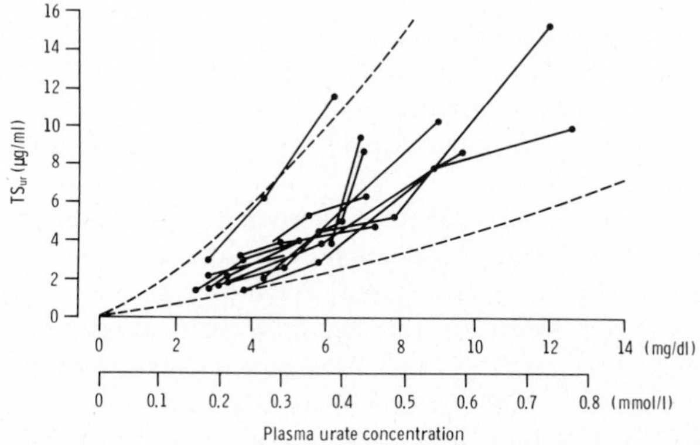

Figure 21.2. Tubular secretion of urate (TS_{ur}), as a function of the plasma urate concentration in normal adults. The dotted lines enclose the 95% prediction confidence limits of TS_{ur}. (Reproduced, by permission, from Steele, 1971).

pletely inhibits urate secretion; some studies in the Cebus monkey, chimpanzee and dog suggest that it also has some effect on urate re-absorption.

It has been generally accepted that the virtually complete re-absorption of filtered urate occurs in the proximal part of the nephron, and that excreted uric acid has been secreted into the distal portion of the nephron. Recent studies suggest that uric acid whch has been secreted by the tubule epithelum may be subsequently re-absorbed. Thus, re-absorptive processes may also occur in the lower nephron, distal to the site of the secretory process, or there may be some bidirectional flux across the same region of the renal tubule. There is a wide gap in our knowledge between what can be deduced from physiological studies in whole animals and in man, even with the help of micro-dissection techniques and stop-flow studies in animals, and with an understanding of events at the molecular level. It is tacitly assumed that the re-absorptive and secretory processes are subserved by discrete carrier mechanisms, but it is possible that the same protein undergoes a conformational change to convert it from a reabsorption into a secretion carrier.

21.1.8. Diet

The dietary purines are almost all in the form of nucleoproteins which are degraded by proteolytic enzymes; the liberated nucleotides are then susceptible to attack by a series of nucleases and phosphodiesterases which are secreted by the pancreas. The nucleotides are converted into nucleosides by various nucleotidases and phosphatases, and may be absorbed as such or converted into free bases by nucleoside phosphorylase. The high guanase and xanthine oxidase activities of the small intestinal mucosa suggest that free guanine, derived from breakdown of nucleoprotein, may be converted into uric acid during the process of absorption. Unabsorbed nucleoprotein will be metabolized by intestinal bacteria with complete degradation of the purine ring. Early experiments with ^{15}N-labelled yeast nucleic acid showed that dietary purines are largely converted directly into uric acid, only a minority being utilized for nucleic acid synthesis.

The total purine content of the diet influences the concentration of uric acid in plasma and in urine. Seegmiller et al. (1961) found that after 7 days on an essentially purine-free diet, groups of normal subjects and patients with gout both showed falls in their serum urate concentrations. The effect on the urinary excretion of uric acid of changing from a Western European or North American diet to a purine-free diet led to a fall in excretion from about 800 to about 600 mg per 24 hours.

The purine content of foods is not necessarily accurately known, so that the construction of low-purine diets is an unreliable procedure. Furthermore, the calculation of purine nitrogen content in relation to unit energy value, as opposed to unit weight, shows that some foods which are traditionally regarded as low purine items can contribute as much dietary purine as meats on an isocaloric basis (Table 21.2). When patients who are taking a purine-free diet ingest graded amounts of AMP, GMP, RNA or DNA, the plasma and urinary uric acid concentrations increase linearly with respect to the amount of purine ingested. Almost all of the purine nitrogen which is administered as AMP and GMP can be accounted for as urinary uric acid, whereas the increase in the excretion of urinary uric acid only accounts for about 25% of the ingested DNA and 50% of the RNA. The rate of

TABLE 21.2.

AVERAGE PURINE NITROGEN CONTENT OF SOME FOODS AND ITS RELATIONSHIP TO ENERGY VALUE

(Data derived from Zöllner and Griebsch, 1974)

	Purine nitrogen (mg/g)	kcalories (per gram)	Purine nitrogen (mg/kcalorie)
Steak (raw)	0.58	1.8	0.33
Chicken (boiled)	0.61	2.0	0.30
Cauliflower (raw)	0.13	0.25	0.52
Cabbage (raw)	0.08	0.25	0.32
Green peas (raw)	0.72	0.64	1.1
Spinach (raw)	0.70	0.24	2.9

hydrolysis of dietary polynucleotides in the intestinal tract appears to be the factor which limits the absorption of dietary purines.

The well documented decrease in the incidence of gout in parts of Europe during and immediately after World War II points to the importance of dietary purine intake in precipitating this disorder in those who are predisposed to it. However, dietary restriction has little place in its practical management.

Proposed developments in the use of the so-called single cell proteins as foods, has stimulated interest in the possible complications of high purine diets. These potential new foodstuffs include yeasts, microfungi and bacteria, all of which contain larger amounts of purine relative to their total protein content than do conventional foods. Their use has been proposed in three contexts: as animal feeds, as food additives in Western countries, and as a major source of dietary protein in areas where there is protein malnutrition. RNA is the main source of purine in these materials, and the risk of producing an epidemic of gout and/or uric acid urolithiasis in the target populations has to be assessed. Bacteria grown in continuous culture may contain as much as 20% RNA on a dry weight basis, the corresponding figures for yeasts and filamentous fungi being 10% and 5% respectively. One gram of dietary RNA increases the urinary uric acid excretion by about 0.8 mmol (130 mg) per 24 hours and the plasma urate concentration by about 0.05 mmol/litre (0.9 mg/dl); the changes attributable to DNA are about half of these values. The amounts of the dietary supplements which are fed should not augment the total dietary purine intake so as to increase the plasma urate concentration and the urinary uric acid excretion above 0.48 mmol/litre (8.0 mg/dl) and 5.9 mmol (1000 mg) per 24 hours respectively. The minimum urine volume should be 1.5 litres per 24 hours. Levels greater than this would carry an unacceptably high risk of increasing the incidence of gout and/or uric acid urolithiasis. The prevalance of hyperuricaemia, gout and uric acid urolithiasis in the target population (see section 21.3.1) needs to be considered before such foodstuffs are generally introduced. The above limits are unlikely to be exceeded if only 2 grams of nucleic acid daily were added to adult human diets ($0.03\ g \cdot kg^{-1} \cdot day^{-1}$), which rarely contain more than this amount of nucleic acid. This corresponds to 10 grams of yeast protein or about 20 grams of algal protein. Although the nucleic acid contents of these products can be reduced by appropriate processing, the possibility of unexpected toxic or allergic reactions associated with other constituents of the microorganism, or derived from the raw materials on which they are grown, requires close attention with careful clinical trials in man. This subject is being kept under review by the WHO Protein Advisory Group (1975).

21.1.9. Pharmacology

Drugs which change the concentration of uric acid in the blood, or its rate of excretion in the urine, do so by altering the rate of uric acid production or by an action on the active transport of uric acid across the renal tubule epithelium. Uricosuric agents increase uric acid excretion by effects on renal tubule transport mechanisms. Drugs which reduce the rate of uric acid production do so by inhibiting xanthine oxidase, which catalyzes the last two reactions of the sequence which leads to uric acid, or by inhibiting one or more of the earlier steps on the pathway of purine biosynthesis de novo. Uric acid production is increased by drugs which accelerate purine biosynthesis de novo, and by cytotoxic drugs or irradiation which destroy tumour tissue, liberating nucleoprotein, the nucleic acid moiety of which is catabolized to uric acid.

21.1.9.1. Drugs which reduce uric acid synthesis

The glutamine antagonists 6-diazo-5-oxo-1-norleucine and azaserine inhibit all three enzymes on the purine biosynthetic pathway which catalyze the transfer of an amino group from the amide group of glutamine (Scheme 21.7). These compounds were introduced as carcinostatic agents; their ability to inhibit purine synthesis de novo was an incidental finding which is clearly demonstrable in gouty patients, but which cannot be exploited for the treatment of gout because of their toxicities. The use of azaserine to specifically block the fourth step on the purine biosynthetic pathway in cells grown in vitro, in order to measure the activity of the earlier steps on the pathway, is referred to in section 21.1.2. The development of more direct approaches to the measurement of the phosphoribosylamidotransferase activity of cells grown in culture, should reduce the need for this indirect approach.

Hadacidine (N-formyl-N-hydroxyglycine), and analogue of L-aspartate, inhibits adenylosuccinate synthetase which catalyzes the conversion of IMP into succinamino-AMP. It has been tried as a carcinostatic agent, but its toxicity contraindicates more general use.

PRPP-amidotransferase is subject to allosteric regulation and inhibition by PRPP and by purine ribonucleotides. Reducing the intracellular concentration of PRPP and increasing the concentration of purine ribonucleotides both promote the conversion of the dimeric into the monomeric form of the enzyme, with consequent reduction in its catalytic activity. It is also inhibited by purine ribonucleotides in a manner which is competitive with respect to PRPP (section 21.1.2).

Several carcinostatic drugs which are purine analogues are converted into ribonucleotides which also inhibit PRPP-amidotransferase. In most cases, their conversion into a ribonucleotide analogue is catalyzed by HGPRT. This reduces the intracellular concentration of PRPP, which diminishes the activity of PRPP-amidotransferase by the allosteric mechanism referred to above. The drugs which inhibit purine synthesis de novo in this way are: 6-mercaptopurine, 6-thioguanine, 8-azaguanine and azathioprine. The last of these is metabolized, at least in part, to 6-mercaptopurine and so it presumably exerts its action as 6-mercaptopurine ribonucleotide. Purine synthesis de novo is not reduced when these drugs are given to patients who are congenitally deficient in HGPRT.

Adenine, 5-amino-4-imidazole carboxamide, 2,6-diaminopurine, allopurinol and orotic acid also reduce de novo purine biosynthesis. They are all converted into the corresponding ribonucleotide, or ribonucleotide analogue, by a phosphoribosyltransferase reaction with consequent consumption of PRPP. Thus PRPP depletion, rather than – or as well as – direct feed-back and pseudofeed-back inhibition of phosphoribosylamidotransferase, would explain the effect of the drugs on purine synthesis de novo.

6-Methylmercaptopurine ribonucleoside, which also inhibits de novo purine synthesis, is converted into the active nucleotide form by adenosine kinase (EC 2.7.1.20). Unlike drugs such as azathioprine, it inhibits de novo purine synthesis in HGPRT deficient cell lines as effectively as in normal cells.

The introduction in 1963 of the xanthine oxidase inhibitor allopurinol (4-hydroxypyrazolo(3,4-d)pyrimidine) for the treatment of hyperuricaemic states in general, and of gout in particular, was a major therapeutic advance. The drug had been investigated in the course of work aimed at developing purine analogues for the treatment of malignant disease, and its powerful inhibitory action on xanthine oxidase, which potentiates the action of 6-mercaptopurine, was already well documented. The knowledge that xanthinuria (congenital xanthine oxidase deficiency) is a relatively benign condition and that the principal biochemical changes produced by allopurinol in man were similar to, but less marked than, those observed in the congenital enzyme deficiency state, encouraged long-term trials of the drug in the treatment of gout.

Allopurinol is a structural analogue of hypoxanthine (Scheme 21.1) and it is oxidized in vivo to oxipurinol (4,6-dihydroxypyrazolo(3,4-d)pyrimidine), which also inhibits xanthine oxidase. Some of the reported Michaelis constants and inhibition constants for human liver and bovine cream xanthine oxidase have been summarized by Wyngaarden and Kelley (1972). Aldehyde oxidase (EC 1.2.3.1) also catalyzes the oxidation of allopurinol.

The effect of allopurinol on the plasma urate concentration and urinary uric acid excretion becomes apparent over the course of a few days; it is maximal after 5 days of treatment, and there is no tendency for the effect to wear off with the passage of time. However, the uric acid levels return to their pretreatment values within 5 days of withdrawing the drug. The biological half-life of allopurinol is about 2 or 3 hours: a small proportion (3 to 10%) is excreted with a renal clearance approximately equal to the glomerular filtration rate; the major part (45 to 65%) is oxidized to oxipurinol, with a portion being converted into allopurinol-1-ribonucleotide, and allopurinol-1-ribonucleoside. Oxipurinol has a longer half life (about 28 hours) and is mainly excreted in the urine. Some is metabolized to oxipurinol-7-ribonucleotide and ribonucleoside and possibly to the 1-ribonucleotide. Early fears that allopurinol ribonucleotide might be incorporated into DNA or RNA have not been substantiated.

Inhibition of purine synthesis de novo is a pharmacological effect of allopurinol which is subsidiary to its main effect on xanthine oxidase activity. The present view is that the conversion of relatively large amounts of allopurinol into allopurinol ribonucleotide reduces the PRPP concentration within the cells, mainly hepatocytes, where purine biosynthesis occurs de novo. The intracellular concentration of PRPP is one of the main determinants of the conformational modification of PRPP-amidotransferase which regulates its activity at physiological substrate concentrations. Allopurinol ribonucleotide is also a pseudofeed-back inhibitor of the enzyme, and presumably replaces or reinforces the actions of its physiological ribonucleotide regulators (AMP and GMP).

The administration of allopurinol is associated with increased activity of erythrocyte orotate phosphoribosyltransferase (EC 2.4.2.10) and orotidine-5′-phosphate decarboxylase (EC 4.1.1.23) when measured in vitro; this is due to an activation or stabilization mechanism, rather than to increased enzyme synthesis or turnover of the enzyme protein. In spite of this, patients taking allopurinol excrete increased amounts of orotic acid and orotidine, and this has been attributed to an overall inhibition of orotidine-5′-phosphate decarboxylase in vivo (Kelley and Beardmore, 1970).

The possible wider biochemical significance of allopurinol is also indicated by the fact that it inhibits purine nucleoside phosphorylase and pyrimidine deoxyribosyltransferase in vitro, and at high concentrations it inhibits urate oxidase (EC 1.7.3.3).

Vessell et al. (1970) reported that allopurinol, like some other drugs, markedly prolonged the plasma half-lives of antipyrine and bishydroxycoumarin in man, and in rats, reduced the activity of drug-metabolizing enzymes, with slight lowering of the level of cytochrome P-450. In spite of these observations, interactions involving allopurinol do not appear to have been a problem in clinical practice, nor does the drug produce serious side-effects. Mild gastrointestinal irritation and erythematous pruritic rashes are sometimes seen; bone marrow depression has been reported but is extremely rare. Hypoxanthine, xanthine, and oxipurinol crystals were demonstrated in the skeletal muscle of patients being treated with allopurinol (Watts et al., 1971a), but there is no indication that its use has been associated with any clinical manifestations of muscle disease.

The formation of xanthine stones as a complication of allopurinol treatment has only been reported occasionally, and in association with the grossly increased rate of purine biosynthesis de novo which occurs in the Lesch–Nyhan syndrome (section 21.6). Unusually high doses of allopurinol may be associated with the precipitation of oxipurinol in the urinary tract. The biochemical effects (Table 21.3) which have been reported in allopurinol-treated patients need not limit its general clinical use. The observation that oxipurinol is excreted more slowly than allopurinol led to the suggestion that most of the therapeutic efficacy of allopurinol was in fact due to its oxidation product, and that the latter might be a better therapeutic agent. This was not borne out by a direct comparison (Chalmers et al., 1968), and may be due to the relatively poor absorption of oxipurinol.

A small daily dose (400 mg) of allopurinol completely abolishes the hyperuric aciduria which is normally associated with the ingestion of nucleic acids, whereas it only reduces endogenous uric acid production by about 45%. This suggests that the dietary and endogenous purine metabolic pools are largely discrete. Oxipurinol, which also inhibits xanthine oxidase, is less well absorbed than allopurinol and does not prevent diet-induced hyperuric aciduria. This has been held to suggest that uric acid production from dietary

TABLE 21.3.

SUMMARY OF THE BIOCHEMICAL EFFECTS OF ALLOPURINOL IN VIVO

(Reports based on animal studies suggesting that allopurinol might produce haemochromatosis have not been substantiated)

1. Decreased blood and urine concentrations of uric acid
2. Increased blood and urine concentrations of hypoxanthine and xanthine
3. Decreased intracellular (erythrocyte) phosphoribosyl pyrophosphate (PRPP)
4. Increased activity of erythrocyte orotate phosphoribosyltransferase (EC 2.4.2.10) and orotidine-5′-phosphate decarboxylase (EC 4.1.1.23)
5. Urinary excretion of 6,8-dihydroxypurine, orotidine and orotic acid
6. Reduced rate of purine biosynthesis de novo
7. Inhibition of tryptophan-2,3-dioxygenase
8. Minute aggregates of hypoxanthine, xanthine and oxipurinol in the muscle fibres of treated gout patients.

purines occurs in the liver rather than in the small intestinal mucosa.

Thiopurinol (4-mercaptopyrazolo(3,4-d)pyrimidine) was developed as a xanthine oxidase inhibitor, and it is an effective hypouricaemic agent in man. Although it only reduces the uric acid excretion in over-producers of uric acid, its administration is not associated with increased production of hypoxanthine or xanthine, indicating that its action is not mediated by xanthine oxidase inhibition. It is not effective in the absence of HGPRT and it has been suggested that it acts only by pseudofeed-back inhibition of purine synthesis de novo. It seems unlikely that thiopurinol will make a great impact on clinical practice.

21.1.9.2. Drugs which increase biosynthesis of uric acid

2-Ethylamino-1,3,4-thiadiazole, which was investigated as a carcinostatic agent, causes marked hyperuricaemia and hyperuric aciduria in man by stimulating purine synthesis de novo. as judged by its effect in enhancing the incorporation of isotopically labelled glycine into urinary uric acid. Its action does not depend on HGPRT because it further enhances the already high rate of purine biosynthesis in children who are congenitally deficient in this enzyme. The drug does not directly alter the enzymatic activity of the biosynthetic pathway or block the inhibition of PRPP-amidotransferase by adenine ribonucleotides. The stimulatory effect of 2-ethylamino-1,3,4-thiadiazole can be reversed in man by nicotinic acid or nicotinamide, and by 6-mercaptopurine or allopurinol, all of which reduce the rate of purine biosynthesis de novo by causing PRPP depletion.

Methylene blue increases the intracellular concentration of PRPP in human erythrocytes in vitro, and the rate of purine biosynthesis de novo in cultured human fibroblasts. This is attributed to accelerated regeneration of $NADP^+$ which increases the activity of the oxidative pathway of glucose metabolism with increased ribose-5-phosphate production; this in turn increases the activity of PRPP synthetase.

Glucose, fructose and mannose also stimulate PRPP synthesis in vitro, and the administration of these sugars, or of xylitol, causes hyperuricaemia and hyperuric aciduria in man and in animals. The effect of fructose on uric acid production has been the most thoroughly studied of these effects in vivo, and it has not been possible to demonstrate the expected changes in erythrocyte PRPP and ribose-5-phosphate levels. This method of sampling the intracellular environment may not necessarily always be valid in studies of purine metabolism, because purine biosynthesis occurs largely in the hepatocyte, and not at all in the erythrocyte.

The mechanism of fructose-induced hyperuricaemia appears to be mainly due to increased degradation of adenine nucleotides (Fox and Kelley, 1972).

Animals which do not normally excrete uric acid because their tissues contain urate oxidase (EC 1.7.3.3) can be made to do so by administering oxonic acid, which inhibits this enzyme.

21.1.9.3. Drugs which increase the renal excretion of uric acid (uricosuric agents)

Kippen et al. (1974) reviewed the pharmacology of the uricosuric drugs and emphasized the possibility that decreased binding of urate by protein in the presence of some uricosuric compounds would augment urate clearance by increasing the filtered urate load. Probenecid, sulfinpyrazone and salicylates have been shown to displace urate from plasma binding sites in equilibrium dialysis experiments in vitro, but there is no direct evidence of similar effects in vivo.

Such drugs may promote either urate excretion or urate retention, depending on the dosage; small doses tend to promote urate retention and large doses to be uricosuric. This dual activity argues against an effect on the protein binding of urate as a major determinant of uricosuric potency. The classification of the drugs which modify uric acid excretion into urate-retaining and uricosuric groups, refers to their pharmacological actions when given in the conventional therapeutic doses.

Probenecid, sulfinpyrazone and large doses of aspirin (more than 4 grams daily) are the most commonly used uricosuric agents; inadequate doses cause urate retention. Phenylbutazone, cortisone and related compounds, and adrenocorticotrophic hormone are also midly uricosuric, and tend to be used in situations where their effects on the serum and urinary uric acid levels may cause diagnostic errors.

The radiocontrast agents such as iopanoic acid and calcium ipodate are powerful uricosuric agents in the doses used in radiological practice, and cause increased uric acid excretion for 5 or 6 days after the test; the uricosuric effects of meglumine iodipamide and sodium diatrizoate are more evanescent. The effects of these powerful uricosuric agents on urine and serum uric acid concentrations should be considered in interpreting the results of uric acid analyses.

Table 21.4 lists other known uricosuric compounds. In addition, substances such as chlorprothixene and the degradation compound 5α,6-anhydro-4-epi-tetracycline, which is formed on prolonged storage of tetracycline, produce proximal renal tubule damage not confined to urate transport. Net increase in renal uric acid clearance could be due to reduced renal tubule re-absorption or to augmented renal tubule excretion of uric acid. It has been suggested, on the basis of the pyrazinamide suppression test, that benziodarone, azopropazone and the radiocontrast agents stimulate renal tubule secretion of uric acid specifically. However, pyrazinamide may enhance renal tubule re-absorption as well as block renal tubule secretion. Thus, it is premature to attempt a rigid classification of

TABLE 21.4.

URICOSURIC SUBSTANCES

This classification of a drug as a uricosuric agent refers to its action when the usual therapeutic dose is given

---

Acetohexamide
6-Azauridine
Azopropazone
Benziodarone
Benzbromarone
Carinamide
Chlorproxithene
Cinchophen
Dicoumarol
Ethylbiscoumacetate
Ethyl-p-chlorophenoxylbutyric acid
Glycine
Halofenate
Meclofenamic acid
p-Nitrophenylbutazone
Orotic acid
Phenylendandione
Phenylbutazone
Probenecid
Phloridzin
Radiocontrast agents:
  iopanoic acid
  meglumine iodipamide
  calcium ipidate
  sodium diatrizoate
Salicylates (doses of more than 4 grams per 24 hours)
Sulfinpyrazone
Zoxazolamine

---

uricosuric drugs into those which block renal tubule re-absorption and those which enhance renal tubule secretion. If, as suggested in section 21.1.7, a carrier protein undergoes a conformational change to convert it from a re-absorption to a secretion carrier, the pharmacological action of uricosuric drugs could depend on their ability to induce such a change.

21.1.9.4. Drugs which decrease the renal excretion of uric acid

Urate retention, which may be sufficient to precipitate an attack of acute gouty arthritis in a patient with otherwise asymptomatic essential hyperuricaemia, is a side-effect of medication with all types of diuretic drugs, and with the salicylates and the antituberculous agents ethambutol and pyrazinamide. Inadequate dosage with uricosuric agents may also exacerbate the hyperuricaemia for which the drug is being given. These effects are usually ascribed to inhibition of urate secretion by the renal tubules, although renal tubule re-absorption may also be affected. Metabolic acidosis due to accumulation of lactic, acetoacetic and β-hydroxybutyric acids is also associated with hyperuricaemia, presumably because these substances compete with uric acid for a common mechanism of active transport across the renal tubule epithelium.

21.1.10. The investigation of purine metabolism in man

The methods which have been used to investigate purine metabolism in man are summarized in Table 21.5. These include studies on cultured fibroblasts and lymphocytes, which have proved necessary to investigate some aspects of the control of purine synthesis and for the diagnosis of certain inborn errors of metabolism. ^{15}N-labelled uric acid has been used to measure pool size and turnover rate, and to assess extrarenal disposal, and ^{14}C-labelled glycine to establish the time course and degree of labelling of urinary uric acid. These studies are exacting and make heavy demands on the time of skilled laboratory personnel. The metabolic pool size and turnover rate of uric acid in normal subjects are about 1.2 grams and 700 mg per 24 hours, respectively, but estimates in patients with gout are quantitatively unreliable because of exchange of labelled urate with tophi.

TABLE 21.5.

SOME METHODS USED IN THE INVESTIGATION OF PURINE METABOLISM IN MAN

Procedure	Key References
1. Measurement of uric acid in urine and plasma	Watts (1974)
2. Measurement of the oxypurines, hypoxanthine and xanthine in both urine and plasma	
(a) as total "oxypurines"	Chalmers and Watts (1968)
(b) by separate measurement of hypoxanthine and xanthine	Chalmers and Watts (1969)
3. Use of the urinary uric acid/creatinine excretion ratio as a test for hyperuricaciduria	Kaufman et al. (1968)
4. Uric acid excretion on a purine-free diet	Seegmiller (1967); Griebsch and Zöllner (1974).
5. Renal clearance of uric acid	Seegmiller (1967)
6. Measurement of tubular secretion of urate by pyrazinamide administration	Steele and Rieselbach (1967)
7. Uric acid pool size and turnover rate	Benedict et al. (1949)
8. Study of the incorporation of isotopically labelled glycine into the urinary uric acid	Benedict et al. (1952)
9. Chemical synthesis and selective degradation of isotopically labelled purines	Korn (1957)
10. Measurement of the extra-renal disposal of uric acid, and the correction of labelled glycine incorporation data for this effect	Seegmiller et al. (1961)
11. Urate-binding plasma α_{1-2}-globulin	Aäkesson and Alvsaker (1971)
(a) immunoelectrophoresis	Alvsaker (1966)
(b) isolation and characterization	Alvsaker and Seegmiller (1972)

TABLE 21.5. (continued)

Procedure	Key References
12. Identification of crystals by polarized light microscopy	Currey (1968) Chayen and Denby (1968) Chalmers et al. (1969c, d) Watts et al. (1971a)
13. Measurement of tissue purines and pyrazolo(3,4-d)-pyrimidines by quantitative high resolution mass spectrometry (integrated ion current technique)	Watts et al. (1971b) Snedden et al. (1970) Snedden and Parker (1971)
14. Measurement of erythrocyte phosphoribosylpyrophosphate (PRPP) concentration	Sperling et al. (1972b, c) Wood et al. (1973) Gordon et al. (1974)
15. Measurement of tissue xanthine oxidase (EC 1.2.3.2)	
(a) by spectrophotofluorimetry	Engelman et al. (1964)
(b) by radiochemical assay	Watts et al. (1965)
16. Measurement of hypoxanthine phosphoribosyltransferase (EC 2.4.2.8) (HGPRT) and adenine phosphoribosyltransferase (EC 2.4.2.7) (APRT)	Seegmiller et al. (1967) Craft et al. (1970) Chow et al. (1970) Sperling et al. (1970) Adams (1973) Schlossberg and Hollander (1973)
17. Measurement of ribose phosphate pyrophosphokinase (EC 2.7.6.1) (PRPP synthetase)	Hershko et al. (1969) Fox and Kelley (1971) Meyskens and Williams (1971) Becker et al. (1973a)
18. Estimation of the rate of purine synthesis de novo in cultured fibroblasts and lymphoblasts by the incorporation of [^{14}C]formate into α-N-formylglycinamide ribonucleotide (FGAR) in the presence of azaserine	Rosenbloom et al. (1968) Boyle et al. (1972)
19. Amidophosphoribosyltransferase (EC 2.4.2.14) activity of cultured lymphoblasts	Wood and Seegmiller (1973) Wood et al. (1973)
20. Methods for the culture of fibroblasts and amniotic cells cloning techniques, and the use of selective tissue culture media	Boyle and Seegmiller (1971) Fujimoto et al. (1971)
21. Immunochemical identification of hypoxanthine phosphoribosyltransferase (EC 2.4.2.8) protein	Arnold and Kelley (1971) Kelley and Meade (1971) Müller and Stemberger (1974) Upchurch et al. (1975) Changas and Milman (1975)

21.2. ANALYTICAL CONSIDERATIONS

21.2.1. Uric acid in blood and urine

All the commonly used means of assaying uric acid depend on its chemical or enzymatic oxidation to allantoin (Scheme 21.4). Chemical methods are based on the reduction of a chromogen to yield a chromophore which is measured spectrophotometrically, and stem from the observation of Frabot in 1904 that an alkaline tungstate solution became intensely blue on the addition of uric acid. Numerous methodologies based on this principle have been published; the earlier literature was reviewed by Peters and Van Slyke (1932), and a later survey (Watts, 1974) revealed an evident need for constant revision of the basic method. This suggests that these means of measuring uric acid are fundamentally unsound when applied to biological fluids. In general, the results of chemical assays of plasma agree closely with those of manual enzymatic spectrophotometric methods, but the susceptibility of the colour development step to chemical interference remains; it is a particularly serious problem in the analysis of urine.

Enzymatic methods of assaying uric acid in biological fluids will probably replace purely chemical methods when the instrumentation and running costs are fully competitive. These methods depend on: following the oxidation of uric acid to allantoin spectrophotometrically; measuring the amount of hydrogen peroxide produced; or determining the oxygen uptake during the reaction. A less satisfactory alternative is to make colorimetric measurements before and after treatment with uricase.

The catalytic activity of uricase is highly specific with respect to the oxidation of uric acid, and the enzyme can be used for the direct measurement of uric acid by observing the decrease in absorbance at 292 nm, without the need for protein precipitation or repeated standardization against uric acid solutions. The differential spectrophotometric method is highly specific and sensitive, but does require good quality instrumentation and highly purified uricase, all of which are relatively expensive.

Methods based on the measurement of the hydrogen peroxide combine the specificity of differential ultraviolet spectrophotometry with the use of simpler colorimeters or spectrophotometers. Some modifications of these methods incorporate fluorometric detection to achieve higher sensitivity.

Methods of assaying uric acid which depend on measuring the uptake of oxygen either polarographically or coulometrically have not gained wide acceptance.

In reviewing methods of measuring uric acid, Watts (1974) concluded that although differential ultraviolet spectrophotometry was an excellent reference method, procedures which depend on measuring hydrogen peroxide production have more potential for widespread application in place of the older colorimetric methods which depend on the reducing properties of uric acid. The manual method of Kageyama (1971) and the automated method of Gochman and Schmitz (1971) are particularly promising, and have the attraction that they utilize the high specificity of uricase, measure a reaction product directly by spectrophotometry in the visible light range, and are economical in their use of expensive reagents.

Advances in high pressure liquid chromatography and in mass spectrometry can be expected to lead to significant improvements in uric acid methodology, especially for the accurate characterization of reference materials with biological matrices (Ismail and Dakin, 1975).

21.2.2. Other purines, nucleosides and nucleotides

The assay of these compounds generally depends upon measurement of their characteristic ultraviolet light absorption after chromatographic separation, supplemented by the use of specific enzymes where these are available. Such assays are unlikely to be needed except for research purposes, but useful compilations of spectral data, and references to analytical methods are found in the source books by Dawson et al. (1969), Colowick and Kaplan (1955–1975) and Sober (1970).

It is sometimes necessary to measure hypoxanthine and xanthine, to confirm the diagnosis of xanthinuria, or in the investigation of patients with the Lesch–Nyhan syndrome who are taking allopurinol.

Enzymatic differential spectrophotometric methods for the measurement of hypoxanthine and xanthine, either together (the "oxypurines"), or separately, in both blood and urine have been published (Table 21.5). The blood for these analyses must be chilled and the plasma immediately separated at 4°C in order to minimize leakage of hypoxanthine from erythrocytes. Hypoxanthine, xanthine, their structural isomers allopurinol and oxipurinol, and uric acid have been measured at the nanogram level by means of quantitative high resolution mass spectrometry (Table 21.5, Procedure 13).

Patients with the Lesch–Nyhan syndrome are sometimes given adenine to correct their megaloblastic anaemia. Xanthine oxidase catalyzes the oxidation of adenine to 2,8-dioxyadenine, which is excreted in the urine and may precipitate in the urinary tract. This possibility requires that the urine be monitored for 2,8-dioxyadenine, and Schulman et al. (1971) described a simple spectrophotometric method of doing this.

21.2.3. Specific enzyme assays which may be needed for the accurate diagnosis of disorders of purine metabolism

21.2.3.1. Hypoxanthine phosphoribosyltransferase (EC 2.4.2.8, HGPRT) and adenine phosphoribosyltransferase (EC 2.4.2.7, APRT)

The activity of HGPRT has to be measured in erythrocytes for the diagnosis of the Lesch–Nyhan syndrome, and in single hair follicles when women are investigated in order to determine if they are carriers of this X-linked inborn error of metabolism.

The activity of HGPRT falls to extremely low or immeasurable levels in patients with the Lesch–Nyhan syndrome, and to a less marked degree in a very small proportion of patients with gout or uric acid urolithiasis. Decreased erythrocyte HGPRT activity is associated with an increase in APRT activity, due to stabilization of the enzyme by PRPP, so that it is useful to measure both enzyme activities. The demonstration of APRT activity in the hair follicle test confirms that enzymatically active cells have been withdrawn from the scalp and the results are expressed as the ratio HGPRT/APRT. A syndrome of familial low erthyrocyte APRT activity has been described, but this is not associated with abnormal purine metabolism.

These enzymes are assayed by incubating the erythrocyte lysate with the appropriate ^{14}C-labelled purine, and saturating amounts of phosphoribosylpyrophosphate and Mg^{2+} in Tris buffer. The radioactive nucleotide is separated from the excess ^{14}C-labelled substrate by an electrophoretic or chromatographic method. Experimental details are given in the references cited in Table 21.5. Thymidine triphosphate (TTP) should be included in the incubation mixture in order to inhibit 5′-nucleotidase when tissues and cells other than erythrocytes are assayed (Adams et al., 1971; Adams, 1973; Adams and Harkness, 1976).

The mean values found for phosphoribosyltransferase activities in human erythrocytes differ between laboratories (Table 21.6), and this reflects the methodological difficulties and the need for each laboratory to establish its own range of reference values. Measurements of HGPRT activity using hypoxanthine as the substrate usually present fewer problems than those which employ guanine. The very low levels of residual enzyme activity which have been reported in some cases of the Lesch–Nyhan syndrome are very difficult to quantitate, and critical appraisal should be directed at the experimentally determined radioactivity measurements rather than to the final derived values. The available methodology is satisfactory for identifying the absent – or virtually absent – HGPRT activity which characterizes the Lesch–Nyhan syndrome. It will also differentiate the somewhat higher values, up to 10% of normal, which are associated with a few cases of gout and urolithiasis with inconstant neurological abnormalities in men. It does not permit quantitative studies aimed at classifying patients on the basis of different HGPRT activities, in the very low range of values found in the Lesch–Nyhan syndrome.

The effects of age and sex on erythrocyte HGPRT and APRT activities have not been thoroughly examined, although Borden et al. (1974) reported that erythrocytes from neonates have higher APRT activity than adult subjects' cells, and that when adult subjects' erythrocytes were fractionated into young and old cells, the young cells had significantly greater APRT activity than the old cells.

The methods of measuring the HGPRT and APRT activities of hair follicles used in the

TABLE 21.6.

REFERENCE VALUES FOR THE PHOSPHORIBOSYLTRANSFERASE ACTIVITIES OF NORMAL HUMAN ERYTHROCYTES

Author	Subjects studied		Purine phosphoribosyltransferase activity (Mean (S.D.) nmol · (mg protein)$^{-1}$ · (hour)$^{-1}$)		
	Number	Sex	Hypoxanthine	Guanine	Adenine
Emmerson and Wyngaarden (1969)	28	Both [a]	70 (15)	82 (24)	15 (5)
Kelley et al. (1969)	32	Not stated	103 (18)	103 (21)	31 (6)
Chow et al. (1970)	26	Not stated	128 (9)	149 (14)	26 (3)
Sperling et al. (1970)	30	Male	51 (6)	113 (22)	10 (2)
Wood et al. (1972)	21	Not stated	71 (9)	–	–
	6	Not stated	–	–	15 (4)
Emmerson and Thompson (1973)	27	Not stated	94 (8)	161 (16)	17 (3)
Itiaba et al. (1973)	51 [b]	Not stated	100 (19)	–	24 (6)
Gordon et al. (1974)	24	Female	94 (8)	–	–
	22	Female	–	–	20 (3)
Müller (1974)	8	Not stated	79 (12)	–	15 (2)
Watts et al. (1974)	20	Both [a]	81 (22)	87 (16)	14 (3)
Allsop and Watts (unpublished) [c]	90	Both [a]	101 (19)	–	21 (7)

[a] No differences detected between male and female subjects

[b] Number of determinations; number of subjects not stated

[c] By the method of Craft et al. (1970) except for the use of a pH 8.0 rather than pH 7.5 buffer

present author's laboratory have been described (McKeran et al., 1975), and attempts to set them up should be checked by comparison with results obtained by skin biopsy and fibroblast culture. Carrier females are mosaics, and two populations of fibroblasts grow out from their skin biopsies. One population ($HGPRT^+$) has normal HGPRT activity; the nuclei of these cells become labelled, as judged by autoradiography when [^{3}H]hypoxanthine is added to the culture medium. The other cell population ($HGPRT^-$) shows only minimal labelling under these conditions (Fujimoto et al., 1968). Cells which lack HGPRT can grow in the presence of concentrations of 6-thiopurine, 6-thioguanine or azaguanine which are lethal to normal cells because they do not convert the drug into its toxic ribonucleotide. Tissue culture media containing these compounds can be used to select against the $HGPRT^+$ cells, and media containing azaserine (to block purine biosynthesis de novo) and hypoxanthine as the only purine source can be used to select against $HGPRT^-$ cells in cultures containing both types of cell (Fujimoto et al., 1971).

21.2.3.2. Ribose phosphate pyrophosphokinase (EC 2.7.6.1, PRPP synthetase)

Increased PRPP synthetase activity is a rare inherited cause of purine overproduction and gout, and two genetically determined variants of the enzyme have been described in association with this functional alteration. A syndrome of hypouricaemia and mental retardation associated with defective PRPP synthetase activity has also been described. For diagnostic purposes, the enzyme is assayed in erythrocyte lysates and the assay involves two steps – PRPP generation from ribose-5-phosphate and ATP, followed by a radiochemical assay of the PRPP produced (Becker et al., 1973a). An alternative method in which the enzyme is assayed in one step by the ribose-5-phosphate-dependent conversion of [^{14}C]-ATP into [^{14}C]AMP was published by Fox and Kelley (1971). Both methods are used in the present author's laboratory, and the one-step method is preferred. Reference values are presented in Table 21.7.

It is, however, recommended that the assay of PRPP-synthetase should only be undertaken by a laboratory in which the assay is being used regularly. In practice, this is likely to be a department in which active research on purine metabolism is in progress. Inexplicable discrepancies have been encountered between the results obtained by the two methods of measuring PRPP-synthetase. These may be related to the presence of unidentified enzyme inhibitors in some cell lysates and not in others.

TABLE 21.7.

REFERENCES VALUES FOR THE ACTIVITIES OF RIBOSE PHOSPHATE PYROPHOSPHOKINASE (EC 2.7.6.1, PRPP SYNTHETASE) IN NORMAL HUMAN ERYTHROCYTES AS REPORTED BY DIFFERENT LABORATORIES

Author	No. of subjects	PRPP synthetase activity (nmol PRPP (mg protein)$^{-1}$ · (hour)$^{-1}$)
Becker et al. (1973a)	28	68 (S.D. 18)
Gordon et al. (1974)	6	41 (S.D. 10)
Allsop and Watts (unpublished) [a]	90	25 (S.D. 7)

[a] By the method of Fox and Kelley (1971).

21.2.3.3. Amidophosphoribosyltransferase (EC 2.4.2.14)

Lymphoblasts and placenta are the only human tissues in which the activity of amidophosphoribosyltransferase has been measured. Wood et al. (1973) described a radiochemical assay of the PRPP-dependent hydrolysis of L-[U-^{14}C]glutamine to L-[U-^{14}C]glutamic acid, which should stimulate further work on the activity of the first specific and rate limiting step on the metabolic pathway of purine biosynthesis de novo. Recent studies (Allsop and Watts, unpublished) have shown that the enzyme is present in unstimulated peripheral blood lymphocytes, the level of activity being 17.5 (S.D. 4.3) mg cell protein per hour based on a total of 45 subjects of both sexes.

21.2.3.4. Xanthine oxidase (EC 1.2.3.2)

Measurements of tissue xanthine oxidase activity are occasionally needed to confirm the diagnosis of xanthinuria (congenital xanthine oxidase deficiency), or in the investigation of the reported association of some cases of gout with increased hepatic xanthine oxidase activity. Spectrophotofluorometric or radiochemical methods are sufficiently sensitive for these purposes (Table 21.8). The enzyme can be studied in human jejunal and hepatic biopsies, or in human milk, and values for the xanthine oxidase activities are summarized in Table 21.8.

TABLE 21.8.

XANTHINE OXIDASE ACTIVITIES OF NORMAL HUMAN LIVER, JEJUNAL MUCOSA AND COLOSTRUM; OTHER TISSUES AND SECRETIONS HAVE NEGLIGIBLE ACTIVITIES (Watts et al. 1965)

Author	Method	Xanthine oxidase activity		
		Liver (pmol substrate · (mg protein)$^{-1}$ · (hour)$^{-1}$)	Jejunum	Colostrum (μmol substrate · ml^{-1} · hour^{-1})
Engelman et al. (1964)	Radiochemical	2550–15200 [a] (Mean = 5650; 6 subjects)	4800–23600 [a] (Mean = 12100; 12 biopsies on 8 subjects)	–
	Fluorometric	40; 127; 149 (Results on 3 subjects)	37–132 [a] (Mean = 80; 8 subjects)	–
Carcassi et al. (1969)	Fluorometric	22,000–58,000 (Mean = 37,000; 12 subjects)	–	–
Riario-Sforza et al. (1969)	Fluorometric	–	6000–32,000 [a] (Mean = 20,000 8 subjects)	–
Oliver et al. (1971)	Radiochemical	–	–	37–125 [a]

[a] Extreme range of values

21.2.3.5. Glucose-6-phosphatase (EC 3.1.3.9)

The diagnosis of type I glycogen storage disease, glucose-6-phosphatase deficiency, requires liver biopsy and direct assay of the enzyme activity. The glycogen content and the activities of the other enzymes, deficiencies of which cause other types of glycogen storage disease, should also be measured. A surgical biopsy is preferable to a needle biopsy in this situation because of the complex biochemical work which is needed. The tissue must be handled very carefully and the finding of a deficiency of more than one enzyme suggests that the tissue has been poorly handled. The diagnostic biochemistry relating to this group of disorders is well reviewed by Ryman (1974).

21.2.3.6. Glutathione reductase (EC 1.6.4.2)

Long (1967) described the identification of the electrophoretically fast-moving variant of glutathione reductase which has increased catalytic activity and which is associated with hyperuricaemia.

21.2.3.7. Adenosine deaminase, purine nucleoside phosphorylase and 5′-nucleotidase

Increased activity of erythrocyte adenosine deaminase (EC 3.5.4.4) in the presence of normal purine nucleoside (inosine) phosphorylase (EC 2.4.1.1) activity was reported for gouty patients by Nishizawa et al. (1975) who also described the analytical methods used. Adenosine deaminase deficiency occurs in combined immunodeficiency disease (Giblett et al., 1972). Purine nucleoside (inosine) phosphorylase deficiency is associated with dysfunction of the T-lymphocytes (Giblett et al., 1975). There is also evidence that some patients with the non-familial adult onset variable type of primary hypogammaglobulinaemia have reduced activity of lymphocyte 5′-nucleotidase (Johnson et al., 1977).

21.2.4. Measurement of erythrocyte phosphoribosylpyrophosphate

The concentration of erythrocyte phosphoribosylpyrophosphate (PRPP) is measured when evidence is sought of excessive PRPP generation as a cause of hyperuricaemia. PRPP synthesis by erythrocyte PRPP synthetase is abolished either by heating the cell lysate or by adding 2,3-diphosphoglyceric acid which inhibits the enzyme; the PRPP is then mea-

TABLE 21.9.

REFERENCE VALUES FOR THE CONCENTRATION OF ERYTHROCYTE PHOSPHORIBOSYLPYROPHOSPHATE (PRPP)

Author	Number and sex of subjects	Erythrocyte phosphoribosylpyrophosphate, mean (S.D.) (nmol per ml packed cells)
Fox and Kelley (1971)	–, Male and female	4.4 (1.8)
Meyskens and Williams (1971)	10, Male and female	3.0 (0.3)
Sperling et al. (1972a, b)	9, Male and female	6.1 (3.1)
Becker et al. (1973a)	24, Not stated	2.8 (0.5)
Allsop and Watts (unpublished) [a]	90, Male and female	17.2 (6.4)

[a] By the method of Gordon et al. (1974); concentration expressed as pmol per mg protein.

sured by its quantitative conversion into nucleotide by adding phosphoribosyltransferase in the presence of a ^{14}C-labelled purine base. Reference values for erythrocyte PRPP levels are presented in Table 21.9. The supply of PRPP is critical for cell replication, it having been shown that the concentration of the metabolite increases within minutes of the application of a mitogenic stimulus to human peripheral blood lymphocytes (Hovi et al., 1975).

21.2.5. Crystal characterization

The demonstration of monosodium urate monohydrate crystals in synovial fluid, or in material obtained from a tophus, is the final proof that a patient suffers from gouty arthritis, and is not an individual with essential hyperuricaemia who has another type of arthritis which resembles gout on clinical grounds. The acute arthritis which may complicate chondrocalcinosis closely resembles gout, but the synovial fluid contains calcium pyrophosphate crystals in this disorder.

Calcium pyrophosphate and monosodium urate monohydrate can be distinguished from one another by examination in a suitable polarizing microscope. They both occur in synovial fluid as thin elongated crystals which appear maximally dark if positioned to lie with the long axis parallel to the planes of polarization of the analyzer and polarizer when these are at 90° to one another ("fully crossed"). They appear maximally bright when placed with the long axis at 45° to the cross of the planes of polarization ("the 45° position"). Thus, calcium pyrophosphate and monosodium urate monohydrate crystals cannot be distinguished by measuring their extinction angles, this being the angle relative to the cross of the planes of polarization at which the crystal appears maximally dark. Figures 21.3 and 21.4 show the appearances of crystals with straight extinction (e.g.

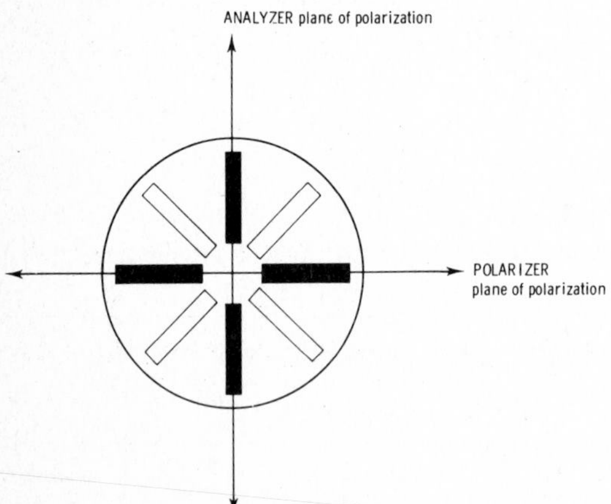

Figure 21.3. Appearance of a crystal which shows straight extinction under polarized light, the polarizer and analyzer being fully crossed, i.e. positioned at 90° with respect to one another. The crystal is maximally dark when it lies parallel to the planes of polarization and maximally bright when lying at 45° to the planes of polarization. Calcium pyrophosphate and monosodium urate monohydrate both have this appearance.

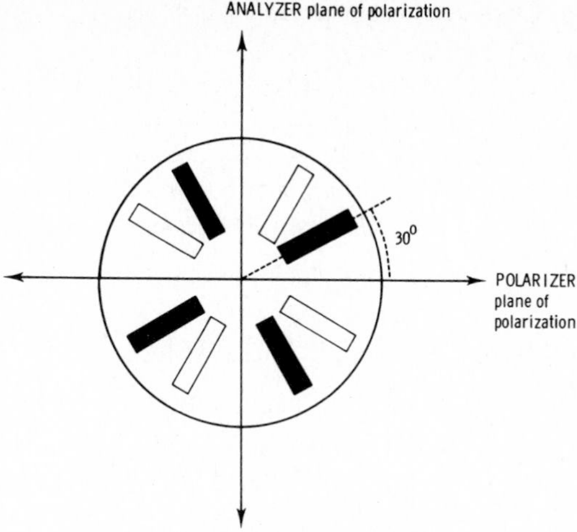

Figure 21.4. Appearance of a crystal which shows asymmetrical extinction under polarized light. In this case, extinction is at 30° to the planes of polarization as with allopurinol.

monosodium urate monohydrate and calcium pyrophosphate) and assymmetrical extinction (e.g. allopurinol) respectively.

Monosodium urate monohydrate and calcium pyrophosphate can be distinguished by their signs of birefringence (Currey, 1968), but the following additional criteria are required for the absolute identification of crystals by optical methods – crystal shape, i.e. the ratio of the dimensions of the three axes of the crystal; extinction angle; refractive index determined by immersion in media of different known refractive indices; the degree of birefringence; the degree of compensation in media of different refractive index (Chayen and Denby, 1968; Watts et al., 1971a). The sign of birefringence and the first two additional criteria serve to distinguish monosodium urate from calcium pyrophosphate where a simple choice has to be made between these two crystals. If the possible identities are more numerous additional criteria are needed, as in the studies of Watts et al. (1971a) in which xanthine, hypoxanthine, uric acid dihydrate, monosodium urate monohydrate, uric acid and oxipurinol monohydrate were identified in muscle biopsies. The technique of quantitative polarized light microscopy has considerable potential in the study of diseases in which crystals are deposited in tissues. It is complementary to ultrasensitive methods of chemical analysis such as quantitative high resolution mass spectrometry (section 21.2.2), as shown by the present author's studies on xanthinuric myopathy (section 21.10).

21.2.6. Urate-binding globulin

Estimation of this plasma protein fraction is needed to identify the cases of gout in which an inherited low plasma concentration of α_{1-2}-urate-binding globulin is associated with the development of gout. The plasma concentration of α_{1-2}-urate-binding-globulin is in the range 15 to 20 mg/dl (calculated from the data of Alvsacker and Seegmiller, 1972).

21.2.7. Immunochemical detection of hypoxanthine phosphoribosyltransferase

Immunochemical methods (Table 21.5, entry 21) are used to detect the presence of catalytically incompetent hypoxanthine phosphoribosyltransferase (EC 2.4.2.8, HGPRT) protein in the Lesch–Nyhan syndrome. In almost all the cases so far examined, the patients' erythrocytes have not contained a detectable amount of protein which cross-reacted with antibodies prepared against human HGPRT, and are described as CRM-negative (Changas and Milman, 1975; Upchurch et al., 1975).

21.3. THE NORMAL CONCENTRATION OF URATE IN PLASMA

Apart from the apparent differences which are attributed to methodological problems, the serum or plasma urate concentration is affected by the following factors: sex, age, pregnancy, genetic constitution, ethnic origin, dietary history, medication and coincidental disease.

21.3.1. Sex, age, genetic and ethnic factors

The serum uric acid concentration is low in both sexes before puberty. Passwell et al. (1974) reported that the mean serum uric acid was 0.21 mmol/litre (3.5 mg/dl) in 50 neonates and infants. Harkness and Nicol (1969) reported a mean value of 0.23 mmol/litre (3.7 mg/dl) and a reference range of 0.09 to 0.40 mmol/litre (1.5 to 6.7 mg/dl) for 171 children of both sexes between 0 and 13 years old. Males show a sharp rise at puberty and reach adult values by 20 years of age; females show a smaller rise at puberty but their plasma concentrations increase after the menopause to the values observed in male subjects. This phenomenon is illustrated in Figure 21.5 which also compares results obtained

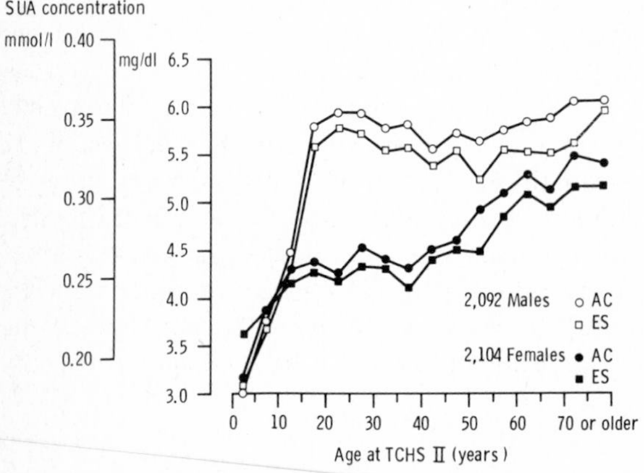

Figure 21.5. The effects of age, sex and different chemical methodology on the mean serum uric acid (SUA) concentration. The sera were analyzed by an enzymatic spectrophotometric (ES) and an automated colorimetric (AC) method. The subjects were 2092 males and 2104 females who participated in the 1962–1965 Tecumseh Community Health Study (Reproduced, by permission, from Dodge and Mikkelsen, 1970).

by an enzymatic spectrophotometric and an automated colorimetric method of analysis. Dodge and Mikkelson (1970) found that an automated colorimetric method more often gave results which were higher than those obtained by an enzymatic spectrophotometric method. Most of the differences were in the range 0.01 to 0.05 mmol/litre (0.1 to 0.9 mg/dl) but differences of more than 0.12 mmol/litre (2.0 mg/dl) were observed in a few cases. These workers used 0.42 mmol/litre (7.0 mg/dl) and 0.36 mmol/litre (6.0 mg/dl) as the upper limits of the ranges of serum uric acid concentration in men and women respectively (Figure 21.6) and classified about 4000 subjects as being normouricaemic or hyperuricaemic on this basis. They found that substitution of the automated colorimetric for the enzymatic spectrophotometric values would have altered the classification of about 6% of the subjects.

The concentration of serum uric acid is a continuous variable and its frequency distribution with respect to age is unimodal, with some skewness due to a small proportion of outlying high values in both sexes (Figure 21.6). This is compatible with the genetic component of the factors which determine the concentration being due to the action of multiple genes rather than to one gene, which if it undergoes a mutation causes hyperuricaemia. This also agrees with the discovery that several different inherited single enzyme defects are associated with hyperuricaemia. The data are usually assumed to have a statistically normal frequency distribution (which is, however, not strictly true), and the reference range of serum uric acid concentration is expressed as two standard deviations about the mean value. On this basis, the upper limit of concentration is usually taken as 0.42 mmol/litre (7.0 mg/dl) and 0.36 mmol/litre (6.0 mg/dl) for men and women respectively (Seegmiller, 1969). These figures may need a slight revision in the upward direction in the future, as analytical performance improves.

Table 21.10 summarizes the results of surveys of serum uric acid concentrations in different parts of the world. It illustrates the differences which have been attributed to the study of different populations, social classes and ethnic groups. The high values in the

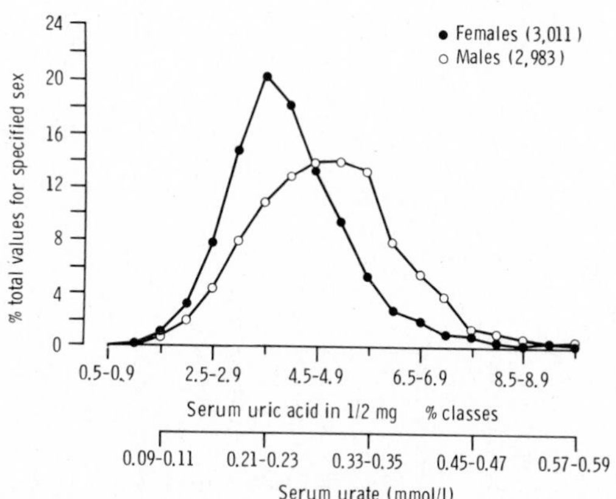

Figure 21.6. The frequency distribution of serum uric acid values. The participants were 2983 males and 3011 females who participated in the 1959–1960 Tecumseh Community Health Study (Reproduced, by permission, from Mikkelsen et al., 1965).

TABLE 21.10.

SERUM URATE CONCENTRATIONS IN DIFFERENT POPULATIONS, SOCIAL AND ETHNIC GROUPS

[After Wyngaarden and Kelley (1972)]

Population, class or group	Males			Females			References
	Number	mean mmol/litre (mg/dl)	S.D. mmol/litre (mg/dl)	Number	mean mmol/litre (mg/dl)	S.D. mmol/litre (mg/dl)	
Population							
Tecumseh, Michigan	2987	0.291 (4.90)	0.083 (1.40)	3013	0.250 (4.20)	0.071 (1.20)	Mikkelsen et al. (1965)
Framingham, Massachusetts [a]	2283	0.305 (5.12)	0.066 (1.11)	2844	0.239 (4.01)	0.056 (0.94)	Hall et al. (1967)
U.S.A.	22	0.316 (5.32)	0.055 (0.93)	18	0.257 (4.32)	0.048 (0.81)	Grayzel et al. (1961)
U.S. Army inductees	817	0.301 (5.06)	0.056 (0.94)	–	– –	– –	Stetten and Hearon (1959)
U.S. prisoners (Caucasian)	90	0.298 (5.01)	0.066 (1.11)	–	– –	– –	Decker et al. (1962)
Denmark	150	0.303 (5.10)	0.071 (1.19)	150	0.238 (4.00)	0.056 (0.94)	Hauge and Harvald (1955)
Wensleydale, England	436	0.265 (4.46)	– –	475	0.220 (3.70)	– –	Popert and Hewitt (1962)
West Germany	265	0.289 (4.86)	0.079 (1.32)	119	0.241 (4.05)	0.077 (1.29)	Zöllner (1963)
Australia (Caucasian) [a]	100	0.331 (5.56)	0.057 (0.95)	100	0.269 (4.52)	0.042 (0.70)	Emmerson and Sandilands (1963)
Social class							
Pittsburgh executives	339	0.341 (5.73)	0.072 (1.21)	–	– –	– –	Dunn et al. (1963)
Oak Ridge National Laboratory Ph.D. scientists	76	0.318 (5.34)	0.073 (1.23)	–	– –	– –	Dunn et al. (1963)
U.S. craftsmen in Pittsburgh and in Oak Ridge National Laboratory	532	0.284 (4.77)	0.067 (1.13)	–	– –	– –	Dunn et al. (1963)
U.S. high school students	138	0.307 (5.16)	– –	–	– –	– –	Cobb (1963)
University of Michigan professors	113	0.337 (5.66)	0.070 (1.17)	–	– –	– –	Brooks and Mueller (1966)
Edinburgh executives	100	0.357 (6.00)	0.052 (0.88)	–	– –	– –	Anumonye et al. (1969)
Ethnic group							
American Negro	154	0.308 (5.17)	– –	–	– –	– –	Long (1970)
North American Indians – Pima	949 [b]	0.291 (4.89)	0.071 (1.19)	–	– –	– –	O'Brien et al. (1966)

TABLE 21.10. (continued)

Population, class or group	Males			Females			References
	Number	mean mmol/litre (mg/dl)	S.D. mmol/litre (mg/dl)	Number	mean mmol/litre (mg/dl)	S.D. mmol/litre (mg/dl)	
Blackfeet	1018 [b]	0.251 (4.22)	0.071 (1.19)	–	–	–	O'Brien et al. (1966)
Haida	237	0.262 (4.41)	0.059 (0.99)	–	–	–	Ford and de Mos (1964)
Filipinos in Seattle	118	0.374 (6.29)	0.077 (1.29)	–	–	–	Decker et al. (1962)
							Healey et al. (1967)
Subgroup I	92	0.345 (5.80)	0.053 (0.89)	–	–	–	Decker et al. (1962)
							Healey et al. (1967)
Subgroup II	26	0.480 (8.07)	0.053 (0.89)	–	–	–	Decker et al. (1962)
							Healey et al. (1967)
Filipinos in Hawaii	60	0.363 (6.10)	0.077 (1.30)	–	–	–	Healey et al. (1967)
Filipinos in Philippines	483	0.309 (5.20)	0.077 (1.30)	–	–	–	Healey et al. (1966)
Hawaiians (full bloods)	49	0.321 (5.40)	0.065 (1.10)	–	–	–	Healey et al. (1966)
Mariana Islanders							
Chamorros (>40 years)	160	0.371 (6.23)	0.090 (1.51)	175	0.303 (5.10)	0.084 (1.41)	Burch et al. (1966)
Carolinians (>40 years)	26	0.432 (7.27)	0.099 (1.67)	29	0.339 (5.70)	0.060 (1.01)	
Polynesians							
Maori (New Zealand)	366	0.420 (7.06)	0.092 (1.54)	381	0.343 (5.77)	0.092 (1.55)	Prior et al. (1966)
Rarotongans	243	0.414 (6.96)	0.083 (1.39)	228	0.355 (5.97)	0.071 (1.20)	
Pukapukans	188	0.419 (7.04)	0.065 (1.10)	191	0.368 (6.18)	0.065 (1.09)	
Australian Aborigines (Aurukun)	82	0.359 (6.03)	0.074 (1.25)	135	0.284 (4.78)	0.073 (1.23)	Emmerson et al. (1969)
Indigenous South Africans (Tswana)	128	0.291 (4.90)	0.065 (1.09)	242	0.265 (4.46)	0.065 (1.09)	Beighton et al. (1973)
S.E. Asia (Thai) [a]	710	0.295 (4.96)	0.054 (0.90)	–	–	–	Flatz (1971)

[a] Colorimetric methods; all other values determined by enzymatic spectrophotometric methods
[b] Males and females about equally distributed in each group

Polynesians are striking. More than 10% of adult male Maoris have gout: many of the Polynesian races eat Western diets and drink alcohol, and suffer from the health problems of Western civilisation – obesity, hypertension and alcoholism. However, the Pukapukans are not Westernised, obese or hypertensive and consume no alcohol, yet they are as hyperuricaemic as the Maoris, 40% of the males having serum urate concentrations greater than 0.42 mmol/litre (7.0 mg/dl). Filipinos have similar concentrations to Europeans and a very low incidence of gout when resident in the Phillipines, but show an increased incidence of gout and hyperuricaemia when they migrate to Hawaii or the U.S.A. This is attributed to dietary factors being superimposed on a genetic predisposition which is not apparent when they reside in the Phillipines, due to their diet being of lower purine content there than in the U.S.A. Similar considerations apply to the difference between the incidence of hyperuricaemia and gout in indigenous African and American negro populations, and to the increasing incidence of gout in Japanese males during the last 20 years. Flatz (1971) noted that body weight, glucose-6-phosphatase deficiency and HbE trait did not seem to influence the serum uric acid concentrations of male Thais, but there was a strong association between low serum uric acid concentrations and the presence of a thallasaemia gene (α or β) or increased osmotic fragility of the erythrocytes.

It has been suggested that women have a higher renal clearance of uric acid than men due to circulating oestrogens. Serum urate concentrations are slightly lower, and urinary uric acid clearances slightly greater, during the first two trimesters of pregnancy than in the non-pregnant state. They revert to non-pregnancy values in the last trimester. Pregnancy toxaemia may be associated with a mild degree of hyperuricaemia.

Hall et al. (1967) analyzed the significance of hyperuricaemia as a risk factor in the development of gout and found that the prevalence of gout increased with the serum uric acid concentration (Table 21.11). The risk of developing gout also increased with the duration of the hyperuricaemia. The small number of subjects in the groups with the highest serum urate concentrations makes it unjustified to compare the proportional incidence of gout in these groups.

TABLE 21.11.

PREVALENCE OF GOUTY ARTHRITIS RELATED TO THE MAXIMUM PLASMA URATE CONCENTRATION IN A POPULATION OF MEAN AGE 58 YEARS

(Data from Hall et al., 1967)

Concentration of uric acid		Men		Women	
mmol/litre	(mg/dl)	No. in group	No. with gout	No. in group	No. with gout
<0.36	(<6.0)	1280	8	2665	2
0.36–0.40	(6.0–6.9)	790	15	151	5
0.42–0.47	(7.0–7.9)	162	27	23	4
0.48–0.53	(8.0–8.9)	40	10	4	0
>0.54	(>9.0)	10	9	1	0

21.3.2. The effects of diet and of medication on the plasma urate concentration

The effects of dietary factors and of drugs on the plasma urate concentration have been reviewed in sections 21.1.8 and 21.1.9 respectively.

21.3.3. The relationship between hyperuricaemia and diseases other than gout or urolithiasis

Population studies show a statistical correlation of gout with: obesity, hypertension, arteriosclerosis, hypertriglyceridaemia, and alcoholism. However, careful epidemiological studies have also shown that hypertension, arteriosclerosis and hypertriglyceridaemia are associated with obesity and not with hyperuricaemia itself. Non-hyperuricaemic and hyperuricaemic populations, matched with respect to body weight, show no excess of hypertension or of hypertriglyceridaemia in the hyperuricaemic group. There is an excess of clinically apparent coronary artery disease in overtly gouty patients, but not among asymptomatic hyperuricaemic subjects.

Such studies do not support the classical teaching that diabetes mellitus and gout are significantly associated. It is likely that confusion has arisen because maturity-onset diabetes is associated with obesity, and patients with overt gout are often overweight. The frequent occurrence of hyperuricaemia in diabetic ketoacidosis is undisputed. It is ascribed to the inhibitory effect of acetoacetate and β-hydroxybutyrate on the renal tubule secretion of uric acid, although depletion of the extracellular fluid volume may be a contributory factor. Hyperuricaemia in this clinical situation is usually transient and of little clinical significance.

Chronic alcoholism and hyperuricaemia are associated with one another, as judged by the results of population studies. Thus, the daily ingestion of 100 ml of ethanol may be associated with hyperuricaemia and increased urinary excretion of uric acid, both of which return to normal after several days abstinence and a normal diet. Several pathophysiological mechanisms are probably involved. Thus, there may be a direct effect on the rate of purine synthesis. Alternatively, increased generation of NADH by the action of alcohol dehydrogenase (EC 1.1.1.1) favours the reduction of pyruvate to lactate, which reaches the kidney and reduces the renal tubule secretion of uric acid, so causing hyperuricaemia. Finally, there is the possibility that illicitly distilled spirits may be contaminated with lead, which produces nephropathy and reduced urate excretion.

Hyperuricaemia is sometimes due to conditions which increase the nucleoprotein turnover. These include: myeloproliferative disorders, reticuloses, multiple myelomatosis, haemoglobinopathies, thalassaemia, secondary polycythaemia (e.g. in cyanotic congenital heart disease), pernicious anaemia, psoriasis, infectious mononucleosis, and widespread metastatic malignant disease. The plasma urate concentration is further increased by vigorous treatment of the malignant conditions with either cytotoxic drugs or irradiation. Gouty arthritis ("secondary gout"), complicating these disorders, occurs most often in the more slowly evolving myeloproliferative disorders, particularly polycythaemia rubra vera and myeloid metaplasia. The figure of 10% incidence previously quoted for myeloproliferative diseases in gouty patients is now probably too high, because more cases of mild primary gout are correctly diagnosed. Gout occurs in between 5 and 9% of patients with polycythaemia rubra vera and less commonly in the other myeloproliferative diseases. Secondary gout does not show the characteristic sex and familial incidence of primary gout, and the plasma concentration and urinary uric acid excretion tend to be higher in secondary gout. Patients with gout secondary to myeloproliferative disease show a gradual rise in the labelling of urinary uric acid from isotopically labelled glycine over a period of about 2 weeks; the isotope content of the urinary uric acid then decreases slowly. This is different from the labelling pattern observed in primary gout, where there is a peak of isotope labelling of the urinary uric acid during the first 2 days after administration of labelled glycine.

Reduced uric acid excretion due to intrinsic renal disease leads to hyperuricaemia, but is rarely associated with gouty arthritis unless the renal disease is itself due to antecedent excessive uric acid synthesis. Urate retention is probably also associated with increased uricolysis (section 21.1.6). The inter-relationship between the disorders of uric acid metabolism and renal disease is discussed in section 21.9.

Hyperuricaemia is also reliably reported in the following conditions: plumbism, Down's syndrome, hypothyroidism, hypoparathyroidism, primary hyperparathyroidism, idiopathic hypercalciuria, nephrogenic diabetes insipidus, hypertension, sarcoidosis, beryllosis and starvation. This appears to be due to reduced renal excretion of uric acid in primary hyperparathyroidism, idiopathic hypercalciuria, hypertension, sarcoidosis, beryllosis and starvation. Structural renal damage, in some cases minor, and particularly affecting renal tubule functions, has been proposed in primary hyperparathyroidism, idiopathic hypercalciuria and hypertension. Plumbism commonly produces more extensive renal lesions, and it is possible that these renal factors may summate with genetic factors to produce overt hyperuricaemia and saturnine gout. The mechanism of the hyperuricaemia in nephrogenic diabetes insipidus is uncertain, but its presence complicates the treatment of the disorder with thiazide diuretics, and allopurinol may be needed also. Lactic acidosis and ketoacidosis have been incriminated as being responsible for renal retention of urate in sarcoidosis and beryllosis, and in starvation respectively. The hyperuricaemia of Down's syndrome, hypothyroidism and hypoparathyroidism lacks any pathophysiological explanation at the present time.

21.4. THE NORMAL URINARY EXCRETION OF URIC ACID

Uric acid production can be roughly measured by the urinary excretion of uric acid which, however, takes no account of the fraction of the total uric acid production which is disposed of by extra-renal mechanisms, or of renal factors which may promote urate retention.

An isocaloric purine-free diet – 10,890 kJoule (2600 kcalories), 70 grams protein, 350 grams carbohydrate, 100 grams fat – is necessary for 5 days before and during the period that the excretion of uric acid is measured. Studies by Gutman and Yü (1957) and Seegmiller et al. (1961) form the basis of the usual recommendation that the urinary uric acid excretion should not exceed 3.62 mmol (600 mg) per 24 hours, when a patient takes a purine-free diet.

The effect of dietary nucleic acids on the urinary uric acid excretion is reviewed in section 21.1.8.

21.5. GOUT

21.5.1. Definition

Gout is the syndrome caused by the crystallization of monosodium urate monohydrate from supersaturated body fluids in vivo. It is merely a complication of hyperuricaemia caused by over-production or under-excretion of uric acid, or by a combination of these factors, and the likelihood of its occurrence increases with the degree and duration of the hyperuricaemia. The term "primary gout" refers to cases which are due to identifiable single enzyme defects and to cases which have no cause identifiable by present methods. "Secondary gout" has an identifiable aetiology other than a single enzyme defect.

21.5.2. Clinical aspects

The synovial membranes of joints, bursae, and tendon sheaths are the favoured sites for crystallization of monosodium urate monohydrate, so that the rheumatological manifestations of the disease dominate the clinical picture. These are: (i) acute painful monoarticular arthritis, in which the joint fluid contains monosodium urate crystals and polymorphonuclear leucocytes; (ii) chronic arthritis due to repeated attacks of acute arthritis, and in which there are deposits of monosodium urate monohydrate around the joints; (iii) tophi, which are chalk-like aggregates of sodium urate embedded in an interstitial matrix and surrounded by a foreign body granuloma with chronic inflammatory reaction; subcutaneous tophi may ulcerate through the skin.

Between 10 and 25% of gouty patients develop uric acid urinary stones, and this is more than 1000 times the incidence in the general population. Renal damage by interstitial deposits of monosodium urate monohydrate is usually due to deposits in the renal pyramids, and these produce a segmental loss of kidney tissue. Sodium urate nephropathy has a poor prognosis, and although it can be prevented or arrested by adequate treatment, the renal damage cannot be reversed. Proteinuria and hypertension occur in 10 to 40% of gouty patients. Before the introduction of allopurinol, which reduces hyperuric aciduria as well as hyperuricaemia, about 25% of gouty patients died from renal failure.

21.5.3. Single enzyme defects which cause gout

The estimate that about 25% of gout patients synthesize and excrete abnormally large amounts of uric acid has been widely accepted. More extensive experience, particularly in Europe as opposed to North America, indicates that this figure is much too high, and reflects a bias in the population of gout patients from which it was derived.

Only a small minority of cases of gout, asymptomatic hyperuricaemia, or uric acid urolithiasis, are associated with an identifiable enzyme defect, even when there is overproduction of uric acid. These enzyme abnormalities are: (i) decreased HGPRT activity; (ii) increased PRPP synthetase activity; (iii) glucose-6-phosphatase deficiency; (iv) increased glutathione reductase activity. Some cases of gout were attributed to increased hepatic xanthine oxidase activity but more recent work shows that this is not so.

21.5.3.1. Decreased HGPRT activity

The virtually complete deficiency of HGPRT which is associated with the Lesch–Nyhan syndrome (section 21.6) is accompanied by gross over-production of uric acid with hyper-uricaemia and hyperuric aciduria. Uric acid urinary stones, hyperuricaemic nephropathy, and gout begin in childhood.

Some mutations of the X-linked gene, which directs the synthesis of HGPRT, leave the enzyme with more residual catalytic activity. Such patients also have recurrent uric acid urolithiasis, and severe gout which may begin in the first or second decade of life. However, their neurological disabilities and mental impairment are much less severe. They have only a few per cent of normal erythrocyte HGPRT activity. The extent to which they contribute to the overall incidence of gout is unknown, but it is unlikely to be more than 0.1% of all cases. Experience has shown that the syndromes of "complete" HGPRT deficiency (Lesch–Nyhan syndrome) and "incomplete" HGPRT deficiency form a continuum, and the degree of neurological deficit does not parallel the residual HGPRT activity, at least as measured in erythrocytes. Intracellular PRPP levels are increased in the HGPRT deficiency syndromes, and the activating effect of this on PRPP-amidotransferase is considered to be responsible for the purine-overproduction which occurs (section 21.1.2).

21.5.3.2. Increased PRPP synthetase activity

Two families have been reported in which uric acid overproduction is associated with increased PRPP synthetase activity. The genetic data are compatible with an X-linked pattern of inheritance in one family (Sperling et al., 1972b), and with an autosomal recessive pattern of inheritance in the other (Becker et al., 1973a, b). The enzyme from the case of Sperling et al. (1972a) was abnormally resistant to inhibition by orthophosphate. This was not so in the cases described by Becker et al. (1973b). The observed increase in PRPP synthetase activity may not be the primary defect in these cases, but may merely reflect decreased activity of an – as yet – unidentified enzyme which alters the concentrations of activators or inhibitors of PRPP synthetase. An analogous situation exists in acute intermittent porphyria, in which the increased activity of δ-aminolaevulic acid synthetase (EC 2.3.1.37) was recognized before the primary defect, a partial deficiency of uroporphyrinogen-I synthetase (EC 4.3.1.8) was identified.

21.5.3.3. Glucose-6-phosphatase deficiency

Hyperuricaemia and gout are well recognized complications of type 1 glycogen storage disease in patients who survive into adult life. Excessive purine biosynthesis and urate retention, due to the abnormal organic acidaemia which occurs in this disease, both contribute to the hyperuricaemia. The purine overproduction is explained as follows: deficiency of glucose-6-phosphatase leaves more glucose-6-phosphate available for metabolism, via the phosphogluconate shunt pathway, with generation of ribose-5-phosphate which is the substrate for PRPP synthetase. Increased PRPP availability increases the activity of PRPP-amidotransferase as described in section 21.1.2.

21.5.3.4. Increased glutathione reductase activity

The increased glutathione reductase activity which is found in association with an electrophoretically fast-moving variant of this enzyme is believed to cause uric acid overproduction by first increasing $NADP^+$ generation from NADPH; this increases phosphogluconate shunt activity, with generation of ribose-5-phosphate and hence of PRPP which activates PRPP-amidotransferase. The sequence of reactions is as follows:

GSSG + NADPH → GSH + $NADP^+$
G-6-P + $NADP^+$ → D-glucono-5-lactone-6-phosphate + NADPH
D-glucono-5-lactone-6-phosphate + H_2O → 6-phospho-D-gluconate
6-phospho-D-gluconate + $NADP^+$ → D-ribulose-5-phosphate
D-ribulose-5-phosphate → ribose-5-phosphate
ribose-5-phosphate + ATP → PRPP + AMP

21.5.3.5. Increased xanthine oxidase activity

Increased hepatic xanthine oxidase activity was reported in gout patients by Carcassi et al. (1969). Rairio-Sforza et al. (1969) and Marcolongo et al. (1974) did not find similar changes in jejunal mucosa. Normal subjects made hyperuricaemic by hypoxanthine or RNA feeding, by fructose-loading or by administration of 2-ethylamino-1,3,4-thiadiazole have increased hepatic xanthine oxidase activity (Marinello et al., 1969; Marcolongo et al., 1974). It is concluded that the changes in xanthine oxidase activity reported by Carcassi et al. (1969) are a non-specific response to increased nucleic acid catabolism.

21.5.3.6. The postulated primary abnormality of phosphoribosylpyrophosphate amidotransferase

The possibility that some cases of uric acid overproduction are due to a primary abnormality of phosphoribosylpyrophosphate amidotransferase, which makes it abnormally resistant to feed-back inhibition by purine ribonucleotides, or abnormally sensitive to PRPP stimulation, has been widely proposed. Such cases have not yet been identified although Becker and Seegmiller (1974) referred to one patient whose fibroblasts showed diminished responsiveness of purine synthetic rate to inhibition by purine bases and who may have had this type of metabolic lesion. Proof of such a postulate would require inhibitor-binding studies and a detailed investigation of the kinetic and allosteric properties of the purified abnormal enzyme isolated from the patient's tissues.

21.5.3.7. The postulated primary abnormality of glutamine metabolism

The suggestion that a deficiency of glutaminase (EC 3.5.1.2) accelerates purine biosynthesis by increasing the intracellular concentration of glutamine, which in turn increases PRPP-amidotransferase activity, has now been abandoned (Becker and Seegmiller, 1974). Pollak and Mattenheimer (1965) found normal glutaminase levels in renal biopsy tissue from four gout patients, and kinetic studies of PRPP-amidotransferase (Holmes et al., 1973a) suggest that the enzyme is fully saturated with glutamine, at the glutamine concentrations found in plasma, so that a further increase in glutamine concentration would be unlikely to increase the activity of the enzyme.

21.5.3.8. Adenine phosphoribosyltransferase deficiency

Four families have been described in which reduced erythrocyte adenine phosphoribosyltransferase (EC 2.4.2.8, APRT) activity was segregating in an autosomal dominant manner. Although some of the patients were hyperuricaemic, there is no evidence for a direct relationship between the APRT deficiency and the hyperuricaemia. Complete APRT deficiency causes the excretion of adenine and 2,8-dihydroxyadenine. The patients present with crystalluria and 2,8-dihydroxyadenine urinary stones in childhood. The stones are radiotranslucent and were confused with uric acid stones on the basis of chemical as well as radiological evidence until special methods (ultraviolet and infrared spectroscopy and mass spectrometry) were used (Cartier and Hamet, 1974; Simmonds et al., 1976).

21.6. THE LESCH–NYHAN SYNDROME

21.6.1. Clinical features

The patients appear normal at birth except for some degree of muscular hypotonia. Choreoathetosis, compulsive self-mutilation, aggressiveness, spasticity, and mental retardation gradually become apparent from the age of about three months. The athetoid movements (torsion dystonia) affect the trunk musculature as well as the limbs and are associated with athetoid dysartharia and dysphagia. Self-mutilation is not associated with sensory neuropathy, congenital indifference to pain or dysautonomia.

The prognosis was formerly governed by the development of urate nephropathy and uric acid stones. These complications, as well as juvenile tophacous gout, are avoided by giving allopurinol from infancy. Allopurinol does not affect the neuropsychiatric manifestations. In some cases. the degree of mental retardation is less than is at first apparent, disability being mainly conditioned by gross motor dysfunction.

The macrocytic anaemia which occurs in the Lesch–Nyhan syndrome can sometimes be corrected by giving adenine. However, adenine has no effect on the neuropsychiatric manifestations even when given from the first weeks of life. Similarly, enzyme replacement by means of an exchange blood transfusion did not alter the clinical state of one 4-year-old patient (Watts et al., 1974). In this study, the level of circulating HGPRT was increased into the lower part of the normal range and exceeded about 10% of the mean reference value for about 100 days. This value is well within the range encountered in patients with partial HGPRT deficiency who do not show self-mutilation, choreoathetosis or severe retardation.

Recent studies have shown that there is some selective impairment of B-lymphocyte function in patients with the Lesch–Nyhan syndrome (Allison et al., 1975). This is not, however, associated with any clinically significant increased liability to infection. It contrasts sharply with the clinical picture in congenital adenosine deaminase deficiency (combined B and T lymphocyte dysfunction), and with that in congenital purine nucleoside (inosine) phosphorylase deficiency (selective T-lymphocyte dysfunction), where the patients' responses to infection are grossly impaired.

21.6.2. Genetics

All of the available data are compatible with the Lesch–Nyhan syndrome being transmitted in an X-linked manner. The affected males do not reproduce because of their physical disabilities and shortened life span due to renal disease. It is not, therefore, possible to apply the classical test for X-linkage, namely, absence of male-to-male transmission. On theoretical grounds, one-third of the cases should be due to new mutations, because the affected males do not reproduce, and this may contribute to the high degree of variability which is observed in the syndrome. Evidence for a case of the Lesch–Nyhan syndrome being the result of a fresh mutation is presented by McKeran et al. (1974, 1975). The clinical picture in the less severely affected cases of the Lesch–Nyhan syndrome forms a continuum with that of patients who present with gout and uric acid stones associated with less reduced levels of HGPRT. Some of these subjects are mildly retarded and have minor neurological abnormalities such as a mild spinocerebellar ataxia. These individuals reproduce, so that it has been possible to demonstrate the absence of male-to-male inheritance in these cases (Kelley et al., 1969).

21.6.3. Diagnosis of the carrier state and prenatal diagnosis

Fibroblast cultures prepared from the mothers of affected boys contain two populations of cells, those with HGPRT ($HGPRT^+$) and those which lack the enzyme ($HGPRT^-$). The numbers of $HGPRT^+$ and $HGPRT^-$ are not exactly equal, as would be predicted from the Lyon hypothesis of random inactivation of the X chromosome, and this inequality has been explained as being due to metabolic cooperation. Subak-Sharpe (1969) defined metabolic co-operation as the phenomenon whereby, when cultured mammalian cells come into contact with one another, their individual metabolism is modified by the exchange of elaborated material. The blood cells do not show similar mosaicism because the growth of $HGPRT^-$ blood cell precursors is impaired, so that the clones of $HGPRT^-$ cells are bred out and ultimately overgrown by cells derived from clones of $HGPRT^+$ cells. This conclusion is based on the study of a family in which the abnormal genes for HGPRT deficiency and glucose-6-phosphate dehydrogenase deficiency were segregating (Nyhan et al., 1970) and on studies of the growth of bone marrow progenitor cells from heterozygotes and affected hemizygotes for complete HGPRT deficiency in tissue culture (McKeran et al., 1975). The expected mosaicism among the bone marrow cells and in the jejunal mucosa of a heterozygote for partial HGPRT deficiency was however observed (McKeran et al., 1975).

Hair follicles display some degree of clonal growth and this property can be used to identify the female carriers of the disorder by virtue of mosaicism of their hair follicles with respect to the presence of HGPRT in the follicle cells (section 21.2.3.1).

It is possible to establish the genetic status of the foetus of female carriers of the abnormal gene by studies on cultured amniotic fluid cells. Affected males show a single population of $HGPRT^-$ cells, carrier females show $HGPRT^+$ and $HGPRT^-$, and normal males and females show a single population of $HGPRT^+$ cells. The use of selective tissue culture media permits selection for either $HGPRT^+$ or $HGPRT^-$ cells in mixed cultures (section 21.2.3.1)

21.6.4. Partial phenocopies of the Lesch–Nyhan syndrome

Hooft et al. (1968) described a girl, who clinically resembled patients of the Lesch–Nyhan syndrome, in whom purine biosynthesis de novo was accelerated but who was normouricaemic; her parents were first cousins. Unfortunately HGPRT activity was not measured in this case. A patient with another apparently inherited disorder of purine metabolism was reported by Nyhan et al. (1969). This boy was grossly hyperuricaemic when he was 4 months old and was mentally retarded and autistic. Purine biosynthesis was accelerated, HGPRT activity was normal but ARPT activity was increased. Coleman et al. (1974) reported gross hyperuricaemia and hyperuric aciduria in a mentally retarded epileptic boy with normal erythrocyte HGPRT activity; the fits were controlled by giving allopurinol.

All of these children appear to have suffered from disorders of purine metabolism, which the early onset of symptoms suggests to have been inborn, but which was different from the Lesch–Nyhan syndrome.

21.6.5. Pathogenesis of the cerebral manifestations of the Lesch–Nyhan syndrome

The neurological disorder in the Lesch–Nyhan syndrome is attributed to impaired neuronal proliferation due to HGPRT deficiency during the perinatal spurt in brain growth. The fundamental pathophysiological abnormality appears to be a failure to conserve guanine as GMP in brain cells, rather than a toxic effect of uric acid, hypoxanthine, xanthine or an unidentified metabolite.

The brain has little capacity for purine synthesis de novo and depends heavily on the HGPRT-catalyzed salvage pathway to supply the GMP necessary for nucleic acid synthesis and for the production of GTP. The translational stage of protein synthesis requires the hydrolysis of GTP as a source of energy. GTP is also needed to convert mannose-1-phosphate into GDP mannose, which participates in glycoprotein synthesis. Brain HGPRT levels increase markedly around the time of birth in animals. The brain cells would be expected to be particularly susceptible to a restricted supply of GMP during the perinatal growth spurt, when nucleoprotein and protein synthesis, and synapse formation are occurring most rapidly.

The neurotransmitters acetylcholine and 5-hydroxytryptamine stimulate guanylate cyclase (EC 4.6.1.2) and therefore the production of cyclic GMP (Weight et al., 1974; Sandler et al., 1975). Lack of GMP, which is the precursor of GTP and hence of cyclic GMP, would therefore be expected to reduce this effect and to impair synaptic transmission with perhaps a specific effect on the function of 5-hydroxytryptamine-mediated neuronal circuits. The presence of HGPRT in well-washed synaptosomes (Gutensohn and Guroff, 1972) also points to a specific role of GMP in neurotransmission. Mizuno and Yugari (1974) reported that L-5-hydroxytryptophan, which is the precursor of 5-hydroxytryptamine, controlled the self-mutilation in four cases of the Lesch–Nyhan syndrome. The postulate that the autoaggressive behaviour in the Lesch–Nyhan syndrome is related to an imbalance of the "ergotrophic" or arousal-sympathetic nervous system and the diencephalic "trophotropic" or quieting-parasympathetic system subserved by 5-hydroxytryptophan, would also accord with the report of increased dopamine-β-hydroxylase (dopamine-β-mono-oxygenase, EC 1.14.17.1) activity in the Lesch–Nyhan syndrome, and with the production of the bizarre pattern of compulsive gnawing, posturing, sniffing and licking in rats and cats by amphetamine (Randrup and Munkvad, 1966; Wallach and Gershon, 1971). Autoaggression has been produced in experimental animals by feeding caffeine or theophylline (Nyhan, 1968; Morgan et al., 1970), which inhibit 3′,5′-cyclic AMP phosphodiesterase (EC 3.1.4.17), the enzyme which catalyzes the hydrolysis of the cyclic nucleotides. The observation of Mizuno and Yugani (1974) was not confirmed by Frith et al. (1976) in a carefully controlled blind trial on one patient.

21.7. PRPP SYNTHETASE DEFICIENCY

Wada et al. (1974) described the case of a boy who had appeared normal at birth but developed fits when he was 3 months old and was severely retarded by 9 months. His bone marrow was megaloblastic; blood, urine and cerebrospinal fluid uric acid concentrations were abnormally low. The PRPP content and PRPP synthetase activity of his erythrocytes were about 50 and 10% of the control values respectively. HGPRT and APRT activities were normal, urinary orotic acid excretion was increased, and there was no abnormal excretion of hypoxanthine and xanthine. Both parents had erythrocyte levels of PRPP synthetase activity which were intermediate between those observed in the control subjects and in the patient.

A different clinical presentation was reported by Valentine et al. (1972) whose 22-year-old female patient had congenital non-spherocyte haemolytic anaemia and erythrocyte PRPP synthetase activity between 20 and 50% of normal. She was not retarded.

21.8. RENAL DISEASE DUE TO DISORDERS OF PURINE METABOLISM

21.8.1. Acute uric acid nephropathy

Patients who are undergoing treatment for widespread malignant disease may suddenly develop oliguria or anuria due to the precipitation of uric acid crystals within the collecting tubules of the kidney as well as in the renal pelves and ureters. The sudden increase in the rate of uric acid production occurs in the context of a complex clinical situation and the factors which determine the occurrence of this complication in some patients, but not in others are obscure. The amount and rate of nucleic acid break-down are important factors, although in the case of leukaemia, the pre-treatment leucocyte count and the incidence of obstructive urinary complications are not closely correlated. Some patients may be predisposed to the complication, either because they are congenital overproducers of uric acid, or because they always secrete a strongly acid urine. Other contributory factors associated with the malignant disease are: metabolic acidosis due to the high level of anaerobic metabolism in tumour tissue and the catabolism of large amounts of tissue protein; dehydration; the use of cytotoxic agents, such as the 2-substituted thiadiazoles which accelerate purine synthesis de novo; and the use of cytotoxic or other drugs which are also uricosuric, e.g. 6-azauridine, the adrenocorticosteroids, methicillin, and large doses of aspirin.

The plasma urate concentration is always high, values greater than 1.90 mmol/litre (20 mg/dl) being common, and this observation should alert the clinician to the possible occurrence of acute uric acid nephropathy as a complication of cancer chemotherapy or irradiation. The urinary uric acid excretion is a more useful index of progress and, were it followed regularly during the course of treatment, would provide a better early guide to the risk of acute uric acid nephropathy developing than occasional measurements of plasma uric acid concentration. Treatment requires bilateral ureteric catheterization to exclude the presence of bilateral impacted radiotranslucent uric acid stones, and the maintenance of an alkaline diuresis. The condition can be avoided by the prophylactic use of allopurinol.

Large doses of radiocontrast media occasionally cause acute oliguric renal failure by virtue of their powerful uricosuric actions, leading to acute uric acid nephropathy.

21.8.2. Chronic urate nephropathy ("gout nephropathy"; "gout nephrosis")

Almost all untreated gouty patients show at least microscopic evidence of renal damage at autopsy. This includes the deposition of monosodium urate crystals in the renal pyramids, chronic inflammatory changes, and arteriosclerosis. Between 20 and 40% of gout patients have proteinuria; a similar proportion have hypertension, and 25% were said to die from renal failure before effective remedies for hyperuricaemia became available. The severity of the gout and of the renal disease generally parallel one another, although occasional patients present with marked renal damage and no history of gouty arthritis, and vice versa. It appears that although the renal damage can be arrested by effectively treating the hyperuricaemia, it cannot be reversed.

It may be difficult to distinguish patients with end-stage renal disease due to primary renal pathology, from cases of advanced chronic urate nephropathy. Hyperuricaemia is a late manifestation in the former patients, who rarely survive long enough to develop tophi and gouty arthritis. Neither the plasma urate concentration nor the endogenous urate clearance correlates with the degree of renal insufficiency, as judged by the plasma urea concentration or glomerular filtration rate. Patients with chronic urate nephropathy have hyperuricaemia, which is disproportionate to the other evidence of renal failure and usually, although not invariably, a history of some other gouty manifestations.

21.8.3. Urolithiasis

Between 10 and 25% of patients with primary gout have urinary stones, and this is more than 1000 times the incidence in the general population. The incidence in secondary gout is even higher – 40%. Most of these stones contain only uric acid, and their formation is favoured by the impaired ability of many gout patients to secrete an alkaline urine, or by the secretion of concentrated urine, as in the tropics. A minority are calcium oxalate stones which grow on a central crystal of uric acid dihydrate by epitaxy. Uric acid urolithiasis may occur in otherwise asymptomatic patients with essential hyperuricaemia. Although uric acid urolithiasis sometimes occurs without increased uric acid excretion, the gouty patient's uric acid excretion should be measured, because this gives a useful indication of the individual subject's predisposition to stone formation. Also, hyperuric aciduria contraindicates the use of uricosuric drugs, such as probenecid and sulfinpyrazone, for the treatment of gout.

Uric acid urinary stones can sometimes be dissolved, or their recurrence after surgery prevented, by maintaining a high rate of urine flow (at least 3 litres per 24 hours) especially at night, and by giving sufficient bicarbonate to keep the urine alkaline. If this regime is adopted, the patient should test the pH of each specimen of urine passed and increase the dose of bicarbonate if the urinary pH falls below about 7.0. Patients who are given allopurinol because of recurrent uric acid urolithiasis should have their urinary uric acid excretion measured to ensure that this remains within the reference range. Particular attention should be paid to the concentration of uric acid and to the pH of the most concentrated (early morning) specimen of urine passed during the 24 hour period.

21.9. PRIMARY RENAL DISEASE AND URIC ACID DISORDERS

21.9.1. Chronic renal failure

This subject has been dealt with (section 21.8.2) in relation to the differential diagnosis of chronic urate nephropathy. Patients on intermittent haemodialysis may be hyperuricaemic for an appreciable length of time between each dialysis, and they sometimes experience attacks resembling acute gouty arthritis. However, these appear to be related to the development of periarticular metastatic calcifications consisting of apatite, rather than to a crystal synovitis due to either monosodium urate monohydrate (gout) or to calcium pyrophosphate (pseudogout, chondrocalcinosis).

21.9.2. Renal tubule re-absorption defects

Hypouricaemia with a correspondingly increased urinary excretion of uric acid may result from an isolated renal tubule re-absorption defect (Praetorious and Kirk, 1950; Simkin et al., 1974) as in the Dalmation coachhound. It may also occur in association with other renal tubule reabsorption defects which, when they co-exist, constitute the Fanconi syndrome.

21.10. XANTHINURIA (CONGENITAL XANTHINE OXIDASE DEFICIENCY)

21.10.1. Definition of the syndrome

Dent and Philpot (1954) proposed xanthine oxidase deficiency as the metabolic lesion to explain their observation that a girl with a xanthine urinary stone had very low levels of uric acid in her blood and urine, but excreted abnormally large amounts of xanthine. This patient was studied again by Dickinson and Smellie (1959) who confirmed the earlier biochemical findings and found that the patient excreted hypoxanthine as well as xanthine. She was also studied by Gibbs et al. (1976) * when she was lactating; both colostrum and milk lacked xanthine oxidase activity, as judged by an ultrasensitive radiochemical assay, thus confirming the original prediction of Dent and Philpot (1954). The milk also contained no immunochemically detectable xanthine oxidase protein, and this is compatible with xanthinuria being due to a no-sense as opposed to a mis-sense mutation (Gibbs et al., 1976). The enzyme defect was first demonstrated by Watts et al. (1964) in a jejunal mucosa biopsy and in liver tissue from a second documented case of the disorder. Chalmers et al. (1969a, c, d) described an additional complication, xanthinuric myopathy, in which hypoxanthine and xanthine crystals form in the skeletal muscles.

The exact status of the earlier cases of xanthine urolithiasis, the first of which was reported by Marcet in 1817, is uncertain owing to lack of chemical evidence. Some may have been cases of xanthinuria, but others were apparently normouricaemic or somewhat hyperuricaemic, and excreted normal amounts of uric acid. Some of the subjects may have been heterozygous for a mutant autosomal gene causing xanthinuria when present in the homozygous state, but the methods were not then available for measuring hypoxanthine and xanthine in body fluids.

21.10.2. Biochemical features of xanthinuria

There are at least 20 well-documented cases of xanthinuria in the literature and it is unlikely that further cases will be reported unless they show some unusual features (Watts, 1976). The diagnosis has been confirmed in 11 cases by direct enzyme assay of one of the following: small intestine mucosa, liver tissue, rectal mucosa, milk, colostrum, mixed leucocytes or platelets. Two sets of sibs with the disorder have been reported.

Urolithiasis occurs in about one-third of the patients, and this complication may begin in infancy or be delayed until adult life. Xanthine stones are usually smooth, round or oval, brownish yellow in colour and soft. They are radiotranslucent and, like other calculi, they may be clinically silent, or cause obstructive uropathy and predispose to recurrent urinary tract infection. Most patients have only had one episode of stone formation.

The majority of cases of xanthinuria are discovered incidentally in patients who are being investigated for other disorders. Hypouricaemia of the order observed in xanthinuria is uncommon, and plasma urate determinations are performed sufficiently frequently to suggest that there is no large residue of undiagnosed cases. Mikkelsen et al. (1965) found no plasma urate concentrations of less than 0.06 mmol/litre (1.0 mg/dl) in 6000 unselected individuals aged 4 years and over.

In xanthinuria, the plasma concentration and urinary uric acid excretion levels are less than 0.06 mmol/litre (1.0 mg/dl) and 0.30 mmol (50 mg) per 24 hours respectively, when the patient is taking an unrestricted diet and the measurements are made by a colorimetric method which depends upon the reduction of phosphotungstic acid. The results of determinations made when the patient is taking a purine-free diet and the analyst uses a differential spectrophotometric enzymatic method, are usually below 0.03 mmol/litre (0.5 mg/dl) and 0.09 mmol (15 mg) per 24 hours respectively. The levels of oxypurines

* We are indebted to the late Professor C.E. Dent, F.R.S. for allowing us to study this patient.

(hypoxanthine plus xanthine) normally present in plasma and urine are: 0.0 to 0.015 mmol/litre (0.0 to 0.25 mg/dl) and 0.07 to 0.13 mmol (11 to 22 mg) per 24 hours respectively. Corresponding values in xanthinuric patients are: 0.03 to 0.05 mmol/litre (0.5 to 0.9 mg/dl) and 0.60 to 3.6 mmol (100 to 600 mg) per 24 hours respectively for plasma and urine. Between 60 and 90% of the total oxypurine excretion is xanthine, and although the ratio of hypoxanthine to xanthine varies in different patients, it is approximately constant for a given individual.

The methods needed to establish the presence of abnormal amounts of hypoxanthine and xanthine in blood and urine, and of deficient tissue xanthine oxidase activity are referred to in section 21.2.2. The diagnosis can be made for routine clinical purposes on the basis of plasma and urine analyses for uric acid and oxypurines. The tissue enzyme activities may be needed, however, if it is proposed to investigate the genetics of the disorder.

21.10.3. Differential diagnosis

Xanthinuria has to be distinguished from other causes of abnormally low plasma urate concentration, i.e. less than 0.12 mmol/litre (2.0 mg/dl). Only allopurinol medication is associated with a decreased urinary uric acid excretion as well as hypouricaemia, but in therapeutic dosage it does not suppress the serum uric acid concentration to the very low levels which are observed in xanthinuria. Table 21.12 summarizes the recognized causes of hypouricaemia. This subject is also reviewed by Ramsdell and Kelley (1973).

Xanthine stones have to be differentiated from other radiotranslucent stones, namely uric acid stones, 2,8-dihydroxyadenine stones, and matrix stones, as well as from aggre-

TABLE 21.12.

CAUSES OF HYPOURICAEMIA (serum uric acid concentration less than 0.12 mmol/litre (2 mg/dl))

1. Reduced xanthine oxidase activity
   - (a) Congenital (xanthinuria)
   - (b) Drug induced (allopurinol)
2. Renal tubule uric acid reabsorption defect
   - (a) Congenital
     - (i) Isolated
     - (ii) Associated with other reabsorption defects in the Fanconi syndrome
   - (b) Drug induced
     - (i) Radiocontrast agents
       - Iopanoic acid (Telepaque)
       - Meglumine iodipamide (Cholografin)
       - Diatrizoate sodium (Hypaque)
     - (ii) Uricosuric agents (including aspirin) in excessive dosage
   - (c) Toxic damage to the renal tubules
3. Neoplastic disease
4. Extensive liver damage (? secondary xanthine oxidase deficiency)
5. Congenital PRPP synthetase deficiency
6. Congenital purine nucleoside phosphorylase deficiency

gates of acid crystals in orotic acidemia, detached renal papillae in renal papillary necrosis, blood clots, and pieces of tumour tissue. Identification may be made by differential spectrophotometry, X-ray diffraction, electrophoresis on paper, or by paper or ion exchange chromatography. Seegmiller (1968) described a procedure which gives unequivocal identification by spectrophotometric demonstration of the xanthine oxidase-catalyzed oxidation of xanthine to uric acid followed by the uricase-catalyzed oxidation of the uric acid.

21.10.4. Renal clearance of oxypurines

The renal clearance of oxypurines (hypoxanthine plus xanthine) is increased to about 80% of the glomerular filtration rate in xanthinuria. This is due to the increased filtered load of the oxypurines (Goldfinger et al., 1965) and not to an associated renal tubule reabsorption defect. Hypoxanthine and xanthine are cleared by the kidneys at about the same rate, and appear to be absorbed and secreted by the tubules (Chalmers et al., 1969a).

21.10.5. Residual xanthine oxidase activity in xanthinuria

Patients with xanthinuria excrete traces of uric acid in their urine even when taking a strict purine-free diet. Isotopically labelled xanthine gives rise to labelling of the uric acid in these subjects, and the administration of allopurinol increases the excretion of hypoxanthine at the expense of xanthine. These observations suggest that the small amount of uric acid which is excreted by xanthinuric patients is formed endogenously. This could be due to the activity of another enzyme or to the metabolic activity of gastrointestinal flora.

The preponderance of xanthine over hypoxanthine in the urine of xanthinuric patients may indicate that the mechanisms concerned have more activity for the first step in the oxidation than for the second. It is also partly explicable by the difference between the turnover rate of hypoxanthine and xanthine metabolic pools in vivo. The hypoxanthine pool is larger and has a greater turnover rate than the xanthine pool, although a larger proportion of the xanthine turnover is converted into uric acid. These observations also reflect the much greater activity of HGPRT with respect to hypoxanthine than to xanthine.

21.10.6. Genetics

Some families show a strict autosomal recessive pattern in inheritance, the presumably heterozygous individuals being completely normal, both clinically and from the point of view of their blood and urine uric acid and oxypurine levels. The xanthine oxidase activities of jejunal mucosa and milk have proved to be normal in two presumably heterozygous subjects from such families. In other families, the pattern is that of an incompletely recessive disorder, in that minor biochemical abnormalities can be detected in the presumably heterozygous individuals. These individuals excrete oxypurines in small amounts which are clearly intermediate between the levels excreted by the affected, presumably homozygous xanthinuric individual, and normal subjects; they have normal plasma and urine uric acid concentrations which may, however, be in the lower part of the normal range. Terhorst (1969) reported a patient with a xanthine stone, oxypurine excretion in the range encountered in complete xanthine oxidase deficiency, but plasma urate concentration and urinary uric acid excretion in the lower part of the normal range. This may be an example of yet another xanthinuric variant, although the authors suggested a renal tubule reabsorption defect. Increased urinary excretion of adenine in a case of xanthinuria has been reported (Castro-Mendoza et al., 1972) but other affected members of the family did not show this phenomenon and its significance is at the present time uncertain.

Another type of heterogeneity in xanthinuria has been claimed on the basis of the observation that some xanthinuric subjects oxidize allopurinol to oxipurinol, which is excreted in the urine, whereas others do not. It seems likely that such oxidation could be due to the action of aldehyde oxidase (EC 1.2.3.1) (Johns et al., 1969) rather than to metabolism of allopurinol by oxidation of a nucleotide analogue as originally suggested by Chalmers et al. (1969b). Further work is needed to establish the significance of the observations from a genetic point of view. A high incidence of consanguineous matings has not been reported in the pedigrees of families in which cases of xanthinuria have occurred. This is compatible with the condition being genetically heterogeneous.

21.11. XERODERMA PIGMENTOSUM

The association of abnormal cutaneous sensitivity to light of wavelength 280 to 310 nm, microcephaly, mental retardation and hypogonadism, is a striking clinical syndrome with an autosomal recessive pattern of inheritance. The skin manifestations progress from erythema, through a stage of multiple hypertrophic pigmented lesions with scarred atrophic telangiectactic areas. Multiple skin cancers develop. The biochemical lesion is deficiency of one of the DNA repair enzymes (EC 6.5.1.1 and 6.5.1.2) and the abnormality can be demonstrated in cultured fibroblasts and amniotic fluid cells. Other DNA repair enzyme defects have been reported in association with abnormal sensitivity to ionizing radiation in, for example, ataxia telangiectasia and Bloom's syndrome.

The effects of these metabolic lesions on the rate of purine biosynthesis and uric acid production have not been investigated, although widespread hyperplastic skin lesions in psoriasis are associated with changes in these functions.

REFERENCES

Aäkesson, I. and Alvsacker, J.O. (1971) The urate-binding alpha 1-2 globulin. Isolation and characterization of the protein from human plasma. European Journal of Clinical Investigation, 1, 281–287.

Adams, A. (1973) The Development, Distribution and Properties of Purine Phosphoribosyltransferase in Mammals. Ph.D. Thesis, University of Edinburgh.

Adams, A., Anderson, J.M., Nicol, A.D. and Harkness, R.A. (1971) The development of hypoxanthine-guanine phosphoribosyltransferase activity in man. Biochemical Journal, 125, 36P.

Adams, A. and Harkness, R.A. (1976) Developmental changes in purine phosphoribosyltransferase in human and rat tissues. Biochemical Journal, 160, 565–576.

Allison, A.C., Hovi, T., Watts, R.W.E. and Webster, A.D.B. (1975) Immunological observations on patients with Lesch–Nyhan syndrome, and on the role of de-novo purine synthesis in lymphocyte transformation. Lancet, i, 1179–1183.

Alvsacker, J.O. (1966) Uric acid in human plasma. V. Isolation and identification of plasma proteins interacting with urate. Scandinavian Journal of Clinical and Laboratory Investigation, 18, 227–239.

Alvsacker, J.O. and Seegmiller, J.E. (1972) Plasma concentrations of the urate-binding alpha 1-2 globulin in patients with different types of primary gout as compared to healthy control subjects. European Journal of Clinical Investigation, 2, 66–71.

Anumonye, A., Dobson, J.W., Oppenheim, S. and Sutherland, J.S. (1969) Plasma uric acid concentrations among Edinburgh business executives. Journal of American Medical Association, 208, 1141–1144.

Arnold, W.J. and Kelley, W.N. (1971) Human hypoxanthine-guanine phosphoribosyltransferase. Purification and subunit structure. Journal of Biological Chemistry, 246, 7398–7404.

Becker, M.A., Meyer, L.J. and Seegmiller, J.E. (1973a) Gout with purine overproduction due to increased phosphoribosylpyrophosphate synthetase activity. American Journal of Medicine, 55, 232–242.

Becker, M.A., Meyer, L.J., Wood, A.W. and Seegmiller, J.E. (1973b) Purine overproduction in man associated with increased phosphoribosylpyrophosphate synthetase activity. Science, 179, 1123–1126.

Becker, M.A. and Seegmiller, J.E. (1974) Genetic aspects of gout. Annual Review of Medicine, 25, 15–28.

Benedict, J.D., Forsham, P.H. and Stetten, DeW., Jr. (1949) Metabolism of uric acid in normal and gouty human studied with aid of isotopic uric acid. Journal of Biological Chemistry, 181, 183–193.

Benedict, J.D., Roche, M., Yü, T.F., Bien, E.J., Gutman, A.B. and Stetten, De. W., Jr. (1952) Incorporation of glycine nitrogen into uric acid in normal and gouty man. Metabolism, 1, 3–12.

Beighton, P., Solomon, L., Soskolne, C.L. and Sweet, B. (1973) Serum uric acid concentrations in a rural Tawana community in Southern Africa. Annals of Rheumatoid Diseases, 32, 346–350.

Borden, M., Nyhan, W.L. and Bakay, B. (1974) Increased activity of adenine phosphoribosyltransferase in erythrocytes of normal newborn infants. Pediatric Research, 8, 31–36.

Boyle, J.A. and Seegmiller, J.E. (1971) Preparation and processing of small samples of human material. In Methods in Enzymology, Vol. 22, Enzyme Purification and Related Techniques (Eds. S.P. Colowick, N.O. Kaplan and W.B. Jakoby) pp. 149–168, Academic Press, London.

Boyle, J.A., Raivio, K.O., Becker, M.A. and Seegmiller, J.E. (1972) Effects of nicotinic acid on human fibroblast purine biosynthesis. Biochimica et Biophysica Acta, 269, 179–183.

Bray, R.C. (1975) Molybdenum iron-sulfur flavin hydroxylases and related enzymes. In Enzymes, Vol. 12, 3rd edn. (Ed. P.D. Boyer) pp. 299–419, Academic Press, New York.

Brooks, G.W. and Mueller, E. (1966). Serum urate concentrations among university professors; relation to drive, achievement and leadership. Journal of American Medical Association, 195, 415–418.

Burch, T.A., O'Brien, W.M., Need, R. and Kurland, L.T. (1966). Hyperuricaemia and gout in the Mariana Islands. Annals of Rheumatoid Diseases, 25, 114–116.

Carcassi, A., Marcolongo, R., Jr., Marinello, E., Raivio-Sforzo, G. and Boggiano, C. (1969) Liver xanthine oxidase in gouty patients. Arthritis and Rheumatism, 12, 17–20.

Cartier, M.P. and Hamet, M. (1974) Une nouvelle maladie metabolique: le deficit complet en adénine-phosphoribosyltransferase avec lithiase de 2,8-dihydroxyadenine. Comptes Rendus Hebdomadaires des Seances de l'Academie des Sciences; D: Sciences Naturelles (Paris), D. 279, 883–886.

Castro-Mendoza, H.J., Cifuentes Delatte, L. and Rapado-Errazti, A. (1972) Una nueva observacion de xantinuria familiar. Revista Clinica Espanola, 124, 341–352.

Chalmers, R.A., Johnson, M., Pallis, C. and Watts, R.W.E. (1969a) Xanthinuria with myopathy (with some observations on the renal handling of oxypurines in the disease). Quarterly Journal of Medicine, 38, 493–512.

Chalmers, R.A., Krömer, H., Scott, J.T. and Watts, R.W.E. (1968) A comparative study of the xanthine oxidase inhibitors allopurinol and oxipurinol in man. Clinical Science, 35, 353–362.

Chalmers, R.A., Parker, R., Simmonds, H.A., Snedden, W. and Watts, R.W.E. (1969b) The conversion of 4-hydroxypyrazolo (3,4-d)pyrimidine (allopurinol) into 4,6-dihydroxypyrazolo(3,4-d)pyrimidine (oxipurinol) in vivo in the absence of xanthine-oxygen oxidoreductase. Biochemical Journal, 112, 527–532.

Chalmers, R.A. and Watts, R.W.E. (1968) An enzymatic spectrophotometric method for the determination of "oxypurines" (hypoxanthine plus xanthine) in urine and blood plasma. Analyst, 93, 354–362.

Chalmers, R.A. and Watts, R.W.E. (1969) The separate determination of xanthine and hypoxanthine in urine and blood plasma by an enzymatic differential spectrophotometric method. Analyst, 94, 226–233.

Chalmers, R.A., Watts, R.W.E., Bitensky, L. and Chayen, J. (1969c) Microscopic studies on crystals in skeletal muscle from two cases of xanthinuria. Journal of Pathology, 99, 45–56.

Chalmers, R.A., Watts, R.W.E., Pallis, C., Bitensky, L. and Chayen, J. (1969d) Crystalline deposits in striped muscle in xanthinuria. Nature (London), 221, 170–171.

Changas, G.S. and Milman, G. (1975). Radioimmune determination of hypoxanthine phosphoribosyltransferase cross reacting material in erythrocytes of Lesch–Nyhan patients. Proceedings of the National Academy of Sciences, 72, 4147–4150.

Chayen, J. and Denby, E.F. (1968) Biophysical Technique as Applied to Cell Biology, Methuen, London, pp. 32–41.

Chow, D.C., Kawahara, F.S., Saunders, T. and Sorensen, L.B. (1970) A new assay method for hypoxanthine-guanine phosphoribosyltransferase. Journal of Laboratory and Clinical Medicine, 76, 733–738.

Cobb, S. (1963) Hyperuricaemia in executives. In Epidemiology of Chronic Rheumatism Vol. 1 (Ed. J.H. Kellgren) pp. 182–186, Blackwell, Oxford.

Coleman, M., Landgrebe, M. and Landgrebe, A. (1974) Progressive seizures with hyperuricosuria reversed by allopurinol. Archives of Neurology, 31, 238–242.

Colowick, S.P. and Kaplan, N.O. (Eds.) (1955–1975) Methods in Enzymology, Vols. I–XXIV. Academic Press, New York and London.

Craft, J.A., Dean, B.M., Watts, R.W.E. and Westwick, W.J. (1970) Studies on human erythrocyte IMP: pyrophosphate phosphoribosyltransferase. European Journal of Biochemistry, 15, 367–373.

Currey, H.L.F. (1968) Examination of joint fluids for crystals. Proceedings of the Royal Society of Medicine, 61, 969–971.

Dawson, R.M.C., Elliott, D.C., Elliott, W.H. and Jones, K.M. (Eds.) (1969) Data for Biochemical Research, 2nd edn. Oxford University Press, London.

Decker, J.L., Lane, J.J., Jr. and Reynolds, W.E. (1962) Hyperuricaemia in a male Filipino population. Arthritis and Rheumatism, 5, 144–155.

Dent, C.E. and Philpot, G.R. (1954) Xanthinuria, an inborn error (or deviation) of metabolism. Lancet, i, 182–185.

Dickinson, C.J. and Smellie, J.M. (1959) Xanthinuria. British Medical Journal, ii, 1217–1221.

Dodge, J.H. and Mikkelsen, W.M. (1970). Observations on the distribution of serum uric acid levels in participants of the Tecumseh, Michigan, Community Health Studies. A comparison of results of one method used at two different times, and of two methods used simultaneously. Journal of Chronic Diseases, 23, 161–172.

Dunn, J.P., Brooks, G.W., Mausner, J., Rodnan, G.P. and Cobb, S. (1963) Social class gradient of serum uric acid levels in males. Journal of American Medical Association, 185, 431–436.

Emmerson, B.T., Douglas, W., Doherty, R.L. and Feigl, P. (1969) Serum urate concentrations in the Australian aboriginal. Annals of Rheumatoid Diseases, 28, 150–156.

Emmerson, B.T. and Sandilands, P. (1963) The normal range of plasma urate levels. Australiasian Annals of Medicine, 12, 46–52.

Emmerson, B.T. and Thompson, L. (1973) The spectrum of hypoxanthine-guanine phosphoribosyltransferase deficiency. Quarterly Journal of Medicine, 42, 423–440.

Emmerson, B.T. and Wyngaarden, J.B. (1969) Purine metabolism in heterozygous carriers of hypoxanthine-guanine phosphoribosyltransferase deficiency. Science, 166, 1533–1535.

Engelman, K., Watts, R.W.E., Klinenberg, J.R., Sjoerdsma, A. and Seegmiller, J.E. (1964) Clinical, physiological and biochemical studies of a patient with xanthinuria and pheochromocytoma. American Journal of Medicine, 37, 839–861.

Fanelli, G.M. and Beyer, K.H. (1974) Uric acid in non-human primates with special reference to its renal transport. Annual Review of Pharmacology, 14, 355–364.

Fanelli, G.M. Jr. and Weiner, I.M. (1973) Pyrazinoate excretion in the chimpanzee. Relation to urate disposition and the actions of uricosuric drugs. Journal of Clinical Investigation, 52, 1946–1957.

Flatz, G. (1971) Genetic and constitutional influences on serum-uric-acid in a tropical rural population. Humangenetik, 11, 83–90.

Ford, D.K. and de Mos, A.M. (1964) Serum uric acid levels of healthy Caucasian, Chinese and Haida Indian males in British Columbia. Canadian Medical Association Journal, 90, 1295–1297.

Fox, I.H. and Kelley, W.N. (1971) Phosphoribosylphosphate in man: biochemical and clinical significance. Annals of Internal Medicine, 74, 424–433.

Fox, I.H. and Kelley, W.N. (1972) Studies on the mechanism of fructose-induced hyperuricaemia in man. Metabolism, 21, 713–721.

Fox, I.H. and Kelley, W.N. (1974) Human phosphoribosyl pyrophosphate (PP-ribose-P) synthetase: properties and regulation. In Advances in Experimental and Medical Biology (Eds. O. Sperling, A. De Vries and J.B. Wyngaarden) pp. 79–86; 463–470, Plenum Press, New York and London.

Frith, C., Johnston, E., Joseph, M.H., Powell, R.J. and Watts, R.W.E. (1976) A double-blind clinical trial of 5-hydroxytryptophan in a case of Lesch–Nyhan syndrome. Journal of Neurology, Neurosurgery and Psychiatry, 39, 656–662.

Fujimoto, W.Y., Seegmiller, J.E., Uhlendorf, B.W. and Jacobson, C.B. (1968) Biochemical diagnosis of an X-linked disease in utero. Lancet, ii, 511–512.

Fujimoto, W.Y., Subak-Sharpe, J.H. and Seegmiller, J.E. (1971) Hypoxanthine-guanine phosphoribosyltransferase deficiency: chemical agents selective for mutant or normal cultured fibroblasts in mixed and heterozygote cultures. Proceedings of the National Academy of Science, 68, 1516–1519.

Gibbs, D.A., Allsop, J. and Watts, R.W.E. (1976) Absence of xanthine oxidase (EC 1.2.3.2) from a xanthine uric patient's milk. Journal of Molecular Medicine, 1, 167–170.

Giblett, E.R., Ammann, A.J., Wara, D.W., Sandman, R. and Diamond, L.K. (1975) Nucleoside-phosphorylase deficiency in a child with severely defective T-cell immunity and normal B-cell immunity. Lancet, i, 1010–1013.

Giblett, E.R., Anderson, J.E., Cohen, F., Pollara, B. and Meuwissen, H.J. (1972) Adenosine-deaminase deficiency in two patients with severely impaired cellular immunity. Lancet, ii, 1067–1069.

Gochman, N. and Schmitz, J.M. (1971) Automated determination of uric acid, with use of a uricase-peroxidase system. Clinical Chemistry, 17, 1154–1159.

Goldfinger, S., Klinenberg, J.R. and Seegmiller, J.E. (1965) The renal excretion of oxypurines. Journal of Clinical Investigation, 44, 623–628.

Gordon, R.B., Thompson, L. and Emmerson, B.T. (1974) Erythrocyte phosphoribosylpyrophosphate concentrations in heterozygotes for hypoxanthine-guanine phosphoribosyltransferase deficiency. Metabolism, 23, 921–927.

Grayzel, A.I., Liddle, L. and Seegmiller, J.E. (1961) Diagnostic significance by hyperuricaemia in arthritis. New England Journal of Medicine, 265, 763–768.

Griebsch, A. and Zöllner, N. (1974) Effect of ribomononucleotides given orally on uric acid production in man. In Advances in Experimental and Medical Biology (Eds. O. Sperling, A. De Vries and J.B. Wyngaarden) pp. 443–449, Plenum Press, New York and London.

Gutensohn, W. (1973) Purification and characterization of a neutral hypoxanthine-guanine-phosphoribosyltransferase (HGPRT). In Advances in Experimental and Medical Biology (Eds. O. Sperling, A. De Vries and J.B. Wyngaarden) pp. 19–22, Plenum Press, New York and London.

Gutman, A.B. and Yü, T.F. (1957) Renal function in gout, with a commentary on the renal regulation of urate excretion and the role of the kidney in the pathogenesis of gout. American Journal of Medicine, 23, 600–622.

Gutman, A.B., Yu, T.F. and Berger, L. (1959) Tubular secretion of urate in man. Journal of Clinical Investigations, 38, 1178–1181.

Gutensohn, W. and Guroff, G. (1972) Hypoxanthine-guanine-phosphoribosyl-transferase from rat brain (purification, kinetic properties, development and distribution). Journal of Neurochemistry, 19, 2139–2150.

Hall, A.P., Barry, P.E., Dawbar, T.R. and McNamara, P.M. (1967) Epidemiology of gout and hyperuricaemia. A long-term population study. American Journal of Medicine, 42, 27–37.

Harkness, R.A. and Nicol, A.D. (1969) Plasma uric acid levels in children. Archives of Diseases of Childhood, 44, 773–778.

Hauge, M. and Harvald, B. (1955) Hereditary in gout and hyperuricaemia. Acta Medica Scandinavica, 152, 247–257.

Healey, L.A., Caner, J.E.Z., Bassett, D.R. and Decker, J.L. (1966a). Serum uric acid and obesity in Hawiians. Journal of American Medical Association, 196, 364–365.

Healey, L.A., Caner, J.E.Z. and Decker, J.L. (1966b) Ethnic variations in serum uric acid Filipino hyperuricaemia in a controlled environment. Arthritis and Rheumatism, 9, 288–294.

Healey, L.A., Skeith, M.D., Decker, J.L. and Banyani-Sioson, P.S. (1967) Hyperuricaemia in Filipinos: interaction of hereditary and environment. American Journal of Human Genetics, 19, 81–85.

Henderson, J.F. (1962) Feedback inhibition of purine biosynthesis in ascites tumour cells. Journal of Biological Chemistry, 237, 2631–2635.

Hershko, A., Razin, A. and Mager, J. (1969) Regulation of the synthesis of 5-phosphoribosyl-1-pyrophosphate in red blood cells of some gouty patients. Biochimica et Biophysica Acta, 184, 64–76.

Holmes, E.W., Jr., MacDonald, J.A., McCord, J.M., Wyngaarden, J.B. and Kelley, W.N. (1973a) Human glutamine phosphoribosylpyrophosphate amidotransferase. Two moleculer forms interconvertible by purine ribonucleotides and phosphoribosyl pyrophosphate. Journal of Biological Chemistry, 248, 144–150.

Holmes, E.W., Jr., Wyngaarden, J.B. and Kelley, W.N. (1973c) Human glutamine phosphoribosylpyrophosphate (PP-ribose-P) amidotransferase: kinetic, regulation and configurational changes. In Advances in Experimental and Medical Biology (Eds. O. Sperling, A. De Vries and J.B. Wyngaarden) pp. 43–53, Plenum Press, New York and London.

Hooft, C., van Nevel, C. and de Schaepdryver, A.F. (1968) Hyperuricosuric encephalopathy without hyperuricaemia. Archives of Diseases of Childhood, 43, 734–737.

Hovi, T., Allison, A.C. and Watts, R.W.E. (1975) Rapid increase of phosphoribosyl pyrophosphate concentration after mitogenic stimulation of lymphocytes. Federation of European Biochemical Societies Letters, 55, 291–293.

Ismail, A.A.A. and Dakin, T.A. (1975) Gas chromatography and characterization of tetraethyl derivatives of uric acid. Journal of Chromatography, 110, 182–186.

Itiaba, K., Banfalvi, M. and Crawhall, J.C. (1973) Metabolism of purines in cultured normal and HPRT-deficient human fibroblasts. Biochemical Genetics, 8, 149–156.

Johns, D.G., Spector, T. and Robins, R.K. (1969) Studies on the mode of oxidation of pyrazolo-(3,4-d)pyrimidine by aldehyde oxidase and xanthine oxidase. Biochemical Pharmacology, 18, 2371–2383.

Johnson, S.M., North, M.E., Asherson, G.L., Allsop, J., Watts, R.W.E. and Webster, A.D.B. (1977) Lymphocyte purine 5′-nucleotidase deficiency in primary hypogammaglobulinaemia. Lancet, i, 168–170.

Kageyama, N. (1971) A direct colorimetric determination of uric acid in serum and urine with uricase-catalase. Clinica Chimica Acta, 31, 421–426.

Kaufman, J.M., Green, M.L. and Seegmiller, J.E. (1968) Urine uric acid to creatinine ratio – a screening test for inherited disorders of purine metabolism. Phosphoribosyltransferase (PRT) deficiency in X-linked cerebral palsy and in a variant of gout. Journal of Pediatrics, 73, 583–592.

Kelley, W.N. and Beardmore, T.D. (1970) Allopurinol: alteration in pyrimidine metabolism in man. Science, 169, 388–390.

Kelley, W.N., Greene, M.L., Rosenbloom, F.M., Henderson, J.F. and Seegmiller, J.E. (1969) Hypoxanthine-guanine phosphoribosyltransferase deficiency in gout. Annals of Internal Medicine, 70, 155–206.

Kelley, W.N. and Meade, J.C. (1971) Studies on hypoxanthine-guanine phosphoribosyltransferase fibroblasts from patients with the Lesch-Nyhan syndrome. Journal of Biological Chemistry, 246, 2953–2958.

Kelley, W.N., Meade, J.C. and Evans, M.C. (1971) Studies on the adenine phosphoribosyltransferase enzyme in human fibroblasts lacking hypoxanthine-guanine phosphoribosyltransferase. Journal of Laboratory and Clinical Medicine, 77, 33–38.

Kelley, W.N. and Wyngaarden, J.B. (1974) Enzymology of gout. Advances in Enzymology, 41, 1–33.

Kippen, I., Whitehouse, M.W. and Klinenberg, J.R. (1974) Pharmacology of uricosuric drugs. Annals of Rheumatoid Diseases, 33, 391–396.

Klinenberg, J.R., Goldfinger, S.E. and Seegmiller, J.E. (1965) The effectiveness of the xanthine oxidase inhibitor allopurinol in the treatment of gout. Annals of Internal Medicine, 62, 639–647.

Korn, E.D. (1957) Purines and Pyrimidines. In Methods in Enzymology (Eds. S.P. Colowick and N.O. Kaplan) pp. 615–642, Academic Press, New York.

Kramp. R.A., Lassiter, W.E. and Gottschalk, C.W. (1971) Urate-2-^{14}C transport in the rat nephron. Journal of Clinical Investigation, 50, 35–48.

Long, W.K. (1967) Glutathione reductase in red blood cells: variant associated with gout. Science, 155, 712–713.

Long, W.K. (1970) Association between glutathione reductase variants and plasma uric acid concentration in a Negro population (abstract). American Journal of Human Genetics, 22, 14a–15a.

Marcet, A. (1817) An Essay on the Chemical History and Medical Treatment of Calculous Disorders. Longman, London.

Mager, J., Hershko, A., Zeitlen-Beck, R., Shoshani, T. and Razin, A. (1967) Turnover of purine nucleotides in rabbit erythrocytes. I Studies in vivo. Biochimica et Biophysica Acta, 149, 50–58.

Marcolongo, R., Marinello, E., Pompucci, G. and Pagani, R. (1974) The role of xanthine oxidase in hyperuricaemic states. Arthritis and Rheumatism, 17, 430–438.

Marinello, E., Carcassi, A., Riaio-Sforza, G., Ciccoli, L. and Marcolongo, R. Jr., (1969) Essetto dei vari sostanse iperucicemizzasti sulla xanthina-ossidarfi patica di soggetti normale. Reumatismo, 21, 310–311.

McKeran, R.O., Andrews, T.M., Howell, A., Gibbs, D.A., Chinn, S. and Watts, R.W.E. (1975) The diagnosis of the carrier state for the Lesch-Nyhan syndrome. Quarterly Journal of Medicine, 44, 189–205.

Meyskens, F.L. and Williams, H.E. (1971) Concentration and synthesis of phosphoribosylpyrophosphate in erythrocytes from normal, hyperuricemic, and gouty subjects. Metabolism, 20, 737–742.

Mikkelsen, W.M., Dodge, H.J. and Valkenberg, H. (1965) The distribution of serum uric acid values in a population unselected as to gout or hyperuricemia: Tecumseh, Michigan, 1959–1960. American Journal of Medicine, 39, 242–251.

Milne, M.D. (1966) Urate excretion. Proceedings of the Royal Society of Medicine, 59, 308–310.

Mizuno, T. and Yugari, Y. (1974) Letter: Self-mutilation in Lesch–Nyhan syndrome. Lancet, i, 761.

Morgan, L.L., Schneiderman, N. and Nyhan, W.L. (1970) Theophylline: induction of self-biting in rabbits. Psychonomic Science, 19, 37–38.

Müller, M.M. (1974) Die Isoenzyme der Purin-Phosphoribosyltransferase im Erythrocytes bei Lesch–Nyhan syndrom. Zeitschrift für Klinische Chemie und Klinische Biochemie (Berlin), 12, 28–32.

Müller, M.M. and Stemberger, H. (1974) Biochemische und immunologische Untersuchungen der Hypoxanthin-Guanin-Phosphoribosyltransferase in den Erythrozyten von Lesch–Nyhan Patienten. Wiener Klinische Wochenschrift, 86, 127–131.

Murray, A.W. (1971) The biological significance of purine salvage. Annual Review of Biochemistry, 40, 811–826.

Nishizawa, T., Nishida, Y., Akaoka, I. and Yoshimura, T. (1975) Erythrocyte adenosine deaminase and purine nucleoside phosphorylase activity in gout. Clinica Chimica Acta, 58, 277–282.

Nyhan, W.L. (1968) In: Seminars on Lesch–Nyhan syndrome (Summary). Federation Proceedings, 27, 1044–1046.

Nyhan, W.L., Bakay, B., Connor, J.D., Marks, J.F. and Keele, D.K. (1970) Hemizygous expression of glucose-6-phosphate dehydrogenase in erythrocytes of heterozygotes for the Lesch–Nyhan syndrome. Proceedings of the National Academy of Sciences, 65, 214–218.

Nyhan, W.L., James, J.A., Teberg, A.J., Sweetman, L. and Nelson, L.G. (1969) A new disorder of purine metabolism with behavioural manifestations. Journal of Pediatrics, 74, 20–27.

O'Brien, W.M., Burch, T.A. and Bunim, J.J. (1966) Genetics of hyperuricaemia in Blackfeet and Pima Indians. Annals of Rheumatoid Diseases, 25, 117–119.

Oliver, I., Sperling, O., Liberman, U.A., Frank, M. and De Vries, A. (1971) Deficiency of xanthine oxidase activity in colostrum of a xanthinuric female. Biochemical Medicine. 5. 279–280.

Passwell, J., Boichis, H., Orda, S. and Buish, M. (1974) Uric acid excretion in infants. Advances in Experimental Medicine and Biology, 41A, 753–758.

Peters, J.P. and Van Slyke, D.D. (1932) Uric acid. In Quantitative Clinical Chemistry, Vol. 2. Methods, 1st edn. pp. 586–596, Williams and Wilkins, Baltimore.

Pollak, V.E. and Mattenheimer, H. (1965) Glutaminase activity in the kidney in gout. Journal of Laboratory and Clinical Medicine, 66, 564–570.

Popert, A.J. and Hewitt, J.V. (1962) Gout and hyperuricaemia in rural and urban populations. Annals of Rheumatoid Diseases, 20, 154–163.

Postlethwaite, A.E. and Kelley, W.N. (1971) Uricosuric effects of radio contrast agents. A study in man of four commonly used preparations. Annals of Internal Medicine, 74, 845–851.

Praetorius, E. and Kirk, J.E. (1950) Hypouricemia: with evidence for tubular elimination of uric acid. Journal of Laboaratory and Clinical Medicine, 35, 865–868.

Prior, I.A.M., Rose, B.S., Harvey, H.P.B. and Davidson, F. (1966) Hyperuricaemia, gout and diabetic abnormality in Polynesian people. Lancet, i. 333–338.

Riario-Sforza, G., Carcassi, A., Bayeli, P.F., Marcolongo, R., Marinello, E. and Montagnani, M. (1969) Attivita xentina-ossidasici nella mucofa digiunale di soggetti gottosi. Bollettino della Societa Italiana di Biologia Sperimentale, 45, 785–786.

Ramsdell, C.M. and Kelley, W.N. (1973) The clinical significance of hypouricemia. Annals of Internal Medicine, 78, 239–242.

Randrup, A. and Munkvad, I. (1966) Role of catecholamines in the excitatory response. Nature (London), 211, 540.

Reem, G.H. (1972) De novo purine biosynthesis by two pathways in Burkitt lymphoma cells and in human spleen. Journal of Clinical Investigation, 51, 1058–1062.

Reem. G.H. (1974) Enzymatic synthesis of phosphoribosylamine in human cells. Journal of Biological Chemistry, 249, 1696–1703.

Rosenbloom, F.M., Henderson, J.F., Caldwell, I.C., Kelley, W.N. and Seegmiller, J.E. (1968) Biochemical bases of accelerated purine biosynthesis de novo in human fibroblasts lacking hypoxanthine-guanine phosphoribosyltransferase. Journal of Biological Chemistry, 243, 1166–1173.

Ryman, B.E. (1974) The glycogen storage diseases. Journal of Clinical Pathology, 27, Suppl. (Royal College of Pathology), 8, 106–121.

Sandler, J.A., Clyman, R.I., Manganiello, V.C. and Vaughan, M. (1975) The effect of serotonin (5-hydroxytryptamine) and derivatives on guanosine 3',5'-monophosphate in human monocytes. Journal of Clinical Investigation, 55, 431–435.

Schlossberg, M.A. and Hollander, V.P. (1973) A rapid radiochemical assay for hypoxanthine-guanine phosphoribosyltransferase. Analytical Biochemistry, 55, 9–15.

Schulman, J.D., Greene, M.L., Fujimoto, W.Y. and Seegmiller, J.E. (1971) Adenine therapy for Lesch–Nyhan syndrome. Pediatric Research, 5, 77–82.

Seegmiller, J.E. (1967) Techniques for evaluating uricosuric agents and inhibitors of uric acid production. In Animal and Clinical Pharmacological Techniques in Drug Evaluation, Vol. 2 (Eds. P.E. Siegler and J.H. Moyer) pp. 729–741, Year Book Medical Publishers Inc, Chicago.

Seegmiller, J.E. (1968) Xanthine stone formation. American Journal of Medicine, 45, 780–783.

Seegmiller, J.E. (1969) Diseases of purine and pyrimidine metabolism. In Duncan's Diseases of Metabolism (Eds. P.K. Bondy and L.E. Rosenberg) pp. 655–774, W.B. Saunders, Philadelphia.

Seegmiller, J.E., Grayzel, A.I., Laster, L. and Liddle, L. (1961) Uric acid production in gout. Journal of Clinical Investigation, 40, 1304–1314.

Seegmiller, J.E., Laster, L. and Stetten, D. Jr. (1955) Incorporation of 4-amino-5-imid-azolecarboxamide-4-C^{13} into uric acid in the normal human. Journal of Biological Chemistry, 216, 653–662.

Seegmiller, J.E., Rosenbloom, F.M. and Kelley, W.N. (1967) Enzyme defect associated with a sex-linked neurological disorder and excessive purine synthesis. Science, 155, 1682–1684.

Simkin, P.A., Skeith, M.D. and Healey, L.A. (1974) Suppression of uric acid secretion in a patient with renal hypouricemia. In Advances in Experimental Medicine and Biology (Eds. O. Sperling, A. De Vries and J.B. Wyngaarden) pp. 723–728, Plenum Press, New York and London.

Simmonds, H.A., Van Acker, K.J., Cameron, J.S. and Snedden, W. (1976) The identification of 2,8-dihydroxyadenine, a new component of urinary stones. Biochemical Journal, 157, 485–487.

Snedden, W. and Parker, R.B. (1971) Determination of volatile constituents of human blood and tissue specimens by quantitative high resolution mass spectrometry. Analytical Chemistry, 43, 1652–1656.

Snedden, W., Parker, R.B. and Watts, R.W.E. (1970) The quantitative high resolution mass spectrometry of human tissue volatiles; the determination of certain purines and purine analagues in the skeletal muscle of gout patients. In Advances in Mass Spectrometry, Vol. 5 (Ed. A. Quayle) pp. 742–745, The Institute of Petroleum, London.

Sober, H.A. (Ed.) (1970) Handbook of Biochemistry and Selected Data for Molecular Biology, 2nd edn. The Chemical Rubber Company, Cleveland, Ohio.

Sorensen, L.B. (1960) The elimination of uric acid in man studied by means of C^{14}-labelled uric acid. Uricolysis. Scandinavian Journal of Clinical and Laboratory Investigations, 12, Suppl. 54, 1–24.

Sperling, O., Boer, P., Persky-Brosh, S., Kanarek, E. and De Vries, A. (1972a) Altered kinetic property of erythrocyte phosphoribosylpyrophosphate synthetase in excessive purine production. European Journal of Clinical and Biological Research, 17, 703–706.

Sperling, O., Eilam, G., Persky-Brosh, S. and De Vries, A. (1972b) Accelerated erythrocyte 5-phosphoribosyl-1-pyrophosphate synthesis. A familial abnormality associated with excessive uric acid production. Biochemical Medicine, 6, 310–316.

Sperling, O., Eilam, G., Persky-Brosh, S. and De Vries, A. (1972c) Simpler method for the determination of 5-phosphoribosyl-1-pyrophosphate in red blood cells. Journal of Laboratory and Clinical Medicine, 79, 1021–1026.

Sperling, O., Frank, M., Ophir, R., Liberman, U.A., Adam, A. and de Vries, A. (1970) Partial deficiency of hypoxanthine-guanine phosphoribosyltransferase associated with gout and uric acid stones. European Journal of Clinical and Biological Research, 15, 942–947.

Steele, T.H. (1971) Control of uric acid excretion. New England Journal of Medicine, 284, 1193–1196.

Steele, T.H. and Rieselbach, R.E. (1967) The contribution of residual nephrons within the chronically diseased kidney to urate homeostasis in man. American Journal of Medicine, 43, 868–875.

Stetten, D. Jr. and Hearon, J.Z. (1959) Intellectual level measured by army classification battery and serum uric acid concentration. Science, 129, 1737.

Subak-Sharpe, J.H. (1969). Metabolic cooperation between cells. In Homeostatic Regulators: A Ciba Foundation Symposium (Eds. G.E.W. Wolstenholme and J. Knight) pp. 276–290, Churchill, London.

Terhorst, B. (1969) Xanthinsteine und Xanthinurie. Einkasuistischen Beitrag. Zeitschrift für Urologie, 62, 37–42.

Upchurch, K.S., Leyva, A., Arnold, W.F., Holmes, E.W. and Kelley, W.V. (1975) Hypoxanthine phosphoribosyltransferase deficiency: association of reduced catalytic activity with reduced levels of immunologically detectable enzyme protein. Proceedings of the National Academy of Sciences, 10, 4142–4146.

Valentine, W.N., Anderson, H.M., Paglia, D.E., Jaffe, E.R., Konrad, P.N. and Harris S.R. (1972) Studies on human erythrocyte nucleotide metabolism. II Nonspherocytic hemolytic anemia, high red cell ATP and ribosephosphate pyrophosphokinase (RPK, EC 2.7.6.1) deficiency. Blood, 39, 674–684.

Vessel, E.S., Passarenti, G.T. and Greene, F.E. (1970) Impairment of drug metabolism in man by allopurinol and nortriptyline. New England Journal of Medicine, 283, 1484–1488.

Wada, Y., Nishimura, Y., Tanabu, M., Yoshimura, Y., Jinuma, K., Yoshida, T. and Arakawa, T. (1974) Hypouricemic, mentally retarded infant with a defect of 5-phosphoribosyl-1-pyrophosphate synthetase of erythrocytes. Tohoku Journal of Experimental Medicine, 113, 149–157.

Wallach, M.B. and Gershon, S. (1971) Induction and antagonism of stereotyped behaviour in cats (abstract). Pharmacologist, 13, 230.

Watts, R.W.E. (1966) Uric acid production with particular reference to the role of xanthine oxidase and its inhibition. Proceedings of the Royal Society of Medicine, 59, 287–292.

Watts, R.W.E. (1972) Disorders of Purine Metabolism. In Eighth Symposium on Advanced Medicine (Ed. G. Neale) Pitman Medical, London.

Watts, R.W.E. (1974) Technical Bulletin No. 31. Determination of uric acid in blood and urine. Annals of Clinical Biochemistry, 11, 103–111.

Watts, R.W.E. (1976) Xanthinuria and xanthine stone formation. In Scientific Foundations of Urology (Eds. D.I. Williams and G.D. Chisholm) Heinemann, London.

Watts, R.W.E., Engelman, K., Klinenberg, J.R., Seegmiller, J.E. and Sjoerdsma, A. (1964) Enzyme defect in a case of xanthinuria. Nature (London), 201, 395–396.

Watts, R.W.E., Gibbs, D.A. and McKeran, R.O. (1975) Some aspects of the use of hair follicles for the biochemical study of inborn errors of metabolism. In Proceedings of the 11th Symposium of the Society for the Study of Inborn Errors of Metabolism (Eds. J. Holton and J.T. Ireland) pp. 27–35, Lancaster Medical and Technical Publishing Co.

Watts, R.W.E., McKeran, R.O., Brown, E., Andrews, T.M. and Griffiths, M.I. (1974) Clinical and biochemical studies on treatment of Lesch–Nyhan syndrome. Archives of Disease in Childhood, 49, 693–702.

Watts, R.W.E., Scott, J.T., Chalmers, R.A., Bitensky, L. and Chayen, J. (1971a) Microscopic studies on skeletal muscle in gout patients treated with allopurinol. Quarterly Journal of Medicine, 40, 1–14.

Watts, R.W.E., Snedden, W. and Parker, R.A. (1971b) A quantitative study of skeletal muscle purines and pyrazolo(3,4-d)pyrimidines in gout patients treated with allopurinol. Clinical Sciences, 41, 153–158.

Watts, R.W.E., Watts, J.E.M. and Seegmiller, J.E. (1965). Xanthine oxidase activity in human tissues and its inhibition by allopurinol (4-hydroxypyrazolo(3,4-d)pyrimidine). Journal of Laboratory and Clinical Medicine, 66, 688–697.

Weight, F.F., Petzold, G. and Greengard, P. (1974) Guanosine 3′,5′-monophosphate in sympathetic ganglia: increase associated with synaptic transmission. Science, 186, 942–944.

WHO Protein Advisory Group (ad hoc Working Group Meeting on Clinical Evaluation and Acceptable Nucleic Acid Levels of SCP for Human Consumption) (1975) Protein Advisory Group Bulletin, 5, 17–26.

Wood, A.W., Becker, M.A. and Seegmiller, J.E. (1973) Purine nucleotide synthesis in lymphoblasts cultured from normal subjects and a patient with Lesch–Nyhan syndrome. Biochemical Genetics, 9, 261–274.

Wood, M.H., Fox, R.M., Vincent, L., Reye, C. and O'Sullivan, W.J. (1972) The Lesch–Nyhan syndrome: report of three cases. Australian and New Zealand Journal of Medicine, 1, 57–64.

Wood, A.W. and Seegmiller, J.E. (1973) Properties of 5-phosphoribosyl-1-pyrophosphate amidotransferase from human lymphoblasts. Journal of Biological Chemistry, 248, 138–143.

Wyngaarden, J.B. and Kelley, W.N. (1978) Gout. In The Metabolic Basis of Inherited Disease (Eds. J.B. Stanbury, J.B. Wyngaarden and D.S. Fredrickson) 4th edn., pp. 916–1010, McGraw-Hill Inc, New York.

Zöllner, N. (1963) Eine einfach Modifikation der enzymatischen der Hannsäurebestimmung. Zeitschrift für Klinische Chemie, 6, 178–182.

Zöllner, N. and Griebsch, A. (1974) Diet and gout. In Advances in Experimental Medicine and Biology

(Eds. O. Sperling, A. De Vries and J.B. Wyngaarden) pp. 435–442, Plenum Press, New York and London.

Zöllner, N., Griebsch, A. and Gröbner, W. (1972) Einfluss verscheidener Purine auf den Hannsäurestoffwechsel. Ernährungs-Umschau, 19, 79–82.

FURTHER READING

Becker, M.A. and Seegmiller, J.E. (1974) Annual Reviews in Medicine, 25, 15–28.

Boyle, J.A. and Seegmiller, J.E. (1971) In Methods in Enzymology, Vol. 22, Enzyme Purification and Related Techniques (Eds. S.P. Colowick, N.O. Kaplan and W.B. Jakoby) pp. 149–168, Academic Press, London.

Bray, R.C. (1975) In Enzymes, Vol. 12, 3rd edn. (Ed. P.D. Boyer) pp. 219–419, Academic Press, New York.

Elliot, K. and Fitzsimons, D.W. (Eds.) (1977) Purine and Pyrimidine Metabolism. Ciba Foundation Symposium 48 (new series), Elsevier/North-Holland Biomedical Press, Amsterdam.

Fanelli, G.M. and Beyer, K.H. (1974) Annual Reviews in Pharmacology, 14, 355–364.

Fox. I.H. and Kelley, W.N. (1971) Annals of Internal Medicine, 74, 424–433.

Kelley, W.N. and Wyngaarden, J.B. (1974) Advances in Enzymology, 41, 1–33.

Kippen, I., Whitehouse, M.W. and Klinenberg, J.R. (1964) Annals of Rheumatic Diseases, 33, 391–396.

McKeran, R.O., Andrews, T.M., Howell, A., Gibbs, D.A., Chinn, S. and Watts, R.W.E. (1975) Quarterly Journal of Medicine, 44, 189–205.

McKeran, R.O. and Watts, R.W.E. (1978) In Recent Advances in Endocrinology and Metabolism (Ed. J.L.H. O'Riordan) Churchill-Livingstone, London.

Müller, M.M., Kaiser, E. and Seegmiller, J.E. (Eds.) (1977) Purine Metabolism in Man. Advances in Experimental Biology and Medicine, Vols. 76A and 76B. Plenum Press, New York.

Murray, A.W. (1971) Annual Reviews of Biochemistry, 40, 811–826.

Nyhan, W.L. (1973) Annual Reviews of Medicine, 24, 41–60.

Seegmiller, J.E. (1967) In Animal and Clinical Pharmacological Techniques in Drug Evaluation, Vol. 2. pp. 729–741, Year Book Publishers, Chicago.

Sperling, O., De Vries, A. and Wyngaarden, J.B. (Eds.) (1974) Advances in Experimental Medicine and Biology, Vols. 41A and 41B. Plenum Press, New York and London.

Steele, T.H. (1971) New England Journal of Medicine, 284, 1192–1196.

Watts, R.W.E. (1972) In Eighth Symposium on Advanced Medicine (Ed. G. Neale) pp. 285–307, Heinemann, London.

Watts, R.W.E. (1974) Annals of Clinical Biochemistry, 11, 103–111.

Watts, R.W.E. (1974) Journal of Clinical Pathology, 27, Suppl. 8, 48–63.

Watts, R.W.E. (1976) In Scientific Foundations of Urology, Vol. 1 (Eds. D.I. Williams and G.D. Chisholm) pp. 310–315, Heinemann, London.

Wyngaarden, J.B. and Kelley, W.N. (1978) In The Metabolic Basis of Inherited Disease, 4th edn. (Eds. J.B. Stanbury, J.B. Wyngaarden and D.S. Fredrickson) McGraw Hill, New York.

Zöllner, N. and Gröbner, W. (1976) Gicht Handbuch der inneren Medicin: Bd 7, Stoffwechselkrankheiten; T3, Springer, Berlin.

ADDENDUM

Some authorities now suggest that only about 1% of patients with primary gout have genuine hyperuric aciduria. Seegmiller et al. (1977) concluded that adenosine inhibits both T- and B-lymphocyte proliferation in adenosine deaminase deficiency. They also proposed that in purine nucleoside phosphorylase deficiency, accumulated inosine inhibits adenosine deaminase raising the concentration of adenosine sufficiently to inhibit the more sensitive T-cells selectively. Cohen et al. (1978) proposed that deoxyadenosine accumulates in adenosine deaminase deficiency and is converted to deoxy-ATP, which inhibits ribonucleotide reductase. Cyclic AMP and S-adenosylhomocysteine have also been proposed as the critical metabolites.

The lymphocyte 5′-nucleotidase activity in different types of primary hypogammaglobulinaemia was studied by Webster et al. (1978).

Allsop and Watts (1978) found that phytohaemagglutinin (PHA)-induced lymphocyte transformation is not associated with a change in the PRPP content of the cells or with changes in the specific activities of either PRPP-amidotransferase or PRPP-synthetase. This suggests that PRPP does not have the specific triggering role in relation to cell replication suggested by Hovi et al. (1975).

The neurotransmitter function of purine nucleotides has been established for ATP in some gastrointestinal autonomic neurones, and more widespread purinergic neurotransmission postulated (Burnstock, 1975).

Allsop, J. and Watts, R.W.E. (1978) The amidophosphoribosyltransferase (EC 2.4.2.14) and ribosephosphate pyrophosphokinase (EC 2.7.6.2) activities, and phosphoribosylpyrophosphate content of unstimulated and stimulated human lymphocytes. Journal of Molecular Medicine, 3, 105–110.

Burnstock, G. (1977) The purinergic nerve hypothesis. In Purine and Pyrimidine Metabolism, Ciba Foundation Symposium 48 (New Series). (Eds. K. Elliot and D. Fitzsimons) Elsevier/North-Holland, Biomedical Press, Amsterdam.

Cohen, A., Hirschhorn, R., Horowitz, S.D., Rubinstein, A., Polmar, S.H., Hong, R. and Martin, D.W. (1978) Deoxyadenosine triphosphate as a potentially toxic metabolite in adenosine deaminase deficiency. Proceedings of the National Academy of Sciences, 75, 472–476.

Seegmiller, J.E., Watanabe, T., Schreier, M.H. and Waldman, T.A. (1977) Immunological aspects of purine metabolism. Advances in Experimental Biology and Medicine. 76A, 412–433.

Webster, A.D.B., North, M., Allsop, J., Asherson, G.L. and Watts, R.W.E. (1978) Purine metabolism in lymphocytes from patients with primary hypogammaglobulinaemia. Clinical and Experimental Immunology, 31, 456–463.

Chapter 22

Vitamins

Hipolito V. Niño

Diagnostic Operations, Biological and Fine Chemicals Division, Beckman Instruments Inc., Fullerton, CA, U.S.A.

CONTENTS

Chemical diagnosis of disease, edited by S.S. Brown, F.L. Mitchell and D.S. Young

22.1. INTRODUCTION

Recent developments in total parenteral nutrition and the better understanding of the interactions between nutrients and drugs, particularly oral contraceptives, have stimulated the study of other conditions in which nutrition affects the care of patients or the health of populations.

Stress and cultural or economic factors influence the quantitative and qualitative composition of the diet, which can produce nutritional deficiencies, imbalances or excess. If these conditions are maintained for some time, they may cause disease or worsen existing disease.

Changes in the environment, especially those contributing to pollution, require continual study to determine the interactions of micronutrients, such as vitamins and trace elements, with pollutants. All these elements and compounds may influence essential physiological functions, although they are present in only minute concentrations in body fluids and tissues.

Historically, the relationship between diet and disease has been recognized by different cultures all over the world. The concept of the vitamin as used today was established by an English biochemist, Sir Frederick Gowland Hopkins, in 1906 to 1912. In 1911 Casimir Funk, a biochemist from Poland working in London, coined the word vitamine, later to be changed to vitamin. The study of the chemistry and physiology of the vitamins parallels the development of modern biochemistry.

Deficiencies of vitamins can often be recognized clinically even when a complete understanding of the mechanisms of action of the vitamins is lacking. This is true for some important vitamins such as A and C. The effect of vitamin D on the prevention of rickets has been known for a number of years. The modern work by DeLuca and his colleagues (1970, 1976) on the biochemical and physiological aspects of vitamin D, represents one of the highlights of contemporary biochemistry, and underlines the importance of vitamins as subjects for basic and clinical research.

Vitamin deficiency, to a varying degree, is a common cause of health impairment all over the world, and results from:

(a) restricted dietary intake (poverty, anorexia, physical deformity, food fads);

(b) decreased absorption (pancreatic and gastrointestinal disease, sprue);

(c) impaired storage or utilization (hepatic disease, renal disease);

(d) increased loss (renal disease);

(e) increased demand (pregnancy, lactation, growth, infection, extensive burns, stress);

(f) metabolic antagonism (selected medications).

On the other hand, toxicity occurs with ingestion of massive doses of vitamins A and D.

Vitamin deficiency is most frequently found as a component of a multiple nutritional deficit; however, under certain conditions a single vitamin deficiency can occur. The early classification of vitamins into fat-soluble and water-soluble, by McCollum and Davis, in 1915 at the University of Wisconsin, is still appropriate (McCollum, 1957). Water-soluble vitamins – those of the B complex and C – are readily absorbed and have a renal threshold. Short-term deficiencies of these vitamins are more likely to develop but they also respond promptly to supplementation. Fat-soluble vitamins (A, D, E, and K) require lipids and bile salts for absorption. They are stored in body tissues and normally are not present in the urine. Considerable time is required before a deficiency develops.

Methods for the measurement of vitamins are unfortunately not frequently available in clinical laboratories. However, increased clinical needs and the better understanding of the biochemical processes in which vitamins are involved have stimulated laboratories to provide analytical services for most vitamins. With modern developments in analytical instrumentation and automation it is foreseeable that in the not too distant future all vitamins will be commonly measured in a modern clinical laboratory.

There is now considerable literature on the diagnostic use of vitamins and only a summary is presented here with key references. This chapter is primarily concerned with practical applications in which the measurement of vitamins, or some of their metabolites, in body fluids contributes to a clinical diagnosis. Some nutritional and haematological aspects of vitamins, with special attention to folate and vitamin B_{12}, are discussed in Chapters 12 and 16 respectively.

A list of further reading is presented to assist in the evaluation of nutritional, clinical, or epidemiological situations in which vitamins play a prominent role. Topics that have been considered in this listing include:

(a) general nutrition in health and disease (Bogert et al., 1973; Goodhart and Shils, 1973; Pike and Brown, 1975);

(b) infant nutrition (Fomon, 1974);

(c) surgical nutrition (Ballinger et al., 1975);

(d) total parenteral nutrition (Fischer, 1976);

(e) effects of oral contraceptives (Butterworth and Sauberlich, 1975; Prasad et al., 1975, 1976; Anderson et al., 1976);

(f) nutrition misinformation (White, 1974);

(g) laboratory evaluation (Demetriou, 1974; Sauberlich et al., 1974; Nino and Shaw, 1976);

(h) population studies (Christakis, 1973; Schaefer, 1963; Sabry, 1973; Ten State Nutrition Survey, USA-DHEW, 1973);

(i) food and nutrition (Farber et al., 1966; Tannahill, 1973; Science, 1975; Eckholm and Record, 1976; Scientific American, 1976).

22.2. VITAMIN A

In 1915 McCollum and Davis described a growth promoting factor for young animals which had been extracted from certain fish oils and animal fats, and named it "fat-soluble A", later to become vitamin A (McCollum, 1957). Yet, deleterious effects on health resulting from its absence in the diet had been observed much earlier. About 1500 B.C. the Egyptians knew how to correct the inability to see in dim light (night blindness), by eating ox liver which is a rich source of vitamin A. Almost 1000 years later, Hippocrates made similar observations and recommendations to cure visual impairment associated with the composition of the diet. The historical attention given to a prominent visual defect can be interpreted as a measure of the magnitude and widespread occurrence of a specific nutritional deficiency.

Today vitamin A deficiency, to various degrees, remains one of the more frequent nutritional problems in developing areas of the world and a major cause of infantile blindness. Even in industrialized countries, nutrition surveys have demonstrated, particularly in young people, a low serum concentration of vitamin A, which is indicative of an inadequate dietary intake or reduced body stores. On the other hand, vitamin A toxicity has been reported in individuals who ingest repeated high doses of the vitamin and in explorers eating the liver of polar bears, which contains a large amount of the vitamin.

22.2.1. Sources and requirements

In nature, vitamin A is present in two forms – provitamin A and preformed vitamin A. Provitamin A occurs mainly in plants and is represented by a group of yellow and orange pigments, the carotenes, of which the more important are the α, β and γ configurations. The α and γ carotenes can be converted into equimolecular quantities of vitamin A; the β yields two molecules of the vitamin. In actual practice, the physiological conversion of the carotenes into vitamin A yields a reduced amount of the vitamin since it is dependent on the intestinal absorption of the carotenes. Dietary protein and lipids are required for the adequate absorption of vitamin A and carotenes. The conversion of carotenes into vitamin A is believed to take place in the intestinal wall and the liver.

Good dietary sources of provitamin A are carrots, beet greens, parsley, apricots, yellow melon, prunes and peaches. Preformed vitamin A is essentially of animal origin. Good dietary sources are whole milk, butter, cheese, eggs, liver, and certain fish oils, e.g. cod liver oil (Roels, 1967).

Requirements for vitamin A are expressed in terms of International Units (I.U.), which have the following equivalents:

1 I.U. = 0.30 μg retinol (vitamin A alcohol);
1 I.U. = 0.34 μg retinyl acetate;
1 I.U. = 0.60 μg all-trans β-carotene.

International units are based on biological activity, not on chemical structure. β-Carotene is the most effective provitamin; one molecule theoretically yields two molecules of vitamin A. Incomplete absorption of carotene and losses by oxidation decrease the effective yield of this conversion.

The recommended daily dietary allowances for vitamin A (National Academy of Sciences, 1974) are as follows:

Infants	1400 I.U.
1 to 3 years	2000 I.U.
4 to 6 years	2500 I.U.
7 to 10 years	3300 I.U.
11 to 14 years	5000 I.U.
over 14 years	5000 I.U.
Pregnancy	5000 I.U.
Lactation	6000 I.U.

Human milk contains about 53 μg/dl vitamin A (176 I.U./dl).

22.2.2. Functions

The role of vitamin A has been identified through recognition of the physiological impairment when deficiency occurs. Progress is being made in the elucidation of the biochemical mechanisms involved, but our present knowledge is still incomplete.

The participation of vitamin A in vision is the best known process and includes the oxidation of retinol to retinal, which is combined with opsin, a protein, to form rhodopsin which acts as a photoreceptor (Wald, 1943, 1953; Wald and Hubbard, 1950, 1957). In deficiency states this conversion is disrupted, causing a decreased adaptation of the retina to low light intensities or to darkness. This results in night blindness, one of the early indicators of the vitamin deficiency. Retinoic acid, an oxidation product of retinol, is not effective in restoring adequate vision. However, when it is given to young vitamin-deficient individuals it stimulates growth. This selective response suggests differences in metabolic function for related molecular structures with vitamin A activity.

Prolonged vitamin deficiency causes xerophthalmia, a term used to describe dryness of the conjunctiva and cornea which is followed by keratomalacia and extensive – usually irreversible – damage to the cornea. Physical disruption of tissues and infection are the ultimate cause of blindness. Continued severe deficiency, which usually involves other nutrients as well, produces a calculated mortality of 25%. It is estimated that vitamin A-related blindness affects about 50,000 to 100,000 infants worldwide per year. Vitamin A deficiency has been identified as a potential cause of sterility and teratogenesis by interfering with spermatogenesis, placental integrity and foetal viability.

There is evidence for other functions of vitamin A in the maintenance of the integrity of cellular and subcellular membrane structures, particularly in the epithelial cells of mucous membranes and as a participant in the biosynthesis of mucopolysaccharides. Vitamin A is also involved in bone growth and in the formation of tooth enamel (McLaren, 1967; Roels, 1967).

22.2.3. Biochemical diagnosis

The liver is the main organ for storage of vitamin A. The measurement of the vitamin content of this organ is possible at present only by tissue biopsy, a rather involved and complex procedure. Measurement of the serum concentration provides the most practical and frequently used way to assess the nutritional and metabolic availability of the vitamin. Early morning fasting specimens are preferable as they are less susceptible to the variability produced by the vitamin A content of recent meals. Repeated determinations are desirable since they can demonstrate an overall picture of the nutritional status of the vitamin, which is not possible with a single determination.

In healthy individuals, the serum concentration of vitamin A correlates fairly well with both the dietary intake and the stores in the liver. A low concentration indicates a decreased dietary intake and reduced liver reserves of vitamin A.

The serum concentration of vitamin A in healthy adults has a range of 400 to 700 μg/litre. Lower limits of acceptable values are 300 μg/litre for children and 200 μg/litre for adults. Serum concentrations of 100 μg/litre or less are an indication of definite deficiency as well as of severe depletion of liver stores (Moore, 1957; Sauberlich et al., 1974). Adult women have a slightly lower serum vitamin A concentration than men, but non-pregnant women taking oral contraceptives present moderately increased values.

Serum carotene measurements are of limited value for the nutritional evaluation of vitamin A. Not all naturally occurring carotenes are absorbed equally nor can all be converted into active forms of vitamin A. The serum concentration has a range in healthy adults that spans from 200 to 2700 μg/litre. A low serum carotene concentration is of diagnostic value in conditions in which acute dietary restrictions prevail, and in gastro-intestinal disease causing malabsorption of nutrients.

The most distinctive clinical symptoms of vitamin A deficiency are night blindness, xerophthalmia, keratomalacia, and follicular hyperkeratosis. All these conditions are associated with a low serum concentration of vitamin A. A decreased serum concentration of vitamin A may also occur with disease of the liver, gastrointestinal tract and pancreas, and in chronic nephritis, chronic infections, and pyrexia.

Vitamin A deficiency can be treated orally with oil-based preparations or emulsions of the vitamin. Intramuscular aqueous dispersions of the vitamin are recommended when it is not possible to administer the vitamin by mouth. Therapeutic doses of 30,000 I.U. daily for a few days, with a total dose of about 500,000 I.U. are recommended for severe deficiency (Moore, 1967). Oil-based intramuscular preparations of vitamin A are not beneficial to the patient.

Vitamin A toxicity results from the ingestion of massive or repeated large doses (50 to 100 times the recommended daily allowance) of the vitamin. In infants, the main symptoms are vomiting, irritability, anorexia, and transient hydrocephalus with a protuberant fontanelle. In adults, reported symptoms of vitamin A toxicity include headaches, drowsiness, restlessness, insomnia, irritability, joint and bone pain, loss of hair, dry skin and fatigue. In toxic states the serum concentration of vitamin A is elevated.

The conversion of carotene into vitamin A can yield enough vitamin to meet nutritional requirements. The conversion may be impeded in patients with hypothyroidism or diabetes mellitus. Hypercarotenaemia, often designated carotenaemia, usually results from the excessive ingestion of carotene-rich foods. This may be associated with hyperlipaemia and is characterized by a high serum carotene concentration and yellow-orange pigmentation of the skin. It does not produce toxicity.

The serum specimens to be used for vitamin A or carotene determinations must be free from haemolysis, protected from light, and analyzed promptly. If absolutely necessary, specimens may be kept frozen (–20°C) for up to 3 weeks. Prolonged storage of specimens in the frozen state increases chromogenicity in most photometric determinations, so producing artificially elevated estimates. Fluorometric determinations are also affected by prolonged frozen storage of the specimens. A laboratory diagnosis of vitamin A deficiency may be complemented by the measurement of serum proteins as an additional indicator of nutritional adequacy, and as a requirement for the mobilization of vitamin A reserves from the liver. Other tests that are of value in the work-up of a vitamin A deficiency include tests of gastrointestinal function and absorption, and tests of pancreatic and liver function. Thyroid function tests are of value in evaluating the possible effect of thyroid hormones on the absorption and utilization of carotenes.

The Carr and Price method for vitamin A in serum was commonly used in most of the early studies of vitamin A in humans. Improved spectrophotometric (Neeld and Pearson, 1963; Roels and Trout, 1972) and fluorometric (Garry et al., 1970; Thompson et al., 1971) methods are currently used by most laboratories. The method of Neeld and Pearson has some advantages of simplicity. The fluorometric methods use a smaller volume of serum but are technically more demanding.

22.3. VITAMIN D

There is no conclusive evidence of rickets in ancient sun-worshipping cultures. The advent of civilization and communal life prompted the clothing of individuals and means of ensuring privacy, thereby restricting their exposure to sunlight. This eventually contributed to the development of rickets, a bone disease affecting mainly infants and children. In the 18th century, the Scots recognized that their children could be protected from rickets by feeding them cod liver oil, a rich source of vitamins A and D. Sir Edward Mellanby (1919) demonstrated the nutritional nature of rickets by the use of cod liver oil in the prevention and cure of the disease. Towards the end of World War I, Huldschinsky (1919) cured children suffering from rickets by exposing them to sunlight or to artificially produced ultraviolet light. By treating cod liver oil with oxygen, McCollum et al. (1922) destroyed the xerophthalmia-preventing factor (vitamin A), without affecting the antirachitic properties of the oil. This rickets-preventing factor was named vitamin D. Steenbock (1924) subsequently irradiated certain foods which then acquired antirachitic properties, through the activation of sterols into active forms of vitamin D. This process was patented and contributed to the initial support of the Wisconsin Alumni Research Foundation (Pike and Brown, 1975). Ten years later, Waddell (1934) demonstrated that vitamin D-active compounds which resulted from the irradiation of sterols from plant origin, e.g. ergocalciferol (vitamin D_2), were different to those originating from animal sources, e.g. cholecalciferol (vitamin D_3). In common usage, the term vitamin D describes all sterols having vitamin activity.

Rickets in children and osteomalacia in adults still occur. Recent reports describe an increased incidence of vitamin D deficiency-related bone disease in sheltered individuals receiving maternal milk or cow's milk not fortified with vitamin D, and in immigrants from the tropics to northern latitudes with decreased sunlight and cool climate requiring abundant clothing. Heavily clothed, lactating Arabian mothers have developed osteomalacia from vitamin D deficiency.

22.3.1. Sources and requirements

Fish liver oils are the only known natural sources having a high concentration of vitamin D. Cod liver oil contains about 100 I.U./g, halibut liver oil about 1200 I.U./g, and bluefin tuna liver oil about 40,000 I.U./g. Other dietary sources include salmon, tuna, and herring with a vitamin concentration ranging from 2 to 3 I.U./g. Cow's milk, eggs, butter, and liver contain from 0.05 to 0.8 I.U./g. The vitamin D content of foods originating from domestic animals is dependent on the exposure to sunlight and the vitamin D content of the animal feed. Most natural sources contain the provitamin as ergosterol or 7-dehydrocholesterol, a cholesterol derivative.

The amount of vitamin D resulting from the irradiation of the sterols in the skin by sunlight provides most, if not all, of the daily vitamin requirement. In situations in which the vitamin must be provided, a daily allowance of 400 I.U. is recommended. One I.U. is equivalent to 0.025 μg cholecalciferol (vitamin D_3), so that 400 I.U. = 10 μg cholecalciferol. Human milk contains 4 to 95 I.U. vitamin D/litre. Cow's milk fortified with synthetic vitamin D (423 I.U./litre at an actual cost of approximately 0.05 cents in U.S.A.) is a widely used source of vitamin D. Supplemental dietary intake of vitamin D in excess of 1200 I.U./day is not recommended. An adequate intake of calcium and phosphorus is also required to ensure adequate bone development.

The recommended daily requirements for calcium are as follows:

infants	360 to 540 mg (9 to 13.5 mmol);
1 to 10 years	800 mg (20 mmol);
10 to 18 years	1200 mg (30 mmol);
pregnant women	1200 mg (30 mmol);
adults	800 mg (20 mmol).

Phosphorus intake should be equivalent to that of calcium. A high dietary phosphorus intake interferes with the absorption of calcium (Omdahl and DeLuca, 1973).

22.3.2. Functions

Like the other fat-soluble vitamins, vitamin D requires adequate lipids in the diet, and normal pancreatic, hepatic, and gastrointestinal function for proper absorption. Chylomicrons containing vitamin D are carried by the lymphatic system to the liver where the vitamin is hydroxylated to 25-hydroxycholecalciferol by calciferol-25-hydroxylase (Ponchon and DeLuca, 1969). 25-Hydroxycholecalciferol is more active than cholecalciferol and it is transported by the same protein, an α_2-globulin, to the kidney where further hydroxylation forms 1,25-dihydroxycholecalciferol which has still higher vitamin D metabolic activity (Omdahl et al., 1971). 1,25-dihydroxycholecalciferol, is believed to be the active form of vitamin D as it affects intestinal absorption of calcium and is actively involved in the mobilization of calcium from bones.

The intestinal absorption of calcium involves active transport requiring sodium ions and energy. This process is enhanced by 1,25-dihydroxycholecalciferol, the biosynthesis of which is regulated by a feed-back mechanism responding to the available calcium. A low calcium concentration increases the synthesis by activation of 25-hydroxycholecalciferol-1-hydroxylase. The biosynthesis of 1,25-dihydroxycholecalciferol is also enhanced by parathormone. A low serum concentration of calcium stimulates the secretion of parathormone, increasing the renal synthesis of 1,25-dihydroxycholecalciferol which in turn stimulates the intestinal absorption and mobilization of calcium from bone. When the serum calcium concentration returns to normal, the secretion of parathormone is reduced and the feed-back mechanism becomes stable.

Thyrocalcitonin (calcitonin), a polypeptide hormone secreted by the C-cells of the thyroid, acts as an antagonist to hypocalcaemia and parathormone secretion. There is a direct relation between the serum calcium concentration and the secretion of calcitonin. This is in opposition to the increased production of parathormone in response to a low serum calcium. The increase of serum calcium concentration that occurs during intestinal absorption stimulates calcitonin secretion which, in turn, inhibits calcium mobilization from bone. It has been suggested that gastric hormones stimulated by calcium could act as regulators of calcitonin secretion. In contrast to parathormone, calcitonin is not vitamin D-dependent. The decrease in bone reabsorption by calcitonin can take place in the presence of vitamin D deficiency or decreased parathormone activity. In vitamin D deficiency, parathormone can prevent the decrease in bone calcium mobilization by calcitonin. It is believed that calcitonin decreases the renal tubular reabsorption of phosphate. Phosphate diuresis is also induced by parathormone.

The interaction of vitamin D, calcium, and phosphorus has been studied by Tanaka and DeLuca (1973) and others. When the serum phosphate concentration is less than 8 mg/dl (2.6 mmol/litre), the synthesis of 1,25-dihydroxycholecalciferol is favoured. When the serum concentration exceeds 8 mg/dl (2.6 mmol/litre) a different metabolite, 24,25-dihydroxycholecalciferol, is formed. Previous observations have demonstrated that 25-hydroxycholecalciferol stimulates the renal tubule reabsorption of phosphate in the presence of parathormone. The 24,25-dihydroxy derivative predominates in hypercalcaemia and the 1,25-dihydroxy derivative in hypocalcaemia. These findings contribute to the understanding of the interactions of calcium, phosphorus, and vitamin D, and in part explain the action of rachitogenic diets containing a low amount of calcium but much phosphorus.

Fat depots are the main sites for storage of vitamin D originating either from intestinal absorption or from the irradiation of skin sterols by sunlight.

The functions of vitamin D parallel those of a hormone. There is a metabolic transformation of physiologically active compounds; the receptor organs are distant from the site of synthesis or activation; and there is ample participation of feed-back mechanisms.

Vitamin D also provides an interesting example of biochemical anthropology, illustrating the adaptation by man of a biological system to meet the demands of civilization.

22.3.3. Biochemical diagnosis

Vitamin D is of diagnostic importance in bone calcification and in the homeostasis of calcium and phosphorus. Magnesium absorption is not vitamin D dependent. Deficiency of this vitamin is the cause of various metabolic disorders which can culminate in rickets in infants and osteomalacia in adults. Radiographic diagnosis of rickets provides conclusive evidence of the disease. There is extensive bone deformity and decreased mineralization, particularly in the epiphyseal region which becomes enlarged and irregular.

Biochemically, rickets is characterized by low serum concentrations of calcium and phosphorus and increased activity of alkaline phosphatase. Previously, the clinical laboratory evaluation of vitamin D function was based on measurements of these compounds before and after vitamin supplementation. More recently, radioisotope competitive binding techniques have facilitated the measurement of vitamin D and of its more active metabolites (Belsey et al., 1974). The serum concentration of 25-hydroxycholecalciferol in healthy adults is 15 to 40 μg/litre with a mean of 25 μg/litre. Hypoparathyroid patients receiving therapeutic doses of vitamin D can achieve a serum concentration of 1250 μg/litre. Certain drugs, e.g. phenytoin and phenobarbitone, by stimulation of the liver microsomal oxidase system, can inactivate vitamin D by oxidation, causing possible hypocalcaemia. A diet that is both quantitatively adequate and well-balanced is essential before evaluation of vitamin D function can be assessed properly.

Serum specimens to be analyzed for 25-hydroxycholecalciferol must be protected from light. No significant changes occur if specimens are kept at 4 °C for a few days. Additional determinations which may contribute to the comprehensive evaluation of vitamin D function include pancreatic, hepatic and gastrointestinal function tests and measurement of serum parathormone and calcitonin concentration. Renal function tests are also important, since the kidney is the site of the formation of 1,25-dihydroxycholecalciferol, which may be decreased in uraemia.

In cases of rickets, treatment is implemented by vitamin D with a therapeutic dose of up to 600,000 I.U., or a series of repeated doses ranging from 50,000 to 100,000 I.U. (O'Reilly et al., 1964; Greaves and Ayres, 1967; Hermodson, 1969). Brickman et al. (1972) used a dose of 100 I.U. (2.7 μg) of 1,25-dihydroxycholecalciferol to treat uraemic patients who failed to respond to high (40,000 I.U.) daily doses of cholecalciferol. Response was evident by an increase of the serum calcium concentration. In these conditions, the therapeutic advantages of 1,25-dihydroxycholecalciferol are demonstrated. However, its high level of activity demands cautious use.

Vitamin D-resistant rickets is a disease of infancy characterized by hypophosphataemia, decreased calcium absorption, possible impairment of vitamin D metabolism, and occasional hypoproteinaemia. It is thought to be essentially a renal phosphate-wasting syndrome. Treatment with high doses of vitamin D (10,000 to 50,000 I.U.) together with oral phosphate, seems to produce better results than treatment with the vitamin alone (Fraser et al., 1973).

The Fanconi syndrome is the term used to describe a renal tubule defect associated with the lack of reabsorption of aminoacids, glucose, and phosphate. The loss of phosphate can lead to rickets or osteomalacia, depending upon the patient's age. The recently discovered highly active vitamin D metabolites are effective in the treatment of this disease.

Vitamin D toxicity is produced by the prolonged ingestion of high doses (3000 to 4000 I.U./day) of the vitamin, and it is more frequently found in infants and children. In adults, the symptoms of toxicity are headache, nausea, vomiting, diarrhoea, weakness and renal insufficiency. If the toxic condition is maintained, deposition of calcium in soft tissues (synovial membrane, kidney, myocardium, pancreas, large arteries, skin, etc.) ensues. Irreversible kidney damage and hypertension are likely to occur.

Infantile idiopathic hypercalcaemia presents a similar picture to that observed in the adult with vitamin D intoxication, but with additional features of mental retardation, failure to thrive, and an "elf-like" expression. The participation of vitamin D in this condition is suspected but has not been fully confirmed (Anderson and Fomon, 1974).

Hypersensitivity to vitamin D can produce toxic-like effects at moderately elevated doses.

Increased concentrations of serum calcium and circulating 25-hydroxycholecalciferol are features of vitamin D toxicity; measurements of these compounds are of value in the diagnosis of vitamin D toxicity, and in monitoring the progress of treatment.

22.4. VITAMIN E

Vitamin E was first described by Evans and Bishop (1922) as a fat-soluble factor capable of preventing foetal resorption and testicular degeneration in experimental animals which had been fed a diet containing rancid fat. Two years later, Sure (1924) designated the new factor as vitamin E. Olcott and Mattill (1931) and Olcott (1935) demonstrated strong antioxidant properties of the vitamin, and identified the compound as an alcohol. Evans et al. (1936) isolated vitamin E from the unsaponifiable fraction of wheat germ oil and named it tocopherol (Greek: tocos = offspring; pheros = to bring; ol = alcohol). The α-. β-, γ- and δ-tocopherols and their corresponding unsaturated tocotrienols have vitamin E activity. The α-tocopherol is the most abundant form in nature and has the most biological activity. The symptoms of vitamin E deficiency in experimental animals do not correspond to those in man. The role of vitamin E in human nutrition is still uncertain. Vitamin E deficiency appears to affect infants and children to a greater extent than adults.

22.4.1. Sources and requirements

Vitamin E is found in plants and it is present in high concentration in seed oils, with the exception of olive, peanut, and coconut oils which are not rich in the vitamin. Tissues from domesticated animals contain small quantities of the vitamin; however, this can be moderately increased by supplementation of the feed with vitamin E. Good dietary sources of vitamin E are wheat germ oil (about 133 mg/dl α-tocopherol), sunflower oil (about 49 mg/dl), cottonseed oil (about 39 mg/dl), palm oil (about 26 mg/dl), and cod liver oil (29 mg/dl). Other sources are almonds (about 27 mg/100 g), peanuts (about 10 mg/100 g) and wheat germ (about 13 mg/100 g).

Human milk contains an average of 40 μg α-tocopherol per gram of lipid; cow's milk contains 11 μg/g of lipid.

Recommended daily dietary allowances for vitamin E are expressed in International Units; 1 I.U. is equivalent to 1.1 mg DL-α-tocopherol (National Academy of Sciences, 1974).

The daily requirement for vitamin E, which is 12 to 15 I.U. for adult, is directly proportional to the polyunsaturated fatty acids (PUFA) in the diet. For infants, a vitamin E/PUFA ratio of 0.4 mg/g is recommended (Anderson and Fomon, 1974); for adults the same ratio is 0.6 mg/g. In healthy individuals a normal blood concentration of vitamin E can be maintained at these ratios (Horwitt, 1962).

22.4.2. Functions

Much information is now available concerning the structural and chemical properties of the tocopherols, yet we do not have a clear or complete picture of the biochemical mechanisms involved with the physiological functions of vitamin E. Despite much research, vitamin E has not been demonstrated to be a co-enzyme. Vitamin E prevents the oxidation of polyunsaturated fatty acids, inhibits the formation of peroxides and free radicals, and prevents the inactivation by oxidation of other important compounds such as vitamins A and C. Free radicals and peroxides interfere with the integrity of cell membranes and the function of other enzyme systems (Tappel, 1962, 1970). Some investigators postulate that the physiological consequences of vitamin E deficiency cannot be explained fully by the peroxidation of lipids, and more specific functions remain to be discovered (Green and Bunyan, 1969).

Vitamin E is stored in adipose tissue. Depletion of the body stores in adults is a very slow process, requiring a few years to produce measurable changes.

22.4.3. Biochemical diagnosis

A clinical entity of vitamin E deficiency is very uncommon in adults. Infants and children are more likely to develop vitamin E deficiency if their diets are low in the vitamin and high in polyunsaturated fatty acids, or if they have impaired intestinal absorption as a result of biliary atresia, steatorrhoea, or cystic fibrosis of the pancreas. A low plasma concentration of α-tocopherol and increased urinary creatine excretion are usual laboratory findings in vitamin E deficiency. Decreased resistance of erythrocytes to haemolysis by hydrogen peroxide is an indirect measure of a low circulating concentration of vitamin E. Haemolysis of erythrocytes is expressed as a percentage of the haemoglobin released from washed erythrocytes after a period of incubation in distilled water and in a dilute solution of hydrogen peroxide. Normal individuals have a haemolysis percentage of less than 10%; values in excess of 20% are indicative of vitamin E deficiency. The index of haemolysis correlates fairly well with the serum concentration of α-tocopherol (Sauberlich et al., 1974).

The normal concentration of vitamin E in serum is 0.8 to 1.1 mg/dl; it may be measured by fluorometric (Hansen and Warwick, 1966) or chromatographic methods. A comprehensive review of vitamin E methodology has been published by Bunnell (1971). Recent and improved methodologies are more specific and free from interference than earlier methods, and produce slightly lower values.

Specimens for vitamin E determinations should be processed promptly and need to be protected from light. Serum specimens can be stored at 4 °C for a few days.

Supplementation of vitamin E to infants may be by oral (4 to 5 I.U./day) or intramuscular (100 mg) routes (Anderson and Fomon, 1974).

There is no evidence that vitamin E crosses the placenta from the mother to the foetus. Unlike the situation with experimental animals, α-tocopherol is not beneficial to patients suffering from muscle disease. Ceroid, an acid fast pigment, has been reported to be present in tissues of individuals considered to be vitamin E deficient. Some infants with severe undernutrition (kwashiorkor) and anaemia, when given a supplement of vitamin E, show a favourable response that is not observed with folate or vitamin B_{12} supplementation. Vitamin E depletion has been observed in astronauts following prolonged space flights (Baker and Frank, 1968).

In recent years, the self-administered uncontrolled supplementation of some vitamins in massive amounts has provided some evidence for the non-toxic nature of vitamin E, even when ingested in great quantity (1 to 2 g/day). The alleged effects of high doses of vitamin E include improved physical performance, augmented sexual drive, and a very long life, but these have not been demonstrated. However, large doses of vitamin E in chicks have produced adverse effects, suggesting that the continuous use of megadoses of vitamin E in humans needs to be investigated.

22.5. VITAMIN K

Dam (1929) in Denmark, observed unexpected haemorrhages in experimental animals which were fed a diet deficient in fat. A few years later, a factor associated with the formation of prothrombin was found to prevent the haemorrhages in animals maintained in similar conditions. This factor was named vitamin K (Danish: koagulation) (Dam et al., 1936; Dam, 1948), and it was isolated by Dam et al. (1939) and McKee et al. (1939) from alfalfa (vitamin K_1) and decomposing fish meal (vitamin K_2) respectively. Vitamins K_1 and K_2 are fat-soluble quinones that differ in chemical structure. Vitamin K_1 is phyloquinone and vitamin K_2 is menaquinone. A synthetic vitamin K, menadione, is water soluble, and has greater biological activity than the naturally occurring forms. A water-soluble factor with vitamin K activity has been isolated from liver (Lev and Milford, 1966) and urine (Wiss and Gloor, 1966).

The biochemical mechanisms involved in the functions of vitamin K are not completely known. Studies by Olson (1970b) and Shah and Suttie (1971) propose a role for vitamin K as a regulating factor in the biosynthesis of polypeptides and proteins related to blood clotting.

22.5.1. Sources and requirements

The daily dietary allowance for vitamin K has not been established. In normal individuals the requirement is satisfied from dietary sources (300 to 400 μg/day) and the bacterial synthesis of the vitamin in the gut. Vitamin K_1 occurs in nature primarily in leafy green vegetables. Good dietary sources include cabbage, broccoli, turnip greens, green tea, spinach, cheese, butter, and liver. Vitamin K_2 is produced by bacterial metabolism of the intestinal flora (*Escherichia coli*) in most animals.

Human milk contains an average of 5 μg/litre of vitamin K, but cow's milk contains as much as 60 μg/litre (Dam et al., 1952). It is estimated that half of the vitamin K requirement for humans is met from plant sources (Rietz et al., 1970).

Based on the amount of vitamin K required to restore the plasma prothrombin time to normal, the estimated exogenous daily requirement of vitamin K is 1 to 2 μg/kg body mass.

Newborn infants frequently present a haemorrhagic tendency associated with a low serum vitamin K concentration. A daily requirement of not more than 5 μg has been estimated. Supplementation of the mother's diet with a high concentration of water-soluble preparations of vitamin K before delivery, or of the newborn infant's feed is not recommended (Anderson and Fomon, 1974).

22.5.2. Functions

The biochemical functions of vitamin K are only partially known. Initial observations on experimental animals suffering from haemorrhagic disease associated with a low dietary fat intake were associated with decreased levels of prothrombin (factor II) (Dam et al., 1936; Quick, 1957). Brinkhous (1940) demonstrated that the blood clotting defect was the result of the lack of vitamin K which decreases the hepatic synthesis of prothrombin; in the next decade other clotting factors, VII, IX, and X, were found to be vitamin K-dependent. The better understood functions of vitamin K relate to the regulation of the biosynthesis of prothrombin and vitamin-dependent clotting factors.

The wide distribution of vitamin K in nature suggests that the vitamin could participate in other important metabolic functions.

Some compounds are antagonists of vitamin K. Dicoumarol was isolated from fermenting sweet clover by Campbell and Link (1941). Its derivatives are used in agriculture as rodenticides, or clinically as anticoagulants. It is believed that the antagonistic action of these compounds results from competition with vitamin K for binding sites which regulate biological activity. The action of vitamin K antagonists is counteracted by phyloquinone and menaquinone, but not by menadione, the synthetic form of the vitamin. Studies by Olson (1970a, b) suggest that the function of vitamin K in the biosynthesis of coagulation proteins occurs in the ribosomes of liver cells.

22.5.3. Biochemical diagnosis

Vitamin K deficiency results in delayed blood clotting. This condition is not commonly found in adults, but newborn infants have low reserves of vitamin K and are likely to develop a short-term deficiency. A low dietary intake of the vitamin, or the use of anticoagulant medication by the mother prior to delivery, may result in haemorrhages which can be prevented by supplementation with vitamin K_1. The administration of high doses of water-soluble vitamin K (menadione) to the mother in labour or to the newborn infant is not recommended. This may cause hyperbilirubinaemia, haemolytic anaemia, kernicterus and possibly death (Committee on Nutrition, 1961). Supplementation of the expectant mother's diet with vitamin K_1 increases the prothrombin activity in the newborn.

The concentration of vitamin K in blood is too low to be measured by available clinical laboratory techniques. The one-stage prothrombin time (Quick, 1939) measures prothrombin activity and the vitamin K-dependent blood clotting factors. Anticoagulant drugs and salicylate compete with vitamin K and increase the prothrombin time. As with deficiency of the other fat-soluble vitamins, vitamin K deficiency may result from gastrointestinal, pancreatic or hepatic disease. The laboratory evaluation of the functions of these organs can assist in the differential diagnosis and the evaluation of blood clotting abnormalities related to vitamin K. If vitamin K deficiency is the main cause of impaired blood clotting, the prothrombin time is promptly restored to normal 1 or 2 days after supplementation is begun. Patients receiving prolonged oral antibiotic or bacteriostatic medication are likely to develop vitamin K deficiency and they should receive supplemental vitamin K.

Large doses of vitamin A administered orally interfere with the utilization of vitamin K. Vitamin K is stored in the liver. The circulating concentration of some fat-soluble vitamins is increased with the use of oral steroid contraceptives. The blood clotting abnormalities observed in some women taking oral contraceptives may be related to the possible influence of the contraceptives on vitamin K metabolism.

Reported signs of vitamin K deficiency include nosebleeds; bleeding peptic ulcers, urinary tract bleeding, cerebral haemorrhage, and ecchymoses resulting from minor bruising. Toxicity from the ingestion of large doses of vitamin K may produce hyperbilirubinaemia and possible haemolytic anaemia in patients with glucose-6-phosphate dehydrogenase deficiency (Halsted, 1976).

The normal prothrombin time is 12 to 15 seconds, which is the time for oxalated or citrated plasma to clot following the addition of factor III (tissue thromboplastin). Bleeding may be apparent when the prothrombin time is about one-third, or less, of the normal value. In vitamin K-deficient individuals, the vitamin should be administered until the prothrombin time is restored to normal.

22.6. THIAMINE (VITAMIN B_1)

Observations made by Takaki in 1887 (cited by Williams (1961)), the medical director of the Japanese navy, contributed to the understanding of the nutritional nature of beriberi, a disease which had been prevalent for 4000 years and was almost endemic in the Orient at that time. He supplemented the Japanese sailor's diet, which was then composed mainly of polished rice, with meat, milk, and whole grains. This resulted in the eradication of the "shipboard" beriberi, which used to affect about one-third of the crews with frequent fatalities. Prior to this, in 1880, van Leent, a Dutch naval medical officer, had noticed a reduced mortality from beriberi when the diet of the Indian crew, composed mainly of rice, was replaced by a European-type of diet. In 1890, Eijkman, physician to a Dutch prison hospital in Java, fed to chickens the food, essentially polished rice, left by patients with beriberi. The chickens developed a beriberi-like polyneuritis which was cured by feeding whole rice. Eijkman, possibly influenced by Pasteur, thought that beriberi was infectious or caused by toxins produced by the carbohydrate in the rice, which could be neutralized by a substance in the husk. Another Dutch physician, Grijns (see Williams, 1961), working at the same hospital in Java, postulated, in 1901, that beriberi was caused by the lack of a certain substance in the polished rice that was present in the whole grain. In 1910, Frazer and Stanton defined beriberi clinically as a metabolic disorder, resulting from the absence of a substance extractable from rice husks that was essential for the nervous tissue. The search for the anti-beriberi factor led Funk (1911) to the establishment of the term and the concept of vitamin. Jansen (1956), working in the same laboratory as Eijkman and Grijns, crystallized a compound with high antineuritic potency from rice husks extracts. Subsequently, Williams, who was exposed as a child to poverty in India and impressed by widespread multiple nutritional deficiencies, began the characterization of the beriberi preventing factor. His experimental work culminated in the synthesis of thiamine (Williams and Cline, 1936). Thiamine is now synthesized economically and is widely used to supplement rice, flour and other grain products. Beriberi still remains a health problem in certain areas of the Orient and in less developed countries. In more affluent societies, thiamine deficiency may occur in alcoholics or in individuals with dietary restrictions or impaired absorption of nutrients.

22.6.1. Sources and requirements

Thiamine is widely distributed in nature, but only a few foods are rich sources of the vitamin. The thiamine content of eggs, fruits, milk, and vegetables rarely exceeds 0.1 mg/100 g. Better sources of the vitamin include whole grains, e.g. sunflower seeds (1.9 mg/100 g), soy beans (1.1 mg/100 g), pinto beans (0.8 mg/100 g), dry oatmeal (0.6 mg/100 g), whole wheat flour (0.5 mg/100 g), lentils (0.4 mg/100 g), peas (0.3 mg/100 g) and meats, e.g. pork (0.5 mg/100 g) and beef heart (0.5 mg/100 g). Bread prepared with thiamine-enriched wheat flour can provide about one-third of the daily thiamine requirement. Loss of thiamine during cooking can vary from 10 to 15% for baked or fried foods, up to 30 to 60% for broiled or roasted meats. Cooking may also destroy thiamine in vegetables.

The International Unit (I.U.) of vitamin B_1 is equivalent to 0.3 μg of thiamine hydrochloride.

The human requirements for thiamine are based on dietary caloric intake. The recommended daily allowance for adults is 0.4 to 0.5 mg/1000 calories (1.0 to 1.5 mg/day) (National Academy of Sciences, 1974). Other recommended daily allowances are: for infants, 0.3 to 0.5 mg; from 1 to 3 years, 0.7 mg; from 4 to 6 years, 0.9 mg; and from 10 to 18 years, 1.2 to 1.5 mg. During pregnancy and lactation 1.3 mg is recommended also.

Human milk contains an average of 16 μg/dl of thiamine, which provides part of the requirements of breast-fed babies.

22.6.2. Functions

Thiamine is activated by ATP phosphorylation in the liver and kidneys to form thiamine pyrophosphate, co-carboxylase, a co-enzyme which participates in a variety of enzyme reactions, some of which are essential for the utilization of carbohydrates.

Thiamine pyrophosphate functions in the oxidative decarboxylation and transfer of two-carbon fragments from α-oxoacids to carboxylic acids. Pyruvic acid is decarboxylated to acetyl co-enzyme A and α-oxoglutaric acid to succinyl co-enzyme A. These reactions also require lipoic acid. Transketolase, which is an important enzyme in plant and animal tissues, requires thiamine pyrophosphate and Mg^{2+} and functions in the transfer and interchange of three, four, five, six and seven carbon sugars to form sedoheptulose-7-phosphate, fructose-6-phosphate and glyceraldehyde-3-phosphate. Measurement of the catalysis by transketolase of the pentose pathway, by following the rate of pentose disappearance, provides a means of assessing the metabolic activity of thiamine pyrophosphate and an individual's nutritional status with respect to thiamine.

22.6.3. Biochemical diagnosis

Beriberi (Singhalese: I can not) is the extreme manifestation of thiamine deficiency. It is found in the Orient but very seldom in the western world. A thiamine intake of 0.2 mg or less per 1000 calories is prone to produce "dry" beriberi, which is characterized by peripheral neuropathy, with hyper- or hyposensitivity, numbness, fatigue, anorexia, constipation, and muscle wasting, particularly in the extremities. Prolonged moderate or severe deficiency results in "wet" beriberi with more accentuated neurological lesions plus cardiovascular involvement. Tachycardia results from minor physical or mental stimulation. Cardiac failure may be caused by moderate physical stress. Oedema is present. Untreated wet beriberi results in paralysis and death.

Beriberi-like symptoms are found in alcoholics who have been drinking for some time, but eating poorly. Tissue reserves of thiamine are depleted in about 2 weeks and symptoms of deficiency are likely to follow. Wernike's encephalopathy is used to describe the clinical manifestations of thiamine deficiency. It includes mental confusion, peripheral neuropathy, and lateral or vertical nystagmus. Administration of glucose may precipitate encephalopathy in deficient individuals, but if the deficiency is not treated, death ensues. Acutely ill patients responding to thiamine therapy (20 to 30 mg/day) may suffer cerebral damage resulting in polyneuritis, retrograde amnaesia, loss of memory, and a tendency to uncontrolled chatting (Korsakoff's syndrome).

Infantile beriberi can occur in the first 4 months of life in the infants of thiamine-deficient mothers. Clinically they present with neuropathies and aphonic (silent) crying. Supplementation of the diet with thiamine enables the infants to recover promptly.

A thermolabile thiamine antimetabolite "thiaminase", which is found in raw fish, competes with thiamine, producing symptoms related to the actual vitamin deficiency (Chastek paralysis in silver foxes). Raw fish consumed in certain oriental diets is believed to interfere with thiamine utilization.

Chemical methods (Hennessey and Cerecedo, 1939; Leveille, 1972) and microbiological methods (Baker and Frank, 1968) are available for the assessment of thiamine metabolism. The biochemical diagnosis is based on the measurement of urinary thiamine and on the activity and the response to thiamine pyrophosphate of transketolase in haemolyzed erythrocytes. The blood pyruvic acid concentration is increased in individuals with thiamine deficiency. However, other conditions, e.g. exercise and anxiety, may also produce a transient increase of pyruvic acid in blood.

Measurement of the concentration of thiamine in serum is of little value in the evaluation of thiamine deficiency.

The urinary concentration of thiamine may be expressed as μg/g creatinine or as μg/24 h. The typical excretion of thiamine in urine is:

1 to 3 years	176 μg/g creatinine
3 to 10 years	120 to 180 μg/g creatinine
10 to 15 years	150 to 180 μg/g creatinine
pregnant women	55 μg/g creatinine
adults	66 μg/g creatinine (100 μg/24 h)

To measure the functional availability of thiamine, the transketolase activity in haemolyzed erythrocyte preparations is determined before and after the addition of thiamine pyrophosphate (Brin, 1967; Chong and Ho, 1970; Nino and Shaw, 1976). The percentage increase in activity is interpreted as follows: 0 to 14%, normal; 15 to 24%, marginal deficiency; over 25%, deficient.

Clinical response by deficient individuals to supplementation of their diets with thiamine correlates well with changes in laboratory measurements. Other tests that should be performed in conjunction with an evaluation of thiamine nutritional status include those for proteins as indicators of general nutrition, gastrointestinal and pancreatic function to evaluate nutrient absorption, and liver function tests to measure possible interference with thiamine phosphorylation.

No toxic effects in man have been reported following the ingestion of massive doses of thiamine. Intravenous or intramuscular injections of thiamine (up to 200 times the recommended daily requirement) have not produced toxicity. Repeated injections of high doses of thiamine to sensitive individuals may produce hypersensitivity which can cause anaphylactic shock.

22.7. RIBOFLAVIN (VITAMIN B_2)

Riboflavin was recognized by Emmett and Luros (1920) as a water-soluble, heat-stable factor with anti-pellagric properties, which was different to the beriberi-preventing factor. In reality, this factor was a combination of B complex vitamins. Warburg and Christian (1933, 1935) identified the first flavoprotein, an oxidative enzyme formed by a protein and a yellow-green fluorescent component. The participation of this component in biochemical oxidation–reduction reactions provided evidence for the function of a vitamin as a coenzyme, which was a significant first step in nutritional biochemistry. Booher (1933) demonstrated that the growth-promoting factor was associated with the yellow-green fluorescent compound. Riboflavin was synthesized independently by Kuhn et al. (1935) and by Karrer et al. (1935).

22.7.1. Sources and requirements

Riboflavin is widely distributed in plant and animal tissues. Good dietary sources of riboflavin are beans (0.2 to 0.3 mg/100 g), cheese (0.4 mg/100 g), egg white (0.3 mg/100 g), milk (0.2 mg/100 g), lean meat (0.2 mg/100 g), beef kidneys (2.6 mg/100 g), heart (1.0 mg/100 g), and liver (3.3 mg/100 g). Human milk contains about 0.04 mg/dl.

The recommended daily allowance of riboflavin is related to the metabolic body size:

children	0.4 to 0.8 mg/day
adults	1.4 to 1.8 mg/day
pregnant women	1.7 mg/day
lactating women	1.9 mg/day

22.7.2. Functions

Riboflavin must be phosphorylated before it is biochemically active. The riboflavin-containing coenzymes are riboflavin-5-phosphate (also known erroneously as flavin mononucleotide) and flavin-adenine-dinucleotide (FAD). These riboflavin coenzymes are essential for various enzymatic oxidative systems including, among many others, amino-acid oxidases, xanthine oxidase and glutathione reductase. Vital functions of cell growth and repair can not take place in the absence of riboflavin coenzymes. They participate in enzymatic oxidation–reduction reactions which are indispensable to cell life. A comprehensive review of flavin-catalyzed enzyme reactions has been published by Neims and Hellerman (1970).

22.7.3. Biochemical diagnosis

Lesions produced by riboflavin deficiency were described in several different countries in the first half of this century, before the vitamin was known. However, it was recognized that the observed pathology was related to a deficiency of a component of the vitamin B complex. Sebrell and Butler (1938, 1939) described riboflavin deficiency in man as a syndrome characterized by seborrhoeic dermatitis about the ears, the nasolabial folds and the scrotum, painful glossitis, angular stomatitis and vascularization of the cornea. Similar findings were reported by Horwitt et al. (1949). A generalized sensation of weakness accompanies riboflavin deficiency. This, however, can also be caused by generalized malnutrition.

Chemical methods (Slater and Morell, 1946) and microbiological (Baker and Frank, 1968; Pearson, 1967) methods are available for the measurement of riboflavin. Blood concentrations of riboflavin have been found to be of limited value for the assessment of riboflavin metabolism. Urine analyses provide a closer indication of riboflavin concentration in body fluids. However, the urine concentration varies with the amount of the vitamin in recent meals: it also may be artificially increased in negative nitrogen balance, with prolonged fasting, and following surgery.

Urinary riboflavin concentrations are usually expressed in terms of μg/g of creatinine. As with thiamine, caution must be exercised in the interpretation of results, and additional tests of renal function may be advisable to rule out renal effects.

Sauberlich et al. (1974) have established reference ranges or values for urinary riboflavin, as follows:

1 to 3 years	$\geqslant$ 500 μg/g creatinine
4 to 9 years	$\geqslant$ 300 μg/g creatinine
10 to 15 years	$\geqslant$ 200 μg/g creatinine
pregnant women	90 to 120 μg/g creatinine
adults	80 μg/g creatinine

A test to evaluate the biochemical activity of riboflavin is based on the response of an FAD-dependent enzyme, such as glutathione reductase in erythrocytes, before and after FAD activation. The difference in absorbance before and after FAD stimulation permits the calculation of an activity coefficient which, if greater than 1.2, is indicative of riboflavin deficiency. This is based on the extent of the FAD unsaturation of the enzyme reaction, which is interpreted as a quantitation of FAD and consequently of riboflavin content (Glatzle et al., 1970; Tillotson and Baker, 1972; Nino and Shaw, 1976).

Deficient individuals respond promptly to riboflavin supplementation with a single dose (25 mg of the sodium salt of riboflavin phosphate) or to repeated daily doses (6 mg) of the vitamin.

Massive oral or intraperitoneal doses of riboflavin have not produced toxic effects in experimental animals, nor has riboflavin toxicity been reported in man. As with other water-soluble vitamins, an increased urinary excretion of the vitamin is usually found after a high intake of riboflavin.

22.8. NIACIN

The discovery of niacin as an essential micronutrient, and of its use in the prevention and cure of pellagra, a nutritional disease with a high prevalance and mortality rate, was one of the more important scientific accomplishments of this century.

There is no evidence that pellagra occurred in the native American population prior to the European discovery of the continent. The introduction of corn from America preceded the appearance of the disease in Europe. In 1735 Gaspar Casal, a Spanish physician, described pellagra as a distinct disease; he named it "mal de la rosa" (Spanish: rose illness). In 1771, Francesco Frapelli, an Italian physician, named the disease pellagra (Italian: rough-sensitive skin).

The nature of the disease was the object of controversy until Goldberger and Wheeler (1915) demonstrated that pellagra was a nutritional disease caused essentially by niacin deficiency. Nicotinic acid (niacin) had previously been discovered in 1867 when it was prepared from nicotine by Huber, a German chemist. Niacin was proved to be a vitamin by Elvehjem et al. (1938) when black-tongue in dogs, the equivalent of niacin deficiency in humans, was cured by nicotinic acid (niacin) prepared from liver extracts. This finding was promptly confirmed by other investigators.

In the first quarter of this century, pellagra reached epidemic proportions in the South of the United States and in other countries. Today pellagra, with different degrees of severity, remains a health problem in isolated areas of the world and it is associated invariably with famine. In more affluent societies, alcoholics or patients with impaired utilization of nutrients may present with symptoms of niacin deficiency.

22.8.1. Sources and requirements

Niacin occurs in foods as a single compound, and it can also be synthesized by the organism from tryptophan. Approximately 60 mg of tryptophan yield 1 mg of niacin. In reality, the rate of conversion is determined by the bioavailability of tryptophan. "Niacin Equivalent" is an expression used to indicate the potential availability of the vitamin in foods. Usually, foods regarded as good sources of niacin are also good sources of thiamine and riboflavin. This dietary relationship contributes to the understanding of pellagra as a niacin deficiency which is compounded by the lack of other B vitamins.

Good dietary sources of niacin are chicken (10.0), soybean (11.1), trout (11.7), and sesame seed (10.2), each expressed as mg/100 g niacin equivalent; also lean beef (46.0), cow's milk (12.4), human milk (9.8), whole eggs (10.8), and wheat flour (7.4) each expressed as mg/1000 calories. The niacin equivalent in mg/1000 calories of corn is 6.7 and of corn grits, 3.0. In some countries where corn which has been treated with lime is consumed in large quantities, no apparent deficiency develops; this is due to the increased bioavailability of niacin induced by the lime treatment. Niacin is fairly stable, and normal cooking produces only minor destruction of the vitamin.

Recommended daily allowances, in mg of niacin equivalents, are as follows:

1 to 3 years	9 mg
pregnant women	16 mg
lactating women	18 mg
adults	14 to 20 mg

The minimum amount of niacin that will prevent pellagra in adults is 4.4 mg/1000 calories, or 9.0 mg if the daily caloric intake is less than 2000 calories (Anderson and Fomon, 1974).

As with most vitamins, synthetic niacin is the most economical source, and it is used for enrichment of some foods. The cost of niacin to satisfy the requirements of an adult is about 5 cents (U.S.) per year. Therefore eradication of pellagra could be achieved at little cost.

22.8.2. Functions

The importance of niacin (nicotinic acid) and its amide (niacinamide or nicotinamide) in metabolic functions was recognized by Warburg and Christian (1933, 1935) before its essential nutritional requirement was known. Niacin is biologically active in two co-enzymes: nicotinamide adenine dinucleotide (NAD) and nicotinamide adenine dinucleotide phosphate (NADP), formerly known as co-enzymes I and II or diphosphopyridine nucleotide (DPN) and triphosphopyridine nucleotide (TPN) respectively. NADH and NADPH are the reduced forms of NAD and NADP. The niacin co-enzymes participate actively in intracellular respiration. NAD participates in reactions involving lactate dehydrogenase (lactate to pyruvate), alcohol dehydrogenase (alcohol to acetaldehyde), glycerolphosphate dehydrogenase and glyceraldehyde-3-phosphate dehydrogenase, among others. NAD and NADP also participate in reactions with glutamic dehydrogenase and isocitric dehydrogenase. The change of glucose-6-phosphate to phosphogluconic acid, and of citric to α-oxoglutaric acid requires the participation of NADP. NADH usually donates hydrogen derived from glycolysis to FAD (section 22.7.2) which transfers it to the cytochrome system where in turn it is transferred to oxygen, forming water. Any decrease in the niacin co-enzymes causes severe interruption in cellular respiration which results in cellular damage. Comprehensive discussions of the functions of the niacin co-enzymes have been published by Chaykin (1967) and Slater et al. (1970).

22.8.3. Biochemical diagnosis

The early symptoms of niacin deficiency are weakness, anorexia, and digestive difficulties – similar symptoms to those occurring with other vitamin B deficiencies. Prolonged deficiency of niacin affects the entire organism, and it is characterized by dermatological, gastrointestinal, and neurological symptoms. Dermatitis, dementia, and death ("the three Ds") describe the chronology of pellagra. Dermatitis, usually bilateral, affects those parts of the body, face, neck, hands, and feet, exposed to light, friction, or heat. The skin becomes hyperkeratotic, sensitive, and hyperpigmented; and in the proximity of moist areas with transitional epithelium (edge of lips, scrotum, anus, vulva) erythema may occur. Secondary infection may appear in prolonged deficiency. The gastrointestinal system is considerably affected. Diarrhoea and malabsorption occur in most cases. The mouth may show cheilosis and fissures; the tongue is sore, inflamed, and may present atrophic fungiform papillae. There is atrophy and inflammation of the small intestine. Painful colitis and rectal discomfort are common complaints. Achlorhydria has been reported in some cases. The initial neurological symptoms are depression, irritability, apathy, neurasthenia, and anorexia. Later in the disease peripheral neuropathy and encephalopathy may occur, resulting in sensory and motor abnormalities, psychosis, mania, convulsions, seizures, and death.

Clinically, symptoms of niacin deficiency may occur in patients with severe malabsorption, diarrhoea, cirrhosis of the liver, neoplasia, and diabetes mellitus. Failure to grow in the young, and anaemia, have been reported in niacin-deficient patients (Sandstead, 1973).

Pellagra was the cause of over 10,000 deaths in the southern United States in 1915. From 1917 to 1918 over 200,000 cases occurred throughout the country. Mental institutions were populated by patients suffering from pellagra-related neurological and psychotic syndromes. A decrease in pellagra-related deaths from 22.4 to 5.1 per 100,000 in the southern United States occurred between 1929 and 1940. The disease also caused many deaths in other areas of the world. The low prevalence of pellagra in countries where corn is a stable dietary constituent is due not only to the lime treatment of corn, but also to the use of coffee and possibly beer, which are adequate sources of niacin.

The biochemical diagnosis of niacin deficiency is based on the measurement of two urinary metabolites: N′-methylnicotinamide and N′-methyl-2-pyridine-5-carboxamide (2-pyridone). These metabolites provide only a partial indication of the niacin nutritional status. Measurement of N′-methylnicotinamide is preferred because of technical simplicity. None of the available methods is completely satisfactory (Carpenter and Kodicek, 1950; Joubert and DeLange, 1962; Pearson, 1966). The range of urinary N′-methylnicotinamide in healthy individuals is 1.6 to 4.3 mg/g creatinine (Schaefer, 1963). Therapeutic doses of niacin, as niacinamide, range from 50 to 250 mg/day for several days, as a supplement to a balanced diet. Nicotinic acid therapy may cause flushing and itching. Prolonged use may result in gastrointestinal hypersensitivity and hepatic irritability.

22.9. VITAMIN B_6

György (1934) described a factor capable of preventing skin lesions in experimental animals maintained on restricted diets; he named this factor vitamin B_6. This factor was identified and later synthesized as pyridoxine. Two additional compounds, pyridoxal and pyridoxamine, were found to have similar properties (Snell et al., 1942; Snell, 1945). Like other B vitamins, vitamin B_6 is phosphorylated to become biologically active, and it functions as a co-enzyme in reactions involving primarily aminoacid metabolism. Vitamin B_6 deficiency is very uncommon, but interest in the vitamin was increased after it was recognized that heat destroyed it in certain canned baby foods, which led to deficiency in babies. The apparent increase in vitamin B_6 requirement in women taking steroid oral contraceptives, and the response to vitamin B_6 supplementation by patients suffering from anaemia which is not responsive to iron or other B-vitamin supplementation also stimulated interest in the role of the vitamin.

22.9.1. Sources and requirements

The distribution of vitamin B_6 in nature is comparable to that of the other B vitamins. Good sources are raw beef liver (0.84 mg/g), raw tuna (0.90), chicken (0.3), bananas (0.5), beans (0.5), walnuts (0.7), wheat bran (0.8), and roasted wheat germ (1.15). Human milk contains about 0.1 mg/dl. Cooking, food processing, and refining may account for losses of 40 to 70% of the food's natural vitamin B_6 content.

The requirement of vitamin B_6 is proportional to the dietary protein. Recommended allowances are as follows:

infants	0.3 mg/day
pregnant or lactating women	2.5 mg/day
adults	1.6–2.0 mg/day

The biological activities of the three forms of the vitamin (pyridoxine, pyridoxal, and pyridoxamine) are practically equal.

22.9.2. Functions

The phosphorylation of pyridoxine, pyridoxal, and pyridoxamine leads to pyridoxal-5-phosphate, the active co-enzyme form of vitamin B_6. Some compounds with structures similar to that of pyridoxine have shown some co-enzyme activity; other analogues (notably 4-deoxypyridoxine) are antimetabolites and cause vitamin B_6 deficiency. Over 50 reactions participating in the metabolism of aminoacids are known to be dependent on pyridoxal-5-phosphate. These include transamination, decarboxylation, cleavage, synthesis, racemization, dehydration, and desulphhydration. The transaminases (aminotransferases) are widely used in clinical diagnosis. The α-amino group from various aminoacids, such as alanine, tryptophan, phenylalanine, and tyrosine is separated and transferred, usually to α-oxoglutarate to complete the nitrogen metabolism. The tricarboxylic acid cycle is the receptor of the aminoacid carboxyl residue where it is metabolized. Pyridoxal-5-phosphate-dependent decarboxylases also performs important functions such as the synthesis of serotonin from 5-hydroxytryptophan. Phosphorylase converts glycogen into glucose-1-phosphate and requires pyridoxal-5-phosphate. The vitamin B_6 co-enzyme also participates in the conversion of tryptophan into niacin. Comprehensive reviews of the co-enzyme functions of vitamin B_6 have been published by Fasella (1967), and McCormick and Wright (1970).

22.9.3. Biochemical diagnosis

Early symptoms of vitamin B_6 deficiency are comparable to those found with the other B vitamins. Data obtained from volunteer subjects maintained on deficient diets show a decrease in the formation of antibodies against typhoid and tetanus. Hypochromic anaemia may also occur. The tryptophan to niacin conversion is interrupted, pellagra-like dermatitis and photosensitivity develop, sensory neuropathy precedes motor disturbances. Irritability, depression, and a "loss of sense of responsibility" may occur. A tryptophan load (3 to 5 g) produces increased excretion of tryptophan metabolites, mainly xanthurenic acid. The urinary concentration of 4-pyridoxic acid, the major metabolite of vitamin B_6, is greatly reduced (Sauberlich and Canham, 1973).

A functional test of vitamin B_6 adequacy is based on the determination, in erythrocyte preparations, of aspartate aminotransferase (AsT) and alanine aminotransferase (AlT) before and after pyridoxal phosphate stimulation. An index is calculated as follows:

$$\text{Erythrocyte} - \text{AsT index} = \frac{\text{E} - \text{AsT with pyridoxal phosphate}}{\text{E} - \text{AsT without pyridoxal phosphate}}$$

$$\text{Erythrocyte} - \text{AlT index} = \frac{\text{E} - \text{AlT with pyridoxal phosphate}}{\text{E} - \text{AlT without pyridoxal phosphate}}$$

For normal individuals, the E-AsT index is less than 1.5, and the Alt index is less than 1.2; the plasma vitamin B_6 concentration is over 50 ng/ml, and the urinary excretion of 4-pyridoxic acid over 0.8 mg/day (Sauberlich et al., 1974).

Deficient patients respond promptly to oral supplementation with 5 to 150 mg/day of pyridoxine hydrochloride. No toxic effects after high or prolonged doses of vitamin B_6 have been reported. Supplementation with vitamin B_6 (5 to 25 mg/day) is recommended for individuals receiving isoniazid for the prophylaxis or treatment of tuberculosis. Penicillamine, semicarbazide, and cycloserine also function as vitamin B_6 antimetabolites and supplementation is indicated when these drugs are administered.

22.10. PANTOTHENIC ACID

In 1938, R.J. Williams (the brother of R.R. Williams, discoverer of thiamine, section 22.6) and his colleagues isolated pantothenic acid from liver and yeast extracts. The pantothenic acid was separated from pyridoxine by adsorption chromatography. Pantothenic acid was not retained by the column (filtrate factor); pyridoxine was retained and selectively eluted (eluate factor). Stiller et al. (1940) later synthesized pantothenic acid.

Pantothenic acid (Greek: pantothen = from all sides) is widely distributed in foods, and its deficiency in humans under natural conditions is not likely to occur. Volunteer subjects maintained on pantothenic acid-free diets plus an antimetabolite developed symptoms similar to those found with other vitamin B deficiencies. These include fatigue, insomnia, nausea, abdominal distress, peripheral neuropathies, and personality changes.

The importance of pantothenic acid originates from its part in co-enzyme A, which is essential for the metabolism of proteins, fats, and carbohydrates (Lipmann and Kaplan, 1946; DeVries et al., 1950). Co-enzyme A also plays an important role in the biosynthesis of cholesterol and adrenocortical hormones. Co-enzyme A interacts with the co-enzymes of thiamine, riboflavin, niacin, and vitamin B_6 as well as with certain minerals like magnesium, phosphorus, and sulphur.

22.11. BIOTIN

Biotin was first described as a protective factor against dermatitis, alopoecia, and the hind leg paralysis which is found in experimental animals fed diets high in raw egg whites (Parsons et al., 1937). Cooked eggs in the diet did not produce any ill effects. Avidin, a protein-carbohydrate, thermolabile compound was found to bind biotin in the intestinal tract, impeding its absorption.

Biotin is widely distributed in nature and its deficiency is unknown in humans. There is evidence of bacterial synthesis of biotin in the intestinal tract. The consumption of a large quantity of raw eggs by humans is not likely to produce a deficiency due to avidin since egg yolk is one of the best natural sources of the vitamin.

Biotin participates in carboxylation reactions involving the conversion of ATP to ADP, or the exchange of carboxyl groups without additional sources of energy (ATP). Biotin-linked enzyme systems have been reviewed by Knappe (1970).

22.12. ASCORBIC ACID (VITAMIN C)

The consequences of ascorbic acid deficiency were recognized long before its nutritional function was known. The Egyptians, the Greeks, and later the soldiers of the Roman Empire, the Spanish explorers, and the Portuguese and English navigators were aware of the lethal effects of scurvy, the disease caused by diets deficient in ascorbic acid. The Spanish explorers brought corn back to Europe, and this eventually contributed to the outbreaks of pellagra. But they also brought potatoes, a good source of ascorbic acid, at a time when scurvy was rampant in Europe. Isolated observations on the effect of ascorbic acid in preventing or curing scurvy were made between 1500 and 1700. Lind (1753), a physician with the British Royal Navy deserves the credit for curing scurvy. He treated scurvy-affected sailors at sea with a diet containing two oranges and a lemon daily – "These they eat with greediness". Prompt recovery permitted the crew to return to normal duties in 6 days. Captain Cook, a friend of Lind, demonstrated that long ocean voyages did not result in scurvy if the crew's diet included fresh vegetables. It took 50 years before Lind's discovery was "officially" recognized. In 1795, the British Admiralty ordered daily rations of fresh citrus juice to all seamen. This gave the British an upper-hand in the Napoleonic Wars. At the time the lemons were called limes and a new term "limeys" was coined to nickname the British sailors (Sebrell and Haggerty, 1967). On the other side of the Atlantic, in 1535, the expedition commanded by Cartier in Newfoundland experienced massive scurvy. It was saved by taking the extract of spruce needles, a rich source of ascorbic acid, provided by the Indians. Scurvy accounted for many lives in the United States during the Gold Rush of the mid 1800s and the Civil War. As late as 1912, scurvy caused the death of Captain Scott and his team when they explored the South Pole.

Ascorbic acid was isolated from oranges, cabbage, and adrenal cortex by Szent-György (1928), Svirbely and Szent-György (1932) and King and Waugh (1932). Ascorbic acid was synthesized independently by Haworth and Hirst (1933), and Reichstein et al. (1933).

Ascorbic acid deficiency remains a health problem for individuals of all ages, in different parts of the world. Availability of qualitatively or quantitatively adequate foods is not as critical as it was in the past: lack of nutrition education, socioeconomic problems, self-neglect, and alcoholism are the modern factors contributing to ascorbic acid deficiency. A comprehensive review of ascorbic acid has been published by Hodges and Baker (1973).

22.12.1. Sources and requirements

Vegetables and fruits are the main natural sources of ascorbic acid. Good sources of ascorbic acid are turnip greens (139 mg/100 g), green peppers (128), broccoli (113), brussel sprouts (102), cauliflower (78), cabbage (47), asparagus (33), green lima beans (29), tomatoes (23), potatoes (20), strawberries (59), oranges (50), lemons (46), and cantaloupe (33). Human milk contains an average of 4.3 mg/dl. Cow's milk, meats, cereal grains, dried fruits, and legumes contain only small amounts of ascorbic acid.

Recommended daily allowances for vitamin C are as follows:

infants	35 mg
1 to 14 years	40 to 45 mg
14 to 60 years	45 to 60 mg; pregnant
	60 mg; lactating
	80 mg

Prolonged storage and cooking decreases the vitamin C content of foods. The use of soda in cooking destroys ascorbic acid.

22.12.2. Functions

The exact biochemical mechanisms of the action of ascorbic acid remain unknown. It is believed to participate in important functions such as an intermediary in oxidation–reduction reactions in cellular respiration, as a reducing compound protecting other important molecules from oxidation, and in the transformation of proline to hydroxyproline in the formation of collagen. It also facilitates the absorption of iron from the intestine and its transfer to ferritin. It may also be involved in increasing resistance to infection, and in other chemical reactions. The widespread cellular damage in scurvy certainly indicates the broad participation of ascorbic acid in maintaining cellular integrity. The body pool of ascorbic acid in well nourished individuals ranges from 600 to 1500 mg.

22.12.3. Biochemical diagnosis

Clinical manifestations of ascorbic acid deficiency are observed after 60 to 90 days of dietary deprivation. Initially, small petechial spots appear in the proximity of hair follicles. Later they become large and ecchymotic. Follicular hyperkeratosis develops in the areas of the body exposed to friction (buttocks, elbows, thighs). Anorexia, weakness, irritability, and joint pain develop. As the deficiency progresses, lesions of the connective tissue appear and the gums are swollen, initially in the proximity of the teeth. Fatigue and weakness are present. By the third month anaemia may develop, the mouth becomes dry, the skin itches, and there may be loss of hair and teeth (Sjögren's syndrome). The plasma albumin concentration is decreased and the concentration of some globulins is increased. Psychological symptoms include depression and hypochondria. Old scars may become haemorrhagic. Death may be sudden from advanced scurvy.

Chemical methods to measure ascorbic acid in plasma or serum are available. Spectrophotometric (Roe and Kuether, 1963) and fluorometric (Deutsch and Weeks, 1965) techniques are commonly used. The method of Lowry et al. (1945) measures total ascorbic acid and has certain advantages. The plasma concentration of ascorbic acid reflects the dietary and metabolic status of the vitamin. Specimens must be protected from deterioration by prompt acidification with trichloroacetic or metaphosphoric acid, and analyzed without delay. Preparations with acid added are stable for about 1 week if they are kept at 4 °C or frozen.

The normal plasma concentration of ascorbic acid is 0.8 to 1.6 mg/dl. A concentration of 0.2 mg/dl or less is indicative of deficiency. Occasionally, a plasma concentration of ascorbic acid of 2.0 to 2.5 mg/dl may occur transiently following the ingestion of large doses of vitamin C. Measurements of ascorbic acid in urine are influenced by the diet and are of limited diagnostic value. The renal threshold of ascorbic acid limits the tubular reabsorption when the plasma concentration reaches about 1.6 mg/dl.

Treatment with 60 to 100 mg of ascorbic acid 3 times a day for a few days produces rapid improvement in deficient individuals. Occasionally the serum cholesterol concentration may increase after treatment, but other studies have demonstrated a reduction in the serum cholesterol concentration, especially if it was high initially (Ginter et al., 1977).

No toxicity due to massive doses (up to 1000 times the daily allowance) of ascorbic acid has been reported. The continual oral ingestion of a large amount of ascorbic acid may produce gastric distress, diarrhoea, and acidification of urine which may encourage the formation of uric acid or phosphate calculi, and possible interference with absorption of other micronutrients. The claims of many health benefits made by advocates (Pauling, 1976) of a large intake of ascorbic acid need to be methodically tested and verified before this controversial subject can be objectively evaluated.

22.13. OTHER COMPOUNDS

Some additional compounds with vitamin or vitamin-like effects in experimental animals have been described. Their roles as vitamins in humans is uncertain. There is no conclusive evidence currently available that they can prevent or cure clinical symptoms allegedly produced by their deficiency. The compounds that have been most studied – all of which are widely distributed in nature – are choline, inositol, bioflavonoids, and carnitine (Goodhart, 1973). Some preparations from natural sources, with presently ill-defined chemical compositions and functional roles, e.g. amygdalin (commonly called Laetrile) have gained popularity and a certain degree of notoriety. They are occasionally considered as vitamins by groups of individuals in their search for the prevention or cure of disease. These substances are discussed here to present a picture of micronutrients that may have some impact on health, and the consequences of the ingestion of preparations of uncertain nutritional value.

22.13.1. Choline

Choline is present in tissues in both free and combined forms. It is a component of lecithin and sphingomyelin and the precursor of acetylcholine, an important neurotransmitter. Choline is recognized to be an essential micronutrient for young animals, including pigs, dogs, chicks, and rats. Choline deficiency in experimental animals produces fatty infiltration of the liver (Best and Huntsman, 1932), and haemorrhagic kidneys (Griffith and Wade, 1939). Choline participates in transmethylation reactions as a methyl donor, in the formation of important biological compounds such as creatine and epinephrine, in the formation of compounds such as N′-methylnicotinamide from niacin, and in interactions with vitamin B_{12}. Some aminoacids like threonine and methionine influence the requirement for choline and the response to its deficiency in young animals (Nino et al., 1954).

Choline deficiency has not been demonstrated in man. Its therapeutic value in humans having similar clinical conditions to those found in experimental animals which have been cured by choline administration, has not been satisfactorily confirmed. A comprehensive review of the functions of choline has been published by Griffith and Dyer (1968).

22.13.2. Inositol

Inositol is a cyclic hexitol which is widely distributed in nature. Animal tissues contain myoinositol (meso inositol = muscle sugar), an isomer found primarily in muscle. The heart contains approximately 1.6 g/100 g, brain 0.9 g/100 g, and skeletal muscle 0.4 g/100 g (Woolley, 1944). Inositol is a component of phospholipids. In plants, inositol is found as phytic acid, the hexaphosphate ester. If it is present in high concentration in the diet, phytic acid complexes with calcium, zinc, iron, and possibly other elements, rendering them unabsorbable and thereby causing deficiency. In experimental animals, inositol counteracts the effects of feeding *p*-aminobenzoic acid, and *p*-aminobenzoic acid prevents a syndrome which is produced by feeding diets high in inositol. This could be the result of the actions of these compounds on the intestinal flora.

Inositol is excreted in an increased amount in the urine of diabetic patients (250 to 350 mg/24 h), in comparison with normal individuals (8 to 144 mg, average 37 mg/24 h) (Daughaday and Larner, 1954). There is evidence for the interaction of glucose and inositol in renal function. An increased amount of inositol is excreted in urine following an intravenous infusion of glucose, possibly as a result of the saturation of the tubular reabsorptive mechanism for glucose. The techniques for determining inositol in body fluids are not entirely satisfactory, so that such measurements are made infrequently.

22.13.3. Bioflavonoids

Rusznyak and Szent-Györgi (1936) observed synergistic potentiation of the effects of ascorbic acid by the addition of citrus fruit and other plant extracts. The active components of the fruit were found to be flavones, and their biological function is related to the decrease of capillary permeability (bleeding), from which arose the now obsolete term of vitamin P. The bioflavonoids (hesperidin, quercitin, and rutin) have been thought, especially by "natural food" addicts, to be effective in preventing or curing many conditions ranging from the common cold, erythroblastosis foetalis, and arthritis, to the effects of ionizing radiation. There is no conclusive evidence that any benefits are derived from the use of bioflavonoids with vitamin C for any of the listed conditions. Shils and Goodhart (1956) have published a comprehensive review on the biological aspects of the flavonoids.

22.13.4. Carnitine

While studying the effects of folate on insect nutrition, Fraenkel et al. (1948) observed that meal worms (*Tenebrio molitor*) did not live beyond 5 weeks if a certain factor was absent from the diet. Using this model as a bioassay, it was found that the factor was present in animal tissues, particularly in meat extracts. The factor was named vitamin B-T, and it proved to be carnitine, a quaternary ammonium compound. The possible metabolic functions of carnitine are as a methyl donor facilitating the transfer of fatty acids to muscle cells, and the stimulation of the oxidation of long chain fatty acids. Urinary excretion of carnitine (approximately 150 mg/24 h) parallels its dietary intake, and in normal individuals the excretion of urinary carnitine is also proportional to that of creatine and creatinine.

22.13.5. Laetrile

Laetrile describes a heterogeneous preparation obtained mainly from apricot (*Prunus armeniaca*) or peach (*Prunus persica*) seeds. The name Laetrile does not characterize a specific chemical or pharmacological compound. The chemical analysis of Laetrile yields as major components: amygdalin, a glycoside of mandelonitrile, and gentobiose, a disaccharide. In aqueous solution, amygdalin may be hydrolyzed enzymatically into glucose, benzaldehyde and hydrocyanic acid. The nitrile group in Laetrile may also be released as hydrocyanic acid in acid media such as gastric hydrochloric acid. Laetrile is claimed by advocates of its efficacy to arrest the proliferation of cancerous cells and cause regression of tumours. No extensive, long-term, controlled studies have been published in which the effectiveness of Laetrile in controlling cancer in humans or experimental animals has been properly evaluated. The available short-term reports do not indicate proved beneficial effects.

Laetrile does not comply with the criteria established to describe a vitamin. It is mentioned here only because of its popular mislabelling as a B vitamin. Establishing the benefits, uselessness or even dangers of Laetrile, will require cautious research before any claims can be substantiated.

22.14. THERAPEUTIC APPLICATIONS OF VITAMINS

Vitamins are normally given to correct specific or multiple nutritional deficiencies. Table 22.1 presents clinical situations where vitamins are used to correct abnormalities of aminoacid metabolism; for convenience the relevant references are presented separately at the beginning of the References section.

22.14.1. Total parenteral nutrition

Total parenteral nutrition represents one of the more significant developments in health care in this century. The progress made in the practical application of this technique also opens new perspectives for the understanding of the biochemical functions of some vitamins as well as other micronutrients, such as trace elements. This is very properly presented by Fischer (1976):

"Parenteral nutrition is in its infancy, and any parenteral nutrition unit should carry a heavy emphasis on research, both into the effects of, and some of the problems with, parenteral nutrition as well as into the development of new forms of parenteral nutrition, particularly for different disease entities. Research, both clinical and experimental, is aided by the presence of a large group of physicians and other medical personnel with the same interest and with cross-fertilization of ideas. A laboratory should be available in which different members of the house and visiting staff may pursue their own ideas in parenteral nutrition, and when possible they should be aided by research assistants housed in the hyperalimentation unit. The resident staff in particular should be encouraged to use the laboratory, as parenteral nutrition and clinical research into its application is one of the more fascinating and more easily available avenues to research open to them at the present time."

22.14.2. Population studies

Nutrition has a direct impact on all individuals in a society. Genetic, geographic, anthropological and social determinants influence the nature and frequency of the diet. This affects the clinical assessment of nutritional status. This chapter deals with individuals as if they were similar. However, ideally all the factors that may influence the state of nutrition should be considered before a diagnosis is made.

In the twentieth century we have learned how to prevent and cure some of man's more devastating ills resulting from inadequate nutrition. However, the social sciences have not always experienced comparable progress, and we have yet to learn how to transfer the newly gained knowledge for the benefit of all mankind. In the last decade, famine has caused deaths (e.g. in Sahel and Bangladesh) in numbers comparable to the epidemics of the Middle Ages. The slums, favelas and barriadas of large prosperous cities are reservoirs of human malnutrition. At the same time, in the more affluent societies, nutritional excesses contribute to the prevalence of degenerative diseases – obesity, hypertension, and cardiovascular disorders – with comparable loss in the quality and length of life.

The increase in population, the progressive depletion of natural resources, and the deterioration of the environment contribute to problems of adequate supply of food for all; this remains one of humanity's long-standing problems and it is extensively discussed in many of the reviews and monographs which are recommended for Further Reading.

To ensure that advances in nutrition are correctly applied, it is necessary to educate

TABLE 22.1. THE VITAMIN-RESPONSIVE DISORDERS OF AMINOACID METABOLISM

(From Scriver and Rosenberg, 1973, with permission)

Vitamin	Disorder	Therapeutic dose	Biochemical basis	Reference [a]
Thiamine (B_1)	Lactic acidosis	5–20 mg	Pyruvate carboxylase deficiency	Brunette et al. (1972)
	Branched-chain aminoacidopathy (MSUD variant)	5–20 mg	Branched-chain oxoacid decarboxylase deficiency	Scriver et al. (1971)
Pyridoxine (B_6)	Infantile convulsions	10–50 mg	Glutamic acid decarboxylase deficiency	Hunt et al. (1954); Scriver and Whelan (1969); Yoshida et al. (1971)
	Hypochromic anaemia	>10 mg	Not known	Horrigan and Harris (1964)
	Cystathioninuria	100–500 mg	Cystathionase deficiency	Frimpter et al. (1963); Frimpter (1965)
	Xanthurenicaciduria	5–10 mg	Kynureninase deficiency	Knapp (1960); Tada et al. (1968)
	Homocystinuria	25–500 mg	Cystathionine synthase deficiency	Mudd et al. (1970); Seashore et al. (1972) Barber and Spaeth (1967)
	Hyperoxaluria	100–500 mg	Glyoxylate; α-oxoglutarate carboligase deficiency	Smith and Williams (1967)
Cobalamin (B_{12})	Juvenile pernicious anaemia	<5 μg	Intrinsic factor deficiency or defective ileal transport	Mohamed et al. (1966); Katz et al. (1972)
	Transcobalamin II deficiency	>100 μg	Deficiency of transcobalamin II	Hakami et al. (1971)
	Methylmalonicaciduria	>250 μg	Defective synthesis of Ad-B_{12} co-enzymes	Rosenberg et al. (1968, 1969); Mahoney et al. (1971)
	Methylmalonicaciduria, homocystinuria and hypomethioninaemia	>500 μg	Defective synthesis of Ad-B_{12} and CH_3-B_{12} co-enzymes	Mudd et al. (1969, 1970); Goodman et al. (1970); Mahoney et al. (1971)
Folic acid	Megaloblastic anaemia	<0.05 mg	Defective intestinal absorption of folate	Luhby et al. (1961); Lanzkowsky (1970)
	Formiminotransferase deficiency	>5 mg	Formiminotransferase deficiency	Arakawa et al. (1963); Arakawa (1970)
	Homocystinuria and hypomethioninemia	>10 mg	N^5,N^{10}-methylenetetrahydrofolate reductase deficiency	Mudd et al. (1972); Freeman et al. (1972); Shih et al. (1972)
	Congenital megaloblastic anaemia	>0.1 mg	Dihydrofolate reductase deficiency	Walters (1967)
Biotin	Propionicacidaemia	10 mg	Propionyl-CoA carboxylase deficiency	Barnes et al. (1970)
Niacin	Hartnup disease	40–200 mg	Defective intestinal and renal transport of tryptophan and other "neutral" amino-acids	Jepson (1972)

[a] Table references are presented separately at the beginning of the References section.

both those who are involved in the production, distribution, and preparation of food, as well as consumers, in the proper nutritional requirements and the means of meeting them.

It is important to recognize that even in affluent societies such as the United States vitamin deficiencies may occur in otherwise healthy individuals. This is especially true for thiamine, niacin and vitamins C and D. Deficiencies are even more common in the sick elderly. Attempts should be made to correct all such deficiencies when the individuals are hospitalized, but this must be associated with education and continual reinforcement when the patients are discharged from the hospital.

REFERENCES

For Table 22.1

Arakawa, T. (1970) Congenital defects in folate utilization. American Journal of Medicine, 48, 594–598.

Arakawa, T., Ohara, K., Kudo, Z., Tada, K., Hayashi, T. and Mizuno, T. (1963) Hyperfolic-acidemia with formiminoglutamic-aciduria following histidine loading. Tohoku Journal of Experimental Medicine, 80, 370–382.

Barber, G.W. and Spaeth, G.L. (1967) Pyridoxine therapy in homocystinuria. Lancet, I, 337.

Barnes, N.D., Hull, D., Balgobin, L. and Gompertz, D. (1970) Biotin-responsive propionicacidaemia. Lancet, II, 244–245.

Brunette, M.G., Delvin, E., Hazel, B. and Scriver, C.R. (1972) Thiamine-responsive lactic acidosis in a patient with deficient low-Km pyruvate carboxylase activity in liver. Pediatrics, 50, 702–711.

Freeman, J.M., Finkelstein, J.D., Mudd, S.H. and Uhlendorf, B.W. (1972) Homocystinuria presenting as reversible "schizophrenia". A new defect in methionine metabolism with reduced methylene-tetrahydrofolate-reductase activity (Abstract). Pediatric Research, 6, 423.

Frimpter, G.W. (1965) Cystathioninuria: nature of the defect. Science, 149, 1095–1096.

Frimpter, G.W., Haymovitz, A. and Horwith, M. (1963) Cystathioninuria. New England Journal of Medicine, 268, 333–339.

Goodman, S.I., Moe, P.G., Hammond, K.B., Mudd, S.H. and Uhlendorf, B.W. (1970) Homocystinuria with methylmalonic aciduria: two cases in a sibship. Biochemical Medicine, 4, 500–515.

Hakami, N., Neiman, P.E., Canellos, G.P. and Lazerson, J. (1971) Neonatal megaloblastic anemia due to inherited transcobalamin II deficiency in two siblings. New England Journal of Medicine, 285, 1163–1170.

Horrigan, D.L. and Harris, J.W. (1964) Pyridoxine-responsive anemia: analysis of 62 cases. Advances in Internal Medicine, 12, 103–174.

Hunt, A.D., Jr., Stokes, J., Jr., McCrory, W.W. and Stroud, H.H. (1954) Pyridoxine dependency: report of a case of intractable convulsions in an infant controlled by pyridoxine. Pediatrics, 13, 140–145.

Jepson, J.B. (1972) Hartnup disease. In The Metabolic Basis of Inherited Disease, 3rd edn. (J.B. Stanbury, J.B. Wyngaarden and D.S. Fredrickson, Eds.) pp. 1486–1503, McGraw-Hill, New York, N.Y.

Katz, M., Lee, S.K. and Cooper, B.A. (1972) Vitamin B_{12} malabsorption due to a biologically inert intrinsic factor. New England Journal of Medicine, 287, 425–429.

Knapp, A. (1960) Uber eine neue hereditare, von Vitamin-B_6 abhangige Storung im Tryptophan-Stoffwechsel. Clinica Chimica Acta, 5, 6–13.

Lanzkowsky, P. (1970) Congenital malabsorption of folate. American Journal of Medicine, 48, 580–583.

Luhby, A.L., Eagle, F.J., Roth, E. and Cooperman, J.M. (1961) Relapsing megaloblastic anemia in an infant due to a specific defect in gastrointestinal absorption of folic acid. American Journal of Diseases of Children, 102, 482–483.

Mahoney, M.J., Rosenberg, L.E., Mudd, S.H. and Uhlendorf, B.W. (1971) Defective metabolism of vitamin B_{12} in fibroblasts from children with methylmalonicaciduria. Biochemical and Biophysical Research Communications, 44, 375–381.

Mohamed, S.D., McKay, E. and Galloway, W.H. (1966) Juvenile familial megaloblastic anemia due to selective malabsorption of vitamin B_{12}. (A family study and review of the literature). Quarterly Journal of Medicine, 35, 433–453.

Mudd, S.H., Edwards, W.A., Loeb, P.M., Brown, M.S. and Laster, L. (1970) Homocystinuria due to cystathionine synthase deficiency: the effect of pyridoxine. Journal of Clinical Investigation, 49, 1762–1773.

Mudd, S.H., Levy, H.L. and Abeles, R.H. (1969) A derangement in B_{12} metabolism leading to homocystinemia; cystathioninemia and methylmalonic aciduria. Biochemical and Biophysical Research Communications, 35, 121–126.

Mudd, S.H., Uhlendorf, B.W., Freeman, J.M., Finkelstein, J.D. and Shih, V.E. (1972) Homocystinuria associated with decreased methylenetetrahydrofolate reductase activity. Biochemical and Biophysical Research Communications, 46, 905–912.

Rosenberg, L.E. (1969) Inherited aminoacidopathies demonstrating vitamin dependency. New England Journal of Medicine, 281, 145–153.

Rosenberg, L.E., Lilljeqvist, A. and Hsia, Y.E. (1968) Methylmalonic aciduria. Metabolic block localization and vitamin B_{12} dependency. Science, 162, 805–807.

Rosenberg, L.E., Lilljeqvist, A., Hsia, Y.E. and Rosenbloom, F.M. (1969) Vitamin B_{12} dependent methylmalonicaciduria: defective B_{12} metabolism in cultured fibroblasts. Biochemical and Biophysical Research Communications, 37, 607–614.

Scriver, C.R., Mackenzie, S., Clow, C.L. and Delvin, E. (1971) Thiamine-responsive maple-syrup-urine disease. Lancet, I, 310–312.

Scriver, C.R. and Whelan, D.T. (1969) Glutamic acid decarboxylase (GAD) in mammalian tissue outside the central nervous system, and its possible relevance to hereditary vitamin B_6 dependency with seizures. Annals of the New York Academy of Sciences, 166, 83–96.

Seashore, M.R., Durant, J.L. and Rosenberg, L.E. (1972) Studies of the mechanism of pyridoxine-responsive homocystinuria. Pediatric Research, 6, 187–196.

Shih, V.E., Salam, M.Z., Mudd, S.H., Uhlendorf, B.W. and Adams, R.D. (1972) A new form of homocystinuria due to $N^{5,10}$-methylene tetrahydrofolate reductase deficiency (Abstract). Pediatric Research, 6, 395.

Smith, L.H., Jr. and Williams, H.E. (1967) Treatment of primary hyperoxaluria. Modern Treatment, 4, 522–530.

Tada, K., Yokoyama, Y., Nakagawa, H. and Arakawa, T. (1968) Vitamin B_6 dependent xanthurenic aciduria (the second report). Tohoku Journal of Experimental Medicine, 95, 107–114.

Walters, T.R. (1967) Congenital megaloblastic anemia responsive to N^5-formyl tetrahydrofolic acid administration. Journal of Pediatrics, 70, 686–687.

Yoshida, T., Tada, K. and Arakawa, T. (1971) Vitamin B_6-dependency of glutamic acid decarboxylase in the kidney from a patient with vitamin B_6 dependent convulsion. Tohoku Journal of Experimental Medicine, 104, 195–198.

For Chapter 22

Anderson, T.A. and Fomon, S.J. (1974) In Infant Nutrition, 2nd edn. (Ed. S.J. Fomon) W.B. Saunders Co., Philadelphia, Pa.

Baker, H. and Frank, O. (1968) Clinical Vitaminology. Interscience Publishers, New York, N.Y.

Belsey, R.E., DeLuca, H.F. and Potts, J.T., Jr. (1974) A rapid assay for 25-OH-vitamin D_3 without preparative chromatography. Journal of Clinical Endocrinology, 38, 1046–1051.

Best, C.H. and Huntsman, M.E. (1932) The effects of the components of lecithin upon deposition of fat in the liver. Journal of Physiology 75, 405–412.

Booher, L.E. (1933) The concentration and probable chemical nature of vitamin G. Journal of Biological Chemistry, 102, 39–46.

Brickman, A.S., Coburn, J.W. and Norman, A.W. (1972) Action of 1,25-dihydroxycholecalciferol, a potent, kidney-produced metabolite of vitamin D, in uremic man. New England Journal of Medicine, 287, 891–895.

Brin, M. (1967) Functional evaluation of nutritional status: thiamine. In Newer Methods of Nutritional Biochemistry, Vol. 3 (Ed. A.A. Albanese) p. 407, Academic Press, New York, N.Y.

Brinkhous, K.M. (1940) Plasma prothrombin; vitamin K. Medicine, 19, 329–416.
Bunnell, R.H. (1971) Modern procedures for the analysis of tocopherols. Lipids, 6, 245–253.
Campbell, H.A. and Link, K.P. (1941) Studies on the hemorrhagic sweet clover disease. IV. The isolation and crystallization of the hemorrhagic agent. Journal of Biological Chemistry, 138, 21–33.
Carpenter, K.J. and Kodicek, E. (1950) The fluorimetric estimation of N^1-methylnicotinamide and its differentiation from coenzyme I. Biochemical Journal, 46, 421–426.
Chaykin, S. (1967) Nicotinamide coenzymes. Annual Reviews of Biochemistry, 36, 149–170.
Chong, Y.H. and Ho, G.S. (1970) Erythrocyte transketolase activity. American Journal of Clinical Nutrition, 23, 261–266.
Committee on Nutrition (American Academy of Pediatrics) (1961) Vitamin K compounds and the water soluble analogues. Pediatrics, 28, 501–507.
Dam, H. (1929) Cholesterinstoffwechsel in Hühnereiern und Hühnehen. Biochemische Zeitschrift, 215, 475–492.
Dam, H. (1948) Vitamin K. Vitamins and Hormones, 6, 27–53.
Dam, H., Dyggve, H., Larsen, H. and Plum, P. (1952) The relation of vitamin K deficiency to hemorrhagic disease in the newborn. Advances in Pediatrics, 5, 129–153.
Dam, H., Geiger, A., Glavind, J., Karrer, P., Karrer, W., Rothchild, E. and Salomon, H. (1939) Isolierung des Vitamins K in hochgereinigter Form. Helvetica Chimica Acta, 22, 310–313.
Dam, H., Schønheyder, F. and Tage-Hansen, E. (1936) CLV. Studies on the mode of action of vitamin K. Biochemical Journal, 30, 1075–1079.
Daughaday, W.H. and Larner, J. (1954) The renal excretion of inositol in normal and diabetic human beings. Journal of Clinical Investigation, 33, 326–332.
DeLuca, H.F. (1976) Recent advances in our understanding of the vitamin D endocrine system, Journal of Laboratory and Clinical Medicine, 87, 7–26.
DeLuca, H.F. and Suttie, J.W. (Eds.) (1970) The Fat-Soluble Vitamins. University of Wisconsin Press, Madison, Wisc.
Deutsch, M.J. and Weeks, C.E. (1965) Microfluorometric assay for vitamin C. Journal of The Association of Official Agricultural Chemists, 48, 1248–1256.
DeVries, W.H., Grovier, W.M., Evans, J.S., Gregory, J.D., Novelli, G.D., Soodak, M. and Lipmann, F. (1950) Purification of coenzyme A from fermentation sources and its further partial identification. Journal of the American Chemical Society, 72, 4838.
Elvehjem, C.A., Madden, R.J., Strong, F.M. and Woolley, D.W. (1938) The isolation and identification of the anti-black tongue factor. Journal of Biological Chemistry, 123, 137–149.
Emmett, A.D. and Luros, G.O. (1920) Water-soluble vitamines. I. Are the antineuritic and the growth-promoting water-soluble B vitamins the same? Journal of Biological Chemistry, 43, 265–280.
Evans, H.M. and Bishop, K.S. (1922) On the existence of a hitherto unrecognized dietary factor essential for reproduction. Science, 56, 650–651.
Evans, H.M., Emerson, O.H. and Emerson, J.S. (1936) The isolation from wheat germ oil of an alcohol, α-tocopherol, having the properties of vitamin E. Journal of Biological Chemistry, 113, 319–332.
Fasella, P. (1967) Pyridoxal phosphate. Annual Reviews of Biochemistry, 36, 185–210.
Fischer, J.E. (1976) Total Parenteral Nutrition. Little, Brown and Company, Boston, Mass.
Fraenkel, G., Blewett, M. and Coles, M. (1948) B_T – a new vitamin of the B-group and its relation to the folic acid group, and other antianaemia factors. Nature, 161, 981–983.
Fraser, D.R., Kooh, S.W., Kind, P.H., Holick, M.T., Tanaka, Y. and DeLuca, H.F. (1973) Pathogenesis of hereditary vitamin D-dependent rickets. New England Journal of Medicine, 289, 817–822.
Funk, C. (1911) On the chemical nature of the substance which cures polyneuritis in birds induced by a diet of polished rice. Journal of Physiology (London), 43, 395–400.
Garry, P.G., Pollack, J.D. and Owen, G.M. (1970) Plasma vitamin A assay by fluorometry and use of a silicic acid column technique. Clinical Chemistry, 16, 766–772.
Ginter, E., Černà, O. Budlovsky, J., Baláž, V., Krubá, F., Roch, V. and Šaško, E. (1977) Effect of ascorbic acid on plasma cholesterol in humans in a long-term experiment. International Journal for Vitamin Nutrition Research, 47, 123–134.
Glatzle, D., Korner, W.F., Christeller, S. and Wiss, O. (1970) Method for the detection of a biochemical riboflavin deficiency. (Stimulation of $NADPH_2$-dependent glutathione reductase from

human erythrocytes by FAD in vitro. Investigations on the vitamin B_2 status in healthy people and geriatric patients). International Journal of Vitamin and Nutrition Research, 40, 166–183.

Goldberger, J. and Wheeler, G.A. (1915) Experimental pellagra in the human subject brought about by a restricted diet. Public Health Reports, 30, 3336–3339.

Goodhart, R.S. (1973) In Modern Nutrition in Health and Disease, 5th edn. (Eds R.S. Goodhart and M.E. Shils) p. 259, Lea and Febiger, Philadelphia, Pa.

Greaves, J.H. and Ayres, P. (1967) Heritable resistance to warfarin in rats. Nature, 215, 877–878.

Green, J. and Bunyan, J. (1969) Vitamin E and the antioxidant theory. Nutrition Abstracts and Reviews, 39, 321–343.

Griffith, W.H. and Dyer, H.M. (1968) Present knowledge of methyl groups in nutrition. Nutrition Reviews, 26, 1–4.

Griffith, W.H. and Wade, N.J. (1939) Choline metabolism. I – The occurrence and prevention of hemorrhagic degeneration in young rats on a low choline diet. Journal of Biological Chemistry, 131, 567–577.

György, P. (1934) Vitamin B_2 and the pellagra-like dermatitis in rats. Nature, 133, 498–499.

Halsted, J.A. (Ed.) (1976) The Laboratory in Clinical Medicine. Saunders, Philadelphia, Pa.

Hansen, L.G. and Warwick, W.J. (1966) A fluorometric micro method for serum tocopherol. American Journal of Clinical Pathology, 46, 133–138.

Haworth, W.N. and Hirst, E.L. (1933) Synthesis of ascorbic acid. Journal of the Society of Chemical Industry, 52, 645–646.

Hennessey, D.J. and Cerecedo, L.R. (1939) The determination of free and phosphorylated thiamine by a modified thiochrome assay. Journal of The American Chemical Society, 61, 179–183.

Hermodson, M.A., Suttie, J.W. and Link, K.P. (1969) Warfarin metabolism and vitamin K requirement in the warfarin-resistant rat. American Journal of Physiology, 217, 1316–1319.

Hodges, R.E. and Baker, E.M. (1973) In Modern Nutrition in Health and Disease, 5th edn. (Eds R.S. Goodhart and M.E. Shils) p. 245, Lea and Febiger, Philadelphia, Pa.

Horwitt, M.K. (1962) Interactions between vitamin E and polyunsaturated fatty acids in adult man. Vitamins and Hormones, 20, 541–558.

Horwitt, M.K., Hills, O.W., Harvey, C.C., Liebert, E. and Steinberg, D.L. (1949) Effects of dietary depletion of riboflavin. Journal of Nutrition, 39, 357–373.

Huldschinsky, K. (1919) Heilung von Rachitis durch kunstliche Hohensone. Deutsche Medizinische Wochenschrift, 45, 712–713.

Jansen, B.C.P. (1956) Early nutritional researchers of beriberi leading to the discovery of vitamin B_1. Nutrition Abstracts and Reviews, 26, 1–14.

Joubert, C.P. and DeLange, J. (1962) A modification of the method for determination of N′-methyl-2-pyridone-carboxylamide in human urine and its application in the evaluation of nicotinic acid status. Proceedings of The Society for Nutrition, South Africa, 3, 60.

Karrer, P., Schopp, K. and Benz, F. (1935) Synthesen von Flavinen IV. Helvetica Chimica Acta, 18, 426–429.

King, C.G. and Waugh, W.A. (1932) The chemical nature of vitamin C. Science, 75, 357–358.

Knappe, J. (1970) Mechanism of biotin action. Annual Review of Biochemistry, 39, 757–776.

Kuhn, R., Reinenrund, K., Weygand, F. and Strobele, R. (1935) Uber die Synthese des Lactoflavins (Vitamin B_2). Chemische Berichte, 68, 1765–1774.

Lev, M. and Milford, A.W. (1966) Water soluble factors with vitamin K activity from pig liver and from fusiformis nigriscens. Nature, 210, 1120–1122.

Leveille, G.A. (1972) Modified thiochrome procedure for the determination of urinary thiamin. American Journal of Clinical Nutrition, 25, 273–274.

Lind, J. (1753) Treatise on Scurvy. Reprinted and edited by C.P. Stewart and D. Guthrie, University of Edinburgh Press, 1953.

Lipmann, F. and Kaplan, N.O. (1946) A common factor in the enzymatic acetylation of sulfanilamide and of choline. Journal of Biological Chemistry, 162, 743–744.

Lowry, O.H., Lopez, J.A. and Bessey, O.A. (1945) The determination of ascorbic acid in small amounts of blood serum. Journal of Biological Chemistry, 160, 609–615.

McCollum, E.V. (1957) A History of Nutrition. Houghton Mifflin Co., Boston, Mass.

McCollum, E., Simmonds, N., Becker, J.E. and Shipley, P.G. (1922) Studies on experimental rickets. XXII. The production of rickets in the rat by diets consisting of essentially purified food substances. Journal of Biological Chemistry, 54, 249–252.

McCormick, D.B. and Wright, L.D. (Eds) (1970) Methods in Enzymology, Vol. 18, Part A. p. 431, Academic Press, New York, N.Y.

McKee, R.W., Binkley, S.G., Thayer, S.A., MacCorquodale, D.W. and Doisy, E.A. (1939) The isolation of vitamin K. Journal of Biological Chemistry, 131, 327–344.

McLaren, D.S. (1967) Effects of vitamin A deficiency in man. In The Vitamins, 2nd edn., Vol. 1 (Eds W.H. Sebrell, Jr. and R.S. Harris) pp. 267–280, Academic Press, New York, N.Y.

Mellanby, E. (1919) An experimental investigation of rickets. Lancet, 2, 407–412.

Moore, T. (1957) Vitamin A. Elsevier, Amsterdam, The Netherlands.

Moore, T. (1967) In The Vitamins, 2nd edn., Vol. 1 (Eds W.H. Sebrell, Jr. and R.S. Harris) Academic Press, New York, N.Y.

National Academy of Sciences (1974) National Research Council, U.S.A. Food and Nutrition Board. Recommended Dietary Allowances. 8th edn., Washington, D.C.

Neeld, J.B. Jr. and Pearson, W.N. (1963) Macro and micro methods for the determination of vitamin A using trifluoroacetic acid. Journal of Nutrition, 79, 454–462.

Neims, A.H. and Hellerman, L. (1970) Flavoenzyme catalysis. Annual Review of Biochemistry, 39, 867–888.

Nino, H.H., Harper, A.D. and Elvehjem, C.A. (1954) Histological differentiation of fatty livers produced by threonine or choline deficiency. Journal of Nutrition, 53, 469–480.

Nino, H.V. and Shaw, W. (1976) Vitamins. In Fundamentals of Clinical Chemistry, 2nd edn. (Ed. N.W. Tietz) W.B. Saunders Co., Philadelphia, Pa.

Olcott, H.S. (1935) Vitamin E. III. Evidence for the presence of a hydroxyl group. The biological utilization of esters. Absorption spectrum. Journal of Biological Chemistry, 110, 695–701.

Olcott, H.S. and Mattill, H.A. (1931) The unsaponifiable lipids of lettuce. II. Fractionation. Journal of Biological Chemistry, 93, 59–64.

Olson, R.E. (1970a) In The Fat-Soluble Vitamins (Eds H.F. DeLuca and J.W. Suttie) University of Wisconsin Press, Madison, Wisc.

Olson, R.E. (1970b) The mode of action of vitamin K. Nutrition Research, 28, 171–176.

Omdahl, J., Holick, M.F., Suda, T., Tanaka, Y. and DeLuca, H.F. (1971) Biological activity of 1,25-dihydroxycholecalciferol. Biochemistry, 10, 2935–2940.

Omdahl, J.L. and DeLuca, H.F. (1973) In Modern Nutrition in Health and Disease, 5th edn. (Eds R.S. Goodhart and M.E. Shils) Lea and Febiger, Philadelphia, Pa.

O'Reilly, R.A., Aggeler, P.M., Hoag, M.S., Leong, L.S. and Kropatkin, M.L. (1964) Hereditary transmission of exceptional resistance to coumarin anticoagulant drugs. The first reported kindred. New England Journal of Medicine, 271, 809–815.

Parsons, H.T., Lease, J.G. and Kelly, E. (1937) LIX. Interrelationship between dietary egg white and the requirement for protective factor in the cure of nutritive disorder due to egg white. Biochemical Journal, 31, 424–432.

Pauling, L. (1976) Vitamin C, The Common Cold, and the Flu. W.H. Freeman Co., San Francisco, California.

Pearson, W.N. (1966) Assessment of nutritional status: biochemical methods. In Nutrition, Vol. 3 (Eds G.H. Beaton and E.W. McHenry) pp. 265–315, Academic Press, New York, N.Y.

Pearson, W.N. (1967) Riboflavin. In The Vitamins, Vol. 7, 2nd edn. (Eds P. Gyorgy and W.N. Pearson) pp. 130–134, Academic Press, New York, N.Y.

Pike, R.L. and Brown, M.L. (1975) Nutrition: An Integrated Approach, 2nd edn. Wiley, New York, N.Y.

Ponchon, G. and DeLuca, H.F. (1969) The role of the liver in the metabolism of vitamin D. Journal of Clinical Investigation, 48, 1273–1279.

Quick, A.J. (1939) Determination of prothrombin. Proceedings of The Society for Experimental Biology and Medicine, 42, 788–789.

Quick, A.J. (1957) Hemorrhagic Diseases. Lea and Febiger, Philadelphia, Pa.

Reichstein, T., Grussner, A. and Oppenauer, R. (1933) Synthese der D- und L-Ascorbinsaure (C-vitamin). Helvetica Chimica Acta, 16, 1019–1023.

Rietz, P., Gloor, U. and Wiss, O. (1970) Menachionone aus menschlicher Leber und Faulschlamm. Internationale Zeitschrift für Vitaminforschung, 40, 351–362.

Roe, J.H. and Kuether, C.A. (1943) The determination of ascorbic acid in whole blood and urine through the 2,4-dinitrophenylhydrazine derivative of dehydroascorbic acid. Journal of Biological Chemistry, 147, 399–407.

Roels, O.A. (1967) In The Vitamins, 2nd edn., Vol. 1 (Eds W.H. Sebrell, Jr. and R.S. Harris) Academic Press, New York, N.Y.

Roels, O.A. and Trout, M. (1972) Vitamin A and carotene. In Standard Methods of Clinical Chemistry, Vol. 7 (Ed. G.R. Cooper) pp. 215–230, Academic Press, New York, N.Y.

Rusznyak, S. and Szent-György, A. (1936) Vitamin P: flanovols as vitamins. Nature, 138, 27.

Sandstead, H. (1973) In Modern Nutrition in Health and Disease, 5th edn. (Eds. R.S. Goodhart and M.E. Shils) p. 596, Lea and Febiger, Philadelphia, Pa.

Sauberlich, H.E. and Canham, J.E. (1973) In Modern Nutrition in Health and Disease, 5th edn. (Eds. R.S. Goodhart and M.E. Shils) p. 210, Lea and Febiger, Philadelphia, Pa.

Sauberlich, H.E., Dowdy, R.P. and Skala, J.H. (1974) Laboratory Tests for the Assessment of Nutritional Status. CRC Press, Cleveland, Ohio.

Schaefer, A.E. (1963) (Executive Director) Manual for Nutrition Surveys, 2nd edn., Interdepartmental Committee on Nutrition for National Defense. (ICNND) National Institutes of Health, Bethesda, Md. U.S. Government Printing Office, Washington, D.C. 20402.

Scriver, C.R. and Rosenberg, L.E. (1973) Amino Acid Metabolism and its Disorders. Saunders, Philadelphia, p. 472.

Sebrell, W.H. and Butler, R.E. (1938) Riboflavin deficiency in man (a preliminary note) Public Health Reports, 53, 2282–2284.

Sebrell, W.H. and Butler, R.E. (1939) Riboflavin deficiency in man (ariboflavinosis). Public Health Reports, 54, 2121–2131.

Sebrell, W.H., Jr. and Haggerty, J.J. (1967) Food and Nutrition. Time-Life Books, New York, N.Y.

Shah, D.V. and Suttie, J.W. (1971) Mechanism of action of vitamin K: evidence for the conversion of a precursor protein to prothrombin in the rat. Proceedings of the National Academy of Sciences, U.S.A., 68, 1653–1657.

Shils, M.E. and Goodhart, R.S. (1956) The Flavonoids in Biology and Medicine. Nutrition Monograph Series No. 2, The National Vitamin Foundation, Inc., New York, N.Y.

Slater, E.C., DeVijlder, J.J.M. and Boers, W. (1970) The binding of NAD^+ and NADP to glyceraldehydephosphate dehydrogenase. Vitamins and Hormones, 28, 315–327.

Slater, E.C. and Morell, D.B. (1946) A modification of the fluorimetric method of determining riboflavin in biological materials. Biochemical Journal, 40, 644–652.

Snell, E.E. (1945) The vitamin B-6 group. IV. Evidence for the occurrence of pyridoxamine and pyridoxal in natural products. Journal of Biological Chemistry, 157, 491–505.

Snell, E.E., Guirard, B.M. and Williams, R.J. (1942) Occurrence in natural products of a physiologically active metabolite of pyridoxine. Journal of Biological Chemistry, 143, 519–530.

Steenbock, J. (1924) The induction of growth promoting and calcifying properties in a ration on exposure to light. Science, 60, 224–225.

Stiller, E.T., Harris, S.A., Finkelstein, J., Keretsztesy, J.C. and Folkers, K. (1940) Pantothenic acid. VIII. The total synthesis of pure pantothenic acid. Journal of the American Chemical Society, 62, 1785–1790.

Sure, B. (1924) Dietary requirements for reproduction. II. The existence of a specific vitamin for reproduction. Journal of Biological Chemistry, 58, 693–709.

Svirbely, J.L. and Szent-György, A. (1932) The chemical nature of vitamin C. Biochemical Journal, 26, 865–870.

Szent-György, A. (1928) Observations on the function of peroxidase systems and the chemistry of the adrenal cortex. Biochemical Journal, 22, 1387–1409.

Tanaka, Y. and DeLuca, H.F. (1973) The control of 25-hydroxy-vitamin D metabolism by inorganic phosphate. Archives of Biochemistry and Biophysics, 154, 566–574.

Tappel, A.L. (1962) Vitamin E as the biological lipid antioxidant. Vitamins and Hormones, 20, 493–510.

Tappel, A.L. (1970) Reactions of vitamin E, ubiquinol and selenoaminoacids and protection of oxidant-labile enzymes. In The Fat-Soluble Vitamins (Eds H.F. DeLuca and J.W. Suttie) pp. 369–374, University of Wisconsin Press, Madison, Wisc.

Thompson, J.N., Erdody, P., Brien, R. and Murray, T.K. (1971) Fluorometric determination of vitamin A in human blood and liver. Biochemical Medicine, 5, 67–89.

Tillotson, J.A. and Baker, E.M. (1972) An enzymatic measurement of the riboflavin status in man. American Journal of Clinical Nutrition, 25, 425–431.

Waddell, J. (1934) The provitamin D of cholesterol. I – The antirachitic efficacy of irradiated cholesterol. Journal of Biological Chemistry, 105, 711–739.

Wald, G. (1943) The photoreceptor function of the carotenoids and vitamins A. Vitamins and Hormones, 1, 195–227.

Wald, G. (1953) The biochemistry of vision. Annual Review of Biochemistry, 22, 497–526.

Wald, G. and Hubbard, R. (1950) The synthesis of rhodopsin from vitamin A_1. Proceeding of the National Academy of Sciences, U.S.A., 36, 92–102.

Wald, G. and Hubbard, R. (1957) Visual pigment of a decapod crustacean: the lobster. Nature, 180, 278–280.

Warburg, O. and Christian, W. (1933) Über das gelbe Ferment und seine Wirkungen. Biochemische Zeitschrift, 266, 377–411.

Warburg, O. and Christian, W. (1935) Co-Fermentproblem. Biochemische Zeitschrift, 275, 112–113.

Williams, R.J., Truesdail, J.H., Weinstock, H.H., Jr., Rohrmann, E., Lyman, C.M. and McBurney, C.H. (1938) Pantothenic acid. II. Its concentration and purification from liver. Journal of the American Chemical Society, 60, 2719–2723.

Williams, R.R. (1961) Toward the Conquest of Beriberi. Harvard University Press, Cambridge, Massachusetts.

Williams, R.R. and Cline, J.K. (1936) Synthesis of vitamin B_1. Journal of the American Chemical Society, 58, 1504–1505.

Wiss, O. and Gloor, U. (1966) Absorption, distribution, storage and metabolites of vitamin K and related quinones. Vitamins and Hormones, 24, 575–586.

Woolley, D.W. (1944) The nutritional significance of inositol. Journal of Nutrition, 28, 305–314.

FURTHER READING

Anderson, K.E., Bodansky, O. and Kappas, A. (1976) Effects of oral contraceptives on vitamin metabolism. Advances in Clinical Chemistry, 18, 248–287.

Ballinger, F.W., Collins, J.A., Drucker, W.R., Dudrick, S.J. and Zeppa, R. (1975) Editorial Subcommittee, Committee on Pre and Postoperative Care. American College of Surgeons. Manual of Surgical Nutrition, Saunders, Philadelphia, Pa.

Bogert, J.L., Briggs, G.M. and Calloway, D.H. (1973) Nutrition and Physical Fitness, 9th edn. Saunders, Philadelphia, Pa.

Butterworth, C.E. and Sauberlich, H. (1975) Effects of oral contraceptive hormones on nutrient metabolism. American Journal of Clinical Nutrition, 28, 333–403 and 28, 519–555.

Christakis, G., Editor (1973) Nutritional assessment in health programs. American Journal of Public Health, 63, Suppl., 1–82.

DeLuca, H.F. and Suttie, J.W. (Eds) (1970) The Fat-Soluble Vitamins, University of Wisconsin Press, Madison, Wisconsin.

DeLuca, H.F. (1976) Recent advances in our understanding of the vitamin D endocrine system. Journal of Laboratory and Clinical Medicine, 87, 7–26.

Demetriou, J.A. (1974) Vitamins. In Clincial Chemistry: Principles and Technics, 2nd edn. (Eds R.H. Henry, D.C. Cannon and J.W. Winkelman) pp. 1371–1420, Harper and Row, Hagerstown, Maryland.

Eckholm, E. and Record, F. (1976) The Two Faces of Malnutrition, Paper 9, Worldwatch Institute, Washington, D.C.

Farber, S.M., Wilson, N.L. and Wilson, R.H.L. (1966) Food and Civilization. C.C. Thomas, Springfield, Ill.

Fischer, J.E. (Ed.) (1976) Total Parenteral Nutrition. Little, Brown, Boston, Mass.

Fomon, S.J. (1974) Infant Nutrition, 2nd edn., Saunders, Philadelphia, Pa.

Goodhart, R.S. and Shils, M.E. (1973) Modern Nutrition in Health and Disease, 5th edn., Lea and Febiger, Philadelphia, Pa.

Nino, H.V. and Shaw, W. (1976) Vitamins. In Fundamentals of Clinical Chemistry, 2nd edn. (Ed. N.W. Tietz) pp. 542–564, Saunders, Philadelphia, Pa.

Pike, R.L. and Brown, M.L. (1975) Nutrition: An Integrated Approach, 2nd edn., Wiley, New York, N.Y.

Prasad, A.S., Lei, K.Y., Oberleas, D., Moghissi, W.S. and Stryker, J.C. (1975) Effect of oral contraceptive agents on nutrients: II. Vitamins. American Journal of Clinical Nutrition, 28, 385–391.

Prasad, A.S., Lei, K.Y., Moghissi, K.S., Stryker, J.C. and Oberleas, D. (1976) Effect of oral contraceptives on nutrients. III. Vitamins B_6, B_{12}, and folic acid. American Journal of Obstetrics and Gynecology, 125, 1063–1069.

Sabry, Z.I. (National Coordinator) (1973) Nutrition Canada, National Survey, Information Canada, Ottawa, Ontario.

Sauberlich, H.E., Dowdy, R.P. and Skala, J.H. (1974) Laboratory Tests for the Assessment of Nutritional Status. CRC Press, Cleveland, Ohio.

Schaefer, A.E. (Executive Director) (1963) Manual for Nutrition Surveys, 2nd edn., Interdepartmental Committee on Nutrition for National Defense (ICNND), National Institutes of Health, Bethesda, Md., U.S. Government Printing Office, Washington, D.C.

Science (1975) Food Special Issue, 188, pp. 501–563.

Scientific American (1976) Food and Agriculture Special Issue, 235, September 1976.

Tannahill, R. (1973) Food in History. Stein and Day, New York, N.Y.

Ten State Nutrition Survey (1968–1970) U.S. Department of Health, Education, and Welfare, Health Services and Mental Health Administration, Center for Disease Control, Atlanta, Ga., DHEW Publication Numbers (HSM) 72–8130 to 72–8134.

White, P.L. (Ed.) (1974) Nutrition Reviews: A Special Supplement – Nutrition Misinformation and Food Fadism, Vol. 32. Nutrition Foundation, New York, N.Y.

ADDENDUM

Since this chapter was originally written, a number of significant papers have been published; these are listed below under their respective headings.

22.15.1. Vitamins, clinical and metabolic aspects

DeLuca, H.F. (1977) Vitamin D Metabolism. Clinical Endocrinology, 7, Suppl., 1S–17S.

Haussler, M.R. and McCain, T.A. (1977a) Basic and clinical concepts related to vitamin D metabolism and action. New England Journal of Medicine, 297, 974–983.

Haussler, M.R. and McCain, T.A. (1977b) Basic and clinical concepts related to vitamin D metabolism and action. New England Journal of Medicine, 297, 1041–1050.

Moran, J.R., and Greene, H.L. (1979) The B vitamins and vitamin C in human nutrition. American Journal of Diseases of Children, 133, 192–199.

New York Academy of Sciences (1975) Second Conference on Vitamin C. (Eds. C.G. King and J.J. Burns) Annals of the New York Academy of Sciences, 258.

New York Academy of Sciences (1977) Food and Nutrition in Health and Disease. (Eds. N.H. Moss and J. Mayer) Annals of the New York Academy of Sciences, 300.

22.15.2. Biochemical diagnosis

Braico, K.T., Humbert, J.R., Terplan, K.L. and Lehotay, J.M. (1979) Laetrile intoxication. New England Journal of Medicine, 238–240.

Coburn, J.W., Brickman, A.S., Sherrard, D.J., Singert, F.R., Wong, E.G.C., Baylink, D.J. and Norman, A.W. (1977) Use of $1,25(OH)_2$-vitamin D_3 to separate 'types' of renal osteodystrophy. European Dialysis and Transplant Association Proceedings, 14, 442–449.

Chertow, B.S., Williams, G.A., Norris, R.M., Baker, G.R. and Hargis, G.K. (1977) Vitamin A stimulation of parathyroid hormone: interactions with calcium, hydrocortisone, and vitamin E in bovine parathyroid tissues and effects of vitamin A in man. European Journal of Clinical Investigation, 7, 307–314.

Dorr, R.T., and Paxinos, J. (1978) The current status of Laetrile. Annals of Internal Medicine, 89, 389–397.

Jubiz, W., Haussler, M.R., McCain, T.A. and Tolman, K.G. (1977) Plasma 1,25-dihydroxyvitamin D levels in patients receiving anticonvulsant drugs. Journal of Clinical Endocrinology and Metabolism, 44, 617–621.

Kanis, J.A., Earnshaw, M., Henderson, R.G., Heynen, G., Ledingham, J.G.G., Naik, R.B., Oliver, D.O., Russell, R.G.G., Smith, R., Wilkinson, R.H. and Woods, C.G. (1977) Correlation of clinical, biochemical and skeletal responses to 1α-hydroxyvitamin D_3 in renal bone disease. Clinical Endocrinology, 7, Suppl., 45S–50S.

Kumar, R., Cohen, W.R., Silva, P. and Epstein, F.H. (1979) Elevated 1,25-dihydroxyvitamin D plasma levels in normal human pregnancy and lactation. Journal of Clinical Investigation, 63, 342–344.

Matsushita, Y., Hasegawa, K., Otomo, S., Morii, H., Okamoto, T., Wada, M. and DeLuca, H.F. (1977) Clinical effects of 25-hydroxycholecalciferol in patients with chronic renal failure. Journal of Nutritional Sciences and Vitaminology, 23, 257–261.

Peck, G.L., Olsen, T.G., Yoder, F.W., Strauss, J.S., Downing, D.T., Pandya, M., Butkus, D. and Arnaud-Battandier, J. (1979) Prolonged remissions of cystic and conglobate acne with 13-cis-retinoic acid. New England Journal of Medicine, 300, 329–333.

Schmidt-Gayk, H., Ritz, E., Mehls, O., Goossen, J. and Forster, P. (1977a) 25-OH-vitamin D in experimental and clinical uremia. Calcified Tissue Research, 22, Suppl., 430–433.

Schmidt-Gayk, H., Grawunder, C., Tschope, W., Schmitt, W., Ritz, E., Pietsch, V. and Andrassy, K. (1977b) 25-hydroxy-vitamin-D in nephrotic syndrome. Lancet, II, 105–108.

Walker, G.S., Peacock, M., Aaron, J., Robinson, P.J.A. and Davison, A.M. (1977) Prophylactic 1α-hydroxyvitamin D_3 therapy in haemodialysis patients. Clinical Endocrinology, 7, Suppl., 125S–130S.

22.15.3. Analytical methodology

Barragry, J.M., Corless, D., Auton, J., Carter, N.D., Long, R.G., Maxwell, J.D. and Switala, S. (1978) Plasma vitamin D-binding globulin in vitamin D deficiency, pregnancy and chronic liver disease. Clinica Chimica Acta, 87, 359–365.

Beckman, A.O., Gallaway, W.S., Kaye, W. and Ulrich, W.F. (1977) History of spectrophotometry at Beckman Instruments, Inc. Analytical Chemistry, 49, 280A–300A.

Bjorkhem, I. and Larsson, A. (1978) A specific assay of vitamin D-3 in human serum. Clinica Chimica Acta, 88, 559–567.

De Leenheer, A.P., De Bevere, V.O., Cruyl, A.A. and Claeys, A.E. (1978) Determination of serum α-tocopherol (vitamin E) by high-performance liquid chromatography. Clinical Chemistry, 24, 585–590.

DeRuyter, M.G.M. and De Leenheer, A.P. (1978) Simultaneous determination of retinol and retinyl esters in serum or plasma by reversed-phase high-performance liquid chromatography. Clinical Chemistry, 24, 1920–1923.

Gilbertson, T.J. and Styrd, R.P. (1977) High-performance liquid chromatographic assay for 25-hydroxyvitamin D_3 in serum. Clinical Chemistry, 23, 1700–1704.

Hansen, L.G., and Warwick, W.J. (1978) An improved assay method for serum vitamins A and E using fluorometry. American Journal of Clinical Pathology, 70, 922–923.

Horst, R.L., Shepard, R.M., Jorgensen, N.A. and DeLuca, H.F. (1979) The determination of 24,25-dihydroxyvitamin D and 25,26-dihydroxyvitamin D in plasma from normal and nephrectomized man. Journal of Laboratory and Clinical Medicine, 93, 277–285.

Jones, G. (1978) Assay of vitamins D_2 and D_3, and 25-hydroxyvitamins D_2 and D_3 in human plasma by high-performance liquid chromatography. Clinical Chemistry, 24, 287–298.

Mason, R.S. and Posen, S. (1977) Some problems associated with assay of 25-hydroxycalciferol in human serum. Clinical Chemistry, 23, 806–810.

Stryd, R.P. and Gilbertson, T.J. (1978) Some problems in development of a high-performance liquid chromatographic assay to measure 25-hydroxyvitamin D_2 and 25-hydroxyvitamin D_3 simultaneously in human serum. Clinical Chemistry, 24, 927–290.

Chapter 23

Toxicology and drug monitoring

Stanley S. Brown and Alexander A.H. Lawson

Division of Clinical Chemistry, Clinical Research Centre, Harrow, Middlesex HA1 3UJ, England and Milesmark Hospital, Dunfermline, Fife KY12 9NR, Scotland.

CONTENTS

Chemical diagnosis of disease, edited by
S.S. Brown, F.L. Mitchell and D.S. Young

23.1. INTRODUCTION

Toxicology is not a new branch of biomedical science. The treatise by Orfila (1815) on Animal, Vegetable and Mineral Poisons, is generally considered to mark the first systematic study of the harmful effects of chemicals on biological systems; but long before his time, a Hindu proverb went "Even nectar is poison if taken to excess" and Shakespeare (Henry IV, part II) wrote "In poison there is physic". These sentiments accord with much of our present knowledge of the toxicities of natural and man-made poisons, and of essential nutrients such as oxygen, water, and salt.

This chapter is concerned with those aspects of clinical toxicology and clinical pharmacology in which chemical analysis or biochemical investigations can afford helpful information in respect of diagnosis or treatment. Only the more common forms of poisoning or drug toxicity are considered here. Even then it must be recognized that "common" must be qualified by the recognition of local, national, or international differences in the prescribing of drugs – and hence of adverse reactions – and in the prevalence of various types of poisoning. Moreover, abreactions to or overdosage of therapeutic agents, and illness resulting from exposure to environmental or industrial toxins and their interactions with drugs (Deer Lodge Conference, 1976), reflect only part of the spectrum of toxicology. Chemical and biochemical assays have important places in the testing for safety of all manner of drugs, food additives, pesticides, insecticides, and the like, but these aspects of toxicology are not relevant to the present context.

Many years ago, Osler wrote "It is the doctor's duty to do all he can to help his patient, but if he cannot do any good, he must at all events do no harm". Unfortunately, iatrogenic illnesses resulting from inappropriate drug dosage or administration, incompatible drug mixtures and inadequate precautions regarding interactions or side-effects are all too common. Modern therapeutics and the correct use of new drugs is an exacting problem for all doctors, as shown by the findings of comprehensive drug surveillance programs which have been established in medical wards (Hurwitz, 1969a; Miller, 1973) and in paediatric units (Boston Collaborative Drug Surveillance Program, 1972). Such studies have included investigations of the side-effects of drug therapy which were experienced by large series of patients, and useful conclusions have been drawn (Lawson and Wilson, 1974). It has been estimated that in the United States up to nine drugs are administered to the average in-patient, compared with six for the average in-patient in Israel and five for the average hospital patient in the United Kingdom. Hurwitz (1969a) has shown, not surprisingly, that older patients tend to receive more drugs and that side-effects increase with the use of more drugs. Studies of this kind have also provided information regarding the number of hospital admissions directly resulting from drug toxicity (Hurwitz, 1969b) and the prevalence of toxicity occurring during therapy (Hoddinott et al., 1967; May et al., 1977). In some countries, official bodies have been set up to monitor drug use, abuse and abreactions, but although valuable information has been gathered in this way (Gross and Inman, 1977; Stewart et al., 1977), the findings are often incomplete and may be based on single observations or poorly documented data. All too often, clinical experience is at variance with the results of what might be called "more scientific" studies, depending on in vitro investigations or animal experiments. This perhaps reflects the differences between individual patients in reponse to recommended dosage regimens, and points to the merit of quantitative drug monitoring in carefully studied patients.

In recent years, the scope and limitations of conventional means of assaying drugs in body fluids have become reasonably well defined (World Health Organization, 1974), with corresponding improvements in methodologies for the measurements of very low concentrations of drugs and, in some cases, of their metabolites (Marks et al., 1973; Wallace et al., 1974; Reid, 1976). Techniques such as gas chromatography and high-performance liquid chromatography, especially when coupled to mass spectrometry, offer high sensitivity and good specificity. Immunoassay and competitive binding methods (Butler, 1973) are, in general, not so specific but present some advantages in the screening or actual analysis of large numbers of specimens. Without doubt, analytical methodology has advanced at a much faster pace than quantitative pharmacology and toxicology. The pioneering efforts of Brodie and his co-workers, more than 30 years ago, in relating blood concentrations of antimalarial, sulphonomide and barbiturate drugs in experimental animals to their pharmacological effects, have proved difficult to extend beyond normal human subjects to patients with overt disease for ethical and other reasons.

The effects of disease on the response to drugs (James, 1974) are most clearly evident in infectious diseases, where the effectiveness of antibiotic therapy has been greatly improved both by the accurate identification of the infecting organism and by a knowledge of its sensitivity to available antibiotics. It is also now accepted that precise diagnosis in the spectrum of disorders resulting in the nephrotic syndrome can greatly increase the predictability of response to corticosteroid treatment (Black et al., 1970). Furthermore, in the accelerated type of hypertension, patients respond better to intravenous diazoxide than to intravenous clonidine, whereas in less severe forms of hypertension the opposite is the case (Mroczek et al., 1973). Quantitative studies of the metabolism of aminopyrine (Hepner and Vesell, 1977) and diazepam (Klotz et al., 1977) in patients with liver disease have recently been performed. All of these examples should encourage the clinical pharmacologist and the clinical chemist in their pursuit of rational chemotherapy (Werner et al., 1975).

23.2. BASIC PRINCIPLES OF PHARMACOKINETICS AND PHARMACOLOGY

Far less is known about the time course of drug transport and transformation, and its relationship to pharmacological and toxic effects, than about the qualitative chemical aspects of metabolism and drug action. This reflects the fact that although the theoretical foundations of pharmacokinetics were laid in the period 1920 to 1940 by the pioneer investigators Widmark, Gehlen, Beccari, Dominguez and Theorell, the first comprehensive review was published less than 20 years ago (Nelson, 1961). It is fair to say that no radically new concepts have emerged in the last decade, but significant advances have stemmed from an increased understanding of the mechanisms of drug absorption and renal handling, and of the relevance of genetic factors and of drug interactions of metabolism (Greenblatt and Koch-Weser, 1975).

Although a good deal is known about the in vitro relationships between pharmacological effects and drug concentrations in body fluids, the corresponding in vivo situation is poorly understood. The overall metabolic and pharmacological picture is very involved, and extrapolation to man from animal species is especially difficult in the field of drug response. It might be expected intuitively that with some drugs at least, there would be a link between blood or tissue concentrations and pharmacological response or therapeutic or toxic effect. In fact, few systematic attempts have been made to put such relationships on a quantitative basis, and Lasagna (1972) has argued that much greater attention should be paid to pharmacokinetic principles in assessing drug action. The reality of differences in tissue responsiveness may be illustrated by the studies of George et al. (1972), who demonstrated that there was a 10-fold variation in response to the β-adrenergic stimulant drug isoprenaline. Moreover, apart from variations in metabolism, there is a 6-fold difference between individual patients in their responses to warfarin (Breckenridge et al., 1971). Some authorities consider that these differences are due to individual variations in the number of specific receptors upon which the drug may act (Rawlins, 1974a).

In the intact mammal the absorption, distribution, biotransformation, and excretion of a given drug is obviously a fully integrated series of processes, but there are immense practical difficulties in establishing a coherent picture of the whole. This is particularly true of studies in man where the most common problem concerns the non-steady-state sequence of reactions which follows a single dose of a xenobiotic. A variety of mathematical methods has been used to tackle the overall problem and to formulate models compatible with experimental data. The most successful of the mathematical approaches in question has proved to be that of compartmental analysis. Atkins (1969) described the scope and limitations of this conceptual technique, and discussed its application to specific examples of drug handling. In spite of the complexity of "the real situation", a number of experimental findings can be usefully rationalized in terms of linear first-order processes interconnecting hypothetical discrete "compartments". These may represent either separate volumes of distribution of a drug, or distinct metabolic states. In the case of drug transport, the first-order rule implies that the kinetics are governed by simple diffusion through membranes; in the case of metabolic turnover, the implication is that reactions proceed at rates which are proportional to the concentrations of the substances concerned. The most widely used models are those in which 1, 2, 3 ... n compartments are interconnected in a straight or in a branching chain; these are the catenary and mamillary systems of compartmental analysis respectively.

For such mathematical exercises to be really meaningful, however, it is desirable that ample experimental data with high analytical precision and chemical specificity are available, and that due allowance is made for biological variation. In practice, these criteria can rarely be strictly met, and most examples of compartmental drug analysis comprise relatively simple models which are consistent with the propositions that, in general, metabolism is mediated by linear enzymic reactions, and that renal excretion is effectively a first-order process. Models involving complex combinations of catenary and mamillary systems have been worked out, but chiefly for physiological species such as calcium, iron, iodine, aminoacids, and glucose, rather than for foreign organic compounds. It is self-evident that the more detailed the general background to a pharmacokinetic problem, and the more powerful the analytical tools for its investigation, the more elaborate may be the corresponding mathematical model.

23.2.1. Metabolic processes

The term "metabolism" properly refers to all of the physical and chemical processes to which a xenobiotic, drug or nutrient is subject in vivo, and these are traditionally summarized (Stolman, 1974) as absorption, distribution, biotransformation and excretion. Many subtle mechanisms of transference are involved in each of these processes and specialist reviews (e.g. Heinz, 1967; Chasseaud, 1972) should be consulted for discussions of passive and active transfer processes.

23.2.1.1. Absorption and distribution

The extent to which a dose of a xenobiotic or drug is absorbed, and the actual rate of absorption, clearly have an important bearing on pharmacological and toxic actions. In both practical and theoretical terms, the most thoroughly investigated of such processes are those governing the pulmonary absorption (and concomitant excretion) of the volatile organic anaesthetics which, in the clinical steady state, display zero-order kinetics. The actual rate of tissue uptake of an anaesthetic agent is largely determined by the partition coefficient between the tissue and arterial blood, but this is a specially simple situation.

Wagner (1961) collected together many references to the percutaneous, parenteral, rectal, and gastrointestinal absorption of drugs, and enumerated formidable lists of physicochemical and biological factors which may influence the kinetics of each process, in addition to the problems of pharmaceutical formulation. Rate-limiting processes governing drug release are an important study in themselves, and there may be large differences in the bioavailability of the active constituent of different preparations of a common drug (Prescott and Nimmo, 1971; Danon et al., 1977).

Goldstein et al. (1974) elaborated some of the pharmacokinetic principles underlying the achievement and maintenance of the therapeutically effective concentration of a drug in vivo. They considered in detail simple cases in which there is zero-, or first-order, drug absorption and first-order elimination, and these provide useful illustrations of the compartmental approach. Absorption may be regarded as instantaneous when one small dose of a drug is given intravascularly. Infusion at a constant rate, corresponding to zero-order absorption, will achieve a plateau concentration in peripheral blood and, in principle, the value can be predicted if the volume of distribution and (first-order) rate constant of elimination are known. Zero-order absorption of solid drugs may also be achieved by sustained release preparations designed for depot use or for oral medication. In general, however, other absorptive processes appear to follow first-order kinetics.

Drug absorption may be reduced if compounds which react with one another are given together; a common example of this in practice is the simultaneous administration of antacids and tetracyclines, which then form insoluble chelates. Obviously malabsorption syndrome from whatever cause may result in variations in response to drugs, but a less well recognized effect on absorption is that many commonly used drugs may undergo metabolism in the gut wall or liver before they ever reach the general circulation. These include tricyclic antidepressants, lignocaine and β-blocking drugs (Rawlins, 1974b), but there are considerable variations in the extent to which this effect occurs from patient to patient.

Following absorption, a foreign compound is distributed, and subsequently re-distributed, among various tissues (Vesell, 1974), and it may be subject to enterohepatic circulation. In the early phase of distribution, tissues such as the heart, brain and kidneys with a rich blood supply are exposed to a high concentration of the substance, but in the later stages, it is distributed into the extracellular fluid and other body tissues, depending upon its lipid solubility, protein binding and affinity for particular cells. The last factor may have an important bearing on individual variation in response to strongly basic drugs such as propranolol and the tricyclic antidepressants (Dollery, 1972). In uraemic patients, there are often abnormalities of protein binding (Reidenberg et al., 1971; Boobis, 1977), and this may explain why such patients are often unduly sensitive to certain drugs.

23.2.1.2. Protein binding

The protein binding of drugs, endogenous substances, and other ligands is a subject of continuing interest, and one on which a variety of elaborate physicochemical techniques have been brought to bear. In drug metabolism, this kind of interaction may result: in combination with receptor proteins, leading to pharmacological activity; with enzymes catalyzing biotransformation; with proteins or lipoproteins of blood plasma or cells, responsible for specific or non-specific transport or storage; or with tissue proteins acting as depot sites. Several of these aspects of protein binding are illustrated by elegant studies, both in vitro and in vivo, of the interaction of warfarin and its principal metabolites with human serum albumin (O'Reilly, 1969; Wilding et al., 1977). Strong binding, and the non-polar character of this drug, account for relatively high concentrations in plasma, low concentrations in urine, and a small volume of distribution. Weak binding, and the more polar character of its metabolites, account for low concentrations in plasma and high concentrations in urine.

Koch-Weser and Sellers (1976) and Vallner (1977) gathered together many hundreds of references to quantitative or semi-quantitative studies of the protein binding of therapeutic agents and other substances, and this, quite apart from work with steroids and related compounds. A few classes of drugs, which are relatively easily assayed, have been studied intensively – the penicillins and other antibiotics, sulpha drugs, salicyclic acid and its derivatives; but the protein binding of highly lipophilic neutral or basic drugs is less well understood (Piafsky and Borgå, 1977).

Many binding studies have been carried out with in vitro systems, and using purified proteins, so that the precise pharmacological and pharmacokinetic significance of the results is largely a matter of speculation. Brodie (1965) was one of the first to discuss the relevance of binding to the rates of drug transfer through biological membranes, and to the concept that protein–drug complexes serve to buffer the level of free drug in the body. The assumption is often made that the free drug, rather than the bound, is the only pharmacologically active fraction, but even in the case of antibacterial substances, with which a valid measure of biological activity is readily obtained, this is a controversial issue.

There is general agreement that, for a given protein solution, the amount of bound drug is some function of drug concentration, the affinities of the binding sites, and their capacities. Although very wide differences in the character of binding of various drugs are known, many drug interactions with albumin appear to involve a small number of binding sites.

Few attempts have been made to demonstrate directly an effect of plasma protein binding on drug distribution or elimination, but the results of some elegant experiments with dicoumarol indicate the potential importance of such effects. This drug is extensively bound to plasma albumin and shows an unusual concentration dependence in binding, which was attributed (Nagashima et al., 1968) to a reversible change of configuration of the protein during the binding process to yield additional binding sites. A remarkably similar concentration dependence was found (Levy and Nagashima, 1969) in the distribution of the drug between liver and plasma, both in vitro (in isolated rat liver perfusion experiments) and in vivo (in intact rats). Furthermore, the first-order elimination rate constant in vivo was found to be dose-dependent, with a minimum value corresponding to that at which the liver/plasma distribution ratio was least. These findings were consistent with the idea that, because of strong protein binding, the rate of hepatic biotransformation and elimination of the drug is a function of its concentration at the liver rather than in the blood.

23.2.1.3. Biotransformations and genetic effects

The two major means of elimination of foreign compounds from the body involve hepatic metabolism and renal excretion. Both processes are involved in the elimination of many drugs, but for lipophilic compounds which have a low renal clearance, hepatic metabolism is the predominant process. The reserve capacities of the kidney and liver for drug processing are large; it has been shown that potentially serious drug accumulation is likely to occur only after the creatinine clearance falls below 25 ml/min (Rawlins, 1974a), and even in severe chronic liver disease, drug metabolism is often preserved to a remarkable degree.

Foreign compounds may be metabolized in many different ways by the liver. The classical routes involve oxidation, reduction, hydrolysis, conjugation with glycine, glucuronic or sulphuric acids, and acetylation (Williams and Parke, 1964). One or other, or a combination of these processes satisfactorily accounts for the biotransformations of an enormous number and variety of substances (Hutson, 1972, 1975). Most conjugation reactions show very little inter-individual variation, but oxidation and acetylation reactions are subject to large differences. Oxidative processes are involved in the metabolism of many common drugs such as barbiturates, tricyclic antidepressants, oral anticoagulants, phenothiazines, phenytoin and benzodiazepines. The variations in oxidation are so marked that it is impossible to predict the degree of metabolism of any of these drugs in any one individual (Smith and Rawlins, 1974). Nutritional status plays an important role in many drug-metabolizing enzyme systems (Campbell and Hayes, 1974).

There is a growing realization of the intrinsic significance of the variation in individual response to a drug as measured by the plasma half-life after a single dose, or by the steady-state plasma concentration after multiple dosage. The experimental design of such studies is not at all simple, and they can only be expected to yield unambiguous results when there is a specific genetic effect (Vesell, 1974) on a particular metabolic step. Thus, it has long been known that there are unusually large person-to-person differences in the metabolism of drugs such as antipyrine, phenylbutazone, and isoniazid. With the last substance, these differences are particularly reproducible, and there is now good evidence (Drayer and Reidenberg, 1977) that slow or rapid inactivation of the drug reflects genetically controlled differences in the speed of hepatic acetylation. Evans and White (1964) showed that sulphamethazine and hydrallazine were also subject to polymorphic acetylation by liver acetyltransferase, but that this did not occur with *p*-aminobenzoate or sulphanilamide, which may possibly be acetylated by extra-hepatic mechanisms. Furthermore (White and Evans, 1968), subjects who were known to be rapid acetylators of sulphamethazine excreted a higher proportion of sulphapyridazine as its acetyl derivative than slow acetylators, but the difference was not clear-cut, and the serum half-life of sulphapyridazine was the same in both rapid and slow acetylators.

In such studies, phenotyping can be carried out by determining the slope of the semilogarithmic plot of plasma concentration after a single dose against time, or by measuring the relative total urinary excretion of unchanged drug and of its acetyl derivative; separate populations of subjects should then be distinguished. Nelson (1965) emphasized that it would be unwise to seek to determine the modality of a population from single determinations of blood concentration in each subject, or from measurements of the overall rates of elimination of drug. If several metabolic steps contribute equally to the observed variations or differences, the operation of a single mutant gene affecting only one process would be unlikely to yield a clear-cut polymodal distribution curve.

Familial studies of drug pharmacokinetics have also proved to be very interesting and instructive. Thus, Motulsky (1965) established the plasma half-life of dicoumarol in the members of several families, and presented evidence that there was a significant correlation in the findings between siblings, but not between them and their parents. Individual differences in metabolism might therefore be attributed to the operation of recessive genes, but it was pointed out that the case was not proved, as environmental as well as genetic factors could have influenced the picture. This point was further investigated by Vesell and Page (1969) who compared the plasma half-life of dicoumarol in sets of identical and fraternal twins given single, oral, therapeutic doses, and in whom the potentially disturbing effects of other drugs and of environmental factors could be ruled out. Between all the subjects taken together there was a 10-fold variation in plasma half-life, but individual values were reproducible. The differences disappeared almost completely in the identical twins, but persisted to some extent in most of the pairs of fraternal twins, and it was considered that these findings did indeed constitute good evidence for genetic control of metabolism. Unfortunately some doubt still remains, because a marked dose-dependence of plasma half-life was demonstrated, together with considerable apparent variations in the rate of gastrointestinal absorption of the drug.

A complementary approach to familial investigations of drug metabolism is exemplified by some pharmacokinetic studies of tricyclic antidepressants. Hammer and Sjöqvist (1967) studied patients on maintenance dosage regimes of desipramine or nortriptyline. They showed that the peak plasma concentrations varied over a 7-fold range and that toxic side-effects were exclusively associated with high values; the plasma half-life, on discontinuing treatment, varied even more widely, but individuals showed a reproducible rate of inactivation when again treated with the drug. It was speculated that such differences might lie at the root of the problems which commonly arise in seeking to establish optimum therapeutic dosage regimes. It was also pointed out that steady-state plasma levels were reduced when phenobarbitone was given concurrently, and that this finding too had obvious therapeutic implications. This, together with evidence showing that there were only small individual variations in the extent of absorption, protein binding, or renal elimination of the antidepressant drugs, suggests that the establishing of steady-state plasma concentrations is mainly determined by the rate of biotransformation. However, the steady-state level of a drug is a function not only of its elimination half-life, but also of its volume of distribution, and the possibility of changes in either or both of these factors must be considered in assessing the meaning of such experiments.

23.2.1.4. pH Dependence of urinary excretion

Studies of drug pharmacokinetics may be incomplete, or even misleading, if account is not taken of the fact that the normal renal excretion of a drug at constant urine volume may be markedly dependent on urinary pH. Several theories of renal tubular function have been propounded to explain this effect: that changes in pH may reverse the direction of an active transport mechanism; that secretion or re-absorption is a passive pH-dependent process. Weiner and Mudge (1964) made an important contribution in gathering the evidence for and against these theories, and developed the theory that organic acids of diverse structure are subject to active tubular secretion, that organic bases participate in a similar but separate mechanism, and that both classes of compound may undergo subsequent tubular re-absorption in which passive back diffusion of the non-ionized fraction of drug across epithelial tissue is the key process, and in which pKa and lipid solubility are therefore prime determinants. These concepts are now widely accepted as rationalizing many of the observed features of tubular action and explain why, in general, the renal clearance of weakly acidic drugs is greater in alkaline urine and that of weakly basic drugs is greater in acid urine.

Milne (1967) indicated the practical importance of the pH-dependent excretion of drugs in the medical management of acute overdosage. Thus, forced acid diuresis would seem to be a logical treatment for quinine, amphetamine, or fenfluramine poisoning, but there are considerable problems and risks in seeking to achieve, and maintain a useful degree of urinary acidification. Analogous difficulties arise in the treatment of aspirin poisoning. Here the rate of excretion of salicylate is considerably increased on instituting forced alkaline diuresis (Brown, 1969) and there is undoubted clinical benefit. Effective alkalinization of the urine requires the infusion of a very large amount of bicarbonate, which in itself is potentially dangerous, and alternative methods of enhancing urinary excretion have therefore been advocated (Morgan and Polak, 1969; Prowse et al., 1970). With other drugs in overdosage, the tendency has been to use forced alkaline diuresis indiscriminately, and in this circumstance its clinical value is less easy to assess. Thus, of the barbiturates (Bloomer, 1966), only phenobarbitone appears to have a low enough pKa and high enough lipid solubility to be subject to significant pH-dependent excretion. It is doubtful if this occurs with the other commonly used barbiturates, with the possible exception of butobarbitone (Mawer and Lee, 1968), but an objective assessment of the problem is beset with the difficulties of distinguishing unchanged drug from metabolites, and of estimating the rates of endogenous biotransformation and excretion.

23.2.2. Physiological factors

It has already been indicated that one of the major problems in drug therapy is that of regulating the dosage of a drug according to the requirements of the individual patient. The equilibrium concentrations of a drug in plasma can vary up to 40- or 50-fold in different patients, because of variations in drug absorption, distribution and elimination (Prescott, 1972), quite apart from the effects of disease and differences in tissue responsiveness.

In any population, response to a drug generally conforms to a unimodal Gaussian type of curve. In other words, the great majority will respond best to the recommended dosage of the drug, and a few others will be resistant to the effects of the drug (Hartshorn, 1970). A further complication is that an individual may respond differently at different times to the same dosage, depending on a number of physiological and other factors, including the mood, the time of day and the attendant circumstances. The more important physiological factors which may alter a patient's response to a drug are now briefly considered; they should be reviewed in the light of the corresponding discussions on Biological Variability in Chapter 1.

23.2.2.1. Age

The infant has a completely different body composition from that of the adult (McCance, 1950) and this affects the blood concentration of a drug and its tissue storage, thereby resulting in a vast difference in the therapeutic response and tolerance. Renal physiology is also different in many ways from an adult and is relatively inefficient (McCance, 1950; Barnett and Vesterdal, 1953; Done, 1964); this may result in the delayed excretion of a drug or an increased susceptibility to kidney damage. The normal infant's liver is also less efficient than that of an adult in metabolizing drugs and this may be another factor which may prolong or increase the effect of any particular drug. Children are extremely susceptible, for example, to the toxic effects of sulphonamides, salicylates, caffeine and many other commonly used preparations (Odell, 1959; Shirkey, 1966).

It is also well known that elderly people tend to be very sensitive to many drugs. Digoxin, for example, must be used with great caution in old people (MacGregor, 1965;

Iisalo and Ruikka, 1974). In addition, the effects of the ageing process on the liver, kidneys and gastrointestinal tract may result in exaggerated or prolonged drug actions, although the evidence for this is contradictory (Brink et al., 1968).

23.2.2.2. Sex

Women are said to be more susceptible to side-effects of drugs than men, although this is not very well substantiated (Hartshorn, 1970). The sex difference is more important in response to sex hormones, which may be given for impotence, various skin diseases and in the treatment of certain types of cancer. The possibility of increasing libido may have to be considered, as criminal acts and sexual offences have resulted from inappropriate hormonal therapy.

23.2.2.3. Pregnancy

During pregnancy, the absorption of drugs may be delayed as the emptying time of the stomach is increased. Special precautions regarding drug therapy must be taken, particularly in the first trimester of pregnancy, to avoid the teratogenic effects of many drugs, and throughout pregnancy in the case of compounds such as pituitary hormones and ergotamine which may alter uterine contractibility or the uterine blood supply. Many therapeutic agents cross the placental barrier and therefore may affect the foetus. Care must also be taken with drug treatment if the mother is breast-feeding because of the excretion of certain drugs in the mother's milk.

23.2.2.4. Race

The best documented variation in response to drugs in different ethnic groups is the anaemia and intravascular haemolysis which may result in Negroes and some Mediterranean peoples in response to certain antimalarial drugs. This arises from a deficiency of glucose-6-phosphate dehydrogenase in the erythrocytes, which does not occur in fair-skinned people of Caucasian origin (Kalow, 1971). Moreover, certain antibiotics such as cephalosporins are said to cause more sensitivity reactions in black women than women of other races.

23.2.2.5. Body mass

The differences in drug responses which may result from variations in body mass are quite obvious. Clearly, small, thin people may be highly sensitive to relatively small doses of a drug, whereas large, obese individuals may require quite large doses in order to obtain a therapeutic response (Hartshorn, 1970).

23.2.2.6. Body temperature

The metabolism of a patient may be much increased in situations of pyrexia and under these circumstances drug action may be shortened. Apart from metabolism, body temperature has a complex effect on drug activity, as it affects both pharmacological and physiological function, the rate of distribution of a drug, its protein binding and excretion (Hartshorn, 1970). In contrast, hypothermia may prolong drug action.

23.2.2.7. *Physiological reserve*

The effects of some drugs may be manifest as an encroachment on the physiological reserve of the patient. For example, in the treatment of hypertension, ganglion blocking drugs and adrenergic blocking drugs may cause severe postural hypotension in patients in the erect position, and particularly when they are exercising, as they no longer have the compensatory mechanisms which normal people use to adjust to activity.

23.2.2.8. *Diurnal steroid variations*

The correct administration of corticosteroid compounds depends upon a proper understanding of the physiological behaviour of endogenous steroids. Because of this diurnal variation it is important to remember that the evening dose of a steroid be kept higher than the morning one in order to achieve an even concentration throughout the 24 hours. This is particularly important in connective tissue disease and rheumatoid arthritis where patients are extremely sensitive to even small changes in steroid concentration.

23.2.2.9. *Time of administration*

All drugs have their characteristic duration of action and obviously the timing and frequency of the dosage of a drug must be organized according to this pharmacological effect. One common and important example is carbimazole in the treatment of hyperthyroidism, which should be administered 8-hourly as nearly as possible and not simply prescribed loosely as "three times daily". Some drugs may be inactivated by certain foods and, therefore, must be given before meals rather than after, whereas others are very liable to cause gastric upset and are better taken after food.

23.2.2.10. *Tolerance*

It is well recognized that patients treated with certain drugs over a long period become tolerant to high blood concentrations and may even become dependent (Takemori, 1974). A good example is afforded by epileptic patients, who may become highly tolerant to barbiturates after prolonged administration. It is not so well appreciated, however, that these same patients may also develop a high degree of tolerance to many other drugs, particularly other hypnotics, as a result of induced synthesis in the liver of microsomal enzymes concerned in drug biotransformation. A similar situation occurs in chronic alcoholics and other chronic drug abusers.

23.3. THE CASE FOR DRUG MONITORING AND SOME EXAMPLES

The marked individual variability of response to a uniform dose of a drug is not surprising in view of the many different factors which have been outlined. The differences which are seen are presumably due to differences in the concentration of active drug at the target site. Much effort in recent years has therefore been devoted to relating the variations in response to the plasma concentration of a drug. Even when there is a high level of compliance by the patient in taking the prescribed dosage regularly, the situation is far from simple. Nevertheless, the plasma concentration may be regarded as an index of the effective concentration of a drug at the site of action, provided that a steady state has been achieved between the various functional organs, that the drug acts reversibly, and that its pharmacological effect is not influenced by its own metabolites. There are, as yet, considerable theoretical and practical limitations to the use of plasma concentrations for the control of individual dosage. Nevertheless, there is little doubt that the effectiveness of and safety of treatment with many drugs could be improved if this field of study were developed. This is particularly the case when it is difficult to assess objectively the clinical response of patients, as in psychiatric illness. Special needs for monitoring may also arise when there is impaired elimination of drugs, as may occur in severe renal or hepatic disease.

Close monitoring of drug therapy is of particular importance, where there is a narrow margin between an effective therapeutic and a toxic dose, and where there is commonly found to be a wide variation in response to normal doses of a drug. Measurement of the plasma concentration of a drug may also be of value in assessing whether failure of therapy is due simply to poor absorption, even if there is little correlation between the plasma concentration and clinical response. This has been found to be of occasional importance in the use of laevodopa (Bianchine et al., 1971). Finally, in research investigations of a new drug in man, measurements of its plasma concentration provide a means of confirming the compliance of participants in the study; this greatly facilitates the proper interpretation and assessment of the effects observed.

Having outlined the case for drug monitoring, it must be recognized that in general clinical practice systematic quantitative measurements are justified for relatively very few drugs – ethanol; salicylate; lithium and tricyclic antidepressants; phenytoin; procaineamide, lignocaine and quinidine; digoxin; and some antibiotics. Suxamethonium is also considered here, even though hypersensitivity reactions are not monitored by measurements of the drug itself.

It must be emphasized once more that in the present state of knowledge, there is often a rather poor correlation between the plasma concentrations of even these drugs and the clinical response, and it is always necessary to relate the reported values to the prevailing clinical situation (Prescott, 1972; Rawlins, 1974a, b). Serial measurements can be of considerable use, however, in two situations. If the clinical response is inadequate and the plasma concentration is low, this suggests either that the patient is not taking the prescribed dosage or that absorption is poor, or that the drug elimination is unexpectedly rapid; appropriate adjustments to the dosage are then made. If toxic features develop, a high plasma concentration will confirm that the dosage should be reduced, and give some indication of the degree to which this should be done.

23.3.1. Ethanol

The metabolism of ethanol and its biological effects (Myerson, 1973), which are also discussed in section 23.5.2, have been investigated more thoroughly, and over a longer period of time, than almost any other drug. Much information has been obtained by traditional methods of assay involving chemical oxidation, but enzymic oxidation is more specific and sensitive, and gas chromatography offers the advantages of speed and simplicity. Any of these techniques can be automated if large numbers of samples are to be analyzed, and different methods should be used in parallel if there is any doubt as to the specificity of an assay in particular circumstances.

Most studies of ethanol metabolism have been concerned with assays of whole blood, since the drug is almost equally distributed between red cells and plasma. Much attention has also been focussed on the relationships between blood alcohol concentration and the urinary excretion or alveolar breath concentration (Dubowski, 1974). Measurements of these ratios may have medicolegal or forensic importance (Wright et al., 1975) but their validity is critically dependent upon the timing and manner of specimen collection and processing, and they are not likely to be relevant to the chemical diagnosis of disease. Care is needed in the handling of ethanol-containing blood specimens because of its volatility and because of the possibility of degradative reactions in vitro. In the last respect, however, ethanol is less labile than glucose. Ethanol is not thought to be a normal product of whole body metabolism nor is it likely that specimens in vitro could form it by metabolic processes.

Medicolegal and toxicological problems apart, the assay of ethanol in single specimens of body fluids may be useful in the diagnosis of alcoholism, and serial monitoring of blood concentrations may be helpful when ethanol is given intravenously for the inhibition of premature labour. Quantitative measurements may also be valuable in the study of interactions of ethanol with other drugs, or of the interaction of drugs with ethanol metabolism (Lieber et al., 1975).

Criteria for the diagnosis of alcoholism were compiled by a Committee of the U.S. National Council on Alcoholism (Kaim, 1972) to establish guidelines for the proper diagnosis and evaluation of this disease. It was emphasized that intoxication is not itself sufficient for the diagnosis of alcoholism; diabetic acidosis, hypoglycaemia, uraemia, impending or completed stroke and other causes of cerebral impairment should be considered. Different criteria of alcoholism were therefore weighted for diagnostic significance and assembled according to type – "Physiological and Clinical", and "Behavioural, Psychological and Attitudinal". The former class included a spectrum of laboratory tests (Table 23.1) of which blood ethanol determinations were assigned the most significant rank of diagnostic level, i.e. the appropriate quantitative finding was "classical, definite, and obligatory" for the diagnosis of alcoholism. In particular, the finding of a blood ethanol concentration of more than 33 mmol/litre (150 mg/dl) without gross evidence of intoxication was indicative of alcoholism. It was pointed out, however, that even with a steady pattern of ethanol consumption, there are likely to be marked fluctuations in the blood concentration during each day; also that quite small amounts of ethanol may evoke aberrant behaviour ("pathological intoxication") in individuals with an idiosyncratic response.

Another aspect of this problem is shown by the results of a British study (Hamlyn et al., 1975) of the usefulness of casual blood ethanol assays in a series of patients with chronic liver disease. About one-third gave a history of heavy drinking and showed histological features of alcoholic hepatitis or steatotis, but only a minority of these patients were found to have measurable blood ethanol concentrations. It was concluded that the chief value of the assay was in the management of alcoholic patients, in whom periodic investigations were useful in monitoring alcohol consumption or detecting relapse from abstinence.

Ethanol infusion has been used over many years for analgesia during labour and as a preinduction analgesic. In some patients, however, ethanol was observed to cause cessa-

TABLE 23.1.

LABORATORY TESTS WHICH CONTRIBUTE MINOR CRITERIA FOR THE DIAGNOSIS OF ALCOHOLISM

(From Kaim et al., 1972)

Criterion	Diagnostic level
(1) Direct	
Blood ethanol concentration at any time of more than 65 mmol/litre (300 mg/dl) or	1
concentration of more than 22 mmol/litre (100 mg/dl) in routine examination	1
(2) Indirect	
Serum osmolarity (reflects blood ethanol concentration): every 22.4 increase over 200 mOsm/litre reflects 11 mmol/litre (50 mg/dl) ethanol	2
Results of ethanol ingestion:	
Hypoglycaemia	3
Hypochloraemic alkalosis	3
Low magnesium concentration	2
Lactic acid increase	3
Transient uric acid increase	3
Potassium depletion	3
Indications of liver abnormality [1]:	
Increase of serum alanine aminotransferase	2
Increase of serum aspartate aminotransferase	3
Increase of sulfobromothalein retention	2
Bilirubin increase	2
Urinary urobilinogen increase	2
Reversal of serum albumin/globulin ratio	2
Blood and blood clotting:	
Anaemia (hypochromic, normocytic, macrocytic, haemolytic with stomatocytosis) low folic acid;	3
Clotting disorders (prothrombin increase, thrombocytopenia)	3
ECG abnormalities (specified)	2
EEG abnormalities (specified)	3
Decreased immune response	3
Decreased response to Synacthen test	3
Chromosomal damage from alcoholism	3

[1] Elevation of serum γ-glutamyltransferase (Rosalki, 1975) might nowadays be added to this listing at diagnostic level 2.

tion of uterine contractions, suggesting that it might suppress the release of oxytocin from the posterior pituitary. On this basis, it was deliberately administered (Fuchs et al., 1967) to patients in premature labour, with some measure of clinical success, so that the manoeuvre is now quite widely used. Few measurements of blood ethanol concentrations have been made in this situation, but it is known that there is very rapid placental transfer of the drug (Waltman and Iniquez, 1972) and a concomitant foetal metabolic acidosis (Mann et al., 1975). It remains to be established whether this complication is important, in comparison with the various risks of prematurity, and whether there are harmful side-effects on foetal hepatic metabolism.

This situation must be distinguished from that obtaining in the "foetal alcohol syndrome" (Mulvihill et al., 1976) which consists of severe pre- and postnatal growth failure with congenital malformation and mental deficiency, in children born to mothers with chronic alcoholism. Cause-and-effect relationship has not yet been established in this condition, but it is plausible that the foetal growth may be susceptible to prolonged exposure to ethanol or to acetaldehyde (Korsten et al., 1975).

23.3.2. Salicylate

Over many years, actual or potential toxic effects of aspirin or other salicylates have been described many times (Moser, 1967; Blacow, 1968). Apart from allergy and hypersensitivity, such effects include various blood disorders, disturbed platelet function and bleeding, gastointestinal haemorrhage, liver damage and hypoglycaemia. At the same time, it has been accepted that optimum plasma salicylate concentrations of around 2.5 mmol/litre (350 μg/ml) are required in the therapy of acute rheumatic fever. Some recent evidence casts doubt on this figure, but most physicians still accept it as reasonable for practical purposes (Mongan et al., 1973). The usefulness of measuring plasma salicylate concentrations is perhaps greater in the case of repeated high dosage, such as occurs commonly in chronic rheumatic disorders. In these circumstances there may be accumulation of the drug, with plasma concentrations of 2- or 3-fold the optimum value, so that chronic salicylate poisoning ensues, the clinical features of which may be difficult to recognize. It is advisable, therefore, to carry out periodic measurements of the plasma salicylate concentrations in these patients.

There is a vast – and still growing – literature on all aspects of metabolism of the salicylates (Davison, 1971). Inter-individual differences in the plateau plasma concentrations of salicylate in patients on chronic therapy are well documented and have been shown to correlate better with the urinary excretion of the principal metabolite, salicylurate, than with the total urinary excretion of salicylate (Gupta et al., 1975). This is consistent with there being important differences between individuals in the rates of capacity-limited biotransformation reactions.

23.3.3. Lithium

Lithium salts, of which the most commonly used is the carbonate (Baldessarini and Lipinski, 1975), are generally considered to be effective in the treatment and prophylaxis of recurrent manic–depressive disorders (Shopsin and Gershon, 1974), although the mechanism of action is still the subject of investigation and speculation (Singer and Rotenberg, 1973; Schou, 1976).

Lithium is readily absorbed from the gastrointestinal tract after oral dosage. Peak plasma concentrations are reached within a few hours, and there is a general distribution throughout the intra- and extra-cellular fluids. It is excreted chiefly through the kidneys, but renal tubular re-absorption occurs if there is inadequate intake of salt. The range of therapeutic plasma concentrations is narrow – about 0.6 to 1.5 mmol/litre (Baastrup et al., 1970) – and side-effects or frank toxicity appear in most cases where the concentration rises above 2.0 mmol/litre. A good example of the value of monitoring in the control of drug therapy was provided by the study by Fry and Marks (1971) of 100 randomly selected patients treated with lithium over several months. Only 36 patients had mean plasma lithium concentrations in the accepted therapeutic range and 34 had values less than 0.6 mmol/litre. Ten had none detectable on at least one occasion, and eight had concentrations of more than 2.0 mmol/litre on at least one occasion.

The more minor side-effects of lithium therapy tend to be related to the dosage regimen and degree of accumulation (Crammer et al., 1974). Thyroid function should be regularly assessed, since goitre and hypothyroidism have been reported in patients on long-term therapy. The features of severe lithium poisoning which may follow chronic, but largely symptomless, toxicity, include oliguria, circulatory failure, pulmonary complications and coma, and there have been cases of fatal overdosage. Forced alkaline diuresis is apparently effective in enhancing the renal clearance of lithium (Forrest, 1975), but haemodialysis may be a more appropriate form of treatment for the most gravely ill patients.

23.3.4. Tricyclic antidepressants

Imipramine and its congeners, the tricyclic antidepressants, have been the drugs of choice in the treatment of depressive illness since their introduction in 1957. They are thought to act by inhibiting re-uptake of transmitter substances into monoaminergic neurones. In overdosage, they have an adverse effect on the myocardium and may cause conduction defects, cardiac arrythmias and infarction which can prove fatal.

With the development, in turn, of sensitive analytical methods, notably isotope derivative techniques for the monomethylated compounds nortriptyline and desmethylimipramine, and gas chromatography and high-performance liquid chromatography for amitriptyline, it has become possible to measure plasma concentrations of these drugs. Such measurements may be useful either to check that psychiatric in-patients or out-patients have actually been taking the prescribed drug, or to monitor drug concentrations when toxic side-effects become manifest (Petit et al., 1977). More interestingly it has been established that there are striking inter-individual differences in the steady-state plasma levels achieved after a multiple dosage regimen.

The tricyclic antidepressants exemplify the pharmacodynamic problems associated with repeated drug dosage. Achievement of a steady-state blood concentration depends upon the dosage – or rather the fraction of each dose which is absorbed – the time interval between doses, the volume of distribution, and the kinetics of biotransformation and excretion. The kinetics may be complicated by changes in distribution accompanying the formation or accumulation of metabolites, while the pharmacological effects may be exerted by one or more metabolites as well as by the parent drug.

At least four independent attempts have been made (Glassman and Perel, 1974) to establish the relationship between the plateau concentrations and the clinical responses of groups of patients. The first such study showed that there was an optimum plasma concentration with a curvilinear relationship indicating poor response at higher or lower levels than the optimum. The second study demonstrated a linear relationship with best response at high concentrations, but the converse of this was found in a third study. The findings of the fourth showed no correlation between these findings. Glassman and Perel considered that these studies demonstrated the difficulty of finding a homogeneous depressive population, and that meaningful responses would only be expected if patients were separated into depressive sub-groups before drug treatment. At the same time, it was possible that there were sufficient inter-individual differences in the character of protein binding of the drugs to invalidate comparisons of total plasma concentrations. Asberg (1974), in a further investigation, did not concede this last point, but considered that heterogeneity of the patient population was indeed an important factor. Studies of small but carefully selected groups of patients, using still more specific analytical methods, confirm that the therapeutic range of concentrations is quite narrow (Biggs and Ziegler, 1977; Kupfer et al., 1977).

In summary, it is not yet possible to define an optimum therapeutic concentration for the treatment of patients suffering from endogenous depression. For nortriptyline (Kragh-Sørensen et al., 1973) the effective therapeutic range is about 160 to 480 nmol/litre (50 to 150 ng/ml); for amitriptyline (Braithwaite et al., 1972), a similar range applies, but it must be recognized that comparable levels of nortriptyline will be found concurrently since this is the principal active metabolite of amitriptyline. If a steady-state is truly achieved, there should be relatively little fluctuation in plasma concentrations of either of these drugs between dosage intervals (Aherne et al., 1977; Montgomery et al., 1977).

23.3.5. Phenytoin

Phenytoin is widely used in the treatment of various types of epilepsy and of cardiac arrythymias, and it may be administered orally or by intramuscular injection. It is subject to hepatic microsomal oxidation, and the conjugates of the *p*-hydroxy derivative so formed are excreted into the bile, re-absorbed, and excreted into the urine. Investigations in epileptic patients (Houghton and Richens, 1974) showed that increasing the daily dose of the drug caused a lengthening of the plasma half-life and a reduction in the ratio of the *p*-hydroxy metabolite to unchanged phenytoin, thus indicating that the hydroxylation reaction was saturable.

Many detailed studies have been carried out (Eadie, 1974; Hvidberg and Dam, 1976) in efforts to establish the pharmacokinetics of phenytoin and of its principal metabolite (Hoppel et al., 1977), and the optimum dosage regimen (Ludden et al., 1977). It has turned out that the metabolism of phenytoin is extremely variable, so that for a given dose there may be large differences in plasma concentrations from patient to patient, and even in the same patient, the values may fluctuate (Baylis et al., 1970; Lund et al., 1971).

It is not surprising that Kutt (1971) found that most failures in therapy were associated with inadequate plasma concentrations of the drug, even when conventional doses were given. Fortunately, there is a close relationship between the plasma concentration and the clinical response, and monitoring therefore provides a very useful aid to control of treatment. The therapeutic range of concentrations is generally taken to be 40 to 80 μmol/litre (10 to 20 μg/ml), above which minor features of toxicity usually occur. Severe overdosage leads to hypotension, coma and respiratory depression.

Long-term therapy with phenytoin has been associated with the development of rickets and osteomalacia, probably due to the induction by phenytoin of liver enzymes involved in the catabolism of vitamin D. For this reason, patients are sometimes required to take regular doses of calciferol.

The practice of treating epileptic patients with combinations of phenytoin and phenobarbitone is commonplace, on the assumption that there is a synergistic effect. Few quantitative studies utilising drug measurements have been carried out to justify this assumption and in experimental animals (Leppik and Sherwin, 1977), the anticonvulsant effects of the two drugs simply appeared to be additive.

23.3.6. Procaineamide, lignocaine (lidocaine) and quinidine

These three cardiac antiarrhythmic drugs may be considered together even though they are chemically dissimilar. In toxic doses, all of these compounds can provoke serious cardiac arrhythmias and hypotension, and it may be very difficult to judge toxicity on a clinical basis. There is a good argument, therefore, for monitoring therapy by appropriately sensitive and specific measurements of plasma concentrations (Prescott, 1972).

The plasma concentrations of procaineamide show a marked individual variation between patients receiving the same dosage of the drug; Koch-Weser and Klein (1971) reported 18-fold differences. The problem is accentuated in the presence of cardiac and renal failure (Prescott, 1972). The optimum therapeutic range of plasma concentration for controlling arrhythmias is 16 to 31 μmol/litre (4 to 8 μg/ml) (Koup et al., 1975) although there is a considerable overlap between the therapeutic and toxic ranges. Toxicity is very likely to occur at concentrations above 48 μmol/litre (12 μg/ml). It is interesting to note that the *N*-acetyl derivative of procaineamide, its principal metabolite, has equal antiarrhthymic potency (Elson et al., 1975).

Plasma concentrations of lignocaine correlate well with its antiarrhythmic properties (Scott and Julian, 1971), but toxicity has been noted at values as low as 8 μmol/litre (2 μg/ml), whereas concentrations as high as 96 μmol/litre (24 μg/ml) have not resulted in adverse effects (Bedynek et al., 1966). The usual therapeutic range is considered to be 4 to 16 μmol/litre (1 to 4 μg/ml). The justification for monitoring plasma concentrations, apart from the individual variations in response mentioned above, may be seen in the demonstration that the plasma clearance is reduced to 30 or 40% of normal in patients with uncomplicated myocardial infarction (Scott and Julian, 1971). This is thought to be due to diminution of cardiac output and reduced liver perfusion; this problem is increased in cardiac failure (Thomson et al., 1971). The dangers of drug accumulation in the therapeutic situation are obvious. Like procaineamide, lignocaine has at least one active metabolite (Halkin et al., 1975).

As with lignocaine, there is a reasonably good correlation between the therapeutic response and the plasma concentration of quinidine. This is particularly the case with oral therapy, and the effective therapeutic range is 6 to 18 μmol/litre (2 to 6 μg/ml); values above 24 μmol/litre (8 μg/ml) are usually associated with toxicity (Smith and Gosselin, 1976). When hypokalaemia is present, however, concentrations as high as 60 μmol/litre (20 μg/ml) have been obtained without untoward effect (Bloomfield et al., 1971). Lack of specificity of methods of assay is almost certainly a contributory factor in differing views (Edwards et al., 1974; Crouthamel, 1975) on the usefulness of plasma concentration measurements.

23.3.7. Digoxin

The standardization of digoxin methodology is intrinsically difficult, but it is a specially important problem because of well-known differences in the bioavailability of digoxin between various preparations (Doherty, 1973), and the consequent need to monitor plasma concentrations so as to achieve reasonably consistent clinical response. Seeming epidemics of digoxin overdosage have occurred (Danon et al., 1977) because of manufacturers changing their formulations of the drug.

The administration of digoxin achieves rapid digitalization in the treatment of congestive heart failure and atrial fibrillation. However, the clinical response is complex, and depends upon acid–base, electrolyte and endocrine status, and the nature of the underlying cardiac disease. It is, therefore, not surprising that there may be considerable overlap in the responses to different drug regimens. Nevertheless, measurement of plasma concentration of digoxin can be in many cases a valuable therapeutic guide (Baylis et al., 1972; British Medical Journal, 1975).

The toxic effects of digoxin are similar to those of digitalis (Smith and Haber, 1973a), but it is more rapidly excreted than the digitalis glycosides (Smith and Haber, 1973b), so that it is less likely to give rise to cumulative effects. At the same time it may be extremely difficult to distinguish by clinical judgement alone under-treatment with digoxin from digitalis-like toxicity. There is general agreement that plasma concentrations of digoxin above 2.5 nmol/litre (2.0 ng/ml) using a radioimmunoassay method of analysis (Smith et al., 1969), or comparable methods, are indicative of toxicity in many cases (Grahame-Smith and Everest, 1969; Bertler and Redfors, 1970; Beller et al., 1971). This is not always so, however, as patients have been described who became toxic only at much higher values (Evered et al., 1970; Smith and Haber, 1970). Furthermore, typical toxicity has been reported in individuals with plasma concentrations as low as 0.5 nmol/litre (0.4 ng/ml) (Fogelman et al., 1971). Measurements of digoxin concentrations have proved helpful in avoiding toxicity (Duhme et al., 1974) and in devising computer-optimized dosage regimens (Sheiner et al., 1975).

23.3.8. Antibiotics

Cycloserine is the only common antibiotic which is presently assayed by purely chemical methods (Protivinsky, 1971). It has a good therapeutic index, and the effects of overdosage on the central nervous system are reversed when the drug is withdrawn.

Microbiological methods have been widely used for the determination of the concentrations of other antibiotics in body fluids, but they have poor specificities when multiple antibiotics are administered. It is also worth noting that similar pharmacokinetic principles apply to these substances as to drugs which are chemically well-defined. Antibiotic concentrations in serum are a direct indication of antibacterial activity, and in severe infections it is desirable to adjust the dosage regimen according to the in vitro assessment of the inhibitory concentrations of the drug. This does not, of course, guarantee that the same concentration will reach the site of infection.

Most antibiotics are eliminated unchanged from the body by renal excretion, so that in conditions of renal impairment accumulation of the drug may occur. This may result in considerable danger in the case of toxic antibiotics such as streptomycin, kanamycin, gentamicin and colistin.

Gentamicin, which is now used commonly in clinical practice, and may cause vestibular damage, has been extensively studied (Hoffbrand et al., 1974). Monitoring of the serum concentration of gentamicin can be used to ensure an adequate peak concentration and to check accumulation since individual variation may occur (Wilson et al., 1973). It has been shown that the cure rate of infections is much improved at a serum concentration above 4 or 5 μg/ml (Jackson and Riff, 1971; Noone et al., 1974), and with Gram-negative infections the concentration should be above 8 μg/ml. Toxic concentrations are as yet poorly defined, but Hewitt (1974) tentatively suggested 12 to 15 μg/ml. These studies have demonstrated that earlier dosage regimens have been too restricted to achieve the optimum therapeutic concentrations and effects.

23.3.9. Suxamethonium (succinylcholine)

Suxamethonium was introduced into clinical anaesthesia in 1951, as a short-acting neuromuscular blocking agent which was particularly suitable for procedures such as endotracheal intubation. Suxamethonium competes with acetylcholine for the receptors of the neuromuscular junction. Acetylcholine is rapidly hydrolyzed by acetylcholinesterase so as to enable muscular contraction to be controlled, but the action of suxamethonium is not terminated until it has been hydrolyzed by plasma cholinesterase. In most individuals, the relaxant action lasts a few minutes, during which time there is apnoea. Within a few years of the introduction of the drug, it was realized (Lehmann et al., 1961) that in a small proportion of patients the administration of suxamethonium resulted in prolonged paralysis of the respiratory muscles and apnoea which lasted for several hours. Fatalities ensued in cases where adequate anaesthetic care was not available.

Prolonged apnoea tended to be associated with low plasma cholinesterase activity due to liver metastases, cirrhosis or acute hepatitis. This explanation was facile, however, and Kalow and his co-workers (Kalow and Gunn, 1959) demonstrated that hypersensitivity to suxamethonium was due not to reduced hepatic synthesis of an active enzyme, but to the presence of an atypical or less catalytically active form. It was shown that the atypical enzyme was genetically determined, and both homozygotes and heterozygotes were identified by an inhibition method of differentiating between the usual and atypical enzymes. With benzoylcholine as substrate, the hydrolysis of which could be followed spectrophotometrically, dibucaine inhibited the usual enzyme by about 80%, but the atypical enzyme by 20%. The percentage inhibition in the presence of dibucaine was referred to as the "dibucaine number". Fluoride has also been widely used to achieve differential inhibition of the variants of the enzyme so that by careful characterization of a plasma specimen with both inhibitors, 10 possible phenotypes can be identified (Lehmann and Liddell, 1969).

Many other methods of assaying cholinesterase activity have been described (Pilz, 1974). The majority measure a secondary effect of the enzymic action such as the liberation of acid, by titrimetric or manometric methods, or else employ a substrate such as thiocholinester, in which the product of the hydrolytic reaction can be detected colorimetrically. Benzoylcholine appears to be the only substrate which offers a direct measure of the hydrolysis of cholinester, and its use is to be preferred for the accurate phenotyping of suxamethonium-sensitive patients and their relatives. The direct measurement of circulating suxamethonium itself, or of its metabolite succinylmonocholine, is not practicable except by radiochemical or biological methods, and they would not be helpful in the clinical situation.

Individuals lacking a gene for the usual enzyme are invariably hypersensitive to suxamethonium. Contrary to popular belief, however, prolonged apnoea may in fact occur in patients with any genotype. The results of five large surveys (Bauld et al., 1974) have shown that approximately one in three of many hundreds of patients investigated because of prolonged apnoea had the usual enzyme. For some of these patients, the usual enzyme had low activity on account of conditions such as metastatic carcinoma, pregnancy, or malnutrition. In patients with a normal activity of the usual enzyme, neuromuscular block may not have been present, but this cannot easily be assessed without peripheral nerve stimulation. The differentiation of central from peripheral causes of apnoea may be difficult. In other patients with a normal activity of the usual enzyme, inappropriately large doses of suxamethonium or of sedative premedication may prolong the response to the drug. The possibility always remains that new genetic variants with reduced catalytic activity may be found, and that such variants, while unable to bind and hydrolyze suxamethonium, could catalyze the hydrolysis of substrates such as benzoylcholine. Such variants would therefore go undetected by present phenotyping methods.

It is doubtful if pre-anaesthetic screening for low cholinesterase activity can be justified, since hypersensitivity to suxamethonium is rare and the management of prolonged apnoea should be straightforward. Patients who demonstrate prolonged apnoea, however, should certainly be followed up by cholinesterase assay and phenotyping, with appropriate family studies (Dewar and Wakefield, 1976). Approximately one in five of relatives of such patients are likely to be at risk and should be issued with a card warning against the administration of suxamethonium.

Although a rare abnormal response to suxamethonium, like other muscle relaxants, may result in malignant hyperthermia (Wolfe et al., 1973), there is no evidence, as yet, to associate this condition with suxamethonium apnoea.

23.4. BASIC PRINCIPLES OF CLINICAL TOXICOLOGY

Several factors may independently influence the toxicity of a given compound in man, quite apart from its chemical nature and physical form. The route of administration –

whether through the skin, lungs, or other organs, by gastric absorption or parenterally – will affect the speed with which a substance is absorbed and distributed, and may profoundly influence the character and rate of metabolism. The period of exposure, and whether it is once-for-all or repeated, will make the difference between acute and chronic poisoning, or a combination of the two.

The agent itself, or a metabolite of it (Mitchell and Jollow, 1975), or both, may give rise to specific toxic lesions (Gillette et al., 1974). Biological or physiological factors, such as the rate of renal or hepatic blood flow, body temperature, or the relative proportion of adipose and lean tissue, may influence toxicity, either directly or indirectly, just as they may influence the pharmacological response to a drug. Genetic factors may increase or diminish the toxic effect and may accelerate or diminish metabolism, depending on the substance in question; acute immunological abreactions may have a genetic basis. Toxic effects may also be modified by the interaction in vivo of the toxic agent with a pre-administered drug, or a xenobiotic substance (Deer Lodge Conference, 1976), or even by chronic dosage with the same agent. There is now a very large literature on such interactions (Morselli et al., 1974) and many different mechanisms may be postulated and recognized in practice: one substance may alter the extent or rate of absorption of another by physicochemical or physiological effects; competition between drugs for carrier or receptor sites may give rise to changes in their volumes of distribution or plasma water concentrations with clinically important consequences (Williams et al., 1976); one drug or foreign compound may stimulate or inhibit the biotransformation of another (Brown, 1975); drugs which affect renal function, by way of modifying urinary flow, or pH, or tubular secretion, may influence the renal clearance of others. The induction of hepatic enzymes, which may be assessed by the urinary excretion of D-glucaric acid (Davidson et al., 1974; March et al., 1974) is a particularly interesting form of interaction. Although this has been relatively little studied in man, in contrast to experimental animals (Parke, 1975; Richens and Woodford, 1976), there is no reasonable doubt that induction may be of clinical significance in certain circumstances (Gelehrter, 1976).

A substance which is administered for therapeutic purposes may elicit toxic effects in normal dosage if there is some inadequacy of the usual mechanism for detoxification or if there is an action on the wrong target system. Therapeutic agents may also be toxic because of accidental or deliberate overdosage; this may give rise to relatively non-specific, but harmful, local reactions, or there may be exaggerated pharmacological effects or specific toxicological lesions.

Substances which are not intended for therapeutic use may have toxic effects of

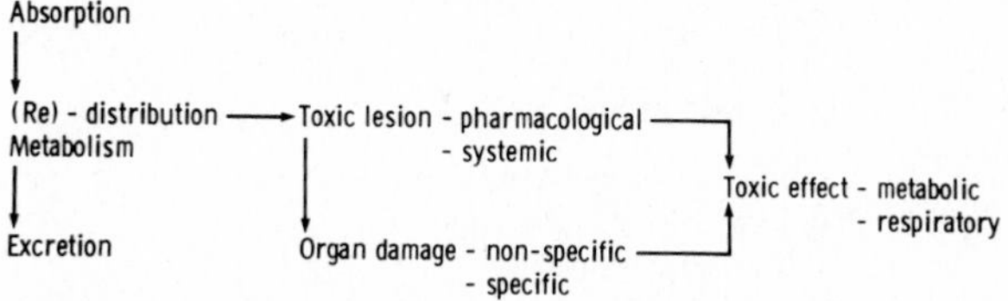

Scheme 23.1. Sequence of steps leading to metabolic or respiratory toxic effects in poisoning or adverse reactions to drugs.

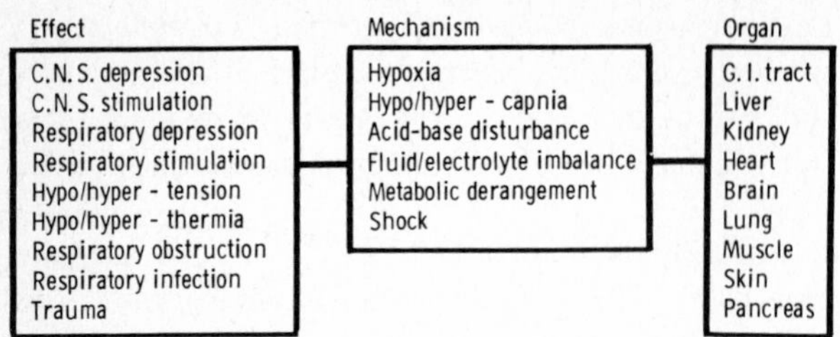

Scheme 23.2. Principal toxic effects, mechanisms and organs involved in different kinds of poisoning.

various kinds. They may be quite non-specific, in the sense that they are generally destructive to tissues by a corrosive or caustic action; they may give rise to specific biochemical lesions, or they may elicit a specific immune mechanism; not least, their toxic effects may be manifested by an indirect form of systemic organ damage. There may of course, be a combination of two or more of these effects, and toxicity may also be manifested by haematological effects. Some drugs, for example, cause over-production or under-production of erythrocytes; others affect their survival or function. Analogous drug-induced changes occur with leucocytes. Toxic effects on platelet function, coagulation and fibrinolysis are also well documented (Dimitrov and Nodine, 1974).

Scheme 23.1 indicates the way in which a primary toxic effect can give rise to organ damage by a non-specific or by a specific mechanism of action. The ensuing organ damage itself may lead to respiratory or metabolic disturbance or a combination of the two, and

TABLE 23.2.

EXAMPLES OF SPECIFIC TOXICITY

Biochemical lesion	Toxic substance
Oxygen transport	
Carboxy/nitric oxide haemoglobin	Carbon monoxide, nitric oxide
Methaemoglobin	Phenacetin
Enzyme inhibition	
Citric acid cycle	Fluoroacetate
Oxidative phosphorylation	Tin alkyls
Fatty acid oxidation	Hypoglycin
Cholinesterase	Organophosphates
Nucleic acid function	
RNA	Actinomycin
DNA	Antimetabolites
DNA	Mutagens, Carcinogens
Cell structure	
Renal tubular necrosis	Mercuric salts
Hepatic necrosis	Carbon tetrachloride
Brain damage	Mercury alkyls
Pulmonary fibrosis	Paraquat

TABLE 23.3.

POISONINGS FOR WHICH THERE ARE SPECIFIC DRUG THERAPIES

(From Locket, 1973; Martindale, 1977)

Toxic substance	Antidote
	Chelating agents
Ferrous iron	Desferrioxamine mesylate
Heavy metals:	
antimony, arsenic, bismuth, gold, mercury	Dimercaprol (BAL)
cadmium, lead, plutonium	Calcium trisodium pentetate; disodium edetate; penicillamine
Cyanide	Cobalt edetate; methaemoglobin (from sodium nitrite, sodium thiosulphate)
	Antagonists
Cholinesterase inhibitors	Pralidoxime salts (PAM); atropine salts
Morphine and its analogues	Nalorphine; levallorphan; naloxone
Pentazocine	Naloxone
Methaemoglobin (drug-induced)	Methylene blue

thence to a variety of clinical features. Different features (Scheme 23.2) are illustrated in the summary descriptions of particular poisonings (section 23.5).

Many examples of specific biochemical lesions have been described (Albert, 1973), and some of these are listed in Table 23.2, but few are commonly seen in clinical practice. Carbon monoxide poisoning, however, was commonly associated with exposure to town (manufactured) gas and can still arise in circumstances where defective appliances burn natural gas or other hydrocarbon fuels with incomplete combustion. Organophosphorus poisoning is associated with the careless use of certain insecticides and herbicides, although their horticultural application is closely controlled in most countries. For these two forms of poisoning, and for a few other special biochemical lesions, there are relatively specific forms of drug treatment (Table 23.3).

Antidotes are not without their own intrinsic hazards (Martindale, 1977), but their use will be indicated more by clinical judgement than by analytical findings, except possibly for iron, lead and other heavy metal poisonings (Locket, 1973). In general clinical practice specific therapies are rarely used, apart from the treatment of carbon monoxide poisoning with oxygen, and narcotic overdosage with nalorphine or its congeners.

23.4.1. The approach to treatment and the role of the laboratory

The role of the laboratory in the management of patients with acute drug overdosage has been a rather controversial one. This has resulted from changes in fashion over the last 40 years in the approach to treatment of poisoned patients (Lawson and Proudfoot,

1971) accompanied by real advances (Table 23.4). Until 1950, the main aims were to achieve precise diagnosis, to use vigorous gastric aspiration and lavage and to seek to provide a specific antidote to the poisoning. Intensive analeptic therapy was strenuously advocated (Koppanyi and Fazekas, 1950). Despite the fact that its use was associated with major side-effects (Dobos et al., 1961; Myschetsky, 1961; Mark, 1967), this treatment enjoyed a prolonged popularity before it fell from favour. The treatment of poisoning then developed along two complementary lines. The major advance was the introduction of the "Scandinavian Method" of intensive supportive treatment (Clemmesen, 1959; Clemmensen and Nilsson, 1961). This form of therapy is now generally accepted as the correct basic approach to the management of poisoned patients. A modern variant of the Scandinavian Method described by Matthew and Lawson (1979) has been shown to be effective in over 95% of poisoned patients.

The second major effort in recent years has been to seek effective means of removing the poison from the body following absorption. Methods to achieve this have included forced diuresis by various techniques (Mawer and Lee, 1968; Maddock and Bloomer, 1968), peritoneal dialysis (Hadden et al., 1969), extracorporeal dialysis (Maddock and Bloomer, 1968), exchange transfusion (Done, 1969) and the passage of blood over ion-exchange resin or coated charcoal absorbants (Weston et al., 1974; Vale et al., 1975). Unfortunately, there have been trends to use this approach far too readily – so much so, that methods of treatment which are not themselves without danger, have been advocated for patients who are only mildly poisoned. Much of the confusion has arisen from attempts to use plasma or blood concentrations to assess the severity of poisoning and to define values for a given substance above which one of these methods of treatment should be instituted (Maher and Schreiner, 1968). This concept failed to take account of the marked individual variations in pharmacological and toxic response which have been discussed earlier. In addition, there was little recognition of the lack of specificity of the analytical methods used in many of the studies and the paucity of information regarding the pharmacological or toxic activities of metabolites of the poison. In view of the success of intensive supportive therapy, it is clear that in the great majority of poisonings these special methods should be reserved only for very seriously ill patients in whom supportive therapy is manifestly inadequate.

TABLE 23.4.

ADVANCES IN THE TREATMENT OF POISONING

(From Matthew and Lawson, 1979)

Year		Mortality (%)
1945	Treatment of shock	25
1948	Maintenance of airway	15
1949	Centralization of treatment	13
1955	Abandoning of analeptic drugs	6
1960	Availability of renal dialysis	2
1965	(Introduction of benzodiazepines)	0.5
	(Introduction of natural gas)	<0.5

In practice there is no doubt that the most important assessment of severity of poisoning is a clinical one. Certainly resuscitation should be started immediately as required, and without waiting for laboratory investigations. For the reasons given above, quantitative measurement of poisons in blood or urine may be misleading as a guide to the severity of the poisoning. It would be wrong, however, to conclude that laboratory investigations are unnecessary in the field of clinical toxicology.

Few poisons produce characteristic features. In practice there is seldom doubt about the diagnosis, as the patient usually gives an indication of having taken a drug overdose or other poison, or else the circumstantial evidence of poisoning is strong. Difficulty arises when there is no such information, and when the physician is faced with the differential diagnosis of an unconscious patient. The importance of rapid screening methods for the qualitative recognition of poisons can be assessed from the fact that in the age group 15 to 50 years, poisoning is likely to be the commonest cause of unconsciousness, second to trauma. Simple rapid screening methods (Berry and Grove, 1973; Blass et al., 1974) are available for approximately 80% of common poisonings using specimens of blood, gastric aspirate or urine as appropriate. If the necessary facilities are readily available and the findings promptly reported, this type of qualitative analysis may be of considerable diagnostic help to the clinician (Goulding and Widdop, 1974). The kinds of poisoning which may in favourable circumstances be detected in this way include salicylate, paracetamol, paraquat, phenothiazines and imipramine, iron, chloroform and its congeners, and carbon monoxide. More elaborate analytical schemes have been described (Deckers and Lewis, 1973; Griffiths et al., 1973; Ehrsson and Knapp, 1974) for a much wider range of poisons, and for dependence-producing drugs (Chruściel and Chruściel, 1975).

In the unusual circumstance that the patient should require one of the forms of treatment to actively remove the poison, it is obvious that chemical analysis may be extremely valuable in making the decision whether or not to proceed. For example, in barbiturate poisoning it is essential to know the type of barbiturate involved. Phenobarbitone and barbitone may be cleared effectively by forced diuresis (Lawson and Proudfoot, 1971) whereas even haemodialysis is ineffective in poisoning with quinalbarbitone, amylobarbitone and pentobarbitone (Hadden et al., 1969). Quantitative measurement is also of importance here, as it is necessary to ascertain that there is a sufficient gradient of drug available to achieve adequate elimination.

In addition to diagnosis of poisoning, chemical analysis may also be of great importance in epidemiological studies as there is an increasing tendency now for patients to take a variety of drugs which makes clinical diagnosis even more difficult. It has been found that up to 26% of patients with acute poisoning now take more than one drug (Matthew and Lawson, 1979). Finally, it will be self-evident that chemical analysis of body fluids or tissues may be of considerable importance in medicolegal matters which sometimes touch upon patient care. Perhaps the most common situation of this kind is the question of drunken driving, but there are many other circumstances which justify a specially rigorous approach to the taking, identification and processing of specimens for toxicological analysis (Temple, 1977).

23.5. PREVALENCE OF ACUTE POISONINGS AND SOME EXAMPLES

The statistics for deaths attributed to poisoning in different countries afford an index of the magnitude of the general problem of acute poisoning. In the United States (Kinney and Melville, 1976), approximately two-thirds of fatal poisonings are currently due to barbiturates, carbon monoxide and ethanol. In the United Kingdom, official statistics (Table 23.5) indicate that in recent years the number of deaths due to poisoning has been comparable to the annual mortality from road traffic accidents. A breakdown of the data by motive ("suicide", "accident", or "intent not determined") and by agent (the substance or class of substance involved) is shown in Table 23.6. The chief group of poisoning agents is the barbiturates and barbiturate-containing preparations, which in 1973 were used in about 60% of all completed suicide attempts which involved drugs. Moreover, in 54% of cases of accidental fatal poisoning and in 64% of cases where it was uncertain whether death was accidental or deliberate, barbiturates were again the agents used. Thus, barbiturates were implicated in 60% of all cases of fatal poisoning involving drugs. More disturbing still, is the fact that there has been little change in the number of deaths resulting from barbiturate poisoning in the past two decades.

Poisoning by aspirin preparations accounted for less than 6% of all poisoning deaths in the United Kingdom in 1973, and this proportion is substantially less than the peak figure of 17% in 1961. A group of drugs which is appearing in the lists with more frequency is the antidepressants, particularly the tricyclic antidepressants. Some 1% of deaths, of which about two-thirds were suicides, were attributed to such drugs.

Although many deaths are certified as being due to single agents, the increasing use of combinations of drugs, e.g. tricyclic antidepressants and barbiturates, antidepressants and tremor controllers, tranquillizers and barbiturates, almost certainly makes these statistics less reliable than they appear at first sight.

A variety of household or industrial chemicals is still used in suicide attempts in the United Kingdom as in other countries, despite the apparent availability of many less

TABLE 23.5.

COMPARISON OF OVERALL STATISTICS FOR DEATHS BY POISONING IN ENGLAND AND WALES, 1972 AND 1973

"Agent" refers to a specified substance or class of substance. (Data for 1972 and 1973 abstracted from Pharmaceutical Journal (1974) 212, 92–96 and (1975) 214, 260–265, respectively).

	1972 Number of agents involved	Number of deaths (all ages)			1973 Number of agents involved	Number of deaths (all ages)		
		Males	Females	Total		Males	Females	Total
Suicide	248	714	1057	1771	330	699	1042	1741
Accident	142	263	305	568	155	255	324	579
Intent not determined	120	221	362	583	143	246	348	594
		1198	1724	2922		1200	1714	2914

TABLE 23.6.

TEN PRINCIPAL AGENTS INVOLVED IN DEATHS BY POISONING (SUICIDE, ACCIDENT OR INTENT NOT DETERMINED) IN ENGLAND AND WALES, 1972 AND 1973

(Data for 1972 and 1973 abstracted from Pharmaceutical Journal (1974) 212, 92–96 and (1975) 214, 260–265 respectively).

	1972 Number of deaths (all ages)			1973 Number of deaths (all ages)		
	Males	Females	Total	Males	Females	Total
Suicide						
Amylobarbitone (and compound preparations)	232	374	606	172	326	498
Pentobarbitone	37	69	106	41	70	111
Barbiturate (not specified)	43	63	106	47	53	100
Aspirin	44	47	91	41	59	100
Salicylate (not specified)	26	29	55	17	25	42
Quinalbarbitone	20	27	47	14	19	33
Phenobarbitone	19	21	40	16	21	37
Amytriptyline	14	28	42	31	33	64
Methaqualone	19	20	39	17	19	36
Paracetamol	8	29	37	16	28	44
Accident						
Amylobarbitone (and compound preparations)	48	87	135	48	88	136
Barbiturate (not specified)	24	29	53	17	33	50
Alcohol	29	14	43	30	17	47
Pentobarbitone	17	18	35	11	17	28
Sodium amytal	13	14	27	6	13	19
Butobarbitone	11	10	21	5	16	21
Carbrital	4	15	19	4	2	6
Aspirin	3	10	13	5	8	13
Methaqualone	4	6	10	5	5	10
Salicylate (not specified)	0	3	3	6	2	8
Intent not determined						
Amylobarbitone (and compound preparations)	61	119	180	47	90	137
Barbiturate (not specified)	24	44	68	19	33	52
Pentobarbitone	18	22	40	17	28	45
Butobarbitone	13	19	32	13	15	28
Amytriptyline	10	9	19	8	7	15
Carbrital	5	10	15	3	3	6
Methaqualone	7	8	15	4	5	9
Salicylate (not specified)	6	9	15	5	3	8
Aspirin	4	10	14	6	8	14
Nitrazepam	5	2	7	3	2	5

bizarre toxic agents. Commonplace domestic or agricultural hazards such as ammonia, corrosive acids, caustic fluids, cleaning agents, disinfectants and weedkillers caused slightly more than 2% of all deaths by poisoning in 1973, and one-third of the deaths involving household poisons were apparently accidental.

The details presented in Table 23.6 do not offer a breakdown of poisoning cases by age groups, but it is clear that a substantial proportion of all cases of fatal accidental poisoning occur among children and young people. Female deaths from poisoning by drugs and chemical agents form almost 60% of all deaths in this manner. Accidental poisoning is more prevalent in the 45 to 64 year age group for females, but for males the age distribution is much wider, spreading across their working lives in the 25 to 64 year age range.

In general, the marked rise in deaths by drug poisoning, whether accidental or deliberate, which occurred in the United Kingdom in the 1960s, coincided with a decline in the number of deaths caused by carbon monoxide (coal-gas) inhalation. The rising trend in fatal poisonings has levelled off, but there is no firm indication of a downward change in the United Kingdom statistics for mortality.

It is likely that these patterns are broadly representative of fatal poisonings in developed countries where many different medicinal agents and industrial and household chemicals are available, and where abuse of ethanol is prevalent.

The proportions of such deaths which occur in hospital – either in spite of or because of treatment for poisoning – are not easy to discover. It is likely that most genuine suicide attempts are completed outside of hospital, whereas most accidental poisonings which have a fatal outcome are treated in hospital. The majority of patients who are admitted to hospital for self-poisoning, however, are not gravely ill even though some present as medical emergencies requiring resuscitation (Table 23.7); their admissions may be due more to the need for psychiatric counselling (Lawson and Mitchell, 1972) than for medical treatment. In the Edinburgh Regional Poisoning Treatment Centre (Matthew et al., 1969), to which all poisoned patients from the conurbation were referred without selection, only 9% of the admissions (approximately 110) in a typical year required supportive measures in the management of unconsciousness and the overall mortality was 0.7%. In only three out of seven fatal cases in this series, was poisoning per se judged to be the cause of death (Table 23.8); concurrent illness or disease, particularly in elderly patients,

TABLE 23.7.

SELF-POISONING IN SHEFFIELD, ENGLAND, 1970

754 Admissions to three major hospitals with casualty departments. (From Smith, 1972)

Unit	Total medical admissions	Total medical emergencies	Cases of self-poisoning	
			% Admissions	% Emergencies
Northern General	2,546	1,018	8.1	20.2
Royal Hospital	2,934	1,170	11.1	27.9
Royal Infirmary	2,562	1,717	8.7	12.9
Total	8,042	3,905	9.4	19.3

TABLE 23.8.

DEATHS IN THE EDINBURGH (SCOTLAND) REGIONAL POISONING TREATMENT CENTRE, 1968

(From Matthew et al., 1969)

Sex	Age (years)	Poison	Cause of death	Comment
M	15	Paraquat	Poisoning	Respiratory failure
F	18	Paracetamol/ ferrous sulphate	Poisoning	Acute massive necrosis of liver
M	41	Orphenadrine	Poisoning	Cardiac arrest
F	77	Barbiturate	Atherosclerosis; diabetes mellitus	
M	78	Coal gas	Cerebrovascular accident	Transient cerebral ischaemic attack before poisoning; blood-stained C.S.F. on admission; died 12 days later
F	about 70	Barbiturate	Chronic uraemia; respiratory infection	Conscious on admission; blood urea 60 mmol/litre (360 mg/dl); extensive pneumonia
M	56	Methaqualone preparation	Acute myocardial infarction	Two previous myocardial infarctions and necropsy evidence of recent infarction; carcinoma of prostate; died after regaining consciousness

was responsible for the remaining deaths. Epilepsy and pregnancy were the most common pre-existing physical conditions in another series of Scottish hospital admissions for poisoning (Table 23.9).

Table 23.10 shows the principal agents which were judged to be the causes of poisoning in the Edinburgh patients, in comparison with the classes of substances which together currently account (Kinney and Melville, 1976) for about 90% of admissions for poisoning to hospitals in the United States. In spite of the separation in space and time of these two series, it is striking that barbiturates head both lists, and this of course is consistent with the statistics for fatal poisoning, discussed above.

TABLE 23.9.

EXISTING PHYSICAL CONDITIONS ASSOCIATED WITH POISONING IN 637 PATIENTS TREATED IN A GENERAL MEDICAL UNIT, 1965–1971

(From Lawson and Mitchell, 1972)

	Trauma	Epilepsy	Pregnancy	Other medical or surgical conditions	Total
Number of patients	8	30	22	116	176

TABLE 23.10.

PRINCIPAL POISONS INVOLVED IN ADMISSIONS TO THE EDINBURGH (SCOTLAND) REGIONAL POISONING TREATMENT CENTRE IN 1968 AND CLASSES OF SUBSTANCES CURRENTLY ACCOUNTING FOR 90% OF ADMISSIONS FOR POISONING TO HOSPITALS IN THE UNITED STATES

(From Matthew et al., 1969 and Kinney and Melville, 1977, respectively)

Edinburgh		United States
Poison	Proportion of admissions (%)	Poisons accounting for 90% of admissions
Barbiturates	26	Barbiturates
Aspirin preparations	14	Non-barbiturate sedatives
Benzodiazepines	12	Salicylates
Methaqualone preparations	10	Tranquillizers
Tricyclic antidepressants	6	Opium alkaloids
Other hypnotic drugs	4	Aliphatic alcohols
Carbon monoxide	4	Carbon monoxide
Phenothiazines	3	Heavy metals
		Cholinesterase inhibitors
		Kerosene
		Naphtha
		Amphetamines

It is interesting to note that the number of annual admissions for poisoning to the Edinburgh Centre in relation to the catchment population corresponds to approximately 1600 per million. This appears to be a high figure, but it accurately reflects the situation for the whole of the United Kingdom, and demonstrates that poisoning is a meaningful part of the general medical case load in British hospitals (Table 23.7). There is little doubt that this is also true in many other countries.

The examples of acute poisoning and overdosage which are now outlined have been selected for the following reasons: because they are commonplace or interesting from the historical viewpoint; because they demonstrate diverse clinical features and different approaches to treatment; or because they are associated with a range of laboratory investigations covering both clinical chemistry and chemical toxicology.

23.5.1. Carbon monoxide poisoning

Carbon monoxide is rapidly absorbed through the lungs and has an affinity for haemoglobin which is 200 to 300 times that of oxygen, so that a low partial pressure of carbon monoxide in air can be dangerous. The toxicity of carbon monoxide has been recognized for many years and is reflected in the official mortality statistics of most countries which use fossil fuels.

The degree of acute exposure to carbon monoxide can be assessed fairly satisfactorily by a variety of methods ranging from differential heat denaturation of oxy- and carboxyhaemoglobin, to gas chromatography of carbon monoxide in whole blood. The only other substance with like properties to carboxyhaemoglobin is nitric oxide-haemoglobin, but other haem proteins – notably cytochrome P-450 – are also capable of binding carbon monoxide. For human subjects in an experimental situation, it has been possible to construct accurate nomograms (Peterson and Stewart, 1970, 1975) relating the proportion of carboxyhaemoglobin in blood to the concentration in air, the alveolar ventilation, and the duration of exposure. At the same time, the classical signs and symptoms of acute carbon monoxide poisoning can be related (Table 23.11) to the blood saturation. However, infants are particularly susceptible to poisoning, and the progression of toxic effects is faster in subjects with pulmonary or cardiovascular disease or anaemia. Adverse effects to the human foetus on chronic exposure to carbon monoxide have been documented (Longo, 1970).

Exposure to quite a low concentration of carbon monoxide in air – little more than 1% – can result in sudden loss of consciousness and fatal cardiac arrhythmia. In this circumstance, or if hypnotic or sedative drugs have been absorbed, the concentration of carboxyhaemoglobin in peripheral blood may be low and not consistent with the clinical picture. The same may be true in a poisoned patient to whom oxygen has been administered before a blood specimen has been taken, but this is an artefact due to the dissociation of carboxyhaemoglobin in vivo. For these reasons, the course of treatment is rarely guided by the assay of carboxyhaemoglobin.

Therapy with oxygen, which is a true pharmacological antidote (section 23.4), constitutes the basis of treatment of poisoning by substantially shortening the biological half-life of carbon monoxide, which is largely excreted unchanged through the lungs. It is doubtful if hyperbaric oxygen therapy offers any real advantage because of the extra lapse of time needed to gain access to and set up the equipment. The treatment and complications of severe poisoning, associated with oedema and prolonged cerebral anoxia,

TABLE 23.11.

ADULT HUMAN RESPONSE TO DIFFERENT CONCENTRATIONS OF CARBOXYHAEMOGLOBIN IN BLOOD

(From Stewart, 1975)

Blood saturation, COHb (%)	Response of healthy adult
<1	Normal range due to endogeneous carbon monoxide production [1]; no known detrimental effect
1–5	Selective increase in blood flow to certain vital organs to compensate for reduction in oxygen-carrying capacity of the blood
6–15	Visual light threshold increased
16–20	Headache; visual-evoked response abnormal
21–30	Throbbing headache; nausea; fine manual dexterity abnormal
31–40	Severe headache, nausea and vomiting, syncope
51–60	Coma; convulsions
>60	Lethal if not treated

[1] i.e. from the catabolism of haem (Coburn, 1973).

have been thoroughly documented (Smith and Brandon, 1970, 1973). Encephalopathy and delayed neuropsychiatric symptoms occur in a large proportion of patients who survive the initial trauma (Ginsburg and Romano, 1976).

Although the features of acute poisoning with carbon monoxide are well defined, there is less agreement on the toxic effects of chronic exposure, due either to cigarette smoking (Astrup, 1973) or to environmental pollution (Stewart, 1975; Lawther, 1975). The fact that there is normal endogeneous production of carbon monoxide from the catabolism of haem (Coburn, 1973) makes it difficult to measure and meaningfully interpret low blood concentrations of carboxyhaemoglobin.

23.5.2. Ethanol intoxication and methanol poisoning

Blood ethanol measurements may be helpful in the investigation of coma associated with road traffic accidents. It is generally accepted that driving performance is impaired when the blood concentration exceeds 11 mmol/litre (50 mg/dl) and several countries have enacted relevant drinking-and-driving legislation. In a series of fatal accidents in Australia (Hossack, 1972), 50% of drivers killed had a blood concentration in excess of 22 mmol/litre (100 mg/dl). The fact that other drugs were also involved in a small number of these cases points to the need for caution in the interpretation of quantitative findings, and a better understanding of the pharmacokinetics of ethanol.

It has long been known that ethanol differs from nearly all other drugs in that, after absorption and distribution is complete, there is a zero-order fall of concentration in blood with time. For most individuals, the rate of fall of blood level is a constant in the range 2 to 5 mmol/litre per hour (10 to 25 mg/dl per hour). This corresponds to the factor β introduced by a pioneer investigator Widmark; β reflects the sum of concurrent redistribution, biotransformation and excretion. Most of an ingested dose of ethanol is oxidized to acetaldehyde by cytoplasmic NAD-linked liver alcohol dehydrogenase, and thus becomes incorporated into the metabolic pool of C_2-compounds. Only a small proportion of the dose is subject to pulmonary or renal excretion as unchanged alcohol, and catabolism to exhaled carbon dioxide is an unimportant pathway. The precise value of β is largely determined by hepatic mass and blood flow (Krebs and Stubbs, 1975), and it is usual to find that chronic alcoholics display high values. Individuals possessing atypical liver alcohol dehydrogenase, which is exceptionally active in vitro, have been found to degrade ethanol at the same rate as individuals with normal liver enzyme (Edwards and Evans, 1967). This may indicate that the availability of NAD may be an important factor in determining the precise value of β. An hepatic microsomal ethanol-oxidizing system has been characterized in experimental animals, but there is controversy (Seixas, 1975) as to whether this pathway is important in the metabolism of ethanol in man.

Many attempts have been made (Plapp, 1975) to increase β in acute alcoholic intoxication by the oral or intravenous administration of substances which might stimulate metabolism. Only large doses of laevulose (fructose) are thought to have a significant effect, which even then is only marginal. The effect may be due to an enhancement of hepatic blood flow, but the availability of laevulose, or of its metabolite D-glyceraldehyde, may increase the normal rate of turnover of reduced NAD and hence speed the oxidation of ethanol. In hepatic disease, as in anoxic states, the administration of large amounts of fructose may cause lactic acidosis (Woods and Alberti, 1972) so that it is doubtful if this therapy is really useful in managing the acute alcoholic crisis.

The metabolism of ethanol may be partially inhibited in vivo, with a consequent reduction in β, by substances – notably disulphiram and cyanamide – which interfere with ethanol metabolism by blocking the further oxidation of acetaldehyde. These substances have found limited clinical application in the treatment of alcoholic patients (Malcolm et al., 1974).

The possibility that methanol may be a minor product of the metabolism of ethanol in vivo has been investigated, but it is doubtful if this pathway is of any practical consequence (Majchrowicz, 1975). On the other hand, there is a sound experimental basis for supposing that there can be a metabolic interaction between the two alcohols, in the sense that ethanol is the preferred substrate for liver alcohol dehydrogenase, so that it can delay the oxidation of methanol in vivo. This effect has an established place in the treatment of methanol poisoning, which is dangerous on account of depression of the central nervous system, severe metabolic acidosis and specific toxicity of the oxidation products for retinal cells.

The oxidation of methanol is catalyzed by liver alcohol dehydrogenase to formaldehyde, and hence to formate, by a number of enzymes including aldehyde oxidase, catalase, peroxidase and xanthine oxidase. Only a small proportion of absorbed methanol is excreted unchanged through the kidneys; nevertheless, the specific detection of methanol in a urine specimen may be helpful in differential diagnosis from diabetic coma, lactic acidosis or renal failure, and it is technically simpler than the assay of formate (Makar et al., 1975).

Since formaldehyde and formate are both substantially more toxic than the parent compound, there is advantage in administering ethanol to achieve a blood concentration of about 22 mmol/litre (100 mg/dl) (Humphrey, 1974), so as to delay the oxidation of methanol. At the same time, of course, acidosis and dehydration must be correctly treated. The most efficient means of eliminating unchanged methanol is by haemodialysis. In a comparative study (Keyvan-Larijarni and Tannenberg, 1974) of haemodialysis and peritoneal dialysis in a small group of poisoned patients, the former technique achieved more rapid falls of serum methanol concentrations than the latter, without mortality or morbidity. The clinical improvement appeared to correlate better with the fall in serum concentration than with changes in ácid–base status.

23.5.3. Acute salicylate poisoning

Salicylate poisoning (Hill, 1973) most commonly arises by ingestion of an overdose of aspirin either accidentally, in children, or deliberately, in young people and adults. Acute or chronic overdosage may also accur in the therapy of rheumatoid arthritis (section 23.3.2) or by percutaneous absorption of salicylic acid in the treatment of dermatoses. Methyl salicylate (oil of wintergreen) is toxic on account of its biotransformation into salicylate. There are many compound preparations of aspirin, in most of which it is the major ingredient.

Salicylate, and its principal metabolite, salicylurate, are excreted in the urine as such, and in conjugated forms (Davison, 1971). The excretion of free salicylate, like that of other acidic drugs, is enhanced in alkaline urine (section 23.2.1.4). Oxidation to gentisic acid and its congeners constitutes a minor pathway of metabolism. The lack of involvement of hepatic mixed function oxidases is likely to account for the paucity of metabolic drug interactions which involve salicylate, and may be associated with a lack of development of pharmacological tolerance. Salicylate is strongly bound by albumin, and other plasma proteins, and drug interactions may occur on account of its displacing less strongly bound drugs such as sulphonamides, from binding sites.

A useful qualitative test for salicylate is afforded by the characteristic colour formed with Fe^{3+} in acid solution. This may be adapted for rapid quantitation of plasma concentrations, since only a small proportion of salicylate circulates as metabolites in peripheral plasma. Salicylurate however, gives a similar colour with Fe^{3+}, so that meaningful quantitation of urinary excretion by this method is not possible. A variety of modern quantitative techniques may be used for salicylate assay, in conjunction with appropriate separation procedures.

The chief toxic effects of salicylate, and their biochemical sequelae, are shown in Scheme 23.3. Salicylate is a powerful central stimulant of respiration and this leads to hypocapnoea and respiratory alkalosis, which is the condition found in most conscious patients admitted to hospital for aspirin overdosage. At the concentration found in severe poisoning, salicylate is also an effective uncoupler of oxidative phosphorylation and inhibitor of other enzymic pathways; this tends to hypercapnoea and metabolic acidosis. It is possible that the liver has an active role in a progression from respiratory alkalosis to metabolic acidosis.

The early literature on acid–base disturbances in salicylate poisoning was often contradictory, and confusion has arisen on three points in particular – firstly, assessment of acid–base status only occasionally included measurements of both respiratory and metabolic components, and the results of isolated estimates of plasma carbon dioxide-combining power are apt to be misleading; secondly, nearly all investigators have used capillary or venous blood samples with attendant difficulties in the collection of specimens or the interpretation of the results; thirdly, generalizations about the pathogenesis of disturbances have been made from findings in acutely poisoned children, or in adults treated with therapeutic doses of aspirin, and the conclusions may not be valid for poisoned

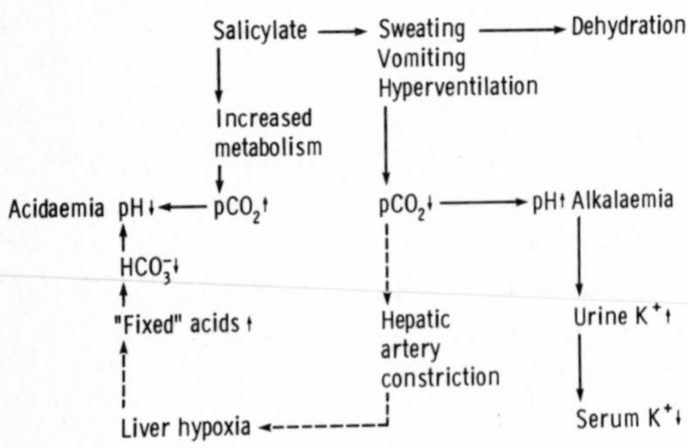

Scheme 23.3. Principal features and biochemical consequences of salicylate poisoning.

adults. In some respects, the features and management of acute salicylate poisoning in children differ from those in adults.

The diagnosis of acute salicylate poisoning is seldom difficult, but the characteristic features of salicylism may be present at quite a low plasma concentration or may not be apparent at all even when the patient has absorbed a large overdose and has quite a high plasma concentration. Quantitative assay is therefore desirable, not so much for diagnosis as for the assessment of the severity of the poisoning. Interpretation, however, requires a knowledge of the lapse of time since ingestion of the overdose and of the acid–base and electrolyte status.

Children are very sensitive to overdosage with salicylate and rapidly become acidaemic. In most adult patients, however, respiratory alkalosis is the dominant disturbance but there is nearly always concurrent metabolic acidosis. The finding of an arterial blood pH below normal is indicative of dangerous poisoning, whether or not the plasma salicylate concentration is high and whether or not consciousness is impaired. Only a small proportion (approximately 1%) of patients are acidaemic on admission to hospital (Proudfoot and Brown, 1969), but this probably reflects the fact that the majority of deaths from salicylate poisoning occur outside hospital. Acute overdosage with salicylates has not been clearly associated with hepatic or renal damage, but since excretion of the drug depends largely on the integrity of renal function, toxic effects may be particularly pronounced in patients with antecedent renal disease.

Hypokalaemia has been reported to be a feature of severe salicylate poisoning, but it is exceptional to find abnormal concentrations of the plasma cations on admission because of concomitant water depletion. The sweating and hyperventilation which characterize salicylate poisoning lead to very large fluid deficits (Lawson et al., 1969) which has an obvious bearing on the role of intravenous fluids in management. Treatment with oral fluids is inadequate for any patient who continues to vomit, or who has marked salicylism, regardless of the plasma salicylate concentration. The correction of dehydration must be an integral part of therapy and this can only be achieved effectively with a regime of intravenous fluid administration. The onset of diuresis may be delayed for 1 or 2 hours, depending on the fluid deficit, but this is not to be viewed with alarm. Patients with plasma salicylate concentrations in excess of 4.3 mmol/litre (600 μg/ml) should be treated by a regime which ensures alkalinization of the urine whether or not symptoms of salicylism are manifest. Effective alkalinization is difficult to achieve, and the marked fall in plasma potassium concentration which is likely to occur reflects not only urinary excretion but shift into the intracellular compartment. It is important to maintain the extracellular potassium concentration near normal, and this requires the addition of large amounts of potassium supplements to the intravenous fluid. Salicylate poisoning therefore presents problems of electrolyte, fluid, and acid–base imbalance similar to those seen in the treatment of diabetic ketosis.

Forced diuresis should be used with caution in the management of acidaemic patients (Proudfoot and Brown, 1969), where the first priority is to normalize the acid–base status. Haemodialysis, rather than forced diuresis, would be required in patients with a history of renal insufficiency.

23.5.4. Acute paracetamol (acetaminophen) poisoning

In therapeutic doses, paracetamol is a safe analgesic and antipyretic drug, but when taken in acute overdosage it can be extremely dangerous. The features of paracetamol poisoning (Scheme 23.4) have been recognized since about 1966. Overdosage is seen commonly in the United Kingdom (Clark et al., 1973) where there is significant mortality, but there are surprisingly few reports from other countries (Rumack and Matthew, 1975; Ferguson et al., 1977).

The most serious and potentially lethal effect of paracetamol overdosage is acute centrilobular necrosis of parenchymal liver cells. Necrotic cells rapidly disappear, leaving areas of reticulin collapse and usually a mild inflammatory reaction, but remarkably complete histological recovery can occur (Portmann et al., 1975). Depending on the lapse of time between the episode of poisoning and the first blood specimen being taken, there may be normal or barely increased serum aspartate or alanine transaminase activities, but in severe poisoning these values increase beyond the measurable range within 12 to 24 hours. This feature is quite characteristic of acute absorption of chemical hepatotoxins, of which the commonest by far are paracetamol and carbon tetrachloride.

Hepatic failure in paracetamol poisoning is likely to lead to metabolic acidosis and hypoglycaemia, and severe disturbance of the blood clotting mechanism. The serum alkaline phosphatase activity is only marginally increased, except in the terminal illness. There is no special advantage in measuring serum γ-glutamyltransferase, even though the activity of this enzyme is commonly increased in hepatic varieties of drug jaundice. The severity of paracetamol poisoning may be gauged from the duration of the prothrombin time, by the highest measured value of serum hydroxybutyrate dehydrogenase activity (Prescott et al., 1971), or by the time taken for the serum transaminase activities to return to normal, which may be several weeks. In experimental paracetamol-induced hepatic necrosis in rats (Dixon et al., 1975), there was a parallel relationship between the serum transaminase activities and the histological extent of necrosis at 24 hours after a relatively large dose of the drug. Furthermore, there was reasonable correlation between the enzyme activities and the grade of necrosis during the next few days of hepatic recovery. These findings confirm the usefulness of knowing the time of ingestion in interpreting clinical enzyme mea-

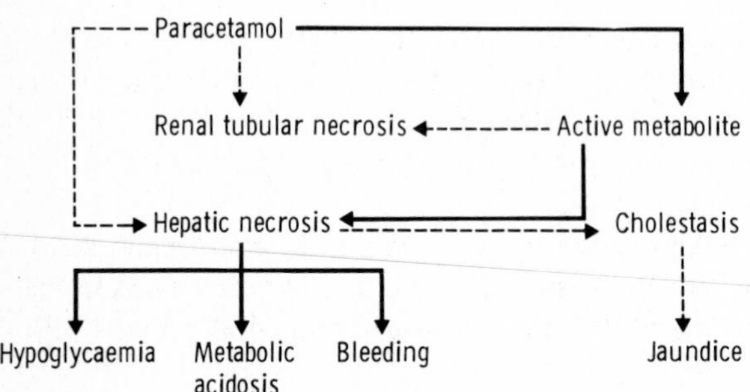

Scheme 23.4. Principal features and biochemical consequences of paracetamol poisoning.

surements, but the possibility of there being acute-on-chronic overdosage must always be considered.

The qualitative detection of paracetamol in plasma, or paracetamol metabolites in urine, may be helpful in the differential diagnosis of liver failure where the aetiology is not known, but here again, there is a possibility that chronic therapeutic dosage may confuse the issue. Traditional means of assaying "total paracetamol" in urine have involved acid hydrolysis and quantitation of the resulting *p*-aminophenol, but there are many pitfalls in performing and interpreting the estimation (Chrastil and Wilson, 1975), and this substance, as such, is only found in urine after a massive overdosage. Free paracetamol in plasma may be extracted and assayed by direct spectrophotometry, but there may be gross interference from other common acidic drugs such as barbiturates or salicylate. Gas chromatography and high-performance liquid chromatography are more satisfactory techniques.

Measurements of the peak plasma concentration of paracetamol may be a useful guide to the prognosis with patients in whom there is moderately severe liver damage and relatively slow increase in serum aminotransferase activities. However, the rate of decrease of the plasma concentration, as measured by the plasma half-life, is more meaningful and is likely to afford an indication for the administration of methionine or cysteamine (Prescott et al., 1971, 1976). Such sulphydryl compounds may protect against liver damage if given rapidly enough after the overdose by inhibiting the formation of an active metabolite (Davis et al., 1976). Paracetamol in therapeutic doses is largely excreted in the urine as phenolic conjugates, but a small proportion is oxidized by a mixed function oxidase to a metabolite which is excreted as a cysteine or mercapturic acid conjugate. Alteration of the availability of hepatic glutathione, by pretreatment with diethyl maleate or cobaltous chloride, alters the extent of experimental hepatic necrosis (Mitchell et al., 1973). The toxic metabolite has not yet been identified; the precise role of hepatic glutathione is still uncertain; and definite indications for therapy with sulphydryl compounds have yet to be formulated. Nevertheless, this approach is likely to replace empirical manoeuvres such as haemodialysis and charcoal haemoperfusion for treatment of paracetamol poisoning (Solomon et al., 1977).

23.5.5. Hypnotic and sedative drug overdosage

The problems of tolerance and of potentiation by ethanol and other drugs (Caldwell and Sever, 1974), and the relative lack of specificity of simple analytical methods, particularly with regard to drug metabolites, make it difficult to interpret measurements of hypnotic or sedative drug concentrations in body fluids. Except in the context of clinical research, therefore, drug assays make little contribution to the management of these kinds of overdosage. In any case, modern drugs such as the benzodiazepines have very favourable therapeutic indices and are relatively innocuous in overdosage (Greenblatt et al., 1977). Because they are so common, however, and because serious medical complications may ensue which require general laboratory support, the principal features of poisoning with barbiturates and with methaqualone, as a typical non-barbiturate hypnotic, are now described.

23.5.5.1. Barbiturate poisoning

The early history of barbiturate poisoning, and of different approaches to treatment, has been summarized by Loennecken (1965). Within one year of the introduction in Germany in 1904 of barbitone (diethylbarbituric acid), cases of suicidal poisoning were reported, and the first review of the symptomology, therapy and prognosis of overdosage was published in 1908. The problem of habituation and the dangers of barbiturate poisoning were also recognized early on – inadequate pulmonary ventilation, obstruction of the respiratory system and aspiration, elimination of the pharyngeal reflexes, renal complications. Treatment was based upon vigorous gastric lavage, oxygen therapy, and stimulus of the cardiovascular system with drugs such as caffeine and camphor: mortality was very high – above 45% – and was not greatly improved by the introduction of central nervous stimulants in the 1930s. In severe poisoning these drugs and the later analeptics might achieve some measure of return of the reflexes, but consciousness was often not regained. Furthermore, analeptic drugs could give rise to serious side-effects including cardiac arrhythmias, convulsions and psychoses (Mark, 1967).

Substantial improvement in mortality was not realized until experience of treating poliomyelitis by assisted ventilation led to the introduction of the Scandinavian approach of the supportive therapy of barbiturate poisoning. Lawson and Proudfoot (1971) have described the extension of the Scandinavian Method to cover emergency treatment – the management of respiratory and circulatory failure, and the prevention of further absorption of the drug – and the general care of hypothermia and rebound hyperthermia, water and electrolyte balance, and infection. This kind of intensive therapy requires a high standard of medical and nursing care. General laboratory support is needed, without special recourse to urgent toxicological analysis since the findings would be unlikely to influence the course of treatment.

In a small minority of patients who prove to be gravely poisoned, it may be justified to perform forced alkaline diuresis or haemodialysis. Exchange transfusion or peritoneal dialysis have also been used to enhance drug elimination, but they are inefficient techniques. However, forced diuresis and haemodialysis have a place in the treatment of severe poisoning by the so-called long-acting barbiturates, provided that the clinical circumstances warrant their use; that there is good qualitative and quantitative analytical evidence of the drug involved; and that there is adequate laboratory monitoring of the patient's electrolyte and acid–base status.

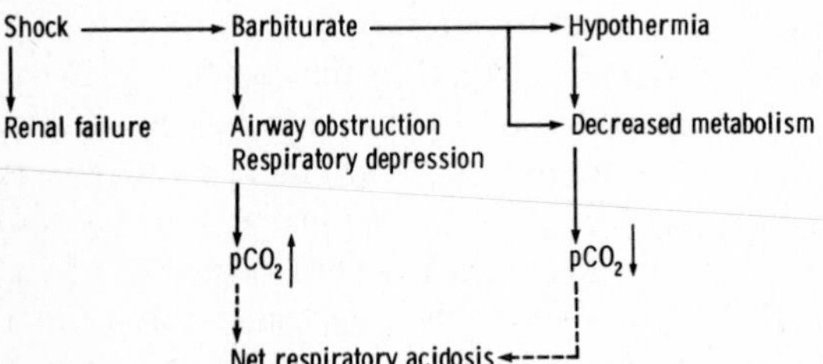

Scheme 23.5. Principal features and biochemical consequences of barbiturate poisoning.

23.5.5.2. Methaqualone poisoning

The history of the use and abuse of methaqualone, and of its chemical toxicology (Brown and Goenechea, 1973), is reminiscent of that of the barbiturates. Methaqualone was introduced into clinical practice about 1960. Clinical trials suggested that it was as effective as other hypnotic–sedative drugs and might have advantages in the treatment of geriatric patients. Preparations of methaqualone base or of the hydrochloride, and compound preparations with a wide variety of other drugs, were marketed vigorously. In some countries, such preparations were available from pharmacists without prescription, and reports of addiction and of fatal overdosage appeared, first in Germany and other European countries, then in Japan and Australia. Methaqualone abuse became widespread in the United States about 1970, and strict legislative control of its use was instituted in 1973. In England and Wales in the early 1970s, poisoning with methaqualone was one of the top ten causes of death from ingested poisons, both in respect to accidents and suicide (Table 23.6).

Although methaqualone was promoted as a non-barbiturate drug, its structure is that of a fused oxopyrimidine. It is now known to be metabolized by hepatic microsomal mixed function oxidation and it is similar to phenobarbitone in its ability to induce hepatic enzymes. Conjugates of most of the ten possible monohydroxy metabolites, and some of the dihydroxy derivatives, have been identified in the urine of humans or experimental animals, but little, if any, unchanged methaqualone is normally excreted.

The slightly unusual physical and chemical properties of methaqualone have facilitated the development of many different methods for its assay of body fluids, but some of them do not readily distinguish methaqualone from its phenolic metabolites (Bailey and Jatlow, 1973) or from other lipophilic drugs which are effectively neutral in character, e.g. glutethimide. As with the barbiturates, the interpretation of quantitative measurements of plasma concentrations in patients after overdosage is difficult because of the ease with which pharmacological tolerance to the drug develops. In principle, the finding of a low concentration in a severely poisoned patient could be helpful since it might exclude the use of an active therapeutic procedure such as haemodialysis; conversely, the finding of a very high concentration might be an indication for such a procedure.

Except for some characteristic neurological signs in less severely poisoned patients, the features and possible complications of methaqualone overdosage are very similar to those associated with barbiturate poisoning. In a large series of patients poisoned with a preparation of methaqualone and diphenhydramine (Matthew et al., 1968), none required artificial ventilation even though some were unconscious for many days. This might perhaps have been due to the respiratory stimulant effect of the antihistamine. Prolonged coma caused by methaqualone, like that due to other drugs, may result in bizarre, but non-specific, increases of serum enzyme activities (Wright et al., 1971). In particular, creatine kinase activity may be increased for many days, and this probably reflects generalized skeletal muscle damage. There is no firm indication that cardiac, renal or hepatic damage may occur as a specific effect of the poisoning.

23.5.6. Paraquat poisoning

Paraquat is a *para*-substituted quaternized derivative of 4,4′-dipyridyl which was synthesized, and subsequently used as a redox indicator, about 40 years ago. Compounds of this type, however, have been known for nearly a century.

As a biochemical reagent, paraquat was known as "methylviologen" because it had the unusual property of being easily reduced to a stable coloured radical-ion. The action of a mild reducing agent on paraquat in neutral aqueous solution gives a green chromophor, which becomes intensely blue on the addition of alkali. This reaction forms the basis of a simple, but highly specific and sensitive, screening test for paraquat in urine. Cation-exchange or high-performance liquid chromatography (Pryde and Darby, 1975) before colour development offers an effective means of concentrating paraquat at the low concentration found in blood plasma, or in urine if a relatively small dose has been absorbed, or if excretion is being followed over a long period of time (Brown, 1971). Diquat, which is sometimes formulated with paraquat and is the only other widely used dipyridyl, undergoes a similar reaction, but the radical-ion has a less intense blue-green colour in alkaline solution.

The herbicidal properties of paraquat were discovered about 1950. For agricultural use, it is formulated as an aqueous concentrate of the dichloride containing spreading agents and other additives. It is likely that these, rather than paraquat itself, are responsible for the local ulcerative effects of the concentrate which are usually seen after accidental ingestion. A stenching agent is now added to at least one commercial formulation to guard against negligent or homicidal abuse, but many cases of poisoning have now been reported in Europe (Hofmann and Frohberg, 1972), North America (Fairshter et al., 1976), Australia (Harrison et al., 1972) and elsewhere (Teare, 1976).

Remarkably little is known about the mechanism of detoxification of paraquat as applied to plants and soils, or about the character of its absorption, distribution or biotransformation in man. Agricultural workers who bear chronic exposure, and continually excrete measurable amounts of paraquat in the urine, apparently suffer no ill effects. In poisoned patients, the detection of a few milligrams only of paraquat in a urine specimen voided within a few hours after ingestion, seems to indicate a good prognosis. The finding of larger amounts, or the continuing excretion for more than a few days, is a grave sign.

Depending on the quantity ingested, and whether or not extensive vomiting occurs, so as to diminish the amount of absorption, symptoms of renal or hepatic damage may occur within a few hours or a few days. Accordingly, great care must be exercised in instituting forced diuresis in an attempt to enhance the urinary excretion of the poison. Pulmonary oedema may supervene, and haemodialysis may then be necessary although there is no real evidence that this technique is of value in enhancing the clearance of paraquat.

Several mechanisms of paraquat toxicity have been proposed (Autor, 1977) on the basis of its electron acceptor properties. Thus it stimulates the rate of oxidation of NADPH in liver cell fractions, and paraquat radical-ion can be oxidized back to paraquat by molecular oxygen, with formation of hydrogen peroxide, and of super-oxide (O_2^-) and hydroperoxy radicals (HO_2^-). Hydrogen peroxide itself or these reactive species, may cause tissue damage as a result of lipid peroxidation. Superoxide dismutase, which is found in most tissues, catalyzes the scavenging of superoxide ($2O_2^- + 2H^+ \rightarrow H_2O_2 + O_2$), and administration of this enzyme has been advocated in the treatment of paraquat toxicity (Fairshter et al., 1976).

The most specific, and potentially lethal, action of paraquat is on the lung. Measurement of arterial pO_2 may give early warning of the development of a diffuse, cellular, intra-alveolar pulmonary fibrosis (Copland et al., 1974); this fibrosis is associated with pulmonary vascular disease. Although renal and hepatic failure in paraquat poisoning may be resolved, there is no firm evidence that lung damage can be reversed. Corticosteroids given systemically and immunosuppressive drugs do not prevent the lung lesion. Dyspnoea and cyanosis become progressively worse in such patients, and death may ensue after a few days or weeks. Oxygen therapy would seem to be mandatory in attempting to treat this stage of paraquat poisoning, but long exposure to high concentrations of oxygen may itself induce pulmonary fibrosis, and such treatment may have a synergistic effect on the action of paraquat. In view of the similarity between the lung pathology caused by paraquat and that arising from oxygen toxicity, combined therapy using superoxide dismutase, D-propranolol and beclomethasone has been used (Davies and Conolly, 1975), but as yet there is no proof that such measures are effective.

The specificity of this action of paraquat is demonstrated by the fact that in man and in experimental animals, high concentrations are found in the kidneys and liver but these organs show no signs of cellular proliferation such as occurs in the lung. In mice (Cagen et al., 1976), liver function is not specially impaired. Further studies of the tissue and species specificity and of the energy-dependent accumulation of paraquat (Rose et al., 1976) are needed to elucidate the mechanisms which underly its toxicity.

23.5.7. Organophosphorus poisoning

A variety of organophosphorus compounds, in many different formulations, is commercially available for pest control. Some, like parathion, are highly toxic to man; others, like malathion, less so. Some require metabolic activation in vivo, but all owe their characteristic toxic effects to the specific inhibition of acetylcholinesterase at the neuromuscular junction. Poisoning is rarely seen in the United Kingdom, but is relatively common in the United States and some other countries (Namba et al., 1971).

Depending on the route of absorption and the dose, the systemic effects of acute poisoning on the central nervous system, the muscles, and the gastrointestinal tract become apparent within an hour or two, and may last for several days. Paralysis due to demyelination of the spinal cord may be irreversible, but its onset may be delayed for several weeks, especially in tri-*o*-cresylphosphate poisoning. By contrast, exposure to organophosphorus compounds can cause death within a few minutes, due to paralysis of the muscles of respiration and depression of the respiratory centre (Koelle, 1975). Chronic poisoning, in the generally accepted sense, does not occur, but continual absorption of sub-toxic doses, which may occur in agricultural workers, will precipitate the features of acute poisoning. Monitoring of the urinary excretion of *p*-nitrophenol in such workers has been advocated as a useful index of absorption of *p*-nitrophenyl-substituted organophosphorus compounds such as parathion.

A more widely applicable test of acute or chronic exposure is afforded by assay of (red cell) acetylcholinesterase or (plasma) cholinesterase. Although the action of these enzymes is not directly related to the symptoms of organophosphorus poisoning, their inhibition undoubtedly reflects the situation in the tissues. Chronic exposure to organophosphorus compounds diminishes the activities of the two enzymes, more quickly for cholinesterase than for acetylcholinesterase. Development of the features of systemic poisoning is accompanied by rapid and substantial inhibition of the two enzymes. When exposure ceases, cholinesterase activity slowly reverts to normal, over 5 or 6 weeks, as the enzyme is re-synthesized by the liver. Acetylcholinesterase activity increases less rapidly, and takes 13 to 17 weeks to return to normal as the red cells are turned over.

Apart from supportive therapy, the treatment of organophosphorus poisoning is based upon two pharmacological principles. Firstly, large doses of atropine tend to reverse the central nervous and muscarinic effects by blocking the action of excess acetylcholine. Secondly, oximes such as pyridine-2-aldoxime (pralidoxime, given as its chloride, methiodide, or methosulphate) specifically detoxify circulating or tissue-bound organophosphorus compounds, and reactivate phosphorylated enzyme so as to reduce the accumulation of acetylcholine. Pralidoxime is rapidly eliminated by the kidney (Swartz and Sidell, 1973), so that repeated dosage may be necessary. Blood specimens for acetylcholinesterase and cholinesterase assays should be taken before the first administration of pralidoxime.

It must be emphasized both that pralidoxime is an adjunct to, and not a substitute for, atropine and that it is not equally antagonistic to all organophosphorus compounds or other cholinesterase inhibitors (Namba et al., 1971).

23.6. CONSPECTUS

There have been great advances in experimental pharmacology and toxicology over the past 20 years. Improvements in analytical chemistry and biochemistry have enabled pharmacokinetics to grow on a sound quantitative basis and have led to better understanding of the molecular basis of many therapeutic and toxic effects. An encouraging number of key findings in experimental animals has been successfully extrapolated to normal human subjects. In spite of many limitations, assays of blood or urine for drugs, or their metabolites, have proved helpful in the general development of rational chemotherapies and for certain drugs, they may be required for the monitoring of a particular patient.

Animals, however, are poor models for human iatrogenic disease, drug overdosage or frank poisoning, especially when there is antecedent or concurrent physical illness. In these contexts, toxicological assays of body fluids have very definite limitations. Their analytical specificities or sensitivities may be inadequate; control investigations are not likely to be feasible; there may be insufficient published data to judge whether the observed concentrations reflect therapeutic, toxic or lethal values. Compilations of such data (e.g. Baselt, 1975; Winek, 1976) should be reviewed critically – we know little enough about the components of variance which make up reference ranges for endogeneous analytes, let alone exogeneous ones. In certain types of poisoning, depending upon the circumstances, a single toxicological analysis may materially assist the diagnosis or prognosis, but serial measurements are likely to be more meaningful. Few cases of poisoning require specific therapy to counteract the poison or active measures to remove it. Most severely poisoned patients are successfully treated by intensive supportive therapy, which requires general clinical laboratory support rather than toxicological analysis.

ACKNOWLEDGEMENTS

We are grateful to Dr. Henry Matthew and other former colleagues of the Edinburgh Regional Poisoning Treatment Centre for stimulating and sustaining our interest in clinical toxicology and drug monitoring.

REFERENCES

Aherne, G.W., Marks, V., Mould, G. and Stout, G. (1977) Radioimmunoassay for nortriptyline and amitriptyline. Lancet, i, 1214.

Albert, A. (1973) Selective Toxicity: the Physico-Chemical Basis of Therapy, 5th edn. Halstead Press, New York.

Asberg, M. (1974) Plasma nortriptyline levels: relationship to clinical effects. Clinical Pharmacology and Therapeutics, 16, 215–229.

Astrup, P. (1973) Carbon monoxide, smoking and atherosclerosis. Postgraduate Medical Journal, 49, 697–706.

Atkins, G.L. (1969) Multicompartment Models for Biological Systems. Methuen, London.

Autor, A.P. (Ed.) (1977) Biochemical Mechanisms of Paraquat Toxicity. Academic Press, New York.

Baastrup, P.C., Poulsen, J.C., Schou, M., Thomsen, K. and Amdisen, A. (1970) Prophylactic lithium: double blind discontinuation in manic-depressive and recurrent-depressive disorders. Lancet, ii, 326–330.

Bailey, D.N. and Jatlow, P.I. (1973) Methaqualone overdose: analytical methodology, and the significance of serum drug concentrations. Clinical Chemistry, 19, 615–620.

Baldessarini, R.J. and Lipinski, J.F. (1975) Lithium salts: 1970–1975. Annals of Internal Medicine, 83, 527–533.

Barnett, H.L. and Vesterdal, J. (1953) The physiologic and clinical significance of unmaturity of kidney function in young infants. Journal of Pediatrics, 42, 99–119.

Baselt, R.C., Wright, J.A. and Cravey, R.H. (1975) Therapeutic and toxic concentrations of more than 100 toxicologically significant drugs in blood, plasma or serum: a tabulation. Clinical Chemistry, 21, 44–62.

Bauld, H.W., Gibson, P.F., Jebson, P.J. and Brown, S.S. (1974) Aetiology of prolonged apnoea after suxamethonium. British Journal of Anaesthesia, 46, 273–281.

Baylis, E.M., Fry, D.E. and Marks, V. (1970) Microdetermination of serum phenobarbitone and diphenylhydantoin by gas-liquid chromatography. Clinica Chimica Acta, 30, 93–103.

Baylis, E.M., Hall, M.S., Lewis, G. and Marks, V. (1972) Effects of renal function on plasma digoxin levels in elderly ambulant patients in domiciliary practice. British Medical Journal, 1, 338–341.

Bedynek, J.L., Jr., Weinstein, K.N., Kah, R.E. and Minton, P.R. (1966) Ventricular tachycardia: control by intermittent intravenous administration of lidocaine hydrochloride. Journal of the American Medical Association, 198, 553–555.

Beller, G.A., Smith, T.W., Abelmann, W.H., Haber, E. and Hood, W.B. (1971) Digitalis intoxication: a prospective clinical study with serum level correlations. New England Journal of Medicine, 284, 989–997.

Berry, D.J. and Grove, J. (1973) Emergency toxicological screening for drugs commonly taken in overdose. Journal of Chromatography, 80, 205–220.

Bertler, A. and Redfors, A. (1970) An improved method of estimating digoxin in human plasma. Clinical Pharmacology and Therapeutics, 11, 665–673.

Bianchine, J.R., Calimlim, L.R., Morgan, J.P., Dujuvne, C.A. and Lasagna, L. (1971) Metabolism and absorption of L-3,4-dihydroxyphenylalanine in patients with Parkinson's disease. Annals of the New York Academy of Sciences, 176, 126–140.

Biggs, J.T. and Ziegler, V.E. (1977) Protriptyline plasma levels and antidepressant response. Clinical Pharmacology and Therapeutics, 22, 269–273.

Black, D.A.K., Rose, G. and Brewer, D.B. (1970) Controlled trial of prednisone in adult patients with the nephrotic syndrome. British Medical Journal, 3, 421–426.

Blacow, N.W. (1968) Is aspirin safe? Pharmaceutical Journal, 200, 325–328.

Blass, K.G., Thibert, R.J. and Draisey, T.F. (1974) A simple, rapid thin-layer chromatographic drug screening procedure. Journal of Chromatography, 95, 75–79.

Bloomer, H.A. (1966) A critical evaluation of diuresis in the treatment of barbiturate intoxication. Journal of Laboratory and Clinical Medicine, 67, 898–905.

Bloomfield, S.S., Romhilt, D.W., Chou, T. and Fowler, N.O. (1971) Quinidine for prophylaxis of arrhythmias in acute myocardial infarction. New England Journal of Medicine, 285, 979–986.

Boobis, S.W. (1977) Alteration of plasma albumin in relation to decreased drug binding in uremia. Clinical Pharmacology and Therapeutics, 22, 147–153.

Boston Collaborative Drug Surveillance Program (1972) Drug surveillance: problems and challenges. Pediatric Clinics of North America, 19, 117–129.

Braithwaite, R.A., Goulding, R., Theano, G., Bailey, J. and Coppen, A. (1972) Plasma concentration of amitriptyline and clinical response. Lancet, i, 1297–1300.

Breckenridge, A., Orme, M.L., Thorgeirsson, S., Davies, D.S. and Brooks, R.V. (1971) Drug interactions with warfarin: studies with dichloral-phenazone, chloral hydrate and phenazone (antipyrine). Clinical Science, 40, 351–364.

Brink, M.F., Speckmann and Balsley, M. (1968) Current concepts in geriatric nutrition. Geriatrics, 23, 113–120.

British Medical Journal (1975) Problems with digoxin (Editorial). British Medical Journal, 1, 49–50.

Brodie, B.B. (1965) Displacement of one drug by another from carrier or receptor sites. Proceedings of the Royal Society of Medicine, 58, Suppl., 946–955.

Brown, S.S. (1969) Clinical chemistry of salicylate poisoning. Annals of Clinical Biochemistry, 6, 13–17.

Brown, S.S. (1971) Paraquat poisoning: clinicopathological conference. Scottish Medical Journal, 16, 410–412.

Brown, S.S. (1975) Metabolic interactions involving drugs or foreign compounds. In Foreign Compound Metabolism in Mammals, Vol. 3 (Ed. D.E. Hathway) pp. 591–630, Chemical Society, London.

Brown, S.S. and Goenechea, S. (1973) Methaqualone: metabolic, kinetic and clinical pharmacologic observations. Clinical Pharmacology and Therapeutics 14, 314–324.

Butler, V.P., Jr. (1973) Radioimmunoassay and competitive binding radioassay methods for the measurement of drugs. Metabolism, 22, 1145–1153.

Cagen, S.Z., Janoff, A.S., Bus, J.S. and Gibson, J.E. (1976) Effect of paraquat (methyl viologen) on liver function in mice. Journal of Pharmacology and Experimental Therapeutics, 198, 222–228.

Caldwell, J. and Sever, P.S. (1974) The biochemical pharmacology of abused drugs: II Alcohol and Barbiturates. Clinical Pharmacology and Therapeutics, 16, 737–749.

Campbell, T.C. and Hayes, J.R. (1974) Role of nutrition in the drug metabolizing enzyme system. Pharmacological Reviews, 26, 171–197.

Chasseaud, L.F. (1972) Transference of radioactively labelled foreign compounds. In Foreign Compound Metabolism in Mammals. Vol. 2 (Ed. D.E. Hathway) pp. 62–162, Chemical Society, London.

Chrastil, J. and Wilson, J.T. (1975) Pitfalls in the estimation of *p*-aminophenol and *p*-chloraniline as products of drug liver metabolism. Biochemical Medicine, 13, 89–97.

Chrusciel, T.L. and Chrusciel, M. (1976) Selected Bibliography on Detection of Dependence-producing Drugs in Body Fluids. WHO, Geneva.

Clark, R., Thompson, R.P.H., Borirakchanyavat, V., Widdop, B., Davidson, A.R., Goulding, R. and Williams, R. (1973) Hepatic damage and death from overdose of paracetamol. Lancet, i, 66–69.

Clemmesen, C. (1959) The treatment of poisoning during the past twenty-five years: a retrospective review. Danish Medical Bulletin, 6, 209–213.

Clemmesen, C. and Nilsson, E. (1961) Therapeutic trends in the treatment of barbiturate poisoning: the Scandinavian method. Clinical Pharmacology and Therapeutics, 2, 220–229.

Coburn, R.F. (1973) Endogeneous carbon monoxide metabolism. Annual Review of Medicine, 24, 241–250.

Copland, G.M., Kolin, A. and Shulman, H.S. (1974) Total pulmonary fibrosis after paraquat ingestion. New England Journal of Medicine, 291, 290–292.

Crammer, J.L., Rosser, R.M. and Crane, G. (1974) Blood levels and management of lithium treatment. British Medical Journal, 3, 650–654.

Crouthamel, W.G. (1975) The effect of congestive heart failure on quinidine pharmacokinetics. American Heart Journal, 90, 335–339.

Danon, A., Horowitz, J., Kaplanski, J. and Glick, S. (1977) An outbreak of digoxin intoxication. Clinical Pharmacology and Therapeutics, 21, 643–646.

Davidson, D.C., McIntosh, W.B. and Ford, J.A. (1974) Assessment of plasma glutamyl transpeptidase activity and urinary D-glucaric acid excretion as indices of enzyme induction. Clinical Science and Molecular Medicine, 47, 279–283.

Davies, D.S. and Conolly, M.E. (1975) Paraquat poisoning – possible therapeutic approach. Proceedings of the Royal Society of Medicine, 68, 442.

Davis, M., Simmons, C.J., Harrison, N.G. and Williams, R. (1976) Paracetamol overdose in man: relationship between pattern of urinary metabolites and severity of liver damage. Quarterly Journal of Medicine, 45, 181–191.

Davison, C. (1971) Salicylate metabolism in man. Annals of the New York Academy of Sciences, 179, 249–268.

Deckers, W.J. and Lewis, L.R. (1973) Evaluation of Screendex – a multireagent system for detection of drug abuse and drug overdose. Clinical Toxicology, 6, 201–210.

Deer Lodge Conference (1976) Proceedings of the Fourth Conference on Clinical Pharmacology, 1976: Environmental Chemicals and Nutrition – Relationship to Metabolism, Action and Toxicity of Drugs. Clinical Pharmacology and Therapeutics, 1977, 22, 623–824.

Dewar, F.M. McK. and Wakefield, G. (1976) Hypersensitivity to suxamethonium in a Suffolk family. British Journal of Anaesthesia, 48, 707–710.

Dimitrov, N.V. and Nodine, J.H. (Eds.) (1974) Drugs and Hematologic Reactions, Proceedings of the 29th Hahnemann Symposium, Grune and Stratton, New York.

Dixon, M.F., Fulker, M.J., Walker, B.E., Kelleher, J. and Losowsky, M.S. (1975) Serum transaminase levels after experimental paracetamol-induced hepatic necrosis. Gut, 16, 800–807.

Dobos, J.K., Phillips, J. and Covo, G.A. (1961) Acute barbiturate intoxication. Journal of the American Medical Association, 176, 268–272.

Doherty, J.E. (1973) Digitalis glycosides: pharmacokinetics and their clinical implications. Annals of Internal Medicine, 79, 229–238.

Dollery, C.T. (1972) Individual differences in response to drugs in man. In Eighth Symposium on Advanced Medicine (Ed. G. Neale) pp. 185–195, Pitman Medical, London.

Done, A.K. (1964) Developmental pharmacology. Clinical Pharmacology and Therapeutics, 5, 432–479.

Done, A.K. (1969) Pharmacologic principles in the treatment of poisoning. Pharmacology for Physicians, 3, 1–10.

Drayer, D.E. and Reidenberg (1977) Clinical consequences of polymorphic acetylation of basic drugs. Clinical Pharmacology and Therapeutics, 22, 251–258.

Dubowski, K.M. (1974) Biological aspects of breath-alcohol analysis. Clinical Chemistry, 20, 294–299.

Duhme, D.W., Greenblatt, D.J. and Koch-Weser, J. (1974) Reduction of digoxin toxicity associated with measurement of serum levels. Annals of Internal Medicine, 80, 516–519.

Eadie, M.J. (1974) Laboratory control of anticonvulsant dosage. Drugs, 8, 386–397.

Edwards, J.A. and Evans, D.A. (1967) Ethanol metabolism in subjects possessing typical and atypical liver alcohol dehydrogenase. Clinical Pharmacology and Therapeutics, 8, 824–829.

Edwards, I.R., Hancock, B.W. and Saynor, R. (1974) Correlation between plasma quinidine and cardiac effect. British Journal of Clinical Pharmacology, 1, 455–459.

Ehrsson, H. and Knapp, D. (1974) Rapid, efficient procedure for extraction of drugs for toxicological analysis. Clinical Chemistry, 20, 1366–1367.

Elson, J., Strong, J.M., Lee, W.-K. and Atkinson, A.J., Jr. (1975) Antiarrhythmic potency of *N*-acetylprocainamide. Clinical Pharmacology and Therapeutics, 17, 134–140.

Evans, D.A.P. and White, T.A. (1964) Human acetylation polymorphism. Journal of Laboratory and Clinical Medicine, 63, 394–403.

Evered, D.C., Chapman, C. and Hayter, C.J. (1970) Measurement of plasma digoxin concentration by radioimmunoassay. British Medical Journal, 3, 427–428.

Fairshter, R.D., Rosen, S.M., Smith, W.R., Glasser, F.L., McRae, D.M. and Wilson, A.F. (1976) Paraquat poisoning: new aspects of therapy. Quarterly Journal of Medicine, 45, 551–565.

Ferguson, D.R., Snyder, S.K. and Cameron, A.J. (1977) Hepatotoxicity in acetaminophen poisoning. Mayo Clinic Proceedings, 52, 246–248.

Fogelman, A.M., La Mont, J.T., Finkelstein, S., Rado, E. and Pearce, M.L. (1971) Fallibility of plasma-digoxin in differentiating toxic from non-toxic patients. Lancet, ii, 727–729.

Forrest, J.A.H. (1975) Forced alkaline diuresis for lithium intoxication. Postgraduate Medical Journal, 51, 189–191.

Fry, D.E. and Marks, V. (1971) Value of plasma-lithium monitoring. Lancet, i, 886–888.

Fuchs, F., Fuchs, A.R., Poblete, V.F., Jr. and Risk, A. (1967) Effect of alcohol on threatened premature labor. American Journal of Obstetrics and Gynecology, 99, 627–637.

Gelehrter, T.D. (1976) Enzyme induction. New England Journal of Medicine, 294, 522–526; 589–595; 646–651.

George, C.F., Conolly, M.E., Fenyvesi, T., Bryant, R.H. and Dollery, C.T. (1972) Intravenously administered isoproterenol sulfate dose–response curves in man. Archives of Internal Medicine, 130, 361–364.

Gillette, J.R., Mitchell, J.R. and Brodie, B.B. (1974) Biochemical mechanisms of drug toxicity. Annual Review of Pharmacology, 14, 271–288.

Ginsburg, R. and Romano, J. (1976) Carbon monoxide encephalopathy: need for appropriate treatment. American Journal of Psychiatry, 133, 317–320.

Glassman, A.H. and Perel, J.M. (1974) Plasma levels and tricyclic antidepressants. Clinical Pharmacology and Therapeutics, 16, 198–200.

Goldstein, A., Aronow, L. and Kalman, S.M. (1974) Principles of Drug Action: the Basis of Pharmacology, 2nd edn. pp. 301–355, Wiley, New York.

Goulding, R. and Widdop, B. (1974) Laboratory toxicology in the district general hospital. Recent Advances in Clinical Pathology, 6, 61–72.

Grahame-Smith, D.G. and Everest, M.S. (1969) Measurement of digoxin in plasma and its use in the diagnosis of digoxin intoxication. British Medical Journal, 1, 286–289.

Greenblatt, D.J., Allen, M.D., Noel, B.J. and Shader, R.I. (1977) Acute overdosage with benzodiazepine derivatives. Clinical Pharmacology and Therapeutics, 21, 497–514.

Greenblatt, D.J. and Koch-Weser, J. (1975) Drug therapy: clinical pharmacokinetics. New England Journal of Medicine, 293, 702–705; 964–970.

Griffiths, W.C., Oleksyk, S.K. and Diamond, I. (1973) A comprehensive gas chromatographic drug screening procedure for the clinical laboratory. Clinical Biochemistry, 2, 124–131.

Gross, F.H. and Inman, W.H.W. (Eds.) (1977) Drug Monitoring. Academic Press, London.

Gupta, N., Sarkissian, E. and Paulus, H.E. (1975) Correlation of plateau serum salicylate levels with rate of salicylate metabolism. Clinical Pharmacology and Therapeutics, 18, 350–355.

Hadden, J., Johnson, K., Smith, S., Price, L. and Giardina, E. (1969) Acute barbiturate intoxication: concepts of management. Journal of the American Medical Association, 209, 893.

Halkin, H., Meffin, P., Melmon, K.L. and Rowland, M. (1975) Influence of congestive heart failure on blood levels of lidocaine and its active monodeethylated metabolite. Clinical Pharmacology and Therapeutics, 17, 669–676.

Hamlyn, A.N., Brown, A.J., Sherlock, S. and Baron, D.N. (1975) Casual blood-ethanol estimations in patients with chronic liver disease. Lancet, ii, 345–347.

Hammer, W. and Sjoqvist, F. (1967) Plasma levels of monomethylated tricyclic antidepressants during treatment with imipramine-like compounds. Life Sciences, 6, 1895–1903.

Harrison, L.C., Dortimer, A.C. and Murphy, K.J. (1972) Fatalities due to the weed-killer paraquat. Medical Journal of Australia, 2, 774–777.

Hartshorn, E.A. (1970) Handbook of Drug Interactions. Francke, Cincinnati.

Heinz, E. (1967) Transport through biological membranes. Annual Review of Physiology, 29, 21–58.

Hepner, G.W. and Vesell, E.S. (1977) Aminopyrine metabolism in the presence of hyperbilirubinaemia due to cholestasis or hepatocellular disease. Clinical Pharmacology and Therapeutics, 21, 620–626.

Hewitt, W.H. (1974) Gentamicin: toxicity in perspective. Postgraduate Medical Journal, 50, Suppl. 7, 55–59.

Hill, J.B. (1973) Current concepts: salicylate intoxication. New England Journal of Medicine, 288, 1110–1113.

Hoddinott, B.C., Gowdey, C.W., Coulter, W.K. and Parker, J.M. (1967) Drug reactions and errors in administration on a medical ward. Canadian Medical Association Journal, 97, 1001–1006.

Hoffbrand, B.E., O'Grady, F.W. and Girdwood, R.H. (1974) Gentamicin: proceedings of a symposium. Postgraduate Medical Journal, 50, Suppl. 7, 1–64.

Hofmann, A. and Frohberg, H. (1972) Gramoxone-Intoxikationen in der Bundesrepublik Deutschland. Deutsche Medizinische Wochenschrift, 1299–1303.

Hoppel, C., Garle, M., Rane, A. and Sjoqvist, F. (1977) Plasma concentrations of 5-(4-hydroxyphenyl)-5-phenylhydantoin in phenytoin-treated patients. Clinical Pharmacology and Therapeutics, 21, 294–300.

Hossack, D.W. (1972) Investigation of 400 people killed in road accidents, with special reference to blood alcohol levels. The Medical Journal of Australia, 2, 255–258.

Houghton, G.W. and Richens, A. (1974) Rate of elimination of tracer doses of phenytoin at different steady-state serum phenytoin concentrations in epileptic patients. British Journal of Clinical Pharmacology, 1, 155–161.

Humphrey, T.J. (1974) Methanol poisoning: management of acidosis with combined haemodialysis and peritoneal dialysis. Medical Journal of Australia, 1, 833–835.

Hutson, D.H. (1972) Mechanisms of Biotransformations. In Foreign Compound Metabolism in Mammals, Vol. 2 (Ed. D.E. Hathway) pp. 328–397, Chemical Society, London.

Hutson, D.H. (1975) Mechanisms of Biotransformation. In Foreign Compound Metabolism in Mammals, Vol. 3 (Ed. D.E. Hathway) pp. 449–549, Chemical Society, London.

Hurwitz, N. (1969a) Predisposing factors in adverse reactions to drugs. British Medical Journal, 1, 536–539.

Hurwitz, N. (1969b) Admissions to hospital due to drugs. British Medical Journal, 1, 539–540.

Hvidberg, E.F. and Dam, M. (1976) Clinical pharmacokinetics of anticonvulsants. Clinical Pharmacokinetics, 1, 161–188.

Iisalo, E. and Ruikka, I. (1974) Serum levels and renal excretion of digoxin in the elderly: a comparison between three different preparations. Acta Medica Scandinavica, 196, 59–63.

Jackson, G.G. and Riff, L.J. (1971) Pseudomonas bacteremia: pharmacologic and other bases for future of treatment with gentiamicin. Journal of Infectious Diseases, 124, Suppl., 185.

James, I.M. (1974) Diseases affecting drug responses. British Journal of Hospital Medicine, 12, 823–836.

Kaim, S.C. (1972) Criteria for the diagnosis of alcoholism: Criteria Committee of the National Council of Alcoholism. Annals of Internal Medicine, 77, 249–258.

Kalow, W. (1971) Topics in pharmacogenetics. Annals of the New York Academy of Sciences, 179, 654–659.

Kalow, W. and Gunn, D.R. (1959) Some statistical data on atypical cholinesterase of human serum. Annals of Human Genetics, 23, 239–250.

Keyvan-Larijarni, H. and Tannenberg, A.M. (1974) Methanol intoxication: comparison of peritoneal dialysis and hemodialysis treatment. Archives of Internal Medicine, 134, 293–296.

Kinney, T.D. and Melville, R.S. (Eds.) (1976) Mechanization, Automation and Increased Effectiveness of the Clinical Laboratory. p. 56, DHEW Publication No. NIH 77–145, Washington D.C.

Klotz, U., Antonin, K.H., Brugel, H. and Bieck, P.R. (1977) Disposition of diazepam and its major metabolite desmethyldiazepam in patients with liver disease. Clinical Pharmacology and Therapeutics, 21, 430–436.

Koch-Weser, J. and Klein, S.W. (1971) Procainamide dosage schedules, plasma concentrations, and clinical effects. Journal of the American Medical Association, 215, 1454–1460.

Koch-Weser, J. Sellers, E.M. (1976) Drug therapy: binding of drugs to serum albumin. New England Journal of Medicine, 294, 311–316: 526–531.

Koelle, G.B. (1975) Anticholinesterase agents. In The Pharmacological Basis of Therapeutics, 5th edn. (Eds. L.S. Goodman, A. Gilman, A.G. Gilman, and G.B. Koelle) pp. 445–466, Macmillan, New York.

Koppanyi, T. and Fazekas, J.F. (1950) Acute barbiturate poisoning: analysis and evaluation of current therapy. American Journal of the Medical Sciences, 220, 559–576.

Korsten, M.A., Matsuzaki, S., Feinman, L. and Lieber, C.S. (1975) High blood acetaldehyde levels after ethanol administration in alcoholics: difference between alcoholic and non-alcoholic subjects. New England Journal of Medicine, 292, 386–389.

Koup, J.R., Jusko, W.J. and Goldfarb, A.L. (1975) pH-Dependent secretion of procainamide into saliva. Journal of Pharmaceutical Sciences, 64, 2008–2010.

Kragh-Sørensen, P., Hansen, C.E. and Asberg, M. (1973) Plasma levels of nortriptyline in the treatment of endogeneous depression. Acta Psychiatrica Scandinavica, 49, 444–456.

Krebs, H.A. and Stubbs, M. (1975) Factors controlling the rate of alcohol disposal by the liver. Advances in Experimental Medicine and Biology, 59, 149–161.

Kupfer, D.J., Hanin, I., Spiker, D.G., Grau, T. and Coble, P. (1977) Amitriptyline plasma levels and clinical response in primary depression. Clinical Pharmacology and Therapeutics, 22, 904–911.

Kutt, H. (1971) Biochemical and genetic factors regulating dilantin metabolism in man. Annals of the New York Academy of Sciences, 179, 705–722.

Lasagna, L. (1972) Drug therapy: hypnotic drugs. New England Journal of Medicine, 287, 1182–1183.

Lawson, A.A.H. and Mitchell, I. (1972) Patients with acute poisoning seen in a general medical unit (1960–1971) British Medical Journal, 4, 153–156 and 760.

Lawson, A.A.H. and Proudfoot, A.T. (1971) In Medical Management of Acute Barbiturate Poisoning (Ed. H. Matthew) pp. 175–193, Excerpta Medica, Amsterdam.

Lawson, A.A.H., Proudfoot, A.T., Brown, S.S., MacDonald, R.H., Fraser, A.G., Cameron, J.C. and Matthew, H. (1969) Forced diuresis in the treatment of acute salicylate poisoning in adults. Quarterly Journal of Medicine, 38, 31–48.

Lawson, D.H. and Wilson, G.M. (1974) Detecting adverse drug reactions. British Journal of Hospital Medicine, 12, 790–798.

Lawther, P.J. (1975) Carbon monoxide. British Medical Bulletin, 31, 256–260.

Lehmann, H. and Liddell, J. (1969) Human cholinesterase (pseudocholinesterase) genetic variants and their recognition. British Journal of Anaesthesia, 41, 235–244.

Lehmann, H., Silk, E. and Liddell, J. (1961) Pseudo-cholinesterase. British Medical Bulletin, 17, 230–233.

Leppik, I.L. and Sherwin, A.L. (1977) Anticonvulsant activity of phenobarbital and phenytoin in combination. Journal of Pharmacology and Experimental Therapeutics, 200, 570–575.

Levy, G. and Nagashima, R. (1969) Comparative pharmacokinetics of coumarin anticoagulants. VI. Effect of plasma protein binding on the distribution and elimination of bishydroxycoumarin by rats. Journal of Pharmaceutical Sciences, 58, 1001–1004.

Lieber, C., Teschke, R., Husvmura, Y. and Decarli, L.M. (1975) Differences in hepatic and metabolic changes after acute and chronic alcohol consumption. Federation Proceedings, 34, 2060–2074.

Loennecken, S.J. (1965) Akute Schlafmittelvergiftung. Schattauer-Verlag, Stuttgart.

Locket, S. (1973) Clinical Toxicology VIII. Antidotes, irrespirable gases, toxic metals and alcohols. The Practitioner, 211, 243–250.

Longo, L.D. (1970) Carbon monoxide in the pregnant mother and fetus and its exchange across the placenta. Annals of the New York Academy of Sciences, 174, 312–341.

Ludden, T.M., Allen, J.P., Valutsky, W.A., Vicuna, A.Y., Nappi, J.M., Hoffman, S.F., Wallace, J.E., Lalka, D. and McNay, J.L. (1977) Individualization of phenytoin dosage regimens. Clinical Pharmacology and Therapeutics, 21, 287–293.

Lund, L., Lunde, P.K., Rane, A., Borga, O. and Sjoqvist, F. (1971) Plasma protein binding, plasma concentrations and effects of diphenylhydantoin in man. Annals of the New York Academy of Sciences, 179, 723–728.

McCance, R.A. (1950) Renal physiology in infancy. American Journal of Medicine, 9, 229–241.

MacGregor, A.G. (1965) Clinical effects of interaction between drugs: review of points at which drugs can interact. Proceedings of the Royal Society of Medicine, 58, Suppl., 943–946.

Maddock, R.K. and Bloomer, H.A. (1968) Limitations of diuresis and dialysis as treatments for sedative intoxication. Clinical Research, 16, 166.

Maher, J.F. and Schreiner, G.E. (1968) The dialysis of poisons and drugs. Transactions of the American Society for Artificial Internal Organs, 14, 440–453.

Majchrowicz, E. (1975) Metabolic correlates of ethanol, acetaldehyde, acetate and methanol in humans and animals. Advances in Experimental Medicine and Biology, 111–156.

Makar, A.B., McMartin, K.E., Palese, M. and Tephly, T.R. (1975) Formate assay in body fluids: application in methanol poisoning. Biochemical Medicine, 13, 117–126.

Malcolm, M.T., Madden, J.S. and Williams, A.E. (1974) Disulfiram implantation critically evaluated. British Journal of Psychiatry, 125, 485–489.

Mann, L.I., Bhakthavathsalan, A., Lium, M. and Makowski, P. (1975) Placental transport of alcohol and its effect on maternal and fetal acid–base balance. American Journal of Obstetrics and Gynecology, 122, 837–844.

March, J., Turner, W.J., Shanley, J. and Field, J. (1974) Values for urinary excretion of D-glucaric acid by normal individuals. Clinical Chemistry, 20, 1155–1158.

Mark, L.C. (1967) Analeptics: changing concepts, declining status. American Journal of the Medical Sciences, 254, 296–302.

Marks, V., Lindup, W.E. and Baylis, E.M. (1973) Measurement of therapeutic agents in blood. Advances in Clinical Chemistry, 16, 47–109.

Martindale: The Extra Pharmacopoeia (1977) 27th edn., (Ed. A. Wade) Chelating Agents and Antagonists. pp. 328–342, Pharmaceutical Press, London.

Matthew, H. and Lawson, A.A.H. (1979) Treatment of Common Acute Poisonings, 4th edn. Churchill Livingstone, Edinburgh.

Matthew, H., Proudfoot, A.T., Brown, S.S. and Aitken, R.C.B. (1969) Acute poisoning: organization and work-load of a treatment centre. British Medical Journal, 3, 489–493.

Matthew, H., Proudfoot, A.T., Brown, S.S. and Smith, A.C.A. (1968) Mandrax poisoning: conservative management of 116 patients. British Medical Journal, 2, 101–102.

Mawer, G.E. and Lee, H.A. (1968) Value of forced diuresis in acute barbiturate poisoning. British Medical Journal, 2, 790–793.

May, F.E., Stewart, R.B. and Cluff, L.E. (1977) Drug interactions and multiple drug administration. Clinical Pharmacology and Therapeutics, 22, 322–328.

Miller, R.R. (1973) Drug surveillance utilizing epidemiologic methods: a report from the Boston Collaborative Drug Surveillance Program. American Journal of Hospital Pharmacy, 30, 584–592.

Milne, M.D. (1967) Drugs, Poisons and the Kidney. In Renal Disease, 2nd edn. (Ed. D.A.K. Black) pp. 546–560, Blackwell, Oxford.

Mitchell, J.R. and Jollow, D.J. (1975) Metabolic activation of drugs to toxic substances. Gastroenterology, 68, 392–410.

Mitchell, J.R., Jollow, D.J., Potter, W.Z., Davis, D.C., Gillette, J.R. and Brodie, B.B. (1973) Acetaminophen-induced hepatic necrosis. I. Role of drug metabolism. Journal of Pharmacology and Experimental Therapeutics, 187, 185–194.

Mongan, E. (1973) Tinnitus as an indication of therapeutic serum salicylate levels. Journal of the American Medical Association, 226, 142–145.

Montgomery, S.A., Braithwaite, R.A. and Crammer, J.L. (1977) Routine nortriptyline levels in treatment of depression. British Medical Journal, 2, 166–167.

Morgan, A.G. and Polak, A. (1969) Acetazolamide and sodium bicarbonate in treatment of salicylate poisoning in adults. British Medical Journal, 1, 16–19.

Morselli, P.L., Cohen, S.N. and Garattini, S. (Eds.) (1974) Drug Interactions. North-Holland, Amsterdam.

Moser, R.H. (1967) Bibliographies on diseases of medical progress; salicylates. Clinical Pharmacology and Therapeutics, 8, 333–345.

Mroczek, W.J., Davidov, M. and Finnerty, F.A., Jr. (1973) Intravenous clonidine in hypertensive patients. Clinical Pharmacology and Therapeutics, 14, 847–851.

Motulsky, A.G. (1965) The genetics of abnormal drug responses. Annals of the New York Academy of Sciences, 123, 167–177.

Mulvihill, J.J., Klimas, J.T., Stokes, D.C. and Risemberg, H.M. (1976) Fetal alcohol syndrome: seven new cases. American Journal of Obstetrics and Gynecology, 126, 937–941.

Myerson, R.M. (1973) Metabolic aspects of alcohol and their biological significance. The Medical Clinics of North America, 57, 925–940.

Myschetsky, A. (1961) The significance of Megimide in the treatment of barbiturate poisoning. Danish Medical Bulletin, 8, 33–36.

Nagashima, R., Levy, G. and Nelson, E. (1968) Comparative pharmacokinetics of coumarin anticoagulants, I. Unusual interaction of bishydroxycoumarin with plasma proteins – development of a new assay. Journal of Pharmaceutical Sciences, 57, 58–67.

Namba, T., Nolte, C.T., Jackrel, J. and Grob, D. (1971) Poisoning due to organophosphate insecticides: acute and chronic manifestations. American Journal of Medicine, 50, 475–492.

Nelson, E. (1961) Kinetics of drug absorption, distribution, metabolism and excretion. Journal of Pharmaceutical Sciences, 50, 181–192.

Nelson, E. (1965) Kinetic considerations in pharmacogenetic studies of drug metabolism. Life Sciences, 4, 949–953.

Noone, P., Parsons, T.M., Pattison, J.R., Slack, R.C.B., Garfield-Davies, D. and Hughes, K. (1974) Experience of monitoring gentamicin therapy during treatment of serious Gram-negative sepsis. British Medical Journal, 1, 477–481.

Odell, G.B. (1959) The dissociation of bilirubin from albumin and its clinical implications. Journal of Pediatrics, 55, 268–279.

O'Reilly, R.A. (1969) Interaction of the anticoagulant drug warfarin and its metabolites with human plasma albumin. Journal of Clinical Investigation, 48, 193–202.

Orfila, M.J.B. (1815) Traite des Poisons Tires Mineral, Vegetal et Animal on Toxicologie Generale sous le Rapports de la Pathologie et de la Medicine Legale. Crochard, Paris. (Quoted by T.A. Loomis (1968) Essentials of Toxicology. p. 3, Kimpton, London.)

Parke, D.V. (Ed.) (1975) Enzyme Induction, Vol. 6, Basic Life Sciences Series. Plenum, New York.

Peterson, J.E. and Stewart, R.D. (1970) Absorption and elimination of carbon monoxide by inactive young men. Archives of Environmental Health, 21, 165–171.

Peterson, J.E. and Stewart, R.D. (1975) Predicting the carboxyhemoglobin levels resulting from carbon monoxide exposures. Journal of Applied Physiology, 39, 633–638.

Petit, J.M., Spiker, D.G., Ruivitch, J.F., Ziegler, V.E., Weiss, A.N. and Biggs, J.T. (1977) Tricyclic antidepressant plasma levels and adverse effects after overdose. Clinical Pharmacology and Therapeutics, 21, 47–51.

Piafsky, K.M. and Borgå, O. (1977) Plasma protein binding of basic drugs. II. Importance of α_1-acid glycoprotein for interindividual variation. Clinical Pharmacology and Therapeutics, 22, 545–549.

Pilz, W. (1974) Cholinesterases. In Methods of Enzymatic Analysis Vol. 2, 2nd edn. (Ed. H.U. Bergmeyer) pp. 831–851, Verlag Chemie, Weinheim.

Plapp, B.V. (1975) Rate-limiting steps in ethanol metabolism and approaches to changing these rates biochemically. Advances in Experimental Medicine and Biology, 56, 77–109.

Portmann, B., Talbot, I.C., Day, D.W., Davidson, A.R., Murray-Lyon, I.M. and Williams, R. (1975) Histopathological changes in the liver following a paracetamol overdose: correlation with clinical and biochemical parameters. Journal of Pathology, 117, 169–181.

Prescott, L.F. (1972) Measurement of plasma drug concentrations as a guide to therapy. In Eighth Symposium on Advanced Medicine (Ed. G. Neale) pp. 196–209, Pitman Medical, London.

Prescott, L.F. and Nimmo, J. (1971) Generic inequivalence – clinical observations. Acta Pharmacologica et Toxicologica, 29, Suppl. 3, 288–303.

Prescott, L.F. Park, J., Sutherland, G.R., Smith, I.J. and Proudfoot, A.T. (1976) Cysteamine, methionine and penicillamine in the treatment of paracetamol poisoning. Lancet, ii, 109–113.

Prescott, L.F., Wright, N., Roscoe, P. and Brown, S.S. (1971) Plasma-paracetamol half-life and hepatic necrosis in patients with paracetamol overdosage. Lancet, i, 519–522.

Protivinsky, R. (1971) Cycloserine. Antibiotics and Chemotherapy, 17, 87–94.

Proudfoot, A.T. and Brown, S.S. (1969) Acidaemia and salicylate poisoning in adults. British Medical Journal, 2, 547–550.

Prowse, K., Pain, M., Marston, A.D. and Cumming, G. (1970) The treatment of salicylate poisoning using mannitol and forced alkaline diuresis. Clinical Science, 38, 327–337.

Pryde, A. and Darby, F.J. (1975) The analysis of paraquat in urine by high-speed liquid chromatography. Journal of Chromatography, 115, 107–116.

Rawlins, M.D. (1974a) Variability in response to drugs. British Medical Journal, 4, 91–94.

Rawlins, M.D. (1974b) Variability of response to drugs in man. British Journal of Hospital Medicine, 12, 803–811.

Reid, E. (1976) Sample preparation in the micro-determination of organic compounds in plasma or urine. Analyst, 101, 1–18.

Reidenberg, M.M., Odar-Cedarlof, I., von Bahr, C., Borgå, O. and Sjoqvist, F. (1971) Protein binding of diphenylhydantoin and desmethylimipramine in plasma from patients with poor renal function. New England Journal of Medicine, 285, 264–267.

Richens, A. and Woodford, F.P. (Eds.) (1976) Anticonvulsant Drugs and Enzyme Inductions. Excerpta Medica, Amsterdam.

Rosalki, S.B. (1975) Gamma-glutamyl transpeptidase. Advances in Clinical Chemistry, 17, 53–107.

Rose, M.S., Lock, E.A., Smith, L.L. and Wyatt, I. (1976) Paraquat accumulation: tissue and species specificity. Biochemical Pharmacology, 25, 419–423.

Rumack, B.H. and Matthew, H. (1975) Acetaminophen poisoning and toxicity. Pediatrics, 55, 871–876.

Schou, M. (1976) Pharmacology and toxicology of lithium. Annual Review of Pharmacology and Toxicology, 16, 231–244.

Scott, D.B. and Julian, D.G. (Eds.) (1971) Lidocaine in the Treatment of Ventricular Arrythmias. Livingstone, Edinburgh.

Seixas, F.A. (1975) Alcohol and its drug interactions. Annals of Internal Medicine, 83, 86–92.

Sheiner, L.B., Halkin, H., Peck, C., Rosenberg, B. and Melmon, K.L. (1975) Improved computer-assisted digoxin therapy: a method using feedback of measured serum digoxin concentrations. Annals of Internal Medicine, 82, 619–627.

Shopsin, B. and Gershon, S. (1974) The current status of lithium in psychiatry. American Journal of the Medical Sciences, 268, 306–323.

Shirkey, H.C. (1966) The innocent child. Journal of the American Medical Association, 196, 418–421.

Singer, I. and Rotenberg, D. (1973) Mechanisms of lithium action. New England Journal of Medicine, 289, 254–260.

Smith, A.J. (1972) Self-poisoning with drugs: a worsening situation. British Medical Journal, 4, 151–159.

Smith, J.S. and Brandon, S. (1970) Acute carbon monoxide poisoning – 3 years' experience in a defined population. Postgraduate Medical Journal, 46, 65–70.

Smith, J.S. and Brandon, S. (1973) Morbidity from acute carbon monoxide poisoning at three year follow-up. British Medical Journal, 1, 318–321.

Smith, R.P. and Gosselin, R.E. (1976) Current concepts about the treatment of selected poisonings: nitrite, cyanide, sulfide, barium, and quinidine. Annual Reviews of Pharmacology and Toxicology, 16, 189–199.

Smith, S.E. and Rawlins, M.D. (1974) Prediction of drug oxidation rates in man: lack of correlation with serum gamma-glutamyl transpeptidase and urinary excretion of D-glucaric acid and 6-β-hydroxycortisol. European Journal of Clinical Pharmacology, 7, 71–75.

Smith, T.W., Butler, V.P., Jr. and Haber, E. (1969) Determination of therapeutic and toxic serum digoxin concentrations by radioimmunoassay. New England Journal of Medicine, 281, 1212–1216.

Smith, T.W. and Haber, E. (1970) Digoxin intoxication: the relationship of clinical presentation to serum digoxin concentration. Journal of Clinical Investigation, 49, 2377–2386.

Smith, T.W. and Haber, E. (1973a) Digitalis: digitalis toxicity. New England Journal of Medicine, 289, 1125–1128.

Smith, T.W. and Haber, E. (1973b) Digitalis: pharmacokinetics and bioavailability. New England Journal of Medicine, 289, 1063–1072.

Solomon, A.E., Briggs, J.D., Knepil, J., Henry, D.A., Winchester, J.F. and Birrell, R. (1977) Therapeutic comparison of thiol compounds in severe paracetamol poisoning. Annals of Clinical Biochemistry, 14, 200–202

Stewart, R.D. (1975) The effect of carbon monoxide on humans. Annual Reviews of Pharmacology, 15, 409–423.

Stewart, R.B., Cluff, L.E. and Philp, J.R. (1977) Drug Monitoring: A Requirement for Responsible Drug Use. Williams and Wilkins, Baltimore.

Stolman, A. (1974) The absorption, distribution and excretion of drugs and poisons and their metabolites. Progress in Chemical Toxicology, 5, 1–99.

Swartz, R.D. and Sidell, F.R. (1973) Effects of heat and exercise on elimination of pralidoxime in man. Clinical Pharmacology and Therapeutics, 14, 83–89.

Takemori, A.E. (1974) Biochemistry of drug dependence. Annual Review of Biochemistry, 43, 15–33.

Teare, R.D. (1976) Poisoning by paraquat. Medicine, Science and the Law, 16, 9–12.

Temple, A.R. (1977) Poison control centers: prospects and capabilities. Annual Review of Pharmacology and Toxicology, 17, 215–222.

Thomson, P.D., Rowland, M. and Melmon, K.L. (1971) The influence of heart failure, liver disease, and renal failure on the disposition of lidocaine in man. American Heart Journal, 82, 417–421.

Vale, J.A., Rees, A.J., Widdop, B. and Goulding, R. (1975) Use of charcoal haemoperfusion in the management of severely poisoned patients. British Medical Journal, 1, 5–9.

Vallner, J.J. Binding of drugs by albumin and plasma protein. Journal of Pharmaceutical Sciences, 66, 447–465.

Vesell, E.S. (1973) Advances in pharmacogenetics. Progress in Medical Genetics, 9. 291–367.

Vesell, E.S. (1974) Relationship between drug distribution and therapeutic effects in man. Annual Review of Pharmacology, 14, 249–270.

Vesell, E.S. and Page, J.G. (1969) Genetic control of the phenobarbital-induced shortening of plasma antipyrine half-lives in man. Journal of Clinical Investigation, 48, 2202–2209.

Wagner, J.G. (1961) Biopharmaceutics: absorption aspects. Journal of Pharmaceutical Sciences, 50, 359–387.

Wallace, J.E., Blum, K. and Singh, J.M. (1974) Determination of drugs in biologic specimens – a review. Clinical Toxicology, 7, 477–495.

Waltman, R. and Iniquez, E.S. (1972) Placental transfer of ethanol and its elimination at term. Obstetrics and Gynecology, 40, 180–185.

Weiner, I.M. and Mudge, G.H. (1964) Renal tubular mechanisms for excretion of organic acids and bases. American Journal of Medicine, 36, 743–762.

Werner, M., Sutherland, E.W., III and Abramson, F.P. (1975) Concepts for the rational selection of assays to be used in monitoring therapeutic drugs. Clinical Chemistry, 21, 1368–1371.

Weston, M.J., Gazzard, B.G., Buxton, B.H., Winch, J., Machado, A.L., Flax, H. and Williams, R. (1974) Effects of haemoperfusion through charcoal or XAD-2 resin on an animal model of fulminant liver failure. Gut, 15, 482–486.

White, T.A. and Evans, D.A.P. (1968) The acetylation of sulfamethazine and sulfamethoxypyridazine by human subjects. Clinical Pharmacology and Therapeutics, 9, 80–88.

Wilding, G., Paigen, B. and Vesell, E.S. (1977) Genetic control of inter-individual variations in racemic warfarin binding to plasma and albumin of twins. Clinical Pharmacology and Therapeutics, 22, 831–842.

Williams, J.R.B., Griffin, J.P. and Parkins, A. (1976) Effect of concomitantly administered drugs on the control of long term anticoagulant therapy. Quarterly Journal of Medicine, 45, 63–73.
Williams, R.T. and Parke, D.V. (1964) The metabolic fate of drugs. Annual Review of Pharmacology, 4, 85–114.
Wilson, T.W., Mahon, W.A., Inaba, T., Johnson, G.E. and Kadar, D. (1973) Elimination of tritiated gentamicin in normal human subjects and in patients with severely impaired renal function. Clinical Pharmacology and Therapeutics, 14, 815–822.
Winek, C.L. (1976) Tabulation of therapeutic, toxic and lethal concentrations of drugs and chemicals in blood. Clinical Chemistry, 22, 832–836.
Wolfe, B.M., Gaston, L.W. and Keltner, R.M. (1973) Malignant hyperthermia of anesthesia. American Journal of Surgery, 126, 717–721.
Woods, H.F. and Alberti, K.G.M.M. (1972) Dangers of intravenous fructose. Lancet, ii, 1354–1357.
World Health Organization (1974) Technical Report Series No. 556: Detection of Dependence-Producing Drugs in Body Fluids. WHO, Geneva.
Wright, B.M., Jones, T.P. and Jones, A.W. (1975) Breath alcohol analysis and the blood/breath ratio. Medicine, Science and the Law, 15, 205–210.
Wright, N., Clarkson, A.R., Brown, S.S. and Fuster, V. (1971) Effects of poisoning on serum enzyme activities, coagulation and fibrinolysis. British Medical Journal, 3, 347–350.

FURTHER READING

Albert, A. (1973) Selective Toxicity: The Physico-Chemical Basis of Therapy, 5th edn. Halstead, New York.
Brown, S.S. (Ed.) (1977) Clinical Chemistry and Chemical Toxicology of Metals. Elsevier/North-Holland Biomedical Press, Amsterdam.
Casarett, L.J. and Doull, J. (1975) Toxicology: The Basic Science of Poisons. Macmillan, New York.
Cluff, L.E. and Petrie, J.C. (Eds.) (1974) Clinical Effects of Interaction Between Drugs. Excerpta Medica, Amsterdam.
Curry, A. (1976) Poison Detection in Human Organs, 3rd Edn. Thomas, Springfield.
Davies, D.S. and Prichard, B.N.C. (Eds.) (1973) Biological Effects of Drugs in Relation to their Plasma Concentrations. Macmillan, London.
Goldstein, A., Aronow, L. and Kalman, S.M. (1974) Principles of Drug Action: The Basis of Pharmacology, 2nd edn. Wiley, New York.
Goodman, L.S. and Gilman, A. (Eds.) (1975) The Pharmacological Basis of Therapeutics. Macmillan, New York.
Lieber, C.S. (Ed.) (1977) Metabolic Aspects of Alcoholism. MTP, Lancaster.
Loomis, T.A. (1974) Essentials of Toxicology, 2nd edn. Kimpton, London.
Matthew, H. (Ed.) (1971) Acute Barbiturate Poisoning. Excerpta Medica, Amsterdam.
Matthew, H. and Lawson, A.A.H. (1979) Treatment of Common Acute Poisonings, 4th edn. Churchill-Livingstone, Edinburgh.
McMahon, F.G. (Ed.) (1974) Drug Induced Chemical Toxicity. Futura, Mount Kisco.
Notari, R.E. (1975) Biopharmaceutics and Pharmacokinetics; An Introduction. Dekker, New York.
Porter, R. and O'Connor, M. (Eds.) (1974) The Poisoned Patient: The Role of the Laboratory, Ciba Foundation Symposium 26. Elsevier, Amsterdam.
Reidenberg, M.M. (Ed.) (1974) Symposium on Individualization of Drug Therapy, Medical Clinics of North America, Vol. 58, No. 5.
Smith, S.E. and Rawlins, M.D. (1973) Variability in Human Drug Response. Butterworths, London.
Sunshine, I. (Ed.) (1975) Methodology for Analytical Toxicology, CRC Press. Cleveland.
Szórády, I. (1973) Pharmacogenetics: Principles and Paediatric Aspects. Akadémiai Kiadó, Budapest.
Vesell, E.S. (Ed.) (1971) Drug Metabolism in Man. Annals of the New York Academy of Sciences, Vol. 179.
Whipple, H.E. (Ed.) (1965) Evaluation and Mechanisms of Drug Toxicity. Annals of the New York Academy of Sciences, Vol. 123.
Wolstenholme, G. and Porter, R. (Eds.) (1967) Ciba Symposium: Drug Responses in Man. Churchill, London.

Chapter 24

Neurogenic amines and secreting tumours

Colin R.J. Ruthven and Merton Sandler

Bernhard Baron Memorial Research Laboratories, Department of Chemical Pathology, Queen Charlotte's Maternity Hospital, Goldhawk Road, London W6 OXG, England

CONTENTS

Chemical diagnosis of disease, edited by
S.S. Brown, F.L. Mitchell and D.S. Young

24.1. INTRODUCTION

The term "monoamines" * embraces a group of weakly basic compounds, usually derived endogenously from aromatic aminoacids and all substrates of the enzyme, monoamine oxidase (EC 1.4.3.4). Whilst many of their functions are unknown, there is good evidence to show that the more intensively studied representatives of the group, dopamine, noradrenaline and 5-hydroxytryptamine, act as neurotransmitters; there is also reason to believe that most of the others, e.g. octopamine, tyramine, etc., play a similar role (Sandler et al., 1976).

Even the catecholamines and 5-hydroxytryptamine, however, the monoamines synthesized in greatest abundance, are present in body fluids in relatively low concentration, so that their metabolic pathways in normal man have, until the recent past, been difficult to quantify. Recent techniques of extreme sensitivity and specificity, particularly gas chromatography and gas chromatography–mass spectrometry have revolutionized the study of this group of compounds and their metabolites and provided considerable data about their physiological variations. As might be expected, most of the information on these themes relates to clinical states associated with hypersecretion and predominantly to the monoamine-secreting tumour; such tumours will accordingly by examined in this chapter in greater detail than other clinical conditions which are associated with disturbed monoamine metabolism.

24.2. THE KEY ROLE OF MONOAMINE OXIDASE

Monoamine oxidase, the enzyme forming the link between the group of its substrates which constitute the subject of this chapter, has been intensively studied in recent years; detailed reviews (e.g. Costa and Sandler, 1972; Sandler and Youdim, 1972; Wolstenholme and Knight, 1976) cover most of the points discussed below.

An insoluble enzyme, located on the outer membrane of the mitochondrion, monoamine oxidase catalyzes the oxidative deamination of monoamines with the production of an aldehyde, hydrogen peroxide and ammonia or a simple alkylamine. In vivo, the aldehyde is then converted either into its corresponding acid or alcohol by the enzymes

---

* Abbreviations commonly used for monoamines and related structures.

A, Adrenaline (epinephrine)
COMT, Catechol-*O*-methyltransferase
DA, Dopamine
DBH, Dopamine-β-hydroxylase
DHMA, 3,4-Dihydroxymandelic acid
DOPA, 3,4-Dihydroxyphenylalanine
DOPAC, 3,4-Dihydroxyphenylacetic acid
5-HIAA, 5-Hydroxyindoleacetic acid
HMPE, 4-Hydroxy-3-methoxyphenylethanol
HMPG, 4-Hydroxy-3-methoxyphenylglycol
5-HT, 5-Hydroxytryptamine
5-HTP, 5-Hydroxytryptophan
HVA, Homovanillic acid
MAO, Monoamine oxidase
NA, Noradrenaline (norepinephrine)
PNMT, Phenylethanolamine-*N*-methyltransferase
VLA, 4-hydroxy-3-methoxyphenyllactic acid
VMA, 4-Hydroxy-3-methoxymandelic acid
VPA, 4-Hydroxy-3-methoxyphenylpyruvic acid

aldehyde dehydrogenase (EC 1.2.1.3) or alcohol dehydrogenase (EC 1.1.1.1; aldehyde reductase) respectively (Scheme 24.1). Apart from the neurotransmitter amines, 5-hydroxytryptophan and the catecholamines, many naturally occurring monoamines, both aliphatic and aromatic, are substrates for monoamine oxidase. Affinity of enzyme for substrate is lowered when a β-hydroxyl group is present in the side chain of monophenolic amines and catecholamines; thus noradrenaline and adrenaline are inferior to dopamine as substrates.

Monoamine oxidase has been identified in all vertebrates in which it has been sought. In man, and indeed in other mammals too, there is high activity in intestine, liver, kidney and salivary glands, and rather less in heart, skin, adrenals, ovaries, uterus and placenta. It is distributed widely, though inhomogeneously, in the central nervous system and in the peripheral sympathetic nervous system, particularly in sympathetic nerve endings. It is also present in tumours which secrete monoamines.

Since the action of iproniazid, a powerful irreversible inhibitor of monoamine oxidase, was first described about 20 years ago, many new and equally efficient irreversible inhibitors of widely differing chemical structure have made their appearance; these include the clinically important pargyline, nialamide and tranylcypromine and isocarboxazid. Although many compounds such as harmine and harmaline, and amphetamine, are reversible competitive inhibitors, this particular action seems to be of little clinical importance.

Although these compounds have been widely employed for the treatment of depressive illness, there are certain well-known dangers associated with their use. Hypertensive crises may supervene after the ingestion of monoamine-containing foods or medicines. Foods containing tyramine are a particular hazard. Monoamine oxidase inhibitors tend nowadays to be rarely employed in the United States, although British psychiatrists still consider them to have a small but useful role in certain categories of depressive illness.

Inhibition of monoamine oxidase in vivo increases the urinary output of amines such as metadrenaline, tyramine, tryptamine, octopamine and synephrine (but not of dop-

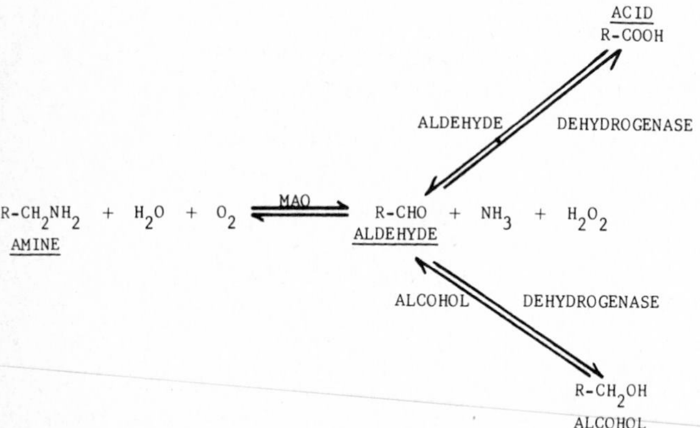

Scheme 24.1. The oxidative deamination of a primary monoamine by monoamine oxidase (MAO) followed by conversion of the resulting aldehyde into the corresponding acid by aldehyde dehydrogenase or into the corresponding alcohol by alcohol dehydrogenase.

amine and noradrenaline, which possess an alternative major pathway of degradation via 3-*O*-methylation). This property forms the basis of a test which has been widely employed for the in vivo assessment of monoamine oxidase activity – the excretion of urinary tryptamine (Sjoerdsma et al., 1959). However, since the output of tryptamine, in common with some other monoamines, e.g. dopamine, is highly dependent on urinary pH (Sandler et al., 1967), the test cannot be considered satisfactory unless the pH is kept constant. This effect, which influences the excretion of certain weak acids, like indoleacetic acid (Milne et al., 1960) or bases, e.g. pethidine (meperidine) (Asatoor et al., 1963) and amphetamine (Beckett et al., 1969), is not observed with compounds such as 5-hydroxyindoleacetic acid, where a specific renal transport mechanism exists (Despopoulos and Weissbach, 1957). None of the numerous other tests of in vivo activity which has been employed, e.g. urinary 5-hydroxyindoleacetic acid output after oral 5-hydroxytryptamine, or infused radioactive adrenaline (Sjoerdsma, 1961) has proved wholly satisfactory.

Perhaps the most useful approach to the measurement of monoamine oxidase activity in clinical practice is by direct assay: the tissue which has been used most widely for this purpose is the blood platelet (Wolstenholme and Knight, 1976). However, it should be pointed out that the properties of monoamine oxidase vary from tissue to tissue and that the platelet enzyme is more atypical than most (Collins and Sandler, 1971). Nevertheless, and even using the convenient but unphysiological kynuramine as substrate, the measurement may be used as a broad indicator of the degree of monoamine oxidase inhibition and of length of time the effect remains after the monoamine oxidase inhibiting drug has been withdrawn. Platelet monoamine oxidase activity may be altered in certain disease states: a decrease has been both claimed and disputed in schizophrenia and iron-deficiency anaemia (Wolstenholme and Knight, 1976), whilst an increase may be present in megaloblastic anaemia (Latt et al., 1968). A decrease has also been detected in platelet monoamine oxidase from patients with migraine (Sandler et al., 1974). Platelet monoamine oxidase is largely monoamine oxidase-B (Wolstenholme and Knight, 1976) and the deficit appears predominantly to be one of monoamine oxidase-B, which is one of the two major multiple forms of the enzyme.

There is a considerable body of evidence to suggest that monoamine oxidase exists in more than one form (Sandler and Youdim, 1972; Wolstenholme and Knight, 1976). Apart from monoamine oxidase-B, another type of enzyme, termed monoamine oxidase-A, has been differentiated by its sensitivity to certain inhibitor drugs. The proportion of each varies from tissue to tissue. Monoamine oxidase-A is more sensitive to the inhibitor clorgyline and monoamine oxidase-B to deprenyl and probably to pargyline. Otherwise, all of the other inhibiting drugs used in clinical practice act equally on both forms.

Noradrenaline, normetadrenaline and 5-hydroxytryptamine appear to be the preferred substrates for type A enzyme and β-phenylethylamine and benzylamine for type B enzyme. Tyramine is a substrate for both forms. Dopamine is a monoamine oxidase-A substrate in the rat but a substrate for the B enzyme in man (Glover et al., 1976). A more complete classification of monoamines in terms of their preference for monoamine oxidase-A or -B is provided by Houslay and Tipton (1974), but the whole classification should probably be considered tentative and there is an increasing number of anomalies

(Glover et al., 1976). Thus Gascoigne et al. (1975) identified a third form of the enzyme in rat brain, resistant to clorgyline but preferring 5-hydroxytryptamine as substrate; they provisionally termed it monoamine oxidase-C; Lyles and Callingham (1975) found evidence of anomalous enzyme activity in rat heart, where phenylethylamine, hitherto considered a substrate for monoamine oxidase-B, appeared to be oxidized by the A variant.

The decrease of monoamine oxidase activity noted in migraine is manifested as a deficit in phenylethylamine-oxidizing ability; when the finding is coupled with the apparent "sensitivity" of some migraine sufferers to phenylethylamine-containing foods, it points to the possibility of this amine playing a role in the pathogenesis of the condition (Sandler et al., 1974). What must be stressed here is that it is no longer sufficient to employ a single substrate, such as kynuramine, when investigating monoamine oxidase status in different diseases; rather, several different ^{14}C-labelled substrates should be used for the assay (Glover et al., 1976), including at least 5-hydroxytryptamine, phenylethylamine, tyramine and dopamine.

Observations of a different kind based on the electrophoretic separation of bands of monoamine oxidase activity from the solubilized enzyme have also been made; each band possesses different substrate and inhibitor specificities (Sandler and Youdim, 1972). These data, however, are difficult to interpret. The present consensus of opinion (Wolstenholme and Knight, 1976) seems to be that multiple forms of monoamine oxidase, whatever method is employed to demonstrate them, depend on the amount of phospholipid which is bound to a single enzyme protein. It is not unlikely that in vivo activity is modulated by this phospholipid. Solubilization procedures (whether employing sonication, a detergent or an organic solvent) are likely to be sufficiently vigorous to interfere with the tertiary structure of the enzyme. Thus the multiple forms which become apparent after electrophoresis are unlikely to reflect the in vivo situation. Nevertheless, one of the electrophoretic bands – the only one to migrate from anode to cathode – possesses much greater affinity for dopamine than the other bands; the possibility of its being a specific "dopamine monoamine oxidase" has not been ruled out (Youdim, 1973).

24.3. CATECHOL-*O*-METHYLTRANSFERASE

Catechol-*O*-methyltransferase (EC 2.1.1.6) specifically catalyzes the transfer of the methyl group of *S*-adenosylmethionine to the oxygen of one or other, but not both, of the ring hydroxyls in compounds possessing a catechol group. It requires the presence of Mg^{2+} or certain other divalent cations for its activity. The enzyme exists in several immunologically distinct forms with molecular masses varying from 11,250 to 37,000 (Creveling et al., 1973).

Methylation of 3,4-dihydroxy compounds takes place more readily in the *meta*- or 3-position than in the *para*- or 4-position. The ratio of isomers formed in vitro can be varied by altering pH, ionic strength, divalent cation and the type and position of substituents on the side-chain (Bohuon and Assicot, 1973). *para*-Methylation has also been observed in vivo. A small quantity of the normal homovanillic acid excretion in the human is made up of this positional isomer (iso-homovanillic acid), and small amounts have been detected in the cerebrospinal fluid (Sandler, 1972a). 4-Hydroxy-3-methoxymandelic acid has not yet been detected in human urine, but both iso-vanillic acid and vanillic acid have been detected after perfusing rat liver with 3,4-dihydroxybenzoic acid (Bohuon and Assicot, 1973). The occurrence of 4-*O*-methylation in patients with catecholamine-secreting tumours has not been demonstrated to date (Sandler, 1972a), but in the light of the evidence mentioned above, it would be unwise to assume that it does not happen.

Catechol-*O*-methyltransferase inhibition has not been studied as intensively as that of monoamine oxidase, no doubt because it has not assumed a similar degree of therapeutic importance. However, a considerable number of catechol-*O*-methyltransferase inhibitors, in vitro and in vivo, have been recorded, although they are mainly competitive. Some of the better known are catechols, polyphenols, catechol flavanoids, tropolones and dopacetamide (Sandler and Ruthven, 1969a).

In contrast to monoamine oxidase, catechol-*O*-methyltransferase is a highly soluble cytoplasmic enzyme, not attached to particulate cellular bodies, although an enzyme has been isolated from rat liver microsomal membrane with similar properties to soluble catechol-*O*-methyltransferase (Creveling et al., 1973). The enzyme is widely distributed in mammalian tissues, including human, the highest concentrations being present in liver with appreciable amounts in brain, peripheral nerve, heart, spleen, thyroid, blood vessels and catecholamine-secreting tumour (Sandler and Ruthven, 1969a). It is highly likely that catechol-*O*-methyltransferase is localized in the region of the sympathetic nerve terminals (Jarrott, 1973). In densely innervated areas, about half the catechol-*O*-methyltransferase activity may be extraneuronal, although in more sparsely innervated tissues, such as heart, kidney and liver, much of the enzyme appears to be non-neuronal (Jarrott, 1973).

From studies of *O*-methylation in intact tissue and in homogenates, it appears that the degree of *O*-methylation at a particular site is governed by the ease with which substrate can be transported through the cell to the enzyme, rather than by availability of enzyme protein or *S*-adenosylmethionine. This ability can vary from tissue to tissue and from species to species (Jarrott, 1973).

The measurement of catechol-*O*-methyltransferase activity, particularly in erythrocytes, has recently assumed added importance following the suggestion that individual differences may be related to the pathogenesis of neurological and psychiatric diseases. Early methods of assay employed either colorimetry, ultraviolet spectroscopy or fluorometry to measure the rate of *O*-methylation of catecholamine or catechol metabolite substrates. Later, simpler and more sensitive radiometric techniques were devised which depended either on the use of labelled noradrenaline or adrenaline as substrate, or the enzymatic transfer of a radioisotopically labelled methyl group from *S*-adenosyl-L-methionine to a catechol: activity was determined by radiometric measurement of the methylated product (Creveling and Daly, 1971). The second approach, applied to human erythrocytes, has been improved by using whole blood (rather than packed cells) and the relatively stable 3,4-dihydroxybenzoic acid as substrate (Raymond and Weinshilboum, 1975). Divalent cations (Ca^{2+}), which inhibit the Mg^{2+} co-factor, are removed with a chelating resin. A novel feature of this method is the addition of partly purified rat liver catechol-*O*-methyltransferase, as an internal standard in order to detect any effect of endogenous inhibitors or activators.

24.4. CATECHOLAMINES

24.4.1. Anatomical considerations

As with measurement of 5-hydroxyindoles (section 24.8), the urinary output of catecholamines and their metabolites has largely been measured diagnostically in the search for tumours which secrete them (Winkler and Smith, 1972). The tumours derive from primitive sympathetic cells in the neural crest (Coupland, 1972). The cells evolve into immature neuroblasts (sympathoblasts) and phaeochromoblasts, which respectively give rise to mature sympathetic ganglion cells and adrenal medullary or paraganglion cells (phaeochromocytes). Phaeochromocytoma, which may be benign or malignant, derives from cells of the second type. Like the carcinoid tumour, it contains granules which possess the ability to reduce chrome salts (chromaffin reaction). This ability, in both cases, stems from a high local concentration of monoamine.

Neuroblasts, the histologically undifferentiated precursors of autonomic ganglion cells, can give rise to the highly malignant neuroblastoma or the more differentiated and relatively benign ganglioneuroma. Transitional forms (ganglioneuroblastoma) exist. Apparent maturation from the more malignant to the benign variant may occasionally be observed. The highly malignant retinoblastoma is related to the neuroblastoma group of tumours and may similarly elaborate catecholamines, although rather less frequently. Any granules these tumours possess, unlike those found in phaeochromocytoma, do not possess the ability to reduce chrome salts. Whilst the phaeochromocytes tend to produce noradrenaline and adrenaline, and the neuroblastoma group dopamine, biochemical lines of demarcation tend to be blurred and, as will be discussed later, there is some degree of overlap. Another group of tumours, the paragangliomas (e.g. carotid body, glomus jugulare and aortic body tumours) which occasionally secrete catecholamines, also tend to be dopamine secretors.

24.4.2. Biosynthesis of catecholamines

Catecholamine-secreting tumours, like carcinoid (section 24.8.1), to some extent reflect their tissue of origin. Their "biochemical profile" is, presumably, not too dissimilar from that of the adrenal medulla, for example, or sympathetic nerve (Gjessing, 1968; Sandler and Ruthven, 1969a).

The initial reaction in the main route of catecholamine biosynthesis (Scheme 24.2) is the hydroxylation of phenylalanine by the enzyme phenylalanine-4-hydroxylase (Kaufman, 1966; Kaufman and Fisher, 1974); this step is not essential so long as tyrosine is available from dietary sources. The next step, the *meta*-hydroxylation of tyrosine to L-3,4-dihydroxyphenylalanine by oxygen and the pteridine requiring enzyme, tyrosine hydroxylase (Kaufman and Fisher, 1974; Numata and Nagatsu, 1975) is essential and probably rate-limiting in catecholamine synthesis. The enzyme, pteridine reductase, may play a part in controlling the action here by regulating the supply of pteridine co-factor. L-3,4-Dihydroxyphenylalanine is decarboxylated to dopamine by the relatively non-specific L-3,4-dihydroxyphenylalanine decarboxylase, sometimes called L-aromatic aminoacid decarboxylase, which is identical to the enzyme promoting the formation of 5-hydroxy-

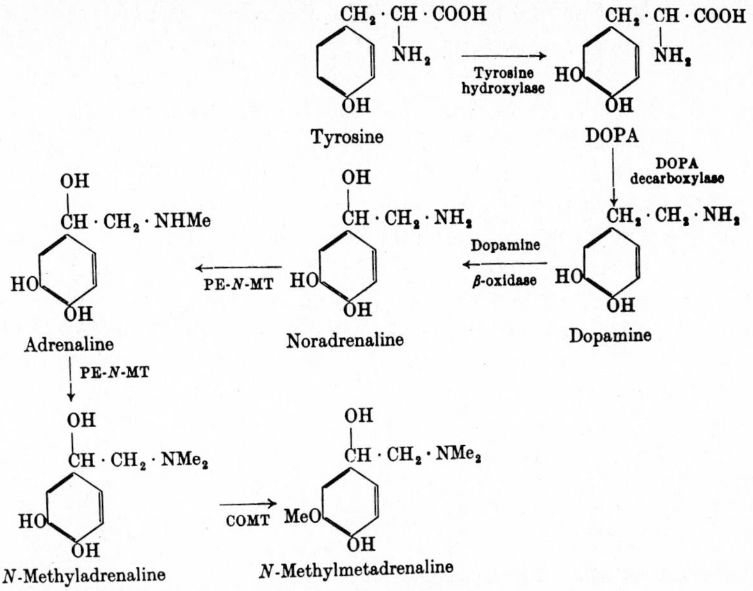

$CH_2 \cdot CH \cdot COOH$ / NH_2 / OH — Tyrosine → (Tyrosine hydroxylase) → $CH_2 \cdot CH \cdot COOH$ / NH_2 / HO / OH — DOPA

DOPA → (DOPA decarboxylase) → $CH_2 \cdot CH_2 \cdot NH_2$ / HO / OH — Dopamine

Dopamine → (Dopamine β-oxidase) → OH / $CH \cdot CH_2 \cdot NH_2$ / HO / OH — Noradrenaline

Noradrenaline → (PE-N-MT) → OH / $CH \cdot CH_2 \cdot NHMe$ / HO / OH — Adrenaline

Adrenaline → (PE-N-MT) → OH / $CH \cdot CH_2 \cdot NMe_2$ / HO / OH — N-Methyladrenaline

N-Methyladrenaline → (COMT) → OH / $CH \cdot CH_2 \cdot NMe_2$ / MeO / OH — N-Methylmetadrenaline

Scheme 24.2. Biosynthesis of the catecholamines (PE-N-MT = phenylethanolamine-*N*-methyltransferase). (Reproduced, with permission, from Sandler, 1970)

tryptamine from 5-hydroxytryptophan (Lovenberg et al., 1962). L-3,4-Dihydroxyphenylalanine may be present in the diet; the broad bean *Vicia faba* contains about 25 g L-3,4-dihydroxyphenylalanine per kg (Sandler, 1972a), although this amount is exceptionally large. It has also been detected in a number of other plants and fungi (Sandler, 1972a). Dopamine, which in recent years has become important in its own right, not just as a precursor of noradrenaline (Hornykiewicz, 1966), is hydroxylated on the β-carbon of the side-chain by the action of dopamine-β-hydroxylase (Kaufman, 1966) to form noradrenaline. This copper-containing mixed function oxidase is located within the catecholamine-containing granules. It has been provisionally characterized as a tetrameric glycoprotein and requires for its activity, ascorbic acid and fumaric acid, as well as ATP, Mn^{2+}, Co^{2+} or Zn^{2+} and molecular oxygen. Dopamine-β-hydroxylase is not inhibited by catecholamines, but is inactivated by chelating agents and excess Cu^{2+} (Sandler and Ruthven, 1969a). Adrenaline, the last major product to be formed in the biosynthetic pathway of the catecholamines, derives from noradrenaline by *N*-methylation. This conversion is effected by methyl group transfer from *S*-adenosylmethionine by the cytoplasmic enzyme, phenylethanolamine-*N*-methyltransferase which has a group specificity for the phenylethanolamine configuration (Axelrod, 1966). Even adrenaline itself can be *N*-methylated further by this enzyme to form *N*-methyladrenaline; this tertiary amine has been identified in the adrenal medulla of several species (Axelrod, 1960). Likewise, 3-*O*-methylated adrenaline (metadrenaline) can be converted into *N*-methylmetadrenaline; this substance has been detected in the urine of normal subjects and, in greater concentration, in urine from patients with phaeochromocytoma (Itoh et al., 1962). Phenylethanolamine-*N*-methyltransferase is inhibited by noradrenaline (Fuller and Hunt, 1965) and even more strongly by adrenaline (Fuller and Hunt, 1967) pointing to regulation both by substrate and product. The adrenal cortex also exerts a regulatory influence through the stimulating action of very high local concentrations of endogenous glucocorticoid (Wurtman, 1966). Phenylethanolamine-*N*-methyltransferase has been detected only in the adrenal medulla, midbrain and heart, so that these tissues are presumably the only sites in the body where significant amounts of adrenaline are normally produced.

24.4.2.1. Alternative pathways of catecholamine biosynthesis

There is little doubt that the biosynthetic pathway just described, first adumbrated by

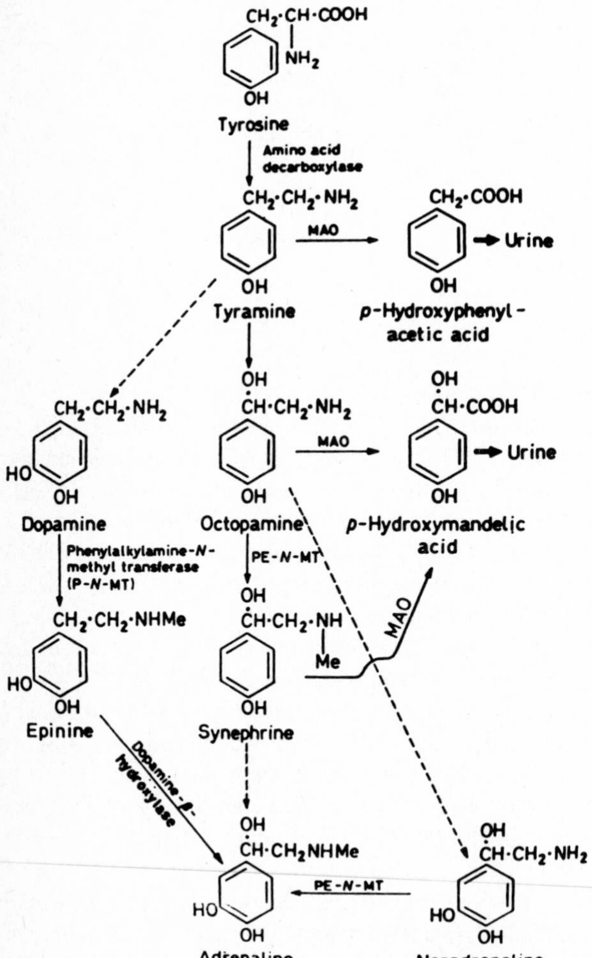

Scheme 24.3. Alternative pathways of catecholamine biosynthesis. (Reproduced, with permission, from Sandler, 1970)

Blaschko (1939), is the major route of catecholamine biosynthesis; however, most of the enzymes involved lack specificity (Sandler and Ruthven, 1969a) so that a number of alternative pathways (Scheme 24.3) are theoretically possible (Axelrod, 1963). Thus, noradrenaline could be formed from tyrosine via *p*-tyramine and octopamine, whilst adrenaline might arise from dopamine via epinine, or from tyrosine via *p*-tyramine, octopamine and synephrine. Another possible biosynthetic pathway to the catecholamines lies by way of *m*-tyrosine (Tong et al., 1971). This reaction might conceivably be catalyzed by known hydroxylating enzymes – phenylalanine hydroxylase, for instance, is known to have some slight action at the *meta*-locus (Coulson et al., 1968). Rat liver and beef adrenal medulla can convert *m*-tyrosine into 3,4-dihydroxyphenylalanine in vitro (Tong et al., 1971), and in vivo the conversion of ingested *m*-tyrosine into dopamine has been reported to occur in rat (Sourkes et al., 1961). However, the present authors have found that the degree of conversion is very small (Sandler et al., 1975).

24.4.3. Metabolism of catecholamines

Sandler and Ruthven (1969a) and Sandler (1970) have reviewed the metabolism of catecholamines (Scheme 24.4).

Noradrenaline and adrenaline share a common metabolic pathway and the analogous degradation route of dopamine only differs from it quantitatively. Catecholamines may be oxidatively deaminated by monoamine oxidase to an aldehyde which may be either further oxidized by aldehyde dehydrogenase (e.g. 3,4-dihydroxymandelic acid is formed from noradrenaline and adrenaline or 3,4-dihydroxyphenylacetic acid from dopamine) or be reduced by aldehyde reductase to an alcohol (e.g. 3,4-dihydroxyphenylglycol from noradrenaline and adrenaline, or 3,4-dihydroxyphenylethanol from dopamine). All of

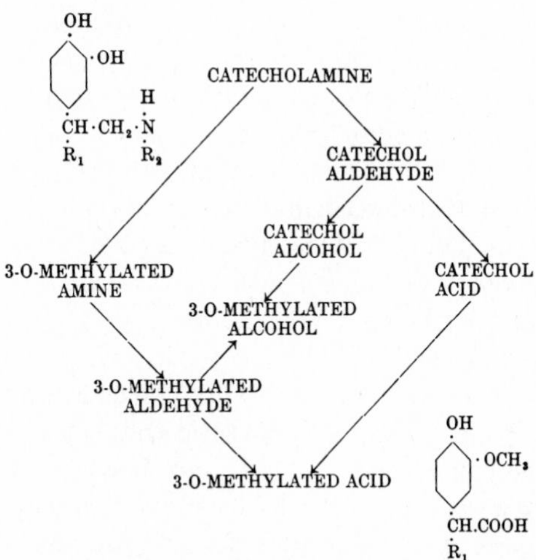

Scheme 24.4. General scheme of catecholamine metabolism: dopamine pathway – R^1 = H, R^2 = H; noradrenaline pathway – R^1 = OH, R^2 = OH; adrenaline pathway – R^1 = OH, R^2 = Me. (Reproduced, with permission, from Sandler, 1970)

these compounds may then be 3-*O*-methylated with catechol-*O*-methyltransferase, the acids forming 4-hydroxy-3-methoxymandelic acid or homovanillic acid respectively, and the alcohols 4-hydroxy-3-methoxyphenylglycol or 4-hydroxy-3-methoxyphenylethanol respectively. Alternatively, the catecholamines may first be 3-*O*-methylated, normetadrenaline being formed from noradrenaline, metadrenaline from adrenaline and 3-methoxytyramine from dopamine. These compounds can then undergo oxidative deamination, and their respective aldehydes (normetadrenaline and metadrenaline give identical aldehydes) may either be oxidized to form 4-hydroxy-3-methoxymandelic acid or homovanillic acid respectively, or reduced to form 4-hydroxy-3-methoxyphenylglycol or 4-hydroxy-3-methoxyphenylethanol.

Qualitative differences between the metabolites of dopamine and the other two catecholamines, noradrenaline and adrenaline, arise from differences in the ease with which they or their derivatives are acted upon by the enzymes responsible for their degradation. Dopamine is a much better substrate for monoamine oxidase than the other catecholamines. Consequently, the formation from it of 3,4-dihydroxyphenylacetic acid is proportionately greater than that of the corresponding acid, 3,4-dihydroxymandelic acid, from noradrenaline and adrenaline. Thus there will be relatively less dopamine available for direct *O*-methylation, resulting in an output of 3-methoxytyramine which is lower than that of the metadrenalines.

Differences in the fate of the unstable intermediate aldehydes formed by oxidative deamination of the catecholamines must also be taken into account: those stemming from phenylethanolamines tend to follow a reductive pathway, whereas the phenylethylamine derivatives are mainly oxidized to the corresponding acid. Thus, whilst 4-hydroxy-3-methoxyphenylglycol is normally excreted at levels about half those of 4-hydroxy-3-methoxymandelic acid, the corresponding alcoholic metabolite of dopamine, 4-hydroxy-3-methoxyphenylethanol, is found in the urine in trace amounts only.

Conjugation is of considerable importance in the metabolism of the catecholamines. Only a small fraction of the total catecholamine production is excreted unchanged – about 3 to 4% of an infused dose of a catecholamine, with about as much again present as sulphate or glucuronide conjugate. 4-Hydroxy-3-methoxymandelic acid and homovanillic acid are found in urine mainly in the free state, but a considerable proportion of 3,4-dihydroxyphenylacetic acid and a greater part of the total metadrenalines, 4-hydroxy-3-methoxyphenylglycol, 3-methoxytyramine and 4-hydroxy-3-methoxyphenylethanol output are present as sulphate and glucuronide conjugates. *N*-Acetylation is a minor metabolic route in man although it may become significant when a large excess of amine is present in the circulation, as in patients with catecholamine-secreting tumours.

Transamination of 3,4-dihydroxyphenylalanine (Scheme 24.5), which is normally a quantitatively unimportant pathway, can also become significant, when the aminoacid is present in tumour effluent. The product, 3,4-dihydroxyphenylpyruvic acid, is partly reduced to 3,4-dihydroxyphenyllactic acid and partly oxidatively decarboxylated to 3,4-dihydroxyphenylacetic acid. These compounds may be 3-*O*-methylated to give 4-hydroxy-3-methoxyphenylpyruvic acid, 4-hydroxy-3-methoxyphenyllactic acid and homovanillic acid respectively. However, in vivo conditions favour prior 3-*O*-methylation of 3,4-dihydroxyphenylalanine to 3-*O*-methyldopa, which is then transaminated to give 4-hydroxy-3-methoxyphenylpyruvic acid, 4-hydroxy-3-methoxyphenyllactic acid and homovanillic acid.

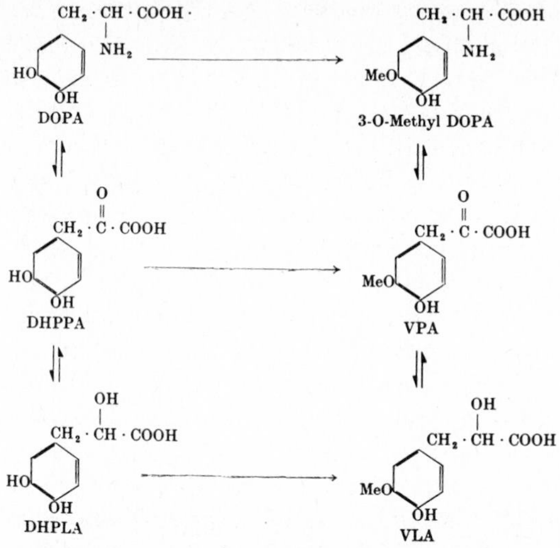

$CH_2 \cdot CH \cdot COOH$ / NH_2 (HO, OH)
DOPA
→
$CH_2 \cdot CH \cdot COOH$ / NH_2 (MeO, OH)
3-O-Methyl DOPA

⇅

$CH_2 \cdot C(=O) \cdot COOH$ (HO, OH)
DHPPA
→
$CH_2 \cdot C(=O) \cdot COOH$ (MeO, OH)
VPA

⇅

$CH_2 \cdot CH(OH) \cdot COOH$ (HO, OH)
DHPLA
→
$CH_2 \cdot CH(OH) \cdot COOH$ (MeO, OH)
VLA

Scheme 24.5. Transamination pathways of L-DOPA metabolism (DHPAA = dihydroxyphenylpyruvic acid; DHPLA = dihydroxyphenyllactic acid; VPA = 4-hydroxy-3-methoxyphenylpyruvic acid; VLA = 4-hydroxy-3-methoxyphenyllactic acid). (Reproduced, with permission, from Sandler, 1970)

24.4.4. Adrenergic mechanisms – a brief history

Some of the observations which eventually led to the discovery of adrenergic neurotransmission were made (Sandler and Ruthven, 1969a) as early as the second half of the last century, although their significance was only recognized slowly. Chemical mediation, as such, in autonomic transmission was postulated by Elliott in 1904, but not conclusively demonstrated for nearly 20 years. At that time, adrenaline, or a closely related substance termed "sympathin", was considered to be the primary neurohormonal agent. It was not until the late 1940s that independent investigations by von Euler and Holtz led to the conclusion that noradrenaline and not adrenaline is the true sympathetic neurotransmitter. Final proof was provided by Peart who demonstrated noradrenaline release directly after stimulating sympathetic nerves (Sandler and Ruthven, 1969a; Blaschko, 1972). The precursors and metabolites of noradrenaline were identified even more recently. The main route in the biosynthesis of noradrenaline and adrenaline was foreshadowed by Blaschko in 1939. By 1957, the sequence of the main steps had been firmly established (Pharmacological Reviews, 1959) although some years were to pass before all of the major enzymes involved were characterized (Pharmacological Reviews, 1966). Until 1957, the catecholamine degradation pathways were unknown. Intravenous perfusion studies showed that a small quantity of catecholamines was excreted unchanged, with an approximately equal amount eliminated as sulphate and glucuronide conjugates (Axelrod, 1959; Kopin, 1972; von Euler, 1972); monoamine oxidase was thought, on exiguous evidence, to be primarily responsible for metabolizing the remainder. However, it was soon discovered that, although the enzyme was involved to some extent, it was not essential for their chemical inactivation (Axelrod, 1959). The key to this problem was provided by two classical observations: Armstrong et al. (1957) found 4-hydroxy-3-methoxymandelic acid to be an important metabolite of adrenaline and noradrenaline and predicted that methylated catecholamines might be its precursor; Axelrod (1957) confirmed this prediction by demonstrating that 3-*O*-methylation is an important route in the metabolism of catecholamines both in vitro and in vivo (Axelrod, 1959). A rapid succession of publications followed, with Axelrod and his colleagues making a major contribution. Within a few years, the main metabolic pathways of the catecholamines were elucidated unequivocally (Axelrod, 1966).

The upsurge of interest in catecholamines following Axelrod's initial observations undoubtedly stimulated a renewed interest in the enzyme systems involved in their biosynthesis and metabolism. Whilst a considerable body of knowledge was already available about L-aromatic aminoacid decarboxylase and monoamine oxidase, the other enzymes responsible (with the exception of the rather ill-defined aldehyde dehydrogenase) had not earlier been identified. However, within a few years tyrosine hydroxylase, dopamine-β-hydroxylase, phenylethanolamine-*N*-methyltransferase and catechol-*O*-methyltransferase had all been characterized, and interest in L-aromatic aminoacid decarboxylase and monoamine oxidase had increased further (Pharmacological Reviews, 1966; Sandler and Ruthven, 1969a). More recent work on these enzymes, focussing on their further characterization, purification, cellular localization and regulatory function in catecholamine biosynthesis, is well summarized in a compilation by Usdin and Snyder (1973).

24.4.5. Physiological role and pharmacological properties of catecholamines

The autonomic nervous system consists of two main subdivisions, sympathetic and parasympathetic, which have contrasting functions. The sympathetic system, which is largely adrenergic, frequently discharges as a unit, particularly during rage and fright. It should be emphasized, however, that apart from these peaks, adrenaline, noradrenaline and dopamine are continually released also, with the level of activity fluctuating in one part of the body compared with another.

The responses to exogenously administered noradrenaline and adrenaline largely mirror those observed on stimulating adrenergic nerves. These actions have been conveniently classified by Koelle (1959) into those on autonomic effector cells (both excitatory and inhibitory), metabolic actions and effects on the central nervous system.

The pharmacological actions of noradrenaline and adrenaline overlap considerably in vivo, although there are differences in their effects on certain complex body functions such as the regulation of blood pressure and heart rate. Peripherally, both amines have a hypertensive action resulting from their respective cardiac and vascular effects. They both increase systolic arterial pressure, but only noradrenaline significantly increases arterial diastolic pressure, adrenaline causing a slight decrease.

The predominant physiological or pharmacological effects produced by the administration of catecholamines or by sympathetic nerve stimulation are given in Table 24.1. Heart rate and cardiac output are increased by adrenaline and decreased by noradrenaline. Blood flow to the skeletal muscles and brain is also increased by adrenaline, while the arterioles and capillaries of the skin are constricted. These actions reflect the physiologi-

TABLE 24.1.

EFFECTS OF CATECHOLAMINES (OR SYMPATHETIC STIMULATION)

(Reproduced, with permission, from Levine and Landsberg, 1974)

	Receptor	Predominant physiologic or pharmacologic effects	Predominant in vivo response
Circulatory effects			
Heart			
Sinus node	β	↑ Rate	↑ Cardiac output
Junctional tissue	β	↑ Conduction velocity	
Myocardium	β	↑ Contractility	
Arteries			
Renal	α	Vasoconstriction	
Splanchnic	α	Vasoconstriction	↓ Local blood flow
Subcutaneous	α	Vasoconstriction	↑ Systemic blood pressure
Mucosal	α	Vasoconstriction	
Cerebral	1	Minimal direct effect	No change in cerebral flow
Coronary	1	Minimal direct effect	↑ Coronary flow (indirect effect)
Skeletal muscle	β	Vasodilatation	↑ Local blood flow ↓ Systematic blood pressure
Veins	α	Vasoconstriction	↑ Venous return ↑ Cardiac output
Juxtaglomerular apparatus	β	↑ Renin secretion	↑ Na^+ reabsorption ↑ Blood pressure
Metabolic effects [1]			
Liver	1	↑ Glycogenolysis	↑ Blood glucose
	1	↑ Gluconeogenesis	↑ Blood glucose
Muscle	β	↑ Glycogenolysis	↑ Blood lactate
	β	↓ Glucose utilization	↑ Blood glucose
Pancreas [2]	α	↓ Insulin secretion	↑ Blood glucose
Adipose tissue	β	↑ Lipolysis	↑ Blood FFA
Visceral effects			
Gastrointestinal tract			
Gastric glands	α,β	↓ Secretion	↓ Gastric acidity, volume
Gastric smooth muscle	β	Relaxation	
Intestinal smooth muscle	α,β	Relaxation	↓ Motility
Intestinal sphincter	α	Contraction	
Lung			
Bronchial smooth muscle	β	Relaxation	Bronchodilatation
Urinary bladder			
Detrusor muscle	β	Relaxation	Inhibits micturition
Trigone, sphincter	α	Contraction	

(continued overleaf)

TABLE 24.1. (continued)

	Receptor	Predominant physiologic or pharmacologic effects	Predominant in vivo response
Eye			
Iris, radial muscle	α	Contraction	Mydriasis
Ciliary muscle	β	Relaxation	Accommodation
Uterus			
Myometrium	α	Contraction	Depends on hormonal milieu
Skin			
Pilomotor muscle	α	Contraction	Piloerection
Sweat glands	α	Secretion	"Adrenergic" sweating

↑ = Increased; ↓ = decreased.

[1] Characterization with regard to receptors is not clearly defined.

[2] β-Receptor effect is to increase insulin secretion, but α effect predominates in vivo.

cal role of these amines. The metabolic effect of a catecholamine on tissues may be stimulatory or depressant, and may involve carbohydrate, lipid, protein and cation metabolism. These compounds initiate energy-mobilizing processes and glycogenolysis in liver and muscle, and gluconeogenesis in liver, resulting in an increase in glucose output. Lipolysis occurs in adipose tissue and cardiac muscle. In the pancreas, insulin secretion is inhibited while amylase secretion is provoked in the salivary glands; in the pineal gland, melatonin secretion is increased. When functioning as metabolic hormones, the catecholamines work by altering the activity of the enzyme, adenyl cyclase, in the nerve cell membrane, modifying synthesis of the product of its action on ATP, cyclic AMP. This "second messenger" stimulates a variety of enzymes in different cells and also alters membrane transport by processes which are unknown but which may be mediated by specific protein kinases (Himms-Hagen, 1972; Mayer, 1973).

So far, discussion has been confined to a description of the peripheral actions of noradrenaline and adrenaline, but dopamine, if less dramatic in its effect, is also known to play a part in controlling sympathetic activity. Its importance in the brain is now unchallenged, but even in the periphery it does not act merely as a precursor in the biosynthetic pathway to noradrenaline. Although dopamine had long been known to possess pharmacological activity similar to, but less potent than, that of noradrenaline and adrenaline, some understanding of its functional role has come more recently. It is the major urinary catecholamine and significant concentrations are present in many tissues including adrenal medulla, sympathetic nerves, heart and lung. In these peripheral tissues, the concentration of dopamine is lower than that of noradrenaline and adrenaline, but in certain highly localized parts of the brain, it is the major catecholamine. Its distribution has been reviewed by Holzbauer and Sharman (1972). Peripherally, dopamine has some specific vasomotor effects, producing an increase in splanchnic and renal blood flow (Goldberg, 1972); but it is in the brain that it performs its most important neurotransmitter role. The discovery that specific pathological and biochemical changes in dopaminergic systems of the brain are present in Parkinson's disease opened a new chapter in the story of dopamine (Hornykiewicz, 1966; Sandler and Ruthven, 1969a; Sandler, 1972a). A profound decrease in dopamine concentration, particularly in the striatum, is thought by many to be the core deficit of this clinical condition. Impairment of dopaminergic transmission and decreased stimulation of dopamine receptors, seems to be primarily linked with the clinical sign of akinesia; it has been suggested that rigidity and tremor derive indirectly from a preponderance of cholinergic input resulting from an absence of normal tonic inhibition by dopamine (Bartholini et al., 1974). Recent observations suggest that central dopaminergic connections are wider than had previously been recognized, extending to septal, hypothalamic and limbic cortical regions of the brain (Fuxe et al., 1974).

24.4.6. Catecholamine receptors

Over the past decade there have been great advances – and a correspondingly vast literature – in our knowledge of events at the adrenergic synapse.

Catecholamine, probably released by exocytosis at the nerve terminal after sympathetic stimulation, elicits a response by interacting with specific sites – adrenergic receptors – on corresponding effector cells. The activating catecholamine is termed an adrenergic agonist while any substance which inhibits this effect is an antagonist or adrenergic blocking agent.

The ultrastructure and precise chemical nature of the receptor is as yet unknown although there has been considerable recent activity in this area of research. Despite the suggestion by Kebabian and his colleagues (1972) that the dopamine-sensitive adenyl cyclase they identified might be the dopamine receptor, rival candidates for the role have been proposed by Snyder and his group, employing radioactive agonists and antagonists as tools in their search (Snyder and Bennett, 1976). So far, however most classification schemes have been pharmacological, based on the effects of certain adrenergic agonists and antagonists. The validity of the approach rests on the assumption that an experimentally induced response accurately imitates the receptor response to an agonist released by sympathetic nerve stimulation. A range of natural and synthetic adrenergic agents, adrenaline, noradrenaline, α-methylnoradrenaline, α-methyladrenaline and isoprenaline, was used by Ahlquist (1948) in his classical experiments which led to the system of adrenergic receptor classification now generally employed. He defined two types of receptor termed α- and β-, a view amply confirmed by subsequent work. Phentolamine and dibenamine are the α-receptor antagonists employed most frequently, whereas propranolol is the most widely used of the β-receptor blockers, a group of drugs with important clinical applications. Noradrenaline acts on α-receptors in many tissues but it stimulates β-receptors in the heart, the overall effect being vasoconstriction combined with bradycardia. Compared with noradrenaline, adrenaline tends to manifest greater β-activity; it elevates systolic blood pressure like noradrenaline but, in contrast, reduces peripheral resistance and produces tachycardia. Both amines are coronary vasodilators.

24.4.7. Regulation of catecholamine biosynthesis

Within the cell, the biosynthetic enzymes are probably situated in close proximity to each other, since intermediates in the synthetic chain do not accumulate. Efficient transfer mechanisms are present: noradrenaline is synthesized within the synaptic vesicle from dopamine which is elaborated outside it. When the noradrenaline is released into the synaptic cleft by exocytosis, the total contents of the vesicle, including dopamine-β-hydroxylase and chromogranin, are extruded (Williams and Munro Neville, 1976), eventually finding their way to the peripheral circulation. Although plasma dopamine-β-hydroxylase has been widely measured in an attempt to obtain some overall index of sympathetic activity, it is generally conceded that the useful clinical information obtained has, on the whole, been disappointing (Geffen, 1974). The assay procedure most commonly used clinically is the colorimetric method of Nagatsu and Udenfriend (1972).

Although the catecholamine biosynthetic sequence in neural and chromaffin tissue is identical, quantitatively there tend to be differences; for example, production is less easily inhibited in adrenal medulla.

The rate of catecholamine production in adrenergic nerves is increased by sympathetic stimulation. The synthetic process is subject to negative feed-back control. When noradrenaline concentration falls below a certain point, an inhibitory action suppressing synthesis may be removed (Bhagat, 1973). In central dopaminergic neurones, it has been claimed that autoreceptors are present, feeding information back to the cell which helps to regulate dopamine biosynthesis (Carlsson, 1974). The regulatory processes appear to act primarily on the rate-limiting enzyme, tyrosine hydroxylase (Udenfriend, 1966), but dopamine-β-hydroxylase is also involved, since a rise in noradrenaline concentration lowers its own production to a greater extent than that of its precursor (Stjärne et al., 1967). Endogenous inhibitors of dopamine-β-hydroxylase may have a regulatory role, while access of substrate to enzyme may also influence the rate of synthesis. This brief account is a gross oversimplification of a complex subject about which our knowledge is still far from complete.

24.4.8. Catecholamine uptake

Circulating and newly-synthesized or released catecholamines are taken up by concentrating mechanisms and bound at various sites in the body, particularly by sympathetic nerves, adrenal gland, heart, spleen and central nervous system. Uptake is a non-destructive process which appears to predominate over degradative termination of noradrenaline and adrenaline action in the tissues. The functional importance of dopamine and 5-hydroxytryptamine uptake processes is much less clear, although they may serve a similar inactivating role after neuronal release. Iversen (1967) has distinguished two uptake mechanisms for noradrenaline and adrenaline, which he termed Uptake_1 and Uptake_2; dopamine and 5-hydroxytryptamine uptake, though similar in many respects, are sensitive to different inhibitors. Uptake_1 is the predominant mechanism – a low-capacity, high-affinity system which operates when the uptake site is exposed to physiologically low concentrations of catecholamines. It transports amines from the extracellular space and across the axonal membrane into the cytoplasm. Here another mechanism transfers free catecholamines into storage vesicles. $Uptake_1$ shows structural preference for derivatives which are not substituted in the *N*-position and displays stereospecificity in favour of L-isomers. $Uptake_2$, a high-capacity, low-affinity system, is extraneuronal and transports amines across membranes in smooth muscle and other postsynaptic cells. It is very rapid, and lacks stereospecificity. It comes into play when the concentration of amine in the tissue rises above a critical point, although it may also function after inhibition of $Uptake_1$ or in tissues where the density of sympathetic innervation is low. It is likely to be important in inactivating circulating noradrenaline and adrenaline (Iversen, 1967, 1973). Uptake processes are capable of creating gradients of amine concentration between binding sites and external media of up to 10,000:1. This physicochemical energy-requiring mechanism operates with the help of ATP and is dependent on Na^+ and K^+ ions and a functioning respiratory chain.

24.4.9. Catecholamine storage

Storage conserves amines by protecting them from enzymatic degradation. It also acts as a reservoir so that a "burst" of amine may be available for release when required. Stores are distributed throughout the body and differ in their specificity towards the different monoamines. They have a finite capacity, but this is rarely saturated. About 90 to 95% of the tissue content of noradrenaline is found in particulate stores (Smith and Winkler, 1972).

Noradrenaline and adrenaline are stored in adrenergic nerves, mainly in the terminals, and also in adrenal medulla and central nervous system. Dopamine has stores of its own in dopaminergic neurones, characteristically in the central nervous system and perhaps in the adrenal medulla (Lishajko, 1968). Noradrenaline stores take up dopamine, but in small amounts compared with noradrenaline. 5-Hydroxytryptamine also has its own stores which are situated in large granules, analogous to chromaffin and mast-cell granules. Blood platelets provide an important store for 5-hydroxytryptamine, as do the enterochromaffin cells of the gut and other tissues, and certain areas of the central nervous system (Garattini and Valzelli, 1965).

As implied earlier, amines are stored within the sympathetic nerve in an internal structure enveloped by a membrane, the storage vesicle; in the adrenal medulla the stores are termed chromaffin granules. The mechanism of storage is not known. Although probably possessing features in common, storage mechanisms are likely to vary according to differences in the amine-specificity of the stores. There may also be differences between catecholamine stores in adrenal medulla and sympathetic nerves. The simple but elegant in vitro experiments of Pletscher and his colleagues (Pletscher et al., 1971) point to the formation of an adenine nucleotide–amine complex of variable proportions within the granule. Binding with membrane lipids may also be a factor in storage, which is more important, perhaps, in nerves than in adrenal medulla. ATP complexes with Mg^{2+} and Ca^{2+} also appear to be closely connected with uptake and storage. Mg^{2+}-dependent ATPase is present in storage granules where it is thought to catalyze the hydrolysis of ATP–amine complexes, facilitating transport processes within the vesicles (Stjärne, 1972; von Euler, 1972).

24.4.10. Catecholamine release on sympathetic stimulation

The normal mechanism of catecholamine release has not been established unequivocally but, as implied earlier, exocytosis appears to be the most likely mechanism, both in adrenal medulla and sympathetic neurone. In this process the amine-containing granule in the chromaffin cell or noradrenergic vesicle in the sympathetic nerve migrates through the cytosol to fuse with the cell membrane. Fusion, which may involve the participation of lysolecithin, is followed by the formation of a single large "pore" at the junction of granule (or vesicle membrane) and cell membrane, allowing all of the contents of the granule or vesicle to escape into the extracellular fluid. The empty vesicle or granule envelope then breaks away from the cell membrane. Biochemical evidence excludes release of the intact granule. All observations point to the granule or vesicle being the site from which noradrenaline or adrenaline is released on nerve stimulation. This action, which appears to require the entry of Ca^{2+} ions into the cell, is also accompanied by an almost stoichiometric outflow of soluble protein. Noradrenaline within the cytosol is not released readily and is unaffected by nerve stimulation. Similarly, neuronal tyrosine hydroxylase and 3,4-dihydroxyphenylalanine decarboxylase, which are found only in the cytosol, are not freed by stimulation, whereas dopamine-β-hydroxylase, which is located in the vesicle, does escape.

In peripheral adrenergic nerves, electron microscopists have distinguished two types of electron-dense vesicle, large and small. These are probably identical with the "heavy" and "light" noradrenergic vesicles, so called because of their sedimentation properties in a density gradient. "Heavy" vesicles are found in nerve cell body, axon and terminal, whilst "light" vesicles are confined to terminal and varicosity. "Heavy" vesicles migrate from cell body down the axon to the nerve terminal where some are transformed into "light" vesicles. "Light" vesicles contain only noradrenaline, although dopamine-β-hydroxylase is probably present attached to the cell membrane. "Heavy" vesicles contain noradrenaline, dopamine-β-hydroxylase and, often, chromogranin "A" and ATP. Both "light" and "heavy" vesicles appear to be discharged at the nerve ending by exocytosis. For a full account of release mechanisms, see Smith and Winkler (1972).

24.4.11. Catecholamine inactivation after release by nerve stimulation

In sympathetic nerves, noradrenaline appears to be released on nerve stimulation from a relatively small store. A larger reserve store exists, and amine is mobilized and transferred from it to the small store when required. Newly synthesized noradrenaline can enter either store. After its release and discharge from the nerve, most of the noradrenaline is taken up again by the nerve and bound once more. A small proportion is *O*-methylated near to the site of release and a further fraction diffuses into the blood stream, mostly to be *O*-methylated by the liver, Noradrenaline also appears to leak continuously from sympathetic nerve granules into the cytoplasm, where much of it is metabolized by monoamine oxidase. Whereas 4-hydroxy-3-methoxymandelic acid and the metadrenalines are the major products of noradrenaline and adrenaline inactivation in the periphery, in the central nervous system, 4-hydroxy-3-methoxyphenylglycol appears to be the major metabolite. However, as in the periphery, homovanillic acid is the main metabolite of

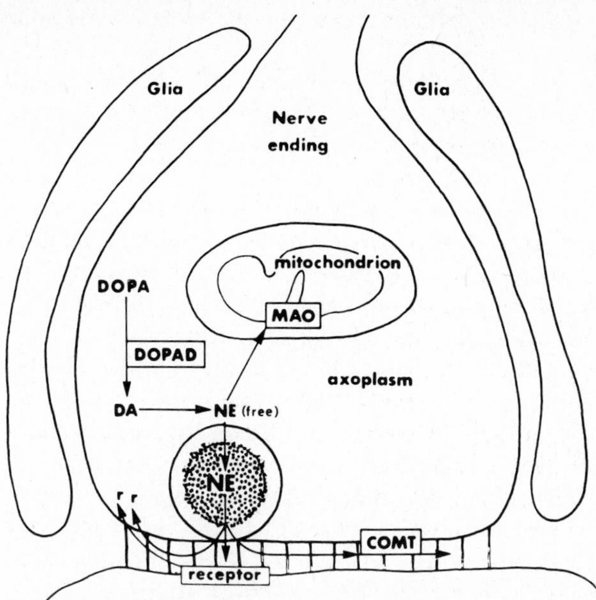

Figure 24.1. Diagram of a noradrenergic synapse with mitochondrial, axoplasmic and synaptic vesicle compartments making synaptic contact with a second neurone. Intersynaptic filaments attach the two synaptic membranes. Monoamine oxidase (MAO) is localized in the mitochondria and may inactivate free noradrenaline (NE) and dopamine (DA). DOPA decarboxylase (DOPAD) is in the axoplasm and may produce DA from DOPA. DA is converted into NE, which can be free or taken up and bound within the synaptic vesicle. These granulated vesicles are ready to release quantal units of NE upon arrival of a nerve impulse. Released NE reacts with the receptor and may be inactivated by re-uptake (r) or by methylation with catechol-*O*-methyltransferase (COMT) (Reproduced, with permission, from de Robertis, 1966).

dopamine in the central nervous system (Sharman, 1973). A representation of a nerve ending and receptor (Figure 24.1) illustrates the intraneuronal biosynthesis, storage and metabolism of noradrenaline, and the fate of the amine following its release on nerve stimulation.

24.4.12. Adrenergic false neurotransmitters

The synthesis, storage and release of noradrenaline are processes that are not wholly specific. Foreign amines which are structurally related to noradrenaline can be formed in vivo and bound in the intra-axonal vesicles, displacing the natural transmitter; they may in turn be released on sympathetic nerve stimulation. The resulting effect on nerve function depends on the amount of natural amine displaced, as well as on the interaction of false transmitter with receptor. The net effect varies considerably, but is usually weaker than that of the physiological transmitter. Although compounds of this type, acting in place of the natural transmitters, have been termed "adrenergic false neurotransmitters" (Kopin, 1968), Baldessarini (Baldessarini and Vogt, 1972) prefers the term "substitute transmitter", thus not excluding a physiological role for certain compounds in this group which are elaborated endogenously.

False transmitters or their precursors can be formed from aminoacids sharing the same biosynthetic pathway as the catecholamines. For example, tyrosine hydroxylase hydroxylates phenylalanine, α-methyltyrosine and metaraminol; 3,4-dihydroxyphenylalanine decarboxylase converts α-methyldopa, *m*-tyrosine, α-methyl-*m*-tyrosine and α-methyl-5-hydroxytryptophan into their corresponding amines. Dopamine-β-hydroxylase hydroxylates amines other than dopamine, e.g. tyramine, α-methyltyramine, *m*-tyramine, α-methyl-*m*-tyramine and α-methyldopamine; and phenylethanolamine-*N*-methyltransferase *N*-methylates β-hydroxylated monoamines other than noradrenaline, including phenylethanolamine, octopamine, *m*-hydroxyphenylethanolamine and α-methylnoradrenaline.

Some, but not all, false transmitters are metabolized in a similar way to the catecholamines. Those with a catechol grouping are *O*-methylated by catechol-*O*-methyltransferase, but the monophenols remain unaltered. α-Methylation of noradrenaline and dopamine shields them from the action of monoamine oxidase but does not alter amine uptake and storage properties. Consequently, unlike other sympathetic amines, two known false transmitters, metaraminol and methyloctopamine have structures which render them invulnerable to the actions of monoamine oxidase and catechol-*O*-methyltransferase, so that they become useful research tools.

24.4.13. Environmental factors modifying catecholamine production

Exercise, "stress", diet and drugs can all modify catecholamine production to a varying extent. It is therefore important to be aware of these effects in order to control them.

24.4.13.1. Exercise

Work and exercise decrease parasympathetic tone and facilitate the flow of sympathetic impulses, which in turn increase plasma noradrenaline concentration and to a lesser extent, that of adrenaline. The magnitude of the response is dependent on the severity of the exercise: there is a significant correlation between oxygen consumption and noradrenaline concentration in arterial blood plasma, the rate of rise increasing logarithmically as work load approaches the limit of endurance. Under these conditions, the concentration of circulating noradrenaline, which can rise, exceptionally, to about 10 μg/litre from a resting level of about 0.1 to 1 μg/litre, may be sufficient to produce significant effects (Häggendal et al., 1970). In contrast to the change in plasma concentration, urinary noradrenaline output does not show a proportional increase with strenuous loads, perhaps because renal and hepatic blood flows are diminished. At lighter loads, the rate of noradrenaline excretion does tend to reflect its concentration in the plasma. However, noradrenaline output is a poor index of exercise stress because of large between- and within-subject variation, and certain other factors connected with work load (Cronan and Howley, 1974). Training may affect noradrenaline excretion (von Euler, 1974).

Exercise produces significant increases in urinary 4-hydroxy-3-methoxymandelic acid output, varying from about 10 to 100 μg/h in subjects doing standardized tests of physical work. The increase is a linear function of the oxygen consumption with an average increase in 4-hydroxy-3-methoxymandelic acid output of 5.5 μg/h for each increase of 1 ml/

min in average oxygen consumption per kg body weight (Neal et al., 1968). Rises in 4-hydroxy-3-methoxymandelic acid excretion rate of about 5 to 10 μg/min have been observed during basketball contests and long-distance skiing (von Euler, 1974). Unexpectedly, virtually no rises in 4-hydroxy-3-methoxyphenylglycol or total metadrenaline outputs were detected after strenuous exercise in which urinary noadrenaline excretion rose 10-fold (Goode et al., 1973).

24.4.13.2. "Stress"

"Stress" is a vague concept which has been linked with responses such as anxiety, unpleasant emotions, emotional tension and anger, aggression, or work accompanied by physical exertion (Levi, 1967a). The urinary excretion of both noradrenaline and adrenaline may be increased, adrenaline particularly so, by anxiety, Both unpleasant stimuli and others such as sexual arousal may provoke increases in urinary catecholamine output. The high temperature and humidity associated with sauna bathing give rise to an average increase of about 50% in mean basal noradrenaline and about 35% in adrenaline excretion although there is considerable variation. 4-Hydroxy-3-methoxymandelic acid output is unchanged (Huikko et al., 1966).

Cold stress, which is particularly important in the neonate, produces an increase in oxygen consumption with an accompanying rise in urinary noradrenaline output (Stern et al., 1965).

The effect of stress promoted by hazardous pursuits on catecholamine metabolism has been the subject of a number of studies. Even the mental stress of normal car driving produces a significant increase in urinary total catecholamine output both in normal subjects and in patients with coronary artery disease (Bellet et al., 1969). Rather erratic changes in excretion pattern of catecholamines and their metabolites were observed in astronauts during stressful training and space flights, possibly because of artefacts arising during specimen collection and storage (Weil-Malherbe et al., 1968). However, the flying of supersonic jet fighters almost doubled the urinary output of 4-hydroxy-3-methoxymandelic acid and homovanillic acid. Interestingly, the rise was highest in experienced pilots, perhaps because their appreciation of the dangers involved was greater than that of young, less experienced fliers (Doležăl et al., 1971). Centrifugation of pilots during training resulted in significant increases of noradrenaline, adrenaline and 4-hydroxy-3-methoxymandelic acid excretion (Goodall and Berman, 1960). Mean urinary 4-hydroxy-3-methoxyphenylglycol output rose by about 25% in pilots involved in aircraft carrier landings made by day, and about 40 to 60% during night landings. To what extent these findings reflect on actual increase in turnover of catecholamines in the central nervous system is still an open question.

24.4.13.3. Dietary and drug interference

Apart from interfering with the assay of catecholamines and their metabolites (section 24.9), dietary constituents and drugs may be potential sources of misleading clinical information. Dietary monoamines are metabolized almost completely in gut wall or liver by sulphate conjugation (Sandler et al., 1975), and by oxidative deamination and *O*-methylation, before reaching the systemic circulation. Thus their ingestion has little effect on urinary excretion of free amines, although metabolite output is affected to a variable extent. Accordingly, free rather than total catecholamine output should be measured when investigating endogenous production. A diet containing certain vegetables or fruits rich in noradrenaline and dopamine, such as bananas, may result in an increased urinary output of normetadrenaline, 4-hydroxy-3-methoxymandelic acid or homovanillic acid. However, rises tend to be relatively small even after considerable intake of the foods in question. Thus the ingestion of four bananas has been reported to increase 4-hydroxy-3-methoxymandelic acid output by only 0.6 mg (Cardon and Guggenheim, 1970). If eaten in any quantity, the broad bean (*Vicia faba*), which is rich in L-3,4-dihydroxyphenylalanine (Sandler, 1972a), is likely to raise urinary homovanillic acid and 3,4-dihydroxyphenylacetic acid excretion to a much greater extent, although the output of noradrenaline is not affected. Apart from the broad bean, the constituents of a normal diet give rise to little change in homovanillic acid output. Obese subjects, presumably on high caloric intake, excrete about 1 to 2 mg/day more of 4-hydroxy-3-methoxymandelic acid than normal individuals (Rath et al., 1967). Coffee and other beverages containing caffeine tend to stimulate the secretion of adrenaline and, to a lesser extent, of noradrenaline; output may be raised by about 80% and 20 to 30% respectively after drinking several cups of coffee. The amine output response may vary considerably at different times in the same individual (Levi, 1967b). Metadrenaline excretion also tends to increase but is not subject to as much variation as that of adrenaline (Cardon and Guggenheim, 1970). Urinary 5-hydroxyindoleacetic acid excretion may be increased by 5-hydroxytryptamine-containing foods. Many edible fruits such as walnuts, bananas and pineapples provide considerable amounts of the substance (Garattini and Valzelli, 1965). Eating about 500 grams of bananas increases urinary 5-hydroxyindoleacetic acid output by about 20 mg/day (Vettorazzi, 1974): 5-hydroxytryptamine-secreting tumours usually manifest with a larger rise. Nevertheless, if a random urine sample is taken for a 5-hydroxyindoleacetic acid screening test at peak excretion after eating bananas, the threshold of sensitivity of the procedure may sometimes be exceeded.

24.4.13.3.1. Drugs. Space permits little more than a brief account of the broad range of drug effects on the sympathetic-adrenal system.

Pletscher (1973) distinguished seven sites of action on adrenergic and tryptaminergic mechanisms – amine biosynthesis, "amine pump", intraneuronal storage, noradrenaline release, nerve terminal structure, catabolism and receptor.

Biosynthesis can be inhibited at each enzymatic step by appropriate drugs. α-Methyl-*p*-tyrosine and *p*-chlorophenylalanine inhibit tyrosine hydroxylase (Spector et al., 1965) and tryptophan hydroxylase (Koe and Weissman, 1966) respectively. L-Aromatic amino-acid decarboxylase is inhibited by such drugs as benserazide (Burkard et al., 1962) or carbidopa (Porter et al., 1962) and dopamine-β-hydroxylase by a variety of drugs including disulfiram; its administration reduces urinary 4-hydroxy-3-methoxymandelic acid excretion to about one-half of its normal value, whilst more than doubling homovanillic acid output (Vesell et al., 1971). It is obviously important to withdraw such a drug before measuring urinary output of these compounds.

Inhibition of the "amine pump", i.e. blocking monoamine uptake at the presynaptic membrane of the monoaminergic nerve terminal, leads to increased amine concentration in the vicinity of the receptor. This delay in amine disposal has the effect of increasing the sensitivity of sympathetically innervated tissues to circulating catecholamines and may have serious consequences in conditions of raised catecholamine production. The onset of a hypertensive crisis has been reported where a pregnant patient with phaeochromocytoma was given the tricyclic antidepressant imipramine, which is a potent "amine pump" inhibitor (Kaufmann, 1974).

Drugs affecting intraneuronal storage may act on the granule membrane or displace catecholamines from, and then occupy, granule stores. Reserpine affects the permeability of this membrane, inhibiting the uptake of 5-hydroxytryptamine, noradrenaline and dopamine, thereby exposing them to degradation by intraneuronal monoamine oxidase. "False transmitters" (section 24.4.12), such as the amines deriving from methyldopa and α-methyl-*m*-tyrosine, replace catecholamines in their store: tyramine releases amine from this store; noradrenaline which is displaced by the action of methyldopa gives rise to an approximately 4-fold increase in the rate of normetadrenaline excretion between 2 and 4 hours after ingesting 0.5 grams of the drug (Stott and Robinson, 1967a).

Noradrenaline release by nerve impulse can be prevented by certain drugs such as bretylium and guanethidine, while another drug in this group, debrisoquine, also inhibits intraneuronal monoamine oxidase. Drugs such as 6-hydroxydopamine, which destroy the structure of nerve terminals and are included in Pletscher's classification, are obviously unsuitable for administration to humans, although they are employed widely in animal experiments.

Of drugs affecting monoamine catabolism, monoamine oxidase inhibitors have been most widely used medicinally. Disulfiram, too, apart from blocking dopamine-β-hydroxylase, also inhibits aldehyde dehydrogenase. This property, which has been employed to bring about an accumulation of acetaldehyde after ethanol ingestion, with unpleasant clinical consequences, has been used in the treatment of alcoholism. Ethanol itself diverts the aldehyde arising from both adrenaline and noradrenaline away from a pathway involving further oxidation to 4-hydroxy-3-methoxymandelic acid towards a reductive pathway, thereby bringing about increased formation of 4-hydroxy-3-methoxyphenylglycol (Davis et al., 1967). Reserpine has a similar effect (Sandler and Youdim, 1968).

Drugs acting on monoamine receptors alter monoamine metabolism by feed-back effects, at least in the central nervous system. Thus, receptor block leads to overproduction of agonist in an effort to overcome it, while receptor stimulation results in decreased synthesis. While such effects may not be as clear-cut in the periphery, they should be borne in mind in that α- and β-adrenergic receptor blocking drugs are widely used in the management of phaeochromocytoma.

24.5. CATECHOLAMINE-SECRETING TUMOURS

It has long been recognized that pressor substances are released into the circulations of patients with phaeochromocytoma. An attempt to demonstrate this fact directly was made more than 50 years ago, although the assay of urinary adrenaline and noradrenaline as a diagnostic aid was only suggested in 1950, noradrenaline having been demonstrated in tumour tissue the previous year. In contrast, the first report of increased urinary excretion of pressor amines in neuroblastoma did not appear until 1957. With hindsight, perhaps, this belated recognition seems surprising, for it was well known that neuroblastoma, like phaeochromocytoma, stems from cells originating in the neural crest (Winkler and Smith, 1972). In sharp contrast with phaeochromocytoma, many patients with neuroblastoma manifest with normal or near normal blood pressure (Voorhess, 1966), and this was perhaps the main factor responsible for delayed recognition of the catecholamine-secreting nature of the tumour.

Once the major pathways of catecholamine biosynthesis and metabolism had been established (Sandler and Ruthven, 1969a), it was soon discovered that catecholamine excretion itself is the tip of the iceberg and that patients with neural tumours excrete considerably greater amounts of amine metabolites. Moreover, there is frequently a clear distinction between the urinary metabolite pattern associated with phaeochromocytoma and that accompanying other neural tumours (Hinterberger and Bartholomew, 1969).

24.5.1. Phaeochromocytoma

24.5.1.1. Incidence, location, sex and age distribution

The early diagnosis of phaeochromocytoma is of great importance; in over 90% of cases it is benign and surgical removal results in complete cure. Nevertheless, if the tumour is undetected, the outcome will almost certainly be fatal. The incidence of phaeochromocytoma is often quoted as being about 0.5% of all persons with hypertension, but this figure, derived from pathological studies on hospital populations, does not give a true impression of its rarity. Less restricted studies point to a frequency of about 0.005%, or about one new case in 1 to 2 million of the population each year. About 80% of tumours are located in the adrenals and about one case in ten of these have bilateral tumours (Gjessing, 1968). The remaining 20% are distributed between the organ of Zuckerkandl, para-aortic bodies, thorax and urinary bladder. The tumour is familial in about 5% of patients, and in this group approximately 40% are bilateral. When the neoplasm is associated with medullary carcinoma of the thyroid (Sipple's syndrome), the incidence of bilateral adrenal tumours rises to about 70%. In the adult, phaeochromocytoma is equally distributed between the sexes, but in children it is found more often in boys than girls (Stackpole et al., 1963). It has its onset at any age, although most cases present between 20 and 50 years of age. Children show a greater tendency than adults to manifest with multiple and extra-adrenal tumours (Stackpole et al., 1963). The neoplasm varies greatly in size, ranging from a few grams to about two kilograms (Montgomery and Welbourn, 1975). Not more than about 10% are malignant (Gjessing, 1968); the figure is probably considerably smaller, if cases are only included which possess secreting metastases at sites not normally occupied by chromaffin tissue.

24.5.1.2. Clinical features

The clinical diagnosis of phaeochromocytoma is difficult; the symptoms and signs, which result directly or indirectly from the pharmacological effects of tumour secretion, may easily be confused with those arising from some other disease. Hypertension is usually the most prominent feature. It is sustained in about 70% of cases and paroxysmal in the remainder. Paroxysms may occur spontaneously or follow a variety of stimuli; they may take place at intervals of a few hours or appear infrequently, lasting for about a minute or persisting for as long as a week. These attacks often produce headache, tachycardia and palpitations, sweating, pallor, nervousness, tremor and, less frequently, other symptoms such as nausea and vomiting. Patients with sustained hypertension often have glycosuria, raised fasting blood glucose concentrations and diabetic glucose tolerance curves. The basal metabolic rate is usually raised, accounting for the concomitant loss of weight. In patients with the rarer predominantly adrenaline-secreting tumour, effects on metabolism are greater than those on the circulatory system, although sometimes hypotension, unaccompanied by hypertension is observed. When hypotension is postural, noradrenaline rather than adrenaline tends to be the predominant amine (Jones et al., 1968). There are other clinical problems to be considered. Circulatory collapse may supervene at operation, during delivery or after injury; cardiovascular complications are frequent and are similar to those observed in severe hypertension. It is not surprising, therefore, that patients with unsuspected phaeochromocytoma are high operative risks and may succumb to relatively minor procedures (Montgomery and Welbourn, 1975).

24.5.1.3. Pharmacological diagnosis of phaeochromocytoma

Diagnosis by pharmacological procedures has largely been superseded. Provocative tests (see below) may trigger the release of catecholamines and precipitate hypertensive crises in affected subjects. Although administration of the α-blocker, phentolamine, is a safer diagnostic procedure, a positive response to it, indicated by a fall in blood pressure a few minutes after injection, may sometimes be seen in normal people or hypertensive subjects without phaeochromocytoma.

24.5.1.3.1. Catecholamine release: initiating factors. One of the most important stimuli initiating an attack may be mechanical pressure which is often able to stimulate the outflow of catecholamines from tumour and sinusoidal spaces. Extra-tumoural catecholamine stores may also be released by reflex action; tilting, for example, can produce an increase in urinary noradrenaline in affected but not in normal subjects (Harrison et al., 1967). Release evoked by various agents – histamine, tyramine and glucagon – has been used in provocative tests for phaeochromocytoma, but all suffer from false-positive or false-negative results. The diagnostic value of the histamine and glucagon tests may be enhanced by measuring urinary catecholamine excretion as well as blood pressure after drug administration. Histamine acts directly on the tumour at high dosage; lower dosage usually induces release of tumour stores indirectly (Winkler and Smith, 1972). In contrast, tyramine acts only by releasing catecholamines from the greatly supplemented peripheral sympathetic stores and not from tumour (Engelman and Sjoerdsma, 1964). The drug is therefore safer to use than histamine or glucagon. Glucagon probably works partly by inducing release from extra-tumoral stores and partly from an effect on the tumour (Winkler and Smith, 1972). Because of their dangers, if the histamine or glucagon tests are used at all, they should be reserved for cases where phaeochromocytoma is strongly suspected clinically but it has not been possible to clinch the diagnosis biochemically.

24.5.1.4. Catecholamine metabolism in tumour tissue

24.5.1.4.1. Biosynthesis. Phaeochromocytoma tumour tissue contains all the enzymes required for catecholamine biosynthesis – tyrosine hydroxylase, 3,4-dihydroxyphenylalanine decarboxylase, dopamine-β-hydroxylase and phenylethanolamine-*N*-methyltransferase (Winkler and Smith, 1972). Their ability to produce L-3,4-dihydroxyphenylalanine, dopamine, noradrenaline and adrenaline from L-tyrosine has been demonstrated in tissue culture cells (Cabana et al., 1964).

Tumour amine concentration can be very high (Winkler and Smith, 1972), suggesting that, compared with adrenal medulla or sympathetic nervous tissue, tyrosine hydroxylase activity in phaeochromocytoma is far less sensitive to feed-back inhibition by catechol compounds. The difference may relate to changes in affinity towards co-factors or to variant forms of the enzyme (Winkler and Smith, 1972). This explanation is not universally accepted; others have claimed that tumour tyrosine hydroxylase has similar substrate and inhibition kinetics, co-factor requirements and intracellular localization as the adrenal medullary enzyme (Waymire et al., 1972).

3,4-Dihydroxyphenylalanine decarboxylase activity is variable, but may be much greater than that of enzyme from human or animal adrenal medulla (Winkler and Smith, 1972), and of the same high order as that of guinea-pig kidney (Lovenberg et al., 1962). Dopamine-β-hydroxylase activity is also variable, higher than that of adrenal medulla in some tumours, and lower in others (Winkler and Smith, 1972). As mentioned earlier (section 24.4.2), phenylethanolamine-*N*-methyltransferase is normally activated by glucocorticoids from the adrenal cortex. However, the glucocorticoid supply to phaeochromocytoma tissue is inferior to that of adrenal medulla, accounting, perhaps, for the relatively low proportion of adrenaline and noradrenaline which is found in many of these tumours (Hermann and Mornex, 1964; Engelman and Hammond, 1968). Nevertheless, large amounts of adrenaline are secreted by the occasional tumour, even when it is situated extra-adrenally (Engelman and Hammond, 1968). This observation has led to the suggestion that an atypical variety of phenylethanolamine-*N*-methyltransferase is present in some tumours, not requiring glucocorticoid for activity (Goldstein et al., 1969).

24.5.1.4.2. Metabolism. As with biosynthesis, all the enzymes required for catecholamine degradation are present in phaeochromocytoma tumour tissue. Monoamine oxidase activity is demonstrable but relatively low (Amar-Costesec et al., 1965); catechol-*O*-methyltransferase has also been clearly demonstrated (Kopin and Axelrod, 1960). The aldehyde dehydrogenase–reductase system (section 24.4.3) has not been identified directly but the presence of one of its components may be inferred from the occurrence of 4-hydroxy-3-methoxyphenylglycol in tumour tissue (Kopin and Axelrod, 1960).

The wide variability of urinary metabolite excretion pattern in patients with phaeochromocytoma (Crout and Sjoerdsma, 1964; von Studnitz, 1966) suggests that major differences may exist in the ability of the tumour to metabolize noradrenaline and adrenaline. However, it should be pointed out that other factors may contribute to these variations, e.g. differences in rate of amine synthesis, storage capacity and site of the tumour in relationship to the liver. Size of tumour has been claimed to be another important variable (Crout and Sjoerdsma, 1964; Crout, 1966). When it is small, with a "low" total content of noradrenaline and adrenaline, the rate of catecholamine turnover tends to be high and the ratio of urinary 4-hydroxy-3-methoxymandelic acid to adrenaline plus noradrenaline low. Conversely, in a large tumour with "high" total content of noradrenaline and adrenaline, the catecholamine turnover rate is often low and the ratio of urinary 4-hydroxy-3-methoxymandelic acid to noradrenaline plus adrenaline high. Thus small tumours (less than 50 grams) tend to secrete relatively more catecholamine than metabolite, while for larger tumours the converse is true. It should be stressed that this difference probably relates to type rather than size of tumour, since slow secretors escape notice in the early stages of their growth. Children with phaeochromocytoma commonly have small tumours (Stackpole et al., 1963). In the adult, sustained hypertension may be associated with small tumours and paroxysmal hypertension with the larger type. However, the concept of functionally different kinds of tumour has been questioned. Tyce and her colleagues (Lauper et al., 1972) could not distinguish any difference between storage cell type observed in small compared with large tumours; others have noted fine structure to be similar and unrelated to clinical picture, in tumours with high or low turnover rates. As Lauper et al. pointed out, errors in calculating turnover rate might arise if one were to include areas of tumour engorged with blood in the total tumour weight used in the calculation.

24.5.1.5. Tumour catecholamines: storage and release

The concentration of catecholamines within a phaeochromocytoma usually exceeds that of the adrenal medulla by a large margin, the variation being very wide and unrelated to tumour size (Hermann and Mornex, 1964). A total content approaching 11 grams of catecholamines has been reported in one tumour (Crout and Sjoerdsma, 1964). Few contain 3,4-dihydroxyphenylalanine or dopamine in significant concentration, although some notable exceptions are on record (Winkler and Smith, 1972).

The high catecholamine content of some tumours has led to conjecture that amine storage is as efficient as in normal adrenal medulla. There is much evidence to suggest that tumour tissue chromaffin granules are essentially similar to those in normal human adrenal medulla. Differences in weight, density, fragility and chemical composition have not been observed. Moreover, the catecholamine/ATP molar ratio in chromaffin granules, which is an index of storage capacity, appears to be identical with that of adrenal medulla (Winkler and Smith, 1972).

Catecholamine release from phaeochromocytoma is likely to differ from the pattern observed in sympathetic nerve endings. It seems unlikely that the tumour possesses the capacity to synthesize sufficient chromogranin to make up for the large deficit which would result if such substantial amounts of catecholamines were associated with it in their release by normal exocytosis mechanisms. After weighing up available information, Winkler and Smith (1972) suggested that the large amounts of catecholamines arising from uncontrolled synthesis in the tumour far exceed the storage capacity of the chromaffin granules, so that diffusion of excess amine through the cytoplasm and across the cell membrane must occur. Therefore the rate of release of amines depends upon the rate of biosynthesis and not upon the store size. Such a mechanism receives further support from the observed reduction in blood pressure in patients with phaeochromocytoma, after receiving the tyrosine hydroxylase inhibitor, α-methyl-p-tyrosine (Jones et al., 1968); a similar reduction is not observed in other hypertensive subjects treated with an equivalent dose of the drug (Winkler and Smith, 1972).

24.5.1.6. Urinary catecholamine and metabolite output in phaeochromocytoma

In phaeochromocytoma, the excretion pattern of urinary catecholamines and their metabolites varies considerably (Sjoerdsma et al., 1966; Marsden and Steward, 1968). The differences are mainly quantitative, apart from a small number of cases where the tumour is dopamine-secreting (von Studnitz, 1966; Jones et al., 1968).

One important variable is the amount of adrenaline secreted. Noradrenaline is usually predominant, although adrenaline content tends to be higher in those cases where tumour catecholamine storage capacity is high (Hermann and Mornex, 1964). Tumour location also tends to influence metabolite excretion pattern, e.g. whether it arises in proximity to organs such as liver and kidney, rich in catechol-*O*-methyltransferase and monoamine oxidase. The particular aggregation of chromaffin cells from which it derives is particularly important in this context. A significantly higher urinary adrenaline excretion may be found in those cases where the tumour is situated in or adjacent to the adrenal medulla. While this finding may bear directly on the need for high local concentrations of glucocorticoid, in order to achieve *N*-methylation mediated by phenylethanolamine-*N*-methyltransferase, the presence of raised amounts of urinary adrenaline in no way rules out an extra-adrenal site of tumour origin. Such tumours, although rare, are well documented (Hermann and Mornex, 1964; Engelman and Hammond, 1968); the phenylethanolamine-*N*-methyltransferase they contain is presumably a non-glucocorticoid requiring variant (section 24.4.2). Nevertheless, the likelihood of a tumour being extra-adrenal is considerably greater when noradrenaline alone is excreted in the urine in excess (Fries and Chamberlain, 1968).

A wide variety of catecholamine metabolites is excreted by patients with phaeochromocytoma. Since its original identification in cases of this type (Armstrong et al., 1957), 4-hydroxy-3-methoxymandelic acid production has been extensively studied (Marsden and Steward, 1968; Hinterberger and Bartholomew, 1969; Voorhess, 1974). Other important metabolites, 4-hydroxy-3-methoxyphenylglycol (Ruthven and Sandler, 1965) and the *O*-methylated amines normetadrenaline and metadrenaline (Sjoerdsma et al., 1966; Marsden and Steward, 1968; Gitlow et al., 1970a) are also present in excess in urine from affected subjects. Minor urinary metabolites (e.g. *N*-methylmetadrenaline) may also be excreted in greater concentration than normal in this condition.

The urinary metabolite pattern derived from catecholamines introduced into the blood stream, whether by injection or phaeochromocytoma, differs from that observed following intracellular release and metabolism. Catecholamines secreted into the circulation rapidly reach organs such as the liver which are rich in catechol-*O*-methyltransferase and monoamine oxidase; there a significant proportion is *O*-methylated, some of this product being further degraded by hepatic conjugation or oxidative deamination. A portion of circulating amine may be taken up and bound at different sites in the body, particularly by adrenal gland, heart, spleen and sympathetic nervous tissue. After equilibration it is slowly released and metabolized.

Noradrenaline is a slightly better substrate for monoamine oxidase than adrenaline, while normetadrenaline is oxidatively deaminated much more readily than metadrenaline. That the urinary ratio of total catecholamines to 4-hydroxy-3-methoxymandelic acid (especially of total metadrenalines to 4-hydroxy-3-methoxymandelic acid) is higher in patients with phaeochromocytoma than normal persons (Crout, 1966; Winkler and

Smith, 1972) presumably reflects the processes just described. It confirms, in particular, that there is direct passage of noradrenaline into the circulating blood – a conclusion supported by direct observation on the plasma of affected subjects and by the profound degree of hypertension which may be associated with a small tumour.

24.5.1.7. Dopamine-secreting phaeochromocytoma

In addition to elaborating noradrenaline and adrenaline, phaeochromocytoma is occasionally dopamine-secreting (Page and Jacoby, 1964; Louis et al., 1972). This property is associated with the excess output of characteristic dopamine metabolites, homovanillic acid (Sankoff and Sourkes, 1963; Page and Jacoby, 1964; Robinson et al., 1964; Sato and Sjoerdsma, 1965; Ruthven and Sandler, 1966; Gitlow et al., 1972), 3-methoxytyramine (Page and Jacoby, 1964; Robinson et al., 1964; Greer et al., 1968) and 3,4-dihydroxyphenylacetic acid (Page and Jacoby, 1964) all of which have been detected. The excretion of increased amounts of *N*-acetyldopamine (Sekeris and Herrlich, 1963), 3,4-dihydroxyphenylacetic acid (Louis et al., 1972) and vanillic acid (Robinson et al., 1964) has also been recorded.

The urinary metabolite pattern of the fully developed case may be almost indistinguishable from that of patients with neuroblastoma (section 24.5.2.4) although high concentrations of adrenaline or metadrenaline should alert the clinician to the correct diagnosis. More commonly, however, the metabolite pattern is that of phaeochromocytoma with a more moderate superimposition of dopamine pathway metabolites (Jones et al., 1968).

The question of a relationship between raised dopamine secretion and malignancy (Robinson et al., 1964) is still unresolved. Certainly, the combination is well documented in phaeochromocytoma (Sankoff and Sourkes, 1963; Ruthven and Sandler, 1966; von Studnitz, 1966; Jones et al., 1968). However, other cases of dopamine-secreting phaeochromocytoma are on record (Page and Jacoby, 1964; Gjessing, 1964; Gitlow et al., 1972) in whom malignancy was not a feature. Conversely, some patients with malignant phaeochromocytoma fail to manifest any overproduction of dopamine, its precursors or metabolites (Sato and Sjoerdsma, 1965). Thus the association remains unproven. Perhaps it is no bad thing to regard all phaeochromocytomas as potentially malignant (Sjoerdsma et al., 1966) and to monitor biochemically, at 3- to 6-monthly intervals, all patients who have had such a tumour removed surgically.

24.5.1.8. Phaeochromocytoma in disguise

A paucity of clinical signs may sometimes serve to disguise the presence of a phaeochromocytoma even when the concentration of circulating catecholamine is considerably elevated and the metabolite excretion raised. Although diagnosis of classical phaeochromocytoma is not difficult, the disease may present in many different ways. Thus it should be considered in the differential diagnosis of acute abdominal pain with shock; fatal cases of this type are on record, with the common feature at autopsy of haemorrhage into a phaeochromocytoma (Huston and Stewart, 1965). Cardiomyopathy, often fatal, may be associated with this tumour. The patient may be normotensive, the only clues being an abnormal glucose tolerance test and symptoms of congestive cardiac failure, associated with high concentrations of circulating and urinary catecholamines (Baker et al., 1972; Garcia and Jennings, 1972).

Phaeochromocytoma of the bladder is rare but unmistakable – once the diagnosis is considered. Apart from local signs of haematuria and dysuria, it is characterized by the appearance of pharmacological signs of catecholamine excess after micturition.

24.5.1.9. Phaeochromocytoma in association with other disorders

The association of phaeochromocytoma with certain diseases of apparently unrelated aetiology is well documented. For instance, the incidence of medullary carcinoma of the thyroid, perhaps associated with circumoral skin neurofibromata (Sipple's syndrome) is 10 times greater in patients with phaeochromocytoma, and these cases show a pronounced familial incidence (Williams, 1965). Phaeochromocytoma may also be associated with certain other carcinomas, e.g. renal carcinoma, ovarian cystadenoma, metastasizing schwannoma of the mediastinum and von Hippel–Lindau's disease (haemangioblastoma of various sites) (Sharp and Platt, 1971).

About 8% of phaeochromocytomas, it has been claimed, occur in association with von Recklinghausen's disease – multiple neurofibromatosis (Hermann and Mornex, 1964). This association prompted the suggestion that meningioma may also secrete catecholamines (Scott, 1974); however, Gabriel and Harrison (1974), who reported a case of this kind, ascribed the overproduction of catecholamines to a secondary effect of raised intracranial pressure from the tumour.

24.5.1.10. Cushing's syndrome associated with phaeochromocytoma

The close anatomical and functional relationship between adrenal cortex and medulla suggests that abnormalities in one may affect the other. Such interactions have indeed been described but are rare. In general, steroid excretion is normal in phaeochromocytoma (Hermann and Mornex, 1964) and the excretion of catecholamines and their metabolites is unaltered in Cushing's syndrome, a condition characterized by corticosteroid hypersecretion. Nevertheless, the association of adrenal cortical hyperplasia with Cushing's syndrome and a medullary tumour secreting catecholamines has occasionally been recognized. Thus the patient described by Meloni et al. (1966) had sustained hypertension and excreted about twice the normal daily amount of total metadrenalines, these values returning to normal when the tumour was removed. In another case (Walters et al., 1962), paroxysmal hypertension and other symptoms of phaeochromocytoma were associated with widespread abdominal tumour metastases. The tumour tissue contained catecholamines (200 μg/g) and there was an associated 2- or 3-fold increase of urinary excretion of catecholamine and 4-hydroxy-3-methoxymandelic acid. Chromaffin granules could not be seen and histologically, the appearance was that of an adrenal cortical tumour. The 17-hydroxycorticoid output was about double. Evidence of active catecholamine secretion from this neoplasm is only indirect and the possibility of a mixed tumour cannot be excluded.

Apart from a known association with phaeochromocytoma (Hermann and Mornex, 1964), Cushing's syndrome may also occur with other neurogenic tumours. Kogut and

Donnell (1961) recorded a case of particular interest in which the syndrome was associated with renal ganglioneuroblastoma without adrenal hyperplasia. Urinary excretion of 17-oxogenic steroids, aldosterone and 4-hydroxy-3-methoxymandelic acid were increased by 4 to 10 times their normal values.

The reason why Cushing's syndrome is occasionally associated with neurogenic tumours is still uncertain although there is a considerable literature on this theme.

24.5.1.11. Adrenal medullary hyperplasia

Over many years, reports have appeared suggesting that symptoms of phaeochromocytoma may develop from hyperplasia of the adrenal medulla, just as Cushing's syndrome may result from hyperplasia of the adrenal cortex. Characteristically, a catecholamine-secreting tumour could not be found at operation or autopsy although clinical, biochemical and pharmacological data had strongly suggested its presence (Carney et al., 1975). Fresh light has now been shed on at least some of these puzzling cases, in the form of convincing evidence for the existence of adrenal medullary hyperplasia as a distinct clinicopathological entity (Visser and Axt, 1975). The patient in question was hypertensive although urinary 4-hydroxy-3-methoxymandelic acid excretion was initially normal and 17-hydroxy- and 17-oxo-steroid outputs were only slightly increased. A complex progression of cardiovascular disasters followed, culminating in a considerably raised output of urinary 4-hydroxy-3-methoxymandelic acid, and a diagnosis of phaeochromocytoma was made. Operation was not feasible and the patient died. At autopsy no tumour could be traced, after extensive search; however, both adrenals were enlarged, containing about twice the normal amount of medullary tissue.

24.5.2. Neuroblastoma group of tumours

24.5.2.1. Occurrence

Neuroblastoma occurs much more frequently in children than in adults, with a peak incidence in the first 2 years of life. Apart from leukaemia and cerebral tumour, it is the commonest neoplasm of childhood, about one case being observed in 10,000 live births. Neuroblastoma is slightly more common in boys than in girls. It is highly malignant, but whether treated or not, survival is more likely if the disease manifests itself in the first year of life. The tumour tends to regress more often than any other human neoplasm, about 5% of cases in children under 2 years resolving spontaneously, suggesting the presence of an immune defence mechanism (Voorhess, 1974). An initially low urinary excretion of homovanillic acid and a rapid return of catecholamine metabolism to normal after therapy, have also been reported to be associated with a better prognosis (Gitlow et al., 1973). Girls tend to survive longer than boys, perhaps because the chances of tumour maturation to the rare but benign ganglioneuroma are greater: ganglioneuroma is more commonly found in girls. A fatal termination is unlikely in children with neuroblastoma who survive more than 2 years after diagnosis (Kinnier Wilson and Draper, 1974). There has been some suggestion that the disease is familial (Voorhess, 1974), although a survey of 2000 patients did not produce any convincing evidence on this point

(Miller et al., 1968). In about two-thirds of the cases in the literature, primary tumours have arisen in the abdomen, divided in origin about equally between adrenal medulla and other sympathetic tissue. The remainder have presented in thoracic or cervical regions of the lymphatic chain and very occasionally in the skull. Patients with neoplasms apparently arising in the neck or thorax tend to have a better prognosis than those whose tumours have an abdominal origin. Skin or liver metastases tend to be favourable prognostic factors even when bone marrow is also involved. The survival rate is extremely low, however, when bone metastases are present (Marsden and Steward, 1968).

24.5.2.2. Clinical features

The diagnosis of tumours in this group by clinical acumen alone is as difficult as for phaeochromocytoma. The symptoms and signs of neuroblastoma vary widely and are often non-specific, e.g. fever, anaemia, weight loss, bone and joint pain, nausea, vomiting and increased sweating. These are often slight until the neoplasm has grown and metastasized extensively. Thus, in about one-third of cases, 1 to 3 months elapse between presenting feature and start of treatment (Kinnier Wilson and Draper, 1974). Abdominal distension, either from primary tumour or secondary deposits in the liver or elsewhere, is usually the first pointer to the disease. Severe diarrhoea may be present, particularly in patients with ganglioneuroma (Smellie and Sandler, 1961; von Studnitz et al., 1963) and these patients may form a well defined subgroup with a presentation not dissimilar to that of coeliac disease (Rosenstein and Engelman, 1963). Hypertension is much less common in neuroblastoma than in phaeochromocytoma. Other features more characteristic of phaeochromocytoma are occasionally present (Montgomery and Welbourn, 1975).

24.5.2.3. Catecholamine metabolism in tumour tissue

24.5.2.3.1. Biosynthesis. There have been fewer studies on catecholamine biosynthetic enzymes in tumours of the neuroblastoma group than in phaeochromocytoma. 3,4-Dihydroxyphenylalanine decarboxylase, for example, does not seem to have been demonstrated. Tyrosine hydroxylase activity is of a similar order to that found in phaeochromocytoma but the enzyme differs in being sensitive to catecholamine inhibition (section 24.5.1.4.1). However, the concentration of noradrenaline in neuroblastoma tumour tissue is usually low compared with phaeochromocytoma (Hinterberger and Bartholomew, 1969; Voorhess, 1974) – too small, in practice, to inhibit tyrosine hydroxylase significantly. The substrate and co-factor requirements of the neuroblastoma enzyme are similar to those of the normal adrenal enzyme (Imashuku et al., 1972). The low tumour catecholamine concentration results from low storage capacity, even though turnover rate is rapid (Käser, 1966). A finding of dopamine and noradrenaline points to the presence of both 3,4-dihydroxyphenylalanine decarboxylase and dopamine-β-hydroxylase in these tumours (Hinterberger and Bartholomew, 1969; Voorhess, 1974). Dopamine-β-hydroxylase has also been demonstrated more directly by the ability of tumour tissue preparations to form noradrenaline and dopamine, although its activity tends to be lower than that of the phaeochromocytoma enzyme (Goldstein et al., 1968a). Information on the presence of phenylethanolamine-*N*-methyltransferase in neuroblastoma tissue is scanty, although von Studnitz (1969) claims to have identified it. Even so, the low concentration of adrenaline in these tumours (Gjessing, 1964; Voorhess, 1974) suggests that activity is very low. If it were an adrenal-type enzyme, it seems unlikely that sufficient glucocorticoid would be available to activate the enzyme.

24.5.2.3.2. Metabolism. In neuroblastoma, there is a paradoxical absence of any severe degree of hypertension; nor are other features of catecholamine overproduction present. The relatively low tumour concentration of noradrenaline (Hinterberger and Bartholomew, 1969; Voorhess, 1974) despite evidence of high production, strongly suggests that most of the amine is metabolized and pharmacologically inactivated within the tumour before reaching the circulation. In support of this thesis is the observation that neural crest tumours in tissue culture readily metabolize noradrenaline to the sulphate conjugate of normetadrenaline.

The formation of this metabolite points to the presence of catechol-*O*-methyltransferase and phenol sulphotransferase in tumour explants. Normetadrenaline has also been identified in neuroblastoma (Page and Jacoby, 1964) and ganglioneuroma (Rosenthal et al., 1969) tumour tissue. The presence of monoamine oxidase and catechol-*O*-methyltransferase has been demonstrated directly in neuroblastoma tissue (Amar-Costesec et al., 1965; Bohuon et al., 1966b).

Because 4-hydroxy-3-methoxymandelic acid is often excreted in greatly increased amount in the urine of patients with neuroblastoma (Hinterberger and Bartholomew, 1969; Gitlow et al., 1970a; Voorhess, 1974), it is not unreasonable to suppose that it is elaborated in tumour tissue. However, there is now evidence to suggest that these tumours secrete 4-hydroxy-3-methoxyphenylglycol rather than 4-hydroxy-3-methoxymandelic acid; this glycol is the main metabolite of noradrenaline in tumour tissue culture, whereas 4-hydroxy-3-methoxymandelic acid generation is minimal (La Brosse, 1970). It seems likely that anaerobic conditions in tumour tissue favour reduction of the intermediate aldehyde deriving from the oxidative deamination of normetadrenaline, so that 4-hydroxy-3-methoxyphenylglycol results. In addition, enzyme studies on both neuroblastoma tumour tissue and cells in culture suggest that aldehyde dehydrogenase activity there is very low (Goldstein et al., 1968b).

Because considerable amounts of urinary 4-hydroxy-3-methoxymandelic acid are often excreted in neuroblastoma, it would appear that 4-hydroxy-3-methoxyphenylglycol or its precursor aldehyde are transformed to 4-hydroxy-3-methoxymandelic acid extra-tumourally, perhaps in liver and kidney (La Brosse, 1970). This conclusion was also reached by Bohuon et al. (1966a) who found that, whereas the concentration of 4-hydroxy-3-methoxymandelic acid is usually greater than that of 4-hydroxy-3-methoxyphenylglycol in neuroblastoma urine, the reverse is usually true for blood. In further support, La Brosse (1970) directly demonstrated the conversion of tritiated 4-hydroxy-3-methoxyphenylglycol into 4-hydroxy-3-methoxymandelic acid in patients with neuroblastoma.

Neuroblastoma tumour tissue has low but approximately equal concentrations of noradrenaline and dopamine; although dopamine concentration in phaeochromocytoma is of a similar order, that of noradrenaline is very high (Hinterberger and Bartholomew, 1969).

Apart from dopamine overproduction, some patients with neuroblastoma excrete 3,4-dihydroxyphenylalanine, and a range of metabolites other than those derived from dopamine, e.g. the 3-*O*-methyl derivative and the transamination metabolites, 4-hydroxy-

3-methoxyphenylpyruvic acid and 4-hydroxy-3-methoxyphenyllactic acid (von Studnitz et al., 1963; Gjessing, 1964). It is possible that the 3,4-dihydroxyphenylalanine-secreting variant is deficient in 3,4-dihydroxyphenylalanine decarboxylase. Tumour catecholamines and metabolites which are characteristic of typical phaeochromocytoma are shown in Table 24.2 in comparison with neuroblastoma.

There are few data concerning the subcellular distribution of catecholamines in neuroblastoma tissue. Winkler and Smith (1972) point out that the undifferentiated neuroblastoma cells do not appear to contain storage granules; as dopamine-β-hydroxylase is normally located in these bodies, it is surprising that the tumours are able to synthesize noradrenaline at all. They suggest that more highly developed cells may also be present which undertake this task or, alternatively, that dopamine-β-hydroxylase can exist in cells unassociated with noradrenaline granules. However, in histologically more differentiated tissue, "secretory" granules have been described (Winkler and Smith, 1972), using combined biochemical, immunological and electron microscopic studies; other workers suggest that some form of catecholamine-storing organelle is indeed present in neuroblastoma, noradrenaline storage resembling that of normal sympathetic tissue (Hörtnagl et al., 1972).

24.5.2.4. Urinary catecholamine and metabolite output in the neuroblastoma tumour group

Biochemically, the neuroblastoma group of tumours differs most dramatically from phaeochromocytoma by the overproduction of dopamine (Page and Jacoby, 1964; Hinterberger and Bartholomew, 1969) and sometimes of 3,4-dihydroxyphenylalanine (Sourkes et al., 1963; Page and Jacoby, 1964), with its associated 3-*O*-methylated derivative, 4-hydroxy-3-methoxyphenylalanine (Greenberg and Gardner, 1960). Transamination

TABLE 24.2.

TUMOUR CATECHOLAMINES AND METABOLITES

Phaeochromocytoma		Other neural tumours
Benign	Malignant (about 1 in 10)	Neuroblastoma, Ganglioneuroblastoma, Ganglioneuroma
High concentration of Noradrenaline Adrenaline (in about 40% in cases) Dopamine (occasionally)	High concentration of Noradrenaline Adrenaline (less frequently than in benign phaeochromocytoma) Dopamine (fairly often)	Low concentration compared with phaeochromocytoma of Noradrenaline Adrenaline (usually minimal) High concentration of Dopamine
Low concentration of Noradrenaline and adrenaline metabolites (usually)	Higher concentration of Noradrenaline and adrenaline metabolites (usually)	High concentration of Noradrenaline and dopamine precursors and metabolites.

metabolites, 4-hydroxy-3-methoxyphenylpyruvic acid (Gjessing and Borud, 1965) and 4-hydroxy-3-methoxyphenyllactic acid (Gjessing, 1964; Gjessing and Borud, 1965) have also been noted in the urine, together with small amounts of dihydroxyphenylpyruvic acid (Gjessing and Borud, 1965). The pattern of urinary excretion commonly observed in phaeochromocytoma is compared in Table 24.3 with that often found in tumours of the neuroblastoma group.

The central biochemical finding, the raised excretion of dopamine, is accompanied by a high urinary excretion of its main metabolites, homovanillic acid (Gjessing, 1964; Hinterberger and Bartholomew, 1969; Gitlow et al., 1970a), 3,4-dihydroxyphenylacetic acid (Gjessing, 1964) and 4-hydroxy-3-methoxyphenylethanol (Gjessing, 1964).

There may be a raised excretion of noradrenaline and occasionally of adrenaline (Page and Jacoby, 1964; Marsden and Steward, 1968; Hinterberger and Bartholomew, 1969), although not in every patient (Sourkes et al., 1963; Marsden and Steward, 1968). The urinary concentration of β-hydroxylated degradation products of noradrenaline is also often considerably increased. Large amounts of 4-hydroxy-3-methoxymandelic acid are likely to be present in neuroblastoma (Gjessing, 1964; Marsden and Steward, 1968; Hinterberger and Bartholomew, 1969; Gitlow et al., 1970a), ganglioneuroblastoma and ganglioneuroma (Gjessing, 1964; Hinterberger and Bartholomew, 1969; Marsden and Steward, 1968). Likewise, there are large increases in excretion of 4-hydroxy-3-methoxyphenylglycol (Gjessing, 1964; Gitlow et al., 1970a) and normetadrenaline (Gjessing, 1964; Marsden and Steward, 1968; Gitlow et al., 1970a). Although 4-hydroxy-3-methoxymandelic acid and homovanillic acid excretions both tend to be raised, to a more consistent degree than other catecholamine metabolites in neuroblastoma, and to considerably higher values than in phaeochromocytoma, cases may occur where 4-hydroxy-3-methoxymandelic acid excretion is normal (Hinterberger and Bartholomew, 1969; Gitlow et al., 1970a).

Biochemically active ganglioneuromas produce a similar metabolite pattern to that of neuroblastoma (Sankoff and Sourkes, 1963); it should be noted that the incidence of non-secreting ganglioneuroma is considerably higher than that of non-secreting ganglioneuroblastoma and neuroblastoma (Käser, 1966). Perhaps the main aim in documenting the minutiae of the processes described is to make finer distinctions in tumour classification possible which can, in turn, be used as guides to prognosis and perhaps, to treatment. Thus one should take note, for instance, of the rise in tyramine output found in some neuroblastoma patients (von Studnitz et al., 1963; Hinterberger and Bartholomew, 1969), suggesting that larger concentrations of tyrosine are trapped by the tumour tissue than can be converted completely into 3,4-dihydroxyphenylalanine. *N*-Acetyltyramine has similarly been detected in the urine of affected subjects (Hinterberger and Bartholomew, 1969), presumably indicating that tyramine production was also raised in these cases. Other evidence of *N*-acetylation is on record: *N*-acetyldopamine (Hanson and von Studnitz, 1965), *N*-acetylnoradrenaline (Herrlich and Sekeris, 1964), *N*-acetylnormetadrenaline and *N*-acetylmetadrenaline (Borud and Gjessing, 1970) have all been identified in neuroblastoma urine. Gjessing (1964) detected such large amounts of vanillic acid in some of these patients that it was unlikely to be dietary in origin. The present authors have investigated a similar case (unpublished observation) and conclude that vanillic acid is derived, at least in part, from tumour catecholamine (see Dirscherl and Thomas, 1966).

TABLE 24.3.

PATTERNS OF URINARY EXCRETION OF MONOAMINES AND THEIR METABOLITES

Abbreviations: 3,4-DHPPA = 3,4-dihydroxyphenylpyruvic acid; DOPA = 3,4-dihydroxyphenylalanine; DOPAC = 3,4-dihydroxyphenylacetic acid; 3OMeDOPA = 4-hydroxy-3-methoxyphenylalanine; HMPE = 4-hydroxy-3-methoxyphenylethanol; HMPG = 4-hydroxy-3-methoxyphenylglycol; *p*-HPLA = *p*-hydroxyphenyllactic acid; MA = metadrenaline; MT = 3-methoxytyramine; *N*-Ac-DA = *N*-acetyldopamine; VA = vanillic acid; VLA = 4-hydroxy-3-methoxyphenyllactic acid; VMA = 4-hydroxy-3-methoxymandelic acid; VPA = 4-hydroxy-3-methoxyphenylpyruvic acid; and in footnote, p. 1219.

Phaeochromocytoma		Other neural tumours
Benign	Malignant (about 1 in 10)	Neuroblastoma, Ganglioneuroblastoma, Ganglioneuroma
Raised excretion of Noradrenaline Adrenaline (in about 40% of cases)	Raised excretion of Noradrenaline Adrenaline (less often than in benign phaeochromocytoma) Dopamine (more often than in benign phaeochromocytoma)	Low excretion (compared with phaeochromocytoma) of Noradrenaline Adrenaline Considerably raised excretion of Dopamine (often)
Raised excretion of Noradrenaline and adrenaline metabolites (MA, VMA, HMPG)	Raised excretion (often higher than in benign phaeochromocytoma) of Noradrenaline and adrenaline metabolites (MA, VMA, HMPG)	Raised excretion (often very high) of Noradrenaline metabolites (VMA and HMPG particularly, usually proportionally less MA)
	When dopamine secreted by the tumour, raised excretion of Dopamine metabolites (HVA, DOPAC MT, and also minor metabolites, VA, *p*-HPLA, *N*-Ac-DA)	Markedly raised excretion of Dopamine metabolites (HVA, DOPAC, MT and also minor metabolites, DOPA, 3OMeDOPA, *N*-Ac-DA, VPA, VLA, *p*-HPLA, 3,4-DHPPA, HMPE, VA).

24.5.2.5. Cystathionine excretion in neuroblastoma

An increased urinary excretion of cystathionine has been found in patients with neuroblastoma (Geiser and Efron, 1968), caused perhaps by pyridoxine deficiency (Gjessing, 1968; von Studnitz, 1970) with which it has been linked in certain other human disease states. Although congenital cystathioninuria is not due directly to pyridoxine deficiency, cystathionine excretion is diminished on giving pyridoxine (Gjessing, 1968). Cystathioninuria is more pronounced in younger patients with neuroblastoma, a finding related perhaps to the increased pyridoxine requirements of infancy.

Whilst a correlation was originally claimed between cystathioninuria and degree of tumour malignancy (Gjessing, 1968), this now seems unlikely (Geiser and Efron, 1968; von Studnitz, 1970). Nor does cystathionine appear in the urine as early in the disease as was once thought (von Studnitz, 1970). Nevertheless, tests for the aminoacid may provide useful diagnostic confirmation (Geiser and Efron, 1968), particularly as raised excretions of 4-hydroxy-3-methoxymandelic acid and cystathionine do not always coincide. Cystathioninuria also occurs in primary liver tumour which must therefore be considered in the differential diagnosis (Gjessing and Mauritzen, 1965).

24.5.3. Catecholamine-secreting tumours in pregnancy

The serious prognosis of phaeochromocytoma during pregnancy and the problems associated with its diagnosis warrant its selection as a topic for special discussion. Records show (Hermann and Mornex, 1964) that, until the early 1960s, this complication of pregnancy carried a mortality of about 50% in both mothers and offspring. However, with the recent improvement in diagnostic procedures, the rate has dropped to about 10% (Sprague et al., 1972). Even though catecholamines appear to cross the placental barrier without special difficulty (Thiery et al., 1967), high concentrations perfusing the foetus still seem to be compatible with life, provided that the tumour is dealt with as expeditiously as possible. This finding contrasts with the situation in the carcinoid syndrome which, from the scanty evidence available, seems to be incompatible with foetal survival (Southgate and Sandler, 1968). The clinical features of phaeochromocytoma in pregnant women are as varied as in the non-pregnant. Perhaps headaches and sweating are more common; otherwise, there is nothing to distinguish the condition during gestation. In fact, diagnosis is rendered more difficult by the possible confusion with pre-eclampsia, which probably occurs in something over 5% of a pregnant population. Many of its clinical features such as sustained hypertension, headache, tachycardia, proteinuria, nausea and vomiting, may overlap with those encountered in phaeochromocytoma. If hypertension is paroxysmal, or sustained but with minimal proteinuria or oedema, there is a greater likelihood of this, admittedly rare, secreting tumour being present. Despite its rarity, however, the otherwise high mortality and the likelihood of cure once a diagnosis is reached, make it worth bearing in mind. Thus, appropriate chemical tests must be used unsparingly if there is a high index of suspicion; pharmacological tests, with their attendant dangers, are quite unacceptable in a gravid patient.

The possibility of congenital neuroblastoma in the foetus is a potential source of error in diagnosis. Catecholamines from the foetus presumably enter the maternal circulation and may produce symptoms in the mother during the last two months of pregnancy similar to those observed in phaeochromocytoma. Six cases are on record of infants from mothers so affected born with raised urinary excretions of 4-hydroxy-3-methoxymandelic acid, 4-hydroxy-3-methoxyphenylglycol and homovanillic acid (Voûte et al., 1970); unfortunately neither catecholamines nor their metabolites were measured in the mothers. It was with this eventuality in mind, therefore, that Zambotti et al. (1975) devised their procedure for the assay of 4-hydroxy-3-methoxyphenylglycol in amniotic fluid obtained by amniocentesis. This approach to the prenatal diagnosis of neuroblastoma must obviously assume greater importance in the future.

From the limited data available, there is no suggestion of any difference between the urinary metabolite pattern of phaeochromocytoma in pregnant compared with non-pregnant subjects. Whilst plasma catecholamine concentrations are usually elevated, it should be borne in mind that plasma catecholamine rises have been claimed during normal pregnancy; Stone et al. (1960) noted a 3-fold increase in adrenaline concentration during the second trimester. However, in severe pre-eclampsia, plasma catecholamine concentrations did not differ from those of normal pregnancy (Swartz et al., 1963). Urinary catecholamine output in the third trimester was similar to that of normal non-pregnant subjects (Zuspan et al., 1967). Noradrenaline output may be marginally raised in toxaemia (Swartz et al., 1963) but the evidence is somewhat slender. A significant rise in output of noradrenaline and adrenaline does occur during the 24 hours following delivery (Zuspan et al., 1967; Zuspan, 1970). 4-Hydroxy-3-methoxymandelic acid and homovanillic acid excretion values are constant throughout pregnancy and do not differ significantly from those of the normal subject, although there may be an increase in urinary 4-hydroxy-3-methoxymandelic acid and serum dopamine-β-hydroxylase just before vaginal delivery (Hashimoto et al., 1974). Thus, on balance, the same criteria may be applied when assessing the results of biochemical tests for phaeochromocytoma in pregnancy as in the non-gravid subject.

24.5.4. Paragangliomas

Although extremely rare, certain catecholamine-secreting tumours are known which arise embryonically from cells of neural origin, but differ from phaeochromocytoma and tumours of the neuroblastoma group in developing from non-chromaffin paraganglionic sites. Those best known derive from the chemoreceptor organs, the carotid and aortic bodies and the glomus jugulare. However, these tumours may not always be entirely devoid of chromaffin cells. A positive chromaffin reaction, for example, was noted in a paraganglioma of the carotid body (Glenner et al., 1962). This tumour elaborated noradrenaline, as did that of Berdal et al. (1962) where a trace of adrenaline was also present. However, only a small proportion of the total are catecholamine-secreting. Tumours of the glomus jugulare may also, on rare occasions, produce considerable amounts of noradrenaline (Tiedge et al., 1964; Parkinson, 1969). Where there is noradrenaline overproduction, diagnostic concentrations of 4-hydroxy-3-methoxymandelic acid are, of course, usually present in the urine. Paragangliomas may be malignant; one such tumour located in the mediastinum was dopamine-secreting, with greatly increased amounts of homovanillic acid present in the urine (Enquist et al., 1974).

24.6. OTHER CONDITIONS ASSOCIATED WITH ABNORMAL CATECHOLAMINE PRODUCTION

24.6.1. Familial dysautonomia

Familial dysautonomia (Riley–Day syndrome) is a rare congenital disorder almost exclusively confined to children of Eastern European Jewish descent. The clinical features are largely those of autonomic dysfunction including postural hypotension, labile hypertension, excessive sweating, etc., although other stigmata of the disease such as lack of pain sensitivity, motor inco-ordination and absence of fungiform papillae of the tongue stem from disorders of other systems.

Certain abnormalities in the urinary excretion pattern of catecholamines and their metabolites appear to be present. Noradrenaline output is reduced but adrenaline excretion is normal. 4-Hydroxy-3-methoxymandelic acid excretion is reduced to a greater extent in homozygotes than heterozygotes and, according to one report, homovanillic acid excretion is raised (Gitlow et al., 1970b) although another (Moses et al., 1967) found it to be normal. These changes can most easily be detected by calculating the 4-hydroxy-3-methoxymandelic acid/homovanillic acid ratio, or better, the 4-hydroxy-3-methoxymandelic acid plus 4-hydroxy-3-methoxyphenylglycol/homovanillic acid ratio, since 4-hydroxy-3-methoxyphenylglycol output, like that of 4-hydroxy-3-methoxymandelic acid, is also decreased (Gitlow et al., 1970b). Total metadrenaline excretion appears to be normal (Gitlow et al., 1970b). The possibility of a defect in catecholamine metabolism suggested by these changes in excretory pattern led to the investigation of serum dopamine-β-hydroxylase activity. However, although mean activity was significantly lower in affected adults, younger patients with dysautonomia did not differ from controls. Moreover, the overall lack of correlation between symptomatology and enzyme activity indicates that the measurement is of little value diagnostically (Freedman et al., 1975). It may be that the catecholamine deficit stems from a depletion of postganglionic sympathetic neurones, or from some dysfunction of the granular vesicle. Alternatively, there may be a failure of the mechanism responsible for the release of amine from adrenal medulla (Pearson et al., 1974).

24.6.2. Hypertension

Although hypertension is the most common clinical feature of phaeochromocytoma, it hardly needs saying that in most patients, this sign derives from other causes. Nevertheless, despite biochemical aids, confusion may occasionally arise; small but significant abnormalities in plasma concentration and urinary excretion of catecholamine may be present in some patients with essential hypertension, although the data are conflicting. Most hypertensives excrete normal (or perhaps marginally increased) quantities of noradrenaline, particularly in the resting state. However, a minority (15 to 20%) excrete significantly increased amounts of amine. Low, normal and high urinary excretions of 4-hydroxy-3-methoxymandelic acid have been claimed, while data on metadrenaline excretion are equally conflicting (Brunjes, 1964; Stott and Robinson, 1967b). A more consistent feature, perhaps, may be an elevation in the ratio of metadrenalines to 4-hydroxy-3-methoxymandelic acid (Brunjes, 1964). The rate of increase of urinary catecholamine excretion on mild exercise is greater in the hypertensive and the absolute output of 4-hydroxy-3-methoxymandelic acid higher (Inoue et al., 1968). Differences have been recorded in urinary excretion of noradrenaline and the plasma concentration in certain hypertensive subgroups (Kuchel et al., 1973). Tilting seems to produce a smaller increase in plasma noradrenaline in hypertensives than normals (Brunjes, 1964), but resting and fasting concentrations of total plasma catecholamines are reported to be almost twice the values of a control population in a group with essential hypertension (Engelman et al., 1970). Plasma dopamine-β-hydroxylase measured by immunoassay and plasma noradrenaline concentration appear to correlate with blood pressure in the resting subject (Louis et al., 1974), but some investigators were unable to find a correlation when dopamine-β-hydroxylase was measured on the basis of enzyme activity (Ogihara et al., 1975). Dopamine-β-hydroxylase determination by immunoassay may thus provide a more sensitive index of sympathetic activity than measurement of enzymic action as such (Louis et al., 1974). However, there is disagreement on this point; other workers claim good correlation between enzymatic and immunological activity of human dopamine-β-hydroxylase, and attribute the disagreement to the use of an immunological assay based on antigen derived from heterologous bovine dopamine-β-hydroxylase rather than from the human enzyme (Stone, 1975). The finding that activity is related to age is another complicating factor which may help to explain these conflicting results (Ogihara et al., 1975).

Dopamine-β-hydroxylase activity has been variously reported as increased or unaltered in essential hypertension (see Stone, 1975). The reported decrease in ratio of urinary dopamine to noradrenaline may stem from an increase in dopamine-β-hydroxylase activity, although it might equally reflect a renal defect (Cuche et al„ 1974), or possibly a local intra-renal increase in dopamine metabolism, since a significant rise in urinary homovanillic acid has been noted in hypertensive subjects compared with normotensives, particularly in those with labile hypertension (Cuche et al., 1975). Most available evidence points, on balance, to a relationship between plasma dopamine-β-hydroxylase activity and hypertension; indeed, some investigators consider the association to be a reliable diagnostic aid, given correct conditions for the enzyme assay (Stone, 1975).

Thus essential hypertension is associated with an elevation in circulating catecholamines and, sometimes, with an increase in the urinary catecholamine excretion. There appear, too, to be changes in plasma dopamine-β-hydroxylase, but whether they are primary or secondary is not known at the present time.

24.6.3. Myocardial infarction

Acute myocardial infarction is accompanied by augmented sympathetic activity and frequently by a rise in urinary excretion and plasma catecholamine concentration. The increases in urinary output are most apparent on the first day after infarction; values have usually returned to normal by the fifth. A direct relationship between degree of elevation and severity of attack is often observed. Cases with a fatal outcome tend to have a higher urinary noradrenaline output and they may also manifest with a raised dopamine excretion (Sznajderman et al., 1974). Urinary noradrenaline excretion may be increased by as much as 8-fold, with up to 4 times the normal output of adrenaline. There is considerable variation, however. Occasionally, the return to normal values can take as long as 3 weeks and may be slower for noradrenaline than for adrenaline (Valori et al., 1967). Heavy smokers with acute myocardial infarction excrete about twice the amount of catecholamine put out by non-smokers with the same disease (Lewis and Boudoulas, 1974). Severe heart failure in infants may also have pronounced effects on catecholamine biochemistry, with 2-fold increases of 4-hydroxy-3-methoxymandelic acid and total metadrenaline output having been reported (Lees, 1966).

Proportionally greater changes in catecholamine concentration are found in plasma than in urine following acute myocardial infarction. Thus it is conceivable that elevated levels of binding protein (Powis, 1975) are present, although this point has never been investigated. Plasma noradrenaline rises are larger than those of adrenaline – up to 16 times the resting level; a 5-fold increase of adrenaline excretion has been recorded (Griffiths and Leung, 1971). The factors responsible for these increases are unknown. The role of the sharp rise in dopamine excretion in this disease is also obscure.

24.6.4. Increased catecholamine production in the absence of secreting tumour

Certain other conditions are known which are not associated with a catecholamine-secreting tumour, but in which the urinary excretion of catecholamines or their metabolites is raised. Hypoxia in children is one example, responsible, perhaps, for the raised plasma noradrenaline and adrenaline concentrations of premature babies (Lees, 1966), and – somewhat more tenuously – for the raised urinary 4-hydroxy-3-methoxymandelic acid excretion of anaemic children (Matsaniotis et al., 1968a). Chronic hypoxia in adults with advanced tuberculosis appears to result in increased 4-hydroxy-3-methoxymandelic acid excretion (Vaccarezza and Ruiz, 1969), as does diabetic ketosis (Assan et al., 1973), in which raised plasma catecholamine concentrations also occur.

Catecholamine excretion appears to be moderately raised in cystic fibrosis (Barbero and Braddock, 1967) although the mechanism is unknown. Changes of this type reported in children with spina bifida (McKibbin et al., 1969) have, however, been disputed (Duckworth et al., 1973). Decreased urinary catecholamine excretion has been noted in children with collagen diseases (Matsaniotis et al., 1968b) although output of 3,4-dihydroxyphenylalanine and its transaminated metabolites was claimed to be raised. Leucine-sensitive hypoglycaemia may be associated with decreased urinary adrenaline excretion (Kinsbourne and Woolf, 1959).

Changes in the urinary excretion of catecholamines and their metabolites have been described in manic–depressive psychosis, but the matter is controversial. 4-Hydroxy-3-methoxymandelic acid excretion may decrease in some depressives but rise several-fold in the manic phase according to Campanini et al. (1970), although in the depressed patients studied by Maas et al. (1973), 4-hydroxy-3-methoxymandelic acid excretion was found to be normal. Some authors hold that 4-hydroxy-3-methoxyphenylglycol excretion drops in severely depressed patients and increases somewhat in mania (Maas et al., 1973). It has been suggested that urinary excretion of 4-hydroxy-3-methoxyphenylglycol, particularly of its sulphate conjugate, reflects noradrenaline turnover in the brain to a greater extent than the periphery, although many consider the evidence to be less than convincing (Bareggi et al., 1974).

Parkinsonism is characterized by a gross depletion of striatal dopamine, although the decrease in urinary dopamine output is equivocal and not accompanied by any abnormaility in the excretion of homovanillic acid or other acidic or alcoholic catecholamine metabolite (Sandler, 1972a). Noradrenaline, adrenaline and 4-hydroxy-3-methoxymandelic acid excretions are likewise unaltered in Huntington's chorea (McNamee et al., 1971).

24.6.5. Malignant melanoma

Malignant melanoma is sometimes accompanied by an increased urinary output of 3,4-dihydroxyphenylalanine and its metabolites (Voorhess, 1970; Hinterberger et al., 1972), particularly when widespread metastases have supervened. The tumours arise from melanin-producing cells of neural crest origin and are thus related embryologically to neuroblastoma and phaeochromocytoma. Because considerable numbers of affected patients have normal 3,4-dihydroxyphenylalanine excretion, chemical tests for it and its metabolites are not as valuable as in the diagnosis of neuroblastoma and phaeochromocytoma. When 3,4-dihydroxyphenylalanine production is increased, however, periodic urinary estimations will assist in monitoring the course of the disease (Voorhess, 1970). Melanin and catecholamine overproduction may occur together in a rare tumour of the jaw which appears in the first few months of life. Doubts about its cellular origin have made for difficulties in classification. However, the finding of a substantial elevation of urinary 4-hydroxy-3-methoxymandelic acid in an affected infant, which fell to normal after tumour extirpation, led to the suggestion that these tumours probably arise embryologically from neural crest tissue; thus the name melanotic neuroectodermal tumour of infancy was proposed (Borello and Gorlin, 1966).

24.7. BIOCHEMICAL DIAGNOSIS OF CATECHOLAMINE-SECRETING TUMOURS

The chemical assay of plasma or urinary catecholamines and their metabolites is a more reliable diagnostic guide to phaeochromocytoma than radiological or pharmacological tests, and is free from their inherent dangers. Whatever other pointers are available, the diagnosis should always be checked biochemically before undertaking surgery.

The choice of metabolite and suitable assay procedure may not be as easy as for the biochemical diagnosis of carcinoid disease (section 24.9). The relevant tests vary in complexity and it is not always practicable or necessary for less specialized or well-equipped laboratories to undertake the full range.

24.7.1. Test selection

It is usually necessary to measure one or two metabolites only to arrive at a reliable diagnosis. When catecholamine-secreting tumours of the neuroblastoma group are suspected, urinary 4-hydroxy-3-methoxymandelic acid and homovanillic acid assays will, in general, suffice. However, if the diagnosis remains in doubt, these measurements should be supplemented by urinary dopamine estimation. Although measurement of total urinary 4-hydroxy-3-methoxyphenylglycol excretion has also been recommended as useful diagnostically (La Brosse, 1970), in our experience, 4-hydroxy-3-methoxyphenylglycol is not increased to as great an extent or as consistently as 4-hydroxy-3-methoxymandelic acid and homovanillic acid.

Opinions differ as to which urinary constituent should be assayed for the diagnosis of phaeochromocytoma. 4-Hydroxy-3-methoxymandelic acid is measured most commonly, no doubt because of the comparative simplicity of its assay procedure. In the present authors' opinion, this advantage outweighs all disadvantages it may possess as a diagnostic aid, although this view is not universally accepted (Crout et al., 1961). Many prefer to assay total metadrenalines, even though the use of a fairly complex ion-exchange column procedure is involved. All agree that if the results of both tests are equivocal, free catecholamines should be measured. Certainly, the "signal-to-noise" ratio is higher for total metadrenaline or catecholamine assay than for 4-hydroxy-3-methoxymandelic acid, and with a small or slowly secreting tumour metadrenaline and catecholamine excretions are more likely to be increased than those of 4-hydroxy-3-methoxymandelic acid.

It is obviously preferable to measure routinely at least two metabolites, e.g. 4-hydroxy-3-methoxymandelic acid and total metadrenalines or 4-hydroxy-3-methoxymandelic acid and catecholamines; this counsel is usually impracticable however, so that the following scheme may be adopted. Carry out 4-hydroxy-3-methoxymandelic acid assay on a 24-hour urine collection. Unless the result approaches the upper limit of normal or strong clinical suspicion remains, no further action is necessary. If marginal values are obtained or compelling clinical pointers to a diagnosis of phaeochromocytoma persist, carry out 4-hydroxy-3-methoxymandelic acid assay on three further 24-hour collections. If equivocal values are still obtained, measure total metadrenalines, and perhaps differential catecholamines too, unless the metadrenaline result is clear-cut. Although it is not an essential test in the preliminary diagnosis of phaeochromocytoma, the estimation of urinary homovanillic acid in established cases may be helpful, in that raised values have been thought by some to be a guide to tumour malignancy (Robinson et al., 1964). Homovanillic acid output should always be measured in cases of suspected neuroblastoma even if the 4-hydroxy-3-methoxymandelic acid excretion is normal.

Laboratories geared to gas chromatographic techniques with electron capture detection have a choice of methods at their disposal. Here, the measurement of differential catecholamines or metadrenalines is likely to be most helpful in cases of suspected phaeochromocytoma and 4-hydroxy-3-methoxymandelic acid and homovanillic acid in diagnosis of tumours of the neuroblastoma group.

Whatever technique is employed, plasma catecholamine estimation is a difficult procedure requiring considerable expertise. It should only be undertaken by laboratories where appropriate skills and specialized equipment are available. With these provisos, it should be stated that such measurements are sometimes able to provide additional information, even when urinary tests are equivocal (Leung and Griffiths, 1974); the assay is particularly helpful when used in conjuction with vena caval sampling. By passing a catheter into the inferior vena cava and estimating catecholamine concentration in samples taken at different levels, the anatomical level of a tumour can often be pinpointed

(Winkler and Smith, 1972), and the technique can be of value in identifying multiple tumours. However, results must be interpreted with some caution since there is evidence that the catecholamine concentration at a particular anatomical site can vary considerably over a short period of time; largely for this reason, the test is of no value in children. In addition, the sampling procedure is not without risks. These considerations make the use of the test as a standard procedure impracticable.

24.7.2. Comments on assay procedures

24.7.2.1. Plasma catecholamines

It has been emphasized that plasma catecholamine estimation is difficult and exacting. The amines are labile and present only in very low concentration in normal plasma (less than 1 μg/litre). Even before the assay stage is reached, losses may occur during blood collection, plasma separation and storage. Carruthers et al., (1970) have made a detailed study of these and other factors, listing the many potential sources of error which may invalidate the result, even when the accuracy of the assay procedure itself is acceptable. Blood samples should therefore be taken as quickly as possible, and the plasma separated, frozen immediately, and stored at –20 °C. Processing should not be delayed more than a few days at most, with minimal thawing and freezing meanwhile. Samples should be thawed singly and not in batches. As venepuncture can increase catecholamine level, when serial sampling is required the blood should be withdrawn through an indwelling venous catheter. Posture (Cryer et al., 1974), time of day, relationship to the last meal, rest, exercise, stress – all may have an effect on the final value. It is desirable, therefore, to control sampling conditions rigorously although this may not always be possible; indeed it may not be critical when monitoring the often large increases in circulating catecholamines observed in phaeochromocytoma.

Fluorometric techniques have been used most widely for the differential measurement of plasma catecholamines. They are rather more protracted (Callingham, 1968; Griffiths et al., 1970; Renzini et al., 1970; Carruthers et al., 1970), but essentially similar in principle to those used for urine, which are described briefly in section 24.7.2.2. Plasma from patients on the antihypertensive drug α-methyldopa cannot be used, because it and its metabolites form interfering fluorophores. In vitro evidence (Carruthers et al., 1970) also points to the possibility of spurious fluorescence derived from plasma taken after treatment with other commonly used drugs such as promethazine and ampicillin, and after ingestion of coffee, tea or cocoa.

A different methodological approach was introduced by Engelman et al. (1970). It involves the use of a double-isotope derivative technique, in which noradrenaline or adrenaline are converted into their [^{14}C]-metadrenaline analogues by incubation with [methyl-^{14}C]*S*-adenosyl-L-methionine and catechol-*O*-methyltransferase in the presence of tracer quantities of [7-^{3}H]noradrenaline. The metadrenalines are oxidized to vanillin, which is counted by a liquid scintillation counter in the double-channel mode. Total catecholamines in the plasma specimen are calculated from the ratio of ^{3}H to ^{14}C. By separating the labelled metadrenalines on a thin-layer chromatogram before conversion into vanillin, noradrenaline and adrenaline can be measured separately (Engelman and Portnoy, 1970; Passon and Peuler, 1973; Cryer et al., 1974). In a modification of this procedure, the metadrenalines are separated electrophoretically and counted without converting them into vanillin (Siggers et al., 1970). These procedures have also been used to estimate dopamine in plasma, urine and gastric juice (Christensen, 1973; Christensen and Brandsborg, 1974). Unfortunately, radioisotopic methods take 2 to 4 days to complete, depending on the modification used; nevertheless, they have the advantage of being more specific and sensitive than fluorometric techniques (Louis and Doyle, 1971).

Gas chromatography, using the highly sensitive electron capture detector, is also potentially suitable for the determination of monoamines. The approach possesses the added advantage of the three catecholamines being measured individually in a single chromatogram. Imai et al. (1973) have described such a method: after deproteinization, the amines are isolated on alumina before elution and chromatography as trifluoracetyl derivatives. A parallel approach is employed in the present authors' laboratory (Weg, unpublished work) using mass fragmentography for extra sensitivity; however, at present, normal plasma concentrations are recorded at the lower limit of detection of the method. The prospect of improving this performance, however, seems good and it is likely that these techniques will become definitive for plasma catecholamine assay.

24.7.2.2. Urinary catecholamines

Although catecholamine assay methods, in general, tend to be complex, the higher concentrations of these compounds in urine make their estimation less demanding and more reliable than plasma procedures. Even so, urinary catecholamines are still the most difficult compounds in this diagnostic group to estimate accurately. A fluorescence screening method described by Hingerty (1957) for the semi-quantitative detection of total urinary catecholamines has been widely used. In spite of its simplicity, it cannot be recommended as it frequently gives rise to false positive reactions originating from the presence of other fluorogen compounds in the urine sample (Hingerty and MacBrinn, 1962). A quantitative procedure should therefore be used, preferably one giving individual values for noradrenaline, adrenaline and dopamine. It is usual to estimate free catecholamine output only rather than total; it can be measured more accurately and tends to provide a better index of endogenous production than measurement of the excretion of free plus conjugated amine (Crout, 1968).

For many years, fluorometric techniques were the only satisfactory methods available. In general, catecholamines are first adsorbed on to alumina or a cation-exchange resin and then eluted. They undergo oxidation and rearrangement in alkali to give fluorescent trihydroxyindole derivatives, which are measured at their characteristic activation/fluorescence wavelengths (Crout, 1961; Weil-Malherbe, 1961; Anton and Sayre, 1962; Crout, 1968). Other methods involve oxidation and condensation with ethylenediamine, to give measurable fluorophores (Weil-Malherbe, 1961; Callingham, 1968). Some of the procedures can be used to estimate dopamine (Sourkes and Murphy, 1961), in addition to noradrenaline and adrenaline; that of Anton and Sayre (1964) is specific for dopamine and 3,4-dihydroxyphenylalanine.

The many variations on this fluorometric approach that have appeared over the years are an indication that none is wholly satisfactory. Although these procedures are highly sensitive, their accuracy and precision is acceptable only if standardized experimental conditions are meticulously observed. They are also highly susceptible to error from interfering sources of fluorescence deriving from reagent impurities and other extraneous material. Reagents must therefore be of the highest purity and all glassware scrupulously cleaned. The stability of fluorescence intensity may be a problem, which can be overcome, however, by stabilizing the fluorophore with dithiothreitol and boric acid (Vaage, 1974).

It would be unwise to attempt to single out a particular fluorometric method for recommendation. Each group of users has its own preference. Quek et al. (1975) have recently assessed critically five alumina–trihydroxyindole methods and, on the basis of the information obtained, have developed what they claim to be a simple, reliable and accurate procedure.

Suitable gas chromatographic methods for urinary catecholamine assay have appeared only recently. Earlier techniques using trimethylsilyl derivatives with flame ionization detection were far too insensitive to allow accurate measurement at normal output concentrations. Electron capture detection after suitable derivatization is essential for accurate and specific differential urinary catecholamine assay. The method in current use in the present authors' laboratory (Wong et al., 1973; Weg, unpublished work) involves the preparation and isothermal gas chromatography of pentafluoropropionyl derivatives of catecholamines previously isolated and concentrated on alumina.

24.7.2.2.1. Metadrenaline assay. The metadrenalines, normetadrenaline and metadrenaline, are excreted largely as acid-labile conjugates. The procedure most widely used for their quantitative estimation in urine is that of Pisano (1960). The amines are freed by acid hydrolysis, adsorbed on to a cation-exchange resin, eluted and oxidized to vanillin which is measured spectrophotometrically. The method will detect a 3- or 4-fold increase in metadrenaline excretion, but a small rise may be missed, particularly if the urine is highly pigmented. A modification of Pisano's method used in our laboratory (Sandler and Ruthven, 1974) avoids this danger. Certain drugs must be excluded, including α-methyldopa (Sandler and Ruthven, 1974) and chlorpromazine (Blumberg et al., 1966) which give spuriously high results, and some radio-opaque dyes containing methylglucamine salts of diatrizoate, which lead to false negative results (Sandler and Ruthven, 1974).

Although the estimation of total rather than individual amines is usually sufficient for diagnostic purposes, differential measurements provide additional information, including some indication of the ratio of noradrenaline to adrenaline in what is secreted by the tumour. A number of differential assay techniques have been described. Paper and thin-layer chromatography (Sandler and Ruthven, 1969b) are relatively simple to perform, but are usually semi-quantitative; considerable patience and practice are required to obtain satisfactory results. Fluorometric procedures for metadrenalines (Smith and Weil-Malherbe, 1962; Anton and Sayre, 1966; Geissbuhler, 1970), although quantitative, are technically more difficult and give rise to similar problems to those encountered in the fluorometric determination of catecholamines. Gas chromatography offers considerable advantages. The procedure of Bertani et al. (1970) involves preliminary separation from neutral and acidic compounds which are also present in hydrolyzed urine samples by adsorption on cation-exchange resin. The metadrenalines are eluted and converted into their trifluoracetyl derivatives, which are analyzed quantitatively by gas chromatography using electron capture detection. A simpler but satisfactory electron capture method has recently been devised in the present authors' laboratory (Nelson et al., 1979) involving solvent extraction of hydrolyzed urine and derivatization of the isolated amines with pentafluoropropionyl anhydride. These methods can also be used to measure the dopamine metabolite, 3-methoxytyramine, and other phenolic amines in urine. The only quantitative methods previously available for 3-methoxytyramine were rather lengthy fluorometric techniques (Geissbuhler, 1970; Käser and Thomke, 1970).

Gas chromatography with electron capture detection has also been used for the quantitation of metadrenaline and 3-methoxytyramine in human plasma (Wang et al., 1974).

24.7.2.2.2. Assay of 4-hydroxy-3-methoxymandelic acid. The urinary excretion of 4-hydroxy-3-methoxymandelic acid is quantitatively greater than that of most other catecholamine metabolites, making it possible to employ assay procedures which are less exacting than those required for accurate measurement of the catecholamines and metadrenalines; for this reason, it is the catecholamine metabolite most commonly measured. A number of screening tests have been devised to measure 4-hydroxy-3-methoxymandelic acid (Sandler and Ruthven, 1966; Gitlow et al., 1970a, c), but in our opinion and that of others (Engelman, 1969), these are unreliable, particularly when the excretion of 4-hydroxy-3-methoxymandelic acid is raised only marginally (Sandler and Ruthven, 1966) or when the urine sample is dilute (Knight et al., 1975). The colorimetric procedure of Mahler and Humoller (1962), for example, was later shown to measure 4-hydroxy-3-methoxymandelic acid plus 5-hydroxyindoleacetic acid (Fleisher et al., 1969), a result which could, in certain circumstances, be dangerously misleading. The screening test of Gitlow et al. (1970a, c) is probably more reliable than most, being largely free from dietary sources of interference except from products containing vanillin (Knight et al., 1975).

4-Hydroxy-3-methoxymandelic acid may be measured semi-quantitatively by paper or thin-layer chromatography or by high-voltage electrophoresis (Sandler and Ruthven, 1966). High-voltage electrophoresis (Lachhein and Schütz, 1967), which may also be used to estimate homovanillic acid and 5-hydroxyindoleacetic acid, requires special equipment; it is semi-quantitative only and may be subject to interference from dietary constituents and drug metabolites.

Although they are somewhat more complex than screening methods, accurate quantitative spectrophotometric procedures, based on the conversion of 4-hydroxy-3-methoxymandelic acid into vanillin (Sandler and Ruthven, 1966), are not technically difficult and generally provide unequivocal results. The method of Pisano et al. (1962) was one of the earliest and probably the simplest technique of this type to be developed, and it is, in our view, the most useful one for the non-specialist laboratory to apply to the diagnosis of catecholamine-secreting tumours (Sandler and Ruthven, 1974). In this context it should be mentioned that Pisano's technique gives falsely low values when large amounts (about 100 mg/24 h) of homovanillic acid are present (Parrad and Bohuon, 1968). Although, in practice, this property does not obscure the diagnosis, it means that some of the published 4-hydroxy-3-methoxymandelic acid values determined by Pisano's method are lower than the true figures in patients in whom homovanillic acid excretion is also high. The method is largely free from dietary interferences; vanillin and vanilla-containing foods may be eaten (Green and Walker, 1970), although it is probably advisable to avoid large amounts of coffee, tea, citrus fruits and bananas. Drug metabolites in general are not a serious source of error. α-Methyldopa does not appear to have any effect but treatment with the cholesterol-lowering agent, clofibrate (Engelman, 1969; Sandler and Ruthven, 1974) and the ingestion of large amounts (3 to 5 g/day) of aspirin (Feldman et al., 1974) give rise to falsely low values. In contrast, the antibacterial drug, nalidixic acid, gives rise to falsely high values (see Sandler and Ruthven, 1974).

With the possible exception of homovanillic acid, gas chromatographic methods have probably been used more for the estimation of 4-hydroxy-3-methoxymandelic acid than for any of the other catecholamine metabolites. Homovanillic acid and 4-hydroxy-3-methoxymandelic acid were among the first of the compounds in this group to be assayed by gas chromatography (Williams and Greer, 1962), being excreted in sufficiently high concentration to make possible their detection by means of flame ionization; electron capture detection was not generally available at that time. The trimethylsilylether/esters or methyl ester/trimethylsilylethers of 4-hydroxy-3-methoxymandelic acid make very satisfactory derivatives for the estimation of urinary 4-hydroxy-3-methoxymandelic acid by flame ionization or macro-argon detection (Karoum et al., 1969). Prior conversion into vanillin (van de Calseyde et al., 1971) appears to be unnecessary. If electron capture detection is available, a method recently devised in the present authors' laboratory may be found convenient. It will measure homovanillic acid as well as 4-hydroxy-3-methoxymandelic acid reliably, at a normal concentration, in the same sample of urine (Weg, unpublished work) and involves solvent extraction, ethyl ester formation and gas chromatography of the pentafluoropropionyl derivative.

24.7.2.2.3. Homovanillic acid assay. Even after its importance for the diagnosis of dopamine-secreting tumours was recognized, urinary homovanillic acid assay was restricted to semi-quantitative procedures based upon paper (Sandler and Ruthven, 1969b, 1974) or thin-layer (Sandler and Ruthven, 1969b) chromatography. Homovanillic acid is chemically less reactive than 4-hydroxy-3-methoxymandelic acid and proved more difficult to assay quantitatively. It was subsequently found that homovanillic acid can be converted into vanillin, although less readily than the metadrenalines or 4-hydroxy-3-methoxymandelic acid. A spectrophotometric method was developed using this reaction (Ruthven and Sandler, 1966), which is suitable for measuring urinary homovanillic acid in both normal and pathological conditions. The procedure is rather time-consuming but provides accurate measurements when facilities for fluorometry or gas chromatography are not available.

Sensitive quantitative fluorometric procedures have been devised for the estimation of homovanillic acid in urine and other biological fluids, involving isolation on an ion-exchange column, elution and oxidation by alkaline potassium ferricyanide, to give a fluorophore which is measured spectrofluorometrically (Sato, 1965; Kahane and Vestergaard, 1971). Aspirin in fairly low dosage (600 to 900 mg) can double the blank readings, and may invalidate the fluorometric method of Sato (Hoeldtke, 1972).

Gas chromatographic assay of urinary homovanillic acid was briefly discussed in the section dealing with 4-hydroxy-3-methoxymandelic acid determination. Trimethylsilyl ether/esters and methyl ester/trimethylsilylethers of homovanillic acid, like those of 4-hydroxy-3-methoxymandelic acid, have good gas chromatographic properties and are suitable derivatives (Karoum et al., 1969). However, now that an electron capture method is available for homovanillic acid (Weg, unpublished work. see section 24.7.2.2.2), an alternative procedure exists which is less subject to interference from other urinary metabolites than methods using silyl derivatives.

24.7.2.2.4. Assay of 3,4-dihydroxyphenylacetic acid. Although paper and thin-layer chromatographic methods for 3,4-dihydroxyphenylacetic acid have been described (Sandler and Ruthven, 1969b), they are at best semi-quantitative and are very susceptible to losses by oxidation. Somewhat more accurate, paper (Millinger and Hvidberg, 1969) and thin-layer (Vidi and Bonardi, 1972) chromatographic methods exist in which a fluorophore derived from 3,4-dihydroxyphenylacetic acid is eluted from paper or a thin-layer plate and measured spectrofluorometrically. A quantitative fluorometric method has been described by Weil-Malherbe and van Buren (1969); 3,4-dihydroxyphenylacetic acid is adsorbed from urine on to an alumina column and, after elution, is coupled with ethylenediamine to form a fluorescent compound. Estimates of urine specimens from control subjects using this method are about twice those obtained by gas chromatography (Weg et al., 1975), perhaps because of interfering fluorescence from unknown urinary constituents (Mellinger and Hvidberg, 1969).

The gas chromatographic estimation of 3,4-dihydroxyphenylacetic acid as its methyl ester/trimethylsilyl ether, after solvent extraction from normal urine (Karoum et al., 1969), is subject to interference from hippuric acid and unidentified material. However, an accurate quantitative gas chromatographic method is now available which employs electron capture detection of the ethyl ester/pentafluoropropionyl ether of 3,4-dihydroxyphenylacetic acid eluted from an alumina column (Weg et al., 1975). It is suited to measuring both free and conjugated (Smith and Weil-Malherbe, 1971) 3,4-dihydroxyphenylacetic acid in normal and pathological urine samples.

24.7.2.2.5. Assay of 4-hydroxy-3-methoxyphenylglycol. 4-Hydroxy-3-methoxyphenylglycol is present in human urine largely as its sulphate ester conjugate, which must be hydrolyzed before assay. Since the free glycol is acid-labile, hydrolysis must be carried out enzymatically. A mixed sulphatase/β-glucuronidase preparation from the snail *Helix pomatia* has been widely used for this purpose although the preparation has recently been found to contain 4-hydroxy-3-methoxyphenylglycol (Sjöquist and Änggård, 1974) in quantities which might introduce serious error to the determination of the small amounts of endogenous substance which are present in tissues, plasma and cerebrospinal fluid. In urine, the error would be less serious, probably not contributing more than a few per cent of normal endogenous 4-hydroxy-3-methoxyphenylglycol levels. In addition to 4-hydroxy-3-methoxyphenylglycol, homovanillic acid and dopamine are present in the sulphatase/β-glucuronidase preparation at concentrations of about 80 and 200 times that of the glycol respectively. However, since free homovanillic acid only is usually measured, contamination from this source is not a serious drawback. Dopamine and homovanillic acid are, in any case, stable to mild acid hydrolysis, so that their conjugates can easily be hydrolyzed when necessary. Sulphatase (type H-1; Sigma) appears to be free from 4-hydroxy-3-methoxyphenylglycol contamination and contains considerably less dopamine and homovanillic acid, but its activity is much lower than the less pure *Helix pomatia* preparation.

Urinary 4-hydroxy-3-methoxyphenylglycol can be estimated spectrophotometrically by oxidizing it to vanillin after enzymatic hydrolysis (Ruthven and Sandler, 1965). The levels detected in normal urine by this method tend to be on the high side of the true values although a modification (Nicholas et al., 1969) gives lower results, agreeing more closely with those found by gas chromatography. The flame ionization detector, or one of equivalent sensitivity, is quite adequate for the measurement of 4-hydroxy-3-methoxy-phenylglycol in normal or pathological urine samples (Karoum et al., 1969). Some authors prefer to oxidize to vanillin before derivatization (Kahane et al., 1970). In our hands, simple preparation of the trimethylsilyl ether of 4-hydroxy-3-methoxyphenyl-glycol itself is perfectly satisfactory.

Electron capture detection may also be used to measure this compound in urine and it is essential for its gas chromatographic assay in plasma, tissue or cerebrospinal fluid. Several different methods are available (Dekirmenjian and Maas, 1970, 1974; Bond, 1972). An electron capture technique for urinary 4-hydroxy-3-methoxyphenylglycol has recently been devised in the present authors' laboratory (Fellows et al., 1975) which compared favourably in speed and simplicity with other quantitative assay procedures. Enzymatically hydrolyzed urine is passed through a column of anion-exchange resin; 4-hydroxy-3-methoxyphenylglycol, which is weakly bound, is eluted and converted into its pentafluoropropionyl derivative for measurement.

24.7.2.2.6. Screening procedures. In concluding this methodological discussion, it is wise to sound a warning note about the use of screening procedures. Some drawbacks of the Hingerty test for urinary catecholamines have already been mentioned, as have the limitations of paper and thin-layer chromatographic and high-voltage electrophoretic techniques for assay of their metabolites. A low-voltage screening test for elevated excretion of 4-hydroxy-3-methoxymandelic acid (Brown et al., 1966) has similar disadvantages. A commercial screening kit for 4-hydroxy-3-methoxymandelic acid marketed in the U.S.A., has given a quite unacceptably high proportion of false positive and false negative results. A test strip designed to detect increased urinary concentrations of 4-hydroxy-3-methoxymandelic acid and metadrenalines as a screening test for neuroblastoma (Leonard et al., 1972) is probably unreliable and too costly to use in a full screening programme.

TABLE 24.4.
URINARY EXCRETION VALUES OF CATECHOLAMINES IN NORMAL SUBJECTS

Age	Noradrenaline (free) (μg/24 h)		Adrenaline (free) (μg/24 h)		Dopamine (free) (μg/24 h)	
	Mean	Range	Mean	Range	Mean	Range
3 months	4	1– 9	–	–	–	–
<1 year	11	5–16	1.3	0.1– 4.3	61	18– 99
1–5 years	19	8–31	3.2	0.8– 9.1	124	48–217
5–15 years	37	19–71	4.8	1.3–10.5	169	80–365
Adult (>15 years)	50	20–90	15	5 –35	300	100–500
	μg/mg creatinine		μg/mg creatinine		μg/mg creatinine	
Adult (>15 years)	0.025	0.01–0.045	0.01	0.003–0.020	0.15	0.05–0.25

TABLE 24.5.

URINARY EXCRETION VALUES OF METHOXY AMINES IN NORMAL SUBJECTS

Age	Total metadrenalines				Age	Free 3-methoxytyramine			
	μg/24 h		μg/mg creatinine			μg/24 h		μg/mg creatinine	
	Mean	Range	Mean	Range		Mean	Range	Mean	Range
<1 year	100	50–200	2	0.1 –5					
0–5 years	200	50–400	1.2 [1]	0.4 –3 [1]	2– 3 years	20	18– 24	0.13	0.07–0.18
5–10 years	300	150–700	1.1	0.2 –3	5– 6 years	34	13– 57	0.10	0.04–0.14
10–15 years	400	200–700	0.7	0.1 –1.8	9–13 years	51	31– 72	0.09	0.05–0.12
Adult (>15 years)	500	250–800	0.4	0.1 –0.8	Adult	88	30–175	0.07	0.02–0.13
Adult (>15 years)	200 [2]	100–450 [2]	0.2 [2]	0.08–0.4 [2]					
Adult (>15 years)	150 [3]	50–250 [3]	0.18 [3]	0.06–0.25 [3]		Total 3-methoxytyramine			
					Adult	300	150–850	0.20	0.07–0.40

[1] 1–5 year value.
[2] Normetadrenaline, free plus conjugated } total.
[3] Metadrenaline, free plus conjugated } total.

24.7.3. Normal ranges

An accurate knowledge of normal urinary excretion values of catecholamines and their metabolites is essential in order to make a reliable biochemical diagnosis of catecholamine-secreting tumour. When interpreting the results of urinary analyses, it is also important to remember that many factors other than the presence of a tumour can influence the excretion of these compounds. Some, such as diet and drugs, exercise, stress and pathological states not associated with secreting tumours have already been discussed. Other factors resulting in changes of excretion include diurnal variation and, for certain compounds – including dopamine, tryptamine and indoleacetic acid – urinary pH and

TABLE 24.6.
URINARY EXCRETION VALUES OF METHOXY ACID METABOLITES IN NORMAL SUBJECTS

Age	4-Hydroxy-3-methoxymandelic acid (free)			
	μg/24 h		μg/mg creatinine	
	Mean	Range	Mean	Range
1–2 day full term	300	50– 500	10	3 –15
1–2 day premature	70	20– 150	10	3 –20
3rd day full term	150	50– 300	7	3 –10
3rd day premature	140	50– 250	15	4 –40
1 week	300	70– 500	15	5 –40
1–6 months	500	100–1000	11	3 –17
6–12 months	1000	200–1500	7	2 –15
1–5 years	1500	500–2500	5	2 –10 [1]
5–10 years	2300	750–3000	3.5	1.5– 7
10–15 years	3300	1000–6000	3	1 – 6
Adult (>15 years)	4000	2000–7000	3	1 – 6
	Homovanillic acid (free)			
	μg/24 h		μg/mg creatinine	
	Mean	Range	Mean	Range
1–2 day full term	350	150– 650	12	5 –20
1–2 day premature	200	30– 400	25	5 –20
3rd day full term	300	150– 500	12	5 –20
3rd day premature	300	100– 450	25	10 –50
1 week	350	100– 650	20	5 –50
1–6 months	500	100–1000	15	3 –40
6–12 months	1000	200–1500	13	3 –30
1–5 years	1500	800–2500	10	3 –20 [1]
5–10 years	3000	1000–6000	7	2 –15
10–15 years	4500	2000–7000	5	1.5–10
Adult (>15 years)	5200	3700–7700	4	1 –7

[1] 0–5 years.

volume (Sandler et al., 1967). Thus, when collecting urine for diagnostic purposes, it is important to standardize these variables whenever possible. Twenty-four-hour specimens are preferable to random urine collections, since they are less subject to alteration by fluctuations in metabolite output. The expression of metabolite excretion in terms of urinary creatinine is not as reliable as the determination of daily excretion, particularly in young children, where creatinine output tends to be very variable (Greenblatt et al., 1976). A combination of protected environment and recumbent posture may bring about some reduction in excretion of catecholamines and their metabolites after several days in hospital. Such variations in catecholamine and metabolite excretion are, in general, too small to give rise to errors when the diagnosis of secreting tumour is in doubt. In the large majority of affected subjects, urinary output of catecholamines and their metabolites is increased several-fold. When values are persistently equivocal, however, or in the face of strong clinical suspicion, shorter urine collection periods following a paroxysm may well reveal the presence of a tumour.

Tables showing mean normal excretion values and ranges, derived from a number of sources and expressed both in terms of 24-hour excretion and creatinine output, have been included to provide a baseline for tumour diagnosis (Tables 24.4, 24.5, 24.6 and 24.7).

TABLE 24.7.

URINARY EXCRETION VALUES OF CATECHOL ACIDS AND METHOXY ALCOHOLS IN NORMAL SUBJECTS

	Age	μg/24 h		μg/mg creatinine	
		Mean	Range	Mean	Range
3,4-Dihydroxyphenylalanine (free)	1–10 years	24	11– 42	0.093	0.035– 0.192
3,4-Dihydroxyphenylalanine (free)	Adult (>15 years)	25	15– 50	0.019	0.008– 0.030
3,4-Dihydroxyphenylacetic acid (free)	Adult (>15 years)	880	330–1850		
3,4-Dihydroxyphenylacetic acid (total)	Adult (>15 years)	1790	1120–2950		
3,4-Dihydroxymandelic acid (free)	Adult (>15 years)	91	36– 178		
4-Hydroxy-3-methoxyphenylethanol (total)	Adult (>15 years)	190	120– 300		
4-Hydroxy-3-methoxyphenylglycol (total)	2–5 days			4.5	3.0 – 5.5
4-Hydroxy-3-methoxyphenylglycol (total)	1 week–1 month			5.0	1.0 –13.0
4-Hydroxy-3-methoxyphenylglycol (total)	Adult (>15 years)	1900	800–3600	1.0	0.3 – 2.0

24.8. INDOLEALKYLAMINES

24.8.1. Anatomical considerations

Although 5-hydroxyindole assays of varying accuracy and specificity have largely been used in clinical practice as an aid to carcinoid tumour diagnosis and for monitoring the response of tumours to treatment, such measurements have also helped to provide an insight into the normal functioning of the cell of origin of the monoamine. Studying the 5-hydroxytryptamine-producing tumour has in fact been virtually the only approach to the gastrointestinal enterochromaffin cell. In many ways, the carcinoid tumour may be considered as the enterochromaffin cell "writ large". 5-Hydroxytryptamine secretion is not a characteristic of all carcinoids. This property appears to some extent to be governed by the site of origin of the neoplasm from the embryonic gut, as shown in Table 24.8. It will be seen that the tumours broadly fall into three clinical groups depending on their origin from fore-, mid- or hind-gut.

The enterochromaffin system (Vialli, 1966) is a diffuse collection of cells, characterized by granules, which, under certain circumstances, reduce silver salts to silver, a property possessed similarly by the carcinoid tumour. This "argentaffin reaction" is made possible by the presence of a high local concentration of 5-hydroxytryptamine within the granule.

Although the clinical spotlight has focussed sharply on the overproduction of 5-hydroxyindoles in carcinoid and related tumours of this system, disturbances of 5-hydroxytryptamine production have also been noted in other disease states. The biochemical changes are, as might be expected, linked to the anatomical distribution of the 5-hy-

TABLE 24.8.

THE CHARACTERISTICS OF CARCINOID TUMOURS DERIVED FROM DIFFERENT EMBRYONIC DIVISIONS OF THE GUT

	Fore-gut	Mid-gut	Hind-gut
Histological structure	Tendency to be trabecular; may differ widely from classical pattern	Characteristic	Tendency to be trabecular
Argentaffin and diazo reactions	Usually negative	Positive	Often negative
Association with the carcinoid syndrome	Frequent	Frequent	None
Tumour 5-hydroxytryptamine content	Low	High	Occasionally raised
Urinary 5-hydroxyindoleacetic acid	High	High	Occasionally raised
5-Hydroxytryptophan secretion	Frequent	Rare	Not detected
Metastases to bone (usually osteoblastic) and skin	Common	Unusual	Common
Association with other endocrine secretion	Frequent	Not described	Not described

droxytryptamine-containing structures. Circulating 5-hydroxytryptamine, for instance, is almost completely localized to the blood platelet and any alteration in blood concentration in disease states or in response to the administration of certain drugs represents a change in platelet amine content (Stacey, 1968). Above all, the proven or suspected role of 5-hydroxytryptamine as one of a growing number of central nervous system transmitters, makes the measurement of its metabolites in the cerebrospinal fluid of considerable importance in the investigation of certain neurological and psychiatric illnesses.

24.8.2. Biosynthesis of 5-hydroxytryptamine

The principal biosynthetic route for the production of 5-hydroxytryptamine (Scheme 24.6) starts from the essential aminoacid, tryptophan, which is hydroxylated to form 5-hydroxytryptophan. The responsible enzyme, tryptophan-5-hydroxylase, which is rate-limiting in the synthesis of 5-hydroxytryptamine, was first identified in carcinoid tumour tissue (Grahame-Smith, 1964a) and shortly afterwards in brain (Grahame-Smith, 1964b). It resembles phenylalanine hydroxylase in its requirement for oxygen, and for a pterin, presumably tetrahydrobiopterin, as co-factor (for review, see Kaufman and Fisher, 1974).

One group of workers has estimated that the 1 to 2% of dietary tryptophan which is normally converted in the body into 5-hydroxyindoles may be expanded to about 60% in carcinoid disease (Sjoerdsma et al., 1956). Such a drain of the essential aminoacid which is normally present in the shortest supply may occasionally result in the superimposition of frank pellagra over the clinical signs of the carcinoid syndrome (Thorson et al., 1958).

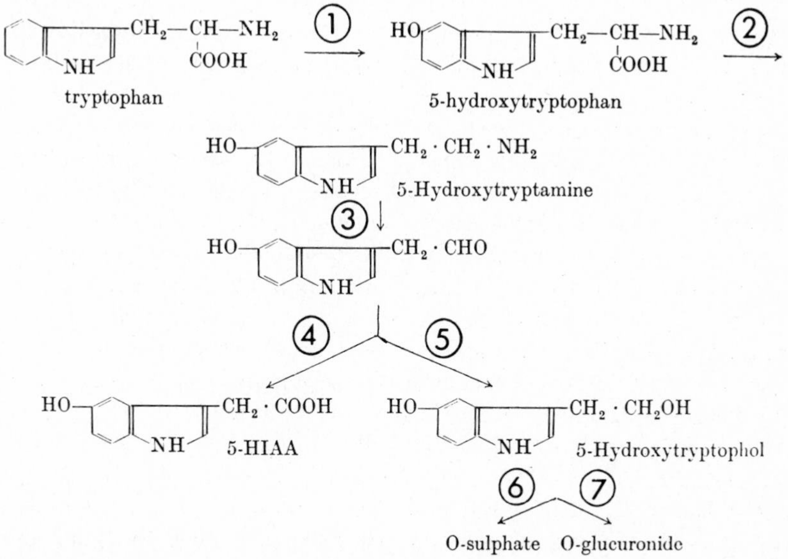

tryptophan ($-CH_2-CH(COOH)-NH_2$, NH) —①→ 5-hydroxytryptophan (HO, $-CH_2-CH(COOH)-NH_2$, NH) —②→

5-Hydroxytryptamine (HO—, $-CH_2 \cdot CH_2 \cdot NH_2$, NH)

③ ↓

HO—, $-CH_2 \cdot CHO$, NH

④ ↙ ↘ ⑤

5-HIAA (HO—, $-CH_2 \cdot COOH$, NH) 5-Hydroxytryptophol (HO—, $-CH_2 \cdot CH_2OH$, NH)

⑥ ↙ ↘ ⑦

O-sulphate O-glucuronide

Scheme 24.6. Biosynthesis and metabolism of 5-hydroxytryptamine. 1, Tryptophan-5-hydroxylase; 2, 5-hydroxytryptophan decarboxylase; 3, monoamine oxidase; 4, aldehyde dehydrogenase; 5, alcohol dehydrogenase; 6, phenol sulphotransferase; 7, UDP-glucuronosyltransferase.

5-Hydroxytryptamine itself is formed from 5-hydroxytryptophan by the action of the pyridoxal-5-phosphate-requiring enzyme, aromatic L-aminoacid decarboxylase, present in high activity in mammalian kidney, liver and gastrointestinal tract (Lovenberg et al., 1962) and in carcinoid tissue (Langemann, 1957).

24.8.3. Metabolism of 5-hydroxytryptamine

24.8.3.1. Major pathway

As implied earlier (Scheme 24.1), the main metabolic pathway for the degradation of 5-hydroxytryptamine involves oxidative deamination by the widely distributed mitochondrial enzyme, monoamine oxidase, resulting in the formation of 5-hydroxyindole-acetaldehyde, which is further oxidized by aldehyde dehydrogenase to 5-hydroxyindole-acetic acid (Scheme 24.6). The aldehyde may also be reduced by aldehyde reductase to 5-hydroxytryptophol, although this route is normally a very minor one, representing not more than about 1% of the substrate. However, certain drugs, such as ethanol and reserpine, possess the ability to divert the intermediate aldehyde from oxidative to reductive pathway (Lancet, 1972), so that considerably larger amounts of 5-hydroxytryptophol may be excreted at the expense of 5-hydroxyindoleacetic acid. Thus the practice of administering ethanol-containing beverages to initiate carcinoid flushing attacks for diagnostic purposes may also on occasion result in a falsely low apparent excretion of 5-hydroxyindole, in that 5-hydroxyindoleacetic acid output is the measurement usually made in this disease.

24.8.3.2. Minor pathways

Apart from the major route of degradation via oxidative deamination, a number of quantitatively minor pathways are known; of these, by far the most intensively studied is that involving the conversion of 5-hydroxytryptamine into melatonin (*N*-acetyl-5-methoxy-tryptamine; Scheme 24.7; for review, see Quay, 1974). Melatonin is elaborated almost solely by the pineal gland where a specific enzyme, 5-hydroxyindole-*O*-methyltransferase, is located. Activity of the *N*-acetylating enzyme is under sympathetic control, being enhanced by β-adrenergic receptor stimulation and retarded by β-blocking agents. Melatonin is the most potent known lightening agent of amphibian skin. However, its function in higher animals is obscure; it appears to have little effect on pigmentary systems, although there is a fairly solid body of evidence pointing to a role in the sexual maturation process. The presence of 5-hydroxyindole-*O*-methyltransferase in some pineal tumours makes it likely that they elaborate large amounts of melatonin (Quay, 1974). However, no specific melatonin overproduction syndrome appears to be on record. While the supporting evidence in man is somewhat exiguous, it is not unlikely that the major degradation route of melatonin is similar to that in the rat – 6-hydroxylation followed by conjugation (Scheme 24.7).

Conjugation of 5-hydroxytryptamine is another minor pathway of interest. Although the question has so far received little attention, it seems likely, to judge from our knowledge of other monoamines (Sandler et al., 1975), that 5-hydroxytryptamine is metabolized by sulphate conjugation when the substance is given orally, to a considerably greater extent than after its parenteral administration or when it is elaborated endogenously.

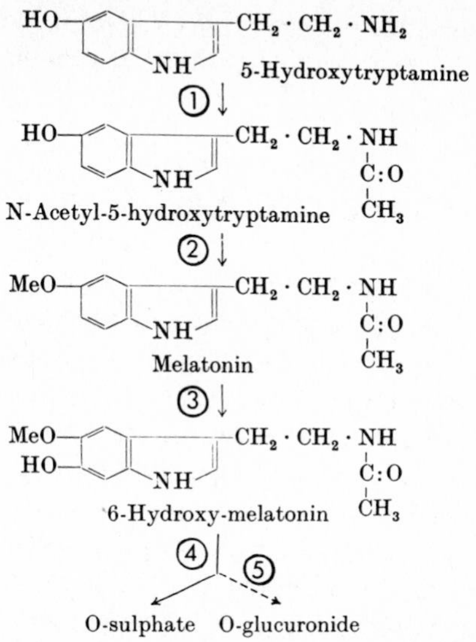

HO–[indole]–$CH_2 \cdot CH_2 \cdot NH_2$ 5-Hydroxytryptamine

① ↓

HO–[indole]–$CH_2 \cdot CH_2 \cdot NH \cdot C{:}O \cdot CH_3$ N-Acetyl-5-hydroxytryptamine

② ↓

MeO–[indole]–$CH_2 \cdot CH_2 \cdot NH \cdot C{:}O \cdot CH_3$ Melatonin

③ ↓

MeO–, HO–[indole]–$CH_2 \cdot CH_2 \cdot NH \cdot C{:}O \cdot CH_3$ 6-Hydroxy-melatonin

④ ↙ ⑤ ↘

O-sulphate O-glucuronide

Scheme 24.7. Biosynthesis and metabolism of melatonin. 1, Serotonin-*N*-acetyltransferase; 2, hydroxyindole-*O*-methyltransferase; 3, indole-6-hydroxylase; 4, phenol sulphotransferase; 5, UDP-glucuronosyltransferase.

One further minor pathway which has been much discussed of late is the *N*-methylation of 5-hydroxytryptamine by an enzyme which has been detected in both the human lung and brain. An overproduction of the potentially hallucinogenic *N,N*-dimethyltryptamine (bufotenine) by this enzyme system has been suggested as one possible aetiological mechanism of schizophrenia, although the supporting evidence is still less than adequate. The status of this enzyme is to some extent unclear. Nevertheless, it is tempting to wonder whether schizophrenia may be, in common perhaps with migraine (Sandler, 1972b), to some extent a pulmonary disease; any psychotomimetic agent elaborated in the lung would be injected directly into the systemic arterial supply and the brain.

Other minor metabolic pathways of the 5-hydroxyindoles, which have yet to prove of clinical importance, include that commencing with the action of a ring-splitting enzyme (Konishi et al., 1971) leading to the formation of a new range of pharmacologically active metabolites (Toda, 1975), 5-hydroxytryptophan transamination and pigment formation from 5-hydroxyindoleacetaldehyde. All 5-hydroxyindoles are easily oxidized and the darkening often observed in acidified carcinoid urine probably derives from oxidation of 5-hydroxyindoleacetic acid.

Like 5-hydroxytryptamine, tryptamine is also produced endogenously in man, although its concentration in brain is considerably lower. Tryptamine presumably derives from tryptophan. However, the mechanism by which it is synthesized is obscure, as this aminoacid is a relatively poor substrate for L-aromatic aminoacid decarboxylase (Lovenberg et al., 1962). Tryptamine is largely metabolized by monoamine oxidase, the major end-product of the intermediate aldehyde being indoleacetic acid. The large amounts of this acid and its glutamine conjugate, in urine from a patient with Hartnup disease

(Jepson, 1972), stem from a specific transport defect; tryptophan and other aromatic aminoacids too, which fail to be absorbed from the small gut, pass into the large intestine where they are decarboxylated by gut flora.

24.9. BIOCHEMICAL DIAGNOSIS OF CARCINOID TUMOUR

Although whole blood 5-hydroxytryptamine is usually raised in carcinoid disease, its estimation is not recommended for the routine diagnosis of carcinoid tumour. It will add little diagnostic information to that obtained from the much simpler urinary 5-hydroxyindoleacetic acid assay. A qualitative screening procedure is available (Sjoerdsma et al., 1955) for detecting 5-hydroxyindoles, which the smaller laboratory may find particularly useful. It utilizes the violet chromophore produced when these compounds are treated with 1-nitroso-2-naphthol in dilute acid containing a trace of nitrite. Urine mixed with this reagent is shaken with ethylene dichloride; the test is positive if a purple colour is seen in the top layer. Urinary concentrations of 5-hydroxyindoleacetic acid down to about 30 mg/litre can be detected in this way. As the urinary 5-hydroxyindoleacetic acid output is considerably higher in most cases of secreting carcinoid, false negatives will rarely occur. A positive test must always be checked by a quantitative estimation of urinary 5-hydroxyindoleacetic acid, since false positives can occur due to the ingestion of certain drugs, such as the expectorant, glyceryl guaiacolate, and foods, especially bananas. Medication should therefore be avoided for some days before performing the test.

Two-way paper chromatography followed by staining with Ehrlich's reagent is a useful procedure for detecting and confirming the presence of an abnormal excretion of urinary 5-hydroxyindoles (Jepson, 1969). It is also valuable for diagnosing the atypical tumour where, in addition to the usual increase in 5-hydroxyindoleacetic acid and its conjugates, considerable amounts of 5-hydroxytryptophan and 5-hydroxytryptamine may be found in the urine. Such atypical carcinoids are characteristically embryonic fore-gut derivatives and the highest output of 5-hydroxytryptophan may be found in the gastric carcinoid tumour, which also secretes histamine, giving rise to the characteristic "geographical" flush (Sandler, 1968).

The quantitative determination of urinary 5-hydroxyindoleacetic acid is the most important chemical method for detecting 5-hydroxyindole-secreting tumours. Most published techniques are modifications of the original colorimetric method of Udenfriend and his colleagues (Udenfriend et al., 1955); 5-hydroxyindoleacetic acid is extracted from urine into ether, back extracted into neutral buffer and reacted with 1-nitroso-2-naphthol. The resulting colour is read spectrophotometrically. This procedure is still widely used and is quite satisfactory for carcinoid diagnosis. The ingestion of large amounts of aspirin should be avoided as its metabolites interfere with the test, to give falsely low results.

Fluorometric methods offer an alternative approach. Most procedures of this type employ the characteristic activation/fluorescence of 5-hydroxyindoles in acid. Contractor (1966) developed a simple but satisfactory fluorometric technique involving prior adsorption of 5-hydroxyindoleacetic acid from urine on to dextran gel. The recently described gas chromatographic procedure of Goodwin et al. (1975) is particularly suited to detecting small fluctuations in 5-hydroxyindoleacetic acid excretion at normal excretion values (i.e. about 1 to 7 mg/24 h).

24.10. CONCLUSION

This presentation has been devoted in greater part to a consideration of the clinical role of the catecholamines, with the indolealkylamines playing a subsidiary role: this division broadly reflects their relative importance in clinical practice. Nevertheless, as was pointed out at the beginning of the chapter, a further array of endogenous monoamine oxidase substrates is distributed discontinuously through the body, although their study has been held back by lack of suitable assay procedures. Recent work (see Sandler et al., 1976) underscores the potential clinical importance of these so-called "trace amines": for example, there appears to be an exceedingly brisk turnover of octopamine in normal subjects, leading to a urinary output of its major metabolite, *p*-hydroxymandelic acid, approaching that of 4-hydroxy-3-methoxymandelic acid; phenylethylamine may well feature in the pathogenesis of some forms of schizophrenia. As is the way with these things, what today is dubbed research may easily form a major share of tomorrow's routine laboratory load. As far as the monoamines are concerned – and despite their vast literature – we are witnessing merely the beginning of an information explosion; this explosion cannot fail to have its fall-out in the field of clinical chemistry.

REFERENCES

Ahlquist, R.P. (1948) A study of adrenotropic receptors. American Journal of Physiology, 153, 586–600.

Amar-Costesec, A., Bohuon, C. and Schweisguth, O. (1965) Activité mono amine oxydase dans les tumeurs de la crête neurale. European Journal of Cancer, 1, 225–231.

Anton, A.H. and Sayre, D.F. (1962) A study of the factors affecting the aluminium oxide-trihydroxyindole procedure for the analysis of catecholamines. Journal of Pharmacology and Experimental Therapeutics, 138, 360–375.

Anton, A.H. and Sayre, D.F. (1964) The distribution of dopamine and dopa in various animals and a method for their determination in diverse biological material. Journal of Pharmacology and Experimental Therapeutics, 145, 326–336.

Anton, A.H. and Sayre, D.F. (1966) Distribution of metanephrine and normetanephrine in various animals and their analysis in diverse biologic material. Journal of Pharmacology and Experimental Therapeutics, 153, 15–29.

Armstrong, M.D., McMillan, A. and Shaw, K.N.F. (1957) 3-Methoxy-4-hydroxy-D-mandelic acid, a urinary metabolite of norepinephrine. Biochimica et Biophysica Acta, 25, 422–423.

Asatoor, A.M., London, D.R., Milne, M.D. and Simenhoff, M.L. (1963) The excretion of pethidine and its derivatives. British Journal of Pharmacology, 20, 285–298.

Assan, R., Dauchy, F. and Boyet, F. (1973) Elevated vanyl-mandelic acid excretion in severe diabetic keto-acidosis. Pathologie et Biologie, 21, 27–31.

Axelrod, J. (1957) *O*-Methylation of epinephrine and other catechols in vitro and in vivo. Science, 126, 400–401.

Axelrod, J. (1959) The metabolism of catecholamines in vivo and in vitro. Pharmacological Reviews, 11, 402–408.

Axelrod, J. (1960) *N*-Methyladrenaline, a new catecholamine in the adrenal gland, Biochimica et Biophysica Acta, 45, 614–615.

Axelrod, J. (1963) The formation, metabolism, uptake and release of noradrenaline and adrenaline. In The Clinical Chemistry of Monoamines (Eds. H. Varley and A.H. Gowenlock) pp. 5–18, Elsevier, Amsterdam.

Axelrod, J. (1966) Methylation reactions in the formation and metabolism of catecholamines and other biogenic amines. Pharmacological Reviews, 18, 95–113.

Baker, G., Zeller, N.H., Weitzner, S. and Leach, J.K. (1972) Pheochromocytoma without hypertension presenting as cardiomyopathy. American Heart Journal, 83, 688–693.

Baldessarini, R.J. and Vogt, M. (1972) Regional release of aromatic amines from tissues of the rat brain in vitro. Journal of Neurochemistry, 19, 755–761.

Barbero, G.J. and Braddock, L.I. (1967) Catecholamines in cystic fibrosis. Lancet, ii, 158.

Bareggi, S.R., Marc, V. and Morselli, P.L. (1974) Urinary excretion of 3-methoxy-4-hydroxyphenylglycol sulphate in rats after intraventricular injection of 6-OHDA. Brain Research, 75, 177–180.

Bartholini, G., Lloyd, K.G. and Stadler, H. (1974) Dopaminergic regulation of cholinergic neurons in the striatum: relation to parkinsonism. In Advances in Neurology, Vol. 5 (Eds. F.H. McDowell and A. Barbeau) pp. 11–17, Raven Press, New York.

Beckett, A.H., Salmon, J.A. and Mitchard, M. (1969) The relation between blood levels and urinary excretion of amphetamine under controlled acidic and under fluctuating urinary pH values using ^{14}C amphetamine. Journal of Pharmacy and Pharmacology, 21, 251–258.

Bellet, S., Roman, L. and Kostis, J. (1969) The effect of automobile driving on catecholamine and adrenocortical excretion. American Journal of Cardiology, 24, 365–368.

Berdal, P., Braaten, M., Cappelen, C. Jr., Mylius, E.A. and Walaas, O. (1962) Noradrenaline–adrenaline producing nonchromaffin paraganglioma, Acta Medica Scandinavica, 172, 249–257.

Bertani, L.M., Dziedzic, S.W., Clarke, D.D. and Gitlow, S.E. (1970) A gas-liquid chromatographic method for the separation and quantitation of normetanephrine and metanephrine in human urine. Clinica Chimica Acta, 30, 227–233.

Bhagat, B. (1973) Role of catecholamines in induction of adrenal tyrosine hydroxylase. In Frontiers in Catecholamine Research (Eds. E. Usdin and S.H. Snyder) pp. 191–193, Pergamon, New York.

Blaschko, H. (1939) The specific action of l-DOPA decarboxylase. Journal of Physiology (London), 96, 50P–51P.

Blaschko, H. (1972) Catecholamines 1922–1971. In Handbook of Experimental Pharmacology, Vol. 33, Catecholamines (Eds. H. Blaschko and E. Muscholl) pp. 1–15, Springer-Verlag, Berlin.

Blumberg, A.G., Heaton, A.M. and Vassiliades, J. (1966) The interference of chlorpromazine metabolites in the analysis of urinary methoxy-catecholamines. Clinical Chemistry, 12, 803–807.

Bohuon, C. and Assicot, M. (1973) Catechol-*O*-methyltransferase. In Frontiers in Catecholamine Research (Eds. E. Usdin and S.H. Snyder) pp. 107–112, Pergamon, New York.

Bohuon, C., Comoy, E. and Amar-Costesec, A. (1966a) Tumeurs des ébauches sympathiques; acides et alcools phénoliques dans le sang. Clinica Chimica Acta, 14, 20–23.

Bohuon, C., La Brosse, E.H., Assicot, M. and Amar-Costesec, A. (1966b) Réflexion sur le dosage de la catéchol-*O*-méthyltransferase et de la monoamine oxydase dans les neuroblastomas. In Neuroblastomas. Biochemical Studies. (Ed. C. Bohuon) pp. 16–22, Springer-Verlag, Berlin.

Bond, P.A. (1972) The determination of 4-hydroxy-3-methoxyphenylethylene glycol in urine and CSF using gas chromatography. Biochemical Medicine, 6, 36–45.

Borello, E.D. and Gorlin, R.J. (1966) Melanotic neuroectodermal tumor of infancy – a neoplasm of neural crest origin. Cancer, 19, 196–206.

Borud, O. and Gjessing, L.R. (1970) *N*-Acetylnormetanephrine and *N*-acetylmetanephrine in urine from patients with neuroblastoma. Clinica Chimica Acta, 27, 552–554.

Brown, W.G., Owens, J.B., Berson, A.W. and Henry, S.K. (1966) Vanilmandelic acid screening test for pheochromocytoma and neuroblastoma. American Journal of Clinical Pathology, 46, 599–602.

Brunjes, S. (1964) Catechol amine metabolism in essential hypertension. New England Journal of Medicine, 271, 120–124.

Burkard, W.P., Gey, K.F. and Pletscher, A. (1962) A new inhibitor of decarboxylase of aromatic amino acids. Experientia, 18, 411–412.

Cabana, B.E., Prokesch, J.C. and Christiansen, G.S. (1964) Study on the biogenesis of catecholamines in pheochromocytoma tissue culture. Archives of Biochemistry and Biophysics, 106, 123–130.

Callingham, B.A. (1968) The catecholamines. Adrenaline; noradrenaline. In Hormones in Blood, Vol. 2, 2nd edn. (Eds. C.H. Gray and A.L. Bacharach) pp. 519–599, Academic Press, London and New York.

Campanini, T., Catalano, A., De Risio, C. and Mardighian, G. (1970) Vanilmandelicaciduria in the different clinical phases of manic depressive psychosis. British Journal of Psychiatry, 116, 435–436.

Cardon, P.V. and Guggenheim, F.G. (1970) Effects of large variations in diet on free catecholamines and their metabolites in urine. Journal of Psychiatric Research, 7, 263–273.

Carlsson, A. (1974) Some aspects of dopamine in the central nervous system. In Advances in Neurology, Vol. 5 (Eds. F.H. McDowell and A. Barbeau) pp. 59–68, Raven, New York.

Carney, J.A., Sizemore, G.W. and Tyce, G.M. (1975) Bilateral adrenal medullary hyperplasia in multiple endocrine neoplasia, type 2. The precursor of bilateral pheochromocytoma. Mayo Clinic Proceedings, 50, 3–10.

Carruthers, M., Taggart, P., Conway, N., Bates, D. and Somerville, W. (1970) Validity of plasma-catecholamine estimations. Lancet, ii, 62–67.

Christensen, N.J. (1973) A sensitive assay for the determination of dopamine in plasma. Scandinavian Journal of Clinical and Laboratory Investigation, 31, 343–346.

Christensen, N.J. and Brandsborg, O. (1974) Dopamine in human gastric juice determined by a sensitive double-isotope-derivative technique. Scandinavian Journal of Clinical Laboratory Investigation, 34, 315–320.

Collins, G.G.S. and Sandler, M. (1971) Human blood platelet monoamine oxidase. Biochemical Pharmacology, 20, 289–296.

Contractor, S.F. (1966) A rapid quantitative method for the estimation of 5-hydroxyindoleacetic acid in human urine. Biochemical Pharmacology, 15, 1701–1706.

Costa, E. and Sandler, M. (Eds.) (1972) Monoamine Oxidases – New Vistas, Advances in Biochemical Psychopharmacology, Vol. 5. Raven, New York.

Coulson, W.F., Henson, G. and Jepson, J.B. (1968) The production of *m*-tyramine from L-phenylalanine by rat-liver preparations. Biochimica et Biophysica Acta, 156, 135–139.

Coupland, R.E. (1972) The chromaffin system. In Handbook of Experimental Pharmacology, Vol. 33, Catecholamines (Eds. H. Blaschko and E. Muscholl) pp. 16–45, Springer-Verlag, Berlin.

Creveling, C.R., Borchardt, R.T. and Isersky, C. (1973) Immunological characterization of catechol-*O*-methyltransferase. In Frontiers in Catecholamine Research (Eds. E. Usdin and S.H. Snyder) pp. 117–119, Pergamon, New York.

Creveling, C.R. and Daly, J.W. (1971) Assay of enzymes of catecholamine biosynthesis and metabolism. In Analysis of Biogenic Amines and their Related Enzymes (Ed. D. Glick) pp. 153–182, Interscience, New York.

Cronan, T.L. III and Howley, E.T. (1974) The effect of training on epinephrine and norepinephrine excretion. Medicine and Science in Sports, 6, 122–125.

Crout, J.R. (1961) Catechol amines in urine. Standard Methods of Clinical Chemistry, 3, 62–80.

Crout, J.R. (1966) Pheochromocytoma. Pharmacological Reviews, 18, 651–657.

Crout, J.R. (1968) Sampling and analysis of catecholamines and metabolites. Anesthesiology, 29, 661–669.

Crout, J.R., Pisano, J.J. and Sjoerdsma, A. (1961) Urinary excretion of catecholamines and their metabolites in pheochromocytoma. American Heart Journal, 61, 375–381.

Crout, J.R. and Sjoerdsma, A. (1964) Turnover and metabolism of catecholamines in patients with pheochromocytoma. Journal of Clinical Investigation, 43, 94–102.

Cryer, P.E., Santiago, J.V. and Shah, S. (1974) Measurement of norepinephrine and epinephrine in small volumes of human plasma by a single isotope derivative method: response to the upright posture. Journal of Clinical Endocrinology and Metabolism, 39, 1025–1029.

Cuche, J.-L., Kuchel, O., Barbeau, A. and Genest, J. (1975) Urinary homovanillic acid, dopamine and noepinephrine excretion in patients with essential hypertension. Canadian Medical Association Journal, 112, 443–446.

Cuche, J.-L., Kuchel, O., Barbeau, A., Langlois, Y., Boucher, R. and Genest, J. (1974) Autonomic nervous system and benign essential hypertension in man. 1. Usual blood pressure, catecholamines, renin, and their interrelationships. Circulation Research, 35, 281–289.

Davis, V.E., Cashaw, J.L., Huff, J.A., Brown, H. and Nicholas, N.L. (1967) Alteration of endogenous catecholamine metabolism by ethanol ingestion. Proceedings of the Society of Experimental Biology, New York, 125, 1140–1143.

de Robertis, E. (1966) Pharmacological Reviews, 18, 413–424.

Dekirmenjian, H. and Maas, J.W. (1970) An improved procedure of 3-methoxy-4-hydroxyphenylethylene glycol determination by gas-liquid chromatography. Analytical Biochemistry, 35, 113–122.

Dekermenjian, H. and Maas, J. (1974) 3-Methoxy-4-hydroxyphenethylene glycol in plasma. Clinica Chimica Acta, 52, 203–210.

Despopoulos, A. and Weissbach, H. (1957) Renal metabolism of 5-hydroxyindoleacetic acid. American Journal of Physiology, 189, 548–550.

Dirscherl, W. and Thomas, H. (1966) Vanillsäure als ein Stoffwechselend-produkt. Revue Roumaine de Biochimie, 3, 47–54.

Doležal, V., Luxa, J. and Perich, F. (1971) Excretion of 3-methoxy-4-hydroxymandelic acid and 3-methoxy-4-hydroxyphenylacetic acid by pilots in relation to flying. Physiologia Bohemoslovaca, 20, 499–507.

Duckworth, T., Bond, P.A., McKibbin, B. and Mitchell, E.C. (1973) Urinary excretion of tyrosine metabolites in spina bifida. Clinica Chimica Acta, 43, 249–255.

Engelman, K. (1969) Principles in the diagnosis of pheochromocytoma. Bulletin of the New York Academy of Medicine, 45, 851–858.

Engelman, K. and Hammond, W.G. (1968) Adrenaline production by an intrathoracic pheochromocytoma, Lancet, i, 609–611.

Engelman, K. and Portnoy, B. (1970) A sensitive double-isotope derivative assay for norepinephrine and epinephrine. Normal resting human plasma levels. Circulation Research, 26, 53–57.

Engelman, K., Portnoy, B. and Sjoerdsma, A. (1970) Plasma catecholamine concentrations in patients with hypertension. Circulation Research, 27, Suppl. I, 141–146.

Engelman, K. and Sjoerdsma, A. (1964) A new test for pheochromocytoma: pressor responsiveness to tyramine. Journal of the American Medical Association, 189, 81–86.

Enquist, R.W., Tormey, D.C., Jenis, E.H. and Warkel, R.L. (1974) Malignant chemodectoma of the superior mediastinum with elevated urinary homovanillic acid. Chest, 66, 209–211.

Fellows, L., Riederer, P. and Sandler, M. (1975) A rapid assay of 4-hydroxy-3-methoxyphenylglycol in urine. Clinica Chimica Acta, 59, 255–257.

Fleisher, M., Dollinger, M.R. and Schwartz, M.K. (1969) Effect of 5-hydroxyindolylacetic acid in the colorimetric determination of urinary vanilmandelic acid. American Journal of Clinical Pathology, 51, 555–558.

Freedman, L.S., Ebstein, R.P., Goldstein, M., Axelrod, F.B. and Dancis, J. (1975) Serum dopamine-β-hydroxylase in familial dysautonomia. Journal of Laboratory and Clinical Medicine, 85, 1008–1012.

Fries, J.G. and Chamberlain, J.A. (1968) Extra-adrenal pheochromocytoma: literature review and report of cervical pheochromocytoma. Surgery (St. Louis), 63, 268–279.

Fuller, R.W. and Hunt, J.M. (1965) Substrate specificity of phenethanolamine *N*-methyl transferase. Biochemical Pharmacology, 14, 1896–1897.

Fuller, R.W. and Hunt, J.M. (1967) Inhibition of phenethanolamine *N*-methyl transferase by its product, epinephrine. Life Sciences, 6, 1107–1112.

Fuxe, F., Goldstein, M., Hökfelt, T., Jonsson, G. and Lidbrink, P. (1974) Dopaminergic involvement in hypothalamic function: extrahypothalamic and hypothalamic control. A neuroanatomical analysis. In Advances in Neurology, Vol. 5 (Eds. F.H. McDowell and A. Barbeau) pp. 405–419, Raven Press, New York.

Gabriel, R. and Harrison, B.D.W. (1974) Meningioma mimicking features of a phaeochromocytoma. British Medical Journal, 2, 312.

Garattini, S. and Valzelli, L. (1965) Serotonin. Elsevier, Amsterdam.

Garcia, R. and Jennings, J.M. (1972) Pheochromocytoma masquerading as a cardiomyopathy. American Journal of Cardiology, 29, 568–571.

Gascoigne, J.E., Williams, D. and Williams, E.D. (1975) Histochemical demonstration of an additional form of rat brain MAO. British Journal of Pharmacology, 54, 274P.

Geffen, L. (1974) Serum dopamine β-hydroxylase as an index of sympathetic function. Life Sciences, 14, 1593–1604.

Geiser, C.F. and Efron, M.L. (1968) Cystathioninuria in patients with neuroblastoma or ganglioneuroblastoma. Its correlation to vanilmandelic acid excretion and its value in diagnosis and therapy. Cancer, 22, 856–860.

Geissbuhler, F. (1970) Dosage fluorométrique de la normétanéphrine, de la métanephrine et de la 3-méthoxytyramine dans l'urine hydrolysée. Clinica Chimica Acta, 30, 143–148.

Gitlow, S.E., Bertani, L.M., Greenwood, S.M., Wong, B.L. and Dziedzic, S.W. (1972) Benign pheochromocytoma associated with elevated excretion of homovanillic acid. Journal of Pediatrics, 81, 1112–1116.

Gitlow, S.E., Bertani, L.M., Rausen, A., Gribetz, D. and Dziedzic, S.W. (1970a) Diagnosis of neuroblastoma by qualitative and quantitative metabolites in urine. Cancer, 25, 1377–1383.

Gitlow, S.E., Bertani, L.M., Wilk, E., Li, B.L. and Dziedzic, S. (1970b) Excretion of catecholamine metabolites by children with familial dysautonomia. Pediatrics, 46, 513–522.

Gitlow, S.E., Dziedzic, L.B., Strauss, L., Greenwood, S.M. and Dziedzic, S.W. (1973) Biochemical and histologic determinants in the prognosis of neuroblastoma. Cancer, 32, 898–905.

Gitlow, S.E., Mendlowitz, M. and Bertani, L.M. (1970c) The biochemical techniques for detecting and establishing the presence of a pheochromocytoma. A review of ten years experience. American Journal of Cardiology, 26, 270–279.

Gjessing, L.R. (1964) Studies of functional neural tumors. VI. Biochemical diagnosis. Scandinavian Journal of Clinical and Laboratory Investigation, 16, 661–669.

Gjessing, L.R. (1968) Biochemistry of functional neural crest tumours. Advances in Clinical Chemistry, 11, 81–131.

Gjessing, L.R. and Borud, O. (1965) Studies of functional neural tumours. VII. Urinary excretion of phenolic-pyruvic acids. Scandinavian Journal of Clinical and Laboratory Investigation, 17, 80–84.

Gjessing, L.R. and Mauritzen, K. (1965) Cystathioninuria in hepatoblastoma. Scandinavian Journal of Clinical Laboratory Investigation, 17, 513–514.

Glenner, G.G., Crout, J.R. and Roberts, W.C. (1962) A functional carotid body-like tumor secreting levarterenol. Archives of Pathology, 73, 230–240.

Glover, V., Sandler, M., Owen, F. and Riley, G.J. (1977) Dopamine is a monoamine oxidase B substrate in man. Nature, 265, 80–81.

Goldberg, L.I. (1972) Cardiovascular and renal actions of dopamine: potential clinical applications. Pharmacological Reviews, 24, 1–29.

Goldstein, M., Gang, H., Anagnoste, B., Goldstein, M.N. and Bohuon, A.C. (1968a) The biosynthesis and metabolism of catecholamines in neuroblastoma tissue cultures and in neuroblastoma tumours. Federation Proceedings, 27, 239.

Goldstein, M., Anagnoste, B. and Goldstein, M.N. (1968b) Tyramine-H^3: deaminated metabolites in neuroblastoma tumours and in continuous cell line of a neuroblastoma. Science, 160, 767–768.

Goldstein, M., Gang, H. and Joh, T.H. (1969) Subcellular distribution and properties of phenylethanolamine-*N*-methyl transferase (PNMT). Federation Proceedings, 28, 287.

Goodall, McC. and Berman, M.L. (1960) Urinary output of adrenaline, noradrenaline and 3-methoxy-4-hydroxymandelic acid following centrifugation and anticipation of centrifugation. Journal of Clinical Investigation, 39, 1533–1546.

Goode, D.J., Dekirmenjian, H., Meltzer, H.Y. and Maas, J.W. (1973) Relation of exercise to MHPG excretion in normal subjects. Archives of General Psychiatry, 29, 391–396.

Goodwin, B.L., Ruthven, C.R.J., Weg, M.W. and Sandler, M. (1975) A specific assay for urinary 5-hydroxyindole-3-acetic acid by gas chromatography. Clinica Chimica Acta, 62, 439–442.

Grahame-Smith, D.G. (1964a) Tryptophan hydroxylation in carcinoid tumours. Biochimica et Biophysica Acta, 86, 176–179.

Grahame-Smith, D.G. (1964b) Tryptophan hydroxylation in brain. Biochemical and Biophysical Research Communications, 16, 586–592.

Green, M. and Walker, G. (1970) Dietary vanillin does not affect the VMA method of Pisano et al. Clinica Chimica Acta, 29, 189–190.

Greenberg, R.E. and Gardner, L.I. (1960) Catecholamine metabolism in a functional neural tumour. Journal of Clinical Investigation, 39, 1729–1736.

Greenblatt, D.J., Ransil, B.J., Harmatz, J.S., Smith, T.W., Duhme, D.W. and Koch-Weser, J. (1976) Variability of 24-hour urinary creatinine excretion by normal subjects. Journal of Clinical Pharmacology, 16, 321–328.

Greer, M., Sprinkle, T.J. and Williams, C.M. (1968) Determination of urinary 3-methoxytyramine, normetanephrine and metanephrine in phaeochromocytoma and neuroblastoma by gas chromatography. Clinica Chimica Acta, 21, 247–253.

Griffiths, J. and Leung, F. (1971) The sequential estimation of plasma catecholamines and whole blood histamine in myocardial infarction. American Heart Journal, 82, 171–179.

Griffiths, J.C., Leung, F.Y.T. and McDonald. T.J. (1970) Fluorimetric determination of plasma catecholamines: normal human epinephrine and norepinephrine levels. Clinica Chimica Acta, 30, 395–405.

Häggendal, J., Hartley, L.H. and Saltin, B. (1970) Arterial noradrenaline concentration during exercise in relation to the relative work levels. Scandinavian Journal of Clinical and Laboratory Investigation, 26, 337–342.

Hanson, A. and von Studnitz, W. (1965) Demonstration of urinary *N*-acetyldopamine in patients with neuroblastoma. Clinica Chimica Acta, 11, 384–385.

Harrison, T.S., Bartlett, J.D. and Seaton, J.F. (1967) Exaggerated urinary norepinephrine response to tilt in pheochromocytoma. New England Journal of Medicine, 277, 725–728.

Hashimoto, Y., Kurobe, Y. and Hirota, K. (1974) Effect of delivery on dopamine-β-hydroxylase activity and urinary vanillyl mandelic acid excretion of normal pregnant subjects. Biochemical Pharmacology, 23, 2185–2187.

Hermann, H. and Mornex, R. (1964) Human Tumours Secreting Catecholamines. Pergamon, Oxford.

Herrlich, P. and Sekeris, C.E. (1964) Identifizierung von *N*-Acetyl-Noradrenalin im Urin eines Patienten mit Neuroblastom. Hoppe-Seyler's Zeitschrift für physiologische Chemie, 339, 249–250.

Himms-Hagen, J. (1972) Effects of catecholamines on metabolism. In Handbook of Experimental Pharmacology, Vol. 33, Catecholamines (Eds. H. Blaschko and E. Muscholl) pp. 363–462, Springer-Verlag, Berlin.

Hingerty, D. (1957) Thirty-minute screening test for phaeochromocytoma. Lancet, i, 766–767.

Hinterberger, H. and Bartholomew, R.J. (1969) Catecholamines and their acidic metabolites in urine and in tumour tissue in neuroblastoma, ganglioneuroma and phaeochromocytoma. Clinica Chimica Acta, 23, 169–175.

Hinterberger, A. Freedman, A. and Bartholomew, R.J. (1972) Precursors of melanin in the blood and urine in malignant melanoma. Clinica Chimica Acta, 39, 395–400.

Hoeldtke, R. (1972) Effect of aspirin on the assay of homovanillic acid in urine. American Journal of Clinical Pathology, 57, 324–325.

Holzbauer, M. and Sharman, D.F. (1972) The distribution of catecholamines in vertebrates. In Handbook of Experimental Pharmacology, Vol. 33, Catecholamines (Eds. H. Blaschko and E. Muscholl) pp. 110–185, Springer-Verlag, Berlin.

Hornykiewicz, O. (1966) Dopamine (3-hydroxytyramine) and brain function. Pharmacological Reviews, 18, 925–964.

Hörtnagl, H., Hörtnagl, H., Winkler, H., Asamer, H., Födisch, H.J. and Klima, J. (1972) Storage of catecholamines in neuroblastoma and ganglioneuroma: a biochemical, immunologic, and morphologic study. Laboratory Investigation, 27, 613–619.

Houslay, M.D. and Tipton, K.F. (1974) A kinetic evaluation of monoamine oxidase activity in rat liver mitochondrial outer membranes. Biochemical Journal, 139, 645–652.

Huikko, M., Jouppila, P. and Kärki, N.T. (1966) Effect of Finnish bath (sauna) on the urinary excretion of noradrenaline, adrenaline and 3-methoxy-4-hydroxy-mandelic acid. Acta Physiologica Scandinavica, 68, 316–321.

Huston, J.R. and Stewart, W.R.C. (1965) Hemorrhagic pheochromocytoma with shock and abdominal pain. American Journal of Medicine, 39, 502–504.

Imai, K., Wang., M.-T., Yoshime, S. and Tamura, Z. (1973) Determination of catecholamines in the plasma of patients with essential hypertension and of normal persons. Clinica Chimica Acta, 43, 145–149.

Imashuku, S., Takada, H., Sawada, T. and Nakamura, T. (1972) Tyrosine hydroxylase activity in neuroblastoma and human adrenal gland. Journal of Laboratory and Clinical Medicine, 80, 190–199.

Inoue, K., Takahashi, E., Adachi, T., Oikawa, R. and Kimura, T. (1968) Urinary excretion of catecholamine derivatives in essential hypertension. Tohoku Journal of Experimental Medicine, 95, 169–176.

Itoh, C., Yoshinaga, K., Sato, T., Ishida, N. and Wada, Y. (1962) Presence of *N*-methyl metadrenaline in human urine and tumour tissue of pheochromocytoma. Nature (London), 193, 477.

Iversen, L.L. (1967) The Uptake and Storage of Noradrenaline in Sympathetic Nerves. Cambridge University Press, London.

Iversen, L.L. (1973) Catecholamine uptake processes. British Medical Bulletin, 29, 130–135.

Jarrott, B. (1973) The cellular localisation and physiological role of catechol-*O*-methyl transferase in the body. In Frontiers in Catecholamine Research (Eds. E. Usdin and S.H. Snyder) pp. 113–115, Pergamon, New York.

Jepson, J.B. (1969) Indoles and related Ehrlich reactors. In Chromatographic and Electrophoretic Techniques, Vol. 1, 3rd edn. (Ed. I. Smith) pp. 243–273, Heinemann, London.

Jepson, J.B. (1972) Hartnup disease. In The Metabolic Basis of Inherited Disease, 3rd edn. (Eds. J.B. Stanbury, J.B. Wyngaarden and D.S. Fredrickson) pp. 1486–1503, McGraw-Hill, New York.

Johnson, A.T. Jr. and Halbert, D. (1974) Congenital neurolastoma presenting as hydrops fetalis. North Carolina Medical Journal, 35, 289–291.

Jones, N.F., Walker, G., Ruthven, C.R.J. and Sandler, M. (1968) α-Methyl-*p*-tyrosine in the management of phaeochromocytoma. Lancet, ii, 1105–1110.

Kahane, Z., Mowat, J.H. and Vestergaard, P. (1970) Gas-chromatographic estimation of 3-methoxy-4-hydroxyphenylglycol after transformation to vanillin methoxime trimethylsilyl ether. Clinica Chimica Acta, 30, 683–687.

Kahane, Z. and Vestergaard, P. (1969) Column chromatographic separation and fluorometric estimation of metanephrine and normetanephrine in urine. Clinica Chimica Acta, 25, 453–458.

Kahane, Z. and Vestergaard, P. (1971) The quantitative estimation of urinary 3-methoxy-4-hydroxy phenylacetic acid (homovanillic acid). Clinica Chimica Acta, 35, 49–52.

Karoum, F., Anah, C.O., Ruthven, C.R.J. and Sandler, M. (1969) Further observations on the gas-chromatographic measurement of urinary phenolic acid indolic metabolites. Clinica Chimica Acta, 24, 341–348.

Käser, H. (1966) Catecholamine-producing neural tumors other than pheochromocytoma. Pharmacological Reviews, 18, 659–665.

Käser, H. and Thomke, E. (1970) Quantitative fluorimetric determination of urinary 3-methoxytyramine. Clinica Chimica Acta, 27, 203–210.

Kaufman, S. (1966) Coenzymes and hydroxylases: ascorbate and dopamine-β-hydroxylase: tetrahydropteridines and phenylalanine and tyrosine hydroxylases. Pharmacological Reviews, 18, 61–69.

Kaufman, S. and Fisher, D.B. (1974) Pterin-requiring aromatic amino acid hydroxylases. In Molecular Mechanisms of Oxygen Activation (Ed. O. Hayaishi) pp. 285–369, Academic Press, New York.

Kaufmann, J.S. (1974) Pheochromocytoma and tricyclic antidepressants. Journal of the American Medical Association, 229, 1282.

Kebabian, J.W., Petzold, G.L. and Greengard, P. (1972) Dopamine-sensitive adenylate cyclase in the caudate nucleus of mammalian brain and its similarity to the "dopamine receptor". Proceedings of the National Academy of Science (U.S.A.), 69, 2145–2149.

Kinnier Wilson, L.M. and Draper, G.J. (1974) Neuroblastoma, its natural history and prognosis: a study of 487 cases. British Medical Journal, 3, 301–307.

Kinsbourne, M. and Woolf, L.I. (1959) Idiopathic infantile hypoglycaemia. Archives of Diseases in Childhood, 34, 166–170.

Knight, J.A., Fronk, S. and Haymond, R.E. (1975) Chemical basis and specificity of chemical screening tests for urinary vanilmandelic acid. Clinical Chemistry, 21, 130–133.

Koe, B.K. and Weissman, A. (1966) *p*-Chlorophenylalanine: a specific depletor of brain serotonin. Journal of Pharmacology and Experimental Therapeutics, 154, 499–516.

Koelle, G.B. (1959) Possible mechanisms for the termination of the physiological actions of catecholamines. Pharmacological Reviews, 11, 381–386.

Kogut, M.D. and Donnell, G.N. (1961) Cushing's syndrome in association with renal ganglioneuroblastoma. Pediatrics, 28, 566–577.

Konishi, N., Noguchi, T. and Kido, R. (1971) The pyrrole ring cleavaging enzyme of 5-hydroxytryptophan. Life Sciences, 10, 431–436.

Kopin, I.J. (1968) False adrenergic transmitters. Annual Review of Pharmacology, 8, 377–394.

Kopin, I.J. and Axelrod, J. (1960) Presence of 3-methoxy-4-hydroxyphenylglycol and metanephrine in phaeochromocytoma tissue. Nature (London), 185, 788.

Kopin, I.J., Pare, C.M.B., Axelrod, J. and Weissbach, H. (1960) 6-Hydroxylation: the major metabolic pathway for melatonin. Biochimica et Biophysica Acta, 40, 377–378.

Kuchel, O., Cuche, J.-L., Hamet, P., Barbeau, A., Boucher, R. and Genest, J. (1973) Catecholamines, cyclic adenosine monophosphate and renin in labile hypertension. In Mechanisms of Hypertension, International Congress Series No. 302. (Ed. M.P. Sambhi) pp. 160–175, Excerpta Medica, Amsterdam.

La Brosse, E.H. (1970) Catecholamine metabolism in neuroblastoma: kinetics of conversion of ^{3}H-3-methoxy-4-hydroxyphenylglycol to ^{3}H-3-methoxy-4-hydroxymandelic acid. Journal of Clinical Endocrinology, 30, 580–589.

Lachhein, L. and Schütz, J. (1967) Einfacher Test auf Phäochromocytome sowie Neuroblastome und Dünndarmcarcinoide, Bestimmung der 3-Methoxy-4-hydroxymandelsäure, 3-Methoxy-4-hydroxyphenylessigsäure und 5-Hydroxyindolessigsäure im Urin mittels Chromatoelektrophorese. Clinica Chimica Acta, 15, 429–434.

Lancet (1972) Leading article – Alcohol addiction: a biochemical approach. Lancet, ii, 24–25.

Langemann, H. (1957) Amino acid decarboxylase and amine oxidase in carcinoid tumour. In 5-Hydroxytryptamine (Ed. G.P. Lewis) pp. 153–157, Pergamon Press, London.

Latt, N., Rippey, J.J. and Stacey, R.S. (1968) Monoamine oxidase activity of platelets. British Journal of Pharmacology, 32, 427P.

Lauper, N.T., Tyce, G.M., Sheps, S.G. and Carney, J.A. (1972) Pheochromocytoma: fine structural, biochemical and clinical observations. American Journal of Cardiology, 30, 197–204.

Lees, M.H. (1966) Catecholamine metabolite excretion of infants with heart failure. Journal of Pediatrics, 69, 259–265.

Leonard, A.S., Roback, S.A., Nesbit, M.E. Jr. and Freier, E. (1972) The VMA test strip: a new tool for mass screening, diagnosis and management of catecholamine-secreting tumours. Journal of Pediatric Surgery, 7, 528–531.

Levi, L. (1967a) Stressors, stress tolerance, emotions and performance in relation to catecholamine excretion. Försvarsmedicin, 3, 192–200.

Levi, L. (1967b) The effect of coffee on the function of the sympathoadrenomedullary system in man. Acta Medica Scandinavica, 181, 431–438.

Levine, R.J. and Landsberg, L. (1974) In Diseases of Metabolism (Eds. P.K. Bondy and L.E. Rosenberg) p. 1190, Saunders, Philadelphia.

Lewis, R.P. and Boudoulas, H. (1974) Catecholamines, cigarette smoking, arrhythmias and acute myocardial infarction. American Heart Journal, 88, 526–528.

Lishajko, F. (1968) Occurrence and some properties of dopamine-containing granules in the sheep adrenal. Acta Physiologica Scandinavica, 72, 255–256.

Louis, W.J. and Doyle, A.E. (1971) The use of a double-isotope derivative plasma assay for noradrenaline and adrenaline in the diagnosis and localisation of phaeochromocytoma. Australian and New Zealand Journal of Medicine, 3, 212–217.

Louis, W.J., Doyle, A.E., Anavekar, S.N., Johnston, C.I., Geffen, L.B. and Rush, R. (1974) Plasma catecholamine, dopamine-beta-hydroxylase and renin levels in essential hypertension. Circulation Research, 34 and 35, Suppl. I, 57–63.

Louis, W.J., Doyle, A.E., Heath, W.C. and Robinson, M.J. (1972) Secretion of dopa in phaeochromocytoma. British Medical Journal, 4, 325–327.

Lovenberg, W., Weissbach, H. and Udenfriend, S. (1962) Aromatic L-amino acid decarboxylase. Journal of Biological Chemistry, 237, 89–93.

Lyles, G.A. and Callingham, B.A. (1975) Evidence for a clorgyline-resistant monoamine metabolizing activity in the rat blood, Journal of Pharmacy and Pharmacology, 27, 682–691.

McKibbin, B., O'Gorman, L. and Duckworth, T. (1969) Catecholamine metabolite excretion in spina bifida. Journal of Clinical Pathology, 22, 687–689.

McNamee, B., Kelvin, A.S. and Turnbull, M.J. (1971) Urinary excretion of some monoamines and metabolites in Huntington's chorea. Scottish Medical Journal, 16, 247–249.

Maas, J.W., Dekermenjian, H. and Jones, F. (1973) The identification of depressed patients who have a disorder of NE metabolism and/or disposition. In Frontiers in Catecholamine Research (Eds. E. Usdin and S.H. Snyder) pp. 1091–1096, Pergamon, New York.

Mahler, D.J. and Humoller, F.L. (1962) A comparison of methods for determining catecholamines and 3-methoxy-4-hydroxymandelic acid in urine. Clinical Chemistry, 8, 47–55.

Marsden, H.B. and Steward, J.K. (1968) Tumours of the sympathetic system. In Tumours in Children, Recent Results in Cancer Research, Vol. 13, pp. 131–170, Springer-Verlag, Berlin.

Matsaniotis, N., Beratis, N. and Economou-Mavrou, C. (1968a) Urinary vanillylmandelic acid (VMA) excretion by chronically anaemic children. Archives of Disease in Childhood, 43, 372–376.

Matsaniotis, N., Danelatos-Athanassiadis, C., Agathopoulos, A., Charokopos, E. and Constantsas, N. (1968b) Urinary excretion of catecholamines by children with collagen diseases. Clinica Chimica Acta, 22, 195–199.

Mayer, S.E. (1973) Metabolic responses of cardiac, skeletal muscle, and fat cells to catecholamines. In Frontiers in Catecholamine Research (Eds. E. Usdin and S.H. Snyder) pp. 351–356, Pergamon, New York.

Mellinger, T.J. and Hvidberg, E.F. (1969) Spectrofluorimetry of dihydroxyphenylacetic acid in urine. American Journal of Clinical Pathology, 51, 559–565.

Meloni, C.R., Tucci, J., Canary, J.J. and Kyle, L.H. (1966) Cushing's syndrome due to bilateral adrenocortical hyperplasia caused by a benign adrenal medullary tumor. Journal of Clinical Endocrinology and Metabolism, 26, 1192–1200.

Miller, R.W., Fraumeni, J.F. and Hill, J.A. (1968) Neuroblastoma: epidemiologic approach to its origin. American Journal of Diseases of Children, 115, 253–261.

Milne, M.D., Crawford, M.A., Girão, C.B. and Loughridge, L. (1960) The excretion of indolylacetic acid and related indolic acids in man and the rat. Clinical Science, 19, 165–179.

Montgomery, D.A.D. and Welbourn, R.B. (Eds.) (1975) The adrenal medulla and adrenalectomy. In Medical and Surgical Endocrinology. pp. 143–162, Edward Arnold, London.

Moses, S.W., Rotem, Y., Jagoda, N., Talmor, N., Eichhorn, F. and Levin, S. (1967) A clinical, genetic and biochemical study of familial dysautonomia in Israel. Israel Journal of Medical Sciences, 3, 358–371.

Nagatsu, T. and Udenfriend, S. (1972) Photometric assay of dopamine-β-hydroxylase activity in human blood. Clinical Chemistry, 18, 980–983.

Neal, C., Smith, C., Dubowski, K. and Naughton, J. (1968) 3-Methoxy-4-hydroxymandelic acid excretion during physical exercise. 24, 619–621.

Nelson, L.M., Bubb, F.A., Lax, P.M., Weg, M.W. and Sandler, M. (1979) An important method for the differential assay of 3-O-methylated catecholamines in human urine using ion-pair extraction and gas chromatography electron capture detection. Clinica Chimica Acta, 92, 235–240.

Nicholas, N.L., Brown, H. and Swander, A.M. (1969) An improved spectrophotometric method for determination of total 3-methoxy-4-hydroxyphenylglycol in urine. Clinical Chemistry, 15, 884–890.

Numata (Sudo), Y. and Nagatsu, T. (1975) Properties of tyrosine hydroxylase in peripheral nerves. Journal of Neurochemistry, 24, 317–322.

Ogihara, T., Nugent, C.A., Shen, S.-W. and Goldfein, S. (1975) Serum dopamine-β-hydroxylase activity in parents and children. Journal of Laboratory and Clinical Medicine, 85, 566–573.

Öhman, U., Granberg, P.-O., Hjern, B. and Sjöberg, H.E. (1974) Pheochromocytoma. Diagnosis, management and follow-up in twenty patients. Acta Chirurgica Scandinavica, 140, 660–666.

Page, L.B. and Jacoby, G.A. (1964) Catecholamine metabolism and storage granules in pheochromocytoma and neuroblastoma. Medicine (Baltimore), 43, 379–386.

Parkinson, D. (1969) Intracranial pheochromocytomas (active glomus jugulare). Journal of Neurosurgery, 31, 94–100.

Parrad, B. and Bohuon, C. (1968) Étude critique du dosage du VMA par la méthode de Pisano – interférence de l'acide homovanillique. Annales de Biologie Clinique, 26, 635–640.

Passon, P.G. and Peuler, J.D. (1973) A simplified radiometric assay for plasma norepinephrine and epinephrine. Analytical Biochemistry, 51, 618–631.

Pearson, J., Axelrod, F. and Dancis, J. (1974) Current concepts of dysautonomia: neuropathological defects. Annals of New York Academy of Sciences, 228, 288–300.

Pharmacological Reviews (1959) Symposium on catecholamines. Pharmacological Reviews, 11, 241–566.

Pharmacological Reviews (1966) Second symposium on catecholamines. Pharmacological Reviews, 18, 1–803.

Pisano, J.J. (1960) A simple analysis for normetanephrine and metanephrine in urine. Clinica Chimica Acta, 5, 406–414.

Pisano, J.J., Crout, J.R. and Abraham, D. (1962) Determination of 3-methoxy-4-hydroxymandelic acid in urine. Clinica Chimica Acta, 7, 285–291.

Pletscher, A. (1973) The impact of monoamine research on drug development. In Frontiers in Catecholamine Research (Eds. E. Usdin and S.H. Snyder) pp. 27–37, Pergamon, New York.

Pletscher, A., Da Prada, M., Berneis, K;H. and Tranzer, J.P. (1971) New aspects on the storage of 5-hydroxytryptamine in blood platelets. Experientia, 27, 993–1002.

Porter, C.C., Watson, L.S., Titus, D.C., Totaro, J.A. and Byer, S.S. (1962) Inhibition of dopa decarboxylase by the hydrazino analog of α-methyldopa.

Powis, G. (1975) The binding of catecholamines to human serum proteins. Biochemical Pharmacology, 24, 707–712.

Quay, W.B. (1974) Pineal Chemistry in Cellular and Physiological Mechanisms. Charles C. Thomas, Springfield, Illinois.

Quek, E.S.C., Buttery, J.E. and De Witt, G.F. (1975) Catecholamines in urine: an evaluation of alumina-trihydroxyindole methods and a description of an improved method. Clinica Chimica Acta, 58, 137–144.

Rath, R., Veselková, A., Vidláková, M. and Mašek, J. (1967) Excretion of vanilmandelic acid by obese women: preliminary report. American Journal of Clinical Nutrition, 20, 457–461.

Raymond, F.A. and Weinshilboum, R.M. (1975) Microassay of human erythrocyte catechol-*O*-methyltransferase: removal of inhibitory calcium ion with chelating resin. Clinica Chimica Acta, 58, 185–194.

Renzini, V., Brunori, C.A. and Valori, C. (1970) A sensitive and specific fluorimetric method for the determination of noradrenaline and adrenaline in human plasma. Clinica Chimica Acta, 30, 587–594.

Robinson, R., Smith, P. and Whittaker, S.R.F. (1964) Secretion of catecholamines in malignant phaeochromocytoma. British Medical Journal, 1, 1422–1424.

Rosenstein, B.J. and Engelman, K. (1963) Diarrhea in a child with a catecholamine secreting ganglioneuroma. Journal of Pediatrics, 63, 217–226.

Rosenthal, I.M., Greenberg, R., Kathan, R., Falk, G.S. and Wong, R. (1969) Catecholamine metabolism of a ganglioneuroma: correlation with electronmicrographs. Pediatric Research, 3, 413–424.

Ruthven, C.R.J. and Sandler, M. (1965) The estimation of 4-hydroxy-3-methoxyphenylglycol and total metadrenalines in human urine. Clinica Chimica Acta, 12, 318–324.

Ruthven, C.R.J. and Sandler, M. (1966) An improved method for the estimation of homovanillic acid in human urine. Clinica Chimica Acta, 14, 511–518.

Sandler, M. (1968) The role of 5-hydroxyindoles in the carcinoid syndrome. In Advances in Pharmacology, Vol. 6B (Eds. E. Costa and M. Sandler) pp. 127–142, Academic Press, New York.

Sandler, M. (1970) Biosynthesis and metabolism of the catecholamines. Schweizerische Medizinische Wochenschrift, 100, 526–531.

Sandler, M. (1972a) Catecholamine synthesis and metabolism in man: clinical implications (with special reference to parkinsonism). In Handbook of Experimental Pharmacology, Vol. 33, Catecholamines (Eds. H. Blaschko and E. Muscholl) pp. 845–899, Springer-Verlag, Berlin.

Sandler, M. (1972b) Migraine; a pulmonary disease? Lancet, i, 618–619.

Sandler, M., Bonham-Carter, S., Cuthbert, M.F. and Pare, C.M.B. (1975) Is there an increase in monoamine-oxidase activity in depressive illness? Lancet, i, 1045–1049.

Sandler, M., Bonham-Carter, S., Goodwin, B.L. and Ruthven, C.R.J. (1976) Trace amine metabolism in man. In Trace Amines and the Brain (Eds. E. Usdin and M. Sandler) pp. 233–281, Dekker, New York.

Sandler, M. and Ruthven, C.R.J. (1966) The measurement of 4-hydroxy-3-methoxymandelic acid and homovanillic acid. Pharmacological Reviews, 18, 343–351.

Sandler, M. and Ruthven, C.R.J. (1969a) The biosynthesis and metabolism of the catecholamines. In Progress in Medicinal Chemistry, Vol. 6 (Eds. G.P. Ellis and G.B. West) pp. 200–265, Butterworth, London.

Sandler, M. and Ruthven, C.R.J. (1969b) Catecholamines, their precursors and metabolites. In Chromatographic and Electrophoretic Techniques, Vol. 1, 3rd edn. (Ed. I. Smith) pp. 714–746, Heinemann, London.

Sandler, M. and Ruthven, C.R.J. (1974) Estimation of catecholamine metabolites in urine. Association of Clinical Pathologists, Broadsheet 82, September.

Sandler, M., Ruthven, C.R.J. and Ceasar, P.M. (1967) Urinary pH and the excretion of biologically active monoamines and their acidic metabolites. Proceedings of 7th International Congress in Biochemistry, Tokyo, p. 971.

Sandler, M. and Youdim, M.B.H. (1968) Promotion of 4-hydroxy-3-methoxyphenylglycol formation in man by reserpine. Nature (London), 217, 771–772.

Sandler, M. and Youdim, M.B.H. (1972) Multiple forms of monoamine oxidase: functional significance. Pharmacological Reviews, 24, 331–348.

Sandler, M., Youdim, M.B.H. and Hanington, E. (1974) A phenylethylamine-oxidising defect in migraine. Nature (London), 250, 335–337.

Sankoff, I. and Sourkes, T.L. (1963) Determination by thin-layer chromatography of urinary homovanillic acid in normal and disease states. Canadian Journal of Biochemistry, 41, 1381–1388.

Sato, T.L. (1965) The quantitative determination of 3-methoxy-4-hydroxyphenylacetic acid (homovanillic acid) in urine. Journal of Laboratory and Clinical Medicine, 66, 517–525.

Sato, T.L. and Sjoerdsma, A. (1965) Urinary homovanillic acid in phaeochromocytoma. British Medical Journal, 2, 1472–1473.

Scott, J. (1974) Meningioma mimicking features of a phaeochromocytoma. British Medical Journal, 3, 174.

Sekeris, C.E. and Herrlich, P. (1963) Nachweis von *N*-Acetyl-dopamin bei einem Fall von Phäochromocytom. Hoppe-Seyler's Zeitschrift für physiologische Chemie, 331, 289–291.

Sharman, D.F. (1973) Metabolites of catecholamines in the cerebrospinal fluid. In Frontiers in Catecholamine Research (Eds. E. Usdin and S.H. Snyder) pp. 1055–1061, Pergamon, New York.

Sharp, W.V. and Platt, R.L. (1971) Familial pheochromocytoma. Association with von Hippel–Lindau's disease. Angiology, 22, 141–146.

Siggers, D.C., Salter, C. and Toseland, P.A. (1970) A double isotope dilution method for differential determination of adrenaline and noradrenaline in plasma. Clinica Chimica Acta, 30, 373–376.

Sjoerdsma, A. (1961) Techniques for measuring monoamine oxidase inhibitory activity in man. Journal of Neuropsychiatry, 2, Suppl. 1, 159–162.

Sjoerdsma, A., Engelman, K., Waldmann, T.A., Cooperman, L.H. and Hammond, W.G. (1966) Pheochromocytoma – current concepts of diagnosis and treatment: combined clinical staff conference at the National Institutes of Health. Annals of Internal Medicine, 65, 1302–1326.

Sjoerdsma, A., Oates, J.A., Zaltman, P. and Udenfriend, S. (1959) Identification and assay of urinary tryptamine: application as an index of monoamine oxidase inhibition in man. Journal of Pharmacology and Experimental Therapeutics, 126, 217–222.

Sjoerdsma, A., Weissbach, H. and Udenfriend, S. (1955) Simple test for diagnosis of metastatic carcinoid (argentaffinoma). Journal of American Medical Association, 159, 397.

Sjoerdsma, A., Weissbach, H. and Udenfriend, S. (1956) A clinical, physiologic and biochemical study of patients with malignant carcinoid (argentaffinoma). American Journal of Medicine, 20, 520–532.

Sjöquist, B. and Änggård, E. (1974) Dopamine, homovanillic acid and 4-hydroxy-3-methoxyphenylglycol in hydrolytic enzyme preparations from *Helix pomatia*. Journal of Neurochemistry, 22, 1161.

Smellie, J.M. and Sandler, M. (1961) Secreting intrathoracic ganglioneuroma. Proceedings of the Royal Society of Medicine, 54, 327–329.

Smith, A.D. and Winkler, H. (1972) Fundamental mechanisms in the release of catecholamines. In Handbook of Experimental Pharmacology, Vol. 33, Catecholamines (Eds. H. Blaschko and E. Muscholl) pp. 538–617, Springer-Verlag, Berlin.

Smith, E.R.B. and Weil-Malherbe, H. (1962) Metanephrine and normetanephrine in human urine: method and results. Journal of Laboratory and Clinical Medicine, 60, 212–223.

Smith, E.R.B. and Weil-Malherbe, H. (1971) On the occurrence of glusulase-hydrolyzable conjugates of 3,4-dihydroxyphenylacetic and homovanillic acids in human urine. Clinica Chimica Acta, 35, 505–507.

Snyder, S.H. and Bennett, J.P. (1976) Neurotransmitter receptors in the brain: biochemical identification. Annual Review of Physiology, 38, 153–175.

Sourkes, T.L., Denton, R.L., Murphy, G.F., Chavez, B. and Saint Cyr, S. (1963) The excretion of dihydroxyphenylalanine, dopamine and dihydroxyphenylacetic acid in neuroblastoma. Pediatrics, 31, 660–668.

Sourkes, T.L. and Murphy, G.F. (1961) Determination of catecholamines and catecholamino acids by differential spectrophotofluorimetry. Methods in Medical Research, 9, 147–152.

Sourkes, T.L., Murphy, G.F. and Rabinovitch, A. (1961) Conversion of DL-*m*-tyrosine to dopamine in the rat. Nature (London), 189, 577–578.

Southgate, J. and Sandler, M. (1968) 5-Hydroxyindole metabolism in pregnancy. In Advances in Pharmacology, Vol. 6B (Eds. E. Costa and M. Sandler) pp. 179–186, Academic Press, New York.

Spector, S., Sjoerdsma, A. and Udenfriend, S. (1965) Blockade of endogenous norepinephrine synthesis by α-methyl-tyrosine, an inhibitor of tyrosine hydroxylase. Journal of Pharmacology and Experimental Therapeutics, 147, 86–95.

Sprague, A.D., Thelin, T.H. and Dilts, P.V. (1972) Phaeochromocytoma associated with pregnancy. Obstetrics and Gynecology, 39, 889–891.

Stacey, R.S. (1968) Some clinical aspects of 5-hydroxytryptamine. Annales Medicinae Experimentalis Fenniae, 46, 498–504.

Stackpole, R.H., Melicow, M.M. and Uson, A.C. (1963) Pheochromocytoma in children. Journal of Pediatrics, 63, 315–330.

Stern, L., Lees, M.H. and Leduc, J. (1965) Environmental temperature, oxygen consumption and catecholamine excretion in newborn infants. Pediatrics, 36, 367–373.

Stjärne, L. (1972) The synthesis, uptake and storage of catecholamines in the adrenal medulla. The effect of drugs. In Handbook of Experimental Pharmacology, Vol. 33, Catecholamines (Eds. H. Blaschko and E. Muscholl) pp. 231–269, Springer-Verlag, Berlin.

Stjärne, L., Lishajko, F. and Roth, R.H. (1967) Regulation of noradrenaline biosynthesis in nerve tissue. Nature (London), 215, 770–772.

Stone, R.A. (1975) Dopamine-beta-hydroxylase – an index of adrenergic function in hypertensive patients. Western Journal of Medicine, 123, 108–114.

Stone, M.L., Piliero, S.J., Hammer, H. and Portnoy, A. (1960) Epinephrine and norepinephrine in pregnancy. Obstetrics and Gynecology, 16, 674–678.

Stott, A.W. and Robinson, R. (1967a) The effect of α-methyldopa on excretion of noradrenaline metabolites. Journal of Pharmacy and Pharmacology, 19, 690–693.

Stott, A.W. and Robinson, R. (1967b) Urinary normetadrenaline excretion in essential hypertension. Clinica Chimica Acta, 16, 249–252.

Swartz, D.P., Box, B. and Stevenson, J.A.F. (1963) Epinephrine and norepinephrine in normal and abnormal pregnancy. Obstetrics and Gynecology, 22, 115–117.

Sznajderman, M., Januszewicz, W. and Wocial, B. (1974) Urinary excretion of dopamine in complicated and uncomplicated myocardial infarction. European Journal of Cardiology, 2, 29–33.

Thiery, M., Derom, R.M.J., van Kets, H.E., de Schaepdryver, A.F., Bernard, P.J., Bekaert, S.A.L., Hooft, C.M.J., Derom, F., Rolly, G. and Roels, H.J.L. (1967) Pheochromocytoma in pregnancy. American Journal of Obstetrics and Gynecology, 97, 21–29.

Thorson, Å., Hanson, A., Pernow, B., Söderström, N., Waldenström, J., Winblad, S. and Wulff, H.B. (1958) Carcinoid tumour within an ovarian teratoma in a patient with the carcinoid syndrome (carcinoidosis). Clinical picture and metabolic studies before and after total resection of tumour. Acta Medica Scandinavica, 161, 495–505.

Tiedge, F., Scheiffarth, F. and Schmid, E. (1964) Über eine Sonderform von hormonal aktivem Tumor des Glomus jugulare-tympanicum. Zeitschrift für Laryngologie, Rhinologie, Otologie und ihre Grenzgebiete, 43, 271–273.

Toda, N. (1975) Analysis of the effect of 5-hydroxykynurenamine, a serotonin metabolite, on isolated cerebral arteries, aortas and atria. Journal of Pharmacology and Experimental Therapeutics, 193, 385–392.

Tong, J.H., D'Iorio, A. and Benoiton, N.L. (1971) Formation of *meta*-tyrosine from L-phenylalanine by beef adrenal medulla. A new biosynthetic route to catecholamines. Biochemical and Biophysical Research Communications, 44, 229–236.

Udenfriend, S. (1966) Tyrosine hydroxylase. Pharmacological Reviews, 18, 43–51.

Udenfriend, S., Titus, E. and Weissbach, H. (1955) The identification of 5-hydroxy-3-indoleacetic acid in normal urine and a method for its assay. Journal of Biological Chemistry, 216, 499–505.

Usdin, E. and Snyder, S.H. (Eds.) (1973) Frontiers in Catecholamine Research. Pergamon, New York.

Vaage, O. (1974) Fluorometric determination of epinephrine and norepinephrine in 1 ml urine introducing dithiothreitol and boric acid as stability and sensitivity-improving agents of the trihydroxyindole method. Biochemical Medicine, 9, 41–53.

Vaccarezza, J.R. and Ruiz, D.C. (1969) The excretion of a urinary metabolite of epinephrine and norepinephrine in tuberculosis. American Review of Respiratory Disease, 100, 398–400.

Valori, C., Thomas, M. and Shillingford, J.P. (1967) Urinary excretion of free noradrenaline and adrenaline following acute myocardial infarction. Lancet, i, 127–130.

van de Calseyde, J.F., Scholtis, R.J.H., Schmidt, N.A. and Leyten, C.J.J.A. (1971) Gas chromatography in the estimation of urinary metanephrine and VMA. Clinica Chimica Acta, 32, 361–366.

Vesell, E.S., Passananti, G.T. and Lee, C.H. (1971) Impairment of drug metabolism by disulfiram in man. Clinical Pharmacology and Therapeutics, 12, 785–792.

Vettorazzi, G. (1974) 5-Hydroxytryptamine content of bananas and banana products. Food and Cosmetics Toxicology, 12, 107–113.

Vialli, M. (1966) Histology of the enterochromaffin cell system. In Handbook of Experimental Pharmacology, Vol. 19 (Ed. V. Erspamer) pp. 1–65, Springer-Verlag, Berlin.

Vidi, A. and Bonardi, G. (1972) Simple quantitative method for determining 3-methoxy-4-hydroxyphenylacetic acid and 3,4-dihydroxyphenylacetic acid in urine. Clinica Chimica Acta, 38, 463–464.

Visser, J.W. and Axt, R. (1975) Bilateral adrenal medullary hyperplasia: a clinicopathological entity. Journal of Clinical Pathology, 28, 298–304.

von Euler, U.S. (1972) Synthesis, uptake and storage of catecholamines in adrenergic nerves, the effect of drugs. In Handbook of Experimental Pharmacology, Vol. 33, Catecholamines (Eds. H. Blaschko and E. Muscholl) pp. 186–230, Springer-Verlag, Berlin.

von Euler, U.S. (1974) Sympatho-adrenal activity in physical exercise. Medicine and Science in Sports, 6, 165–173.

von Studnitz, W. (1966) Chemistry and pharmacology of catecholamine secreting tumors. Pharmacological Reviews, 18, 645–650.

von Studnitz, W. (1969) Phenylethanolamine-*N*-methyltransferase and neuroblastoma. Enzymologia Biologica et Clinica, 10, 45.7.

von Studnitz, W. (1970) Cystathioninuria in children with neuroblastoma with and without metastasis. Acta Pediatrica Scandinavia, 59, 80–82.

von Studnitz, W., Käser, H. and Sjoerdsma, A. (1963) Spectrum of catecholamine biochemistry in patients with neuroblastoma. New England Journal of Medicine, 269, 232–235.

Voorhess, M.L. (1966) Functioning neural tumors. Pediatric Clinics of North America, 13, 3–18.

Voorhess, M.L. (1970) Urinary excretion of DOPA and metabolites by patients with melanoma. Cancer, 26, 146–149.

Voorhess, M.L. (1974) Neuroblastoma – pheochromocytoma; products and pathogenesis. Annals of the New York Academy of Sciences, 230, 187–194.

Voûte, P.A. Jr., Wadman, S.K. and van Putten, W.J. (1970) Congenital neuroblastoma. Symptoms in the mother during pregnancy. Clinical Pediatrics, 9, 206–207.

Walters, G., Wyatt, G.B. and Kelleher, J. (1962) Carcinoma of the adrenal cortex presenting as a pheochromocytoma: report of a case. Journal of Clinical Endocrinology and Metabolism, 22, 575–580.

Wang, M.-T., Imai, K., Yoshioka, M. and Tamura, Z. (1974) Determination of 3-methoxytyramine, normetanephrine and metanephrine in human plasma by gas chromatography. Chemical and Pharmaceutical Bulletin, 22, 970.

Waymire, J.C., Weiner, N., Schneider, F.H., Goldstein, M. and Freedman, L.S. (1972) Tyrosine hydroxylase in human adrenal and pheochromocytoma: localization, kinetics and catecholamine inhibition. Journal of Clinical Investigation, 51, 1798–1804.

Weg, M.W., Ruthven, C.R.J., Goodwin, B.L. and Sandler, M. (1975) Specific gas chromatographic measurement of urinary 3,4-dihydroxyphenylacetic acid. Clinica Chimica Acta, 59, 249–251.

Weil-Malherbe, H. (1961) The fluorimetric estimation of catecholamines. Methods in Medical Research, 9, 130–146.

Weil-Melherbe, H., Smith, E.R.B. and Bowles, G.R. (1968) Excretion of catecholamines and catecholamine metabolites in Project Mercury pilots. Journal of Applied Physiology, 24, 146–151.

Weil-Malherbe, H. and van Buren, J.M. (1969) The excretion of dopamine and dopamine metabolites in Parkinson's disease and the effect of diet thereon. Journal of Laboratory and Clinical Medicine, 74, 305–318.

Williams, C.M. and Greer, M. (1962) Diagnosis of neuroblastoma by quantitative gas chromatographic analysis of urinary homovanillic and vanilomandelic acid. Clinica Chimica Acta, 7, 880–883.

Williams, E.D. (1965) A review of 17 cases of carcinoma of the thyroid and phaeochromocytoma. Journal of Clinical Pathology, 18, 288–292.

Williams, K. and Munro Neville, A. (1976) Biochemical abnormalities in some human neoplasms. (4) Tumours of the adrenal gland. In Scientific Foundations of Oncology (Eds. T. Symington and R.L. Carter) pp. 98–107, Heinemann, London.

Winkler, H. and Smith, A.D. (1972) Phaeochromocytoma and other catecholamine-producing tumours. In Handbook of Experimental Pharmacology, Vol. 33, Catecholamines (Eds. H. Blaschko and E. Muscholl) pp. 900–933, Springer-Verlag, Berlin.

Wolstenholme, G.E.W. and Knight, J. (Eds.) (1976) Monoamine Oxidase and Its Inhibition. Elsevier/North-Holland Biomedical Press, Amsterdam.

Wong, K.P., Ruthven, C.R.J. and Sandler, M. (1973) Gas chromatographic measurement of urinary catecholamines by an electron capture detection procedure. Clinica Chimica Acta, 47, 215–222.

Wurtman, R.J. (1966) Control of epinephrine synthesis in the adrenal medulla by the adrenal cortex hormonal specificity and dose-response characteristics. Endocrinology, 79, 608–614.

Youdim, M.B.H. (1973) Multiple forms of mitochondrial monoamine oxidase. British Medical Bulletin, 29, 120–122.

Zambotti, F., Blau, K., King, G.S., Campbell, S. and Sandler, M. (1975) Monoamine metabolites and related compounds in human amniotic fluid: assay by gas chromatography and gas chromatography–mass spectrometry. Clinica Chimica Acta, 61, 247–256.

Zuspan, F.P. (1970) Urinary excretion of epinephrine and norepinephrine during pregnancy. Journal of Clinical Endocrinology, 30, 357–360.

Zuspan, F.P., Nelson, G.H. and Ahlquist, R.P. (1967) Alterations of urinary epinephrine and norepinephrine. The antepartum, intrapartum and postpartum periods. American Journal of Obstetrics and Gynecology, 99, 709–721.

FURTHER READING

Blaschko, H. and Muscholl, E. (Eds.) (1972) Handbook of Experimental Pharmacology, Vol. 33, Catecholamines. Springer-Verlag, Berlin.

Costa, E., Gessa, G.L. and Sandler, M. (Eds.) (1974) Serotonin – New Vistas, Advances in Biochemical Psychopharmacology, Vols. 10 and 11. Raven, New York.

Costa, E. and Sandler, M. (Eds.) (1968) Biological Role of Indolealkylamine Derivatives, Advances in Pharmacology, Vol. 6, Parts A and B. Academic Press, New York.

Costa, E. and Sandler, M. (Eds.) (1972) Monoamine Oxidases – New Vistas, Advances in Biochemical Psychopharmacology, Vol. 5, Raven, New York.

Erspamer, V. (Ed.) (1966) 5-Hydroxytryptamine and Related Indolealkylamines, Handbook of Experimental Pharmacology, Vol. 19. Springer-Verlag, Berlin.

Gjessing, L.R. (1968) Biochemistry of functional neural crest tumours. Advances in Clinical Chemistry, 11, 81–131.

Johnston, J.P. (1968) Some observations upon a new inhibitor of monoamine oxidase in brain tissue. Biochemical Pharmacology, 17, 1285–1297.

Montgomery, D.A.D. and Welbourn, R.B. (1975) The adrenal medulla and adrenalectomy. In Medical and Surgical Endocrinology. pp. 143–162, Edward Arnold, London.

Quay, W.B. (1974) Pineal Chemistry in Cellular and Physiological Mechanisms. Charles C. Thomas, Springfield, Illinois.

Sandler, M. and Ruthven, C.R.J. (1969) The biosynthesis and metabolism of the catecholamines. In Progress in Medicinal Chemistry (Eds. G.P. Ellis and G.B. West) pp. 200–265, Butterworth, London.

Usdin, E. and Sandler, M. (Eds.) (1976) Trace Amines and the Brain. Dekker, New York.

Usdin, E. and Snyder, S.H. (Eds.) (1973) Frontiers in Catecholamine Research. Pergamon, New York.

Wolstenholme, G.E.W. and Knight, J. (Eds.) (1976) Monoamine Oxidase and Its Inhibition. Elsevier/North-Holland Biomedical Press, Amsterdam.

Chapter 25

Cancer

Morton K. Schwartz and Donald S. Young

Department of Biochemistry, Memorial Hospital for Cancer and Allied Diseases, New York, NY 10021 and Department of Laboratory Medicine, Mayo Clinic, Rochester, MN 55901, U.S.A.

CONTENTS

Chemical diagnosis of disease, edited by
S.S. Brown, F.L. Mitchell and D.S. Young

25.1. INTRODUCTION

The early diagnosis and treatment of cancer generally leads to a better prognosis. The inadequacy of both history and physical examination in enabling an early diagnosis to be made has prompted the extensive use of ancillary aids such as clinical laboratory tests, X-rays and other elaborate diagnostic procedures.

For many years clinical laboratory tests that are specific for cancer have been sought. This has generally been unsuccessful although for a few tumours, characterized by unusual metabolites, it is now possible to detect the presence of a neoplasm. Even in these situations it is not possible to identify the site of the tumour, whether it is benign or malignant, the presence or absence of metastases, or the severity of the disease. It is unwise to make a judgement on the presence or absence of a tumour solely on findings from a clinical laboratory, because of the far reaching consequences of such a decision. Undoubtedly, laboratory tests do have a role in certain diagnostic situations, but the major role may lie in monitoring the response to treatment by following the change in concentration or activity of a constituent that has been clearly associated with the presence of tumour.

While the following discussion is largely concerned with the association of a change in test values with particular tumours it is rare in clinical practice to have a situation in which malignant disease, at least in an advanced state, is not complicated by other manifestations of disease. Thus cachexia and fever are frequent complications. Encephalopathy, dermatomyositis and osteoarthropathy are also commonly associated with malignant disease even though the cause is frequently unexplained (Bondy, 1976). The presence of a tumour may lead to obstruction of various organs, such as the ureter, gastrointestinal tract and bile-duct, each of which can be associated with a group of signs and symptoms which are characteristic of the obstruction but not of cancer. Tumours may also lead to haemorrhage with a resulting anaemia. Certain tumours may secrete hormones, and others may present with hypercalcaemia or hyperglycaemia.

Bodansky (1975) emphasized the requirement for blood tests for the diagnosis of cancer. These should depend on the release of material from the tumour, or reaction of the tumour on surrounding tissue releasing substances into the circulation. Moreover, the test should give an indication of the clinical status of the patient, being capable of indicating an increase or decrease in the size of the tumour as this occurs with growth, or response to treatment. To these requirements should be added others of sensitivity, specificity, simplicity and short analytical time. Few of our current tests meet these criteria, although to some extent the concentration of human chorionic gonadotrophin in choriocarcinoma, lysozyme in myelomonocytic leukaemia, and monoclonal γ-globulins in myelomatosis does correlate with tumour mass (Cooper, 1976). It should also be noted that while a single test may not be of value in indicating the presence of a tumour, a combination of tests when used with discriminant analysis may provide greater certainty in the laboratory diagnosis of a tumour.

Few of the current diagnostic tests are able to pinpoint the site of a tumour, but it is possible in certain instances, when there is a strong suspicion that a particular organ is involved, to use certain tests on the arterial and venous blood perfusing it to confirm or disprove the suspicion.

25.2. ENZYMES

Increased activities of certain enzymes in serum are commonly found in malignant disease. No enzyme is specific for cancer and the presence of increased activity of an enzyme in serum is not diagnostic of cancer, or indicative of its site or the presence or absence of metastases. Many of the enzymes that have been associated with cancer are common to many tissues. Others are confined to a few tissues.

There are probably several mechanisms for the increased activities of serum enzymes in cancer. The tumour may produce large quantities of enzyme, as exemplified by the production of alkaline phosphatase in osteogenic sarcoma. Blockage of duct systems, such as the pancreatic or biliary duct, through which an enzyme passes as it is eliminated from the body, may cause regurgitation of the enzyme into the blood stream. Metastatic tumours may cause induction of enzymes, e.g. alkaline phosphatase and 5′-nucleotidase, in the liver. Altered permeability of tumour cell membranes may cause leakage of enzyme to the blood stream. Rapid turnover of cells may also allow the release of enzyme into the blood-stream as the cells die or are destroyed.

Alteration of renal function, as frequently occurs in advanced malignant disease, may affect the rate of excretion of enzymes eliminated by the kidney. The presence of abnormal quantities of endogenous or exogenous activators or inhibitors in the blood stream may also affect the metabolism of the enzymes, and hence their activities.

25.2.1. Organ-specific enzymes

Of the various schemes that have been proposed for classification of enzymes, that which considers cellular enzymes as either organ-specific or general metabolic enzymes is most useful for the discussion of enzymes related to cancer.

25.2.1.1. Acid phosphatase

Measurement of the activity of serum acid phosphatase (EC 3.1.3.2) was one of the first laboratory tests to be used for the diagnosis of cancer. It has been used for almost 40 years in the evaluation of carcinoma of the prostate. Up to 90% of patients with carcinoma of the prostate with skeletal metastases have increased activity of acid phosphatase in their serum. When metastases have occurred to soft tissues only, the incidence of increased acid phosphatase activity is lower and the maximum values are less than when bone metastases are present. Enzyme activity is elevated in only 24% of patients without metastases. Many studies have demonstrated that activity is not increased in benign prostatic hypertrophy or prostatitis. However, the low incidence of increased serum enzyme activity in early prostatic cancer has meant that measurement of serum acid phosphatase activity is relatively poor in providing assistance in the differential diagnosis of prostatic diseases.

The substrate used for the measurement of acid phosphatase activity may influence the results in different diseases. Thus, when phenylphosphate is used instead of β-glycerophosphate, increased activity may be observed in Paget's disease, hyperparathyroidism, myeloproliferative disorders and Gaucher's disease. Increased activity is more often observed in malignant disease other than prostatic carcinoma when phenylphosphate is used in place of β-glycerophosphate. While Fishman et al. (1956) have observed a greater incidence of increased tartrate-inhibitable acid phosphatase activity than that of total acid phosphatase in cases of carcinoma of the prostate, our experience has failed to convince us that tartrate inhibition is useful as a clinical laboratory tool. Marshall and Amador (1969) even question the utility of any acid phosphatase measurements in the diagnosis of carcinoma of the prostate. They demonstrated convincingly that clinicians are able to make the diagnosis of carcinoma of the prostate without any measurements of the enzyme.

There is some dispute as to whether serial determinations of acid phosphatase can indicate exacerbation or remission of a neoplasm. In patients who have been successfully treated by orchiectomy or stilboestrol administration, high activity may persist in spite of a successful clinical response. Extensive metastases have also been observed when there are only small increases in the serum enzyme activity. Assay of acid phosphatase in serum obtained from bone marrow aspirates from the posterior superior iliac crest has been advocated as useful for the staging of prostatic carcinoma. In several cases this has demonstrated more advanced disease than was initially supposed (Reynolds et al., 1973). Indeed, serum acid phosphatase activity may be normal with a localized tumour and bone marrow enzyme activity may be increased. Bone marrow blood acid phosphatase may be greatly increased in the presence of metastases to bone. Increased bone marrow aspirate acid phosphatase is not specific for prostatic carcinomas, as increased activity has been observed in various anaemias, and in leukaemia, multiple myeloma and oat cell carcinoma.

When serum of healthy adults is fractionated by disc electrophoresis on polyacrylamide gel three to five acid phosphatase isoenzymes are observed. Electrophoresis of homogenates of prostatic tissue or the serum of patients with prostatic carcinoma has revealed additional isoenzymes. This technique requires further evaluation as a diagnostic aid in cancer of the prostate. A radioimmunological technique has now been developed for human prostatic acid phosphatase which can detect as little as 0.1 ng of phosphatase protein in 0.1 ml serum with an error of 5% on duplicate analysis (Cooper and Foti, 1974). This technique also warrants further investigation in the diagnosis of prostatic carcinoma.

The isoenzyme composition of acid phosphatase differs between normal and leukaemic leucocytes (Schapira, 1973). The isoenzyme composition of leukaemic cells in spleen and bone marrow is different from that of the acid phosphatase of lymphosarcoma.

25.2.1.2. Alkaline phosphatase

Assays of serum alkaline phosphatase (EC 3.1.3.1) have been useful in evaluation of cancer of bone or liver and cancer that has metastasized to these tissues. In primary tumours of bone, as well as in metastatic disease of bone, alkaline phosphatase activity is increased when the tumour is primarily osteoblastic. With breast carcinoma, most bony metastases are osteolytic, and alkaline phosphatase activity is usually within the normal range or only slightly increased. In prostatic carcinoma most of the metastatic lesions are osteoblastic, and the serum alkaline phosphatase activity is elevated to 4 or 10 times the upper limit of normal. During successful treatment, there may be an elevation in the serum alkaline phosphatase activity, presumably related to the repair of bone. These elevations have been referred to as the "paradoxical rise" in serum alkaline phosphatase. Serial alkaline phosphatase measurements have proved useful in monitoring the response of osteogenic sarcomata to therapy (Rosen, 1975). Changes in enzyme activity may occur prior to clinical evidence of response, or lack of response, to the drug and permit changes in the chemotherapeutic regime earlier than would otherwise have been possible. The magnitude of the increase in serum alkaline phosphatase activity that typically occurs with various neoplastic diseases which affect bone is illustrated in Table 25.1.

Modest increases in the activity of serum alkaline phosphatase are observed in about 40% of patients with multiple myeloma. Greater increases are observed in most patients with parathyroid adenoma or carcinoma. Alkaline phosphatase activity may also be greatly increased in non-neoplastic disease of the bone such as rickets and Paget's disease.

More than 90% of patients with extrahepatic obstruction of the bile ducts demonstrate increases in serum alkaline phosphatase activity to more than twice the upper limit of

TABLE 25.1.

INCREASES IN SERUM ALKALINE PHOSPHATASE ACTIVITY IN CASES WITH TUMOURS AFFECTING BONE

(Reproduced, by permission, from Schwartz, 1973)

Cancer type	Number	Percent of cases within				
		Normal range	1.1–1.9× normal	2.0–3.9× normal	4.0–6.0× normal	More than 6× normal
Osteogenic sarcoma						
(a) blastic	18	0	39	39	11	11
(b) lytic	16	50	25	19	6	0
Parathyroid	39	3	15	20	31	31
Breast with metastases	40	23	53	18	3	5
Prostate with metastases	29	14	35	17	10	24
Multiple myeloma	23	57	43	0	0	0

normal. The exact mechanism for the increase is not understood but it is presumed to be related to pressure transmitted from the obstructed bile duct to the liver. In infiltrative disease of the liver such as leukaemia, reticulum cell sarcoma or Hodgkin's disease, alkaline phosphatase activity may be markedly increased and directly related to the extent of liver involvement. In one study of patients with intrahepatic metastases the mean alkaline phosphatase activity in individuals without a palpable liver was 1.2 times the upper limit of normal; when the liver was palpable at the costal margin it was 1.8 times the upper limit, and in those with the liver palpable at the umbilicus or below, the mean activity was 3 times the upper limit of normal.

In another study of patients thought to have liver metastases but whose liver was normal on laparotomy, 32% demonstrated increased serum alkaline phosphatase activity, whereas 81% of patients with a single nodule of tumour, and 83% of patients with tumour in either one or both lobes, had increased serum alkaline phosphatase activity. The incidence of increased alkaline phosphatase activity was greater than that of increased retention of bromosulphthalein or increased bilirubin concentration or alanine aminotransferase activity. Aminotransferase activity was increased in only 18% of patients with an isolated nodule or larger metastasis in one lobe and 56% of those with extensive metastases. In patients with primary liver cancer, increase in alkaline phosphatase activity is found more often than increase in retention of bromosulphthalein, or activity of aspartate or alanine aminotransferase or bilirubin concentration, and even α-foetoprotein concentration. Increased activity of alkaline phosphatase has been observed in as many as 86% of these patients (Almersjö et al., 1974).

Recently there has been considerable interest in the isoenzymes of alkaline phosphatase and the so-called "Regan isoenzyme" in the serum of patients with cancer. In 1968, Fishman and his associates identified an unusual alkaline phosphatase isoenzyme in the serum and malignant tissue of a patient with carcinoma of the lung. They named the isoenzyme the Regan isoenzyme after the patient in whom it was detected. Investigations have demonstrated that the isoenzyme is identical to the heat-stable, L-phenylalanine-sensitive alkaline phosphatase of human placenta in its electrophoretic mobility before and after neuraminidase treatment, and in its reaction with antiserum prepared against placental alkaline phosphatase. In several studies the Regan isoenzyme, determined by heat stability, has been observed in from 7 to 10% of patients with different forms of cancer. Cadeau et al. (1974), using the heat-stability properties of the isoenzyme, found it in 15% of women with cancer of the breast and genitourinary tract. Ovarian and pancreatic carcinomas appear to have the highest incidence of Regan isoenzyme activity. The isoenzyme has been described as a carcinoplacental antigen and the amount of the isoenzyme reflects the clinical status of the patient (Fishman, 1974). Nevertheless, patients with early cervical carcinoma tend to have a higher incidence of the placental isoenzyme than patients with advanced disease. This situation also pertains with carcinoma of the uterus (Kellen et al., 1976).

Regan isoenzyme has also been reported in the serum of patients with stage IV Hodgkin's disease and poorly differentiated lymphoma. However, with a sensitive immunochemical assay, Regan isoenzyme has been detected in almost all healthy adults that have been studied and in as high a proportion of patients with malignant disease. Only 10% of the cancer patients showed increased quantities of the isoenzyme – a figure comparable to the incidence of Regan isoenzyme activity as determined by traditional methods. The increase varied from 3 to 300 times the average normal value (Usategui-Gomez et al., 1973).

An alkaline phosphatase variant differing from the Regan isoenzyme has been observed in the serum of 6 of 21 patients with hepatoma (Portugal et al., 1970). All of these patients had α-foetoprotein in their serum. The variant was not found in any of 16 cases in whom the α-foetoprotein test was negative. Higashino et al. (1975) have identified a different variant in other patients with hepatocellular carcinoma. It was only observed in advanced cases. In other studies of cancer patients it has been shown that the Regan isoenzyme is not related to the presence in serum of carcinoembryonic antigen, chorionic gonadotrophin or placental lactogen (Sussman et al., 1974).

Another alkaline phosphatase variant, similar in all respects to the Regan isoenzyme except for an additional sensitivity to leucine, has been found in sera of patients with cancer of the lung, pancreas and bile duct (Fishman, 1974). Yet another variant which is inhibited to a lesser degree by heat or phenylalanine than the Regan isoenzyme, and which during electrophoresis migrates anodally at a somewhat more rapid rate than the normal liver isoenzyme, has been found in the serum of 8 of 10 patients with hepatocellular carcinoma (Fishman, 1974). Additional isoenzymes of alkaline phosphatase have been observed on electrophoresis of serum from individual patients with adrenal carcinoma, metastasizing ventricular carcinoma, lung cancer, carcinoma of the pancreas and islet cell tumour (Schwartz, 1973). Alkaline phosphatase isoenzyme variants have also been observed in some cancer-related benign diseases including familial polyposis, ulcerative colitis and some types of hepatic cirrhosis (Nathanson and Fishman, 1971). Despite the association of alkaline phosphatase isoenzyme variants with malignant disease, and the claim that sequential measurements may indicate the clinical state and the response to therapy of cancer patients, such measurements have not gained general clinical acceptance.

Since serum alkaline phosphatase activity may be elevated in either bone or liver disease, it is important to establish the source of the elevated serum enzyme activity. Electrophoresis, heat stability, the use of specific chemical inhibitors and immunochemical techniques may be used to differentiate the tissue origin. It is relatively simple to differentiate between intestinal or kidney alkaline phosphatase on the one hand and enzyme from either bone or liver on the other, but separation and differential identification of the bone enzyme from liver alkaline phosphatase is more subtle and difficult. In our experience, the measurement of 5′-nucleotidase is a simple and precise method of establishing whether bone or liver is the source of increased alkaline phosphatase activity.

25.2.1.3. 5′-Nucleotidase

5′-Nucleotidase (EC 3.1.3.5; 5′-ribonucleotide phosphohydrolase) specifically catalyzes the hydrolysis of 5′-nucleotides. The test is useful in confirming the presence of liver disease when the serum alkaline phosphatase activity is increased and skeletal surveys indicate the presence of bony metastases. In some patients, the 5′-nucleotidase increase may be the only indicator of liver involvement and it may be elevated at a time when other biochemical tests of liver function and liver scan or physical palpation fail to suggest metastases to the liver. Serum 5′-nucleotidase activity may increase earlier than that of alkaline phosphatase. The magnitude of the increase may also be greater for 5′-nucleotidase than alkaline phosphatase. In neoplastic hepatic disease, without skeletal metastases, 5′-nucleotidase measurement may be a more sensitive indicator of hepatic metastases than alkaline phosphatase activity.

25.2.1.4. Leucine aminopeptidase

Leucine aminopeptidase (EC 3.4.11.1; L-leucyl-peptide hydrolase) was originally considered a specific marker for pancreatic carcinoma, but it is now considered to be an indicator of liver involvement both by metastatic disease and a variety of liver diseases including hepatitis and biliary calculi. Like 5′-nucleotidase, leucine aminopeptidase is able to provide an indication as to whether an elevated serum alkaline phosphatase activity is of skeletal or liver origin. However, it is incapable of differentiating whether an elevation is due to a benign or malignant tumour. Leucine aminopeptidase is widely distributed in the tissues of the body and increased activity has been observed in the serum and urine of patients with a wide variety of disseminated cancers, although many of the elevations are attributable to involvement of the liver.

Two major isoenzymes of leucine aminopeptidase have been observed in normal serum. These are designated X, which migrates on electrophoresis in the region of α_2-globulin, and Y which migrates in the β-globulin region; a small amount of a third isoenzyme, designated Z, is found at the point of sample application. In cancer patients there is a difference in the ratio of the Y to X component from that observed in healthy individuals. The Y component increases during exacerbation of the disease and decreases during remissions. In most patients with cancer the Y/X ratio is increased regardless of the presence or absence of liver disease. This also occurs even when the total leucine aminopeptidase activity is normal. An abnormal ratio has also been observed in individuals with liver disease but without cancer (Phillips and Manildi, 1970).

25.2.1.5. Amylase

Cancer of the pancreas is one of the most malignant forms of cancer. About one individual in 10,000 gets this disease each year in the United States. Treatment is most effective when the disease is recognized early and consequently there is a need for effective and specific biochemical tests as diagnostic tools and aids in following the disease. Although measurements of serum amylase (EC 3.2.1.1) have been made for over 100 years in the evaluation of pancreatic disease, they have not been of much value in the diagnosis of carcinoma of the pancreas. Serum amylase activity is increased in many disorders which are not directly related to cancer though sometimes associated with it. From 8 to 40% of patients with cancer of the pancreas have increased serum amylase activity (Schwartz and Fleisher, 1970). The low incidence is presumed to be due to a failure of the serum enzyme activity to increase until the tumour causes at least partial occlusion of the pancreatic duct. In many cases this means that the tumour must be quite large before an increase in enzyme activity can be detected.

Serum amylase activity may also be increased in individuals with non-pancreatic cancer. Thus, following perforation of a gastric ulcer, or intestinal obstruction, leakage of amylase may occur into the peritoneal cavity from which it is absorbed; this is reflected in increased serum activity. With renal insufficiency, the urinary excretion of amylase is impaired and serum activity will be increased as a consequence. In advanced liver disease, which may or may not be caused by cancer, the ability of the liver to synthesize amylase may be impaired, and the total serum amylase activity may be reduced as most of the normal serum activity originates from the liver. Isoenzyme measurement has had little use in determining the presence of tumours, although a unique isoenzyme has been observed in the serum of several patients with pancreatic carcinoma (Shimamura et al., 1975).

Although urinary amylase activity is directly related to serum amylase activity in healthy individuals, and in patients with pancreatic tumours who have normal renal function, some workers feel that urine amylase measurements are more useful than serum assays. In one study, only 11% of patients with pancreatic tumours had abnormal serum activity, but 26% excreted greater than normal activities in their urine (Gambill and Mason, 1964).

Less than a normal response to pancreozymin-secretin stimulation, or a test meal of skimmed milk and corn oil, has been observed in the duodenal aspirate from patients with pancreatic cancer. In one study, a depressed amylase response was observed in 12 of 16 patients with cancer of the head of the pancreas. It is not known how early in the disease the depressed response develops, but presumably the response becomes progressively impaired as the amount of functioning exocrine pancreatic tissue is reduced. This occurs with replacement by tumour or when the tumour occludes the pancreatic duct.

25.2.1.6. Lipase

Measurements of serum lipase (EC 3.1.1.3) are no more effective than amylase measurements in pin-pointing a tumour of the pancreas. However, urinary lipase has been observed to be abnormally low in patients with a carcinoma of either the body or the tail of the pancreas (Pfeffer et al., 1967).

In healthy individuals, pancreozymin-secretin stimulation causes an increase of 2 to 10 times in the duodenal fluid lipase activity. In some patients with carcinoma of the pancreas the increase is less than this; indeed no increase at all may occur in response to the hormone stimulation, yet the lipase secretion increased normally in other patients with cancer of the pancreas (Warnes et al., 1972).

25.2.1.7. Gamma-glutamyltransferase

Gamma-glutamyltransferase (EC 2.3.2.1; γ-glutamyltranspeptidase) is a sensitive indicator of liver damage. The activity of the enzyme is increased in the serum of patients with liver metastases or primary liver tumours, but not in patients with cancer not associated with liver metastases. Its activity is also increased in a large variety of conditions such as alcoholism, malabsorption, biliary obstruction, hepatitis, myocardial infarction, neurological diseases and in response to many drugs that are inducers of hepatic microsomal enzymes. This extreme sensitivity to other conditions, including the ingestion of a small quantity of alcohol (ethanol), may militate against its use in evaluation of metastases to the liver. Nevertheless, Aronsen et al. (1970) claim that γ-glutamyltransferase is the single best enzymatic test for identifying the presence of liver tumours.

A comparison of serum 5′-nucleotidase and γ-glutamyltransferase measurements in patients with cancer has shown that the increase in γ-glutamyltransferase activity may be greater than the increase of 5′-nucleotidase although the increase in activity does not occur earlier (Korsten et al., 1974). Gamma-glutamyltransferase is more sensitive to drug-induced hepatotoxicity than 5′-nucleotidase, so that one of its major applications may be in the differentiation of causes of increased activity of other enzymes in serum. A change in the activity of serum γ-glutamyltransferase activity in a patient with cancer may indicate the development of hepatic metastases, particularly when the change occurs concomitantly with changes in the amount of carcinoembryonic antigen. The magnitude of a change in a person with known metastases may be correlated with a change in the size of the tumour (Munjal et al., 1976).

25.2.2. Non organ-specific enzymes

These enzymes have been described as ubiquitous enzymes because of their wide tissue distribution. They also serve a variety of metabolic functions and are affected by many different diseases.

25.2.2.1. Sulphatases

Aryl sulphatase is an enzyme found in stomach, colon and a variety of other tissues. The enzyme exists as three isoenzymes, designated A, B, and C which may be differentiated by their substrate specificities. Aryl sulphatase B has been observed in higher concentration in colon cancer tissue than in the homologous normal colon tissue. In the urine of these patients, the excretion of the isoenzyme correlates with the extent of the disease (Dzialoszynski et al., 1966). Thus, activity is observed in the urine of more patients with Dukes' C and D lesions (75%) than with either stage A (28%) or B (55%), but the usefulness of these determinations has still to be substantiated.

Normal aryl sulphatase activity has been reported in 40% of specimens of tumours from patients with cancer of the colon in one study (Morgan et al., 1975). All of the patients who responded to treatment with 5-fluorouracil demonstrated normal sulphatase activity in their tumours.

The ability of breast carcinomatous tissue to sulphurylate steroids has been proposed as a test for the likelihood of response of the tumour to hormone ablative surgery. Patients in whom breast cancer tissue did not contain the sulphotransferase required for sulphurylation of dehydroepiandrosterone and oestradiol rarely responded to bilateral adrenalectomy. All of 30 patients lacking the enzyme failed to respond to ablation therapy, whereas 21 of 29 patients with the enzyme experienced a remission (Dao, 1972). There was apparently no relationship between the sulphatase and sulphotransferase activity, and 87% of tumour tissues which were capable of sulphating steroids also contained sulphatase activity.

25.2.2.2. Glycolytic enzymes

Warburg demonstrated prior to 1930 that neoplastic tissue had high aerobic and anaerobic glycolytic rates. Oxygen consumption is generally higher than in normal tissue. Anaerobic glycolysis is also higher in neoplastic tissue than normal tissue in the same organ (Bodansky, 1975).

Glycolytic enzyme activity of tumour tissue usually is higher than in surrounding normal tissue. From the few studies that have been performed, the increased glycolytic capacity of neoplastic tissue appears to be limited by phosphofructokinase (Shonk et al., 1965). Serum activity of glycolytic enzymes is increased in a large proportion of patients with cancer that has metastasized to the liver. Activity is usually normal in patients with early cancer.

Measurement of serum glycolytic enzymes is of most value in following the course of cancer or the growth or regression of a tumour, and in determining the effectiveness of various types of treatment. Because one enzyme may be affected to a greater extent than others in different disease situations it is important to measure several different enzymes. It is possible that isoenzyme measurements may have even greater usefulness.

(a) *Lactate dehydrogenase* (EC 1.1.1.27). About 70% of patients with metastases to the liver have increased serum activity of lactate dehydrogenase (Tan et al., 1963). In patients with tumours of various tissues without hepatic metastases, increased serum enzyme activity has been observed in 20 to 60% of cases, depending on the organ involved. The lower incidence is found in patients with carcinoma of the head, neck or oesophagus, and the higher incidence in patients with cancer of the breast.

In cancer tissue there is usually a preponderance of the LD_5 isoenzyme (Table 25.2). This has been observed in tumours of the breast, uterus, prostate, brain, stomach, lung, bowel, thyroid, pancreas and ovary (Goldman et al., 1964). An absolute increase in the M component has been found in malignant tumours of each of these tissues. In benign tumours, the isoenzyme pattern is the same as in normal tissue. The ratio of LD_5 to LD_1 in carcinoma of the breast is 6 times that observed in fibroadenoma. In most cases of carcinoma of the prostate, the ratio is greater than one whereas the converse is characteristic of benign hypertrophy. Latner et al. (1966) have demonstrated that LD_5 activity is increased in the cervical epithelium in the preinvasive stage of carcinoma of the cervix.

The shift towards an increase in the LD_5 isoenzyme in malignant tumour tissue appears to be especially marked in tumours of the digestive and genital tracts. LD_5 is more capable than LD_1 of converting pyruvate into lactate at high pyruvate concentrations. This replenishes NAD, which is required as a hydrogen acceptor in the oxidation of triose phosphate produced earlier in the glycolytic cycle (Bodansky, 1975).

TABLE 25.2.

RELATIVE PROPORTIONS OF LACTATE DEHYDROGENASE AND ITS PRINCIPAL ISOENZYMES IN MALIGNANT TISSUES

(Reproduced, by permission, from Bodansky, 1975)

Tissue	Ratio, cancer/normal		
	Total activity	LD-5	LD-1
Stomach	0.88	2.76	0.37
Colon	1.89	2.45	1.26
Lung	1.96	2.29	1.33
Breast	5.07	7.33	2.56

In most patients in whom total serum lactate dehydrogenase activity is increased, the proportion of LD_5 activity is also increased, but the change is not as marked as in the tumour tissue itself. LD_3 and LD_4 activities may also be increased at the expense of the two fastest migrating isoenzymes. A small proportion of patients may demonstrate abnormal patterns of serum lactate dehydrogenase activity, although the total enzyme activity is still within normal limits. The isoenzyme pattern in serum may vary with the stage of the disease and also with its response to treatment.

In lymphocytic leukaemia and lymphosarcoma, total serum lactate dehydrogenase activity is increased in about 60% of patients. The increase is mainly due to fractions 2 and 3 which predominate in normal and leukaemic lymphocytes. In chronic and acute myeloid leukaemia the third fraction is most marked in serum, although LD_5 is the most abundant isoenzyme in normal granulocytes, but myeloblasts are high in LD_1 and low in LD_5. In Hodgkin's disease, total lactate dehydrogenase activity is often increased in serum. This is mainly attributable to increased LD_2 or LD_3. Lactate dehydrogenase activity may be increased in the serum of more than 90% patients with acute leukaemia, but the increase may not be correlated with the white cell count. The increase in lactate dehydrogenase activity in serum is less marked in chronic leukaemia than in acute leukaemia. Enzyme activity may rise several weeks before a relapse occurs, but it also falls prior to remissions.

(b) *Fructose diphosphate aldolase* (EC 4.1.2.13). Serum total aldolase activity is increased in many patients with malignant disease. The magnitude of the increase generally correlates well with the mass of the tumour. Thus, increases are found in 70% of patients with gastrointestinal cancer and 75% of patients with tumours that have metastasized to the liver. Enzyme activity is increased in 45% of patients with cancer of the head, neck, oesophagus or breast. The incidence is about 62% in patients with cancer of the lung (Bodansky, 1975). The increase is not specific for malignant disease and may be found in many other diseases. However, the ratio of fructose diphosphate aldolase activity to that of fructose phosphate aldolase may be used to provide greater assurance that increased activity in serum is caused by a tumour. The ratio is about 2.8 in healthy individuals and 1.3 in acute hepatitis (similar to the ratio of 1 to 2 in normal liver). In primary hepatoma it may be greater than 18, and in cancer without liver metastases 12, but when the liver is also involved the ratio decreases to about 7.

Aldolase exists as three isoenzymes: A in muscle, B in liver and C in brain and nerve tissue. Primary tumours of the liver contain aldolase A and not the B of normal liver. Serum of patients with cancer contains a greater proportion of muscle variant aldolase, and this isoenzyme is found in foetal brain and liver. In malignant tissue, the isoenzymes tend to revert to the foetal form. While meningiomas contain aldolase A, gliomas only contain the C isoenzyme of normal brain tissue.

(c) *Glucosephosphate isomerase* (EC 5.3.1.9). Glucosephosphate (phosphohexose) isomerase activity is more often increased in the serum of patients with malignant disease than any other "ubiquitous" enzyme. The enzyme activity is increased in the serum of more than 80% of patients with cancer and metastases in the liver. It is also increased more commonly than other enzymes in carcinoma of the gastrointestinal tract, head, neck and oesophagus, lung and breast (Schwartz, 1973). The increased enzyme activity is not detected in the early stages of tumour growth, but as the tumour grows there is generally a good correlation between the serum activity and the size of the tumour. Glucosephosphate isomerase activity may be increased in various diseases such as tuberculosis, infectious hepatitis, heart diseases and leukaemia.

25.2.2.3. Miscellaneous enzymes

The incidence of increased activity in serum of several common enzymes is summarized in Table 25.3 (Bodansky, 1975). It is apparent that glucosephosphate isomerase is the most sensitive indicator of the presence of a tumour and the aminotransferases the least sensitive. Much of the usefulness in making serum enzyme measurements in patients with malignant disease is in following the progress of the disease. Increased activity of enzymes in serum generally reflects the amount of tumour tissue rather than specific invasion of the liver. When enzyme assays are employed to monitor a tumour's response to therapy, several different enzymes should be measured as not all enzymes may respond.

(a) *Aryl hydrocarbon hydroxylase.* Aryl hydrocarbon hydroxylase is an enzyme involved in the metabolism of polycyclic carcinogens. The white male population in the United States may be characterized as to its ability to induce aryl hydrocarbon hydroxylase activity in peripheral lymphocytes. Individuals may have high, intermediate or low inducibility. High inducibility has been observed in 9.4% of healthy controls but 30% of patients with cancer of the bronchus: low inducibility has been observed in 4.0% of cancer patients but 45% of controls. Intermediate inducibility was observed in 66% of cancer patients and 46% of healthy controls (Kellerman et al., 1973). Further study is required to determine if aryl hydrocarbon hydroxylase measurement can be used to characterize individuals with a high risk of cancer.

(b) *Lysozyme* (EC 3.2.1.17). Lysozyme (muramidase) hydrolyzes β-1,4 links between N-acetylmuramic acid and N-acetylglucosamine residues in mucopolysaccharides or mucopolypeptides. Increased activity of the enzyme in serum has been observed in leukaemia and in generalized carcinomatosis. Activity is highest in patients with monocytic leukaemia, but it is also high in patients with acute myelomonocytic leukaemia and to a lesser extent in both acute and chronic myelocytic leukaemia. Activity is normal in patients with acute leukaemia and slightly reduced in chronic lymphocytic leukaemia.

TABLE 25.3.

INCIDENCE OF INCREASED SERUM ENZYME ACTIVITIES IN PATIENTS WITH CANCER

GPI, glucosephosphate isomerase; ALS, fructosediphosphate aldolase; LD, lactate dehydrogenase; ASP, aspartate aminotransferase; ICD, isocitrate dehydrogenase; MD, malate dehydrogenase; GTD, glutathione reductase; ALT, alanine aminotransferase. (Reproduced, by permission, from Bodansky, 1975)

Tissue	Number of Patients	GPI	ALS	LD	ASP	ICD	MD	GTD	ALT
Gastrointestinal tract	119	74	70	53	35	40	37	30	19
Head, neck, oesophagus	88	51	45	21	16	21	10	15	9
Lung	126	72	62	53	15	24	25	28	–
Breast	57	70	45	60	–	40	40	35	–
Metastases to liver	284	84	75	69	51	53	62	47	44

Urinary lysozyme excretion is increased in the same patients. There is a relationship between leucocyte and serum lysozyme activity and between the leucocyte count and serum lysozyme activity. The ratio of serum lysozyme to white cell count is similar for acute leukaemic patients and healthy controls. In chronic lymphocytic and myelocytic leukaemia the ratio is reduced. In one study, the mean ratio in acute myelocytic leukaemia was 3 times that of controls, 12 times that of controls in acute monomyelocytic leukaemia and 8 times that of controls in acute monocytic leukaemia (Wiernik and Serpick, 1969).

Increased lysozyme activity in cerebrospinal fluid occurs when the protein concentration is increased and therefore this finding is not diagnostic of a tumour of the central nervous system.

Urinary lysozyme excretion in patients with the nephrotic syndrome, cadmium poisoning and some other chronic renal diseases, as well as in patients with sarcoidosis and chronic infections, is greater than in healthy individuals. The excretion is much increased in patients with certain forms of leukaemia. In patients with high serum enzyme activity there is usually high urinary enzyme activity but there is a poor correlation between the two sets of activity. Nevertheless, the urinary excretion is greatest in patients with acute monocytic leukaemia, but it is also increased in individuals with acute myelomonocytic leukaemia.

During the transition from a variety of myeloproliferative disorders to acute myeloblastic or acute myelomonocytic leukaemia, there may be a striking increase in both serum and urine muramidase activity. As with the increased activity observed in these fluids in generalized carcinomatosis, multiple myeloma or Hodgkin's disease, this may reflect overproduction of the enzyme as the result of proliferation of cells in the tumours or other tissues.

(c) *Other enzymes.* Tan et al. (1963) demonstrated increased activity of serum glutathione reductase in almost two-thirds of their patients. Chretien et al. (1973) observed increased serum alkaline ribonuclease activity in patients with adenocarcinoma, whereas normal activity occurred in patients with sarcomas or melanomas. Alpha-1,4-glucosidase activity in serum may be increased in patients with cancer. Its measurement has proved useful in the early diagnosis of breast cancer (Gamklou and Schersten, 1973) and may have much wider application in the diagnosis of cancer because increased activity has not been found in diseases other than cancer.

Prolyl hydroxylase is involved in the synthesis of collagen. The activity of the enzyme is increased in the serum of up to 70% of all patients with hepatocellular carcinoma. Activity of the enzyme in serum may be increased in premalignant states (Baillie et al., 1975). When measured in conjunction with α-foetoprotein it is possible to detect all patients with hepatocellular carcinoma (McGee et al., 1975). The enzyme has been demonstrated histochemically in breast tumour cells, but the importance of this as a diagnostic tool has still to be assessed (Neville and Cooper, 1976). The activity of sialyltransferase, which catalyzes the incorporation of sialic acid onto the galactose residue of desialyated fetuin, is higher in breast and colonic neoplasms than in normal tissues (Bosmann and Hall, 1974). This is also reflected in the plasma of patients with malignant disease. In one study, the mean plasma value in patients with malignant disease was almost twice the value in healthy individuals (Kessel and Allen, 1975).

Changes in the plasma sialyltransferase activity are correlated with the clinical course of the malignant disease. The highest enzyme activity occurs in patients with liver or lung metastases. The normal plasma enzyme activity arises from liver cells. Henderson and Kessel (1977) have postulated that liver metastases could promote enzyme release from normal liver cells by stimulating lysis of these cells. The enzyme lacks diagnostic specificity for cancer, as activity in serum may be increased in a variety of acute and chronic non-neoplastic liver diseases and rheumatoid arthritis.

Adenosine deaminase activity is increased in the serum of a large proportion of patients with malignant disease. However, the increase is related more to the growth of the tumour and the clinical state of the patient than to the presence of a tumour per se. Serum ornithine carbamoyltransferase activity is increased in patients with liver tumours but not to the extent observed in acute hepatitis. Cholinesterase activity is reduced, as in other liver diseases, and its measurement has no diagnostic specificity for cancer (Bodansky, 1975). It should be noted that the isoenzyme composition of enzymes elaborated by tumours is very often more like foetal than adult enzyme in composition. Thus, an increase in the proportion of the BB isoenzyme of creatine kinase may be observed in the serum of patients with cancer.

Ronquist et al. (1977) have shown in a small series that adenylate kinase activity is consistently raised in the spinal fluid of patients with malignant brain tumours. No activity was detected in spinal fluid of healthy individuals or patients with benign tumours. Whether this test is as useful as it appears to be initially will only be proved with time and more extensive studies.

25.2.3. Enzymes in fluids other than blood

Increased activity of 6-phosphogluconate dehydrogenase and β-glucuronidase has been observed in vaginal fluid of women with carcinoma of the cervix, but increased activity has also been observed in many other conditions. Glucosephosphate isomerase has also been suggested as an enzyme that can indicate the presence of a cervical tumour, but it, too, may be increased by many benign conditions (Schwartz, 1973).

High enzyme activity in pleural and other effusions is suggestive of an underlying malignancy. Lactate dehydrogenase has been studied both with regard to total activity and isoenzyme composition to demonstrate the malignant nature of an effusion.

25.3. HORMONES

For almost 80 years there has been great interest in the role of hormones in tumour growth and the possible use of hormones in the treatment of cancer. However, the modern development of immunological techniques was required before detailed studies could be made.

25.3.1. Polypeptide hormones

Excess secretion of some hormones may produce readily recognizable clinical syndromes, yet the excess secretion of other hormones may be accompanied by no obvious clinical features. The hormones secreted by tumour tissue appear to be structurally and immunologically similar to those secreted by normal endocrine tissues. Vaitukaitis (1976) has established several criteria that identify the secretion of hormones from non-endocrine sources. These include: (a) a greater concentration of the hormone in the tumour than surrounding tissue; (b) demonstration of the hormone within the tissue; (c) disappearance of the hormone after removal of the tumour; (d) a difference between the arterial and venous concentrations of the hormone across the tissue; and (e) production of the hormone by the tumour tissue in vitro.

Different tumours may secrete different hormones (Table 25.4). Thus, corticotrophin is often secreted by tumours of the lung, whereas calcitonin is more characteristic of adenocarcinoma of the stomach. Several mechanisms have been postulated to explain the high concentration of hormones in tumours. These include: (a) non-specific trapping of serum hormones by the tumour; (b) random and non-random depression of the genome; (c) amine and precursor uptake with decarboxylation; and (d) cell hybridization.

None of these theories has been substantiated and arguments have been produced against each of them.

25.3.1.1. Corticotrophin

Carcinomas of the lung (50% of the total) are the tumours most commonly associated with production of corticotrophin (ACTH), with tumours of the pancreas (10%) and thymus (10%) often also responsible for corticotrophin production (Odell, 1974). The corticotrophin appears to be identical to that secreted by the pituitary gland except that the ectopic hormone has a greater reactivity with the C-terminal directed antibody. Lung tumours may contain a big form of corticotrophin with low immunological activity. Subcomponents of corticotrophin, e.g. N-terminal fragments, may also be produced by tumours. The increased secretion of corticotrophin produces a high plasma concentration of the hormone and an increased plasma cortisol concentration. A hypokalaemic alkalosis may occur, together with hypertension, oedema and hyperglycaemia (Bodansky, 1975; Vaitukaitis, 1976), but the clinical manifestations vary with the size of the tumour and the age of the patient.

TABLE 25.4.

ECTOPIC HUMORAL SYNDROMES

(Reproduced, by permission, from Vaitukaitis, 1976 and Durie and Salmon, 1975)

Ectopic hormone	Tumour most commonly associated
Calcitonin	Lung, stomach
Enteroglucagon	Kidney
Prolactin	Lung, kidney
Thyroid stimulating hormone	Lung, breast
Corticotrophin	Lung, pancreas, thymus
Parathormone	Lung, kidney, lymphoma
Antidiuretic hormone	Lung
Chorionic somatomammotrophin	Lung
Growth hormone	Stomach, lung
Chorionic gonadotrophin	Trophoblast, stomach, ovaries, pancreas, hepatoma

25.3.1.2. Melanocyte stimulating hormone

The plasma concentration of β-melanocyte stimulating hormone (MSH) is high in patients who secrete ectopic corticotrophin. The hormone secreted by the tumour is structurally different from the pituitary hormone, but is nonetheless responsible for the increased skin pigmentation observed in 10 to 33% of patients with the ectopic corticotrophin syndrome (Vaitukaitis, 1976). The frequency of ectopic β-melanocyte stimulating hormone secretion is probably comparable with that of corticotrophin as most patients with ectopic production of corticotrophin also secrete increased melanocyte stimulating hormone. Its isolated production by neoplasms has also been reported (Odell, 1974).

25.3.1.3. Parathormone

Hypercalcaemia is commonly associated with bone metastases, but may also be observed in the absence of bone involvement. Certain tumours are capable of elaborating a material with similar properties to parathormone, while lacking identical immunological characteristics. In patients with non-parathyroid tumours, the concentration of parathormone-like activity in serum is less than in patients with hyperparathyroidism at the same serum calcium concentration (Bodansky, 1975). The hypercalcaemia resulting from the secretion of parathormone-like material by a neoplasm originates from bones, but it may be associated with a low or normal concentration of phosphorus in the serum. Tumours of the lungs, breast, kidneys and bladder have been demonstrated to secrete parathormone-like material. Other less common sites are ovary, bladder and pancreas although isolated cases affecting other organs have been reported. The parathormone isolated from the rare tumours of the parathyroid gland appears to be immunologically similar to the hormone secreted by the normal gland.

In not all patients with malignant tumours and hypercalcaemia has it been possible to demonstrate increased serum parathormone-like activity. In these cases it has been postulated that the tumour elaborates either a parathyrotrophic agent that acts on the parathyroid gland or in some way causes prostaglandin E_2 to be secreted in an increased amount. Patients with carcinoma and hypercalcaemia do have higher serum and urine concentrations of prostaglandins than other individuals. The cells of patients with multiple myeloma have been demonstrated to produce an osteoclast activating factor which is capable of causing bone reabsorption. Some tumours can synthesise Vitamin-D like sterols (stigmasterol and 17-hydroxysitosterol), and increased concentrations have been observed in plasma and breast tissue (Gordan et al., 1966) but this has not been confirmed by other investigators (Woodhead and Walker, 1976).

25.3.1.4. Antidiuretic hormone

Antidiuretic hormone (ADH)-like activity has been reported in tumours of the lung, duodenum and pancreas (Bodansky, 1975). Oat-cell carcinoma of the bronchus is the most common cause of ectopic antidiuretic hormone production. Other cases of inappropriate secretion of antidiuretic hormone arise from the secretion of neurophysin by tumours. It should be noted that the syndrome of inappropriate secretion of antidiuretic hormone (Bartter's syndrome) may also occur in severe lung disease and in some diseases of the brain.

25.3.1.5. Chorionic gonadotrophin

Human chorionic gonadotrophin (hCG) is not normally detectable in serum except during pregnancy; its presence at other times is suggestive of a tumour. In men with testicular tumours, high concentrations of the hormone in the urine have been reported (Hobson, 1965). This is more common with choriocarcinoma (90%) than teratoma (29%) or embryonal carcinoma (21%); it is even less common with other testicular tumours.

In women, chorionic gonadotrophin excretion is high with a hydatidiform mole and in the presence of choriocarcinoma of the uterus. The excretion of chorionic gonadotrophin may also be high in patients with choriocarcinoma of the ovaries and the rare choriocarcinoma of other organs. Adenocarcinomas of the stomach, ovary, pancreas and hepatomas are the other tumours most often associated with ectopic secretion of chorionic gonadotrophin (Vaitukaitis, 1976). The incidence of hormone secretion is up to 40% in some of these types of tumours. In some of these tumours the α- or β-subunits of the hormone may be identified, and the specific subunit may be quantified. Measurement of the hormone may be used to follow the progress of the disease or the response of the tumour to therapy.

Secretion of follicle stimulating hormone and luteinizing hormone by neoplasms is rare.

25.3.1.6. Growth hormone

Increased serum growth hormone (hGH) as a result of ectopic secretion is rare but has been observed in tumours of the lung. Gastric tumours may also cause an increased growth hormone concentration. Treatment of the tumours causes a reduction in the growth hormone concentraton.

25.3.1.7. Chorionic somatomammotrophin

A high serum concentration of chorionic somatomammotrophin (hCS) has been observed in patients with some tumours of the ovary and testis, but an increased concentration has also been observed in patients with tumours of the lung. The hormone is normally not detectable in the serum of non-pregnant women.

25.3.1.8. Prolactin

Serum prolactin is increased in some women with cancer of the breast. Indeed, the basal serum concentration may be higher in women with a family history of breast cancer (Henderson et al., 1975). Many tumours of the pituitary gland secrete prolactin.

25.3.1.9. Insulin

Many of the tumours that cause hypoglycaemia are mesotheliomas or fibrosarcomas. Less frequently they are adrenal carcinomas or hepatomas. Often the tumours are benign. Hypoglycaemia may be caused by insulin-like material rather than by insulin itself because it may occur without any increase in material reacting against anti-insulin antibodies. Hypoglycaemia may occur solely as a result of increased activity of the Cori cycle in the liver in patients with cancer (Holroyde et al., 1975). A high blood glucose concentration may be caused by increased secretion of glucagon from the α-cells of the pancreas. Alpha-cell tumours are rare but should be considered in patients with hyperglycaemia in whom a diagnosis of diabetes mellitus can be excluded.

25.3.1.10. Gastrin

The Zollinger–Ellison syndrome is produced by secretion of gastrin peptides in the pancreas. These peptides differ only slightly in chemical composition from normal gastrin but are powerful gastric secretagogues, and the serum gastrin concentration is considerably above that found in healthy individuals.

25.3.1.11. Other polypeptide hormones

Many other hormones are produced by ectopic tissue. The hormones or materials with hormone-like activity include somatostatin in pancreatic cells, calcitonin in the C cells of the thyroid gland or mammary or bronchial tumours, erythropoietin in certain renal and other tumours, thyrotrophin in women with hydatidiform moles or choriocarcinoma and men with testicular teratocarcinoma.

Tumours of the endocrine glands are discussed elsewhere in this book. The features are generally of hypersecretion of the normal hormones produced by the gland, but without the normal regulatory mechanisms operating.

Although serum or urine is usually examined to determine the presence of a tumour, cerebrospinal fluid has been studied to determine extension of pituitary tumours outside the pituitary fossa. While patients with neurological diseases, or with a pituitary tumour confined to the pituitary fossa, had a low concentration of anterior pituitary hormones, the hormone concentrations were higher in patients with suprasellar extension (Jordan et al., 1976).

25.3.2. Steroid hormones

25.3.2.1. Urinary steroids

Steroid metabolism may be altered by tumours of several different tissues. Cancer of the breast is the most studied disease but many other neoplasms can affect steroid metabolism. However, the use of individual steroid analyses in diagnosing a tumour or predicting responsiveness of hormone-dependent tumours to adrenalectomy, hypophysectomy or chemotherapy has not been very successful. This lack of success is undoubtedly due in part to the effects of age, body mass, emotional stress of hospitalization, and extent of the illness upon hormone excretion, as well as to the relatively large analytical error associated with steroid analyses.

In women patients with breast cancer, the excretion of corticosteroid sulphate is increased in approximately one-third of the patients with either localized or metastatic disease. The same proportion of patients with colonic cancer shows the same results. The excretion of free cortisol is usually unaffected by the presence of cancer (Rose et al., 1975). The increased corticosteroid sulphate and cortisol sulphate excretion probably arises both from increased cortisol production and increased sulphurylation of the steroid, which might occur in some tumour cells, as well as in the liver and adrenal glands.

In an attempt to improve the prediction of tumour responsiveness to therapy, Bulbrook et al. (1960) have used a group of urinary steroid measurements with discriminant function analysis. This was a development of their earlier work which indicated that urinary aetiocholanolone excretion tended to be higher, and urinary 17-hydroxycorticosteroid excretion lower, in patients with breast cancer who had a successful response to adrenalectomy or hypophysectomy. The Bulbrook discriminant D is given by

D = 80–80 (17-OHCS) + Aetiocholanolone

when 17-hydroxycorticosteroid (17-OHCS) excretion is measured in milligrams per 24 hours and aetiocholanolone in micrograms per 24 hours. The more positive the discriminant, the more favourable is the probable response to ablative surgery. Using this discriminant in over 200 patients with metastatic breast cancer, Atkins et al. (1968) showed that of the patients with positive discriminants treated by hypophysectomy, 47% responded successfully and 23% failed to respond. Of the patients with negative discriminants only 11% responded well and 67% were failures (Table 25.5). The Bulbrook discriminant is generally of little value in early breast cancer.

Moore et al. (1968) have developed another discriminant based on the change in 17-hydroxycorticosteroid excretion and 17-oxosteroid excretion in response to corticotrophin administration. Using this, they were able to identify, in a small series, 80% of the responders and 75% of the non-responders to treatment.

Other discriminants have been proposed and include the mass excretion ratio (mg/24 h) of urinary 11-deoxy-17-oxosteroids to 17-hydroxycorticosteroids and a combination of the aetiocholanolone and oestradiol excretions with the patient's age. The latter has been used to differentiate between benign and malignant disease. In a small series, 14 of 18 patients with benign breast tumours had a negative discriminant whereas all 7 patients with malignant disease had a positive discriminant.

A combination of urinary steroid measurements with discriminant analysis has been used to differentiate between benign prostatic disease and prostatic carcinoma. Approximately 80% of patients with prostatic cancer had a positive discriminant and 90% with benign prostatic hypertrophy had a negative discriminant. Another discriminant for evaluation of patients with lung cancer involves the measurement of urinary androsterone, aetiocholanolone and 17-hydroxycorticosteroids. Approximately 90% of patients with inoperable cancer had a negative discriminant and the same proportion of controls had a positive discriminant.

TABLE 25.5.

RESPONSE OF PATIENTS WITH POSITIVE OR NEGATIVE BULBROOK DISCRIMINANTS TO ADRENALECTOMY OR HYPOPHYSECTOMY

(Reproduced, by permission, from Atkins et al., 1968)

	Number	Success (%)	Intermediates (%)	Failure (%)
Response to hypophysectomy				
Positive discriminants	47	47	30	23
Negative discriminants	46	11	22	67
Response to adrenalectomy				
Positive discriminants	47	32	19	49
Negative discriminants	56	13	32	55

Reports are conflicting about the relationship of the excretion of total and individual oestrogens to the presence of breast cancer. However, De Guili and De Guili (1973) found a higher total excretion in men with breast cancer and Dao et al. (1973) have noted higher values of the individual oestrogens in male breast cancer patients.

25.3.2.2. Plasma steroids

Wan et al. (1968) have determined the concentration of dehydroepiandrosterone and androsterone sulphate in plasma of women with breast cancer. The plasma concentration of dehydroepiandrosterone was less in patients with advanced disease than in benign disease. In male patients with breast cancer the plasma concentrations of oestrone, 17β-oestradiol, and oestriol are higher than in age-matched healthy individuals (Calabresi et al., 1976).

With tumours of the endocrine glands, the plasma concentration of the hormones elaborated in the gland is usually high and unresponsive to normal inhibitory measures.

25.3.3. Hormone receptors

The binding of oestrogen to macromolecular components (receptor protein) has received wide attention as a possible indicator of response to ablative hormone surgery. In vivo and in vitro studies have shown that human breast cancer tissue often accumulates more oestrogen than normal breast tissue. Folca et al. (1961) first demonstrated a link between the hormone responsiveness of breast cancer and the ability of such tumours to concentrate oestrogen. These workers initially demonstrated that patients who responded to ablative surgery had a greater uptake of oestrogen than patients who did not respond. In vivo studies of uptake of the hormone by tissues are limited because of possible radiation hazards, the expense of the large amount of radioactive hormone required and the many uncontrolled factors that can affect the metabolism and excretion of hormones. In vitro uptake of tritiated oestradiol was later determined in tissue slices of breast cancers. In the most comprehensive evaluation of radioactive oestradiol uptake in breast tumour published to date (McGuire et al., 1975), almost 50% of the patients possessed oestrogen receptor protein in their tumours, studied as tissue cytosol. Just over another 3% demonstrated equivocal results while the remainder were negative for the protein. Less than 6% of the patients without receptors responded to therapy whereas more than 54% of those with receptors responded. The incidence of oestrogen receptor protein in other studies has been similar. It should be noted that a small proportion (5%) of individuals with benign breast lesions or normal breast tissue demonstrate the presence of oestrogen receptor protein (Rosen et al., 1975). The binding in tumour tissue is not related to the presence of metastases or the number of carcinoma cells in the specimens studied.

Jensen et al. (1971) demonstrated that the oestrogen receptor protein could be separated from other proteins in an 8S sucrose density gradient peak. Wittliff et al. (1971) have determined that the average binding capacity of receptor positive malignant tissue is 43.0 ± 5.3 (S.E.) fmol/mg protein. Tumours considered negative had an average binding capacity of less than 2 fmol/mg protein. In an unselected population, a range of 0 to 612 fmol of oestrogen binding protein per mg cytosol protein has been observed in one study of 64 primary and metastatic human breast tumours. The specific 8S protein binding activity was not detected in any specimen containing less than 9.0 fmol/mg protein of the oestrogen binder.

The majority of patients with oestrogen receptor-positive tumours appears to benefit from endocrine therapy, whereas only about 10% of receptor negative patients have a therapeutic response. Unfortunately, endocrine responsive tumours constitute only from 20 to 40% of treated cases although the success rate can be improved by selecting for treatment only those patients with positive oestrogen receptor protein in their tumour.

Measurement of progesterone receptors in addition to oestrogen receptors provides a better indication of probable tumour response to hormone therapy, than measurement of oestrogen receptor alone (McGuire, 1976). Of 236 human breast tumours analyzed, only 8% of the oestrogen receptor negative tumours contained progesterone receptor whereas 62% of the oestrogen receptor-positive tumours contained the progesterone receptor. The best therapeutic response could be anticipated by those tumours that demonstrated both receptors.

Prolactin receptors have also been studied histoenzymatically in breast tumours. It is even believed that prolactin is the primary hormone in initiation of breast cancer growth (Pearson et al., 1969). In a series of 50 patients, 16 exhibited prolactin dependency, of which 10 were only prolactin dependent. Of the other tumours, 4 showed oestrogen dependency and one was only androgen dependent (Salih et al., 1973). In patients with testosterone dependency, the majority responds favourably to antiandrogen therapy. Some breast tumours exhibit dependency on growth hormone or a variety of different hormones.

While hormone receptors are present in other tissues they have not been extensively studied in relation to malignant disease of these organs.

25.4. POLYAMINES

The diamine putrescine [NH_2–$(CH_2)_4$–NH_2] and the polyamines spermidine [NH_2–$(CH_2)_3$–NH–$(CH_2)_4$–NH_2] and spermine [NH_2–$(CH_2)_3$–NH–$(CH_2)_3$–NH–$(CH_2)_4$–NH_2] are widely distributed in growing tissue. These compounds are believed to regulate RNA synthesis. Putrescine is formed from arginine via agmatine and from ornithine through the action of ornithine decarboxylase. This enzyme has a wide tissue distribution, and liver and tumour tissue are rich sources of the enzyme. The enzyme has a short half-life and its activity responds rapidly to hormonal stimulation. In rats, at least, activity is increased by growth hormone, testosterone, oestradiol and cortisone. In response to increased ornithine decarboxylase activity there are parallel increases in the synthesis of polyamines and RNA. Spermidine and spermine are formed from putrescine following its reaction with compounds such as adenosylmethionine. The polycationic nature of the polyamines causes them to form complexes with other compounds such as nucleic acid.

There are no known degradation pathways for polyamines, so that augmented synthesis causes accumulation of the compounds in cells. On release of the amines from the cells, and especially with the release due to increased turnover of cells, the concentrations of the polyamines rise in plasma and their urinary excretions are also increased. The amines in urine are normally present as conjugates. The ranges of normal excretion of the polyamines per day in the urine of healthy individuals are 2.7 ± 0.5 mg for putrescine, 3.4 ± 0.7 mg for spermine and 3.1 ± 0.6 mg for spermidine. In patients with cancer, the urinary excretion is increased 5- to 10-fold, but the excretion fluctuates with the clinical state of the patient and his response to treatment. Surgical removal of a tumour always leads to a reduction in the excretion of polyamines.

Increased polyamine excretion appears to be characteristic of malignant disease (Table 25.6). Thus, excretion has been reported to be increased in leukaemia, and in cancer of the ovaries, lung, colon, rectum, genitourinary tract including prostate, kidney, testes and bladder. Excretion is also increased in patients with malignant melanoma. In all instances there has been good correlation between the urinary excretion of polyamines and the clinical course of the disease. However, not all patients with malignant disease exhibit increased excretion of polyamines. Thus, in a study of patients with prostatic malignancy, only 31 of 44 urine specimens showed an increased excretion. Only one out of 10 patients with histological grade I tumours demonstrated an increased excretion, whereas 30 out of 34 with more advanced malignant disease demonstrated increased excretion. There is a low incidence of false-positives. In this same study, one patient out of 5 with benign prostatic hypertrophy had an increased excretion of polyamines.

In healthy individuals spermidine is present in blood serum at a concentration of 0.32 ± 0.07 μmol/litre whereas spermine and putrescine are normally not detected. In all 18 patients with cancer who were studied, spermidine was detected in the serum at a concentration between 0.44 and 3.30 μmol/litre. The highest value was observed in a patient with mediastinal choriocarcinoma. Sixteen of the 18 patients had values greater than 2 standard deviations above the mean value of normal controls. In these cancer patients, putrescine was not detected in the blood and spermine was only found in 3 patients at a concentration of from 0.14 to 0.28 μmol/litre. Therefore, if it is possible to measure only one polyamine the measurement of spermidine is probably of most value as an aid to the

TABLE 25.6.

POLYAMINE EXCRETION IN PATIENTS WITH NON-MALIGNANT AND MALIGNANT CONDITIONS (mean values in mg/24 h)

(Reproduced, by permission, from Fujita et al., 1976)

Condition	Number	Putrescine	Spermidine	Spermine	Total
Healthy individuals	56	4.2	1.1	3.4	8.7
Nontumor patients	72	5.2	1.6	3.8	10.6
Blood cancers	4	17.1	10.8	15.9	43.8
Solid tumors	46	10.0	2.8	4.4	17.2
Stomach	26	10.7	3.5	5.6	19.8
Lung	4	6.2	2.0	3.3	11.5
Pancreas	4	10.7	1.9	1.9	14.5
Colon	2	6.5	2.4	5.4	14.3
Gallbladder	2	21.4	5.1	2.7	29.2
Oesophagus	2	17.7	1.3	2.1	21.1
Uterus	4	5.9	1.8	3.1	10.8

diagnosis of cancer. Russell et al. (1975) have postulated that spermidine is the best marker of tumour-cell destruction whereas putrescine is the marker for cell proliferation.

The clinical utility of polyamine assays as markers for screening or diagnostic and therapeutic monitoring programmes is subject to the development of good analytical methods. Currently, aminoacid or gas chromatographic analytical techniques are used. These procedures require initial acid hydrolysis of the specimens and have a low throughput. A radioimmunoassay has been described for free spermine with a sensitivity of 200 pg and a precision of about 15%. Spermidine cross-reacts to an extent of about 22% and putrescine to 1%. With this technique, healthy individuals had a serum concentration of 28 ± 6 μg/litre, and each of 8 cancer patients had a serum concentration of from 3 to 14 times the mean value in healthy individuals. In the patients the mean value was 159 μg/litre (standard deviation, ±40 μg/litre).

Increased concentrations of spermine and spermidine have been detected in the spinal fluid of patients with neuromeningeal leukaemia (Rennert et al., 1977).

25.5. TUMOUR-ASSOCIATED ANTIGENS

In recent years, a relationship of the cancer cell to an embryonic state has become widely accepted. Analysis of foetal enzymes and antigens in body fluids has been used in an attempt to detect the presence of tumours and to understand the relationship of foetal macromolecules to malignant disease. While certain tumour-associated enzymes and hormones may have metabolic effects, the oncofoetal antigens probably have none. The development of sensitive radioimmunoassays capable of detecting material in the nanogram range has permitted the introduction of these assays for primary detection of cancer and then for following the course of the disease. However, considerable care should be exercised in applying these assays to the detection of tumours because of the ramifications that a false-positive or -negative value may have on the future management of a patient.

25.5.1. Carcinoembryonic antigen

Carcinoembryonic antigen (CEA) of the human digestive system was first described by Gold and Freedman (1965). The antigen, which is a protein–polysaccharide complex, is found in foetal intestine, liver and pancreas during the first 6 months of gestation, and in human cancer tissue from the colon, pancreas or liver. Subsequent studies have shown that the antigen may be present in the serum of individuals with either gastrointestinal or other malignancies, in extracts from such tumours and in extracts of the foetal gastrointestinal tract. CEA may be detected in the serum of healthy individuals. The upper limit of normal varies with the method. CEA immunoreactivity has also been detected in urine, faeces and intestinal secretions of both cancer patients and normal individuals (Go, 1976).

CEA is a glycoprotein with molecular mass of about 200,000. It is associated with cell membranes. Although a high concentration of CEA in serum could perhaps arise from decreased degradation of circulating CEA or as a result of induction of synthesis in the liver by some stimulus from cancer cells, there is abundant evidence that CEA arises in the cancer cells themselves. The CEA detected in urine and other body fluids should probably be described as CEA-like material because the molecular mass of the protein is quite different from that of CEA itself. In the urine, the molecular mass varies from 12,000 to 50,000, although that in cyst fluid from the breast is similar to the serum CEA.

Healthy individuals have a serum CEA concentration of less than 2.5 μg/litre when determined by the most widely used Hansen technique. About 3% of pregnant women have values greater than this, but generally serum CEA concentration is unaffected by sex, age or circadian influences. The presence or absence of a family history of cancer also has no influence (Go, 1976).

In a review of carcinoembryonic antigen, Martin et al. (1976) have reiterated the lack of specificity of CEA in indicating the presence of a tumour in the gastrointestinal tract. Thus, above normal CEA activity in serum may be detected in inflammatory disease of the bowel, collagen disease, pancreatitis, chronic lung diseases such as bronchitis or pulmonary emphysema in chronic heavy smokers, in liver disease and polyps of the gastrointestinal tract. Tumours of the bladder, head and neck, reproductive tract, breast and neuroblastomas may also give rise to positive tests in the serum. However, normal concentrations of CEA have been reported in more than two-thirds of Dukes' A and almost half of Dukes' B stage tumours of bowel, and in many poorly differentiated tumours. Increased CEA activity may occur in as many as 68% of patients with lung cancer. A value of more than 6 times the upper limit of normal is usually associated with a bad prognosis (Vincent et al., 1975).

In general, the amount of circulating CEA varies with the stage of the cancer (Table 25.7). A large proportion of patients with early colonic cancer has a normal concentration of circulating CEA, but if the tumour spreads to adjacent tissue or metastasizes to other organs the serum CEA concentration increases. With surgery to remove a tumour of the colon, the serum CEA concentration usually decreases, but a fall to within the normal range does not necessarily imply complete removal of the tumour. The new concentration of CEA reaches a plateau in from 7 to 30 days after surgery. If the tumour recurs, the serum CEA concentration begins to rise again. Similar decreases in CEA concentration

TABLE 25.7.

PLASMA CARCINOEMBRYONIC ANTIGEN IN PATIENTS WITH CANCER

(Reproduced, by permission, from Schwartz, 1976)

Extent of disease	Number of patients	Percent of patients with values		
		less than 5 ng/ml	5–25 ng/ml	greater than 25 ng/ml
Previously treated and no clinical evidence of disease	143	68	30	2
No known metastases	208	70	28	2
Regional metastases	108	59	34	·6
Distant metastases	231	34	45	21

occur with other forms of therapy also, although transient increases as a result of tumour necrosis may occur shortly after chemotherapy is started (Bagshawe et al., 1973). Serial measurement of CEA activity is now accepted practice in many centres for monitoring the response to treatment of malignant disease. Go (1976) indicates that the correlation between the response to chemotherapy and the serum CEA concentration is fair. He also has observed that CEA activity may decrease preterminally and that some tumours may cause death even without producing CEA. Some chemotherapeutic agents may also affect CEA production without affecting the growth of the tumour. In patients with carcinoma of the colon or rectum, a high preoperative CEA concentration is often associated with a greater incidence of recurrence of the tumour than when the CEA concentration is low (Zamcheck et al., 1975). A high postoperative value is frequently associated with recurrences of a tumour (Wang et al., 1975).

The incidence of abnormal serum CEA concentrations in a variety of malignant and other diseases is illustrated in the data of Schwartz (1976) shown in Table 25.8. Another study has shown that CEA concentrations in serum were increased in 90% of cases with pancreatic carcinoma, 60% of metastatic breast cancer patients and 35% of patients with other tumours (Martin et al., 1976). However, the incidence of values above the accepted upper limit of normal ranged from 29 to 45% in patients with diverticulitis, colonic polyps or ulcerative colitis – all of which may be regarded as premalignant conditions. The serum CEA concentration in patients with ulcerative colitis varies with the clinical state of the disease, tending to rise with exacerbations and decline with remissions. The CEA concentration is also increased in some patients with regional ileitis, cholecystitis, peptic ulcer, gastritis, pancreatitis and liver disease in the absence of known tumours. In about 20% of women with benign conditions of the breast, e.g. cysts or mastitis, the serum CEA concentration may be increased.

TABLE 25.8.

PLASMA CARCINOEMBRYONIC ANTIGEN IN PATIENTS WITH MALIGNANT OR OTHER DISEASE

(Reproduced, by permission, from Schwartz, 1976)

Disease	Number of patients	Percent of patients with values less than	
		2.5 ng/ml	5.0 ng/ml
Cancer			
Colon and rectum	544	28	51
Lung	181	24	49
Pancreas	55	9	40
Stomach	79	39	71
Breast	125	55	73
Leukaemia, lymphoma, etc.	150	66	89
Pulmonary emphysema	49	43	90
Alcoholic cirrhosis	120	30	77
Ulcerative colitis	146	69	87
Pancreatitis	95	47	78

Schwartz (1976) has observed a significantly increased concentration of CEA in serum in only about one-quarter of the patients that he has studied with leukaemia, lymphoma, Hodgkin's disease or multiple myeloma. In all instances, the increased concentration was quite small. He also observed similar small changes in less than 20% of the patients with malignant melanoma or sarcoma. In these patients there was no correlation between the serum CEA concentration and the extent of the disease.

In general, measurements of CEA concentration and enzyme activity should be considered complementary in the diagnosis of primary and metastatic tumours. Simultaneous measurements of CEA with other tumour-associated antigens also leads to greater confidence in the biochemical determination of the presence of a tumour. Alterations in the serum concentration of CEA or enzyme activity may antedate the clinical confirmation of cancer by many weeks or months.

CEA activity has been measured in many different body secretions with the hope of localization of the site of a tumour. CEA activity is normally high in colonic secretions and to a lesser extent in pancreatico-biliary secretion. CEA activity in colonic lavage specimens is higher in patients with cancer of the colon than in healthy individuals. The CEA content of pancreatic juice cannot be used as a discriminant to differentiate cases of carcinoma of the pancreas from other causes of pancreatic disease (Go, 1976). Two-thirds of patients with bladder cancer have increased CEA-like activity in their urine and the frequency of abnormal CEA values can be correlated with the extent and grade of the tumour. However, infections of the urinary tract may also be associated with increased urinary CEA activity, and seminal fluid is also known to contain CEA.

An isomeric form of CEA, CEA-S, has been described which has been identified in 80% of patients with cancer of the digestive tract and in 86% of patients with colonic cancer. Edgington et al. (1975) have also observed a higher incidence of increased CEA-S antigen than increased CEA in patients with gastrointestinal cancer, and an absence of the CEA-S antigen in patients with benign gastrointestinal disease compared with a 10% incidence of increased CEA. The incidence of increased CEA-S antigen concentration is low in cirrhosis of the liver and increased CEA-S is much less common than increased CEA in breast cancer and lung cancer. Thus, CEA-S measurements appear to have greater specificity and sensitivity in determining the presence and site of a tumour.

When used in conjunction with other clinical laboratory tests and with a history and physical examination, measurement of CEA is of considerable value in providing confirmation of the presence of a tumour. The test is perhaps of most value in monitoring the response of a tumour to therapy. In no situation should the test be thought of as a screening test for malignant disease because of the significant incidence of both false-positive and false-negative results that may be observed.

25.5.2. Alpha-foetoprotein

Alpha-foetoprotein is synthesized by developing liver, beginning at least as early as the sixth week of gestation. The antigen is an α_1-globulin and should properly be designated α_1-foetoprotein instead of just α-foetoprotein, as an α_2-foetoprotein has also been identified. The serum α-foetoprotein concentration reaches a maximum about the thirteenth week of pregnancy. It then decreases rapidly to less than 2% of the maximum at 34 to 36 weeks of pregnancy. At birth, the concentration may still be as much as 20 to 30 mg/litre, but this rapidly decreases in the first few weeks of extrauterine life, when synthesis ceases. A small increase in the serum α-foetoprotein concentration may be observed in individuals after age 60 years (Massayeff et al., 1974). The half-life of α-foetoprotein is about 3.5 days. The same foetal protein is produced by hepatomas and occurs in the serum of patients with primary liver cancer (Abelev, 1971).

The presence of α-foetoprotein is useful diagnostically in determining the presence of hepatocellular cancer or teratoblastomas. The choice of method to determine α-foetoprotein has influenced the results reported in various studies of liver tumours (Table 25.9). The radioimmunoassay procedure that is now widely used is about 40,000 times more sensitive than the original agar-gel immunodiffusion procedure. The incidence of positive α-foetoprotein values in patients with hepatocellular carcinoma is almost 90% but with the radioimmunoassay procedure the incidence of false-positives is almost 20%. With the sensitive radioimmunoassay procedure positive values may be observed in patients with viral and chronic active hepatitis, alcoholic cirrhosis, ulcerative colitis and in up to 20% of cases of carcinoma of other tissues, even without metastases to the liver. The highest incidence of false-positives occurs with tumours of the pancreas, biliary tract and stomach (Neville and Cooper, 1976). In most of these tumours, the α-foetoprotein titre is only moderately increased. Such false-positives are not observed with the gel diffusion technique. The false-positive values have been attributed to the regeneration of liver, although it is also possible that a low concentration of circulating α-foetoprotein may be associated with genetic or nutritional factors. The serum α-foetoprotein concentration in patients with primary liver cancer does not correlate significantly with conventional liver function tests.

Alpha-foetoprotein occurs in the serum of patients with embryonal malignant teratoblastomas of the testes and ovary, but not usually in the serum of patients with other embryonal tumours (seminomas, neuroblastomas, or Wilm's tumours). The serum α-foetoprotein concentration appears to be directly related to the size of the tumour and its measurement is useful in following the course of the disease. Teratomas with a normal α-foetoprotein concentration generally respond well to therapy. While 50% of cases with teratoma have been reported to have an increased concentration of α-foetoprotein in serum

TABLE 25.9.

INCIDENCE OF POSITIVE ALPHA-FOETOPROTEIN DETERMINATIONS BY GEL DIFFUSION AND RADIOIMMUNOASSAY

(From data cited by Schwartz, 1976)

	Gel diffusion	Radioimmunoassay
Primary liver cancer	70	88
Miscellaneous cancers	0	8
Hepatitis	0	45
Cirrhosis	0	47
Miscellaneous diseases	0	31

by the agar-gel precipitation technique, as many as 80% have abnormal concentrations by immunoradioautography.

The incidence of increased α-foetoprotein concentrations is extremely low in the absence of a liver or embryonic tumour. Thus, in only 0.5% specimens from patients with non-hepatic benign lesions is a positive test for α-foetoprotein likely to occur with the radioimmunoassay procedure. As a result, the measurement and detection of α-foetoprotein in a non-pregnant woman is one of the most tumour-specific assays that is currently available. Raised α-foetoprotein concentrations may occur before the presence of a tumour can be detected by other means; successful therapy leads to a decrease in the concentration. However, as with carcinoembryonic antigen (section 25.5.1) a sudden marked decrease in concentration of α-foetoprotein may also occur shortly before death.

25.5.3. Other tumour-associated antigens

While carcinoembryonic antigen and α-foetoprotein are the two tumour-associated antigens that have been most widely studied, many additional antigens have been detected. Some of these antigens have been observed only intracellularly and have not, as yet, been detected in body fluids. There is still an active search for both organ- and tumour-specific antigens. Most of those that appear initially to have considerable specificity ultimately fail to withstand the test of time. Those that currently appear promising include pancreatic oncofoetal antigen (section 25.5.3.10) and the various colonic antigens described by Goldenberg et al. (1976).

25.5.3.1. Gamma-foetoprotein

Two foetoproteins with γ-globulin electrophoretic mobility have been observed in human tumours. They have been designated γ-foetoprotein-1 and γ-foetoprotein-2. The latter has been discovered only recently and occurs in breast tumours, but also in non-cancerous breast tissue. The term γ-foetoprotein, applied in previous studies of the antigen, refers to what would now be designated γ-foetoprotein-1. This protein does not occur in the serum of healthy people, pregnant women, or patients with non-neoplastic disease. It was also absent from as many as 179 normal tissue specimens and was present in only 2% of non-cancerous diseased organs studied (Edynak et al., 1972). Yet, the antigen has been detected in 110 of 153 carcinomas, 21 of 24 sarcomas, 23 of 28 leukaemic blood specimens and 15 of 20 benign tumours. Another study has indicated that the antigen occurs in the serum of about 11% of patients with cancer. The incidence is about 13% in breast cancer, 20% in sarcoma and in about 55% of patients with acute lymphoblastic leukaemia.

Antibody to the γ-foetoprotein-1 antigen has been observed in 8 of 1518 cancer patients. Highly sensitive versions of tests for both the γ-foetoprotein-1 antigen and its antibody are required before their usefulness in the diagnosis of cancer can be properly assessed.

25.5.3.2. Alpha$_2$H-foetoprotein

This protein is detectable in foetal liver and serum up to the end of the second postnatal month. Measurement of the antigen has had greatest application in the diagnosis of tumours in children after age 3 months. Serum activity is detectable in a large proportion of children with nephroblastomas, neuroblastomas, teratomas, hepatomas, and cerebral tumours, but it is also detectable in from 30 to 50% of patients with cholangiocarcinomas, myeloma, lymphoma or acute leukaemia. Almost 40% of the cirrhotic patients studied also had a positive assay. The incidence of positive tests is greater in chronic leukaemia than in healthy controls (Neville, 1973). In adults, the antigen is occasionally detected in association with regenerating liver tissue or inflammatory liver diseases.

25.5.3.3. Beta-S-foetoprotein

This protein, which normally disappears from serum by the seventh postnatal month, has been observed in increased amount in the serum of patients with a variety of liver diseases including hepatocarcinoma, cholangiocarcinoma and cirrhosis. Increased amounts have also been observed in the serum of patients with gastric carcinoma, leukaemia and lymphoma (Neville, 1973).

25.5.3.4. Leukaemia-associated antigens

Leukaemia-associated antigens are derived from tumour cell membranes. They have been detected in the serum of about one-third of patients with leukaemia and also in some patients with Hodgkin's disease. The value of measuring the antigens has still to be determined because their concentration does not necessarily decline during remissions (Harris et al., 1971).

25.5.3.5. Non-specific cross-reacting antigen

Non-specific cross-reacting antigen (NCA) is a β-globulin that has been extracted from carcinomas of the colon. The antigen is probably the same as that also known as NGP (normal glycoprotein), CEX, CEA-2 or BCGP (von Kleist and Burtin, 1969). It is a glycoprotein that is situated at the surface of invasive cells and in intraglandular deposits. It has been found in normal lung, spleen, stomach and colonic mucosa, in circulating mononuclear cells, and also in cancerous tissue, especially that of the gastrointestinal tract. This antigen shows the same immunologic identity as carcinoembryonic antigen but forms a precipitin ring closer to the antibody than carcinoembryonic antigen on immunodiffusion.

25.5.3.6. Membrane tissular antigen

This protein, also called membrane tissular autoantigen, migrates as an α-globulin on electrophoresis. It is a glycoprotein and has a different antigenic relationship from carcinoembryonic antigen and non-specific cross-reacting antigen. It has been found in tumours of the colon and rectum and in hepatic metastases. It also occurs in foetal colon (Burtin, 1974).

25.5.3.7. Tissue polypeptide antigen

Tissue polypeptide antigen has been isolated from human neoplasms and placenta. The antigen is present in the serum of most cancer patients, regardless of the type or site of the tumour. For many cancers, 4 of every 5 patients will have an increased concentration of the antigen, but as many as 36% of patients with benign diseases may also have increased antigen in their serum. The incidence appears to be highest in infections of the liver, lower respiratory tract and urinary tract. However, in cancer patients the antigen concentration persists at a high level whereas it is usually transient in patients with non-malignant disease. About 1% of healthy individuals have an increased serum concentration of tissue polypeptide antigen (Lundstrom et al., 1973).

Measurement of tissue polypeptide antigen appears to be of value in both diagnosis and follow-up of patients with cancer. Improvements in the test procedure have enabled Schwartz (1976) to increase the incidence of antigenaemia that he has observed in cancer patients from 70% to 88%.

25.5.3.8. T-Globulin

In 1970 Tal and Halperin proposed the assay of serum "T-globulin" as a cancer diagnostic procedure. The test is based on the assumption that cancer cells contain a unique glycolipid in their membranes which serves as a hapten to produce a cancer-specific protein antibody (T-globulin). The assay is carried out by immunoelectrophoresis. In the original study of more than 500 patients, negative results were obtained in 163 of 164 patients without cancer and positive results were obtained in 337 of 350 patients with cancer. However, a later study has shown many positive tests in patients with benign diseases so that the test can not be recommended in its present state of development (Tal et al., 1973).

Pregnancy-associated macroglobulin may be related to T-globulin. Its serum concentration is increased in many malignant diseases and its concentration correlates well with the extent and severity of the malignant disease so that it may be used to monitor response of a tumour to therapy.

25.5.3.9. Foetal sulphoglycoprotein antigen

This antigen occurs in the gastric juice of the foetus and has been detected in the gastric juice of 96% patients with gastric carcinomas. It may have a common antigenic determinant with carcinoembryonic antigen. The antigen is found in the cells of the gastric carcinoma and in the superficial cells of the mucosa close to the tumour. Unfortunately, from the viewpoint of differential diagnosis, the antigen is also found in 14% of individuals with gastric ulcers. This greatly exceeds the incidence of malignant change supervening on a gastric ulcer. Further, the test can not be used to monitor therapy as the amount of foetal sulphoglycoprotein antigen in the gastric juice does not necessarily decline, even with successful treatment (Neville, 1973).

25.5.3.10. Pancreatic oncofoetal antigen

Banwo et al. (1974) recently described an antigen in foetal pancreas and adult pancreatic tumours. The test appears to have great specificity for these tissues, and the antigen is absent from the serum of patients with cancer of the gastrointestinal tract, pancreatitis, and jaundice not caused by a pancreatic tumour.

25.5.4. Tumour-associated antibodies

Almost all patients with nasopharyngeal cancer and Burkitt's lymphoma have circulating antibodies to Epstein–Barr virus-associated antigens. With other, but similar, tumours the incidence of high titres is much less. The value of the titre of the antibodies can be correlated to some extent with the stage of the disease and its clinical course. Antibodies to antigens associated with herpes simplex virus have been identified with cervical cancer and squamous cell carcinoma of the head and neck. Antibodies to antigens in some tumours, e.g. melanoma and osteosarcoma, have also been described, but many healthy individuals give positive reactions so that the specificity of the antigens requires refinement. However, serial antibody determinations may be useful in assessing both the prognosis of the disease and its response to treatment (Herberman, 1976).

25.5.5. Immunological diagnostic procedures

Various immunological procedures, e.g. for cancer basic protein or the MEM (macrophage electrophoretic mobility) test, have been devised for the diagnosis of cancer (Field and Caspary, 1970; Pritchard et al., 1973). These tests, and those for immune responsiveness to tumour or virus associated antigens, are beyond the scope of this Chapter.

25.6. PROTEINS

Neoplastic disease is usually associated with a reduction in the total plasma protein concentration unless the disease is specifically associated with the accumulation of a paraprotein. Most of the reduction is due to a decrease in the albumin concentration because there frequently is a significant increase in the concentration of both α-globulin and fibrinogen. The magnitude of the increase of the α_1-globulin, and to a lesser extent of the α_2-globulin, may vary with the severity of the disease. The concentrations of β- and γ-globulins may increase slightly in advanced cancer. These responses are not specific for the type of cancer and are generally associated with chronic metabolic or infectious diseases.

It should be noted that the α_1- and α_2-globulins are mainly composed of acute phase reactants. Most of these specific proteins are affected by cancer (section 25.6.1.2), although they are also affected by conditions such as bacterial infections which may be superimposed on the basal state of cancer patients. Ablin et al. (1973) observed an increase in the concentration of α_2- and β-globulins in the serum of patients with carcinoma of the prostate. The increase in α_2-globulin is not due to the presence of α_2-macroglobulins, and Cooper et al. (1976) also confirmed that the increased α_2-globulin in patients with colonic cancer is also not due to the presence of macroglobulins. They were unable to demonstrate an increased β-globulin concentration in these patients.

The decreased serum albumin observed in many cancer patients is thought to be due to decreased synthesis of the protein. Toporek (1973) has demonstrated that tumours may contain a substance that suppresses albumin synthesis. The low levels in patients with gastric carcinoma may also be a result of loss through the tumour into the gastrointestinal tract (Jarnum and Schwartz, 1960).

Fahey and Boggs (1960) have shown that in acute leukaemia there is usually a decrease in the concentration of albumin but no effect on the concentration of β-globulin. The γ-globulin concentration is increased in acute myeloblastic, but not lymphoblastic, leukaemia, whereas the α_2-globulin is increased in the latter disease. In chronic leukaemia the plasma albumin concentration is often normal but the γ-globulin is decreased in lymphocytic leukaemia and increased in myelocytic leukaemia. In Hodgkin's disease the albumin concentration is reduced but α-globulin is increased. In patients with malignant melanoma, the albumin concentration is also reduced. Changes in all cases are influenced by the stage of the disease. In patients with meningeal leukaemia the concentration of albumin in cerebrospinal fluid is usually increased whereas that of prealbumin is reduced below normal. The ratio of the concentration of albumin in the cerebrospinal fluid to that in the serum is increased (Rothman et al., 1964).

The total protein concentration in the serum of patients with multiple myeloma may be very high because of the presence of the myeloma protein.

25.6.1. Specific proteins

Measurement of total protein, or even of the major globulin fractions, in serum is an insensitive technique and not specific for cancer. However, some changes are observed in the concentration of individual serum proteins that are of value in determining the nature of a tumour.

25.6.1.1. Immunoglobulins

The concentration of IgA is raised in the serum of some women with breast cancer and the concentration of IgG is significantly reduced in comparison with healthy controls (Roberts et al., 1975). In most cases the serum IgG concentration still fell within the normal range, but in some it was reduced below the accepted lower limit of normal. Meyer et al. (1973) demonstrated that women with a high concentration of serum IgA responded better to treatment than those in whom it was normal. The changes in immunoglobulin concentration were not related to the age of the patients or the stage of the disease. Although serum IgA concentration is increased in patients with hepatocellular carcinoma (Akdamar et al., 1972), the changes in patients with breast cancer were unrelated to the presence of hepatic metastases. The concentration of IgM in the serum of women is unaffected by the presence of a breast tumour even though breast cancerous tissue contains more IgM than benign or normal breast tissue. The amount of IgA is reduced in malignant breast tissue (Roberts et al., 1973). Treatment of a breast tumour by mastectomy and irradiation does not alter the concentration of the immunoglobulins in serum. Mander et al. (1975) have observed no change in the concentration of IgE in the serum of patients with breast cancer although its concentration may be greatly increased in the serum of patients with gastrointestinal cancer.

Ablin et al. (1972) have observed a reduction in the serum IgG concentration of men with carcinoma of the prostate and have suggested that such reductions may be related to the impaired ability of an individual with malignant disease to produce antibodies. Depression of heterophile antibody activity has indeed been observed in tumours of the breast and large bowel (Thomas and Fox, 1973).

Excluding cancer of haematopoietic tissues, the concentration of the immunoglobulins is often normal in the serum of patients with malignant disease (Table 25.10). However, Hughes (1971a) found increased concentrations of IgA and IgG in the serum of men with carcinoma of the skin or lungs. He also observed increased IgA in the serum of patients

TABLE 25.10.

SERUM IMMUNOGLOBULIN CONCENTRATIONS IN MALIGNANT DISEASE

0, no change from normal; +, increased and –, decreased compared with sex-matched healthy controls. (Reproduced, by permission, from Hughes, 1971)

Site of tumour	IgG		IgA		IgM		Ratio IgA/IgG	
	Male	Female	Male	Female	Male	Female	Male	Female
Skin	+	0	+	0	0	0	0	0
Lung	+	+	+	0	0	0	0	0
Mouth, larynx, gut	0	0	+	+	0	0	+	+
Colon and rectum	0	0	+	+	0	0	+	+
Uterus		0		+		0		+
Sarcoma	0	0	0	0	+	0	0	0
Melanoma	0	0	0	0	0	+	0	0
Ovary		0		0		–		0
Benign tumors		0		0		0		0
Ulcerative colitis	+	0	+	0	0	0	0	0

with cancer of the mouth, gastrointestinal tract or uterus, and in these patients the ratio of IgA to IgG was significantly increased. Edwards et al. (1977) have confirmed an increased ratio of IgA to IgG in the serum of patients with gastrointestinal carcinoma. IgM concentration is increased in the serum of women with melanoma.

Mander et al. (1975) found increased serum IgE in individuals with cancer of the colon, stomach or oesophagus, although other investigators have demonstrated both high and low concentrations of serum IgE in cancer (Jacobs et al., 1972; Serrou et al., 1975).

Iio et al. (1977) demonstrated a decreased mean serum IgE concentration in patients with chronic lymphocytic leukaemia. The rate of synthesis is reduced but the half-life of the protein is prolonged. In Hodgkin's disease, IgE concentration is increased.

Immunoglobulin A is the predominant immunoglobulin in tracheobronchial secretion and its concentration is increased both in the serum of patients with lung cancer and in the bronchial washings of patients with carcinoma of the lung (Mandel et al., 1976).

(a) *Multiple myeloma.* Multiple myeloma is essentially malignant disease of the plasma cells. Tumour cells may be localized in a small area of bone marrow or they may be widely disseminated. The overall incidence of the disease in the population is 1% in people over age 70 years. The most common forms of myelomatosis affect IgG, IgA or Bence Jones protein. More than 90% of patients with a malignant immunocytoma exhibit suppressed formation of normal immunoglobulins, and a single sharp band on electrophoresis of above 10 g/litre. With a benign immunocytoma the immunoglobulin concentration is rarely increased, and only a small proportion of people have suppression of formation of normal immunoglobulins. With myeloma affecting IgG, the concentration of the protein is usually higher than when IgA is affected.

Bence Jones protein has been detected in the urine of up to 65% of patients with multiple myeloma. It may also be excreted by patients with macroglobulinaemia, other neoplastic diseases and a few non-neoplastic diseases. The structure of the protein is discussed in detail elsewhere (Chapter 6).

Macroglobulinaemia may occur with uncontrolled proliferation of lymphocytoid cells which synthesize immunoglobulin IgG. Abnormal serum proteins may occur with lymphomas and leukaemia, more often when it affects lymphocytes than other cells (Bodansky, 1975).

25.6.1.2. Acute phase reactants

Alpha$_1$- and alpha$_2$-globulins are mainly composed of the acute phase reactant proteins which are synthesized in the liver. Many members of this group of proteins are increased in the serum of patients with cancer. However, many conditions that are unrelated to cancer, but which in some situations could be superimposed on underlying malignancy, are associated with an increase in the concentration of the acute phase reactants. These conditions include major surgery, acute and chronic infections, thermal injury and various inflammatory and degenerative diseases.

(a) *Alpha$_1$-antitrypsin.* Increases in the concentration of α_1-antitrypsin in serum have been observed in patients with cancer of the lung, colon, rectum, stomach and in patients with transitional tumours of the bladder. Alpha$_1$-antitrypsin concentration is also increased in patients with metastatic tumours. The concentration is linked to some extent to the size of the tumour.

Trypsin inhibitory capacity in the serum of patients with lung cancer is, on average, twice the value in healthy individuals, regardless of the type of cancer. Harris et al. (1976) observed that patients with abnormal sputum cytology, but with no clinical evidence of lung cancer, had both normal α_1-antitrypsin activity and trypsin inhibitory capacity. However, it should be noted that in patients with the non-MM phenotypes, serum α_1-antitrypsin activity is less in patients with abnormal sputum cytology than in patients with the MM phenotype.

(b) *Haptoglobin.* Serum haptoglobin concentration is often increased in the presence of tumours. This has been confirmed for colorectal, ovarian and renal neoplasms. In metastatic colorectal tumours, the increase in haptoglobin usually occurs with a rise in the plasma carcinoembryonic antigen. Measurement of haptoglobin, because of its simplicity, might serve as a substitute for the latter measurement in following the progress of the disease (Cooper et al., 1976). In primary colorectal tumours, a high serum haptoglobin concentration may occur without a corresponding increase in the carcinoembryonic antigen concentration.

In general, serum haptoglobin concentration is only slightly increased when a tumour is localized. Highest values are observed in individuals in whom metastases have developed in the skeleton and lung. The haptoglobin concentration is frequently normal in individuals with liver metastases (Nyman, 1959). The serum haptoglobin concentration is usually increased in patients with lymphomas, leukaemia, Hodgkin's disease and myeloma (Owen et al., 1964).

The mechanism for the increase in haptoglobin concentration has not been completely established. It is unlikely that decreased removal from the circulation, or increased release from stores, could be responsible (Mueller et al., 1971) so it is presumed that a tumour releases a factor that causes increased synthesis of haptoglobin in the liver, the only known site of its synthesis. The presence of such a factor has not been confirmed but support for its existence is suggested by the reported correlation between tumour size and concentration of haptoglobin. Unlike the situation pertaining with many biochemical tumour markers, the concentration of haptoglobin does not necessarily decrease following surgical removal of a bowel cancer (Ward et al., 1977) but a sustained increase above the previous concentration following surgery may indicate local recurrence or metastases.

As haptoglobin is influenced by many factors these should be eliminated as causes of an increased serum concentration before a diagnosis of malignancy is considered. When the history, clinical findings and other investigations suggest the possibility of a tumour, measurement of haptoglobin can provide help in following the progress of the disease.

Haemopexin, also concerned with the binding of haem, shows the same non-specific variations in serum in response to inflammatory disease and malignancy as does haptoglobin.

(c) *Caeruloplasmin.* The concentration of caeruloplasmin is increased in a variety of conditions besides cancer. These include chronic infections, rheumatoid arthritis, ankylosing spondylitis, pregnancy and the ingestion of oral contraceptives containing oestrogens (Hughes, 1972). Because copper is transported bound to caeruloplasmin, both copper and caeruloplasmin concentrations tend to increase and decline together. Shifrine and Fisher (1976) demonstrated that the ratio of serum copper to caeruloplasmin remains constant, at least in patients with osteosarcoma. The concentration of caeruloplasmin is increased in most types of cancer. While a wide range of values is often found, the mean value is significantly increased in carcinoma of the breast in women, cancer of the mouth and gut, and in haematopoietic malignancies.

(d) *Transferrin.* In contrast to the change in serum caeruloplasmin concentration in malignant disease, the concentration of transferrin is decreased. This is not diagnostic of a malignant disease, since transferrin concentration is also decreased in chronic infections, chronic liver disease, uraemia and malnutrition – all conditions that may occur independently, or be associated with advanced cancer. Hughes (1972) has specifically identified cancer of the mouth, gastrointestinal tract and haematopoietic tissues as being associated with a low serum transferrin concentration. A wide range of serum transferrin values has been found in patients with cancer; the cause of the change has not yet been established as to whether it is due to decreased synthesis or increased catabolism of the protein.

(e) *Orosomucoid.* Serum orosomucoid (α_1-acid glycoprotein) concentration appears to have the same sensitivity as other acute phase reactants in indicating the presence of a tumour. It is subject to the same factors that affect the concentration of the other acute phase reactants, e.g. inflammatory disorders and infections. The concentration of orosomucoid is highest when metastases have occurred, and the concentration is related to the overall mass of tumour (Ward et al., 1977). Multiple myeloma has been reported to be associated with a low concentration of orosomucoid (Bacchus, 1965).

(f) *Prealbumin.* Cancer is often associated with a decreased concentration of serum prealbumin. This may be as much associated with the presence of a tumour, because the degree of depression of the concentration is the same with an uncomplicated primary tumour as with a tumour with widespread metastases. Both the fall in the concentration occurring with a tumour and the increase following chemotherapy take place slowly.

(g) *Protein-bound hexoses and hexosamines.* The serum concentration of these compounds is increased in many inflammatory, infectious and neoplastic states. The magnitude of the increase is usually comparable in the different diseases, yet the change from normal can be correlated to some extent with the severity of the disease. The concentration of protein-bound hexoses and hexosamines varies in many different diseases; their measurement does not have any special diagnostic benefits in malignant disease.

25.6.1.3. Group-specific (Gc) protein

Gc protein consists of three components. In patients with cancers of lymphatic tissue other than lymphatic leukaemia, there is both a statistically significant increase in the concentration of the protein in serum and also an alteration in the relative frequencies of the three groups or components (Hughes, 1971b). For most cancers, the concentration of Gc protein in serum does not differ from that in healthy controls, and even in patients with cancers of lymphatic tissue the increase is slight.

25.6.1.4. Milk proteins

(a) *Casein.* Casein is a constituent of human milk. Secretion of the protein is under the control of prolactin. Casein is present in the serum of all lactating women but is not usually found during pregnancy. It may be detected in a small proportion of healthy men and non-pregnant or non-lactating women. The serum concentration of casein is high in women with untreated breast tumours, but it may decrease to an undetectable concentration in about one-half of the women who have been treated. The serum concentration tends to be higher when the tumour is more advanced at the time of its treatment. With local recurrence or more distant metastases following treatment, the serum concentration may increase to a very high value. The serum casein concentration is raised in individuals with lung cancer and in about one-half of the patients with tumours of the gastrointestinal tract. In these cases the increase is modest. There appears to be no correlation between the histological nature of a tumour and the serum casein concentration (Hendrick and Franchimont, 1974).

Further study is required to determine if measurements of serum casein can be used to monitor the response of tumours to therapy or to predict the possibility of recurrences. In many respects casein serves as a tumour marker or antigen and it is possible that repeated measurements may be as useful as repeated measurements of other tumour antigens in following progress of the disease.

(b) *Lactoferrin.* Patients with leukaemia have a higher serum lactoferrin concentration than healthy individuals (Bennett and Mohla, 1976). The compound is present in circulating monocytes, as well as in milk. Its measurement is probably of more value in evaluating leukaemia than breast cancer.

25.6.1.5. Complement

Serum total complement activity is increased in patients with acute leukaemia, Hodgkin's disease and sarcoma (Lichtenfeld et al., 1976). In all three conditions the C_9 component is considerably increased, and C_3 and C_7 are less frequently affected. The cause of these changes is at present not understood, but the observation by Edwards et al. (1977) that the concentration of C_3 in blood leaving the tumour is higher than in the general circulation suggests a locally produced tumour effect.

25.6.2. Urinary proteins and peptides

Rudman et al. (1969) described the excretion of peptides of molecular mass from 5000 to 8000 and proteins of molecular mass from 12,000 to 50,000 in at least 15% of patients with cancer. These compounds are different from those found in the urine of healthy individuals and are more common in the urine of patients with cancer during the last 6 months of their lives. The presence of the peptides and proteins is associated with a poor prognosis. The peptides are rich in glycine, alanine and proline; some also contain hexose and hexosamine. Rudman et al. (1976) also described glycoproteins, not present in normal plasma, in the urine of patients with leukaemia and cancer. The origin of these compounds is presumed to be the tumour tissue. At least one of these glycoproteins disappears from the urine with remissions or successful treatment of leukaemia.

25.7. LIPIDS

25.7.1. Plasma lipids

The plasma concentration of non-esterified fatty acids has been reported to be higher in patients with cancer than in healthy individuals. The concentration varies with the severity of the disease and with its response to therapy (Mueller and Watkin, 1961), yet similar alterations may be observed in patients with other debilitating diseases.

Serum lipoproteins are reportedly decreased in patients with advanced breast cancer or gynaecological tumours. Alpha-lipoproteins, phospholipids, and cholesterol are reduced in the serum of individuals with malignant tumours. The changes are unrelated to the extent of the disease or type of treatment.

25.7.2. Urinary cholesterol

Increased urinary excretion of non-esterified cholesterol has been reported in women with carcinoma of the steroid-producing glands, and in men with testicular or prostatic cancer. The mean excretion in well individuals is 0.65 ± 0.18 mg/24 h, but in most patients with adenocarcinoma of the prostate the excretion exceeds 1.2 mg/24 h (Acevedo et al., 1973). Increased excretion also occurs in patients with choriocarcinoma, teratocarcinoma and embryonal cell carcinoma of the testes and in patients with metastatic carcinoma of the testis and prostate. Normal values are observed in patients with testicular seminomas. In general, the abnormal values appear to correlate with the clinical course of the disease. Hyperexcretion of cholesterol has been observed in some patients with hyperplasia of the prostate, other forms of cancer, and in some healthy individuals over 45 years of age. Increased excretion may also be observed with Cushing's syndrome and diabetic ketoacidosis. Generally, a normal urinary excretion of non-esterified cholesterol occurs in women with neoplastic diseases unrelated to the steroid-producing glands and their target organs (Acevedo et al., 1975). Normal values are also observed in women with neoplasms other than of the ovaries and body of the uterus and in diseases such as endometriosis of these organs. The majority of women with carcinoma of the cervix (including those with tumour in situ) and carcinoma of the endometrium, excrete increased quantities of non-esterified cholesterol, with the concentration correlating well with the clinical status of the patient. Changes in concentration may be used to monitor changes in the patient's clinical state and response to therapy.

25.8. TRACE AND OTHER ELEMENTS

Trace elements have been implicated both in causing cancer, e.g. with arsenic or mercury compounds, and in preventing or curing the disease. Trace element measurements have been used to monitor the progress of tumours.

25.8.1. Zinc

Both the serum concentration and the concentration of zinc in erythrocytes, granulocytes and leucocytes of patients with cancer of the bronchus and colon are reduced compared with the same measurements in healthy individuals. At the same time, the urinary zinc excretion is increased up to 3 times the normal value. Molybdenum excretion is reduced and a urinary zinc/molybdenum ratio of greater than 300 has been described as indicative of advanced cancer (Pfeilsticher, 1965). Malignant tissue from a prostate gland has a higher zinc content than normal tissue, but tissue from liver, kidney or lung that contains tumour metastases has a higher zinc content than either the corresponding normal tissue or the tumour itself (Schwartz, 1975). Low concentrations of zinc are observed in both primary liver tumour tissue and hepatic metastases of tumours with primary sites elsewhere (Kew and Mallett, 1974). However, high concentrations of zinc have been reported in tumour tissue from the lung and breast (Mulay et al., 1971), and in osteogenic sarcoma.

It should be noted that the amount of zinc that has been reported in different tumours is very variable. Probably little credence should be attached to the use of zinc measurements in determining the presence of a neoplasm.

Zinc deficiency is associated both with delayed wound healing and impaired growth of tumours in experimental animals. The relationship of the effect on cancer growth in humans has still to be determined.

25.8.2. Copper

More than 95% of the serum copper is present in caeruloplasmin. The concentration of this protein is frequently increased in the serum of cancer patients and accordingly the serum copper concentration is increased.

In patients with leukaemia, the serum copper concentration is increased when the disease is active, but it declines to normal in remissions or in response to therapy (Hrgovcic et al., 1968). Serum copper measurements have been used to provide an index of response to radiotherapy or chemotherapy. A rise of the concentration in a treated individual often antedates clinical relapse by as much as 1 to 6 months. The magnitude of the increase in serum copper in patients with leukaemia appears to be correlated with the severity of the disease. The changes occur regardless of the type of leukaemia. Similar changes have been observed in patients with Hodgkin's disease, although normal values have been observed in some patients. Some patients with reticulum cell sarcoma also demonstrate increased serum copper concentration.

In most of these conditions, the increased serum copper concentration is attributable to an increase in the concentration of the circulating caeruloplasmin. However, when liver disease is present, part of the increase may be caused by impaired biliary excretion of the copper. The source of the increased serum copper is not yet clear, and the increased concentration has been postulated to arise from the breakdown of tumour tissue, but more probably it arises from tissue stores. Its purpose may be to fill the requirements of the rapidly metabolizing malignant tissue for increased enzyme activity (Hoch-Ligeti, 1969).

Serum copper concentrations are increased in cancer of many different organs. This has been described for bronchogenic carcinoma, squamous cell carcinoma of the larynx, osteosarcoma, cervical and other cancers of the reproductive system, and bladder cancer. In one study, an increase was found in 43 of 71 patients with lung cancer. In another study, all 23 patients with breast cancer had an increased serum copper concentration. The average increase was 2.8 times the normal upper limit, yet other studies have not confirmed such an increase in all patients (Schwartz, 1975). In cervical and bladder cancers, the increased serum copper concentration can be correlated with the stage of the disease and its response to treatment.

Higher concentrations of copper have been found in cancerous breast and laryngeal tissue than in the corresponding healthy tissue. In breast neoplasms the average increase was 2.3 times the concentration in healthy tissue.

25.8.3. Calcium

Hypercalcaemia may be observed in as many as 10% of patients with malignant disease, but the incidence varies with the population studied. Thus, it is most common in patients with carcinoma of the bronchus or with tumours of the breast or bladder (Heath, 1976). The majority of patients with hypercalcaemia have metastases, often to bone (Myers, 1960). The associated biochemical features include hypophosphataemia, decreased renal tubular reabsorption of phosphorus with increased reabsorption of calcium (Heath, 1976). Increased serum alkaline phosphatase activity with a low serum albumin and high globulin may also be observed.

In a small proportion of cases, parathyroid hormone is secreted by the tumour itself. In other cases the tumour secretes an immunologically different form of parathyroid hormone. In some instances a parathyrotrophic agent secreted by the tumour has been postulated as the cause of parathyroid hyperplasia and hypercalcaemia. In other cases, parathyroid adenomata appear to occur concurrently with non-parathyroid malignancy (Kaplan et al., 1971). In other cases prostaglandin E_2, and vitamin D-like sterols secreted by the cells of patients with multiple myeloma, have been proposed as possible causes of hypercalcaemia.

25.8.4. Other trace elements

The manganese content of malignant breast tissue is higher than that of normal tissue, and that of osteogenic sarcoma is higher than that of normal long bone (Mulay et al., 1971). The tin content of some malignant tissues has been reported to be less than in healthy tissue, but the cobalt concentrations of malignant tumours of bone and healthy bone are similar.

Deficiencies of certain trace elements have been linked with cancer. The cancer death rate in several countries has been related inversely to the dietary selenium intake. The blood selenium concentration reflects this also, being low in individuals from those countries where the incidence of breast cancer is high. Prolonged industrial exposure to certain trace elements, e.g. nickel and beryllium, may lead to a higher incidence of cancer than in people not exposed to the same amounts of these elements.

Many patients with malignant disease have a low serum iron concentration. The reticuloendothelial stores of iron are increased as is typical of the anaemia of chronic disease.

25.9. MISCELLANEOUS COMPOUNDS

25.9.1. Tryptophan metabolites

The excretion of tryptophan metabolites, e.g. kynurenine and 3-hydroxykynurenine, tends to be higher in some patients with tumours of the bladder than in healthy individuals. In response to a loading dose (2 grams) of tryptophan, the excretion of kynurenine was increased in cancer patients with abnormal metabolism to a level substantially greater than in healthy individuals or cancer patients with normal metabolism. The different responses have been attributed to increased activity of tryptophan pyrrolase and reduced activity of kynureninase in the liver of patients with abnormal metabolism. Musajo and Benassi (1964) observed abnormal tryptophan metabolism in 30% of patients with bladder tumours, 49% of patients with extra-bladder tumours, 59% of patients with kidney tumours and 15% of patients with non-neoplastic urologic diseases.

The excretion of tryptophan metabolites after a loading dose of tryptophan is higher in approximately 70% of patients with Hodgkin's disease than in healthy individuals (Crepaldi and Parpajola, 1964). About 50% of patients with breast cancer excrete abnormal quantities of tryptophan metabolites after tryptophan loading. The excretion of metabolites is greater in patients with metastases than others (DeGeorge and Brown, 1970). Davis et al. (1973) demonstrated that patients with breast cancer who display abnormal tryptophan metabolism excrete reduced quantities of aetiocholanolone. The reduced androgen excretion may be interlinked with the altered oestrogen metabolism that often accompanies breast cancer and is known to affect tryptophan pyrrolase activity in the liver.

25.9.2. Fucose

Fucose is a component of glycoproteins, the concentration of which is often increased in the serum of patients with malignant disease. Bodansky (1975) has summarized the studies of serum fucose in breast cancer and concluded that as 73% of patients with breast cancer had an increased concentration, and 23% of patients without malignant disease also had an increased concentration, the test has little discriminatory value.

25.9.3. Aminoacids

Changes in plasma or urinary aminoacids occur with neoplastic diseases but are not characteristic of them. Serum tryptophan concentration is increased in malignant disease. Urinary hydroxyproline excretion may be increased with tumours that have metastasized to bone, and it has been alleged to be greater in the presence of osteoblastic than osteolytic lesions. The greatest excretion occurs with primary tumours of bone. The increased excretion of hydroxyproline may be related to increased reabsorption of mature bone or new bone formation. Urinary hydroxyproline excretion may also be increased when soft tissue metastases are present (Guzzo et al., 1969). In many instances an increased urinary hydroxyproline to creatinine ratio may antedate clinically- or radiologically-evident bone metastases. A decreasing ratio of hydroxyproline to creatinine has been used to follow successful response of tumours to chemotherapy.

Leukaemic patients excrete greater quantities of aspartate, threonine and serine than healthy individuals during periods of active disease, but during remission the leukaemic patient excretes a normal quantity of aminoacids. The increased excretion tends to be quite small, but is greater in patients with acute lymphoblastic leukaemia than acute myelogenous leukaemia. Excretion of aminoacids is increased with chemotherapy, presumably due to the destruction of malignant cells and impaired reutilization of the aminoacids (Wiseman et al., 1976). The high turnover and destruction of leukaemic cells with release of DNA may be responsible for the increased excretion of β-aminoisobutyric acid that is also observed in leukaemia (Killman et al., 1961).

Patients with liver carcinoma have mild increases in the concentration of taurine in their plasma. Patients with extensive hepatic infiltration have shown increased plasma concentrations of sarcosine and hydroxyproline, which are barely detectable in normal plasma (Balis et al., 1962).

25.9.4. Purines

Uric acid concentration tends to be higher in both serum and urine of patients with acute leukaemia and chronic granulocytic leukaemia, although it is less common with chronic lymphocytic leukaemia. Increased excretion of uracil may be observed in patients with chronic myelocytic leukaemia. 5-Ribosyluracil excretion may also be increased.

Hyperuricaemia is quite common in patients with cancer due to the rapid turnover of cells. N(2),N(2)-dimethylguanosine, 1-methylinosine and pseudouridine occur largely in transfer RNA but to a lesser extent in ribosomal RNA. Increased transfer RNA methylase activity occurs with neoplastic growth and increased urinary excretion of the nucleosides has been observed in patients with cancer of the breast and other tissues (Tormey et al., 1975). The excretion of N(2),N(2)-dimethylguanosine was increased in as many as 57% of patients with metastatic breast tumours and in 44% with local lymph node involvement. The incidence of increased 1-methylinosine excretion was 44% and 33% in the two groups, and that of pseudouridine was 25% in both groups. The excretion of these compounds may revert to normal with successful therapy.

Increased concentrations of N(2),N(2)-dimethylguanosine and 1-methylinosine may be detectable in the plasma of patients with acute leukaemia or breast cancer (Levine et al., 1975).

25.9.5. Ferritin

An increased serum ferritin concentration is observed in patients with Hodgkin's disease, leukaemia and myeloma. It is believed that the effect is caused by inhibition of the release of iron from the reticuloendothelial cells (Jones et al., 1973). The concentration is very high (up to 25 times normal) in patients with myelomonocytic leukaemia, presumably as a consequence of the high content of ferritin in monocytes. The serum ferritin concentration is increased in most forms of cancer but it is usually higher with cancer of parenchymal organs than cancer of the gastrointestinal tract (Niitsu et al., 1975).

It has been postulated that tumour cells produce an acidic "carcinofoetal" isoferritin, but acidic isoferritins are not restricted to malignant tissue, and the normal serum ferritin consists of three component isoferritins. The ferritin from malignant tissue may contain an additional isoferritin to those found in normal tissue. The tumour-specific ferritin is also present in early foetal ferritins (Alpert et al., 1973).

Jacobs et al. (1976) found that patients with a high serum ferritin concentration have a higher tumour recurrence rate during the 4 years following treatment of the tumour.

25.10. PRODUCTS OF TUMOUR METABOLISM

25.10.1. Pheochromocytoma, pheochromoblastoma, ganglioneuroma and neuroblastoma

The biochemical features of these tumours are considered in detail in Chapter 24. In summary, the plasma concentration of norepinephrine is usually increased in patients with pheochromocytoma; the concentration of epinephrine is less frequently increased. The urinary excretions of catecholamines and 3-methoxy-4-hydroxymandelic acid and 3-methoxy-4-hydroxyphenylglycol are increased in patients with pheochromocytoma; in patients with pheochromoblastoma the urinary excretion of homovanillic acid is also increased. Hypercystathioninuria and hypomethioninuria have also been reported with large amounts of N-acetylated dopamine in the urine (Bodansky, 1975).

In the majority of patients with neuroblastoma the urinary excretion of dopamine is increased. Dihydroxyphenylalanine and dihydroxyphenylacetic acid excretions are also increased. The excretion of homovanillic acid is increased in a smaller proportion of patients, but that of 3-methoxy-4-hydroxymandelic acid is increased in almost all patients. Epinephrine and norepinephrine excretion usually is unaffected by neuroblastomas or ganglioneuromas. Goldstein et al. (1972) have indicated that serum dopamine-β-hydroxylase activity may be increased in many patients with neuroblastoma. Cystathionine excretion may be greatly increased in patients with neuroblastoma, especially when widespread metastases are present.

25.10.2. Melanoma

The urine of patients with generalized melanoma contains both indolic melanogens, derived from 5,6-dioxyindole, and phenolic melanogens which have been studied more frequently. Dihydroxyphenylalanine excretion is increased in patients with melanoma. The excretion of other catechols may also be increased. 5-S-cysteinyldopa has been observed in the urine of patients with melanoma (Agrup et al., 1975). Its measurement can be used to monitor changes in the state of the patient's response to therapy. Excretion of homovanillic acid is generally normal when a melanoma is benign or confined to the skin, but when the melanoma is disseminated, the excretion of the acid is increased (Trapeznikov et al., 1975).

25.10.3. Carcinoid

The characteristic biochemical findings in the body fluids of patients with the carcinoid syndrome include an increased concentration of 5-hydroxytryptamine (serotonin) in the blood and 5-hydroxyindoleacetic acid in the urine. 5-hydroxytryptamine excretion in the urine is also increased. The urinary excretion of histamine may also be increased.

25.11. POPULATION SCREENING

The usefulness of several of the biochemical tests discussed above in the detection of breast cancer has been discussed by Coombes et al. (1977). Their population consisted of patients with metastases as well as those with localized tumours. In the former group serum ferritin, C-reactive protein, carcinoembryonic antigen, acid glycoprotein, total alkaline phosphatase, sialyltransferase, and urinary hydroxyproline/creatinine ratio were increased in more than one-half of the patients (Table 25.11). Ferritin, C-reactive protein, and carcinoembryonic antigen were increased in more than 80%. The incidence of biochemical abnormalities was comparable with results obtained by physical means for detecting metastases.

The biochemical tests were much less effective in detecting cancer without metastases. Only 22% of the patients had an increased value of any of the seven parameters found effective in detecting metastases. Many of the biochemical tests lack specificity for cancer and can be affected by a wide variety of other diseases. Yet, when taken in conjunction with measurement of tumour products, they are capable of detecting most cases of advanced cancer. However, the combination of available biochemical tests lacks the sensitivity required to screen a well population for early disease.

Biochemical tests, in general, lack the sensitivity to detect a malignancy before a patient becomes aware that he has a medical problem. The most useful test is the occult

TABLE 25.11.

FREQUENCY (%) OF ABNORMALITIES IN PLASMA OF VARIOUS TUMOUR MARKERS IN 17 PATIENTS WITH METASTATIC BREAST CANCER

(Reproduced, by permission, from Coombes et al., 1977)

Carcinoembryonic antigen	81
Ferritin	88
Alkaline phosphatase (total)	64
Sialyltransferase	56
Acid glycoprotein	75
C-Reactive protein	87
Pregnancy associated macroglobulin	35
α_1-Antitrypsin	31
Haemopexin	19
Haptoglobin	38
Caeruloplasmin	38
Lysozyme	0
Calcitonin	11
Human chorionic gonadotrophin	5
Alkaline phosphatase (placental)	0
α-Lactalbumin	0

blood test for gastrointestinal bleeding. Although the presence of blood is not diagnostic of malignant disease, the test is sensitive to small amounts of blood, which may be an early sign of cancer or other serious disease of the gastrointestinal tract.

For all screening programmes, the costs must be balanced against the yield of useful diagnostic information. At the present time, the only biochemical test that might be considered cost beneficial is the occult blood test. Even then proper preparation of the patient and handling of the specimen is required to minimize the incidence of false-negative results.

Currently the role of biochemical tests in cancer is much better established for following the progress of the disease, and its response to therapy, than in establishing a diagnosis. Even though the patient's history and physical examination are insensitive tools in detecting early cancer it appears that it will be some time before they will be supplanted by biochemical screening tests.

REFERENCES

Abelev, G.I. (1971) Alpha-foetoprotein in ontogenesis and its association with malignant tumors. Advances in Cancer Research, 14, 295–358.

Ablin, R.J., Gonder, M.J. and Soanes, W.A. (1972) Levels of immunoglobulins in the serum of patients with carcinoma of the prostate. Neoplasma, 19, 57–60.

Ablin, R.J., Gonder, M.J. and Soanes, W.A. (1973) Serum proteins in prostatic cancer. 1. Relationship between clinical stage and level. Journal of Urology, 110, 238–241.

Acevedo, H.F., Campbell, E.A., Saier, E.L., Frich, J.C., Jr., Merkow, L.P., Hayeslip, D.W., Bartok, S.P., Grauer, R.C. and Hamilton, J.L. (1973) Urinary cholesterol – V. Its excretion in men with testicular and prostatic neoplasms. Cancer, 32, 196–205.

Acevedo, H.F., Campbell, E.A., Frich, J.C., Jr., Merkow, L.P., Hayeslip, D.W. and Gilmore, J. (1975) Urinary cholesterol – VII. The significance of the excretion of nonesterified cholesterol in patients with uterine carcinomas. Cancer, 36, 1459–1469.

Agrup, G., Agrup, P., Andersson, R., Falck, B., Hansson, J.A., Jacobsson, S., Rorsman, H., Rosengren, A.-M. and Rosengren, E. (1975) Urinary excretion of 5-S-cysteinyldopa in patients with primary melanoma or melanoma metastasis. Acta Dermatologica, 55, 337–341.

Akdamar, K., Epps, A.C., Maumus, L.T. and Sparks, R.D. (1972) Immunoglobulin changes in liver disease. Annals of the New York Academy of Sciences, 197, 101–107.

Almersjö, O., Bengmark, S., Hafström, L. and Rosengren, K. (1974) Accuracy of diagnostic tools in malignant hepatic lesions. A comparative study using serum tests, angiography, scintiscanning and laparotomy. American Journal of Surgery, 127, 663–668.

Alpert, E., Coston, R.L. and Drysdale J.W. (1973) Carcino-foetal human liver ferritins. Nature, 242, 194–196.

Aronsen, K.F., Nosslin, B. and Pihl, B. (1970) The value of γ-glutamyl transpeptidase as a screen test for liver tumour. Acta chirurgica Scandinavica, 136, 17–22.

Atkins, H., Bulbrook, R.D., Falconer, M.A., Hayward, J.L., MacLean, K.S. and Schurr, Ph.H. (1968) Ten years' experience of steroid assays in the management of breast cancer. Lancet, II, 1255–1260.

Bacchus, H. (1965) Serum seromucoid and acid mucopolysaccharide in malignant neoplastic diseases. Cancer, 18, 1285–1291.

Bagshawe, K.D., Rogers, G.T., Searle, F. and Wilson, H. (1973) Blood carcinoembryonic antigen, Regan isoenzyme, and human chorionic gondatrophin in primary mediastinal carcinoma. Lancet, I, 210–211.

Baillie, J., Al Adnani, M.S., Patrick, R.S., Kirrane, J.A. and McGee, J.O.D. (1975) The expression of prolyl hydroxylase and collagen by premalignant and malignant hepatocytes. Journal of Medical Microbiology, 5, 23.

Balis, M.E., Salser, J.S. and Brown, G.B. (1962) Amino acid levels in malignancy. Cancer Chemotherapy Reports, 16, 487–489.

Banwo, O., Versey, J. and Hobbs, J.R. (1974) New oncofoetal antigen for human pancreas. Lancet, I, 643–645.

Bennett, R.M. and Mohla, C. (1976) A solid-phase radioimmunoassay for the measurement of lactoferrin in human plasma: variations with age, sex and disease. Journal of Laboratory and Clinical Medicine, 88, 156–166.

Bodansky, O. (1975) Biochemistry of Human Cancer, Academic Press, New York.

Bondy, P.K. (1976) Systemic effects of neoplasia. In Scientific Foundations of Oncology (Eds. T. Symington and R.L. Carter) Heinemann, London.

Bosmann, H.B. and Hall, T.C. (1974) Enzyme activity in invasive tumors of human breast and colon. Proceedings of the National Academy of Sciences, 71, 1833–1837.

Bulbrook, R.D., Greenwood, F.C. and Hayward, J.L. (1960) Selection of breast-cancer patients for adrenalectomy or hypophysectomy by determination of urinary 17-hydroxycorticosteroids and aetiocholanolone. Lancet, I, 1154–1157.

Burtin, P. (1974) Membrane antigens of the colonic tumors. Cancer, 34, 829–834.

Cadeau, B.J., Blackstein, M.E. and Malkin, A. (1974) Increased incidence of placenta-like alkaline phosphatase activity in breast and genitourinary cancer. Cancer Research, 34, 729–732.

Calabresi, E., De Guili, G., Becciolini, A., Giannotti, P., Lombardi, G. and Serio, M. (1976). Plasma estrogens and androgens in male breast cancer. Journal of Steroid Biochemistry, 7, 605–609.

Chretien, P.B., Matthews, W. and Twomey, P.L. (1973) Serum ribonucleases in cancer – Relation to tumor histology. Cancer, 31, 175–179.

Coombes, R.C., Powles, T.J., Gazet, J.C., Ford, H.T., Sloane, J.P. and Lawrence, D.J.R. (1977) Biochemical markers in human breast cancer. Lancet, I, 132–134.

Cooper, E.H. (1976) The nature of cancer. Annals of Clinical Biochemistry, 13, 467–470.

Cooper, E.H., Turner, R., Geekie, A., Neville, A.M., Goligher, J.C., Graham, N.G., Giles, F.-R., Hall, R. and MacAdam, W.A.F. (1976) Alpha-globulins in the surveillance of colorectal cancer. Biomedicine, 24, 171–178.

Cooper, J.F. and Foti, A. (1974) A radioimmunoassay for prostatic acid phosphatase. 1. Methodology and range of normal male serum values. Investigative Urology, 12, 98–102.

Crepaldi, G. and Parpajola, A. (1964) Excretion of tryptophan metabolites in different forms of haemoblastosis. Clinica Chimica Acta, 9, 106–117.

Dao, T.L. (1972) Ablation therapy for hormone-dependent tumors. Annual Review of Medicine, 23, 1–18.

Dao, T.L., Morreal, C. and Nemoto, T. (1973) Urinary estrogen excretion in men with breast cancer. New England Journal of Medicine, 298, 138–140.

Davis, H.L., Jr., Brown, R.R., Leklem, J. and Carlson, I.H. (1973) Tryptophan metabolism in breast cancer. Correlation with urinary steroid excretion. Cancer, 31, 1061–1064.

DeGeorge, F.V. and Brown, R.R. (1970) Differences in tryptophan metabolism between breast cancer patients with and without cancer at other sites. Cancer, 26, 767–770.

De Guili, G. and De Guili, S. (1973) In Characterization of Human Tumors (Eds. W. Davis and C. Maltoni) pp. 213–217, Excerpta Medica, Amsterdam.

Durie, B.G. and Salmon, S.E. (1975) Cellular kinetics, staging, and immunoglobulin synthesis in multiple myeloma. Annual Reviews of Medicine, 26, 283–288.

Dzialoszynski, L.M., Kvoll, J.L. and Frohlich, A. (1966) Arylsulphatase activity of some malignant tumors. Clinica Chimica Acta, 14, 450–453.

Edgington, T.S., Astarita, R.W. and Plow, E.F. (1975) Association of an isomeric species of carcinoembryonic antigen (CEA-S) with neoplasia of the gastrointestinal tract. New England Journal of Medicine, 293, 103–107.

Edwards, A.J., Lee, M. and Harcourt, G. (1977) Serum immunoglobulins and C_3 complement concentrations in malignancy. Clinical Oncology, 3, 65–73.

Edynak, E.M., Old, L.J., Vrana, M. and Lardis, M.P. (1972) A fetal antigen associated with human neoplasia. New England Journal of Medicine, 286, 1178–1183.

Fahey, J.L. and Boggs, D.R. (1960) Serum protein changes in malignant diseases. 1. The acute leukemias. Blood, 16, 1479–1490.

Field, E.J. and Caspary, E.A. (1970) Lymphocyte sensitisation: an in-vitro test for cancer. Lancet, II, 1337–1341.

Fishman, W.H. (1974). Perspectives on alkaline phosphatase isoenzymes. American Journal of Medicine, 56, 617–650.

Fishman, W.H., Bonner, C.D. and Homburger, F. (1956) Serum "prostatic" acid phosphatase and cancer of the prostate. New England Journal of Medicine, 255, 925–933.

Fishman, W.H., Inglis, N.I., Strolbach, L.L. and Krant, M.J. (1968) A serum alkaline phosphatase isoenzyme of human neoplastic cell origin. Cancer Research, 28, 150–154.

Folca, P.J., Glascock, R.F. and Irvine, W.T. (1961) Studies with tritium labelled hexoestrol in advanced breast cancer. Comparison of tissue accumulation of hexoestrol with response to bilateral adrenalectomy and oophorectomy. Lancet, II, 796–798.

Fujita, K., Nagatsu, T., Maruta, K., Ito, M., Senba, H. and Miki, K. (1976) Urinary putrescine, spermidine and spermine in human blood and solid cancers and in experimental gastric tumor of rats. Cancer Research, 36, 1320–1324.

Gambill, E.E. and Mason, H.L. (1964) Urinary amylase in patients with pancreatic carcinoma. Journal of the American Medical Association, 188, 824–826.

Gamklou, R. and Schersten, T. (1973) Activity of alpha-1,4-glucosidase in serum from patients with malignant tumor. Cancer, 32, 298–301.

Go, V.L.W. (1976) Carcinoembryonic antigen: clinical application. Cancer, 37, 562–566.

Gold, P. and Freedman, S.O. (1965) Demonstration of tumor specific antigens in human colonic carcinomata by immunological tolerance and absorption techniques. Journal of Experimental Medicine, 121, 439–462.

Goldenberg, D.M., Pant, K.D. and Dahlman, H.L. (1976) Antigens associated with normal and malignant gastrointestinal tissues. Cancer Research, 36, 3455–3463.

Goldman, R.D., Kaplan, N.O. and Hall, T.C. (1964) Lactate dehydrogenase in human neoplastic tissue. Cancer Research, 24, 389–399.

Goldstein, M., Freedman, L.S., Bohoun, A.C. and Guerinot, F. (1972) Serum dopamine-β-hydroxylase activity in neuroblastoma. New England Journal of Medicine, 286, 1123–1125.

Gordan, G.S., Cantino, T.J., Erhardt, L., Hansen, J. and Lubich, W. (1966) Osteolytic sterol in human breast cancer. Science, 151, 1226–1228.

Guzzo, C.E., Pachas, W.N., Pinals, R.S. and Krant, M.J. (1969) Urinary hydroxyproline excretion in patients with cancer. Cancer, 24, 382–387.

Harris, C.C., Cohen, M.H., Conner, R., Primack, A., Saccomanno, G. and Talamo, R.C. (1976) Serum alpha$_1$-antitrypsin in patients with lung cancer or abnormal cytology. Cancer, 38, 1655–1657.

Harris, R., Viza, D., Todd, R., Phillips, J., Sugar, R., Jennison, R.F., Marriott, G. and Gleeson, M.H. (1971) Detection of human leukaemia associated antigens in leukaemic serum and normal embryos. Nature, 233, 556–557.

Heath, D.A. (1976) Hypercalcaemia and malignancy. Annals of Clinical Biochemistry, 13, 555–560.

Henderson, B.E., Gerkins, V., Rosario, I., Casagrande, J. and Pike, M.C. (1975) Elevated serum levels of estrogen and prolactin in daughters of patients with breast cancer. New England Journal of Medicine, 293, 790–795.

Henderson, M. and Kessel, D. (1977) Alterations in plasma sialyltransferase levels in patients with neoplastic disease. Cancer, 39, 1129–1134.

Herberman, R.B. (1976) Immunologic approaches to the diagnosis of cancer. Cancer, 37, 549–561.

Hendrick, J.C. and Franchimont, P. (1974) Radio-immunoassay of casein in the serum of normal subjects and of patients with various malignancies. European Journal of Cancer, 10, 725–730.

Higashino, K., Ohtani, R., Kudo, S., Hashinotsume, M., Hada, T., Kang, K.-Y., Ohkochi, T., Takahashi, Y. and Yamamura, Y. (1975) Hepatocellular carcinoma and a variant alkaline phosphatase. Annals of Internal Medicine, 83, 74–78.

Hobson, B.M. (1965) The excretion of chorionic gonadotrophin by men with testicular tumours. Acta Endocrinologica (Copenhagen), 49, 337–348.

Hoch-Ligeti, C. (1969) Laboratory Aids in Diagnosis of Cancer. Thomas, Springfield, Ill.

Holroyde, C.P., Gabzuda, T.G., Putnam, R.C., Paul, P. and Reichard, G.A. (1975) Altered glucose metabolism in metastatic carcinoma. Cancer Research, 35, 3710–3714.

Hrgovcic, M., Tessmer, C.F., Minckler, T.F., Mosler, B. and Taylor, G.H. (1968) Serum copper levels in lymphoma and leukemia: special reference to Hodgkin's disease. Cancer, 21, 743–755.

Hughes, N.R. (1971a). Serum concentration of γG, γA, and γM immunoglobulins in patients with carcinoma, melanoma and sarcoma. Journal of the National Cancer Institute, 46, 1015–1028.

Hughes, N.R. (1971b) Serum group-specific (Gc) protein concentrations in patients with carcinoma, melanoma, sarcoma and cancer of haematopoietic tissues as determined by radial immunodiffusion. Journal of the Cancer Institute, 46, 665–675.

Hughes, N.R. (1972) Serum transferrin and caeruloplasmin concentrations in patients with carcinoma, melanoma, sarcoma and cancers of haematopoietic tissues. Australian Journal of Experimental Biology and Medical Sciences, 50, 97–107.

Iio, A., Strober, W., Broder, S., Polmar, S.H. and Waldmann, T.A. (1977) The metabolism of IgE in patients with immunodeficiency states and neoplastic conditions. Journal of Clinical Investigation, 59, 743–755.

Jacobs, A., Jones, B., Ricketts, C., Bulbrook, R.D. and Wang, D.Y. (1976) Serum ferritin concentration in early breast cancer. British Journal of Cancer, 34, 286–290.

Jacobs, D., Houri, M., Landon, J. and Merrett, T.G. (1972) Circulating levels of immunoglobulin E in patients with cancer. Lancet, II, 1059–1061.

Jarnum, S. and Schwartz, M. (1960) Hypoalbuminemia in gastric carcinoma. Gastroenterology, 38, 769–776.

Jensen, E.V., Block, G.E., Smith, S., Kyser, K. and De Sombre, E.R. (1971) Estrogen receptors and breast cancer response to adrenalectomy. National Cancer Institute Monographs, 34, 55–70.

Jones, P.A.E., Miller, F.M., Worwood, M. and Jacobs, A. (1973) Ferritinaemia in leukaemia and Hodgkin's Disease. British Journal of Cancer, 27, 212–217.

Jordan, R.M., Kendall, J.W., Search, J.L., Allen, J.P., Paulsen, C.A., Kerber, C.W. and Vanderlaan, W.P. (1976) Cerebrospinal fluid hormone concentration in the evaluation of pituitary tumors. Annals of Internal Medicine, 85, 49–55.

Kaplan, L., Katz, A.D., Ben-Isaac, C. and Massry, S.G. (1971) Malignant neoplasms and parathyroid adenoma. Cancer, 28, 401–407.

Kellen, J.A., Bush, R.S. and Malkin, A. (1976) Placenta-like alkaline phosphatase in gynecological cancers. Cancer Research, 36, 269–271.

Kellerman, G., Shaw, C.R. and Luyten-Kellerman, M. (1973) Aryl hydrocarbon hydroxylase inducibility and bronchogenic carcinoma. New England Journal of Medicine, 289, 934–937.

Kessel, D. and Allen, J. (1975) Elevated plasma sialyltransferase in the cancer patient. Cancer Research, 35, 670–672.

Kew, M.C. and Mallett, R.C. (1974) Hepatic zinc concentrations in primary cancer of the liver. British Journal of Cancer, 29, 80–83.

Killman, S.-A., Rubini, J.R., Cronkite, E.P. and Bond, V.P. (1961) Urinary excretion of beta-amino-isobutyric acid (BAIBA) in leukemia and polycythemia vera. Acta Haematologica, 25, 81–97.

Korsten, C.B., Persijn, J.P. and Van der Silk, W. (1974) The application of the serum γ-glutamyltranspeptidase and the 5′-nucleotidase assay in cancer patients: a comparative study. Zeitschrift für klinische Chemie und klinische Biochemie, 12, 116–120.

Latner, A.L., Turner, D.M. and Way, S.A. (1966) Enzyme and isoenzyme studies in preinvasive carcinoma of the cervix. Lancet, II, 814–816.

Levine, L., Waalkes, T. and Stolbach, L. (1975) Serum levels of N^2,N^2-dimethylguanosine and pseudouridine as determined by radioimmunoassay for patients with malignancy. Journal of the National Cancer Institute, 54, 341–343.

Lichtenfeld, J.L., Wiernik, P.H., Mardincy, M.R. Jr. and Zarco, R.M. (1976) Abnormalities of complement and its components in patients with acute leukemia, Hodgkin's disease and sarcoma. Cancer Research, 36, 3678–3680.

Lundstrom, R., Bjorklund, B. and Eklund, G. (1973) A tissue-derived polypeptide antigen: its relation to cancer and its temporary occurrence in certain infectious diseases. In Immunological Techniques for Detection of Cancer (Ed. B. Bjorklund) Bonniers, Stockholm.

Mandel, M.A., Dvorak, K.J., Worman, L.W. and De Cosse, J.J. (1976) Immunoglobulin content in the bronchial washings of patients with benign and malignant pulmonary disease. New England Journal of Medicine, 295, 694–698.

Mander, A.M., Bolton, P.M., Davidson, J.M., Newcombe, R.G., Fifield, R. and Keyser, J.W. (1975) IgE serum levels in cancer patients, Lancet, I, 396–397.

Marshall, G. and Amador, E. (1969) Diagnostic usefulness of serum acid β-glycerophosphatase in prostatic disease. American Journal of Clinical Pathology, 51, 551–554.

Martin, E.W. Jr., Kibbey, W.E., DiVecchia, L., Anderson, G., Catalano, P. and Minton, J.P. (1976) Carcinoembryonic antigen: clinical and historical aspects. Cancer, 37, 62–81.

Massayeff, R., Gilli, J., Krebs, B., Bonet, C. and Zrihen, H. (1974) In Alpha-Foetoprotein, Proceedings of the International Congress, p. 313. Inserm, Paris.

McGee, J.O'D., Baillie, J., Al Adnani, M.S. and Patrick, R.S. (1975) The use of serum prolyl hydroxylase as a diagnostic tool in human hepatocellular cancer. Journal of Medical Microbiology, 8, p. 23.

McGuire, W.L. (1976) Conference on Biochemical Actions of Progesterone and Progestins. New York Academy of Sciences, May 5–7, 1976.

McGuire, W.L., Carbone, P.P., Sears, M.E. and Escher, G.C. (1975) In Estrogen Receptors in Human Breast Cancer (Eds. W.L. McGuire, P.P. Carbone and E.P. Vollmer) pp. 1–7, Raven Press, New York.

Meyer, K.K., Mackler, G.L. and Beck, W.C. (1973) Increased IgA in women free of recurrence after mastectomy and radiation. Archives of Surgery, 107, 159–161.

Moore, F.C., Woodrow, S.E., Aliapoulios, M.A. and Wilson, R.D. (1968) Carcinoma of the Breast. A Decade of New Results with Old Concepts. Little, Brown, Boston, Mass.

Morgan, L.R., Gillen, L.E., Maddux, B.E. and Krementz, E.T. (1975) Arylsulfatase in colon-rectal carcinoma and response to 5-fluorouracil. Proceedings of the American Association for Cancer Research, 16, 190.

Mueller, W.K., Handschumacher, R. and Wade, M.E. (1971) Serum haptoglobin in patients with ovarian malignancies. Obstetrics and Gynecology, 38, 427–435.

Mueller, P.S. and Watkin, D.M. (1961) Plasma unesterified fatty acid concentrations in neoplastic disease. Journal of Laboratory and Clinical Medicine, 57, 95–108.

Mulay, I.L., Roy, R., Knox, B.E., Suhr, N.H. and Delaney, W.E. (1971) Trace metal analysis of cancerous human tissues. Journal of the National Cancer Institute, 47, 1–13.

Munjal, D., Chawla, P.L., Lokich, J.J. and Zamchek, N. (1976) Carcinoembryonic antigen and phosphohexose isomerase, gamma glutamyl transpeptidase and lactate dehydrogenase levels in patients with and without liver metastases. Cancer, 37, 1800–1807.

Musajo, L. and Benassi, C.A. (1964) Aspects of disorders of the kynurenine pathway of tryptophan metabolism in man. Advances in Clinical Chemistry, 7, 63–135.

Myers, W.P.L. (1960) Hypercalcaemia in neoplastic disease. Annals of Surgery, 80, 308–318.

Nathanson, L. and Fishman, W.H. (1971) New observations on the Regan isoenzyme of alkaline phosphatase in cancer patients. Cancer, 27, 1388–1497.

Neville, A.M. (1973) Human tumor antigens and their potential usefulness in modern medicine. In Immunological techniques for detection of cancer (Ed. B. Bjorklund) Bonniers, Stockholm.

Neville, A.M. and Cooper, E.H. (1976) Biochemical monitoring of cancer. Annals of Clinical Biochemistry, 13, 283–305.

Niitsu, Y., Kohgo, Y., Yokota, M. and Urushizaki, I. (1975) Radioimmunoassay of serum ferritin in patients with malignancy. Annals of the New York Academy of Sciences, 259, 450–452.

Nyman, M. (1959) Serum haptoglobin: methodological and clinical studies. Scandinavian Journal of Clinical and Laboratory Investigations, II, Suppl. 39.

Odell, W.D. (1974) Humoral manifestations of nonendocrine neoplasms – ectopic hormone production. In Textbook of Endocrinology, 7th edn. (Ed. R.H. Williams) pp. 1105–1116, Saunders, Philadelphia, Pa.

Owen, J.A., Smith, R. and Radanyi, R. (1964) Serum haptoglobin in disease. Clinical Science, 26, 1–6.

Pearson, O.H., Llerna, O., Llerna, L., Molina, A. and Balter, T. (1969) Prolactin-dependent rat mammary cancer: a model for man? Transactions of the American Association of Physicians, 82, 225–238.

Pfeffer, R.B., Dishman, A., Cohen, T., Tesler, M. and Aronson, A.R. (1967) Urinary lipase excretion in pancreatic and hepatobiliary disease. Surgery, Gynecology and Obstetrics, 124, 1071–1074.

Pfeilsticher, K. (1965) Spurenelemente in Organen und Urin bei Krebs. Zeitschrift für klinische Chemie und klinische Biochemie, 3, 145–150.

Phillips, R.W. and Manildi, E.R. (1970) Elevation of leucine aminopeptidase in disseminated malignant disease. Cancer, 26, 1006–1012.

Portugal, M.L., Azevedo, M.S. and Manso, C. (1970) Serum alphafetoprotein and variant alkaline phosphatase in human hepatocellular carcinoma. International Journal of Cancer, 6, 383–387.

Pritchard, J.A.V., Moore, J.L., Sutherland, W.H. and Joslin, C.A.F. (1973) Evaluation and development of the macrophage electrophoretic mobility (MEM) test for malignant disease. British Journal of Cancer, 27, 1–9.

Rennert, O.M., Lawson, D.L., Shukla, J.B. and Miale, T.D. (1977) Cerebrospinal fluid polyamine monitoring in central nervous system leukemia. Clinica Chimica Acta, 75, 365–369.

Reynolds, R.D., Greenberg, B.R., Martin, N.D., Lucas, R.N., Gaffney, C.N. and Hawn, L. (1973) Usefulness of bone marrow serum acid phosphatase in staging carcinoma of the prostate. Cancer, 32, 181–184.

Roberts, M.M., Bass, E.M., Wallace, I.W.J. and Stevenson, A. (1973) Local immunoglobulin production in breast cancer. British Journal of Cancer, 27, 269–275.

Roberts, M.M., Bathgate, E.M. and Stevenson, A. (1975) Serum immunoglobulin levels in patients with breast cancer. Cancer, 36, 221–224.

Ronquist, G., Frithz, G., Ericsson, P. and Hugosson, R. (1977) Malignant brain tumours associated with adenylate kinase in cerebrospinal fluid. Lancet, I, 1284–1286.

Rose, D.P., Fahl, W.E. and Liskowski, L. (1975) The urinary excretion of corticosteroid sulfates by cancer patients. Cancer, 36, 2060–2063.

Rosen, G. (1975) The development of an adjuvant chemotherapy program for the treatment of osteogenic sarcoma. In Frontiers of Radiation Therapy and Oncology, Vol. 10 (Ed. J. Vaath) pp. 115–133, Karger, Basel.

Rosen, P.P., Menendez-Botet, C.J., Nisselbaum, J.S., Urban, J.A., Mike, V., Fracchia, A. and Schwartz, M.K. (1975) Pathological review of breast lesions analyzed for estrogen receptor protein. Cancer Research, 35, 3187–3194.

Rothman, A.R., Carbone, P.P., Rieselbach, R. and Freireich, E.J. (1964) Paper electrophoresis of cerebrospinal fluid proteins in patients with meningeal leukemia. Cancer, 17, 798–802.

Rudman, D., Chawla, R.K., Henrickson, L.J., Vogler, W.R. and Sophianopoulos, A.J. (1976) Isolation of a novel glycoprotein (EDC-1) from the urine of a patient with acute myelocytic leukemia. Cancer Research, 36, 1837–1846.

Rudman, D., Del Rio, A., Akgun, S. and Frumin, E. (1969) Novel proteins and peptides in the urine of patients with advanced neoplastic disease. American Journal of Medicine, 46, 174–187.

Russell, D.H., Durie, B.G.M. and Salmon, S.E. (1975) Polyamines as predictors of success and failure in cancer chemotherapy. Lancet, II, 797–799.

Salih, H., Flax, H., Brander, W. and Hobbs, J.R. (1973) Prolactin dependence in human breast cancer. Lancet, I, 1103–1105.

Schapira, F. (1973) Isozymes and cancer. Advances in Cancer Research, 18, 77–153.

Schwartz, M.K. (1973) Enzymes in cancer. Clinical Chemistry, 19, 1–22.

Schwartz, M.K. (1975) Role of trace elements in cancer. Cancer Research, 35, 3481–3487.

Schwartz, M.K. (1976) Biochemical and immunochemical markers associated with cancer. Clinical Bulletin: Memorial Sloan-Kettering Cancer Center, 6, 62–68.

Schwartz, M.K. and Fleisher, M. (1970) Diagnostic biochemical methods in pancreatic disease. Advances in Clinical Chemistry, 11, 113–159.

Serrou, B., Dubois, J.B. and Robinet-Levy, M. (1975) IgE serum levels in cancer patients. Lancet, I, 396.

Shifrine, M. and Fisher, G.L. (1976) Ceruloplasmin levels in sera from human patients with osteosarcoma. Cancer, 38, 244–248.

Shimamura, J., Fridhandler, L. and Berk, J.E. (1975) Specific detection of abnormally high levels of pancreatic isoamylase in urine. Gastroenterology, 68, 985.

Shonk, C.E., Arison, R.N., Koven, B.J., Majima, H. and Boxer, G.E. (1965) Enzyme patterns in human tissues. III. Glycolytic enzymes in normal and malignant tissues of the colon and rectum. Cancer Research, 25, 206–213.

Sussman, H.H., Weintraub, B.D. and Rosen, S.W. (1974) Relationship of ectopic placental alkaline phosphatase to ectopic chorionic gonadotropin and placental lactogen. Cancer, 33, 820–823.

Tal, C. and Halperin, M. (1970) Presence of serologically distinct protein in serum of cancer patients and pregnant women: an attempt to develop a diagnostic cancer test. Israel Journal of Medical Sciences, 6, 708–716.

Tal, C., Raychandhyri, A., Herberman, R.B. and Buncher, C.R. (1973) Simplified technique for the T-globulin cancer test. Journal of the National Cancer Institute, 51, 33–43.

Tan, C.O., Cohen, J., West, M. and Zimmerman, H.J. (1963) Serum enzymes in disease. XIV. Abnormality of levels of transaminases and glycolytic and oxidative enzymes and of liver functions as related to the extent of metastatic carcinoma of the liver. Cancer Research, 16, 1373–1387.

Thomas, G.G. and Fox, M. (1973) Depression of immune responsiveness in breast and large bowel tumours as measured by heterophile antibody activity. British Journal of Surgery, 60, 352–355.

Toporek, M. (1973) Effects of whole blood or albumin from tumor-bearing rats on liver protein synthesis. Cancer Research, 33, 2579–2583.

Tormey, D.C., Waalkes, T.P., Ahmann, D., Gehrke, C.W., Zumwalt, R.W., Snyder, J. and Hansen, H. (1975) Biological markers in breast carcinoma. I. Incidence of abnormalities of CEA, HCG, three polyamines and three minor nucleosides. Cancer, 35, 1095–1100.

Trapeznikov, N.N., Raushenbakh, M.O., Ivansova, V.D. and Yovorsky, V.V. (1975) Clinical evaluation of a method of quantitative determination of homovanillic acid for the estimation of degree of tumor dissemination process in melanoma of the skin. Cancer, 36, 2064–2068.

Usategui-Gomez, M., Yeager, F.M. and Fernadez de Castro, A. (1973) A sensitive immunochemical method for the determination of the Regan isoenzyme in serum. Cancer Research, 33, 1574–1577.

Vaitukaitis, J.L. (1976) Peptide hormones as tumor markers. Cancer, 37, 567–572.

Vincent, R.G., Chu, T.M., Fergen, T.B. and Ostrander, M. (1975) Carcinoembryonic antigen in 228 patients with carcinoma of the lung. Cancer, 36, 2069–2076.

von Kleist, S. and Burtin, P. (1969) Isolation of a fetal antigen from human colonic tumours. Cancer Research, 29, 1961–1964.

Wang, D.Y., Bulbrook, R.D., Thomas, B.S. and Friedman, M. (1968) Determination of solvolysed sulphate esters of dehydroepiandrosterone and androsterone in human peripheral plasma by gas-liquid chromatography. Journal of Endocrinology, 42, 567–578.

Wang, D.Y., Bulbrook, R.D., Hayward, J.L., Hendrick, J.C. and Franchimont, P. (1975) Relationship between plasma carcinoembryonic antigen and prognosis in women with breast cancer. European Journal of Cancer, 11, 615–618.

Ward, A.M., Cooper, E.H., Turner, R., Anderson, J.A. and Neville, A.M. (1977) Acute-phase reactant protein profiles: an aid to monitoring large bowel cancer by CEA and serum enzymes. British Journal of Cancer, 35, 170–178.

Warnes, T.W., Timperly, W.R., Hine, P. and Kay, G. (1972) Pancreatic alkaline phosphatase and tumor variant. Gut, 13, 513–519.

Wiernik, P.H. and Serpick, A.A. (1969) Clinical significance of serum and urinary muramidase activity in leukemia and other hematological malignancies. American Journal of Medicine, 46, 330–343.

Wiseman, C., McGregor, R.F. and McCredice, K.B. (1976) Urinary amino acid excretion in acute leukemia. Cancer, 38, 219–224.

Wittliff, J.L., Hilf, R., Brooks, W.F. Jr., Savlov, E.D., Hall, T.C. and Orlando, R.A. (1971) Specific estrogen-binding capacity of the cytoplasmic receptor in normal and neoplastic breast tissues of humans. Cancer Research, 32, 1983–1992.

Woodhead, J.S. and Walker, D.A. (1976) Assay of parathyroid hormone in human serum and its uses. Annals of Clinical Biochemistry, 13, 549–554.

Zamcheck, N., Doos, W.G., Prudente, R., Lurie, B.B. and Gottlieb, L.S. (1975) Prognostic factors in colon carcinoma: correlation of serum carcinoembryonic antigen level and tumor histopathology. Human Pathology, 6, 31–45.

FURTHER READING

Bodansky, O. (1975) Biochemistry of Human Cancer. Academic Press, New York.

Busch, H. (Editor). Methods in Cancer Research, Vols. 1–13. Academic Press, New York.

Fishman, W.H. (1974) Perspectives on alkaline phosphatase isoenzymes. American Journal of Medicine, 56, 617–650.

Go, V.L.W. (1976) Carcinoembryonic antigen: clinical application. Cancer, 37, 562–566.

Hall, T.C. (Ed.) (1974) Paraneoplastic Syndromes. Annals of the New York Academy of Sciences, 230, 1–577.

Herberman, R.B. (1976) Immunologic approaches to the diagnosis of cancer. Cancer, 37, 549–561.

Hoch-Ligeti, C. (1969) Laboratory Aids in Diagnosis of Cancer. Thomas, Springfield, Ill.

Horton, J. and Hill, G.J. II (Eds.) (1977) Clinical Oncology. Saunders, Philadelphia, Pa.

McKerns, K.W. (Ed.) (1974) Hormones and Cancer. Academic Press, New York.

Neville, A.M. and Cooper, E.H. (1976) Biochemical monitoring of cancer. Annals of Clinical Biochemistry, 13, 283–305.

Odell, W.D. (1974) Humoral manifestations of nonendocrine neoplasms – ectopic hormone production. In Textbook of Endocrinology, 7th edn (Ed. R.H. Williams) pp. 1105–1116, Saunders, Philadelphia, Pa.

Schapira, F. (1973) Isozymes and cancer. Advances in Cancer Research, 18, 77–153.

Schwartz, M.K. (1973) Enzymes in cancer. Clinical Chemistry, 19, 1–22.

ADDENDUM

Continued experience with the measurement of enzymes in body fluids has confirmed their general non-specificity as markers for malignant disease. The sensitivity of radioimmunoassay appears to allow greater certainty in the diagnosis of prostatic cancer when compared with the enzymatic measurement of prostatic acid phosphatase. Yet the studies to date have not used optimum enzymatic procedures nor studied enough patients with diseases other than malignant disease of the prostate to truly evaluate its utility. Nevertheless, it continues to offer promise as a screening test for prostatic cancer. Further study of other enzymes have generally failed to confirm possible utility in the diagnosis of cancer.

However, both α-2- and α-3-fucosyltransferase activities in serum and galactosyltransferase, especially its isoenzyme II, have been advocated recently as being useful measurements for monitoring cancer treatment and perhaps diagnosis. DNA polymerase activity is high in the immature blood cells of patients with acute leukaemias, and this also appears to be true for lymphocyte deoxynucleotidyltransferase activity. The measurement of serum glycylproline p-nitroanilidase activity may be of interest because unlike the activity of most enzymes which increases in malignant disease that of this enzyme and glycylproline β-naphthylamidase is reduced as in the serum of healthy neonates (Fujita et al., 1977). Markel (1978) has recently reviewed the application of enzyme measurements in clinical oncology.

From studies of both normal and malignant tissues, Odell et al. (1977) have developed the view that ectopic peptide synthesis is associated with all neoplasia. These investigators have demonstrated that normal tissues contain small amounts of immunoreactive hormones indicating that the genetic information for such peptide translation is not totally repressed in normal cells. Repression is even less effective in malignant cells. In another recent review, Tashima (1977) has discussed the higher incidence of cancer in patients with congenital endocrine syndromes or acquired endocrinopathies and patients who have received hormone therapy. He reiterates the usefulness of endocrine manipulation in the treatment of many forms of cancer. While some studies (McGuire et al., 1977) continue to demonstrate the greater response to endocrine therapy of patients with breast cancer that contains both oestrogen and progesterone receptors than oestrogen receptors, only progresterone receptor activity is infrequently measured even in major cancer centres.

As with many other cancer diagnostic tests, the early promise of many tumour markers has not been confirmed, being often less specific for cancer, and especially the site of cancer, than originally suggested. They may still have a role in the monitoring of the response to treatment although this too has to be confirmed. New tumour markers continue to be discovered, including some that appear to have a greater degree of organ specificity than carcinoembryonic antigen or α-foetoprotein (Herberman, 1979). Application of CEA tests to screening of individuals for the presence of cancer has proved discouraging because of the large number of false-positive results (Williams et al., 1977; Chu and Murphy, 1978). While the presence of antigen–antibody complexes is not diagnostic of cancer, the studies of Rossen (1978) suggest that the Clq binding test will prove of value in following patients whose cancers have been treated and their tumours suppressed below the threshold of detection by conventional diagnostic procedures.

Chu, T.M. and Murphy, G.P. (1978) Carcinoembryonic antigen: evaluation as screening assay in non-cancer clinics. New York State Journal of Medicine, 78, 879–882.

Fujita, K., Hirano, M., Tokunaga, K., Nagatsu, I., Nagatsu, T., and Sakakibara, S. (1977) Serum glycyl-proline p-nitroanilidase activity in blood cancer. Clinica Chimica Acta, 81, 215–217.

Herberman, R.B. (1979) Immunodiagnosis of cancer. In Clinical Biochemistry of Cancer (Ed. M. Fleisher) American Association for Clinical Chemistry, Washington D.C.

Markel, S.F. (1978) Clinical enzymology in cancer. Critical Reviews in Clinical Laboratory Sciences, 9, 85–104.

McGuire, W.L., Horwitz, K.B., Pearson, O.H., and Segaloff, A. (1977) Current status of estrogen and progesterone receptors in breast cancer. Cancer, 39, 2934–2947.

Odell, W., Wolfsen, A., Yoshimoto, Y., Weitzman, R., Fisher, D., and Hirose, F. (1977) Ectopic peptide synthesis: a universal concomitant of neoplasia. Transactions of the Association of American Physicians, 90, 204–225.

Rossen, R.D. (1978) Detection of antigen–antibody complexes in cancer patients. Antibiotics and Chemotherapy, 22, 5–15.

Tashima, C.K. (1977) Defining the endocrine and metabolic aspects of cancer. Geriatrics, 32, 53–69.

Williams, R.R., McIntire, K.R., Waldmann, T.A., Feinleib, M., Go, V.L.W., Kannel, W.B., Dawber, T.R., Castelli, W.P., and McNamara, P.M. (1977) Tumor-associated antigen levels (carcinoembryonic antigen, human chorionic gonadotropin, and alpha-fetoprotein) antedating the diagnosis of cancer in the Framingham study. Journal of the National Cancer Institute, 58, 1547–1551.

Subject index

A

B

D

E

F

G

H

I

J

K

L

M

Measles, 602

P

Q

R

S

T

U

V

W

X

Z